Essentials of Neonatal Ventilation

P.K. Rajiv
DCH, MD

Fellowship in Neonatology (Australia), Prime Hospitals and Clinics, Burjuman Centre, Dubai, United Arab Emirates (ex Professor of Neonatology Amrita Institute of Medical Sciences, Kochi, Kerala, India)

Dharmapuri Vidyasagar
MD, FAAP, FCCM, PhD(Hon)

Professor Emeritus Pediatrics, Division of Neonatology, University of Illinois at Chicago, Chicago, IL, United States

Satyan Lakshminrusimha
MD, FAAP

Professor and Dennis and Nancy Marks Chair of Pediatrics, Pediatrician-in-Chief, UC Davis Children's Hospital, University of California, Davis, Sacramento, CA, United States

Foreword by
Richard A. Polin
MD

William T. Speck, Professor of Pediatrics, College of Physicians and Surgeons, Columbia University, New York, NY, United States

Director, Division of Neonatology, Morgan Stanley Children's Hospital of New York-Presbyterian, New York, NY, United States

ELSEVIER

ELSEVIER

RELX India Pvt. Ltd.
Registered Office: 818, Indraprakash Building, 8th Floor, 21, Barakhamba Road, New Delhi-110001
Corporate Office: 14th Floor, Building No. 10B, DLF Cyber City, Phase II, Gurgaon-122 002, Haryana, India

Essentials of Neonatal Ventilation, 1e, P.K. Rajiv, Dharmapuri Vidyasagar, Satyan Lakshminrusimha

ISBN: 978-81-312-4998-7
e-Book ISBN: 978-81-312-4999-4

First Printed in India 2019, Reprinted 2020

Notice
Practitioners and researchers must always rely on their own experience and knowledge in evaluating and using any information, methods, compounds or experiments described herein. Because of rapid advances in the medical sciences, in particular, independent verification of diagnoses and drug dosages should be made. To the fullest extent of the law, no responsibility is assumed by Elsevier, authors, editors or contributors in relation to the adaptation or for any injury and/or damage to persons or property as a matter of products liability, negligence or otherwise, or from any use or operation of any methods, products, instructions, or ideas contained in the material herein.

Content Strategist: Sheenam Aggarwal
Content Project Manager: Ayan Dhar
Cover Designer: Milind Majgaonkar
Production Executive: Dhan Singh

Typeset by: Thomson Digital
Printed in India by EIH Limited-Unit Printing Press, IMT Manesar, Gurgaon, Haryana.

Contributors

Thouseef Ahmed, MD
Specialist Neonatologist, NMC Hospital, Dubai, United Arab Emirates

Said A. Al-kindi, BHSc, MD, DCH, MRCPCH, FRACP
Armed Forces Hospital, Muscat, Sultanate of Oman

Namasivayam Ambalavanan, MD
Professor of Pediatrics, University of Alabama at Birmingham, Birmingham, AL, United States

K. Shreedhara Avabratha, MD, DNB (Pediatrics)
Professor, Dept of Pediatrics, Fr.Muller Medical College, Mangaluru, Karnataka, India

Rakhi Balachandran, MD
Amrita Institute of Medical Sciences and Research Centre, Amrita Vishwa Vidyapeetham, Kochi, Kerala, India

Jeya Balaji, MD
Fellowship in Neonatology, Professor, Department of Pediatrics and Neonatology, Velammal Medical College and Research Institute, Madurai, Tamil Nadu, India

Dushyant Batra, MRCPCH
Nottingham University Hospitals NHS Trust, Nottingham, United Kingdom

Catherine C. Beaullieu, MD
UT Health McGovern Medical School, Houston, TX, United States

Nagamani Beligere, MD, MPH
Associate Professor, University of Illinois Medical Center, Chicago, IL, United States

Anita Bhandari, MD
University of Pennsylvania, Children's Hospital of Philadelphia, Philadelphia, PA, United States

Vineet Bhandari, MD, DNB, DM
Professor and Division Chief, Drexel University College of Medicine, St. Christopher's Hospital for Children, Philadelphia, PA, United States

Rama Bhat, MD, FAAP
Professor Emeritus Pediatrics, University of Illinois, Chicago, IL, United States

Manoj Biniwale, MBBS, MD, MRCP, MRCPCH, FAAP
Keck School of Medicine of USC, LAC+USC Medical Center, Los Angeles, CA, United States

John P. Breinholt, III, MD
UT Health McGovern Medical School, Houston, TX, United States

Ilia Bresesti, MD
"V. Buzzi" Children's Hospital, Milan, Italy

Bert Bunnell, ScD, FAIMBE
Biomedical Engineering, University of Utah, Salt Lake City, UT, United States

Dinesh K. Chirla, MD, DM, MRCPCH, CCST
Rainbow Children's Hospital, Hyderabad, Telangana, India

Swarup K. Dash, MD, DNB
Senior Neonatologist, Latifa Women and Children Hospital, DHA – Dubai, United Arab Emirates

Narendra Dereddy, MD, FAAP
Associate Professor, University of Central Florida, Associate Medical Director, Neonatology at Advent Health Hospital for Children, Orlando, FL, United States

Ramasubbareddy Dhanireddy, MD
University Distinguished Professor, Professor of Pediatrics, Obstetrics and Gynecology, University of Tennessee Health Science Center, Memphis, TN, United States

Vikramaditya Dumpa, MD, FAAP
NYU Winthrop Hospital, Mineola, NY, United States

Khaled El-Atawi, Mb.Bch, M.Sc., PhD, iFAAP, FRCPCH (Pediatrics) & M.Sc. (HCM)
Consultant Neonatologist, Latifa Women and Children Hospital, DHA – Dubai, United Arab Emirates

Mahmoud Saleh Elhalik, MD, DCH, ABP, FAAP, FRCPCH
Latifa Women and Children Hospital, Dubai, United Arab Emirates

Ahmed Zakaria Elmorsy, Mb.Bch, M.Sc. (Pediatrics)
Senior Neonatologist, Latifa Women and Children Hospital, DHA – Dubai, United Arab Emirates

Kimberly S. Firestone, MSc, RRT
Akron Children's Hospital, Akron, OH, United States

Regan E. Giesinger, MD, FRCPC
University of Iowa, Iowa City, IA, United States

Hariram M., MD, DCH
Consultant Neonatologist

Helmut D. Hummler, MD, MBA
University of Ulm, Germany and Sidra Medicine, Weill Cornell Medicine-Qatar, Doha, Qatar

Contributors

Abbas Hyderi, MD, FRCPC, FAAP
University of Alberta, Stollery Children's Hospital, Edmonton, AB, Canada

Lucky Jain, MD, MBA
Richard W. Blumberg Professor and Chair of Pediatrics, Chief Academic Officer, Children's Healthcare of Atlanta

Jegen Kandasamy, MD
University of Alabama at Birmingham, Birmingham, AL, United States

Martin Keszler, MD, FAAP
Brown University, Women and Infants Hospital, Providence, RI, United States

Abrar A. Khan, MD
Latifa Women and Children Hospital, Dubai, United Arab Emirates

Junaid Muhib Khan, MD, FRCP, FAAF, FAAP, CMQ
Al-Rahba Hospital/Johns Hopkins Medicine International, Abu Dhabi, United Arab Emirates

Sai Sunil Kishore M., MD (Pediatrics), DM (Neonatology)
Mycure Hospital, Visakhapatnam, Andhra Pradesh, India

G. Ganesh Konduri, MD
Professor of Pediatrics and Chief of Neonatology Division, Muma Endowed Chair of Neonatology, Children's Research Institute, Medical College of Wisconsin, Children's Hospital of Wisconsin, Milwaukee, WI, United States

Mathew Kripail, MD
Consultant Neonatologist

Raman Krishna Kumar, MD, DM
Amrita Institute of Medical Sciences and Research Centre, Amrita Vishwa Vidyapeetham, Kochi, Kerala, India

Praveen Kumar, DCH, MD
Associate Chair, Department of Pediatrics, Visiting Professor of Pediatrics, University of Illinois, Children's Hospital of Illinois, Peoria, IL, United States

Satyan Lakshminrusimha, MD, FAAP
Professor and Dennis and Nancy Marks Chair of Pediatrics, Pediatrician-In-Chief, UC Davis Children's Hospital, University of California, Davis, Sacramento, CA, United States

Laurance Lequier, MD, FRCPC
Stollery Children's Hospital, University of Alberta, Edmonton, AB, Canada

Gianluca Lista, MD, PhD
"V. Buzzi" Children's Hospital, Milan, Italy

Suzanne M. Lopez, MD
UT Health McGovern Medical School, Houston, TX, United States

Mohamed M A Soliman, MBBCh, MSc, MRCPCH, EPIC
Specialist Paediatrics and Neonatology, National Research Centre, Giza, Egypt

Manoj N. Malviya, MBBS, MRCP (UK)
Khoula Hospital, Muscat, Sultanate of Oman

Mark C. Mammel, MD, FAAP
Professor of pediatrics, University of Minnesota Medical Center, Saint Paul, MN, United States

Prakash Manikoth, MBBS, DCH, MRCP (UK), FRCPCH
The Royal Hospital, Muscat, Sultanate of Oman

Bobby Mathew, MRCP
Assistant Professor of Pediatrics, Jacobs School of Medicine and Biomedical Sciences, University at Buffalo, NY, United States

Patrick J. McNamara, MB, BCh, BAO, MRCP, MRCPCH
Professor and Division Chief of Neonatology, Stead Family Children's Hospital, University of Iowa, Iowa City, IA, United States

Rafique Memon, Md(Ped)
Fellowship Neonatology, Specialist Pediatrician, NMC Speciality Hospital, Dubai, United Arab Emirates

Srinivas Murki, MD, DM
Fernandez Hospital, Hyderabad, Telangana, India

K.Y. Ashok Murthy, BE
Mg Director, Erkadi Medical Systems

Durga P. Naidu, MD
Children's Heart Clinic of Louisiana, Lafayette, LA, United States

Arun Nair, MBBS, MD (Paed), DCH, MRCP, FRCPCH, FRACP
Waikato Hospital, Hamilton; Auckland University, Auckland, New Zealand

Jayasree Nair, MD
Assistant Professor of Pediatrics, Jacobs School of Medicine and Biomedical Sciences, University at Buffalo, Buffalo, NY, United States

Elaine Neary, MD, PhD
The Hospital of Sick Kids, Toronto, ON, Canada

Josef Neu, MD
Professor of Pediatrics, University of Florida Health Shands Children's Hospital, Gainesville, FL, United States

Donald M. Null, MD
University of California, Davis; UC Davis Children's Hospital, Sacramento, CA, United States

Nalinikant Panigrahy, MD, DNB
Rainbow Children's Hospital, Hyderabad, Telangana, India

Merlin Pinto, MD
Fellowship in Neonatology (Canada), NIDCAP certified Professional, MetroHealth Hospital, Case Western Reserve University, Cleveland, OH, United States

P.K. Rajiv, DCH, MD
Fellowship in Neonatology (Australia), Prime Hospitals and Clinics, Burjuman Centre, Dubai, United Arab Emirates (ex Professor of Neonatology Amrita Institute of Medical Sciences, Kochi, Kerala, India)

Aiman Rahmani, MD, MBA, FAAP
Chief Medical Officer Consultant, Division of Neonatology, Clinical Professor, Faculty of Medicine, United Arab Emirates University, Abu Dhabi, United Arab Emirates

Manimaran Ramani, MBBS, MD
University of Alabama at Birmingham, Birmingham, AL, United States

Rangasamy Ramanathan, MD, FAAP
Professor of Pediatrics at the Keck School of Medicine and Division Chief, Director of Neonatal Respiratory therapy program, Program director, Neonatal Perinatal Fellowship Program, University of Southern California, Los Angeles, CA, United States

P. Syamasundar Rao, MD, FAAP, FACC, FSCAI
Professor of Pediatrics, Division of Pediatric Cardiology, UT Health McGovern Medical School, Houston, TX, United States

Maura Helena Ferrari Resende, MD
Clinical Fellow, The Hospital for Sick Children, Toronto, ON, Canada

Rakesh Sahni, MD
Professor of Pediatrics, Columbia University College of Physicians and Surgeons, New York-Presbyterian Morgan Stanley Children's Hospital, Columbia University Medical Center, New York, NY, United States

Mitali Sahni, MD
Fellow in Neonatal-Perinatal Medicine, St. Christopher's Hospital for Children, Drexel University College of Medicine, Philadelphia, PA, United States

Marwa al Sayyed, MBBS, MSc
Neonatal Registrar, NMC speciality Hospital, Dubai, United Arab Emirates

Bernard Schoonakker, MRCPCH
Nottingham University Hospitals NHS Trust, Nottingham, United Kingdom

Craig Smith, MRCPCH
Nottingham University Hospitals NHS Trust, Nottingham, United Kingdom

Augusto Sola, MD
Director Medico Ejecutivo, SIBEN, Por los recién nacidos

Howard Stein, MD, FAAP
Promedica Toledo Children's Hospital, University of Toledo Health Science Campus, Toledo, OH, United States

RoseMary S. Stocks, MD, PharmD
Department of Otolaryngology, Head and Neck Surgery, University of Tennessee Health Sciences Center, Memphis, TN, United States

Sreeram Subramanian, MD, DM
Consultant, Paramitha Children's Hospital; NEOBBC Children's Hospital, Hyderabad, Telangana, India

Gautham Suresh, MD, DM, MS, FAAP
Section Head and Service Chief, Neonatology, Professor of Pediatrics, Texas Children's Hospital, Baylor College of Medicine, Houston, TX, United States

Ru-Jeng Teng, MD
Children's Research Institute, Medical College of Wisconsin, Children's Hospital of Wisconsin, Milwaukee, WI, United States

Vikrum A. Thimmappa, MD
Department of Otolaryngology, Head and Neck Surgery, University of Tennessee Health Sciences Center, Memphis, TN, United States

Jerome W. Thompson, MD, MBA
Department of Otolaryngology, Head and Neck Surgery, University of Tennessee Health Sciences Center, Memphis, TN, United States

David A. Todd, FIMLS, MSc, PhD, MBBS
Centenary Hospital, Canberra, ACT, Australia

Kirtikumar Upadhyay, MD, FAAP
University of Tennessee Health Science Center, Memphis, TN, United States

Karunakar Vadlamudi, MD
Stollery Children's Hospital, University of Alberta, Edmonton, AB, Canada

Payam Vali, MD
University of California, Davis; UC Davis Children's Hospital, Sacramento, CA, United States

Máximo Vento, MD, PhD
University and Polytechnic Hospital La Fe Valencia, València, Spain

Sudeep Verma, MD, FNB
KIMS-Institute of cardiac Sciences, Secunderabad-Hyderabad, Telangana, India

Dharmapuri Vidyasagar, MD, FAAP, FCCM, PhD(Hon)
Professor Emeritus Pediatrics, Division of Neonatology, University of Illinois at Chicago, Chicago, IL, United States

Koert de Waal, PhD, FRACP
John Hunter Children's Hospital, Newcastle, NSW, Australia

Mark F. Weems, MD, FAAP
University of Tennessee Health Science Center, Memphis, TN, United States

Jen-Tien Wung, MD
Professor of Pediatrics, Columbia University College of Physicians and Surgeons, Columbia University Medical Center, New York, NY, United States

Hakam Yaseen, MD, CES (Paed), DUN (Neonat) [France], CCST (UK), FRCPCH [UK]
University of Sharjah, Medical Director (CMO), University Hospital Sharjah (UHS), Sharjah, United Arab Emirates

Foreword

Since the late 1960s, there has been considerable debate about the best way to provide respiratory support for preterm infants with RDS. Early attempts to ventilate infants met with limited success and survivors often suffered from chronic lung disease. In the early 1970s, Gregory et al. reported success in using CPAP to care for preterm infants with RDS; however, despite its simplicity, there was little interest in using that technology. As ventilators increased in sophistication (and complexity), noninvasive ventilation was viewed as a modality that could supplement invasive ventilation, but not as a primary mode. Furthermore, the randomized clinical trials of surfactant suggested that most premature infants with RDS should be intubated and administered surfactant. The pendulum began to swing back toward noninvasive ventilation in the last decade as randomized clinical trials demonstrated that early application of CPAP was better than routinely intubating infants and given surfactant. In 2018, the choices for respiratory support are even greater. Not only are there newer generation of ventilators, but the choices for noninvasive support commonly include nasal intermittent positive pressure ventilation and high-flow nasal cannula. This textbook, *Essentials of Neonatal Ventilation*, edited by Rajiv, Satyan, and Vidysagar, offers clinicians a complete source for the latest developments in respiratory care of critically ill newborn infants. This book is a unique addition because of its comprehensive nature and practical approach to respiratory care. The authors for each chapter are leaders in their fields. It is noteworthy that the book also addresses complications of mechanical ventilation (e.g., bronchopulmonary dysplasia) and includes sections on common neonatal problems, ECMO and nursing care. The editors should be congratulated on assembling such a wonderful book.

Richard A. Polin, MD
William T. Speck, Professor of Pediatrics,
College of Physicians and Surgeons,
Columbia University, New York, NY, United States

Director, Division of Neonatology, Morgan Stanley
Children's Hospital of New York-Presbyterian, New York,
NY, United States

Preface

The evolution of assisted ventilation in newborn intensive care has made a unique paradigm shift. Noninvasive ventilation, a significant milestone in the 1970s, has made a comeback in the current decade. Newer methods of synchronization, gentle ventilation, and permissive hypercapnia using both invasive and noninvasive modes are the standard of care in neonatal intensive care today. This book is a Herculean attempt to standardize and optimize ventilatory care at the bedside. Each chapter is written by international experts in the field, hoping to ignite a path to the successful resolution of the pulmonary dysfunction, without lung and brain morbidity. Technologies of promise of the future are incorporated, and noninvasive monitoring and assessment are given significant emphasis. The neonatal intensivist is currently exposed to a huge arena of ever-evolving technologies. The bedside practitioner will find this book helpful in knowing the benefits and limitations of these technologies and support neonatal gas exchange without compromising neurodevelopmental outcome.

More advanced technology is not always better. Simple techniques such as nasal CPAP with noninvasive monitoring have great outcomes in preterm and term infants with lung injury. This book gives great emphasis to this basic technology.

The chapters are designed to evolve from the basics to applied physiology and graduate through the assisted ventilation technologies. A section on cardiac issues in respiratory care, nutritional support, and ancillary care is deliberately magnified for the intensivist to manage accurately and objectively a critical neonate with respiratory distress.

This book with E-Book facilities of videos on critical chapters supplemented by lecture presentations would prove to be a handy and reliable bedside companion for all NICUs all over the world. The presentations and illustrations are provided to assist in education of a new generation of neonatal providers. We gratefully acknowledge the authors for contributing to these chapters, and providing videos and illustrations to enhance the book.

P.K. Rajiv
Dharmapuri Vidyasagar
Satyan Lakshminrusimha

Acknowledgments

Rajiv gratefully acknowledges the didactic teaching of his fellow teacher Dr. Elizabeth John, whose extreme sensitivities to the adjustment of CPAP up or down still ring a bell in his ears. This singular caution to optimize continuous positive airway pressure or positive end-expiratory pressure laid the foundation of his strategy in any critical lung disease. This was the fulcrum of his success in neonatal ventilation in the last 30 years.

Rajiv acknowledges the heartfelt help of his teachers Dr. Vidyasagar, Dr. Georg Simbrunner, Dr. Ramanathan, Dr. Martin Keszler, and Dr. Dhanireddy for teaching him and for being authors of many chapters and reviewing many more of them. Dr. Vidyasagar was the first to agree to the concept of this book many years ago and has been the guiding light in the evolution of this book. Rajiv's close associates Dr. Prakash, Dr. Arun, and Dr. David Todd gave him exceptional chapters at a short notice. His junior associates Dr. Nalinikant and Dr. Srinivas provided very unique, well-researched chapters. He is indebted to coeditor Satyan who joined the team in 2016 for his immortal illustrations and editorial stewardship. His illustrations offer an additional tool for neonatal providers to educate students and parents.

Rajiv also thanks his team members Iftekar, Jason, and Sherly for uncompromising secretarial and artwork. He further thanks Dr. Karunakar, his associate, for responding to the perennial demands of perfection of the chapters, without any hesitation.

This book is a unique joint effort of a highly talented provider-publisher team. Last but not the least, Rajiv thanks his wife Bindoo for silently bearing with him all the timeless lapses at home while he was playing Archimedes for the development of this book.

Dr. Vidyasagar gratefully acknowledges his mentors, Dr. Thomas Boggs, Dr. Jack Downes, and Dr. Victor Chernick who introduced him to neonatal ventilation. He thanks his wife Dr. Nagamani Beligere for her support all through his career. His children Sahana, Sadhana, and Sanjay and grandchildren Kavi, Anika, and Maaya have been the source of his energy.

Satyan thanks his children (Ananya, Aniruddha, and Arun for posing as models during their neonatal period for his illustrations) and his wife Veena Manja, MD, MSc, for her unrelenting support. He expresses gratitude to his parents, sisters, parents-in-law, teachers, and mentors for supporting and guiding him throughout his career.

All the editors sincerely appreciate the exceptional support by Mr. Ayan Dhar and Ms. Sheenam Aggarwal at Elsevier India. Above all, the editors are thankful to all the babies and their parents who contributed to our understanding of neonatal physiology and the functioning of assisted ventilation.

P.K. Rajiv
Dharmapuri Vidyasagar
Satyan Lakshminrusimha

Contents

Contents

Contents

Section VIII: General Issues

Online supplementary materials

Please visit MedEnact (https://www.medenact.com/Home) to access the videos and lecture PPTs.

Section | I |

Introduction and History of Ventilation

Chapter | **1** |

Introduction

This book was conceived several years ago, when there appeared to be a distinct lacuna of comprehensive bedside ventilatory management guides in neonatal care history. Currently, there are excellent textbooks to refer to and obtain broad concepts on the approach to providing respiratory assistance to a baby in distress, but a detailed evidence-based book on bedside management is missing. In this book we attempted to provide the readers an evidence-based practice bedside guidelines. In doing so, we sought the contributions from the most experienced leaders in the field. This book is an honest attempt to get the world's best pioneers in each area to contribute their signature chapters of their research to give the neonatal intensivist, detailed bedside ventilation navigation in critical situations. We earnestly hope readers will find these guidelines useful in managing critically ill neonates.

This book is divided into eight sections. Here are some of the highlights of these sections. **Section I** reviews the history of neonatal ventilation. **Section II** deals with basic chapters covering embryology and physiology of pulmonary disease, with the time frame from extreme prematurity at the limits of viability to dysmorphology in the full-term infant. The delivery process and golden first hour are addressed in detail, due to its long-term impact on respiratory and neurological morbidity.

Section III deals with the *basics of neonatal ventilation* and evolves through the genesis of lung injury to lung mechanics. The chapters on ventilator give deep insight to the reader on the limitations and benefits of its application. The chapters progress to the provision of mechanical ventilation and its attendant complications, which are again discussed in detail.

Section IV is an in-depth analysis in real time of the various *respiratory care devices* currently available for the neonate. These chapters give an operating framework and the bedside navigation in critically ill babies with trouble shooting algorithms by authentic authors.

Section V is the heart of this book with *comprehensive bedside management guidelines* of the common respiratory conditions faced in neonatal intensive care. They offer detailed flowcharts, algorithms, and case scenarios in complicated respiratory care management. There is a separate chapter on the management of the 23–25 weeks' gestation babies: "micropremies"—a challenge for any intensivist.

Section VI deals in-depth for all the *common cardiac conditions* complicating respiratory care. Management of shock and cyanotic heart disease, PDA, and arrhythmias are discussed. Functional echo is comprehensively discussed as it is evolving as the new standard of care.

No ventilator support will be successful without strong ancillary support. **Section VII** details all critical aspects of *ancillary care* of the ventilated neonate, including monitoring, infection control, nutrition, and procedures.

It is heartening to note that there is emergence of an increasing number of neonatal intensive care units (NICUs) to improve survival among low- and middle-income countries (LMCs). Ventilatory support is an essential part of the neonatal intensive care. Proper ventilator care requires a combination of skilled personnel, appropriate equipment, and ancillary support which are the prerequisites for optimal outcome but are difficult to fulfill in some LMCs. Several chapters in the book offer guidelines to assist pioneers in LMCs in establishing ventilatory support in their prospective units and teach physicians, trainees, and nurses.

Besides the rich evidence-based content of the book, it has several unique features to help the practitioner better manage infants requiring ventilatory care. This book is *digitally enhanced* with illustrations and *videos* linked to their respective chapters and *lecture PowerPoint* to most chapters of this book to give the intensivist a 360-degree comprehension of neonatal ventilation.

This book is intended for neonatologists, intensivists, postgraduates (residents and fellows), respiratory therapists, and neonatal nurses as a ready bedside reckoner for urgent consult.

We thank all the authors for their contributions to this book. Because of our goal to make this book reader-friendly, the authors were burdened with additional tasks of preparing video clips and PowerPoint presentation of their chapters. We sincerely thank them for complying with our requests and making the *book very unique in its presentation*. We hope the readers will find these educational tools valuable in their practice.

I want to thank my secretarial staff Mr. Iftekar, Mr. Jason, and Mrs. Serly for their sincere commitment to the development of this book. We thank ELSEVIER publisher and its staff Ayan Dhar and Sheenam Aggarwal for their innovation, receptivity and patience during the publication of this book.

Warm regards,
P.K. Rajiv MBBS, DCH, MD
Fellowship in Neonatology (Australia)
(*formerly Professor of Neonatology*)
Amrita Institute of Medical Sciences
Kochi, Kerala, India
Prime Hospitals and Clinics
Dubai, United Arab Emirates

Dharmapuri Vidyasagar MD, FAAP, FCCM
Professor Emeritus Pediatrics
Division of Neonatology
University of Illinois at Chicago
Chicago, IL, United States

Satyan Lakshminrusimha MD, FAAP
Dennis and Nancy Marks Chair of Pediatrics
Professor of Pediatrics
University of California, Davis
Sacramento, CA, United States

Chapter | 2 |

Evolution of Neonatal Ventilation a Retrospective View

Dharmapuri Vidyasagar, PhD (Hon)

Introduction

The author of this article is fortunate to have personally seen the evolution of improved neonatal intensive care and neonatal ventilation in the United States over last half century [1]. He along with Dr. George F. Smith, a geneticist and Head of the Department of Pediatrics at the Illinois Masonic Hospital and Professor at the University of Illinois, Chicago, were interested in medical history and organized a symposium on "Historical Perspective of Perinatal Medicine in 1980." Many giants in the field of neonatology participated in this symposium. The proceedings were supported and published by the Mead Johnson, Nutritional Division in two volumes (Fig. 2.1A–B); however, they were not copyrighted [2]. Fortunately, later they were placed on the website "Neonatology on the Web" **created by Dr. Ray Duncan** of Mount Sinai Hospital, Los Angeles. The two volumes on the Internet are readily available for interested readers at the website [3] (permission to reproduce figures by personal communication).

These books contain valuable historical information that would have been lost but for the ingenious method of placing the proceedings on the web. I am grateful to Dr. Duncan for this innovative method of preserving the historical volumes. The material from these books in part form the basis of the current chapter.

The history of assisted ventilation of a newborn is closely intertwined with evolution of neonatology. Therefore, it would be appropriated first to review the evolution of the specialty of neonatology then delve into the evolution of neonatal ventilation.

The story of development of neonatology and respiratory care of a newborn, particularly of the premature babies, has been told by several authors in the past [1,4–10].

The chapter is written from the perspective of both a witness and participant of these developments over the past 50 years. Following narration is based on the above referenced material. The material related to the development of neonatal ventilation is based on several reports [4–8] and three major symposia: Ross symposium in 1968, Paris symposium in 1969, and the Chicago symposium in 1980 [2].

(A)

NEONATAL and
PERINATAL
MEDICINE

Volume 1: Neonatal Medicine

edited by
George F. Smith, M.D.
Dharmapuri Vidyasagar, M.D.

Recent Advances
in
Neonatal and
Perinatal Medicine

Edited by George F. Smith, MD
and Dharmapuri Vidyasagar, MD
Published by Mead Johnson
Nutritional Division, 1980

This Book Was Not Copyrighted

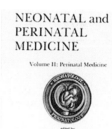

NEONATAL and
PERINATAL
MEDICINE

Volume II: Perinatal Medicine

edited by
George F. Smith, M.D.
Dharmapuri Vidyasagar, M.D.

Introduction
1. Perinatal Medicine .... Nicholas M. Nelson
2. Perspectives in Neonatology .... Thomas E. Cone, Jr.
3. Thermoregulation in the Newborn Infant .... Leo Stern

(B)

THE CONTENTS OF THE SYMPOSIUM

Introduction
1. Perinatal Medicine .... Nicholas M. Nelson
2. Perspectives in Neonatology .... Thomas E. Cone, Jr.
3. Thermoregulation in the Newborn Infant .... Leo Stern
4. Neonatal Feeding .... Martin H. Greenberg
5. The Nutrition of Premature Infants .... Lewis A. Barness
6. Neonatal Jaundice: A Selected Retrospective ..... Lawrence M. Gartner
7. The Rise and Fall of Rh Disease .... A. Zipursky
8. Nursing in Neonatology .... Mitzi L. Duxbury
9. Maternal Bonding: An Overview .... Roberto Sosa
10. The Obstetric View of Premature Labor .... M. Yusoff Dawood
11. Birth Asphyxia .... Phillip J. Goldstein
12. Infectious Diseases of the Newborn Infant -- Historical Perspectives ..... Jerome O. Klein
13. Immunobiology of the Fetus and Newborn -- Historical Perspectives and Recent Advances Aditya Kaul and George F. Smith
14. Researches in Perinatal Circulation .... John Lind
15. Assisted Ventilation in Newborn Infants .... Mildred T. Stahlman
16. The Treatment of Hyaline Membrane Disease ...... Victor Chernick
17. Retrolental Fibroplasia: A Medical and Legal Tragedy ..... Richard L. Day
18. Historical Perspectives and Recent Advances of Neonatal Monitoring ..... Dharmapuri Vidyasagar
19. Biochemical Monitoring .... Parvin Justice, Shanta Nath, and Dharmapuri Vidyasagar
20. Congenital Abnormalities and Genetic Concepts in Neonatology ..... George F. Smith
21. Neonatal Surgery: Historical Perspectives and a Glimpse of the Future ..... Kevin C. Pringle
22. The Impact of Regionalization on Neonatal Outcome ..... L. Joseph Butterfield
23. The Developmental Outcome of Premature Infants ..... Lula O. Lubchenco
24. Maternity and Infant Care Services in Chicago Retrospectus: Our Legacy, Our Challenge Donald Dye and Karen Tarpey
25. Julius Hess, M.D. .... Alwin C. Rambar
26. William Harvey in Perinatal Perspective .... Billy F. Andrews
27. Soranus of Ephesus: Who Was He and What Did He Do? ..... T. N. K. Raju
28. Some Famous "High Risk" Newborn Babies .... T. N. K. Raju

Fig. 2.1 (A) Images of the cover pages of two volumes of symposium; Historical Perspectives and Recent Advances in Neonatal and Perinatal Medicine held in Chicago 1980, published by Mead Johnson Nutritional Division. Columbus OHIO. (B) The list of contents and presenters of two volumes. Note the list of illustrious personalities who participated in the symposium. Neonatology on the web. Available from: http://www.neonatology.org/classics/mj1980/ [3].

The development of neonatology

Until the mid-20th century, the primary care of newly born infants was provided by the obstetricians. In the mid-20th century, pediatricians began to take care of the newborn. The premature babies were viewed as a medical curiosity and exhibited for public view at various exhibitions [11]. However, the excellent scientific work of many investigators, both in the United States and Europe, led to better understanding of physiology and pathology of the mature term newborn and premature babies. These studies showed that a premature newborn required special thermal and nutritional care. These understandings lead to the development of premature care centers. Dr. Julius Hess in Chicago [12] was the leading authority on premature care in those days [13]. In 1914, he opened the first 24-bed premature care center at the Sarah Morris Hospital of Michael Reese Hospital (now defunct). Dr. Hess (Fig. 2.2) was the head of Department of Pediatrics at University of Illinois, Chicago and the head of pediatrics at Michael Reese hospital. He along with the help of his nurse Evelyn Lundeen provided the state of the art care of its time for premature babies. With their expert care, they showed increased survival of premature babies.

The Chicago Board of Health had established several centers in the city for the care of premature babies. Premature babies born in the community hospitals were mandated to be transported to one of these centers, if they survived the first 24 h after birth. Dr. Hess developed an incubator with the help of an engineer, "the Hess incubator" (Fig. 2.3) [14]. He also developed a transport incubator (Fig. 2.4), which could be plugged into taxis of Chicago for electric power for transportation of the babies to premature care centers within Chicago.

Both Dr. Hess and nurse Lundeen wrote several papers and books [13] on the care of premature babies, mainly on care of the newborn, particularly the premature babies and their feedings. With these advances, the care of the premature infants in Chicago improved greatly. Indeed, the premature care center at the Sarah Morris Hospital gained national and international fame. It became the center of academic learning in premature baby care for doctors and nurses from around the world.

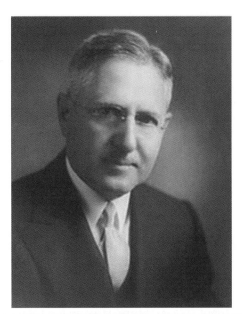

Fig. 2.2 Photograph of Dr. Julius Hess (1876–1953) Who was In-Charge of the Premature Care Center at Sarah Morris Hospital/Michael Reese Hospital in Chicago. Neonatology on the web. Available from: http://www. neonatology.org/classics/mj1980/ [3].

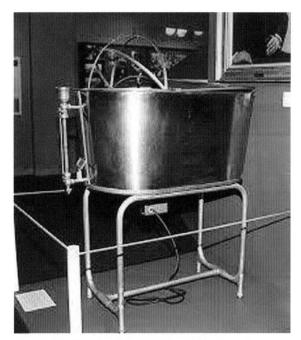

Fig. 2.3 The Hess Incubator Designed for Care of Premature Babies, Developed by Dr. Hess With the Help of an Engineer. Neonatology on the web. Available from: http://www.neonatology.org/classics/mj1980/ [3].

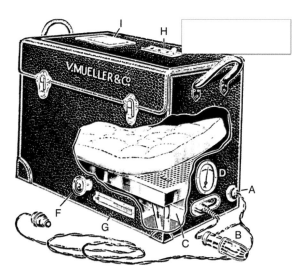

Fig. 2.4 The Hess Transport Incubator. Dr. Hess also developed a portable incubator for transporting babies from community hospitals to designated Premature Care Centers in Chicago. Note: the incubator had an adopter to be connected to taxis of Chicago for power during transport. Neonatology on the web. Available from: http://www.neonatology.org/classics/mj1980/ [3].

The birth of modern neonatal intensive care unit (NICU)

In October 1960, Dr. Loius Gluck established the first known neonatal intensive care unit (NICU) at Yale-New Haven Hospital, United States. Prior to this time, premature infants were often isolated in small cubicles and had little direct contact with doctors and parents because of fear of infections. With focus on hand washing, Dr. Gluck's design for NICU took shape with the help of US$ 3 million from a benefactor whose premature grandson he had saved [15]. It was set up as a one big open room, filled with newborns in their incubators. This development had a profound influence on the subsequent direction of care of the sick newborn, including premature babies in the United States and rest of the world.

The birth of a new specialty: neonatology—the newborn medicine

The scientific basis of newborn care improved significantly with the work of several physiologists: the work of Joseph Barcroft brought new understanding of the fetus [16,17];

Dr. Geoffrey Dawes in Oxford, England [18–20] and investigators in the laboratories of Julius Comroe, United States studied neonatal physiology extensively. Dr. Clement Smith, Professor of Pediatrics at Harvard Medical School, published his book on the physiology of a newborn infant [21]. These seminal developments in understanding of the fetal and neonatal physiology laid the foundation for the clinicians to develop an evidence-based neonatal care in coming decades.

Dr. Alexander Schaffer [22] was the first one to coin the term *Neonatology* as the science of newborn medicine and *Neonatologist* as one practicing neonatal medicine in the preface to his book *Diseases of the Newborn* (published by Saunders in 1960). It is interesting to note that in a short span of 15 years of coining the term *Neonatology, it became* an established Board Certifiable Pediatric subspecialty. The first *Neonatal–Perinatal Medicine* specialty board examination was conducted in 1975. The author was one of the 355 candidates certified at the first board examination.

The growth of neonatology continued by leaps and bounds from 1970 onward (Fig. 2.5). The scientific exploration of neonatal illnesses and developing evidence-based therapeutic interventions also grew exponentially leading to steady decrease in neonatal mortality rates (NMR) as shown in Fig. 2.5.

Fig. 2.5 highlights the advances made in different areas of neonatology during the 20th century and also shows the impact of these developments on steady decline of NMR in the United States and the United Kingdom. It shows development in six major areas of neonatology: (1) improved thermal care, (2) improved nutrition, (3) improved nursing care and opening of premature care centers and NICUs, (4) prevention of infections, (5) improved care of infants in respiratory distress and finally, (6) improved perinatal care and resuscitation in the delivery room and ventilation. In the past century, these improvements have resulted in increased neonatal survival.

The evolution of ventilator care of the newborn

As prematurity was the major contributing factor to high NMR and the respiratory problems particularly hyaline membrane disease (HMD) was the major cause of NMR, they received greatest attention in basic and clinical research. These investigative efforts were further boosted with the tragic death of prematurely born son of the then President Kennedy.

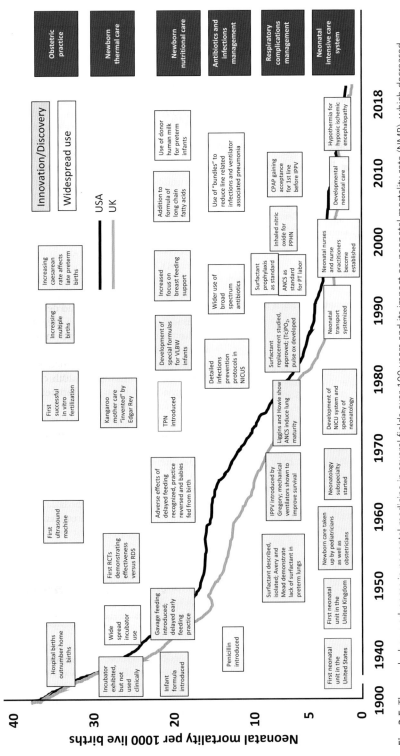

Fig. 2.5 The graph shows advances in neonatal medicine in several fields over 100 years and its impact on neonatal mortality rate (NMR), which decreased steadily in the United Kingdom and the United States (from: Born Too Soon published by March of Dimes/WHO 2014). *CPAP*, Continuous positive airway pressure; *NICU*, neonatal intensive care unit; *TPN*, total parental nutrition.

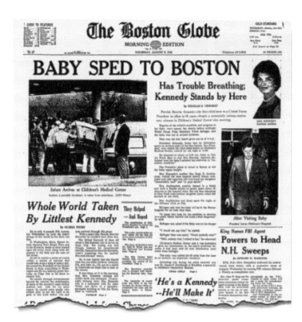

Fig. 2.6 The News of Death of Prematurely Born Baby Kennedy Printed in Boston Globe.

On August 7, 1963, Jacqueline Kennedy, wife of President Kennedy, gave birth to a premature baby (34-week GA, birth weight of 2.1 kg) [2] (Fig. 2.6, Boston Globe News item) in Boston who developed breathing difficulties, now what is known as the HMD. Usher's regime [3], infusion of 10% dextrose water with NaHCO$_3$ was the only known treatment for HMD. Neonatal ventilator care was not available even for the President's baby in the United States in 1963. Moreover, sending the President's baby to neighboring Canada where neonatal ventilation was available was not an option. The baby died after 2 days on August 9, 1963. The death of President Kennedy's baby was a day for national mourning. As the story of demise of baby Kennedy unfolded HMD, a disease of premature babies, became known to all in America. It was estimated that in 1960s about 25,000 babies died of HMD annually in the United States. With the death of baby Kennedy, the interest in research on disease HMD accelerated. The interest in newborn care increased.

Oxygen therapy

Prior to use of any form of assisted ventilation, administration of oxygen was the *only* available therapy for infants requiring delivery room resuscitation and infants in respiratory distress. The use of oxygen in the treatment of neonates with respiratory distress has been reported for more than a century. In 1907, Budin recommended oxygen "supplied through a funnel, the large opening of which is placed beside the infant's face," for the treatment of cyanotic episodes in newborns [23]. In the 1930s, Hess developed an incubator capable of delivering approximately 40% oxygen for extended periods of time [12,23]. By the 1940s, a commercially available incubator capable of providing a high concentration of oxygen facilitated the liberal use of oxygen for the treatment of cyanosis, apnea, and periodic breathing of newborns.

Throughout this time, oxygen administration was guided by the clinical observations of skin color, as well as the respiratory rate, regularity, and work of breathing. It wasn't until the 1960s and 1970s that the technology of microsampling of blood gases was available [24]. In 1980s, noninvasive methods of transcutaneous oxygen [25] and CO$_2$ monitoring became available. Pulse oximetry [26] became available in 1980s for more precise monitoring of oxygen saturation in the blood. It remains the standard method of monitoring blood oxygenation in a newborn.

The overall goal of oxygen therapy was to achieve adequate oxygenation using the lowest concentration of inspired oxygen. However, achieving this goal is complicated due to a number of factors. Routine administration of oxygen to all premature infants led to the catastrophic results of the development of retinopathy of prematurity (ROP) and related blindness [24,27]. However, a study to curtail oxygen therapy was associated with increased cerebral palsy [28–32].

Despite over 75 years of routine oxygen administration to newborn infants, administering optimal level of oxygenation and monitoring—one that avoids the detrimental effects of hypoxia on the one hand, and those caused by hyperoxia on the other hand—has been very difficult [33]. Current recommendations for oxygen saturation targets are different between the United States and Europe. The European recommendations are to keep the target oxygen saturations between 90% and 94% for premature infants requiring supplemental oxygen [34]. The American Academy of Pediatrics states that the ideal target oxygen saturation is not known and in some preterm infants, 91%–95% target may be safer than 85%–89% [33].

In order to achieve the goals of neonatal oxygen therapy, we need to develop and evaluate appropriate devices of oxygen delivery systems. The clinicians today need to have an adequate knowledge of the use of oxygen delivery equipment, and have the training on the concepts of neonatal oxygenation and equipment used to monitor the effects of oxygen therapy.

Usher regime

Prior to the introduction of neonatal ventilation in late 1950s and early 1960s, Dr. Robert Usher of Montreal, Canada after extensive studies in premature infants with HMD showed that they suffer from metabolic acidosis and hyperkalemia [35]. To counteract these changes he proposed a treatment regime of administering $NaHCO_3$ in 10% dextrose to infants in respiratory distress [35]. This therapy became known as Usher regime resulted in significant (50%) reduction of mortality in infants with HMD. The Usher regime was one of the major milestones in the treatment of HMD prior to initiation of assisted ventilation.

At this point, a retrospective view of experience with neonatal ventilation and neonatal ventilators is in order.

History of neonatal ventilation

Several reviewers have stated that it is difficult to time exactly when ventilation of the newborn was initiated and probably occurred in the late 1950s and 60s [10,36,37]. Downes in an editorial [38] refers to the work of Smythe and Bull from South Africa to have used successful long-term neonatal ventilation in infants afflicted with tetanus. These infants were treated with D-tubocurarine, tracheostomy, and ventilation; and the mortality was reduced from nearly 100% to 20%. However, these infants had normal lungs [38]. Initial reports of mechanical ventilation of newborns with pulmonary insufficiency were reported by Benson et al. and Donald et al. in 1958 [39,40]. The first highly successful use of mechanical ventilation in premature infants with HMD was reported by Maria Delivoria-Papadopoulos in 1965 [41–43]. In this series, out of 20 infants with severe HMD, 7 survived (35%) and 6 of them were neurologically intact. Since then, several other investigators reported use of assisted ventilation in HMD with increasing success. Some used positive pressure ventilation, including Strang and Reynolds in London [44], Thomas et al. at Stanford [45], and de Heese et al. in Cape Town [46]. Historically, negative pressure ventilation was designed earlier in 1889 by Alexander Graham Bell [47,48]. He presented a paper to the American Association for the advancement of science in Montreal on the use of ventilator for newborn babies and was "met with little enthusiasm." The design and device are preserved at The Alexander Graham Bell museum in Nova Scotia, Canada [49]. Later in 1960s, Dr. Stahlman in Nashville, Tennessee [50], and Stern in Montreal, Canada [51] used negative pressure ventilation (Fig. 2.7) to treat babies with RDS. Chernick and Vidyasagar in Winnipeg, Canada [52,53] modified negative pressure ventilator to create

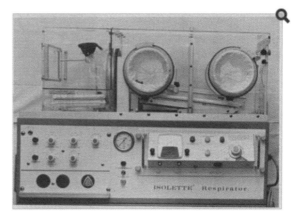

Fig. 2.7 Photograph of Air-Shield Negative Pressure Respirator. Note the respirator has two arts: the closed chamber wherein the baby's body is placed with the head lays outside open to atmospheric pressure. An adjustable sleeve around the neck seals the body chamber. The incubator is fitted with a vacuum creator underneath the body. Turning the knobs in front allow to create desired negative pressure and adjust the respiratory cycle (operated by vacuum creating machine and a solenoid valve underneath the body).

constant negative distend pressure (similar to continuous positive airway pressure [CPAP]) without an endotracheal tube with success in the management of respiratory failure in newborn.

Readers should note that negative pressure ventilation is no more in use as we have developed several simpler noninvasive methods of ventilation (see chapter on noninvasive ventilation in this book). However, the use of negative pressure respirator to support babies in respiratory distress remains an important phase in the history of neonatal ventilation.

Ross symposium on neonatal intensive care

In 1968, a conference was organized on neonatal intensive care in Vermont by Ross laboratories. Several aspects of neonatal intensive care including design of these units and ventilation techniques were discussed at the conference [54]. Several leading neonatologists of the time from the United States and Canada participated in this conference. The conference was intended to share the experiences of different units and learn the problems of neonatal intensive care units of the day. Presentations by various speakers showed the impact of intensive care on improved survival, complications, and long-term intact survival of babies cared in their respective units.

Survival with assisted ventilation was highest among infants with tetanus neonatorum who had no lung disease. It reversed the 80% mortality in tetanus prior to assisted ventilation to 80% survival with assisted ventilation. Survival rate in RDS although improved was still at 28%. The results of assisted ventilation in other respiratory conditions were not so encouraging. At the end Dr. Lucey, the chairman of the conference, summarized the conference as follows: "Now that you have read the proceedings of this conference some will be frustrated and discouraged. Others will be encouraged to try to improve the care in their own nurseries. Hopefully this conference will have supplied with early but firm data to encourage you in these efforts and warn you of the problems involved" and cautioned "whereas intensive care is effective we still do not have a clear idea about the key elements of success. The construction of a new nursery or the purchase of a blood gas machine and respirator do not an intensive care nursery make!". The key elements are intelligent personnel or as one participant put it "people who care intensely" (Dr. Nick Nelson of Harvard).

This is one of the earliest reports on the impact of modern neonatal intensive care including the results of neonatal ventilation.

In 1969, another conference solely on assisted ventilation was organized in Paris by Professor Alex Minkowski. In this symposium, clinician researchers from different countries shared their experiences with neonatal ventilation. Representatives from France, Belgium, England, South Africa, Finland, Canada, and the United States participated in the symposium. A review of published proceedings in Biology of the Neonate (current name of this journal is "Neonatology") shows the struggles faced by the clinician researchers of the day in finding the right ventilator for the user in newborn, the optimal time for initiating ventilation, monitoring babies on ventilation, and improving outcomes at this time [55–58].

In writing the summary of the symposium, Dr. Paul Swyer from Toronto, Canada who conducted the meeting *raised the big question: whether neonatologists should continue to provide assisted ventilation! (Perhaps, more aggressively) or whether the possible complications outweighed neonatal ventilation.*

However, the efforts to improve the clinical practice of providing assisted ventilation to the sick newborn continued.

The introduction of CPAP in managing infants with HMD by Gregory et al. in 1967 was a major breakthrough in neonatal respiratory management [59]. Using this approach he showed a significant improvement in survival of infants with HMD (16 of the 20 infants survived—including 10 less than 1500 g) [59].

Introduction of surfactant therapy in HMD/RDS

The invention of CPAP and the discovery [60–64] and production of surfactant further reduced mechanical complications of ventilation in preterm newborns [65,66].

In 1959, Avery and Mead [63] reported that the low surface tension in the lining of the lung permits stability of the alveoli at end expiration. Lacking such material, immature infants and infants dying with HMD, surface tension was higher than expected. They speculated that deficiency of surface-active material might be significant in the pathogenesis of HMD. This article was cited 376 times in the period 1961–77.

In 1980, Fujiwara et al. from Japan reported successful use of an artificial surfactant in 10 preterm infants severely ill with HMD [67,68]. Following instillation of artificial surfactant, alveolar–arterial gradients decreased, the levels of inspired oxygen and peak inspiratory pressures decreased, and radiological abnormalities resolved. All survived. Raju et al. [69] reported that replacement therapy with surfactant in a randomized trial significantly improved oxygenation, reduced complications of neonatal ventilation such as air-leak syndromes (pneumothorax and pulmonary interstitial emphysema), and improved survival without BPD.

Soon after multiple randomized clinical trials of surfactant replacement therapy substantiating improvement in survival of infants with RDS treated with surfactant [70]. These studies led to FDA approval of a surfactant "Survanta" for clinical use in 1993. Introduction of surfactant in the treatment of RDS remains a major milestone in the history of neonatology

The modern neonatal ventilators

Prior to 1970s, neonatologists had to use modified adult ventilators providing intermittent positive pressure ventilation. However, these ventilators could not match the physiologic pattern of breathing at higher rates. Ventilators designed specifically for the newborn appeared during mid-1970s–90s. Dr. Sola in this book discusses currently available ventilators incorporated with various functional modalities for use by the clinician. Goldsmith et al. [71] describe the milestones of technological developments in designing ventilators specifically for the newborns and premature infants—starting from the modified adult ventilators to current highly sophisticated incorporation of space age technology into ventilators used currently in the NICUs.

The rhetoric question raised at the Paris symposium in 1969 regarding the value of assisted ventilation has been answered by the continued efforts to improve technological, perinatal, and neonatal therapeutic advances to treat babies with HMD. Undoubtedly, assisted ventilation has improved overall survival of tiniest babies with HMD (24% mortality among extremely preterm infants <29 weeks of gestation and 2.9% mortality among moderately preterm infants, 29–33 weeks of gestation) [72], but the persistence of associated complications of ventilator-induced lung injury continue to vex the clinician and stimulate further research.

Summary

In summary technological innovations—*the likes of Hess incubator*—of early 20th century were the precursors of modern incubators. The premature care centers of early 20th century were the beginning of modern neonatal intensive care units. The evolution of incubator care of the premature infants, combined with the extensive basic and clinical research on fetal and neonatal physiology in the last century, gave birth to the subspecialty of neonatology.

Modern ventilatory care evolved from earlier efforts to save babies dying of neonatal tetanus. Similar earlier efforts to ventilate premature babies with lung disease (HMD) were discouragingly poor. Persistent and continued efforts

to develop ventilators to match neonatal physiology combined with modern space age microprocessors resulted in the modern neonatal ventilators. It was also realized that machines alone do not make an intensive care. It is the people (skilled nurses/doctors/respiratory therapists, support staff) who care "intensively" and make the intensive care unit.

With these principles of care the outcome results of modern ventilation in the premature newborn, supplemented with surfactant therapy, nutritional support and nursing care are exceedingly high even in the extreme premature babies (over 92% survival at 28 weeks) [73].

Today, it is estimated that in the United States alone 65,000 babies are ventilated annually [74]. Further, with global efforts of technology transfer to the developing countries, the practice of neonatal ventilator support particularly of the premature baby is widely used even in low- and middle-income countries [75]. While these developments are a very nice welcome, the novice should be cautioned in venturing into this territory without the expertise or the total organizational support needed for the operation of neonatal ventilation.

However, long-term ventilation is associated with pulmonary morbidity (CLD/BPD). Experts in the field have discussed various preventive aspects of ventilator-induced lung injury in this book. *Prevention of ventilation-induced lung injury (VILI) remains the major challenge for the future generation of neonatologists.* A summary of evolution of neonatal ventilation is shown in Fig. 2.8.

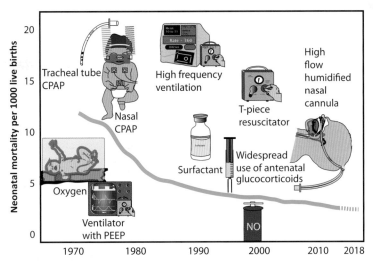

Fig. 2.8 Graph Showing Neonatal Mortality Rate and Various Innovations in Neonatal Respiratory Care. *CPAP*, Continuous positive airway pressure. Copyright: Satyan Lakshminrusimha.

References

[1] Vidyasagar D. "Half a century of evolution of neonatology: a witness's story": Dr. K. C. Chaudhuri Lifetime Achievement Award Oration delivered at AIIMS, New Delhi on 7th September 2014. Indian J Pediatr 2015;82(12):1117–1125.

[2] Smith GF, Vidyasagar D. Historical review and recent advances in neonatal and perinatal medicine. Mead Johnson Nutritional Division, Evansville, IN; 1983.

[3] Neonatology on the web. Available from: http://www.neonatology.org/classics/mj1980/.

[4] Butterfield LJ. Historical perspectives of neonatal transport. Pediatr Clin North Am 1993;40(2):221–239.

[5] Obladen M. History of neonatal resuscitation. Part 1: Artificial ventilation. Neonatology 2008;94(3):144–149.

[6] Raju TN. History of neonatal resuscitation. Tales of heroism and desperation. Clin Perinatol 1999;26(3):629–640.

[7] Vidyasagar D. Editorial: advances in neonatology—III. Indian J Pediatr 2015;82(1):44–45.

[8] Vidyasagar D. Editorial: advances in neonatology—II. Indian J Pediatr 2014;81(6):568–569.

[9] Vidyasagar D. Editorial: advances in neonatology. Indian J Pediatr 2014;81(5):464–465.

[10] Philip AG. The evolution of neonatology. Pediatr Res 2005;58(4):799–815.

[11] Silverman WA. Incubator-baby side shows (Dr. Martin A. Couney). Pediatrics 1979;64(2):127–141.

[12] Dunn PM. Perinatal lessons from the past. Julius Hess, MD, (1876–1955) and the premature infant. Arch Dis Child Fetal Neonatal Ed 2001;85(2):F141–F144.

[13] Hess JH. Experiences gained in a thirty year study of prematurely born infants. Pediatrics 1953;11(5):425–434.

[14] Raju TN. An extant Hess incubator on display. Pediatrics 2001;107(4):805.

[15] Fountain N. Louis Gluck, 73, pediatrician who advanced neonatal care. New York Times, 1997, Dec 15.

[16] Barcroft J, Barron DH, Cowie AT, Forsham PH. The oxygen supply of the foetal brain of the sheep and the effect of asphyxia on foetal respiratory movement. J Physiol 1940;97(3):338–346.

[17] Barcroft J, Kennedy JA, Mason MF. Oxygen in the blood of the umbilical vessels of the sheep. J Physiol 1940;97(3):347–356.

[18] Dawes GS. Foetal and neonatal physiology—a comparative study of the changes at birth. Chicago: Year book Medical Publishers Inc; 1968.

[19] Dawes GS. Pulmonary circulation in the foetus and new-born. British medical bulletin 1966;22(1):61–65.

[20] Ardran G, Dawes GS, Prichard MM, Reynolds SR, Eyatt DG. The effect of ventilation of the foetal lungs upon the pulmonary circulation. J Physiol 1952;118(1):12–22.

[21] Smith CA, Nelson NM. The physiology of the newborn infant. Springfield, IL, 1976.

[22] Schaffer AJ, Avery ME, Taeusch HW. Schaffer's diseases of the newborn. W.B. Saunders, Philadelphia, PA; 1984.

[23] Walsh BK, Brooks TM, Grenier BM. Oxygen therapy in the neonatal care environment. Respir Care 2009;54(9):1193–1202.

[24] Kinsey VE, Arnold HJ, Kalina RE, Stern L, Stahlman M, Odell G, et al. PaO_2 levels and retrolental fibroplasia: a report of the cooperative study. Pediatrics 1977;60(5):655–668.

[25] Huch A, Huch R. Transcutaneous, noninvasive monitoring of pO_2. Hosp Pract 1976;11(6):43–52.

[26] Severinghaus JW, Honda Y. History of blood gas analysis. VII. Pulse oximetry. J Clin Monit 1987;3(2):135–138.

[27] James S, Lanman JT. History of oxygen therapy and retrolental fibroplasia. Prepared by the American Academy of Pediatrics, Committee on Fetus and Newborn with the collaboration of special consultants. Pediatrics 1976;57(Suppl. 2):591–642.

[28] Silverman WA, Blodi FC, Locke JC, Day RL, Reese AB. Incidence of retrolental fibroplasia in a New York nursery. AMA Arch Ophthalmol 1952;48(6):698–711.

[29] Silverman WA. The lesson of retrolental fibroplasia. Sci Am 1977;236(6):100–107.

[30] Silverman WA. Oxygen and retrolental fibroplasia in neonates. Public Health Rep 1969;84(1):16–17.

[31] Genn MM, Silverman WA. The mental development of ex-premature children with retrolental fibroplasia. J Nerv Ment Dis 1964;138:79–86.

[32] Silverman W. A cautionary tale about supplemental oxygen: the albatross of neonatal medicine. Pediatrics 2004;113:394–396.

[33] Cummings JJ, Polin RA. Committee on Fetus and Newborn. Oxygen targeting in extremely low birth weight infants. Pediatrics 2016;138(2):e20161576.

[34] Sweet DG, Carnielli V, Greisen G, Hallman M, Ozek E, Plavka R, et al. European Consensus Guidelines on the management of respiratory distress syndrome—2016 update. Neonatology 2016;111(2):107–125.

[35] Usher R. Reduction of mortality from respiratory distress syndrome of prematurity with early administration of intravenous glucose and sodium bicarbonate. Pediatrics 1963;32:966–975.

[36] Daily WJ, Sunshine P, Smith PC. Mechanical ventilation of newborn infants. V. Five years' experience. Anesthesiology 1971;34(2):132–138.

[37] Daily WJ, Meyer HB, Sunshine P, Smith PC. Mechanical ventilation of newborn infants. 3. Historical comments and development of a scoring system for selection of infants. Anesthesiology 1971;34(2):119–126.

[38] Downes JJ. Mechanical ventilation of the newborn. Anesthesiology 1971;34(2):116–118.

[39] Benson F, Celander O, Haglund G, Nilsson L, Paulsen L, Renck L. Positive-pressure respirator treatment of severe pulmonary insufficiency in the newborn infant; a clinical report. Acta Anaesthesiol Scand 1958;2(1):37–43.

[40] Donald I, Kerr MM, Macdonald IR. Respiratory phenomena in the newborn; experiments in their measurement and assistance. Scott Med J 1958;3(4):151–164.

[41] Delivoria-Papadopoulos M, Swyer PR. Assisted ventilation in terminal hyaline membrane disease. Arch Dis Child 1964;39:481–484.

[42] Delivoria-Papadopoulos M, Levison H, Swyer PR. Intermittent positive pressure respiration as a treatment in severe respiratory distress syndrome. Arch Dis Child 1965;40(213):474–479.

[43] Swyer PR, Levison H. The current status of the respiratory distress syndrome of the newly born. Can Med Assoc J 1965;93:335–342.

[44] Adamson TM, Collins LM, Dehan M, Hawker JM, Reynolds EO, Strang LB. Mechanical ventilation in newborn infants with respiratory failure. Lancet 1968;2(7562):227–231.

[45] Thomas DV, Fletcher G, Sunshine P, Schafer IA, Klaus MH. Prolonged respirator use in pulmonary insufficiency of newborn. JAMA 1965;193:183–190.

[46] de Heese HV, Harrison VC, Klein M, Malan AF. Intermittent positive pressure ventilation in hyaline membrane disease. J Pediatr 1970;76(2):183–193.

[47] Woollam CH. The development of apparatus for intermittent negative pressure respiration. (2) 1919–1976, with special reference to the development and uses of cuirass respirators. Anaesthesia 1976;31(5):666–685.

[48] Woollam CH. The development of apparatus for intermittent negative pressure respiration. Anaesthesia 1976;31(4):537–547.

[49] Stern L. Results of artificial ventilation in the newborn. Biol Neonate 1970;16(1):155–163.

[50] Stahlman MT, Malan AF, Shepard FM, Blankenship WJ, Young WC, Gray J. Negative pressure assisted ventilation in infants with hyaline membrane disease. J Pediatr 1970;76(2):174–182.

[51] Stern L, Ramos AD, Outerbridge EW, Beaudry PH. Negative pressure artificial respiration: use in treatment of respiratory failure of the newborn. Can Med Assoc J 1970;102(6):595–601.

[52] Chernick V, Vidyasagar D. Continuous negative chest wall pressure in hyaline membrane disease: one year experience. Pediatrics 1972;49(5):753–760.

[53] Vidyasagar D, Chernick V. Continuous positive transpulmonary pressure in

hyaline membrane disease: a simple device. Pediatrics 1971;48(2):296–299.

[54] Problems of neonatal intensive care units. Report of the fifty-ninth Ross Conference on Pediatric Research. Lucey JF, editor. 1969: Ross Laboratories; 1969.

[55] Swyer PR. Patient monitoring during artificial ventilation. Biol Neonate 1970;16(1):88–91.

[56] Swyer PR. Results of artificial ventilation. Experience at the Hospital for Sick Children, Toronto. Biol Neonate 1970;16(1):148–154.

[57] Swyer PR. Methods of artificial ventilation in the newborn (IPPV). Biol Neonate 1970;16(1):3–15.

[58] Swyer PR. Symposium on artificial ventilation. Summary of conference proceedings. Biol Neonate 1970;16(1):191–195.

[59] Gregory GA, Kitterman JA, Phibbs RH, Tooley WH, Hamilton WK. Treatment of the idiopathic respiratory-distress syndrome with continuous positive airway pressure. N Engl J Med 1971;284(24):1333–1340.

[60] Avery ME. Surfactant deficiency in hyaline membrane disease: the story of discovery. Am J Respir Crit Care Med 2000;161(4 Pt. 1):1074–1075.

[61] Avery ME. Chevalier Jackson Lecture: in quest of the prevention of hyaline membrane disease. Ann Otol Rhinol Laryngol 1977;86(5 Pt. 1):573–576.

[62] Brumley GW, Hodson WA, Avery ME. Lung phospholipids and surface tension correlations in infants with and without hyaline membrane disease and in adults. Pediatrics 1967;40(1):13–19.

[63] Avery GB. Recent concepts of pulmonary hyaline membrane disease. Med Ann Dist Columbia 1962;31:92–94.

[64] Avery ME. Recent increase in mortality from hyaline membrane disease. J Pediatr 1960;57:553–559.

[65] Halliday HL. History of surfactant from 1980. Biol Neonate 2005;87(4):317–322.

[66] Obladen M. History of surfactant up to 1980. Biol Neonate 2005;87(4):308–316.

[67] Fujiwara T, Adams FH. Surfactant for hyaline membrane disease. Pediatrics 1980;66(5):795–798.

[68] Fujiwara T, Maeta H, Chida S, Morita T, Watabe Y, Abe T. Artificial surfactant therapy in hyaline-membrane disease. Lancet 1980;1(8159):55–59.

[69] Raju TN, Vidyasagar D, Bhat R, Sobel D, McCulloch KM, Anderson M, et al. Double-blind controlled trial of single-dose treatment with bovine surfactant in severe hyaline membrane disease. Lancet 1987;1(8534):651–656.

[70] Seger N, Soll R. Animal derived surfactant extract for treatment of respiratory distress syndrome. Cochrane Database Syst Rev 2009;(2):CD007836.

[71] Goldsmith JP, Karotkin E, Suresh G, Keszler M. Assisted ventilation of the neonate: evidence-based approach to newborn respiratory care. Saunders Elsevier, St. Louis, MO; 2016.

[72] Walsh MC, Bell EF, Kandefer S, Saha S, Carlo WA, D'Angio CT, et al. Neonatal outcomes of moderately preterm infants compared to extremely preterm infants. Pediatr Res 2017;82(2):297–304.

[73] Stoll BJ, Hansen NI, Bell EF, Shankaran S, Laptook AR, Walsh MC, et al. Neonatal outcomes of extremely preterm infants from the NICHD Neonatal Research Network. Pediatrics 2010;126(3):443–456.

[74] Clark RH. The epidemiology of respiratory failure in neonates born at an estimated gestational age of 34 weeks or more. J Perinatol 2005;25(4):251–257.

[75] Vidyasagar D, Singhal N. Neonatal ventilator care in resource limited countries. In: Goldsmith JP, Karotkin E, editors. Assisted ventilation of the neonate. Philadelphia: Elsevier; 2011. p. 521–530.

Section | II |

Lung Development and Interventions in the Prenatal and Perinatal Period

Chapter | 3 |

Pathophysiology of Fetal Lung Development

Bobby Mathew, MBBS, MRCP, Lucky Jain, MD, MBA, Satyan Lakshminrusimha, MD

CHAPTER POINTS

- Fetal lung development is a highly complex developmental process orchestrated by genetic, hormonal, and physical factors.
- Lung development proceeds from 4 weeks of gestation through childhood in five continuous but overlapping stages
- Specific disorders are associated with derangements, insults and exposures at various developmental stages and following preterm birth.
- Studies in animal models have significantly advanced our understanding of the molecular mechanisms of lung development.
- Recent studies with stem cells hold promise to further our knowledge towards development of potential therapeutic interventions in this vulnerable patient population.

Introduction

The primary function of the respiratory system is oxygenation and removal of carbon dioxide from the blood. This is accomplished through a highly complex system of airways and blood vessels that are closely related from an anatomical, functional, and developmental perspective. Gas exchange between the atmospheric air and the blood occurs across the double-layered alveolar–capillary membrane. The lungs consists of extensive airway conducting system, with many different specialized epithelial lining cells, neuroendocrine cells, and an expansive gas exchange zone composed of intricately arranged pulmonary epithelial cells and capillaries. Fetal lung development is a highly complex developmental process orchestrated by genetic, hormonal, and physical factors. This chapter briefly describes the development of the lungs, the disorders associated with derangements at various developmental stages, and the effects of exposure to adverse intrauterine environment from various insults during gestation and following preterm birth [1].

Embryology

The lungs develop from the primitive foregut endoderm and the surrounding mesoderm. All of the three germ layers give origin to the different tissues of the lung. The pulmonary epithelium is derived from the endoderm. The pulmonary vasculature, the cartilage, the airway, and vascular smooth muscle and connective tissues are of mesodermal origin. The neural innervation of the lung is of ectodermal origin. Reciprocal mesenchymal–epithelial inductive interactions are mediated through direct cell-to-cell contact, soluble factors, and spatiotemporal- and concentration-dependent activation of different growth factors and genes lead to coordinated development of the lungs. Mesenchyme influences epithelial growth and morphology, patterning of ductal branching, and activates specific patterns of epithelial cytodifferentiation and functional activities [2]. Fetal lung development proceeds from 4 weeks of gestation through childhood in five continuous but overlapping stages (Fig. 3.1 and Table 3.1).

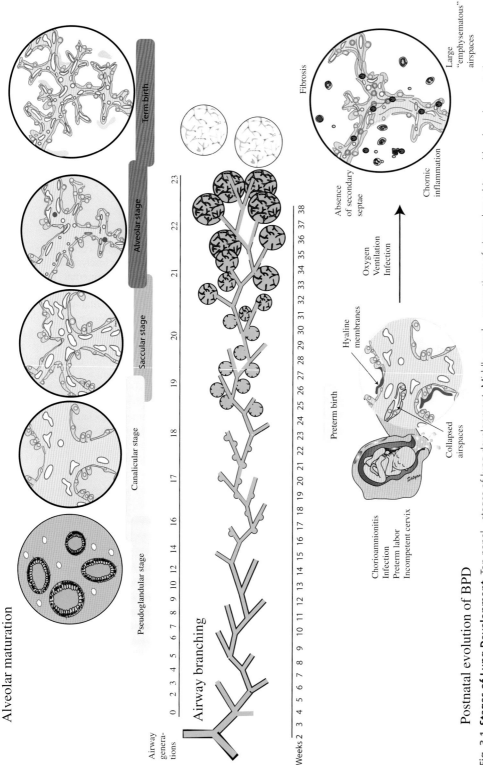

Alveolar maturation

Airway branching

Postnatal evolution of BPD

Fig. 3.1 Stages of Lung Development. Top panel—stages of lung development. Middle panel—generations of airway branching with advancing gestation. Bottom panel—factors leading to preterm birth, and postnatal factors leading to the pathological changes associated with bronchopulmonary dysplasia. *BPD*, Bronchopulmonary dysplasia. Copyright: Satyan Lakshminrusimha.

Table 3.1 Stages of lung development and timing based on postmenstrual age (PMA)

Stages	Weeks (PMA)	Main events	Examples of anomalies resulting from disruption at this stage
Embryonic	5–9	Tracheobronchial branching	Tracheoesophageal fistula, esophageal atresia, pulmonary agenesis/aplasia.
Pseudoglandular	6–17	Elongation and repetitive branching of airways and pulmonary vascular development	Bronchogenic cysts, pulmonary hypoplasia, tracheobronchomalacia, intralobar pulmonary sequestration, alveolar capillary dysplasia, congenital diaphragmatic hernia and pulmonary vascular lymphangiectasis
Canalicular	16–26	Differentiation of type I and II cells, surfactant and lung liquid production; alveolar–capillary interface begins to form	Pulmonary hypoplasia, alveolar capillary dysplasia
Saccular	24–38	Formation of air sacs and better apposition of alveolar and capillary membranes	Bronchopulmonary dysplasia following preterm birth
Alveolar	36 weeks to postnatal age (2–8 years)	Secondary septa formation and fusion and thinning of double-capillary network	

Disruption of each stage can lead to specific congenital or developmental anomalies of the lung.

Embryonic stage

This stage extends from 5 to 9 weeks of postmenstrual age (PMA). The major events during the embryonic stage are the formation of the lung bud and the development of the major airways to the level of segmental bronchi. At 28 days of gestation a group of cells in the ventral foregut endoderm are committed to become respiratory epithelial progenitors by localized expression of the homeobox gene Nkx2-1 [3]. At 5 weeks of PMA, these cells give rise to lung buds that appears as a ventral outpouchings from the primitive gut endoderm and grows into the surrounding mesoderm anterior to and parallel to the developing esophagus. The trachea is formed by the fusion of lung buds by 6 weeks of PMA. Epithelial cells (endodermal origin) invade the surrounding mesoderm and undergo a series of branching giving rise to the tracheobronchial tree. By the 7th week of PMA, bifurcation of the lung buds occurs, two on the left and three on the right. In the subsequent week, a further round of branching occurs which gives rise to segmental branches, 8–9 on the left and 10 on the right and establishes the bronchopulmonary segments of the lung. The separation of trachea and esophagus is complete by the end of this stage. The pulmonary artery branches from the sixth aortic arch and the pulmonary veins emerging from the left atrium are established. Perturbations in development during this stage can lead to tracheoesophageal fistula, esophageal atresia, and pulmonary agenesis/aplasia.

Pseudoglandular stage

This stage extends from 6 to 18 weeks of PMA. During this stage the developing lungs assumes a glandular appearance with multiple branching epithelial tubes surrounded by abundant mesenchyme. The main event that occurs during this stage is the elongation and repetitive branching of the airways, differentiation of the epithelial linings of the respiratory tree, and the development of airway smooth muscle and cartilage. Branching morphogenesis is tightly controlled temporally and spatially with proximal–distal (P–D) patterning, resulting in generation of proximal epithelial progenitors giving rise to neuroendocrine, mucociliary, and basal cells of the conducting airways and distal epithelial progenitors yielding pneumocytes in the periphery of the lungs [4–6]. The P–D patterning is brought about by differential expression of transcription factors, Sox2 in the proximal airway lining cells and Sox 9 in the distal epithelium of the lungs [7,8]. The cartilage extends into the segmental bronchi and smooth muscle to the respiratory bronchioles. Vascular development during this stage includes the development of pulmonary arterial system in parallel to the airway branching and the pulmonary veins and lymphatics extending into the interlobular septa. Closure of the pleuroperitoneal cavity occurs during this stage. Breathing movements are first noted around 10 weeks of PMA. Congenital abnormalities during this stage of development include bronchogenic cysts, pulmonary hypoplasia, tracheobronchomalacia, intralobar pulmonary sequestration, alveolar capillary dysplasia, congenital diaphragmatic hernia, and pulmonary vascular lymphangiectasis.

Canalicular stage

This stage extends between 16 and 26 weeks of gestation. Canalization of the lung parenchyma with increasing pulmonary capillary network, formation of the air blood barrier, differentiation of the epithelial cells in the lung are the main events in this stage. The alveolar lining cells—the type 1 and 2 alveolar cells appear in the second half of this stage. The lumen of the airways enlarge, with thinning of the alveolar septa and an exponential increase in development of the capillary bed with greater apposition of the airway and the vasculature resulting in the formation of the immature yet functional air–blood barrier. The conducting airways are lined by fully differentiated ciliated cells, submucosal glands, smooth muscle, and cartilage as far distally as in the mature lung. Respiratory bronchioles and alveolar ducts develop during this stage. The epithelial cells secrete fetal lung fluid and the alveolar type 2 cells begin to produce surfactant. Infants born toward the end of this stage have severe respiratory insufficiency but can survive with surfactant replacement therapy and intensive care. Abnormalities associated with this stage of lung development are pulmonary hypoplasia due to impairment of the thoracic cavity or loss of fetal lung fluid as in oligohydramnios and alveolar capillary dysplasia.

Saccular stage

This stage extends between 24 and 38 weeks of gestation. Formation of alveolar ducts and saccules occurs by the expansion and dilation of the terminal clusters of the acinar tubules. Intersaccular and interductal septa develop which contain a double capillary network. Greater apposition of the capillaries and the type 1 alveolar epithelial cells with fusion of the basal lamina of the type 1 alveolar epithelial cells and the endothelium of the capillary results in the formation of alveolar–capillary membrane. Further maturation of the type 2 alveolar epithelial cells occurs as evidenced by increase in number and size of the lamellar bodies and increase in amounts of tubular myelin in the airspaces.

Alveolar stage

The alveolar stage of lung development extends from 36 weeks of PMA to 2 years postnatal and is characterized by the maturation of the alveolar–capillary membrane and the formation of secondary septa, which divide the terminal saccules into alveolar ducts and alveoli. The alveolar septum is thick and contains a double capillary network at the beginning of this stage. Development of secondary septa/crests with further lengthening, thinning, and fusion of the double capillary network leads to closer apposition of the alveolar capillary interface and increase in surface area for gas exchange and the formation of the mature alveolus. Alveolarization occurs in two phases. The initial phase in the first 2 years of life of rapid increase in alveolar numbers with decreased volumetric expansion is termed bulk alveolarization. This is followed in childhood through young adolescence by a period of slower increase in number and increased growth of the alveoli resulting in increased lung volumes [9,10]. At term gestation, the mature lung has approximately 150 million alveoli and this increases to about 480 million by adulthood.

Pulmonary vascular development

The pulmonary vascular system consists of the pulmonary arterial and venous systems and pulmonary lymphatics. Converse to what was believed earlier, vascular morphogenesis starts early in the embryonic phase with the development of a primitive vascular plexus around the lung bud [11]. The pulmonary vasculature develops form mesodermal progenitor cells, which are committed to endothelial lineage with specific markers, such as VGFR2, CD31, and Sox17. The two major processes through which pulmonary blood vessels develop are vasculogenesis and angiogenesis. Vasculogenesis involves the de novo formation of blood vessels through primitive endothelial cells forming tubes or sinusoids. Angiogenesis is the process by which new vessels are formed by sprouting or branching from preexisting vessels. The main pulmonary artery is formed by vasculogenesis and so are the blood vessels at periphery of the lung. Angiogenesis accounts for the formation of the proximal pulmonary arteries and veins [12]. The development of the pulmonary arterial system closely mirrors the airway system. All the preacinar arteries and veins are formed by the end of the pseudoglandular stage. In the canalicular stage, there is a rapid increase in blood vessel formation and closer apposition of the blood vessels to the pulmonary epithelium. During the saccular and alveolar stages, fusion of the basement membrane of the alveolar epithelial cells to the pulmonary endothelial cell further decreases the diffusion distance and increases the efficiency of gas exchange of the alveolar–capillary membrane. Alveolar and pulmonary vascular development is exceedingly interdependent processes and perturbation of pulmonary vascular development leads to impairment of alveolarization [13–15].

Transcription factors and growth factors in lung development

Lung development is dependent on interactions between the epithelium and the mesenchyme and modulated by multiple signaling pathways. Several transcription factors, growth factors, and their receptors with specific temporal and spatial profiles play vital role in different stages of lung development. The role of different factors in lung development has been elucidated by gain or loss of function studies in null, mutant, and transgenic mouse models. The progenitors for the future respiratory tract are first identified around 28-day gestation by localized expression of homeobox gene Nkx2-1 in a subset of cells in the ventral foregut endoderm. NKX2-1/Thyroid transcription factor (TTF1) is a key regulator involved in all stages of lung development from the embryonic stage through to alveolarization in the postnatal period. In experimental animals, disruption of NKX2-1 results in nonseparation of the trachea from the esophagus, severe lung hypoplasia, impairment of branching morphogenesis and epithelial differentiation, and abnormalities in surfactant homeostasis [16,17]. In the earliest stage of development, Forkhead box A1 and 2 (FOXA) is expressed in the ventral foregut endoderm at the initiation of lung bud formation along with the NKX2-1. Mutation of the Foxf1 is the underlying genetic abnormality in alveolar–capillary dysplasia [18,19]. Fibroblast growth factors (FGF) regulate an array of functions, including migration, cellular proliferation, and differentiation. FGF10, a mitogen, and chemoattractant for the epithelium and its receptor FGFR2IIIb play an important role in the branching morphogenesis. FGF10 deficient mice have arrested development at the stage of the trachea with no pulmonary branching [20,21]. Sonic hedgehog (Shh) plays an important role in epithelial mesenchymal signaling with deficiency leading to decreased cell proliferation and increased apoptosis and overexpression resulting in mesenchymal hypercellularity and smaller lungs with dysfunctional alveoli [22,23]. Other genes and transcription factors, such as HOX, Myc, GATA, Wnts, BMPs, play crucial roles in the branching morphogenesis [24–28]. Elastogenesis is critical for secondary septation in the stage of alveolarization. Elastin deposition occurs at the sites of interalveolar septa formation. Platelet-derived growth factor, a key chemoattractant for myofibroblasts, FGF18, retinoic acid have an important role in elastogenesis, secondary septation, and alveolarization. Retinoic acid upregulates tropoelastin gene expression and mRNA expression of FGF18, PGDF, and its receptors. Vitamin A deficiency has been shown to delay alveolar development, and supplementation results in increasing number of alveoli in rat pups [29]. Vitamin A supplementation has been shown to decrease mortality

and the risk of bronchopulmonary dysplasia in preterm infants [30]. Remodeling of the extracellular matrix is brought about by the matrix metalloproteinases (MMP2 and MMP14) and the tissue inhibitors of metalloproteinases (TIMP). Low levels of MMP2 in tracheal secretions were found to be associated with an increased risk of bronchopulmonary dysplasia in preterm infants [31].

Vascular endothelial growth factor (VEGF) plays a major role both in blood vessel formation and alveolarization (Fig. 3.2). In experimental animals, ablation of the VEGF gene caused abnormal spatial organization of blood vessels, severe cardiovascular abnormalities, and in utero death. VEGF-mediated angiogenesis is brought about in part through nitric oxide. In newborn mice, treatment with VEGF inhibitor SU5416 decreased lung endothelial nitric oxide synthase (eNOS) activity resulting in right ventricular hypertrophy (RVH) and decreased radial alveolar count (RAC). Inhaled nitric oxide treatment prevented the development of RVH and improved the RAC [32]. VEGF expression is tightly controlled during lung development, as seen in experimental studies in mice; overexpression of VEGF resulted in pulmonary vascular leak and hemorrhage alveolar inflammation and death [33]. Other important mediators of pulmonary vascular development include epidermal growth factor (EGF), transforming growth factor, angiopoietins, BMPs platelet-derived growth factors, and transcription factors such as HIF, Hox, Fox, and Sox that play a critical role in lung development.

Maturation of pulmonary surfactant system

Pulmonary surfactant is synthesized and secreted by the type 2 alveolar cells. Type 2 cells are first recognized in the late canalicular stage. In utero, type 2 cells secrete only small amounts of surfactant even at term gestation. Surfactant synthesis and secretion are tightly regulated by hormonal, physical, and chemical stimuli. Regulation of type 2 alveolar epithelial cells, maturation, and surfactant release are influenced by late-term elevations of intracellular cyclic 3′-5′ adenosine monophosphate (cAMP), cortisol, thyroid hormone, catecholamines, and through stimulation of beta adrenoceptors and natriuretic peptide receptors [34,35] (Fig. 3.3). Lamellar bodies, the storage form of surfactant, first appear in the fetal lungs between 20 and 24 weeks of gestation. The surfactant pool size of preterm infants with RDS is about 10 mg/kg as compared to 100 mg/kg in term infants [36]. The rate of synthesis and clearance of surfactant is about 10-fold less than in the adult [37]. However, birth even at extreme preterm gestation, the surfactant system is turned on and these infants are able to

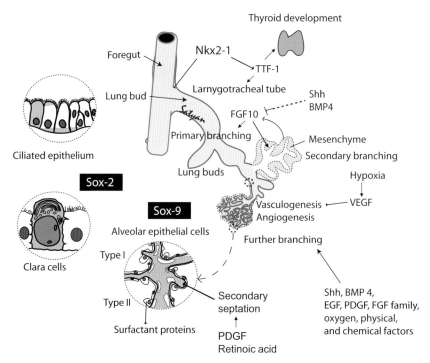

Fig. 3.2 Development of the Respiratory System —Role of Genes, Growth Factors and Transcription Factors. Localized expression of NKX2-1 on the endodermal cells on the ventral surface of the primitive foregut commits them to respiratory cell lineage. At 5-week PMA, lung buds appear as two ventral outpouchings and grow into the surrounding mesoderm. Positive signaling by fibroblast growth factor 10 (FGF 10) and negative signaling by Sonic Hedgehog (Shh), bone morphogenetic protein 4 (BMP4), Sprouty 2 (spry2) facilitate primary and secondary branching. Further branching is facilitated by Shh, BMP4, spry2, transforming growth factor β (TGFβ), epidermal growth factor (EGF), platelet-derived growth factor (PGDF), and fibroblast growth factors (FGFs). PGDF and retinoic acid (RA) have important role in secondary septation and alveolarization. Thyroid transcription factor-1 (TTF-1) and GATA-6 are important in cell differentiation and the development of the surfactant system. Forkhead homolog 4 (HFH-4) plays an important role in differentiation of ciliated epithelial cell lineage. Differential expression of the Sox2 and Sox9 leads to the proximal distal patterning of airway development. *VEGF*, Vascular endothelial growth factor. Copyright: Satyan Lakshminrusimha.

produce though lower but adequate amounts of surfactant by 4–7 days of life without the need for further exogenous surfactant replacement therapy [38]. Changes in composition of surfactant also occur with advancing gestation, and are the basis of tests for lung maturity in fetus, such as lecithin to sphingomyelin (*L:S*) ratio [39]. The phospholipid composition of the surfactant also changes with gestation with an increase in content of phosphatidylcholine and the ratio of phosphatidylglycerol to phosphatidylinositol [40]. The presence of phosphatidylglycerol in the amniotic fluid is considered as positive test for lung maturity. The preterm lung is also deficient in surfactant proteins (SPs) [41,42]. The decreased level of SPs in the preterm decreases its efficiency at improving the lung compliance and increases the susceptibility to inactivation. SP-A and SP-D are water-soluble collectins, decreased levels of which lead to impairment of host defense from decreased phagocytic and opsonization functions [43]. SP-B and SP-C are hydrophobic

peptides associated with surfactant phospholipids and are stored in the lamellar bodies. SP-B is absolutely critical to surfactant function, as it is an essential for synthesis, assembly and functioning of surfactant, and deficiency leads to death in the newborn period. They have antiinflammatory and antioxidant properties, and a lower level in preterm infants translates to increased susceptibility to infection, inflammation, and hyperoxia-mediated lung injury [44].

Intrauterine exposures and its effect on lung development

Smoking

The fetus is indirectly exposed to many environmental pollutants through the transplacental route. Maternal smoking

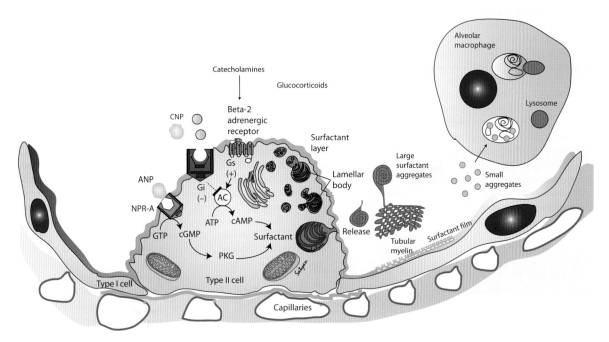

Fig. 3.3 Control of Surfactant Secretion. Catecholamines act through the adenylyl cyclase stimulate surfactant secretion. ANP at lower doses binds to the NPR-A receptor and stimulates surfactant release. At higher doses, ANP also binds to the NPR-C receptor and inhibits beta-2 agonist stimulation of surfactant release. *CNP*, C-type natriuretic peptid. Copyright: Satyan Lakshminrusimha.

during pregnancy has been the most extensively studied among toxic exposures to the fetus. Cigarette smoking in pregnancy leads to premature birth, poor intrauterine growth, and increases perinatal mortality. Nicotine in cigarette smoke crosses the placenta and through binding to the nicotinic acetylcholine receptors in the developing lung leads to long-term structural and functional abnormalities. In animal models, antenatal nicotine exposure is associated with decreased alveolar septation, elastin content, and lung volume and increased lamellar bodies and collagen [45,46]. Abnormalities in lung function include decrease in functional residual capacity, forced expiratory volume and compliance [47,48]. Abnormalities in airways with increased number airways of smaller diameter result in increased resistance to airflow [49]. This translates to an increased incidence of lower respiratory illness, such as reactive airways disease and asthma in childhood [50].

Intrauterine growth restriction (IUGR)/maternal undernutrition

Intrauterine growth restriction (IUGR) results from multiple etiologic factors, disorders of abnormal placental function, decreased fetal perfusion resulting in deficient oxygen and nutrient delivery, maternal undernutrition, systemic

illness, exposures to drugs and toxins or from factors intrinsic to the fetus. In animal models, fetal growth restriction has been shown to decrease the overall lung volume, the alveolar surface area and increase the thickness of the alveolar–capillary membrane resulting in decreased diffusing capacity [51–53]. In a maternal hyperthermia model of IUGR in fetal sheep, decreased pulmonary alveolar and vascular growth and endothelial dysfunction were shown to be the underlying mechanisms for pulmonary hypertension. In a retrospective study of infants' ≤28 weeks gestation at birth with moderate to severe BPD, birth weight below 25th percentile was found to be an independent predictor for pulmonary hypertension [54]. Studies in animal models have also shown an increased risk of development of pulmonary hypertension and cardiac dysfunction with age in IUGR [55].

Chorioamnionitis

Ascending infection from the lower genital tract spreads to the amniotic cavity through the choriodecidual plane. Common etiologic agents causing chorioamnionitis and precipitating preterm labor are *Ureaplasma*, *Mycoplasma*, and *Fusobacterium*. Studies of intraamniotic injections with bacterial products, such as lipopolysaccharide (LPS) or proinflammatory cytokines (IL-1 Beta IL-1 alpha), lead to increase in pulmonary surfactant, lung maturation, and improved compliance [56,57]. This functional maturation is brought about at the expense of structural lung development with decrease in the number and increase in size of the alveoli leading to decreased surface area for gas exchange [58]. Intraamniotic injection of LPS in fetal sheep leads to hypertrophy of the smooth muscle and fibroblast proliferation in the adventitia resulting in pulmonary vascular remodeling and increased pulmonary vascular resistance contributing to the development of pulmonary hypertension [59,60]. The effect of chorioamnionitis on long-term pulmonary outcomes is not well established. However, the available evidence in preterm infants with chorioamnionitis suggests an increased risk of bronchopulmonary dysplasia in newborn period and reactive airways disease in childhood [61,62].

Physical factors: lung liquid and fetal breathing movements

Lung fluid is secreted by the epithelial cells by active transport of chloride ions into the lumen of the lung. The near term fetal lung in sheep secretes about 4–5 mL/kg/h of fetal lung fluid and the lungs contain about 25–40 mL/kg body weight, which is approximately equal to or slightly higher than the functional residual capacity of the term lung. The intraluminal pressure in the lungs is higher than the intraamniotic pressure by about 2 mmHg and fetal lung fluid drains intermittently with breathing movements into the amniotic cavity (Fig. 3.4). This distending pressure is vital and promotes the development of the lungs in the fetus. Moessinger et al. have demonstrated that the loss of fetal lung fluid results in lung hypoplasia in fetal lambs [63]. Oligohydramnios as it occurs in fetuses with renal agenesis (Potter's syndrome), preterm prelabor rupture of membranes leads to an increased risk of pulmonary hypoplasia and the risk increases with the time and duration of oligohydramnios. The increased volume of fetal lung liquid causes lung hyperplasia, and this is the basis of the fetal endoluminal tracheal occlusion (FETO) procedure in fetuses with antenatal diagnosis of congenital diaphragmatic hernia. (NCT02710968 and others at clinicaltrials.gov).

Fetal breathing movements are required for optimal lung development. In human fetuses, breathing movements start around 10-week gestation and the frequency increases with advancing gestation. At term gestation, breathing movements occur about 30% of the time. In utero transection of the phrenic nerve during in utero development on day 24.5 in rabbit fetus resulted in hypoplastic lungs [64].

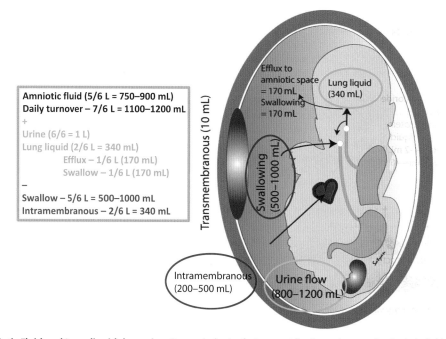

Fig. 3.4 Amniotic Fluid and Lung liquid dynamics. *Green*—indicates factors contributing to increase in amniotic fluid. *Red* indicates factors depleting amniotic fluid. Fetal lung liquid is the second most important contributor to amniotic fluid volume (the primary contributor being fetal urine). The volumes are shown as fractions with a denominator of 6 for ease. Copyright: Satyan Lakshminrusimha.

Peristaltic contractile activity of the airway propagates distal movement of the lung fluid, expansion of the lung buds, and promotes lung growth and development. Restriction of chest cavity impairs lung growth. This could result from extrinsic restriction, as it occurs with abnormalities of chest shape, for example, thoracic dystrophies, severe kyphoscoliosis or congenital diaphragmatic hernia, lung masses/cysts, or effusions.

In preparation for postnatal gas exchange, the alveolar epithelium shifts from a fluid secreting to a reabsorbing membrane (Fig. 3.5). This is brought about through changes in transmembrane transport channels, humoral factors, and changes in oxygen tension. The effects of these are also modified by the gestational age at birth, labor, and mode of delivery. During late gestation, an increase in circulating catecholamines and elevation in intracellular cAMP levels result in maturation of the pulmonary epithelium preparing the lungs for surfactant secretion and fluid clearance. At the onset of labor, active transcellular movement of sodium from the lumen to the interstitial space and further into the pulmonary lymphatics and to the venous system is facilitated by the epithelial sodium channel (ENaC) on the luminal side and the sodium potassium ATPase (Na,K-ATPase) and sodium potassium chloride cotransporter (NaKCC1) on the basolateral membrane [65]. This effect is blocked by the sodium channel blocker amiloride [66]. ENaC knockout mice have delayed alveolar

fluid clearance in the newborn period with improvement on rescue with αENaC transgene [67]. Epinephrine causes lung fluid resorption through beta adrenergic pathway and this effect is blocked by propranolol [68]. Thyroid hormone and glucocorticoids play a key role in advancing the absorptive response of the pulmonary epithelium to catecholamines [69]. Exposure to prenatal steroids has been shown to increase the levels of αENaC mRNA in the fetal rat lungs [70]. The increase in PaO_2 as seen following birth inhibits fluid secretion in lung explants from late gestation but not in early gestations [71]. However, this effect can be induced at earlier gestation on treatment with thyroid or steroid hormones. Preterm premature rupture of membranes leads to fetal lung maturation as evidenced by rapid acceleration of the rate of increased L/S ratio to levels seen with lung maturity.

Glucocorticoids

Glucocorticoids induce accelerated maturation of the lung with thinning of the alveolar wall and fusion of the double capillary network and maturation of the surfactant system resulting in decreased severity of respiratory distress syndrome in infants born preterm. However, this also causes inhibition of vascular development and earlier termination of the septation leading to fewer and larger alveoli with decrease in lung surface area for gas exchange [72,73].

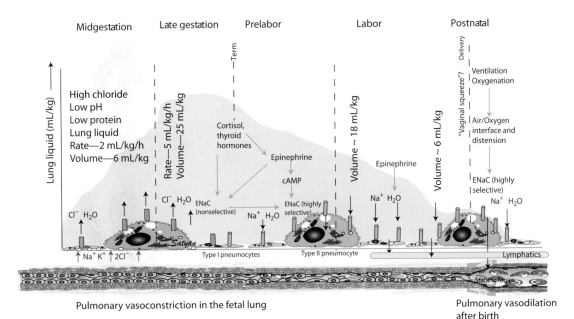

Fig. 3.5 Changes in lung liquid volume during various phases of gestation, term birth, and postnatal period. Factors contributing to secretion and resorption of lung liquid are shown. The vertical axis represents lung liquid volume in mL/kg. *cAMP*, Cyclic 3'-5' adenosine monophosphate; *ENaC*, epithelial sodium channel. Copyright: Satyan Lakshminrusimha.

Expectant mothers with threatened preterm labor before 34 weeks of gestation are routinely given a single course of antenatal steroids. Infants born 24 h to 7 days following complete course of antenatal steroids have decreased severity of respiratory distress syndrome intraventricular hemorrhage and mortality. However, infants whose mothers received multiple courses of antenatal steroids had decreased birth weight, length, and head circumference with no improvement in neonatal morbidities [74].

Premature birth and oxygen exposure

The fetal lung develops in a hypoxemic environment. Low oxygen tension promotes optimal fetal lung development through hypoxia inducible factor (HIF) and its effect on VEGF. Extremely preterm infants born toward the end of the canalicular stage of lung development are capable of surviving with intensive care, surfactant replacement therapy, and assisted ventilation. The gas exchange units at this stage consist of terminal clusters of acinar tubules, alveolar ducts, and saccules and a primitive alveolar–capillary membrane. Exposure to hyperoxia and ventilator-induced lung injury are inevitable consequences of extreme preterm birth. Inhibition of VEGF (due to hyperoxia) leads to impairment of both vascularization and alveolarization. Exposure to hyperoxia also causes oxidative stress-mediated lung damage, which overwhelms the immature antioxidant capabilities of the preterm lungs that lead to the development of bronchopulmonary dysplasia and long-term pulmonary morbidity in survivors of preterm birth.

Conclusions

Arrest of lung development, intrauterine/perinatal and postnatal infections, and iatrogenic lung injury remains the cause of major morbidity and mortality in infants born extremely preterm. Current treatment modalities are targeted at decreasing ventilator-induced lung injury, optimizing nutrition, prevention and treatment of infections, gastroesophageal reflux, which cause impaired lung development and deterioration of lung function. Timely and effective antenatal care, minimizing noxious exposures, and ensuring adequate fetal and postnatal growth can to a degree mitigate the developmental consequences to the lung of preterm birth. Studies in animal models have significantly advanced our understanding of the molecular mechanisms of lung development. However, significant gaps in our knowledge remain. Inaccessibility to the lung during fetal development has limited our ability to study their role in human lung development. The emerging field of study using induced pluripotent stem cells (iPSCs) offers the potential to recapitulate the molecular mechanisms in vitro. Further advances in these techniques is likely to provide an in vitro model to study lung development and derangements associated with disease states, design new drugs, and develop lung tissue that can used for transplant in patients with end-stage lung disease.

References

[1] Jobe A, Whitsett J, Abman S. Fetal and neonatal lung development: clinical correlates and technologies for the future. Cambridge University Press, New York, USA; 2016.

[2] Minoo P, King RJ. Epithelial-mesenchymal interactions in lung development. Annu Rev Physiol 1994;56:13–45.

[3] Lazzaro D, Price M, de Felice M, Di Lauro R. The transcription factor TTF-1 is expressed at the onset of thyroid and lung morphogenesis and in restricted regions of the foetal brain. Development 1991;113(4):1093–1104.

[4] Morrisey EE, Hogan BL. Preparing for the first breath: genetic and cellular mechanisms in lung development. Dev Cell 2010;18(1):8–23.

[5] Varner VD, Nelson CM. Cellular and physical mechanisms of branching morphogenesis. Development 2014;141(14):2750–2759.

[6] Metzger RJ, Klein OD, Martin GR, Krasnow MA. The branching programme of mouse lung development. Nature 2008;453(7196):745–750.

[7] Tompkins DH, Besnard V, Lange AW, Keiser AR, Wert SE, Bruno MD, et al. Sox2 activates cell proliferation and differentiation in the respiratory epithelium. Am J Respir Cell Mol Biol 2011;45(1):101–110.

[8] Rockich BE, Hrycaj SM, Shih HP, Nagy MS, Ferguson MA, Kopp JL, et al. Sox9 plays multiple roles in the lung epithelium during branching morphogenesis. Proc Natl Acad Sci 2013;110(47):E4456–E4464.

[9] Tschanz SA, Salm LA, Roth-Kleiner M, Barre SF, Burri PH, Schittny JC. Rat lungs show a biphasic formation of new alveoli during postnatal development. J Appl Physiol 2014;117(1):89–95.

[10] Burri PH. Structural aspects of postnatal lung development—alveolar formation and growth. Biol Neonate 2006;89(4):313–322.

[11] Schachtner SK, Wang Y, Scott Baldwin H. Qualitative and quantitative analysis of embryonic pulmonary vessel formation. Am J Respir Cell Mol Biol 2000;22(2):157–165.

[12] deMello DE, Sawyer D, Galvin N, Reid LM. Early fetal development of lung vasculature. Am J Respir Cell Mol Biol 1997;16(5):568–581.

[13] Thebaud B, Ladha F, Michelakis ED, Sawicka M, Thurston G, Eaton F, et al. Vascular endothelial growth factor gene therapy increases survival, promotes lung angiogenesis, and prevents alveolar damage in hyperoxia-induced lung injury: evidence that angiogenesis participates in alveolarization. Circulation 2005;112(16):2477–2486.

[14] Jakkula M, Le Cras TD, Gebb S, Hirth KP, Tuder RM, Voelkel NF, et al. Inhibition of angiogenesis decreases alveolarization in the developing rat lung. Am J Physiol Lung Cell Mol Physiol 2000;279(3):L600–L607.

[15] Bhatt AJ, Pryhuber GS, Huyck H, Watkins RH, Metlay LA, Maniscalco WM. Disrupted pulmonary vasculature and decreased vascular endothelial growth factor, Flt-1, and TIE-2 in human infants dying with bronchopulmonary dysplasia. Am J Respir Crit Care Med 2001;164(10 Pt 1):1971–1980.

[16] Kimura S. Thyroid-specific enhancer-binding protein role in thyroid function and organogenesis. Trends Endocrinol Metab 1996;7(7):247–252.

[17] DeFelice M, Silberschmidt D, DiLauro R, Xu Y, Wert SE, Weaver TE, et al. TTF-1 phosphorylation is required for peripheral lung morphogenesis, perinatal survival, and tissue-specific gene expression. J Biol Chem 2003;278(37):35574–35583.

[18] Miranda J, Rocha G, Soares P, Morgado H, Baptista MJ, Azevedo I, et al. A novel mutation in FOXF1 gene associated with alveolar capillary dysplasia with misalignment of pulmonary veins, intestinal malrotation and annular pancreas. Neonatology 2013;103(4):241–245.

[19] Sen P, Yang Y, Navarro C, Silva I, Szafranski P, Kolodziejska KE, et al. Novel FOXF1 mutations in sporadic and familial cases of alveolar capillary dysplasia with misaligned pulmonary veins imply a role for its DNA binding domain. Hum Mutat 2013;34(6):801–811.

[20] Sekine K, Ohuchi H, Fujiwara M, Yamasaki M, Yoshizawa T, Sato T, et al. Fgf10 is essential for limb and lung formation. Nat Genet 1999;21(1):138–141.

[21] Arman E, Haffner-Krausz R, Gorivodsky M, Lonai P. Fgfr2 is required for limb outgrowth and lung-branching morphogenesis. Proc Natl Acad Sci 1999;96(21):11895–11899.

[22] Pepicelli CV, Lewis PM, McMahon AP. Sonic hedgehog regulates branching morphogenesis in the mammalian lung. Curr Biol 1998;8(19):1083–1086.

[23] Litingtung Y, Lei L, Westphal H, Chiang C. Sonic hedgehog is essential to foregut development. Nat Genet 1998;20(1):58–61.

[24] Hyatt BA, Shangguan X, Shannon JM. FGF-10 induces SP-C and Bmp4 and regulates proximal-distal patterning in embryonic tracheal epithelium. Am J Physiol Lung Cell Mol Physiol 2004;287(6):L1116–L1126.

[25] Rajagopal J, Carroll TJ, Guseh JS, Bores SA, Blank LJ, Anderson WJ, et al. Wnt7b stimulates embryonic lung growth by coordinately increasing the replication of epithelium and mesenchyme. Development 2008;135(9):1625–1634.

[26] Krumlauf R. Hox genes in vertebrate development. Cell 1994;78(2):191–201.

[27] Moens CB, Auerbach AB, Conlon RA, Joyner AL, Rossant J. A targeted mutation reveals a role for N-myc in branching morphogenesis in the embryonic mouse lung. Genes Dev 1992;6(5):691–704.

[28] Okubo T, Knoepfler PS, Eisenman RN, Hogan BL. Nmyc plays an essential role during lung development as a dosage-sensitive regulator of progenitor cell proliferation and differentiation. Development 2005;132(6):1363–1374.

[29] Massaro GD, Massaro D. Postnatal treatment with retinoic acid increases the number of pulmonary alveoli in rats. Am J Physiol 1996;270(2 Pt 1):L305–L310.

[30] Darlow BA, Graham PJ. Vitamin A supplementation to prevent mortality and short- and long-term morbidity in very low birth weight infants. Cochrane Database Syst Rev 2011;(10):CD000501.

[31] Danan C, Jarreau PH, Franco ML, Dassieu G, Grillon C, Abd Alsamad I, et al. Gelatinase activities in the airways of premature infants and development of bronchopulmonary dysplasia. Am J Physiol Lung Cell Mol Physiol 2002;283(5):L1086–L1093.

[32] Tang JR, Markham NE, Lin YJ, McMurtry IF, Maxey A, Kinsella JP, et al. Inhaled nitric oxide attenuates pulmonary hypertension and improves lung growth in infant rats after neonatal treatment with a VEGF receptor inhibitor. Am J Physiol Lung Cell Mol Physiol 2004;287(2):L344–L351.

[33] Le Cras TD, Spitzmiller RE, Albertine KH, Greenberg JM, Whitsett JA, Akeson AL. VEGF causes pulmonary hemorrhage, hemosiderosis, and air space enlargement in neonatal mice. Am J Physiol Lung Cell Mol Physiol 2004;287(1):L134–L142.

[34] Chander A, Fisher AB. Regulation of lung surfactant secretion. Am J Physiol 1990;258(6 Pt 1):L241–L253.

[35] Mathew B, D'Angelis CA, Lakshminrusimha S, Nickerson PA, Sokolowski JJ, Kumar VHS, et al. Natriuretic peptide C receptor in the developing sheep lung: role in perinatal transition. Pediatr Res 2017;82(2):349–355.

[36] Torresin M, Zimmermann LJ, Cogo PE, Cavicchioli P, Badon T, Giordano G, et al. Exogenous surfactant kinetics in infant respiratory distress syndrome: a novel method with stable isotopes. Am J Respir Crit Care Med 2000;161(5):1584–1589.

[37] Jacobs H, Jobe A, Ikegami M, Jones S. Surfactant phosphatidylcholine source, fluxes, and turnover times in 3-day-old, 10-day-old, and adult rabbits. J Biol Chem 1982;257(4):1805–1810.

[38] Jackson JC, Palmer S, Truog WE, Standaert TA, Murphy JH, Hodson WA. Surfactant quantity and composition during recovery from hyaline membrane disease. Pediatr Res 1986;20(12):1243–1247.

[39] Gluck L, Kulovich MV, Borer RC Jr, Brenner PH, Anderson GG, Spellacy WN. Diagnosis of the respiratory distress syndrome by amniocentesis. Am J Obstet Gynecol 1971;109(3):440–445.

[40] Hallman M, Kulovich M, Kirkpatrick E, Sugarman RG, Gluck L. Phosphatidylinositol and phosphatidylglycerol in amniotic fluid: indices of lung maturity. Am J Obstet Gynecol 1976;125(5):613–617.

[41] Snyder JM, Mendelson CR. Induction and characterization of the major surfactant apoprotein during rabbit fetal lung development. Biochim Biophys Acta 1987;920(3):226–236.

[42] Ross GF, Ikegami M, Steinhilber W, Jobe AH. Surfactant protein C in fetal and ventilated preterm rabbit lungs. Am J Physiol 1999;277(6 Pt 1):L1104–L1108.

[43] Crouch EC. Collectins and pulmonary host defense. Am J Respir Cell Mol Biol 1998;19(2):177–201.

[44] Ikegami M, Whitsett JA, Martis PC, Weaver TE. Reversibility of lung inflammation caused by SP-B deficiency. Am J Physiol Lung Cell Mol Physiol 2005;289(6):L962–L970.

[45] Collins MH, Moessinger AC, Kleinerman J, Bassi J, Rosso P, Collins AM, et al. Fetal lung hypoplasia associated with maternal smoking: a

morphometric analysis. Pediatr Res 1985;19(4):408–412.

[46] Sekhon HS, Jia Y, Raab R, Kuryatov A, Pankow JF, Whitsett JA, et al. Prenatal nicotine increases pulmonary alpha7 nicotinic receptor expression and alters fetal lung development in monkeys. J Clin Invest 1999;103(5): 637–647.

[47] Milner AD, Marsh MJ, Ingram DM, Fox GF, Susiva C. Effects of smoking in pregnancy on neonatal lung function. Arch Dis Child Fetal Neonatal Ed 1999;80(1):F8–14.

[48] Hayatbakhsh MR, Sadasivam S, Mamun AA, Najman JM, Williams GM, O'Callaghan MJ. Maternal smoking during and after pregnancy and lung function in early adulthood: a prospective study. Thorax 2009;64(9):810–814.

[49] Wongtrakool C, Roser-Page S, Rivera HN, Roman J. Nicotine alters lung branching morphogenesis through the alpha7 nicotinic acetylcholine receptor. Am J Physiol Lung Cell Mol Physiol 2007;293(3):L611–L618.

[50] Neuman A, Hohmann C, Orsini N, Pershagen G, Eller E, Kjaer HF, et al. Maternal smoking in pregnancy and asthma in preschool children: a pooled analysis of eight birth cohorts. Am J Respir Crit Care Med 2012;186(10):1037–1043.

[51] Lechner AJ. Perinatal age determines the severity of retarded lung development induced by starvation. Am Rev Respir Dis 1985;131(4): 638–643.

[52] Maritz GS, Cock ML, Louey S, Suzuki K, Harding R. Fetal growth restriction has long-term effects on postnatal lung structure in sheep. Pediatr Res 2004;55(2):287–295.

[53] Kalenga M, Tschanz SA, Burri PH. Protein deficiency and the growing rat lung. I. Nutritional findings and related lung volumes. Pediatr Res 1995;37(6):783–788.

[54] Check J, Gotteiner N, Liu X, Su E, Porta N, Steinhorn R, et al. Fetal growth restriction and pulmonary hypertension in premature infants with bronchopulmonary dysplasia. J Perinatol 2013;33(7): 553–557.

[55] Rueda-Clausen CF, Morton JS, Davidge ST. Effects of hypoxia-induced intrauterine growth restriction on cardiopulmonary structure and function during adulthood. Cardiovasc Res 2009;81(4):713–722.

[56] Kallapur SG, Willet KE, Jobe AH, Ikegami M, Bachurski CJ. Intra-amniotic endotoxin: chorioamnionitis precedes lung maturation in preterm lambs. Am J Physiol Lung Cell Mol Physiol 2001;280(3):L527–L536.

[57] Bachurski CJ, Ross GF, Ikegami M, Kramer BW, Jobe AH. Intra-amniotic endotoxin increases pulmonary surfactant proteins and induces SP-B processing in fetal sheep. Am J Physiol Lung Cell Mol Physiol 2001;280(2):L279–L285.

[58] Willet KE, Jobe AH, Ikegami M, Newnham J, Brennan S, Sly PD. Antenatal endotoxin and glucocorticoid effects on lung morphometry in preterm lambs. Pediatr Res 2000;48(6):782–788.

[59] Kallapur SG, Bachurski CJ, Le Cras TD, Joshi SN, Ikegami M, Jobe AH. Vascular changes after intra-amniotic endotoxin in preterm lamb lungs. Am J Physiol Lung Cell Mol Physiol 2004;287(6):L1178–L1185.

[60] Polglase GR, Hooper SB, Gill AW, Allison BJ, Crossley KJ, Moss TJ, et al. Intrauterine inflammation causes pulmonary hypertension and cardiovascular sequelae in preterm lambs. J Appl Physiol (1985) 2010;108(5):1757–1765.

[61] Lowe J, Watkins WJ, Edwards MO, Spiller OB, Jacqz-Aigrain E, Kotecha SJ, et al. Association between pulmonary ureaplasma colonization and bronchopulmonary dysplasia in preterm infants: updated systematic review and meta-analysis. Pediatr Infect Dis J 2014;33(7):697–702.

[62] Kumar R, Yu Y, Story RE, Pongracic JA, Gupta R, Pearson C, et al. Prematurity, chorioamnionitis, and the development of recurrent wheezing: a prospective birth cohort study. J Allergy Clin Immunol 2008;121(4). 878–84 e6.

[63] Moessinger AC, Harding R, Adamson TM, Singh M, Kiu GT. Role of lung fluid volume in growth and maturation of the fetal sheep lung. J Clin Invest 1990;86(4):1270–1277.

[64] Wigglesworth JS, Desai R. Effect on lung growth of cervical cord section in the rabbit fetus. Early Hum Dev 1979;3(1):51–65.

[65] Hummler E, Barker P, Gatzy J, Beermann F, Verdumo C, Schmidt A, et al. Early death due to defective neonatal lung liquid clearance in alpha-ENaC-deficient mice. Nat Genet 1996;12(3):325–328.

[66] O'Brodovich H, Hannam V, Seear M, Mullen JB. Amiloride impairs lung water clearance in newborn guinea pigs. J Appl Physiol (1985) 1990;68(4):1758–1762.

[67] Hummler E, Barker P, Talbot C, Wang Q, Verdumo C, Grubb B, et al. A mouse model for the renal salt-wasting syndrome pseudohypoaldosteronism. Proc Natl Acad Sci 1997;94(21):11710–11715.

[68] Olver RE, Ramsden CA, Strang LB, Walters DV. The role of amiloride-blockable sodium transport in adrenaline-induced lung liquid reabsorption in the fetal lamb. J Physiol 1986;376:321–340.

[69] Barker PM, Markiewicz M, Parker KA, Walters DV, Strang LB. Synergistic action of triiodothyronine and hydrocortisone on epinephrine-induced reabsorption of fetal lung liquid. Pediatr Res 1990;27(6): 588–591.

[70] Champigny G, Voilley N, Lingueglia E, Friend V, Barbry P, Lazdunski M. Regulation of expression of the lung amiloride-sensitive Na⁺ channel by steroid hormones. EMBO J 1994;13(9):2177–2181.

[71] Barker PM, Gatzy JT. Effect of gas composition on liquid secretion by explants of distal lung of fetal rat in submersion culture. Am J Physiol 1993;265(5 Pt 1):L512–L517.

[72] Tschanz SA, Damke BM, Burri PH. Influence of postnatally administered glucocorticoids on rat lung growth. Biol Neonate 1995;68(4):229–245.

[73] Willet KE, Jobe AH, Ikegami M, Kovar J, Sly PD. Lung morphometry after repetitive antenatal glucocorticoid treatment in preterm sheep. Am J Respir Crit Care Med 2001;163(6):1437–1443.

[74] Murphy KE, Hannah ME, Willan AR, Hewson SA, Ohlsson A, Kelly EN, et al. Multiple courses of antenatal corticosteroids for preterm birth (MACS): a randomised controlled trial. Lancet 2008;372(9656): 2143–2151.

Chapter | **4** |

Transition in the Delivery Room: Current NRP Recommendations

Máximo Vento, MD, PhD

CHAPTER POINTS

- Both anticipation and debriefing are vital for a good resuscitation.
- Keep the delivery room at 26°C.
- The team should have a leader, taking care of the respiratory airways, and caregivers taking care of monitoring and providing drugs if necessary.
- Allow for delayed cord clamping at least 1 min except in an extreme emergency when stripping of the cord could be performed by the obstetrician in 20 seconds.
- Initiate pulse oximetry monitoring immediately after birth.
- Initiate respiratory support with noninvasive ventilation (bag & mask; nasal route) with a rhythm of 30 breaths per minute.
- Use of oxygen:
  - In term infants and preterm infants with a gestational age of >32 weeks, use an inspired fraction of oxygen (FiO_2) of .21
  - In preterm infants with 28-32 weeks' gestation use an initial FiO_2 of 0.21-0.3
  - In preterm infants <28 weeks' gestation use an initial FiO_2 of 03
  - titrate FiO_2 according to SpO_2 and heart rate response
- If drug (epinephrine) administratie

Introduction

The achievement of a significant reduction in maternal and child mortality in the last 25 years has been widely acknowledged. However, it is striking that the reduction in mortality in the neonatal period (<28 days after birth) has lagged significantly as compared with the postneonatal mortality (>28 days and 5 years of age) [1]. Worldwide 130 million babies are born every year and approximately 2.8 million of newborn infants die during the neonatal period, and 73% of these deaths occur during the first week of postnatal life and represent early neonatal deaths (ENND). Out of these ENND, almost 40% die in the first hours as a consequence of birth-related complications. Birth asphyxia still represents 11% of ENND in high-income countries but reaches 30%–40% in low-income countries, especially in rural areas [2,3].

Overall, 10% of all newborn infant require some form of intervention in the first minutes after birth (Fig. 4.1). Newborn infants undergo complex respiratory and cardiocirculatory changes during fetal-to-neonatal transition, and failure to achieve these changes represents the most frequent cause of postnatal maladaptation. Therefore, the essential goal of neonatal resuscitation is ventilation of the lungs as opposed to the adult resuscitation focusing on cardiac activity [4]. Breathing initiates a sequence of events that lead to increased oxygenation, decreased pulmonary vascular resistance (PVR), increased pulmonary blood flow, and closure of intra- and extracardiac shunts in the first minutes after birth [5].

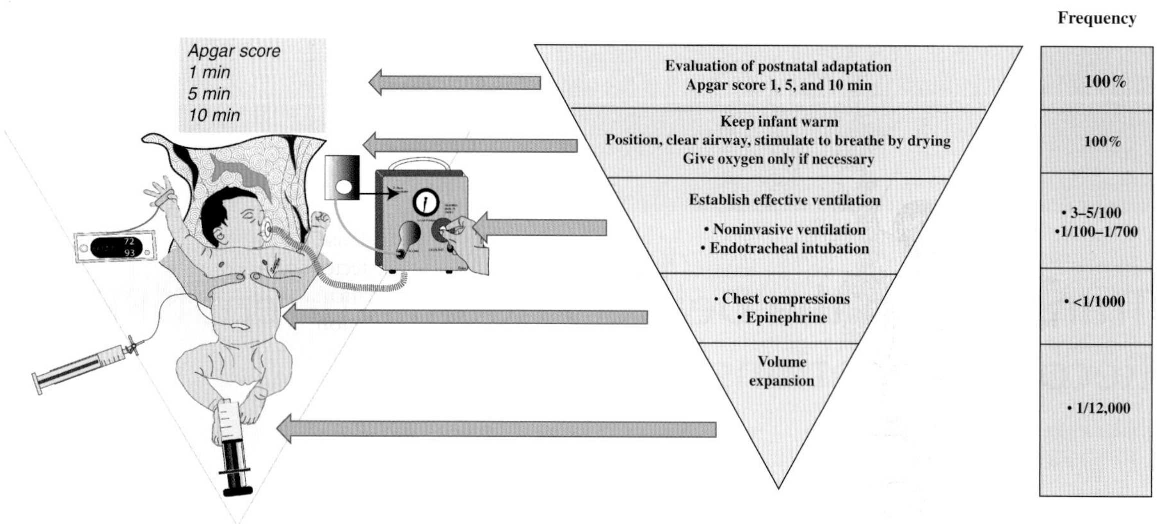

Fig. 4.1 Frequency of the Different Interventions Performed in the Delivery Room in the Newborn infant. Modified from Vento M, Saugstad OD. Resuscitation of the term and preterm infant. Semin Fetal Neonatal Med 2010;15:216–222 [6]. Copyright: Satyan Lakshminrusimha.

Physiologic changes in the fetal-to-neonatal transition

Fetal circulation

In the fetus, gas exchange does not occur in the lungs but in the placenta. Deoxygenated blood from the systemic circulation reaches the placental circulation via the umbilical arteries where gas exchange takes place and returns oxygenated via the umbilical vein to the fetal arterial circulation. The fetal circulation is designed in such a way that the preferential streaming of oxygenated blood is directed to brain and myocardium due to the presence of intracardiac (*foramen ovale*) and extracardiac (*ductus arteriosus*) shunts. Hence, the oxygenated blood bypasses the hepatic circulation via the *ductus venosus*, and reaches the right atrium via the inferior vena cava and the left atrium across the *foramen ovale*. Oxygenated blood reaches the left ventricle and is ejected into the aorta, thus reaching myocardium and brain. In addition, deoxygenated blood coming from the lower part of the body reaches the right auricle via inferior vena cava and is ejected by the right ventricle through the pulmonary artery. The high PVR drives the right ventricular output to the descending aorta via the *ductus arteriosus*. Thus, the deoxygenated blood is directed to the placenta. Of note, during fetal life the lung only receives 16% of the combined ventricular output [7,8] (Fig. 4.2).

Fetal gas exchange

During gestation, gas exchange is driven by the differential partial pressures of oxygen and carbon dioxide between the mother and fetus blood across the placental intervillous space. The fetal arterial partial pressure of oxygen (P_aO_2) *in utero* at the end of gestation is approximately 25–30 mmHg (3.0–3.5 kPa). Immediately after birth, P_aO_2 rises to 80–90 mmHg (10.5–12.0 kPa) and stays within this range until the adult life. Despite the great difference in P_aO_2, oxygen delivery to tissue does not substantially differ between the fetus and the newborn. First, the fetus is endowed with fetal-type hemoglobin that has a greater affinity for oxygen and provides with increased oxygen saturation (SpO_2) for a given P_aO_2. In addition, the cardiac output in the fetus is significantly greater than during infancy or childhood (250–300 mL/kg/min). Moreover, venous return coming from the placenta is redirected to organs with high oxygen needs *ex utero*. At the end of gestation the intervillous partial pressure of oxygen reaches 45–48 mmHg, and these values correspond to an SpO_2 of 50%–60% in the fetus [9,10].

Antioxidant defenses and surfactant production during fetal life

The genes that express the enzymatic machinery responsible for the synthesis of surfactant, antioxidant enzymes, and sulfur disulfide couples only get activated late in gestation preparing the fetus for aerobic respiration. Experimental studies in rabbits have shown that antioxidant enzymes

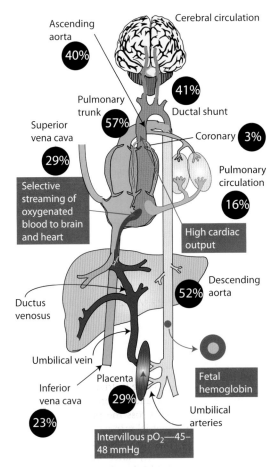

40%

41%

Ascending aorta

Cerebral circulation

Pulmonary trunk

Ductal shunt

57%

Superior vena cava

Coronary 3%

29%

Pulmonary circulation

16%

Selective streaming of oxygenated blood to brain and heart

High cardiac output

Descending aorta

52%

Ductus venosus

Umbilical vein

Inferior vena cava

Placenta

Fetal hemoglobin

29%

23%

Umbilical arteries

Intervillous pO₂—45–48 mmHg

Fig. 4.2 Diagram Representing Fetal Circulation. Copyright Satyan Lakshminrusimha.

such as superoxide dismutases (SOD), catalase (CAT), and glutathione peroxidases (GPx) develop in the last weeks of gestation [11] paralleling the maturation pattern of surfactant. Moreover, pulmonary surfactant contains substantial amounts of these antioxidant enzymes to help prevent oxidative damage to lung structures by reactive oxygen species (ROS) [12]. In addition, the limiting enzyme for the synthesis of glutathione (GSH) is γ-cystathionase which converts cystathionine in ʟ-cysteine and is not expressed until late in gestation. GSH is a ubiquitous tripeptide (γ-glutamyl-cysteinil-glycine) present in the cytoplasm of the cells and the most relevant cytoplasmic nonenzymatic antioxidant. Under normal conditions, two molecules of reduced GSH can combine to form a disulfide bond (GS═SG) and reduce ROS with two electrons. GSH is also the main determinant of the redox status of cell cytoplasm. Remarkably, studies performed in preterm infants have shown that the expression of γ-cystathionase also occurs late in gestation

rendering ʟ-cysteine a conditionally essential amino acid for extremely preterm infants [13,14].

Surfactant is a complex macroaggregate of phospholipids and specific proteins that has tensioactive and anti-infective properties. Surfactant drastically reduces alveolar surface tension opposing to alveolar collapse during the expiratory phase of respiration, promoting the acquisition of a lung function residual capacity, and also contributing to the lung's defense system. Surfactant synthesis and secretion are first detected in the human fetus type II pneumocytes in the canalicular stage of lung development at 20–22 weeks of gestation. However, secretion of surfactant into the amniotic fluid is detectable only after 30–32 weeks of gestation. Consequently, babies born before 32 weeks of gestation are at a greater risk of developing respiratory distress syndrome secondary to surfactant deficiency [15,16].

Transition in the delivery room

Cardiorespiratory changes in the first minutes after birth in the term infant

Immediately after birth, term babies cry and initiate respiratory efforts. Ventilation causes immediate dilatation of the pulmonary vessels, the right ventricular output is redirected toward the pulmonary circulation, and oxygenated venous blood returns to the left atrium via pulmonary veins providing left ventricular preload. Circulatory changes lead to closure of the intra- and extracardiac shunts. Few minutes after birth, the newborn baby establishes an adult-type circulation with two circuits in parallel, pulmonary and systemic, without admixture of oxygenated and deoxygenated blood [17]. During the first breaths, term infants generate very high inspiratory and expiratory pressures with a mean of (−) 50 cmH₂O during inspiration and +60 to 70 cmH₂O during expiration [18]. In addition, at the end of expiration braking maneuvers such as closure of the glottis avoid alveolar collapse by keeping a positive end-expiratory pressure (PEEP). The negative hydrostatic pressure created during inspiration constitutes the physical force that thrusts the fluid filling the lung to the surrounding tissue and contributes to lung aeration [19,20]. The surfactant layer expands on the alveolar surface acting as a tensioactive factor that counteracts the elastic recoil forces that tend to collapse the alveoli during expiration. The gas remaining at the end of expiration in the lung constitutes the functional residual capacity (FRC). FRC notably enhances gas exchange and reduces the amount of pressure needed to open the lung in the following inspiratory movements. Hence, after initial lung expansion and establishment of FRC, subsequent respirations in the newborn infant will only need to reach negative thoracic pressures of -20 to -25 cmH$_2$O to allow sufficient air to reach the alveolar space and achieve stable gas exchange. Such negative intrathoracic pressures can be accomplished with gentle contractions of the diaphragm [20].

Consequences of preterm birth on postnatal adaptation

Circumstances surrounding the preterm delivery are somewhat different. Both the immaturity of the thoracic cage and the weakness of the thoracic muscles hinder the achievement of high negative intrathoracic pressures during inspiration and the enhanced elastic recoil and lack of surfactant that prompt lung collapse during expiration. The consequences are the limitation of lung aeration and fluid reabsorption during inspiration and the tendency toward atelectasis during expiration and avoidance of the establishment of FRC. Altogether, these circumstances hamper effective gas exchange and lead to respiratory insufficiency with tendency to hypoxemia and hypercarbia. Therefore, one of the principal efforts of the caregivers in the delivery room (DR) is to establish an effective ventilation and oxygenation, especially in the very preterm infants (<32 weeks of gestation) [16].

Oxidative stress during the fetal-to-neonatal transition

Even with a mature antioxidant defense system and breathing room air, the burden of oxygen free radicals generated during the fetal-to-neonatal transition will inevitably cause an oxidative stress in the immediate postnatal period. In experiments performed with term rat pups, it was shown that normal deliveries cause oxidative stress as evidenced by a significant reduction of the reduced to oxidized (GSH/GSSG) GSH ratio in isolated hepatocytes [21]. GSH, the most relevant nonenzymatic antioxidant, is further reduced in the fetal-to-neonatal transition when rat pups are reoxygenated with higher oxygen concentrations and proapoptotic and proinflammatory pathways are secondarily activated in brain and lung [22,23]. However, offspring of pregnant mice delivered and kept in a low oxygen atmosphere mimicking *in utero* milieu (FiO$_2$ = 0.14) exhibited an increased GSH/GSSG ratio in lung on day 1 and in the brain on day 7 after birth as compared with pups born in room air (FiO$_2$ = 0.21). The activation of the NRF-2-related antioxidant genes was significantly increased in lung and brain. Apparently, a smooth transition from the lower oxygen milieu *in utero* to the relatively hyperoxic milieu *ex utero* seemed to be protective [24].

Studies in a hypoxic piglet model of hypoxia-reoxygenation showed that the use of pure oxygen caused not only

an increased concentration of extracellular glycerol in the brain striatum but also increased matrix metalloproteinases in lung, liver, heart, and brain compared with the use of room air. Interestingly, there is clear dose-dependent oxygen toxicity, and elimination of biomarkers of oxidative damage caused to protein and DNA significantly correlated to the FiO$_2$ provided during resuscitation [25]. Translating these findings in experimental animals into the clinical setting would imply avoiding targeting high saturations too rapidly in preterm infants after birth. Stabilization with high oxygen concentrations is not only toxic to the lungs but also to different organs such as heart, liver, and brain.

Current NRP recommendations

International guidelines have set up algorithms to guide caregivers in the DR and to take decisions when difficulties in postnatal adaptation arise. The most relevant clinical parameters that need to be assessed immediately after birth by caregivers are breathing, heart rate (HR), and peripheral oxygen saturation measured by pulse oximetry (SpO$_2$) [26]. Fig. 4.3 summarizes the resuscitation flow diagram.

Anticipation

Information provided by the obstetric team before birth is important to anticipate the necessary personnel and material needed and design the best strategy for an effective resuscitation. Ideally, at every delivery there should be at least one caregiver responsible for the newly born with the adequate skills to assess the infant's status, initiate resuscitation, apply positive pressure ventilation, perform endotracheal intubation (ET) and chest compressions, and administer medication. Of note, most of the babies (but not all) requiring active resuscitation are to be identified before birth allowing for the recruitment of a team of skilled professionals under the leadership of an expert neonatologist and briefing of the expected difficulties according to the type and circumstances of the delivery [28]. The Delivery Room Intensive Care Unit (DRICU) concept recommends that referral centers, where high-risk pregnancies are centralized, trained caregivers as well as monitoring and ventilatory devices should be available round the clock all year through to provide optimal resuscitation [29]. Interventions that have proven to improve outcomes of extremely preterm low birth weight (ELBW) infants should be considered before birth. Such interventions include the following:

1. The use of tocolytics to prevent preterm birth to allow fetal maturation.
2. Transfer to a regional referral center with expertise in the treatment of ELBW infants.

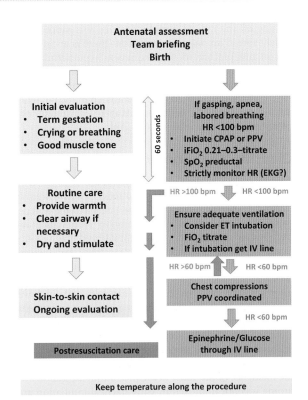

Fig. 4.3 Flow Diagram of the Interventions Performed in the Delivery Room According to the Infant's Clinical Status and Response Following the ILCOR 2015 Guidelines [27].

3. Antibiotics in case of preterm rupture of membranes to avoid fetal infections.
4. Antenatal steroids to mature fetal lung.
5. Magnesium sulfate administered to the mother shortly before birth as an efficacious neuroprotective drug to the fetus [26].

Initial steps in stabilization: assessment and intervention

Newborn infants should be evaluated in the DR in the first 60 s after birth during the so-called "golden minute." Gestational age, the presence of spontaneous breathing or crying and good tone and active movements should be immediately assessed. Cord clamping should be delayed between 30 and 60 s in all babies unless immediate resuscitation is needed. The benefits of placental transfusion in babies that require active resuscitation are being actively investigated in translational animal models and clinical trials. The time of birth should be recorded when the body of the baby is expelled from the *introitus* or uterine incision [30]. Babies at term who breathe or cry spontaneously and vigorously and have a good tone (flexed extremities) should be briefly dried with a warm towel, gently stimulated and immediately put in skin-to-skin contact with the mother and covered with a warm blanket. Importantly, baby's head should be slightly hyperextended to facilitate breathing and if oral secretions are adverted, they could be wiped with gauze. Breastfeeding should be promoted immediately after birth. Approximately after one 1 h vitamin K and erythromycin eye drops should be administered [31].

Delayed cord clamping or umbilical cord milking

Delayed cord clamping (DCC) for at least 60 s after birth is now recommended for term infants. It provides an additional blood volume that increases hemoglobin concentrations at 24–48 h and iron stores at 3–6 months. However, DCC is associated with an increased rate and intensity of neonatal hyperbilirubinemia and the need for phototherapy [32]. The driving forces for blood flow from the placenta to the baby are respiratory movements, crying, and uterine contractions, and these factors play a more important role than time to cord clamping. Physiology-based cord clamping has recently emerged whereby the timing of cord clamping should be based on the infant's physiology rather than time [26]. DCC in preterm infants increases blood volumes by up to 25%, especially after vaginal birth. Moreover, if the blood flow is allowed for 180 s, there is a substantial reduction in intraventricular hemorrhage (IVH), necrotizing enterocolitis (NEC), and/or need for transfusion while no negative side effects for mother of infant have been described [33]. Umbilical cord milking (UCM) from the placental end of the cord toward the baby can be a valid alternative to delayed cord clamping and especially useful for preterm infants who need resuscitation. UCM is achieved by stripping the cord toward the infant 2–4 times before it is clamped. UCM is performed within 20 s and allows for an earlier access for resuscitation. In preterm infants, UCM increases superior vena cava flow, right ventricular output, blood pressure, and urine output and hemoglobin concentration. However, no differences with DCC have been found in relation to death, cardiovascular stability, IVH, and long-term neurodevelopmental outcomes. Despite these potential benefits, ILCOR 2015 recommended against the routine use of DCC or UCM for infants born at ≤28 weeks of gestation considering that the available evidence was still too weak to openly recommend these techniques. However, they supported both techniques on an individual basis or in a research setting. In the latter years after the publication of the guidelines, new and supportive information has been reported. In a recent meta-analyses, seven randomized controlled trials (RCTs) comparing immediate UCM in preterm infants <33 weeks with immediate cord clamping were analyzed and showed that UCM reduced the risk of IVH of all grades and chronic lung disease. Moreover, UCM offered advantages over delayed cord clamping in newborn infant that were deemed too unstable and were at highest risk of severe IVH and death. However, although some studies have shown similar long-term follow-up outcomes in babies undergoing DCC, UCM, or immediate cord clamping, they were not adequately powered for neurodevelopmental follow-up. Further ongoing trials will soon provide us with relevant information in this regard [34].

Heart rate monitoring

Bradycardia (HR <100 bpm) is probably the most reliable clinical sign that informs the caregiver on the severity of neonatal depression. Persistence of low HR indicates the need for chest compression and administration of epinephrine, while a rapid increase in HR reveals successful ventilation and a better prognosis [6,35]. Traditionally, HR has been assessed by auscultation. More recently, HR is routinely assessed using a pulse oximeter and a reference range put together in healthy term and preterm babies not needing resuscitation at birth [36]. However, HR estimate by auscultation and/or pulse oximetry may be inaccurate, and detection of HR by pulse oximeter can be delayed by several minutes. New ECG devices easy to adhere to the newborn's skin, giving accurate readings in few seconds, are being developed and will be routinely used in the future. Meanwhile, according to ILCOR 2015 HR monitoring by auscultation and/or pulse oximetry still remains crucial to inform of the infant's response to resuscitation [27].

Temperature control

Maintaining newly born babies within a normothermic range (36.5–37.5°C) is a strong recommendation because hyper- and/or hypothermia has been associated with negative outcomes, especially in preterm infants [37]. Term newborn infants should be resuscitated under a radiant heater. ELBW infants are especially prone to heat loss and therefore during resuscitation the room temperature should be kept at 23–25°C, and babies should be wrapped in a polyethylene bag without being dried and with a thermal mattress underneath. However, there is an inherent risk for hyperthermia with the use of exothermic mattresses in addition to plastic covers. Hyperthermia increases the risk of subsequent adverse neurological outcome. If babies need ventilation, the gas source should also be heated and humidified because cold gases may be injurious to the lungs. Once the babies are adequately protected from heat loss, skin-to-skin contact and kangaroo care can be safely performed in babies >30 weeks of gestation [27]. In asphyxiated term or near-term infants, therapeutic hypothermia should be initiated within 6 h after birth. Although evidence for turning off the radiant heater is lacking, this procedure is widely spread among neonatologists. There is an inherent risk in this practice to provoke severe hypothermia with severe negative consequences, and frequent or continuous monitoring of core body temperature is important. Therefore, hypothermia should only be initiated in the DR when infants' meet clinical, neurological, and electrophysiological criteria recommended in RCTs [38].

Clearing the airway

Routine suction of the upper airways should be avoided for it may stimulate a vagal reflex and induce bradycardia. In addition, repeated suctioning of the trachea in the absence of secretions can deteriorate pulmonary compliance and oxygenation and reduction in cerebral blood flow velocity. Contrarily, in the presence of secretions there is an increase in respiratory resistance and subsequent increase in work of breathing [28]. Distressed fetuses, however, can pass meconium into the amniotic fluid that can pass into the lower respiratory airway if fetus gasps as a response to hypoxia. Meconium aspiration syndrome occurs when meconium aspirated into the lower respiratory airways causes obstruction and severe respiratory failure and frequently persistent pulmonary hypertension with severe hypoxemia. In RCTs, the incidence of mortality in the meconium aspiration syndrome was not improved by early tracheal intubation and suctioning neither in vigorous nor in nonvigorous newborn infants with meconium-stained amniotic fluid. Therefore, intubation and aspiration of the trachea immediately after birth is not further recommended despite the presence of meconium-stained amniotic fluid [39,40].

Normal oxygen saturation ranges in the delivery room

Whenever resuscitation is anticipated, the use of a pulse oximeter with a preductal location (right hand or wrist) to inform about cerebral oxygen saturation (SpO_2) has become a standard of care. Reliable SpO_2 and HR are achieved after 90–120 s after birth [31]. Of note, assessment of the infant's color has been withdrawn from the initial evaluation because of the lack of reliability, although tongue inspection has been proposed as an alternative for deliveries in rural areas of developing countries [41,42].

Oxygen toxicity limits the use of color for the stabilization of term or preterm infants. The relative hypoxia *in utero* followed by a sudden increase in the oxygen availability to tissues after birth causes a physiologic oxidative stress. However, during severe ischemia reperfusion in perinatal asphyxia or as a consequence of the immaturity of the lungs and antioxidant defenses in preterm infants, a burst of oxygen free radicals is generated. Free radicals cause significant direct damage to tissue/organs and trigger a generalized

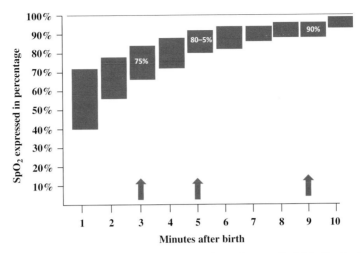

Fig. 4.4 **Centiles of Preductal Oxygen Saturation Measured by Pulse Oximetry (SpO$_2$) in the First Minutes After Birth According to Dawson et al.** [43].

inflammatory response with deleterious consequences [23]. To avoid the negative consequences of hypo- or hyperoxia, recommended ranges for SpO$_2$ and HR for the first 10 min after birth have been defined (Figs. 4.4 and 4.5) [43,44]. These centile charts were developed retrieving oxygen saturation and pulse from healthy term and preterm babies not needing resuscitation after birth. Keeping the newly born term or preterm infants within the 10th–90th centile of these charts provides with the best available reference to optimize oxygen supplementation [36,43]. DR caregivers should adjust FiO$_2$ every 15–30 s according to the pulse oximeter readings, increasing or decreasing FiO$_2$ by 0.1 every 15–30 s to keep SpO$_2$ within the chosen centiles for a given time after birth. It is extremely important to keep HR always above 100 bpm avoiding bradycardia. Persistent bradycardia requires the assessment of an adequate mask positioning and adjustment, evaluation of chest excursions, and rapid increase of FiO$_2$. The lack of response after performing these maneuvers requires immediate

Oxygen supplementation in term and preterm infants

Traditionally, 100% oxygen was systematically used for resuscitation irrespective of gestational age or severity of depression [6]. In a meta-analysis performed including more than 2000 asphyxiated patients, it was shown that the use of 100% oxygen upon resuscitation significantly increased mortality as compared to the use of room air [47]. Since 2010 ILCOR guidelines recommend the initial use of room air in the resuscitation of term and near term in the first minutes and oxygen titration according to the infant's response [28].

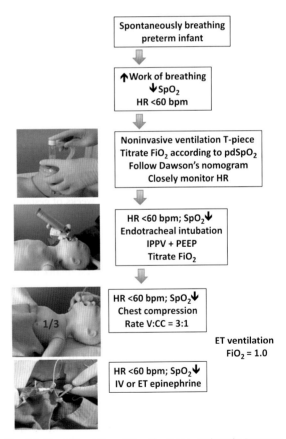

Fig. 4.5 **Flow Chart Describing the Interventions in Preterm Infants With Severe Depression at Birth Based on ILCOR 2015 guidelines and experts' recommendations** [27,45,46].

the mask and an adequate chin lift are necessary. The rim of the mask should be placed on the tip of the chin and the mask should cover both mouth and nose, but not the eyes. Apparently, the best hold is achieved by the OK-rim-hold (thumb and index finger form a C-shape) technique (Figs. 4.7 and 4.8) [65].

Endotracheal intubation and/or laryngeal mask

ET is indicated when noninvasive ventilation is rendered ineffective, when chest compressions are performed or in special situations such as diaphragmatic hernia [28]. The

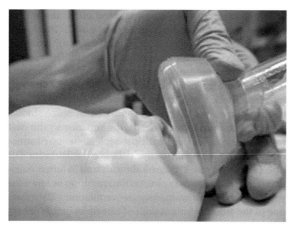

Fig. 4.7 Photograph Showing the Positioning of the Face Mask [64].

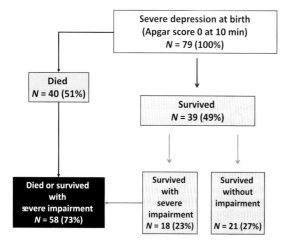

Fig. 4.8 Outcomes After Extremely Severe Depression at Birth With Apgar Score 0 at 1, 5, and 10 min and Ulterior Moderate Body Hypothermia [66].

ILCOR 2015 guidelines do not recommend routine tracheal intubation for meconium suctioning even in depressed infants born through meconium-stained amniotic fluid [27]. Successful tracheal intubation immediately increases HR and air entry can be assessed by auscultation over both lung fields. In addition, CO_2 detectors can be used to confirm that the tracheal tube is in the right position. A positive detection of CO_2 exhalation accompanied by a good cardiac output confirms placement of the tube, and a negative test result strongly suggests esophageal intubation. Occasionally, low lung perfusion can give a negative result despite the tube being in the trachea. A Cochrane review in 2014 did not find any studies specifically addressing this issue and therefore the pretended advantages of using CO_2 detectors rely on the individual experience of caregivers or teams [67].

The increasing use of noninvasive ventilation has substantially reduced the need for ET both in the DR and in the NICU and subsequently the opportunity to learn and the skills of providers. ET is considered the most difficult technique to teach and learn in neonatal resuscitation. In this scenario the use of laryngeal mask (LM) has been suggested as a valid alternative to access the lower respiratory airways, especially in late preterm and term infants. Several RCTs in late preterm and term infants have evidenced the feasibility, efficacy, and safety of using the LM to resuscitate late preterm (>34 weeks of gestation) and term infants when mask ventilation rendered ineffective and ET was not feasible or unsuccessful. Studies comparing resuscitation with LM versus bag and mask ventilation showed a greater resuscitation rate with LM. Moreover, the total ventilation time was shorter with LM than with bag and mask, and the success with the first attempt was 98.5% with a short insertion time of <10 s. In addition, the use of LM has also been compared with ET and no differences in successfully performing the technique and in the clinical recovery of depressed neonatal patients in the DR have been found. Therefore, it has been concluded that LM is a valid alternative when ET is not feasible or the providers have not acquired or maintained the necessary skills to successfully and rapidly perform ET [68–70].

Circulatory support

Chest compressions (CC) are indicated when HR remains <60 bpm despite adequate ventilation and oxygen supplementation for 30 s. As ventilation is the mainstay of neonatal resuscitation, before initiating CC the resuscitating team should ensure that effective ventilation is being performed without increase in HR [28]. The aim of CC is to improve cerebral and myocardial perfusion. The former improves neurological outcome and the latter increases the likelihood of a faster return of spontaneous circulation (ROSC). The quality of CC depends upon the rate, the ratio CC to ventilation, and applied force by the provider. Although increased rate would be apparently more efficient as shown in mathematical modeling or in experimental studies with manikins or piglet models, increasing and unavoidable fatigue in the provider render higher rates ineffective. Therefore, during the process of CC, although respirations, HR, and SpO$_2$ should be closely monitored, reassessed, and coordinated, compressions should be continuously performed as interruptions will compromise maintenance of systemic and coronary perfusion and worsen prognosis [71]. ILCOR 2015 guidelines recommend to deliver CC on the lower third of the sternum and to a depth of approximately one-third of the anterior–posterior diameter of the chest using both thumbs to compress the sternum and the rest of the fingers encircling the thorax and supporting the back. The rate compression to ventilation should be 3:1 allowing the chest to re-expand during relaxation for a total of 90 compressions and 30 ventilations/min. Oxygen supplementation during CC has not been studied in the human. Experiments in animal models have shown different results regarding the levels of oxidative stress biomarkers or histological damage to organs such as CNS, heart, or lung. Of note, none of the studies showed an advantage in the use of 100% oxygen during CC. However, from a clinical point of view, when during resuscitation the provider has reached the stage of needing CC to overcome bradycardia, it seems prudent to use effective ventilation and increase oxygen concentration to try to achieve ROSC. However, when the HR recovers, high FiO$_2$ should be rapidly weaned based on preductal SpO$_2$ to avoid additional oxidative damage [27].

Drugs: epinephrine

Only seldom are drugs used during resuscitation. Drugs are indicated when the newborn infant remains bradycardic and profoundly hypoxemic despite being adequately ventilated through an endotracheal tube with 100% oxygen and receiving chest compressions. Under these circumstances, administration of epinephrine and/or volume expansion may be indicated [6]. The use of bicarbonate, naloxone, or vasopressors is not currently considered part of the acute resuscitation but can, under special circumstances, be used in the postresuscitation [72,73].

Epinephrine causes an intense peripheral vasoconstriction, thus increasing aortic flow pressure gradient. During chest compression, oxygenated blood pumped by the left ventricle is redirected toward the dilated coronary arteries with less pressure gradient contributing to mitochondrial ATP synthesis, activation of myocardial contractions, and ROSC [45]. Intravenous administration, and especially through the umbilical vein which is easily accessible, is the preferred and the most efficacious route for epinephrine administration during neonatal resuscitation.

Following the principles of DRICU of providing maximal care in the DR, a group of neonatal providers should be available for complex resuscitations involving drugs. One neonatal provider secures the airway, one provides chest compressions, and another gains access to the umbilical vein [29,74]. Another accessible route is via endotracheal tube. Of note, the plasma concentration achieved is lower and the time to reach the peak concentration is slower as compared to the intravenous route. Notwithstanding, it is a valid alternative when the patient is severely bradycardic and there is no intravenous line accessible. Finally, the last possible alternatives are the intraosseous or the intramuscular access. However, there is very limited information and most of the caregivers are not comfortable with these techniques and prefer the tracheal route. Remarkably, the intramuscular route causes significant tissue damage at the site of injection [45]. The current recommendations indicate that epinephrine should be repeated every 3–5 min if the HR remains bradycardic (<60 bpm) [74]. Occasionally, repeated and high doses of epinephrine are needed to overcome a severe neonatal depression. The consequence is a generalized vasoconstriction causing hypertension and tachycardia. Moreover, vasoconstriction reduces blood flow in renal and mesenteric territories, elevation of pulmonary arterial pressure, and increase myocardial oxygen consumption. All these complications may lead to long-term morbidities such as intestinal perforation, renal insufficiency, or persistent pulmonary hypertension. Finally, an imbalance of various neurotransmitters has been described reducing the threshold for seizures [28].

Volume expansion

Volume expansion should be provided when evidence or suspicion of blood loss is present and the infant does not overcome bradycardia despite the application of other resuscitative measures. As mentioned it is mandatory that the resuscitation team early anticipates the need for a peripheral or central (cord vein) route for volume administration. An isotonic crystalloid solution or blood may be considered for volume expansion. The recommended dose is 10 mL/kg, which may need to be repeated. Remarkably, when resuscitating premature infants, it is reasonable to avoid giving volume expanders too rapidly because rapid infusions of large volumes could cause IVH [74].

Ethical considerations

When should resuscitation not be initiated?

Resuscitation efforts after delivery are not indicated under certain circumstance in which there is no possibility of survival. Although infrequent, caregiver in the DR may have to confront this situation. In such cases, initiation of neonatal resuscitation is not ethical and should not be offered. The most frequent circumstance is extreme prematurity. To date, newborn infants <22 weeks of gestation do not have a chance of survival as opposed to previous guidelines that put the limit at 23 weeks and birth weight of 400 g. However, limiting the resuscitation efforts based on the gestational age frequently depends on the traditions or beliefs in different countries or cultures and guidelines may vary from one country to another. Moreover, assessment of gestational age may also incur errors that may preclude resuscitation in a baby who is really within an acceptable gestational age for initiating resuscitation maneuvers. Therefore, caregivers in the DR confronted with a baby around 22 weeks of gestational should also consider other factors such as physical maturity, heartbeat, or reactivity before deciding not to initiate resuscitation. Other cases include chromosomal abnormalities and severe congenital malformations. In cases where there is uncertainty about survival or a high risk of severe morbidity, the parents should be included in decisions regarding resuscitation plans. It is very relevant that each hospital has its own statistical information regarding these different clinical conditions. This facilitates neonatologist to provide parents with accurate and homogenous information. In these cases, after appropriate prenatal counseling, the parent's desires should be taken into account to guide resuscitation efforts [74].

When should resuscitation be withdrawn?

The current international neonatal resuscitation guidelines uniformly suggest ceasing resuscitation efforts after 10 min of effective resuscitation that includes ventilation, chest compressions, and the use of intravenous epinephrine without achieving ROSC. The ILCOR 2015 guidelines indicate that the outcome of infants with Apgar of zero at 10 min was "almost universally poor" and supported the cessation of resuscitation at 10 min of no detectable heartbeat [27]. Similar recommendations are indicated by the European Resuscitation Council and the American Heart Association [45,46,74]. This guidance is based on previously published retrospective data that revealed that

babies with 0 Apgar score at 10 min resuscitated for more than 10 min either died or had severe neurodevelopmental impairment [75,76]. However, the improvement in resuscitation and postresuscitation care and the introduction of therapeutic hypothermia have drastically changed the prognosis of extremely depressed newly born babies. Fig. 4.6 summarizes the outcomes of babies who had Apgar score of 0 at 10 min and were transferred to the NICU and treated with therapeutic hypothermia. Out of a total of 79, 21% of these infants survived without neurological impairment while 23% had poor outcomes, and 51% of them died [66]. These numbers, however, should be analyzed with caution as they refer only to babies who made it to the NICU and not to those who died in the DR.

Outcomes of severely depressed extremely preterm infants showed a completely different scenario. In a recent review study, outcome of preterm infants <28 weeks of gestation with severe depression were analyzed. Only 0.6% of infants with an Apgar score of 0 at 1 min survived to the NICU and 0.09% were discharged from the hospital. Remarkably, none of the infants with an Apgar score of 0 at 5 min survived [77]. Ethical considerations are extremely important when taking the decision to continue or withdraw resuscitation procedures in the DR. The "best interest" of the infant should always be a priority. If survival would imply severe limitations in life's quality or assuring only a very short survival, it is generally considered ethical to withhold or withdraw resuscitation efforts. In the case of an uncertain prognosis as it frequently happens, either withholding or withdrawing is ethically equivalent. However, withholding treatment has the advantage of retrieving additional information in the NICU that will allow better judgment of the infants' prognosis. Parents should be always informed about ongoing resuscitation and should give their consent regarding withdrawal of therapeutic efforts. However, when the resuscitation team has already decided that withholding resuscitation is medically unacceptable it would be arguable if the parents should give their consent for ceasing therapeutic efforts [78]. It is important to communicate with the parents and involve them in the decision-making process to provide family-centered care in the DRNICU.

References

[1] Lehtonen L, Gimeno A, Parra-Llorca A, et al. Early neonatal death: a challenge worldwide. Semin Fetal Neonat Med 2017;22:153–160.

[2] World Health Organization/UNICEF/UNFPA/World Bank/United Nations Population Division. Trends in maternal mortality: 1990-2013. Geneva: WHO; 2014.

[3] Lawn JE, Blencowe H, Oza S, et al. Every newborn: progress, priorities, and potential beyond survival. Lancet 2014;384:189–205.

[4] Kattwinkel J. Textbook of neonatal resuscitation. 6th ed. Elk Grove Village, IL: American Academy of Pediatrics; 2011.

[5] Hooper SB, te Pas AB, Lang J, et al. Cardiovascular transition at birth: a physiological sequence. Pediatr Res 2015;77:608–614.

[6] Vento M, Saugstad OD. Resuscitation of the term and preterm infant. Semin Fetal Neonatal Med 2010;15:216–222.

[7] Murphy PJ. The fetal circulation. Cont Educ Anaesth Crit Care Pain 2005;5:107–112.

[8] Gao Y, Raj JU. Regulation of pulmonary circulation in the fetus and newborn. Physiol Rev 2010;90:1291–1335.

[9] Schneider H. Oxygenation of the placental-fetal unit in humans. Respir Physiol Neurobiol 2011;178:51e8.

[10] Vento M, Teramo K. Evaluating the fetus at risk for cardiopulmonary compromise. Semin Fetal Neonatal Med 2013;18:324–329.

[11] Frank L, Groseclose EE. Preparation for birth into an O_2-rich environment: the antioxidant enzymes in the developing rabbit lung. Pediatr Res 1984;18:240e4.

[12] Davis JM, Auten RL. Maturation of the antioxidant system and the effects on preterm birth. Semin Fetal Neonatal Med 2010;15:191–195.

[13] Viña J, Vento M, García-Sala F, et al. L-Cysteine and glutathione metabolism are impaired in premature infants due to cystathionase deficiency. Am J Clin Nutr 1995;61:1067–1069.

[14] Martín JA, Pereda J, Martínez-López I, et al. Oxidative stress as a signal to up-regulate gamma-cystathionase in the fetal-to-neonatal transition in rats. Cell Mol Biol (Noisy-le-grand) 2007;53(Suppl.). OL1010-7.

[15] Mendelson CR, Boggaram V. Hormonal control of the surfactant system in fetal lung. Annu Rev Physiol 1991;53:415–440.

[16] Sweet DG, Carnielli V, Greisen G, et al. European Consensus Guidelines on the Management of Respiratory Distress Syndrome—2016 Update. Neonatology 2017;111:107–125.

[17] Vali P, Mathew B, Laskhminrusimha S. Neonatal resuscitation: evolving strategies. Matern Health Neonatol Perinatol 2015;1:4.

[18] Vyas H, Field D, Milner AD, et al. Determinants of the first inspiratory volume and functional residual capacity at birth. Pediatr Pulmonol 1986;2:189–193.

[19] Siew ML, Wallace MJ, Kitchen MJ, et al. Inspiration regulates the rate and temporal pattern of lung liquid clearance and lung aeration at birth. J Appl Physiol 2009;106:1888–1895.

[20] Hooper SB, Te Pas AB, Kitchen MJ. Respiratory transition in the newborn: a three-phase process. Arch Dis Child Fetal Neonatal Ed 2016;101:F266–F271.

[21] Pallardo FV, Sastre J, Asensi M, et al. Physiological changes in glutathione metabolism in foetal and newborn rat liver. Biochem J 1991;274:891–893.

[22] Gelfand SL, Vento M, Sastre J, et al. A new model of oxidative stress in rat pups. Neonatology 2008;94:293–299.

[23] Torres-Cuevas I, Parra-Llorca A, Sánchez-Illana A, et al. Oxygen and oxidative stress in the perinatal period. Redox Biol 2017;12:674–681.

[24] Escobar J, Cubells E, Enomoto M, et al. Prolonging in utero-like oxygenation after birth diminishes oxidative stress in the lung and brain of mice pups. Redox Biol 2013;1:297–303.

[25] Saugstad OD, Sejersted Y, Solberg R, et al. Oxygenation of the newborn: a molecular approach. Neonatology 2012;101:315–325.

[26] Manley BJ, Owen L, Hooper SB, et al. Towards evidence-based resuscitation of the newborn. Lancet 2017;389:1639–1648.

[27] Perlman JM, Wyllie J, Kattwinkel J, et al. Part 7: neonatal resuscitation: 2015 International Consensus on cardiopulmonary resuscitation and emergency cardiovascular care science with treatment recommendations. Circulation 2015;132(Suppl. 1):S204–S241.

[28] Kattwinkel J, Perlman JM, Aziz K, et al. Part 15: neonatal resuscitation: 2010 American Heart Association Guidelines for Cardiopulmonary Resuscitation and Emergency Cardiovascular Care. Circulation 2010;122(Suppl. 3):S909–S919.

[29] Vento M, Aguar M, Leone TA, et al. Using intensive care technology in the delivery room: a new concept for the resuscitation of extremely preterm neonates. Pediatrics 2008;122:1113–1116.

[30] Saugstad OD, Robertson NJ, Vento M. A critical review of the 2015 International Liaison Committee on Resuscitation treatment recommendations for resuscitating the newly born infant. Acta Paediatr 2016;105:442–444.

[31] Pino-Vazquez A, Ruiz-Campillo CW, Sánchez-Mateos M. Pasos iniciales en reanimación neonatal. In: Iriondo-Sanz M, Grupo de Reanimación Neonatal de la Sociedad Española de Neonatología, editors. 4th ed. Madrid: Ergón Editores; 2017. p. 59–69.

[32] McDonald SJ, Middleton P, Dowswell T, et al. Effect of timing of umbilical cord clamping of term infants on maternal and neonatal outcomes. Cochrane Database Syst Rev 2013;7:CD004074.

[33] Rabe H, Diaz-Rossello JL, Duley L, et al. Effect of timing of umbilical cord clamping and other strategies to influence placental transfusion at preterm birth on maternal and infant outcomes. Cochrane Database Syst Rev 2012;8:CD003248.

[34] Katheria AC, Lakshminrusimha S, Rabe H, et al. Placental transfusion: a review. J Perinatol 2017;37:105–111.

[35] Saugstad OD, Ramji S, Rootwelt T, et al. Response to resuscitation of the newborn: early prognostic variables. Acta Paediatr 2005;94:890–895.

[36] Dawson JA, Kamlin CO, Wong C, et al. Changes in heart rate in the first minutes after birth. Arch Dis Child Fetal Neonatal Ed 2010;95:F177–F181.

[37] Lyu Y, Shah PS, Ye XY, et al. Association between admission temperature and mortality and major morbidity in preterm infants born at fewer than 33 weeks' gestation. JAMA Pediatr 2015;169:e150277.

[38] Jacobs SE, Berg M, Hunt R, Tarnow-Mordi WO, Inder TE, Davis PG. Cooling for newborns with hypoxic-ischaemic encephalopathy. Cochrane Database Syst Rev 2013;1:CD003311.

[39] Vain NE, Szyld EG, Prudent LM, et al. Oropharyngeal and nasopharyngeal suctioning of meconium-stained neonates before delivery of their shoulders: multicentre, randomised controlled trial. Lancet 2004;364(9434):597–602.

[40] Chettri S, Adhisivam B, Bhat BV. Endotracheal suction for nonvigorous neonates born through meconium stained amniotic fluid: a randomized controlled trial. J Pediatr 2015;166:1208–1213.e1.

[41] Dawson JA, Ekström A, Frisk C, et al. Assessing the tongue colour of newly born infants may help to predict the need for supplemental oxygen in the delivery room. Acta Paediatr 2015;104:356–359.

[42] Vento M. What does the colour of the tongue tells us in the delivery room? Acta Paediatr 2015;104:329–330.

[43] Dawson JA, Kamlin CO, Vento M, et al. Defining the reference range for oxygen saturation for infants after birth. Pediatrics 2010;125:e1340–e1347.

[44] Dawson JA, Vento M, Finer NN, et al. Managing oxygen therapy during delivery room stabilization of preterm infants. J Pediatr 2012;160:158–161.

[45] Kapadia VS, Wyckoff MH. Epinephrine use during newborn resuscitation. Front Pediatr 2017;5:97.

[46] Sawyer T, Umoren RA, Gray MM. Neonatal resuscitation: advances in training and practice. Adv Med Educ Pract 2016;8:11–19.

[47] Saugstad OD, Ramji S, Soll RF, et al. Resuscitation of newborn infants with 21% or 100% oxygen: an updated systematic review and meta-analysis. Neonatology 2008;94:176–182.

[48] Torres-Cuevas I, Cernada M, Nuñez A, et al. Oxygen supplementation to stabilize preterm infants in the fetal to neonatal transition: no satisfactory answer. Front Pediatr 2016;4:29.

[49] Ezaki S, Suzuki K, Kurishima C, et al. Resuscitation of preterm infants with reduced oxygen results in less oxidative stress than resuscitation with 100% oxygen. J Clin Biochem Nutr 2009;44:111–118.

[50] Vento M, Moro M, Escrig R, et al. Preterm resuscitation with low oxygen causes less oxidative stress, inflammation, and chronic lung disease. Pediatrics 2009;124:e439–e449.

[51] Kapadia VS, Chalak LF, Sparks JE, et al. Resuscitation of preterm neonates with limited versus high oxygen strategy. Pediatrics 2013;132:e1488–e1496.

[52] Tataranno ML, Oei JL, Perrone S, et al. Resuscitating preterm infants with 100% oxygen is associated with higher oxidative stress than room air. Acta Paediatr 2015;104:759–765.

[53] Wang CL, Anderson C, Leone TA, et al. Resuscitation of preterm neonates by using room air or 100% oxygen. Pediatrics 2008;121:1083–1089.

[54] Rabi Y, Lodha A, Soraisham A, et al. Outcomes of preterm infants following the introduction of room air resuscitation. Resuscitation 2015;96:252–259.

[55] Oei JL, Saugstad OD, Lui K, et al. Targeted oxygen in the resuscitation of preterm infants, a randomized clinical trial. Pediatrics 2017;139. pii: e20161452.

[56] Oei JL, Vento M, Rabi Y, et al. Higher or lower oxygen for delivery room resuscitation of preterm infants below 28 completed weeks gestation: a meta-analysis. Arch Dis Child Fetal Neonatal Ed 2017;102:F24–F30.

[57] Oei JL, Finer NN, Saugstad OD, Wright IM, Rabi Y, Tarnow-Mordi W, et al. Outcomes of oxygen saturation targeting during delivery room stabilisation of preterm infants. Arch Dis Child Fetal Neonatal Ed. 2018 Sep;103(5):F446–F454.

[58] Schmoelzer GM, Kumar M, Pichler G, et al. Non-invasive versus invasive respiratory support in preterm infants at birth: systematic review and meta-analysis. BMJ 2013;347:f5980.

[59] O'Donnell CP, Davis PG, Lau R, et al. Neonatal resuscitation 2: an evaluation of manual ventilation devices and face masks. Arch Dis Child Fetal Neonatal Ed 2005;90: F392–F396.

[60] Iriondo M, Thió M, Burón E, et al. A survey of neonatal resuscitation in Spain: gaps between guidelines and practice. Acta Paediatr 2009;98: 786–791.

[61] Roehr CC, Gröbe S, Rüdiger M, et al. Delivery room management of very low birth weight infants in Germany, Austria and Switzerland—a comparison of protocols. Eur J Med Res 2010;15:493–503.

[62] Mann C, Ward C, Grubb M, et al. Marked variation in newborn resuscitation practice: a national survey in the UK. Resuscitation 2012;83:607–611.

[63] Hawkes CP, Ryan CA, Dempsey EM. Comparison of the T-piece resuscitator with other neonatal manual ventilation devices: a qualitative review. Resuscitation 2012;83:797–802.

[64] Guinsburg R, de Almeida MFB, de Castro JS, et al. T-piece versus self-inflating bag ventilation in preterm neonates at birth. Arch Dis Child Fetal Neonatal Ed 2018;103:F49–F55.

[65] Fuchs H, Schilleman K, Hummler HD, te Pas AB. Techniques and devices to improve noninvasive ventilation in the delivery room. Neoreviews 2012;13:e353.

[66] Harrington DJ, Redman CW, Moulden M, et al. The long-termo utcome in surviving infants with Apgar zero at 10 minutes: a systematic review of the literatura and hospital-based cohort. Am J Obstet Gynecol 2007;196(463):e1–e5.

[67] Schmölzer GM, Roehr CC. Techniques to ascertain correct endotracheal tube placement in neonates. Cochrane Database Syst Rev 2014;9:CD010221.

[68] Zhu XY, Lin BC, Zhang QS, et al. A prospective evaluation of the efficacy of the laryngeal mask airway during neonatal resuscitation. Resuscitation 2011;82:1405–1409.

[69] Trevisanuto D, Cavallin F, Nguyen LN, et al. Supreme laryngeal mask airway versus face mask during neonatal resuscitation: a randomized controlled trial. J Pediatr 2015;167:286–291.e1.

[70] Yang C, Zhu X, Lin W, et al. Randomized, controlled trial comparing laryngeal mask versus endotracheal intubation during neonatal resuscitation—a secondary publication. BMC Pediatr 2016;16:17.

[71] Solevåg AL, Schmölzer GM. Optimal chest compression rate and compression to ventilation ratio in delivery room resuscitation: evidence from newborn piglets and neonatal manikins. Front Pediatr 2017;5:3.

[72] Wyllie J, Niermeyer S. The role of resuscitation drugs and placental transfusion in the delivery room management of newborn infants. Semin Fetal Neonatal Med 2008;13:416–423.

[73] Sáenz P, Brugada M, de Jongh B, Sola A, Torres E, Moreno L, Vento M. A survey of intravenous sodium bicarbonate in neonatal asphyxia among European neonatologists: gaps between scientific evidence and clinical practice. Neonatology 2011;99:170–176.

[74] Wyckoff MH, Aziz K, Escobedo MB, Kapadia VS, Kattwinkel J, Perlman JM, et al. Part 13: neonatal resuscitation: 2015 American Heart Association guidelines update for cardiopulmonary resuscitation and emergency cardiovascular care. Pediatrics 2015;136(Suppl. 2):S196–S218.

[75] Wyllie J, Bruinenberg J, Roehr CC, et al. European resuscitation council guidelines for resuscitation 2015: Section 7. Resuscitation and support of transition of babies at birth. Resuscitation 2015;95:249–263.

[76] Jain L, Ferre C, Vidyasagar D, et al. Cardiopulmonary resuscitation of apparently stillborn infants: survival and long-term outcome. J Pediatr 1991;118:778–782.

[77] McGrath JS, Roehr CC, Wilkinson DJ. When should resuscitation at birth cease? Early Hum Dev 2016;102:31–36.

[78] Haines M, Wright IM, Bajuk B, et al. Population-based study shows that resuscitating apparently stillborn extremely preterm babies is associated with poor outcomes. Acta Paediatr 2016;105:1305–1311.

Chapter | 5 |

Sustained Lung Inflation

Gianluca Lista, MD, PhD, Ilia Bresesti, MD

CHAPTER POINTS

- Transpulmonary pressure following the first breaths plays an important role in fluid removal from the lung at birth.
- Sustained inflation (SI), in which an initial inflating pressure is held for a prolonged duration may assist in lung fluid clearance and establishment of functional residual capacity (FRC).
- Data from experimental animal studies suggest that SI results in uniform lung aeration, better lung function, and stable cerebral oxygen delivery when compared to conventional ventilation.
- In randomized clinical trials (Italian SLI trial and international SAIL trial), some safety concerns arose. SLI trial demonstrated a higher but nonsignificant incidence of pneumothorax in very preterm infants (25–29 weeks gestation). Preliminary data from the SAIL trial showed an excess of early deaths (<48 h of age) in the SI arm (7.5% vs. 1.4%) but no difference in pneumothorax and intraventricular hemorrhage in extremely preterm infants (23–26 weeks gestation) who required resuscitation at birth.
- Further studies of this promising technique evaluating differences in mortality and long-term outcomes are needed.

Physiology of the respiratory transition after birth

In the physiological transition from intra- to extrauterine life, aeration of the lung and clearance of fetal lung liquid from the alveoli are crucial steps during initial adaptation of the newborn, especially in the preterm infant, whose lungs are immature and extremely fragile. Therefore, facilitating the neonatal adaptation while minimizing lung injury is an enormous challenge for the neonatologist.

The respiratory transition is usually recognized as a three-phase process [1], which reflects the three physiological status of the lung during transition to extrauterine life.

In the first phase of the respiratory transition, the lungs are fluid-filled, and for this reason no gas exchange can occur. Immediately after birth, the term infant usually takes a few deep breaths, which generate a large tidal volume and trigger a cascade of physiological events promoting the clearance of the fluid from the lungs and the establishment of pulmonary gas exchanges. All these changes are critical for initiating postnatal circulation and for the achievement of an early and adequate functional residual capacity (FRC).

The mechanism of lung fluid reabsorption and lung aeration at birth has been recently clarified, as the activation of epithelial sodium channels could not completely explain the rate of fluid clearance observed at birth in healthy newborns. Experimental studies, in fact, showed that the transpulmonary pressure following the first breaths can overcome the airflow resistance, and is indeed the main determinant of the fluid removal from the lung.

During the second phase, lung fluid should be prevented from reentering the lung. In order to maintain the lung volume without a continuous opening and closing of the alveoli, endogenous surfactant and positive end-expiratory pressure (PEEP) play an important role in reducing surface tension and preventing alveoli collapse, respectively.

The third phase, then, is characterized by the initiation of gas exchange and the subsequent establishment of cardiorespiratory homeostasis.

While all these transitions are made by the full-term healthy newborn by himself within a few minutes after birth, preterm infants must deal with several physiological impairments to properly aerate the lung. These include a high compliance of the chest wall and a weak respiratory musculature, ineffective function of epithelial channels, structural immaturity of the lungs, and insufficient surfactant composition, production, and storage. Accordingly, almost all extremely preterm babies require respiratory support during neonatal transition [2].

When infants fail to create the transepithelial pressure gradient necessary for the lung liquid clearance, applying positive pressure to the airways helps in achieving this goal. After a preterm infant has cleared the liquid from the lungs, gas exchange becomes possible in the recruited alveoli. This liquid, however, initially remains in the surrounding interstitial tissues with a great risk of reentering the alveoli and interfering with gas exchange. For this reason, maintaining a constant distending pressure in the airway using continuous positive airway pressure (CPAP) is important in this early phase to avoid losing the acquired FRC.

Definition and rationale for sustained inflations

As we have previously mentioned, preterm infants, especially those of extremely low gestational age, are not capable of generating a subatmospheric pressure around the distal airways.

These infants, however, need a more uniform lung aeration to avoid wide and dangerous ventilation–perfusion mismatches, which are responsible for the ineffective increase in pulmonary blood flow and heart rate after birth.

The standard practice to promote lung aeration is intermittent positive pressure ventilation (IPPV) with PEEP and/or CPAP in apneic or spontaneously breathing infants, respectively.

However, to date the best method to favor lung aeration while avoiding harmful trauma to the fragile preterm lung still remains under investigation.

Using large transpulmonary peak pressure with short inflation times certainly contributes to heterogeneity of lung aeration, but could result in overdistention and injury to already aerated regions [3]. This is the reason why an alternative approach has been proposed. It is the so-called "sustained inflation" (SI), in which an initial inflating pressure is held for a prolonged duration (15–20 s) using the physiological time constant of the lungs.

Several decades ago, Boon et al. [4], studying the formation of FRC and tidal volume in asphyxiated intubated neonates, demonstrated that 13–32 cmH$_2$O was the necessary pressure to move air from trachea to distal airways. In the same period, Vyas et al. [5] described the effects of prolonged inflations (5 s) in the same population, and showed that time, rather than pressure, was responsible for the establishment of an adequate FRC.

Although these initial findings were of great interest, SI remained understudied for many years.

Recently, there is a renewed interest in this technique and its potential effects on premature babies.

What literature says

Experimental animal studies

Several studies were conducted on animals about the effects of SI, both in asphyxiated and premature models. In these experiments, SI seems to provide satisfactory results in improving respiratory transition, contributing in establishing FRC and in enhancing gas exchange immediately after birth.

Using preterm rabbit model, te Pas et al. [3] demonstrated that a combination of SI and PEEP was the most effective to uniformly aerate the lung and fully recruit an adequate FRC. Moreover, they also showed that using longer inspiration times contributes significantly in the uniformity of lung aeration. Sobotka et al. [6] demonstrated better lung function in lamb model treated with SI and more stable cerebral oxygen delivery without adverse circulatory effects.

Klingenberg et al. [7] found that in asphyxiated lambs an initial SI lasting 30 s shortens the time necessary to recover adequate heart rate, blood pressure, and oxygenation when compared with standard duration inflations.

Human studies

van Vonderen et al. [8] observed that SI was not effective unless the preterm infants were spontaneously breathing. As most of the FRC gain occurs when the baby breathes, the role of spontaneous breathing and active glottis adduction appears to be crucial to make SI effective. Similar results are described by Lista et al. [9] using respiratory function monitoring.

The use of near-infrared spectroscopy (NIRS) during SI has led to interesting results, which highlight the need for further studies including physiological and clinical outcomes in premature babies.

Fuchs et al. [10] used NIRS to measure preductal arterial oxygen saturation and cerebral tissue oxygenation in a group of preterm infants treated with SI and compared results with a group of preterm infants requiring CPAP only. Increase in cerebral oxygen saturation in the SI group was almost as rapid, suggesting that the intrathoracic pressure increase imposed by SI does not affect gas exchange and brain perfusion.

Schwaberger et al. [11] randomized 40 preterm infants comparing the effects of SI with "standard" respiratory care on cerebral blood volume. It remained essentially unchanged in the SI-treated infants, while decreased in the first 15 min after birth in the control group with no adverse neurological effects.

A few observational studies have been conducted comparing outcomes of preterm infants treated with SI with a control group. Even if these studies are not homogeneous in terms of population, definition of SI, respiratory management in the control group, and main outcomes, they showed the feasibility and safety of treating preterm infants with SI. Moreover, although they are all limited by the use of historical controls, they suggest essential preliminary data for the design of randomized controlled trials (RCTs).

Randomized clinical trials

Given the lack of a standardized definition of SI in terms of duration, peak pressure to apply, and number of inflations to perform, there is no homogeneity in the use of SI itself in all of the RCTs currently available. To date, there are five published RCTs of SI in preterm neonates, the results of which can be used to assume a provisional conclusion on its efficacy and safety. The recently concluded multicenter international trial, the SAIL trial [12], compared IPPV and SI in extremely preterm infants with BPD and death as primary outcomes (details below).

One of the main concerns that has arisen in regard to SI is the safety of this maneuver, and specifically the risk for air leaks.

In the Italian SLI trial (Lista et al.) [13], there was a higher but nonsignificant incidence of pneumothorax in very preterm infants (25–29 weeks of gestational age) who underwent SI, in respect to the control group. Similar findings in a population of late preterm infants characterized the study of Mercadante et al. [14]. In both these trials, SI was performed regardless of respiratory status, and infants belonging to the SI arm received this procedure prophylactically. Nevertheless, of note, in the SLI trial the incidence of pneumothorax occurred at a median age of 70 h. It is possible, then, that other factors influenced the incidence of air leaks (i.e., surfactant administration timing). It must be underlined that if SI is effective, it dramatically changes lung mechanics and therefore neonatologists have to be very careful in setting the respiratory parameters. Theoretically, it is possible that the caregivers may not have paid enough attention to this issue and this could explain the tendency toward increased incidence of air leaks and pneumothorax in the following days. In addition, the last Cochrane Review [15] did not mention in the main results any concerns about air leaks or pneumothorax related to SI.

Harling et al. [16] enrolled 52 preterm infants to receive either a 5-s SI or a 2-s conventional lung inflation (IPPV). They collected bronchoalveolar lavage fluid immediately after intubation and after 12 h, and then they measured cytokine concentration. They did not find any significant differences between the two groups, neither in cytokine levels nor in other clinical outcomes (mortality, BPD).

te Pas and Walther randomized 207 preterm infants comparing two DR protocols. SIs (10-s inflation with 20 cmH$_2$O, which could be increased to 25 cmH$_2$O for another 10 s depending on individual response) were delivered with a T-piece via nasopharyngeal tube, and nasal CPAP was started after 1–2 SIs. In the control group, infants were treated with IPPV via self-inflating bag and facemask, and CPAP was not used in the DR. The primary outcome was the need for mechanical ventilation in the first 72 h of life, which was significantly lower in the SI group. Surfactant was administered less in the SI arm, and moderate–severe BPD rate seemed to favor the SI-treated infants. However, as these protocols were a package of interventions, it is difficult to isolate the individual effect of SI on clinical outcomes [17].

Two systematic reviews about the use of SI in preterm infants have been recently published [15,18].

Schmolzer et al. found a significant reduction in the intubation and need of mechanical ventilation rate in the first 72 h of life in SI groups, with no differences in mortality, BPD rate, IVH, or air leaks.

The last Cochrane Review did not find any significant difference in terms of mortality or BPD, but only in the duration of MV, which was shortened in the SI group. The authors concluded suggesting caution in the interpretation of this result, as it could be influenced by study characteristics other than the intervention.

Preliminary data from the SAIL trial showed an excess of early deaths (<48 h of age) in the SI arm (7.5% vs. 1.4%) but no difference in pneumothorax and intraventricular hemorrhage in extremely preterm infants (23–26 weeks gestation) who required resuscitation at birth. DSMB upon review halted the trial for harm after recruiting 460 infants (out of a total desired sample of 592). The detailed analysis of the early mortality causes still needs to be clarified in order to understand which could be the possible link between SI and early death. Anyway long-term outcome (death and BPD occurrence) were similar between SI and control group. According to the results of the SAIL trial and the SLI trial, it seems that further researches are warranted to better understand the effect of SI and its use in delivery room management of preterm infants with signs of RDS or at risk of respiratory failure.

Current recommendations

Given the current evidence available, SI seems to be a promising technique to optimize neonatal transition after birth. However, it must be considered still an experimental therapy, as there is insufficient data to advocate its use in clinical settings. The latest ERC guidelines on neonatal resuscitation argue against the routine use of initial SI for preterm infants without spontaneous respiration immediately after birth, but allow SI to be considered in individual clinical circumstances or research settings [19]. However, they recommend maintaining the initial pressure for 2–3 s for the first five positive pressure inflations during resuscitation.

Despite the lack of strong evidence, we suggest some key practical points for performing SIs in the delivery room. The parameters are chosen according to those set in clinical studies.

- **Peak pressure**: It would be desirable to start with 20–30 cmH$_2$O according to gestational age.
- **Duration of SI**: It ranges from 5 to 20 s. Animal studies have shown that inflations lasting less than 5 s are not effective to clear the fluid from the lungs.
- **Number of SIs**: There is no consensus about it. Most clinical studies have performed 1–3 SIs, with different approaches in terms of delivered pressure (same peak pressure for the all SIs or progressively increased peak pressures from 20 to 25 cmH$_2$O if no response was obtained after the first maneuver).
- **Time between SIs**: Even if there is lack of evidence regarding this aspect, it is reasonable to suggest to leave enough time between one SI and the next one to observe the infant's response. However, observation time should be limited to avoid

reducing the efficacy of the second SLI due to airway obstruction.

- **Monitoring of SI's efficacy**: Verifying the effects of SI in real time remains quite challenging in the delivery room. As chest expansion could be difficult to evaluate, the efficacy of the SI maneuver should be judged based on heart rate and SpO$_2$ response. The routine use of devices targeted at the measurement of respiratory patterns and tidal volume and/or end-tidal CO$_2$ may be helpful to verify the efficacy of this intervention as well.

It is indeed clear that further evidence from well-designed RCTs is needed to determine in more detail how, and in which clinical circumstances, SI should be used.

Unresolved issues about SI

At present, there are still several aspects of SI that need to be better clarified in order to recommend the use of this maneuver as a routine care procedure.

- What is the ideal and safest SI peak to deliver?
- What is the ideal duration of SI?
- What is the optimal number of SIs to perform?
- Might we use different parameters for different GA?
- Should SI be used as a prophylactic or rescue maneuver?
- What is the role of spontaneous breathing on the efficacy of SI?
- How can the SI maneuver be monitored and how can it be tailored to individual response?
- What is the best interface to deliver SI?
- Should surfactant replacement therapy be administered prior to, or after, SI?
- Is SI use feasible in asphyxiated infants?
- How can we minimize the risk of air leak related to SI?
- What are the effects of SI on tissue oxygenation (cerebral, pulmonary, cardiac, etc.)?
- Does SI have a significant impact on relevant clinical outcomes (death, BPD, etc.)?

Online Supplementary Material

Please visit MedEnact to access the video on SLI.

References

[1] Hooper SB, Te Pas AB, Kitchen M.J. Respiratory transition in the newborn: a three-phase process. Arch Dis Child Fetal Neonatal Ed 2016;101:F266–F271.

[2] Aziz K, Chadwick M, Baker M, Andrews W. Ante- and intra-partum factors that predict increased need for neonatal resuscitation. Resuscitation 2008;79:444–452.

[3] te Pas AB, Siew M, Wallace MJ, Kitchen MJ, Fouras A, Lewis RA, et al. Establishing functional residual capacity at birth: the effect of sustained inflation and positive end-

expiratory pressure in a preterm rabbit model. Pediatr Res 2009;65:537–541.

[4] Boon AW, Milner AD, Hopkin IE. Lung expansion, tidal exchange, and formation of the functional residual capacity during resuscitation of asphyxiated neonates. J Pediatr 1979;95:1031–1036.

[5] Vyas H, Field D, Milner AD, Hopkin IE. Determinants of the first inspiratory volume and functional residual capacity at birth. Pediatr Pulmonol 1986;2:189–193.

[6] Sobotka KS, Hooper SB, Allison BJ, Te Pas AB, Davis PG, Morley CJ, et al. An initial sustained inflation improves the respiratory and cardiovascular transition at birth in preterm lambs. Pediatr Res 2011;70:56–60.

[7] Klingenberg C, Sobotka KS, Ong T, Allison BJ, Schmolzer GM, Moss TJ, et al. Effect of sustained inflation duration; resuscitation of near-term asphyxiated lambs. Arch Dis Child Fetal Neonatal 2013;98:F222–F227.

[8] van Vonderen JJ, Hooper SB, Hummler HD, Lopriore E, te Pas AB. Effects of a sustained inflation in preterm infants at birth. J Pediatr 2014;165:903–908.e1.

[9] Lista G, Cavigioli F, La Verde PA, Castoldi F, Bresesti I, Morley CJ. Effects of breathing and apnoea during sustained inflations in resuscitation of preterm infants. Neonatology 2017;111:360–366.

[10] Fuchs H, Lindner W, Buschko A, Trischberger T, Schmid M, Hummler HD. Cerebral oxygenation in very low birth weight infants supported with sustained lung inflations after birth. Pediatr Res 2011;70:176–180.

[11] Schwaberger B, Pichler G, Avian A, Binder-Heschl C, Baik N, Urlesberger B. Do sustained lung inflations during neonatal resuscitation affect cerebral blood volume in preterm infants? A randomized controlled pilot study. PLoS One 2015;10:e0138964.

[12] Foglia EE, Owen LS, Thio M, Ratcliffe SJ, Lista G, Te Pas A, et al. Sustained Aeration of Infant Lungs (SAIL) trial: study protocol for a randomized controlled trial. Trials 2015;16:95.

[13] Lista G, Boni L, Scopesi F, Mosca F, Trevisanuto D, Messner H, et al. Sustained lung inflation at birth for preterm infants: a randomized clinical trial. Pediatrics 2015;135:e457–e464.

[14] Mercadante D, Colnaghi M, Polimeni V, Ghezzi E, Fumagalli M, Consonni D, et al. Sustained lung inflation in late preterm infants: a randomized controlled trial. J Perinatol 2016;36:443–447.

[15] Bruschettini M, O'Donnell CP, Davis PG, Morley CJ, Moja L, Zappettini S, et al. Sustained versus standard inflations during neonatal resuscitation to prevent mortality and improve respiratory outcomes. Cochrane Database Syst Rev 2017;7:CD004953.

[16] Harling AE, Beresford MW, Vince GS, Bates M, Yoxall CW. Does sustained lung inflation at resuscitation reduce lung injury in the preterm infant? Arch Dis Child Fetal Neonatal Ed 2005;90:F406–F410.

[17] te Pas AB, Walther FJ. A randomized, controlled trial of delivery-room respiratory management in very preterm infants. Pediatrics 2007;120:322–329.

[18] Schmolzer GM, Kumar M, Aziz K, Pichler G, O'Reilly M, Lista G, et al. Sustained inflation versus positive pressure ventilation at birth: a systematic review and meta-analysis. Arch Dis Child Fetal Neonatal Ed 2015;100:F361–F368.

[19] Wyllie J, Bruinenberg J, Roehr CC, Rudiger M, Trevisanuto D, Urlesberger B. European Resuscitation Council Guidelines for Resuscitation 2015: Section 7. Resuscitation and support of transition of babies at birth. Resuscitation 2015;95:249–263.

Section | III |

Applied Physiology, and Ventilator Support: General Considerations

Chapter | 6 |

Introduction to Lung Mechanics

Jegen Kandasamy, MD, Namasivayam Ambalavanan, MD

CHAPTER POINTS

- Overview of respiratory mechanics
- Mechanics of the respiratory pump
- Elastic and resistive properties of the respiratory system
- Respiratory mechanics in disease

Introduction

The primary function of the respiratory system is translation of neural output into mechanical events that allow air to flow in and out of the lungs and facilitate gas exchange at the alveolar–vascular interface [1]. The conversion of force generated by respiratory muscles into pressure changes across the respiratory system is dependent on the mechanical characteristics of the respiratory system. Tidal changes in lung volume are created by stretching elastic components in the respiratory system, and resistive elements in the airway and lung tissue are overcome to create flow of air through the respiratory tree. This chapter will detail the mechanical characteristics of the respiratory system, their interactions with one another, and their role in the function of the neonatal respiratory system during various disease states.

Overview of respiratory mechanics

The mechanical elements of the respiratory system can be described as consisting of a pump and a load. The pump is made up of structures in the thoracoabdominal wall including the ribs, sternum, and the muscles of inspiration and expiration. The load that the respiratory pump acts on consists of the elastic and resistive properties of the chest wall, lungs, and airways. Elastic recoil of the chest wall and the lungs are opposing forces that determine the resting (end-expiratory) volume of the respiratory system (Fig. 6.1). At this point of the respiratory cycle, the inwardly directed elastic recoil of the lung is balanced by the elastic recoil of the chest wall which is directed outward to create a small negative intrapleural pressure (P_{pl}) of -3 to -6 cm H_2O with respect to the atmospheric pressure (P_{atm}) which is assumed to be zero in this setting. The volume of air left in the alveoli at the end of normal expiration largely depends on the magnitude of this negative P_{pl} (see Section: Elastic properties of the respiratory system).

In this resting state, the pressure at the airway opening (P_{ao}) as well as the alveolar pressure (P_{al}) are both at equilibrium with P_{atm} and therefore zero as well. During inspiration, the respiratory muscles contract to expand intrathoracic volume. This outward chest wall movement

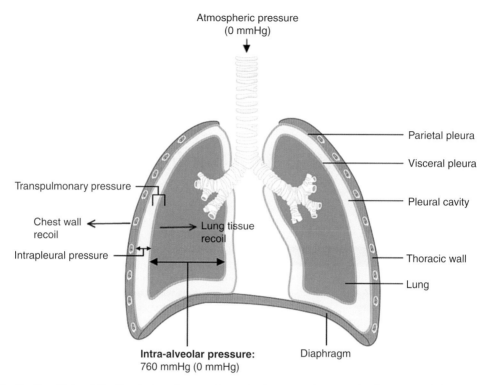

Atmospheric pressure
(0 mmHg)

Parietal pleura

Visceral pleura

Transpulmonary pressure

Pleural cavity

Chest wall
recoil

Lung tissue
recoil

Intrapleural pressure

Thoracic wall

Lung

Intra-alveolar pressure:
760 mmHg (0 mmHg)

Diaphragm

Fig. 6.1 The Resting State of the Respiratory System. Atmospheric pressure is assumed to be 0 mmHg in lung mechanics. Functional residual capacity is generated by the negative intrapleural pressure created by the opposing recoils of the chest wall and the lung.

decreases P_{pl} further and expands the alveoli and terminal airways. This creates a pressure differential between P_{ao} (which remains zero) and P_{al} (which is now negative) that drives air into the lungs. At the end of inspiration, the respiratory muscles relax and the chest wall collapses inward. This increases P_{pl} back to its baseline and releases the expansionary force placed on the alveoli that recoil back toward their resting volume. The positive P_{al} created in this process overcomes the resistance to flow created by the terminal airways and forces air out of the lungs, thereby completing the cycle and returning the respiratory system to its resting state [2–4].

The pressure differential that opens the alveoli $(P_{al} - P_{pl})$ and the driving pressure for airflow $(P_{ao} - P_{al})$ are both required to create the volume and airflow changes necessary to permit normal respiration. The total pressure that is required to drive respiration—referred to as the transpulmonary pressure (P_{tp})—is traditionally $P_{alv} - P_{pl}$ (difference between alveolar pressure and pleural pressure), but as we can more readily measure alveolar opening pressure (P_{ao}) but not P_{alv}, which approximates P_{alv} at end inspiration, P_{tp} is usually estimated $P_{ao} - P_{pl}$ (difference between airway opening pressure and intrapleural pressure).

Physical principles of respiratory mechanics

The mechanical properties that determine lung volume and airflow changes through the respiratory system during inspiration and expiration in the manner described earlier are elastance, conductance, and inertance [5]. Elastance is the tendency of a hollow organ to recoil to its initial size after removal of the distending pressure. Elastance of the entire respiratory system includes the elastance of the chest wall and that of the lungs. Compliance is the reciprocal of elastance and measures distensibility. It is defined as the change in volume (V) of a hollow organ per unit change in the distending pressure (P).

$$\text{Compliance } (C) = \Delta V / \Delta P$$

Respiratory conductance represents the instantaneous amount of airflow in the lungs (Q), defined as the volume of air moved per unit time (t) per unit amount of pressure difference between the airway opening and the alveoli. Resistance, which measures the impedance to airflow offered by the tissues of the respiratory system, is the reciprocal of conductance.

$$\mathrm{Re\,sistance}\ (R) = \Delta P/(dV/dt) = \Delta P/Q$$

The total pressure difference that is required to overcome inertia during motion in the respiratory system and accelerate airflow is called total respiratory inertance.

$$\mathrm{Inertance}\ (I) = \Delta P/dQ/dt$$

Very minimal pressure is required to accelerate airflow through the respiratory tract. Respiratory system inertance becomes a significant factor only when respiratory frequency is as high as those used in high-frequency ventilation; during tidal breathing and conventional ventilation, this factor can be safely ignored [6].

Lung mechanics can be highly heterogeneous and vary in different regions, especially during disease states. However, a single-compartment model can be used to simplify the various concepts of lung mechanics [7]. In one such model (Fig. 6.2), the alveolar compartment (with a volume of V) is represented by a pair of canisters that slide against each other and are connected to each other by a spring with elastic recoil of E and a resistive element R_t. The spring represents the elastic recoil (elastance) stored in the respiratory system when it is stretched beyond its resting volume. This recoil is used by the respiratory system for lung deflation during expiration which is usually passive during normal tidal breathing and does not require additional work by the respiratory pump. R_t represents the resistance to airflow offered by the tissues that make up the lungs and the chest wall (viscous resistance). Inflow to this system is through a tube that represents the airways and offers its own resistance (R_{aw}) to airflow.

The pressures required to overcome elastance (P_{el}) and resistance (P_{res}) and allow ventilation to proceed during each breath can be obtained by rearranging and adding the first two equations mentioned previously.

$$P_{total} = P_{el} + P_{res} = V/C + R*Q$$

P_{tp} which was described in the previous section and P_{total} represent the same entity, namely the pressure that needs to be generated by the respiratory pump to overcome respiratory system elasticity and resistance (offered by the airways as well as lung tissue) and allow ventilation to proceed unimpeded. These mechanical concepts can be summed up into one equation, which is referred to as the equation of motion for the respiratory system.

$$P_{tp} = P_{ao} - P_{pl} = P_{el} + P_{res} = E*V \text{ (pressure required to}$$
overcome elastance$) + R_t * Q$ (pressure required to overcome viscous or tissue resistance$) + R_{aw} * Q$ (pressure required to overcome airway resistance)

or more simply,

$$P_{tp} = E*V + R_t *Q + R_{aw} *Q$$

Airflow in the respiratory system is terminated when P_{ao} equilibrates with P_{al}. The time taken for this pressure equilibration to be achieved determines the rate of emptying and filling of alveoli and therefore determines the duration of a single breath. If all respiration was passive and the lung an ideal single-compartment model, the rate of filling or emptying of the lung can be determined using its compliance and resistance to calculate the time constant of the respiratory system (τ) [8].

$$\tau = C \times R = \Delta V/\Delta P * \Delta P/Q = \Delta V/Q$$

In other words, τ is the rate of change of volume for a given airflow rate within the idealized respiratory system. Based on this model, lung inflation and deflation is an exponential process that is 63% complete after one τ, 87% complete after two τ, and almost fully complete after three time constants (95%) have elapsed (Fig. 6.3). Smaller τ

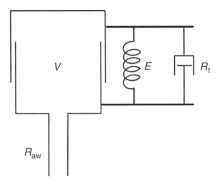

Fig. 6.2 **An Idealized Single-Compartment Model of the Respiratory System.** V represents lung volume, E represents elastance of the lung, and R_t and R_{aw} represent resistance of the lung tissue and airway, respectively.

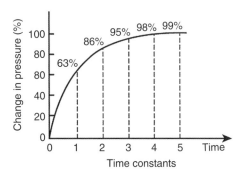

Fig. 6.3 **Changes in Lung Pressure for Every Time Constant That Elapses in a Single Breath.**

values allow for quicker $P_{ao} - P_{al}$ equilibration and completion of the respiratory cycle and correspondingly faster respiratory rates. Studies have shown that the respiratory rates of various animal species correlate closely with their τ values. Larger mammals have longer τ and slower respiratory rates and smaller bird species have shorter τ and faster rates [9]. The τ varies in infants with various respiratory diseases. Knowledge of these variations can help clinicians determine the appropriate inspiratory time (I-time) and respiratory rate that will permit lung inflation and deflation to be fully complete with every breath. Since inspiration is an active process, it is not strictly a linear time-invariant model and time constants often overestimate the time lungs take to inflate.

Energy is expended for the work of the respiratory pump that moves air through the respiratory system. The total work (force × displacement) done by the respiratory system over a single breath can be derived from the pressure required (the force component) to effect changes in the volume of the respiratory system (the displacement component). Assuming that work of breathing is constant for every breath, work of breathing per minute can be calculated if the respiratory rate (RR) is known [5].

Clinical scenario 1

A 7-day-old 26-week gestational age (GA) newborn infant who is being mechanically ventilated is noted to have metabolic acidosis on the latest blood gas. The nurse also tells you that the infant has been hypotensive and responded minimally to vasopressors. When you review the previous blood gases you notice that in the last 4 h the infant had respiratory acidosis and that his ventilator rates were increased to correct this, without much success. You notice the flow waveform on the ventilator that is shown in Fig. 6.4A. What is the cause of this infant's worsening blood gases, how can this be confirmed, and what corrective and preventive measures can be taken?

Answer

The ventilator waveform depicts incomplete emptying of the lungs during expiration (Fig. 6.4B). As discussed earlier, any increase in the time constant can increase the time required to complete exhalation. Mucus plugs can obstruct endotracheal tubes (ETTs), increase airway resistance, and increase τ values. If respiratory rates are increased without ensuring that the inspiratory time:expiratory time (I:E) ratio is appropriate to allow expiration to be complete, breaths can "stack" and cause air trapping in the lungs. This can create increased positive pressure on the mediastinal

structures, such as the right heart, and reduce venous filling and cardiac output leading to metabolic acidosis. Paying attention to the ventilator flow waveforms to ensure that adequate time is being provided for exhalation to be complete will allow for quicker detection of this phenomenon. Other clues could be a measured positive end-expiratory pressure (PEEP) on the ventilator that is higher than the "set" PEEP (so-called "auto"-PEEP), and chest X-ray findings of flattened diaphragms and horizontally aligned ribs that indicate overdistended lungs. Decreasing the I-time can increase lung emptying and tidal volume changes and decrease the hypercarbia and respiratory acidosis. When lungs are overdistended, increasing lung emptying will also relieve right heart pressure and improve cardiac output and oxygenation.

Work of breathing/minute = work of breathing/breath
*RR = $\Delta P * \Delta V * RR$

As illustrated in Fig. 6.5, energy is required for work done to overcome elastic forces (portion ABCA) and resistive forces during inspiration (ADCA) as well as for resistive work during expiration (ACEA). Most of the work required to overcome the frictional airway and tissue resistive forces is dissipated as heat. Under conditions of normal tidal breathing, the expiratory phase is non-energy requiring and passive. However, during pathologic states, such as airway obstruction that lead to flow limitation, expiration can require active contraction of the abdominal wall and internal intercostal muscles, a process that consumes energy and increases work of breathing, as is often noted in infants with bronchopulmonary dysplasia (BPD) [10].

Newborn infants have high respiratory rates and work of breathing due to their smaller body sizes [11]. They have high body surface area to volume ratios due to which they lose heat excessively through the convective and evaporative routes, a phenomenon that is more severe in prematurely born infants. Increased metabolic rates are therefore necessary to generate more heat to maintain their body temperature. To sustain such high metabolic rates, their oxygen consumption needs be increased, which requires increased minute ventilation (tidal volume × RR). Since their small lung volumes prevent them from being able to greatly increase their tidal volume, newborn infants achieve higher minute ventilation by breathing at faster rates which increases their work of breathing significantly. However, when corrected for such high metabolic rates, newborn infants have similar work of breathing when compared to adults [12].

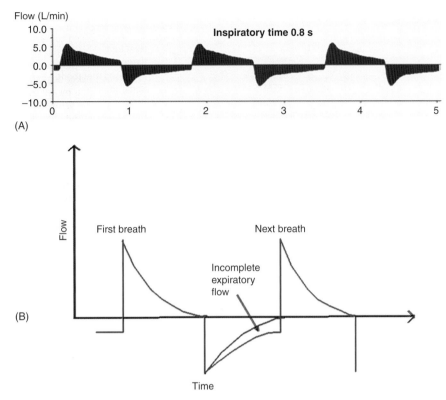

Fig. 6.4 (A) and (B) show a waveform with incomplete expiration that when unrecognized can lead to auto-PEEP.

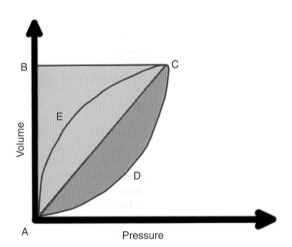

Fig. 6.5 A Typical Dynamic Pressure–Volume (PV) Plot That Illustrates Work of Breathing. The area shaded in *gray* (ADCA) represents the work done to overcome resistance during inspiration, while the *yellow-shaded areas* represent work done to overcome elastic forces during inspiration (ABCA) and to overcome resistive forces during expiration (ACEA). Also, note that lung volumes at any given pressure are higher during expiration than inspiration (hysteresis).

Mechanics of the respiratory pump

All the mechanical work that is required for breathing is performed by the structures that make up the respiratory pump which is comprised of the inspiratory and expiratory muscles that act like levers and the skeletal and connective tissue structures of the thoracoabdominal cage that function like a fulcrum around which respiratory motion occurs (Fig. 6.6).

Muscles of inspiration

These include the diaphragm and the external intercostal muscles. The diaphragm is the primary generator of the pressure changes required for inspiration. Its muscle fibers originate from the lumbar spine, the xiphoid process of the sternum, and lower six rib pairs and insert into a central tendon that is pulled downward and forward during contraction of the diaphragm. This downward motion of the diaphragm increases the anteroposterior and vertical dimensions of the thorax, generates negative P_{pl}, and causes air to flow into the lungs [13]. The area of the lowermost rib cage that is in direct contact with the diaphragm is called the appositional area.

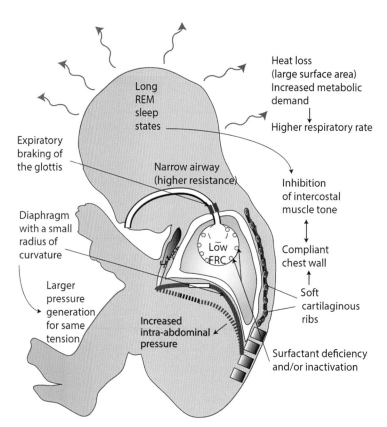

Fig. 6.6 Mechanics of Neonatal Breathing Compared to Breathing in Older Children and Adults. Copyright: Satyan Lakshminrusimha.

The larger this area, the greater is the ability of the diaphragm to expand intrathoracic volume. A larger zone of apposition also allows the increased intra-abdominal pressure generated by the downward diaphragmatic movement to be transmitted more efficiently to the chest wall. This effect "splints" the chest wall and increases its outward motion during inspiration [14]. The tension generated by a muscle fiber is directly proportional to its initial length. Diaphragmatic flattening, often caused by overdistended lungs, shortens the diaphragmatic muscle fibers and decreases its contractile strength.

At birth, the diaphragm has a low muscle mass and is composed of fewer fatigue-resistant fast-oxidative fibers (10% at 24 weeks, 20% at term gestation) compared to the adult (60%), though its dimensions increase rapidly with postnatal growth and body weight gain [1,15,16]. Therefore, the newborn's diaphragm has low contractile strength. Despite these disadvantages the newborn's diaphragm can generate pressures that are adequate for tidal breathing. During the first several breaths after birth, negative intrapleural pressures as high as 100 cm H_2O are achieved when the newborn cries. In addition, tidal P_{pl} swings during normal respiration are similar in magnitude (5–7 cm H_2O) to that

generated by older infants and adults [17]. This is made possible by the mechanical laws that govern the motion of contractile spherical structures. For a given radius of curvature (r), the pressure generated (P) by a spherical structure with wall tension (T) is given by the law of Laplace as follows:

$$P = 2T/r$$

According to this principle, the pressure generated by the newborn's diaphragm with its small radius of curvature is higher for any given wall tension than the adult's diaphragm whose radius of curvature is larger. In addition, any such pressure generated by the neonatal diaphragm is also applied to a proportionally smaller thoracic area when compared to older children and adults. Recent studies have also shown that muscle fiber composition does not always correlate well with diaphragmatic fatigability and that the neonatal diaphragm can indeed generate high pressures when required [9]. In the absence of other pathology, these factors allow the diaphragm of even the most premature infant to function without being fatigued for long periods of time. Therefore, diaphragmatic function is usually not a limiting factor in the neonatal respiratory system.

58

The external intercostal muscles run between ribs and slope downward and anteriorly. Due to their course in the intercostal spaces and the angular inclination of the ribs in the thoracic cage, external intercostal muscle activity is greatest in the dorsal portions of the anterior intercostal spaces. During contraction, they elevate the ribs and pull them to a more anterior position to increase the lateral and anteroposterior diameters of the thorax. This stabilizing action of the intercostal muscles minimizes the inward collapse of the highly compliant neonatal chest wall with diaphragmatic contraction. They also reduce diaphragmatic shortening and improve its mechanical efficiency [18]. However, in the newborn, the intercostal muscles run a shorter distance from their origin on the upper rib to their insertion to the lower rib reducing their length and therefore their contractility when compared to adults. In addition, newborns, especially premature infants, spend 80% of their sleep in the rapid eye movement (REM) phase; they also sleep longer (>18–20 h/day). During this sleep phase, intercostal muscle tone is subjected to both phasic and tonic inhibition which causes these muscles to become inactive and significantly decreases chest wall stability and movement in the newborn [19].

Muscles of expiration

Expiration is mostly passive. However, during conditions that cause airflow obstruction, the muscles of the abdominal wall—the internal and external oblique as well as the rectus and transversus abdominis—contract to raise intra-abdominal pressure and push up the diaphragm to cause forced expiratory flow [20]. The internal intercostal muscles which run between ribs in the opposite direction to the external intercostals also contract to cause the ribs to move downward and inward to decrease thoracic volume. Their contraction also stabilizes the chest wall and prevents it from moving forward when expiration is actively forced [18].

Chest wall

At birth, the ribs articulate at almost right angles to their corresponding vertebral bodies. This creates a circular thoracic configuration in which the diaphragm is flatter and operates over a less efficient portion of its force–length curve. The rounded shape of the infant thorax also leads to a decreased surface area of the zone of apposition. Due to this, there is inefficient transmission of intra-abdominal pressure that is generated during inspiration to the thorax. In addition, the newborn's chest wall is made of pliable ribs, thin muscles, and is primarily cartilaginous rather than skeletal in composition. These features are even more pronounced at lower GAs, which causes the preterm newborn's chest wall to be highly compliant and paradoxically move inward when P_{pl} becomes more negative during inspiration. Therefore, the premature infant's inspiratory

muscles need to work harder to generate additional negative pressure in the intrapleural space to achieve adequate tidal volumes. The newborn attempts to improve chest wall stability during such conditions by recruiting the accessory muscles of inspiration, such as the scalene muscles, sternomastoids, and alae nasae. The active contraction of these muscles is responsible for the characteristic signs of respiratory distress that are often noted in young infants, such as sternal and intercostal retractions and head bobbing [21]. This abnormally high chest wall compliance (C_{cw}) is one of the most important factors that prevent premature infants from being able to establish normal lung function. C_{cw} slowly decreases in infancy and lung compliance (C_l) which is low at birth increases with age. C_{cw} and C_l become nearly equal by 2 years of age [22].

Clinical scenario 2

The nurse taking care of a mechanically ventilated infant informs you during morning rounds that turning him to the prone position improves the infant's oxygenation. The student physician on rounds with you wants to know the physiologic mechanism behind this phenomenon. While you both are at the infant's bedside you notice that the infant's oxygen saturation is decreasing again and he requires increased ventilator settings to improve his oxygenation. Why would prone positioning cause only a transient improvement of this infant's oxygenation?

Answer

Newborn infants have a thin anterior abdominal wall musculature that can accommodate a large volume without generating much intra-abdominal pressure. In addition, the lower appositional area of the diaphragm reduces intra-abdominal pressure transmission to the diaphragm. These two factors lead to insufficient expansion of the lower ribs and decrease the mechanical efficiency of inspiration. In the prone position, the protuberant infant's abdomen is effectively splinted, leading to increased intra-abdominal pressure generation that causes increased diaphragmatic efficiency and improved ventilation overall. Additionally, the superior (anterior) diaphragm moves better in the supine position when compared to the inferior (posterior) diaphragm, but perfusion is preferentially directed to the dependent portions of the lungs (the inferior regions). This creates increased ventilation–perfusion (mismatch) and decreased oxygenation. When the infant is turned to the prone position, the posterior diaphragmatic portion is now able to move better leading to better ventilation and perfusion, though any such effect is likely to be transient since prolonged prone position will tend to lead to better perfusion in the anterior (and now inferior) regions of the lung. A recent study of prone positioning (which is commonly done for infants in neonatal intensive care units) showed that there are no consistent short- or long-term benefits from this practice for infants with respiratory distress syndrome (RDS) [23].

Elastic properties of the respiratory system

Elastic properties of the alveoli, chest wall, and airways determine changes in lung volume for a given amount of pressure in the respiratory system [24]. The slope of a pressure–volume (PV) curve between P_{tp} measurements made in a lung that is distended to various known volumes of air represents the *static* compliance of the lung (C_l). Slopes of PV plots of lung volumes against transthoracic pressure (the difference between P_{pl} and P_{atm}) represent the compliance of the chest wall (Fig. 6.7). Similarly, the slope of a plot of the difference between P_{ao} and P_{atm} against lung volumes represents the compliance of the entire respiratory system (C_{rs}) [25]. C_{l-dyn} measurements can closely approximate static compliance measurements. PV plots are available on most modern ventilators and can be useful to calculate *dynamic* compliance of the lung (C_{l-dyn}) in the ventilated infant [26,27].

For any given pressure on a dynamic PV plot, lung volume is always greater during deflation than during inflation (Fig. 6.2). This implies that lung compliance is greater during expiration than inspiration. This phenomenon is called hysteresis and is commonly observed in nonlinear systems, such as the lungs, which have different mechanical properties during different states of operation. Hysteresis can be exaggerated in the preterm newborn due to abnormally high expiratory air trapping within the lungs [28]. This is because negative P_{pl} is required during end-expiration to

maintain the patency of smaller airways that lack the cartilaginous support available in the walls of the larger airways. Since premature infants cannot generate adequate negative P_{pl} due to their high C_{cw}, they are often unable to maintain smaller airway patency in the dependent regions of the lung during end-expiration. This leads to incomplete expiration and increases lung closing volumes (maximal lung volume at which airway closure can be detected in the dependent parts of the lungs). This process can worsen further at higher breathing frequencies since expiratory time is reduced at such high frequencies leading to increased air trapping.

Functional residual capacity (FRC) of the lung is defined as the volume of air that is in communication with the upper airway at end-expiration. FRC is low in preterm infants, since they are unable to create negative P_{pl} which is also required to establish an adequate FRC [29,30]. The low FRC of preterm infant lungs causes them to operate at a significant mechanical disadvantage. As shown in Fig. 6.8, dynamic PV plots of the normal lung assume a sigmoidal shape. Therefore, the slope of these plots is highest (and compliance is optimal) when lungs are inflated and deflated within the range of their FRC. Underinflation and atelectasis (low FRC) or air trapping and overexpansion (high FRC) both cause C_{l-dyn} to shift to the ends of the sigmoidal curve where it is low.

Preterm infants use several corrective measures that attempt to limit FRC loss. These include post-inspiratory activation of the diaphragm which can terminate expiration before it is complete, high respiratory rates with a short expiratory time that increases alveolar air trapping even in

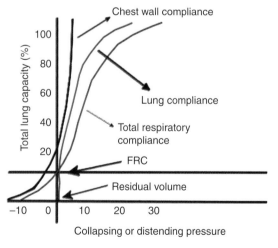

Fig. 6.7 Static Pressure–Volume Curves of the Newborn Respiratory System. Lung compliance is very low and chest wall compliance is much higher than in adults. Respiratory system compliance which is the sum of these two compliances is low.

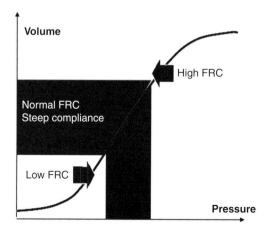

Fig. 6.8 Pressure–Volume Curves at Different Levels of FRC. Underinflated lungs and overdistended lungs both lead to poor lung compliance.

nondependent areas as well as expiratory braking of the glottis that generates additional PEEP and is responsible for the characteristic grunting that is associated with premature infant breathing [31].

The pattern of low FRC and higher closing volumes seen in premature infants is the inverse of that seen in older children and adults and is associated with clinical consequences that include atelectasis, increased ventilation–perfusion mismatch, and hypoxia. Lung compliance corrected for FRC is referred to as *specific* compliance. Specific compliance increases rapidly in the days after the newborn is born and approaches adult values, as intra-alveolar pulmonary fluid is resorbed and replaced by air [32]. Specific compliance values are much lower in pre-term infants than in older infants and adults despite their low FRCs since their lung compliance is disproportionately lower.

While low FRC is usually the cause for their abnormally low C_{l-dyn}, premature infants ventilated at high respiratory rates can also have increased, rather than decreased FRC, as the cause for decreased dynamic lung compliance. This is because their developing lungs are still immature and have high heterogeneity of time constant values in different regions and air trapping can occur in regions of the lung with longer time constants, a phenomenon referred to as frequency dependence of dynamic compliance.

In addition to these dynamic factors, physical components of the lung architecture also play a major role in determining lung compliance. These include surface tension forces in the alveoli, interstitial and intra-alveolar fluid content (which is usually not a major influence on lung compliance beyond the first several hours to days of life), and the amount of elastic connective tissue in the lung. At birth, the airways and the alveoli of the lung contain a larger amount of elastic tissue with correspondingly higher amounts of collagen and elastin. With postnatal growth and maturation, connective tissue volume in the lung decreases and alveolar membranes become thinner which allows the lung to become more compliant [33].

The most important determinant of lung compliance is the physical force of surface tension (ST). The alveolus can be considered a spherical structure with an air–fluid interface covering its interior surface. At this interface, the polar molecules of water that line the alveolar epithelium are attracted more strongly to each other than to the molecules of the gases in the air that they interface with. This can lead to alveolar contraction and volume reduction that can become severe enough to cause lung atelectasis. Based on the law of Laplace discussed earlier, an alveolus with radius *r* would require a distending pressure that is equal to ST/*r* to counteract these inward-directed surface tension forces. As can be deduced from this relationship, the smaller the alveolar size, the higher the pressure that is required to keep

it open. This surface tension effect causes the alveoli to have a strong tendency to collapse when their radius is small, a state that exists during expiration. Therefore, unopposed surface tension forces would cause alveoli to become atelectatic at end-expiration. At the beginning of inspiration, these collapsed alveoli would require high pressures to be generated through increased work by the respiratory pump to air to reopen and allow gas exchange to be carried out (Fig. 6.9).

The increased work of breathing that is required to overcome surface tension–induced atelectasis can overwhelm the respiratory system and lead to respiratory failure [24]. Type II alveolar epithelial cells produce a surface-active phospholipid called surfactant that counteracts and reduces the effects of surface tension in the alveoli and terminal airways. Its structure has hydrophilic ends that coat the surface of water molecules and prevent cohesive forces from bringing them closer to each other and lower surface tension. As the alveoli reduce in size during expiration, surfactant molecular density increases and its effectiveness increases when surface tension effects are at their highest in the air–fluid interface that lines the alveolar inner surface. In addition, when the alveoli expand during inspiration, surfactant function is reduced, leaving residual surface tension that is required to prevent alveolar overdistension.

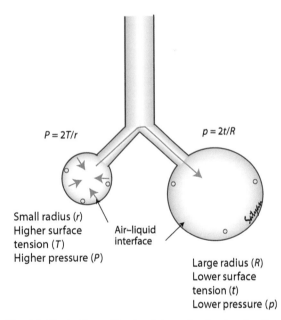

$P = 2T/r$

$p = 2t/R$

Small radius (*r*)
Higher surface tension (*T*)
Higher pressure (*P*)

Air–liquid interface

Large radius (*R*)
Lower surface tension (*t*)
Lower pressure (*p*)

Fig. 6.9 Illustration of Laplace's Law. An alveolus of radius *r* requires a distending pressure equal to surface tension (*T*)/*r* to counteract inward-directed surface tension forces. Smaller the alveolar size, the higher the pressure that is required to keep it open. Copyright: Satyan Lakshminrusimha.

Clinical scenario 3

A premature female newborn born at 26 weeks GA who is currently 3 days old and was stable on the ventilator until this morning suddenly develops abdominal distension. Her chest X-ray is unchanged since the last film, but an abdominal plain film shows moderate pneumoperitoneum and portal venous air. She has never been fed enterally. While you are considering the diagnosis of spontaneous intestinal perforation (SIP), her nurse informs you that she now has poor chest rise, decreased saturations, and metabolic acidosis. She requires increased mean airway pressure and vasopressors to improve her respiratory and hemodynamic status. What principle of respiratory mechanics could best explain this scenario?

Answer

C_{CW} also forms part of the total respiratory system compliance. Airway pressure (P_{aw}), C_l, and C_{CW} determine P_{pl} according to the following equation:

$$P_{pl} = P_{aw} * (C_l/C_l + C_{CW})$$

Therefore, in situations where P_{aw} is constant but C_{CW} is low and C_l is unchanged, P_{pl} is increased. Since P_{pl} is transmitted to mediastinal structures, this can lead to increased pressure on the right side of the heart, decreased venous return, and metabolic acidosis. At least 50% of intra-abdominal pressure is transmitted upward through the diaphragm to the thorax which can decrease chest wall movement and cause decreased C_{CW} [3,34]. This is most likely the phenomenon that caused poor chest wall movement in the premature infant in this scenario. Infants with abdominal distension and increased intra-abdominal pressure from any cause (common examples include NEC, SIP, postsurgical states after repair of CDH, omphalocele, or gastroschisis) are prone to this issue. Therefore, such infants should be monitored for signs of respiratory and hemodynamic compromise and treated accordingly by increasing P_{aw} and correction of their hemodynamic status if required.

Deficiency of surfactant leading to increased surface tension within the alveoli and the highly pliant chest wall that is unable to prevent the resultant alveolar collapse are the primary causes of the decreased FRC and the resultant RDS that is often seen in prematurely born infants in the first several days after birth [35]. Atelectotrauma (alveolar injury caused by repeated expansion of collapsed alveoli) can inactivate the small volume of surfactant that is available in their lungs [36]. Lung function impairment due to these factors can be attenuated by two major interventions: administration of exogenous surfactant, or the application of continuous positive airway pressure (CPAP) to minimize loss of FRC and to prevent atelectotrauma and surfactant inactivation.

Resistive properties of the respiratory system

Unlike compliance which can be static or dynamic, resistance—which represents the impediment to *airflow* offered by the airways and lungs—is relevant only as a dynamic mechanical property of the respiratory system. When respiratory system resistance (R_{rs}) is increased, the $P_{ao} - P_{al}$ pressure differential needs to be greater to allow airflow into the alveoli. Generation of this increase in pressure differential increases the work of breathing; 80% of R_{rs} in adults is due to the frictional resistance of the airways while lung tissue (viscous) resistance is responsible for the remainder. Due to their thicker alveolar walls, denser pulmonary connective tissue, and increased interstitial and alveolar fluid, viscous resistance is a higher fraction of R_{rs} in the newborn (up to 40%).

In newborn, 60% of R_{rs} resides in the airways. The nasal passages are the major site of airway resistance (R_{aw}) in the newborn (60%). Alae nasal muscle contraction leading to nasal flaring is often seen in infants with respiratory distress who attempt to decrease R_{rs} through this mechanism. Almost all the remainder of R_{aw} is attributable to the glottis (10%) and the proximal generations of the trachea–bronchial tree (20%). Though newborn infants have lower specific resistance (R_{rs}/FRC) when compared to adults, their narrow airways make them prone to significant airflow limitation even with minor airway obstructions. Despite their smaller individual size, the distal and smaller airways have a large total surface area which causes R_{aw} to decrease to negligible levels in these airway generations (10% of R_{aw}) [37].

Airflow through the respiratory tract can be visualized as layers of concentric cylinders that create frictional shear stress as they move past each other at varying velocities. Such flow can be smooth and streamlined (laminar) with reduced friction between the various layers of airflow or more chaotic (turbulent) with increased frictional loss of airflow kinetic energy to heat. The tendency of airflow across the respiratory conduit to be laminar or turbulent depends on several properties—the density (ρ) and viscosity (μ) of the air, the radius of the airway (r), and the velocity of the airflow (v)—that are used to derive the Reynolds' number (Re):

$$Re = 2 \rho r v/\mu$$

Higher Re values (>2000) lead to turbulent airflow, while lower values (<2000) create conditions conducive to laminar flow. Based on these parameters, denser and less viscous gas moving at a faster velocity through a large respiratory tract increases turbulent airflow [24]. Since very low flow velocities are generated in the smaller newborn airway tree, airflow can be (and usually is) laminar in the neonatal airway. However, in addition to increased resistance created by turbulent flow, R_{rs} can also be high even during laminar conditions. Airway resistance to laminar airflow (R) can be derived using Poiseuille's law:

$$R = 8\mu L/\pi r^4$$

According to this law, airflow resistance increases with airway length (L) and air viscosity and decreases with the fourth power of the airway's radius [25]. This relationship between R_{aw} and airway radius is the predominant determinant of impedance to airflow in the respiratory system. Since the neonatal airway is about half the diameter of an adult airway, its resistance is at least 16 times higher (about 19–30 cm H_2O/L/s compared to 1–2 cm H_2O/L/s in the adult) [37]. Airway radius is significantly lowered during mechanical ventilation of the newborn infant since physical constraints make it necessary to use ETTs with very small internal diameters (ID) for these infants. The significant increase in R_{aw} created by ETTs with IDs less than 3.5 mm can cause difficulty in weaning infants from respiratory support. In addition, assessment of spontaneous breathing ability using ETT-CPAP to assess extubation readiness could lead to infants being misclassified as being at risk for failure since they need to work harder to overcome the resistance created by the ETT than they would have to if they were placed on another type of noninvasive support, such as nasal CPAP [38,39].

High flow rates through narrow conduits can lead to turbulent flow that causes increased resistance. This is often noted in premature infants who are intubated with ETTs whose ID is 3.0 mm or less. Flow rates greater than 5 and 10 L/min cause turbulent flow in 2.5 and 3.0 mm ETTs, respectively. The increased resistance created by these high flow rates could also interfere with weaning infants off the respiratory support. Therefore, flow rates should be routinely monitored in infants intubated with tubes smaller than 3.0 mm ID. Since the resistance of the ETT is proportional to its length, cutting long ETTs whose standard length is usually 14.5 cm to a shorter length also decreases resistance in ventilated infants. For example, the standard depth of insertion for a preterm infant who weighs 0.5 kg would be 6.5 cm. Shortening the length of the 14.5 cm ETT to 7 cm would lower the resistance of this ETT by 50%, as the length is reduced by 50% [38].

R_{rs} is also dependent on lung volume and is greater during inspiration than during expiration. This is despite the increased movement of air through the airways during inspiration that proportionally increases resistance by creating conditions that favor turbulent flow. This is also because of the outsized effects of airway radius on laminar flow resistance due to Poiseuille's law. Lung expansion during inspiration increases the support offered by the connective tissue that holds the airways open, increasing their radii and leading to exponentially lowered R_{aw} during inspiration. During expiration the airway radius decreases and the exponential increase in R_{aw} can lead to increased air trapping, a risk that is especially increased in infants with meconium aspiration syndrome (MAS) or chronically intubated infants who are predisposed to excessive mucus plugging of their airways due to reduced mucociliary clearance. In these conditions, increased predisposition to air leak syndromes is often noted when airway resistance is abnormally increased by a ball-valve mechanism that permits air to flow in but not out. Based on similar principles, increasing PEEP can cause alveoli and airways to remain larger in size at end-expiration and lower airway resistance; this has been amply demonstrated in studies of mechanically ventilated infants as well as adults [40,41].

Another strategy to decrease R_{aw} is by reducing the density of the air moving through the respiratory tract. A mixture of helium and oxygen (heliox) which is less dense than air has been shown to cause airflow to be more laminar and reduce R_{aw} in infants with RDS and BPD and shorten the number of days these infants required mechanical ventilation, but no long-term benefits were noted [42].

Respiratory mechanics in disease states

Respiratory mechanics and their implications for several common and important disease states in both term and preterm newborn infants have been the subject of several studies. A summary of their findings is provided in this section (Table 6.1).

Transient tachypnea of the newborn

Successful adaptation to postnatal life requires clearance of excess fluid that fills the alveoli and airways in the first few hours to days after birth. Infants born with immature respiratory epithelial Na^+ transport due to decreased expression of epithelial Na^+ channels often have difficulty in switching their respiratory epithelial function from fluid secretion to fluid reabsorption. This results in fluid-filled alveoli, poor alveolar gas exchange, hypoxemia, tachypnea, and respiratory distress that is usually self-resolved and is referred to as transient tachypnea of the newborn (TTN) [43]. As would be expected with such pathology, these infants have reduced lung compliance and lower tidal volumes. They maintain a near-normal minute ventilation by increasing their respiratory rate. Their respiratory system resistance is similar to that of normal term infants [44,45].

Table 6.1 Lung Mechanics Alterations in Common Neonatal Lung Disorders

Disorder	Compliance	Resistance	Implications
Transient tachypnea of the newborn	Reduced	Normal	Rapid respiratory rate
Meconium aspiration syndrome	Reduced	Increased	Air trapping, air leak syndromes
Respiratory distress syndrome	Reduced	Normal	Rapid respiratory rate, atelectasis
Bronchopulmonary dysplasia	Reduced (often reduced alveolar compliance but increased airway compliance)	Increased	

Meconium aspiration syndrome

Aspiration of large amounts of meconium because of hypoxia-induced intrauterine stress can cause increased R_{aw} during the first 48 h of life. A secondary consequence of airway obstruction in MAS is alveolar atelectasis and decreased lung compliance. Air trapping, which is also a feature of MAS, can lead to regions of overdistended alveoli in the lung. Therefore, lung volume in MAS is variable and lung compliance could be low due to either atelectasis or overdistension. R_{aw} is typically increased significantly which offsets any decrease in lung compliance and causes the expiratory time constant to increase [46]. The infant with MAS is therefore at high risk for alveolar overdistension, "auto"-PEEP, and air leak syndromes secondary to volutrauma. In addition, surfactant administration has been shown to increase $C_{l\text{-dyn}}$, decrease R_{aw}, and reduce mean airway pressures that are required to ventilate these infants, thus improving lung function significantly [47].

Clinical scenario 4

A 6-h old 30-week GA male mechanically ventilated infant is being given surfactant. You are discussing his management at the bedside with the resident on call who tells you that she is aware that the infant could be at risk of a pneumothorax after surfactant therapy and wants to know if there are any warning signs she should look for and if there are interventions that could help minimize this infant's risk. What would your answer be?

Answer

Surfactant administration improves lung compliance which leads to an increased change in lung volume for a given amount of mean airway pressure. Hence, if the mean airway pressure provided to the infant after surfactant administration is left unchanged, lung compliance improvements lead to higher tidal volumes. This can lead to barotrauma, volutrauma, and air leak syndromes in the mechanically

ventilated infant after surfactant administration. Clinically, these changes in lung mechanics can be detected by monitoring the infant for increased chest rise or the ventilator-measured exhaled tidal volume changes. Once these changes are identified, mean airway pressures provided should be reduced to minimize the risk for these complications. In addition, since compliance is increased while resistance is unchanged, expiratory time constant increases after surfactant administration which could lead to air trapping. Thus, reducing I-time and/or respiratory rate, as well as monitoring oxygen saturation changes to promptly decrease the inspired oxygen concentration may become necessary. If volume-targeted ventilation rather than pressure-limited ventilation is used, these manual adjustments may not be required since inspiratory pressure is tailored to achieve tidal volumes and will decrease as compliance improves and the desired tidal volumes can be delivered at lower pressures. However, dynamic PV curves found on most modern ventilators are not useful to monitor changes in lung compliance with surfactant administration because these graphics are reset to zero lung volume at the beginning of each breath and will usually not change shape even if compliance improves [2,3].

Respiratory distress syndrome

Approximately 50% of infants with birth weight less than 1.5 kg develop RDS, depending on their gestational immaturity [48]. RDS is primarily a disease of the distal airspaces and is caused by decreased surfactant secretion by the immature Type II alveolar epithelial cells. Its deficiency leads to decreased lung compliance by increasing the inward recoil force created by intra-alveolar surface tension. This increases the tendency of the alveoli to become atelectatic during expiration and reduces lung FRC.

A study of 20 preterm infants showed that body weight–adjusted lung compliance in these infants soon after birth was 0.40 ± 0.14 mL/cm H_2O/kg, and improved by 45% to 0.58 ± 0.17 mL/cm H_2O/kg within 3 h after surfactant was administered [32]. Changes in lung compliance also correlated significantly with higher pulmonary arterial oxygen content showing that surfactant administration improves ventilation–perfusion matching by allowing atelectatic lung regions to reopen at lower inspiratory pressures. While R_{rs} was found to be unchanged in this study when measured 3 h after the surfactant was given, acute increase in R_{rs} should be expected immediately after administration of a surfactant dose. Therefore, a transient increase in inspiratory time and/or mean airway pressures may be required during this period [1].

Another strategy to increase lung compliance in infants with RDS is by increasing mean airway pressure to shift lung inflation from the lower (flatter) portion of the PV loop to the middle (optimal performance portion). This can be achieved in the spontaneously breathing preterm infant through the application of CPAP or PEEP. The SUPPORT study, a large clinical trial of 1316 infants, compared the effectiveness of early intubation with surfactant delivery to application of CPAP at birth. Infants who received early CPAP needed intubation less frequently and required mechanical ventilation for a shorter duration in the 1st week of life suggesting that CPAP application improved lung mechanics in the short term better than surfactant administration. However, these advantages for early CPAP may not be clinically significant as these two approaches were found to be equally effective in reducing the long-term outcome of death or BPD in these infants [49].

Bronchopulmonary dysplasia

The pathophysiology of BPD has undergone remarkable changes over time in the era of near-universal antenatal maternal steroid and postnatal surfactant administration. Classic BPD was usually noted in infants with high degree of mechanical ventilation and supplemental oxygen requirements and was the result of cystic changes and interstitial fibrosis in large areas of the lungs in affected infants. The newer form of BPD is now often seen in infants who had mild or no requirement for mechanical ventilation in the first several weeks of life. Chest radiography in such infants usually reveals uniformly hazy and low lung volumes reflective of arrested alveolar and vascular development that leads to fewer and larger terminal air spaces [50].

While increased R_{aw} and airflow obstruction was a consistent and persistent feature in the mechanics of lungs of infants with classic BPD, infants with new BPD also show abnormally high R_{rs} at 10 days of life, but then improve with age and normalize their R_{rs} by term GA [51,52]. Low C_{rs} values at 10 days of life in prematurely born infants correlated positively with low forced expiratory airflows indicative of airway obstruction at 2 years of life [52]. This could be because preterm infants are born with low alveolar compliance but high airway compliance [1]. Chronic overdistension of these compliant airways due to the high pressures

required to adequately distend the low-compliance alveoli could cause severe distortion of the airways in these infants, predisposing them to subsequently develop BPD [53].

C_L is low at birth but increases by 0.17 mL/cm H_2O/week in preterm newborn infants beyond 28 weeks GA. By term postmenstrual age, lung compliance in most prematurely born infants reaches mean (SD) values of 2.5 (0.07) mL/cm H_2O [54]. A study of 74 infants that included 23 infants with moderate or severe BPD as well as 12 infants with mild BPD (mean GA of 26 weeks) and 39 infants without BPD who served as controls (mean GA of 31 weeks) found that the former groups had lower FRC and specific C_{rs} on day 3 after birth when compared to the control group. The lowest FRC and specific C_{rs} values were noted in the infants with moderate/severe BPD. Contrary to its hypotheses, the study also found that all infant groups continued to increase their FRC and compliance, with the highest increase compared to baseline values noted in the moderate/severe BPD group. Thus, infants who later develop BPD had severe lung functional abnormalities in their early postnatal life [55]. Other studies have also shown reduced FRC and C_{rs} at 14 and 28 days of life for infants who later develop BPD when compared to gender and GA matched controls without BPD [56]. This evidence suggests that studies of lung function could help identify in early identification and risk stratification of infants at highest risk for BPD.

Infants with BPD have low FRC at birth, but this lung capacity as well as C_{rs} tend to normalize during their infancy and are close to values obtained from normal term infants by 2 years of age [57]. However, they develop airway abnormalities that increase R_{aw} especially during expiration, in their smaller peripheral airways which then continue to be persistent into early infancy and later childhood years. Spirometric measurements from 28 infants with a history of BPD (GA 26.4 ± 2.1 weeks, mean ± SD) at 68.0 ± 35.6 weeks postnatal age showed that when compared to term infants without respiratory disease they had decreased forced expiratory volume in 0.5 s (FEV$_{0.5}$; 76.3 ± 19.6%), forced expiratory flow at 75% of expired forced vital capacity (FEF75; 59.5 ± 30.7%), and FEF(25–75) (74.0 ± 26.8%) along with increased FRC (107.9 ± 25.3%), residual volume (RV, 124.5 ± 42.7%), and RV/total lung capacity (RV/TLC, 128.2 ± 35.3%) indicative of increased air trapping in these infants at almost 2 years postnatal age [58]. FEF at 25% of forced vital capacity (FEF$_{25-75}$) was reduced in ex-preterm young adolescents born and this decrease was noted in those with previous history of BPD as well as those without this diagnosis (Anand et al 2003) [59].

Finally, the widely used NICHD BPD definitions use the degree of oxygenation impairment and need for supplemental oxygen to classify the severity of lung function impairment seen in infants, reflecting the importance of poor early developmental alveolarization in the pathogenesis of this disease. However, the role played by airway abnormalities in causing respiratory symptoms has been poorly recognized until recently. A study of 55 infants of GA between 23 and 30 weeks measured their lung function at 6 and 18 months postnatal age. When compared to published normative data, infants with BPD had lower maximal flow at functional capacity (V'_{max}FRC), $FEV_{0.5}$ and mid-expiratory flow (MEF_{50}) at 6 months and lower $FEV_{0.5}$ and MEF_{50} at 18 months. While there were differences in these measures between infants who had respiratory symptoms versus those who did not, there were no differences in these airflow obstruction indicators between infants diagnosed with mild BPD and those with moderate or severe [60]. In addition, a recent meta-analysis found decreased FEV_1 even in preterm infants without a diagnosis of BPD (−7.2%) as well as more severe reductions in infants with BPD at 36 weeks PMA (−19%) when compared to term controls [61]. This evidence suggests that early life diagnosis and classification of BPD severity may not carry prognostic importance in predicting risk for later-life obstructive lung disease in prematurely born infants. Every infant who is born prematurely is potentially at risk for later-life lung impairment and should be monitored for symptoms, such as wheezing with early assessments of airway obstruction by tests, such as spirometry to optimize care.

Clinical scenario 5

On morning rounds, you are asked to help with ventilator settings for two intubated patients: a 4-day-old infant with RDS and a 6-month old with BPD both of whom have had a poor clinical course during the night with hypoxia and

hypercarbia noted on their AM blood gases. How would you make use of the differences between their respiratory mechanics to help you choose appropriate settings on the ventilator for each of these infants?

Answer

Young preterm infants with RDS (and TTN) have decreased lung compliance but low-normal airway resistance. Their time constants are therefore very short. Typical compliance and resistance values in intubated preterm infants with RDS are 0.0006 L/cm H_2O and 50 cm H_2O/L/s, respectively, giving these infants an average expiratory time constant of 0.03 s. This implies that their alveoli can be emptied and filled to near-completion in 0.15–0.2 s. These mechanical properties of their respiratory system allow the clinician to use faster rates by using short I-times while also allowing expiration to be fully complete before the next breath begins. A typical lung-protective ventilation strategy for these infants would be to use low pressure, low tidal volume, and high rates with short I-times. Their short time constants also make these infants well-suited for high-frequency ventilation strategies [62]. Older infants with BPD (and younger infants with MAS) have poor lung compliance and high airway resistance. Typical values for these parameters are 0.001 L/cm H_2O and 150 cm H_2O/L/s for infants with BPD, giving them longer time constant of 0.15 s compared to infants with RDS. Due to this, these infants often have difficulty in completing expiration when they are ventilated with fast rates. An ideal strategy to minimize the risk for hypercarbia in these infants would be to use slow rates with longer breaths and expiratory times that are adequate to allow their lungs to empty completely and to minimize the risk for air trapping [63].

References

[1] Mortola JP. The neonatal neuromechanical unit: generalities of operation. In: Rimensberger PC, editor. Pediatric and neonatal mechanical ventilation: from basics to clinical practice. Berlin, Heidelberg: Springer; 2015. p. 27–42.

[2] Couser RJ, Ferrara TB, Ebert J, Hoekstra RE, Fangman JJ. Effects of exogenous surfactant therapy on dynamic compliance during mechanical breathing in preterm infants with hyaline membrane disease. J Pediatr 1990;116(1):119–124.

[3] Dimitriou G, Greenough A, Laubscher B. Appropriate positive end expiratory pressure level in surfactant-treated

preterm infants. Eur J Pediatr 1999;158(11):888–891.

[4] Traeger N, Panitch HB. Tests of respiratory muscle strength in neonates. NeoReviews 2004;5(5):e208.

[5] West JB. A web-based course of lectures in respiratory physiology. Adv Physiol Educ 2011;35(3):249–251.

[6] Lanteri CJ, Petak F, Gurrin L, Sly PD. Influence of inertance on respiratory mechanics measurements in mechanically ventilated puppies. Pediatr Pulmonol 1999;28(2):130–138.

[7] Bates JHT. Lung mechanics: an inverse modeling approach. 1st ed. New York, NY: Cambridge University Press; 2009.

[8] Melo e Silva CA, Ventura CEGdS. A simple model illustrating the

respiratory system's time constant concept. Adv Physiol Educ 2006;30(3):129.

[9] Mortola JP. Respiratory physiology of newborn mammals: a comparative perspective. Baltimore: The Johns Hopkins University Press; 2001.

[10] Kurzner SI, Garg M, Bautista DB, Sargent CW, Bowman CM, Keens TG. Growth failure in bronchopulmonary dysplasia: elevated metabolic rates and pulmonary mechanics. J Pediatr 1988;112(1):73–80.

[11] Mortola JP. Some functional mechanical implications of the structural design of the respiratory system in newborn mammals. Am Rev Respir Dis 1983;128(2 Pt. 2):S69–S72.

[12] Gagliardi L, Rusconi F. Respiratory rate and body mass in the first three years of life. Arch Dis Child 1997;76(2):151.

[13] The chest wall and the respiratory pump. In: Wilson TA, editor. Respiratory mechanics. Cham: Springer International Publishing; 2016. p. 19–42.

[14] Mead J. Functional significance of the area of apposition of diaphragm to rib cage. Am Rev Respir Dis 1979;119(2 Pt. 2):31–32.

[15] Gaultier C. Respiratory muscle function in infants. Eur Respir J 1995;8(1):150–153.

[16] Rehan VK, Laiprasert J, Wallach M, Rubin LP, McCool FD. Diaphragm dimensions of the healthy preterm infant. Pediatrics 2001;108(5):E91.

[17] Mantilla CB, Sieck GC. Key aspects of phrenic motoneuron and diaphragm muscle development during the perinatal period. J Appl Physiol 2008;104(6):1818–1827.

[18] De Troyer A, Kirkwood PA, Wilson TA. Respiratory action of the intercostal muscles. Physiol Rev 2005;85(2):717.

[19] Muller NL, Bryan AC. Chest wall mechanics and respiratory muscles in infants. Pediatr Clin North Am 1979;26(3):503–516.

[20] Vassilakopoulos T. Control of ventilation and respiratory muscles. In: Spiro SG, Silvestri GA, Agustí A, editors. Clinical respiratory medicine. 4th ed. Philadelphia, PA: W.B. Saunders; 2012. p. 50–62. [chapter 6].

[21] Weaver AA, Schoell SL, Stitzel JD. Morphometric analysis of variation in the ribs with age and sex. J Anat 2014;225(2):246–261.

[22] Papastamelos C, Panitch HB, England SE, Allen JL. Developmental changes in chest wall compliance in infancy and early childhood. J Appl Physiol 1995;78(1):179.

[23] Vendettuoli V, Veneroni C, Zannin E, Mercadante D, Matassa P, Pedotti A, et al. Positional effects on lung mechanics of ventilated preterm infants with acute and chronic lung disease. Pediatr Pulmonol 2015;50(8):798–804.

[24] West JB. Respiratory physiology: the essentials. Philadelphia, PA: Lippincott Williams & Wilkins; 2005.

[25] Levitzky MG. Mechanics of breathing. 8th ed. Pulmonary physiology. New York, NY: The McGraw-Hill Companies; 2013. [chapter 2].

[26] Kano S, Lanteri CJ, Duncan AW, Sly PD. Influence of nonlinearities on estimates of respiratory mechanics

using multilinear regression analysis. J Appl Physiol 1994;77(3):1185–1197.

[27] Airen M, Panitch HB. Infant pulmonary mechanics during tidal breathing. NeoReviews 2004;5(5):e194.

[28] Escolar JD, Escolar A. Lung hysteresis: a morphological view. Histol Histopathol 2004;19(1):159–166.

[29] Hutten GJ, van Eykern LA, Latzin P, Thamrin C, van Aalderen WM, Frey U. Respiratory muscle activity related to flow and lung volume in preterm infants compared with term infants. Pediatr Res 2010;68(4):339–343.

[30] Neumann RP, von Ungern-Sternberg BS. The neonatal lung: physiology and ventilation. Paediatr Anaesth 2014;24(1):10–21.

[31] Eber E, Midulla F. ERS handbook of paediatric respiratory medicine. Lausanne: European Respiratory Society; 2013.

[32] Baraldi E, Pettenazzo A, Filippone M, Magagnin GP, Saia OS, Zacchello F. Rapid improvement of static compliance after surfactant treatment in preterm infants with respiratory distress syndrome. Pediatr Pulmonol 1993;15(3):157–162.

[33] Zeltner TB, Burri PH. The postnatal development and growth of the human lung. II. Morphology. Respir Physiol 1987;67(3):269–282.

[34] Wauters J, Claus P, Brosens N, McLaughlin M, Hermans G, Malbrain M, et al. Relationship between abdominal pressure, pulmonary compliance, and cardiac preload in a porcine model. Crit Care Res Pract 2012;2012:6.

[35] Sardesai S, Biniwale M, Wertheimer F, Garingo A, Ramanathan R. Evolution of surfactant therapy for respiratory distress syndrome: past, present, and future. Pediatr Res 2017;81(1–2):240–248.

[36] Veldhuizen RA, Tremblay LN, Govindarajan A, van Rozendaal BA, Haagsman HP, Slutsky AS. Pulmonary surfactant is altered during mechanical ventilation of isolated rat lung. Crit Care Med 2000;28(7):2545–2551.

[37] Bielsky MD, Alan R. A practice of anesthesia for infants and children. 4th ed. Anesthesiology, vol. 112. p. 256–257.

[38] Keszler M, Abubakar K. Physiologic principles. 6th ed. Assisted ventilation of the neonate. Philadelphia, PA: Elsevier; 2017. p. 8.e33–30.e33 [chapter 2].

[39] Davis PG, Henderson-Smart DJ. Extubation from low-rate

intermittent positive airway pressure versus extubation after a trial of endotracheal continuous positive airway pressure in intubated preterm infants. Cochrane Database Syst Rev 2001;4:CD001078.

[40] de Waal KA, Evans N, Osborn DA, Kluckow M. Cardiorespiratory effects of changes in end expiratory pressure in ventilated newborns. Arch Dis Child Fetal Neonatal Ed 2007;92(6):F444–F448.

[41] Guerin C, Fournier G, Milic-Emili J. Effects of PEEP on inspiratory resistance in mechanically ventilated COPD patients. Eur Respir J 2001;18(3):491–498.

[42] Colnaghi M, Pierro M, Migliori C, Ciralli F, Matassa PG, Vendettuoli V, et al. Nasal continuous positive airway pressure with heliox in preterm infants with respiratory distress syndrome. Pediatrics 2012;129(2):e333–e338.

[43] Guglani L, Lakshminrusimha S, Ryan RM. Transient tachypnea of the newborn. Pediatr. Rev 2008;29(11):e59.

[44] Benito Zaballos MF, Pedraz Garcia C, Salazar V, Villalobos A. Pulmonary function in newborn infants with transitory tachypnea and pneumothorax. An Esp Pediatr 1989;31(3):210–215.

[45] Helve O, Andersson S, Kirjavainen T, Pitkänen OM. Improvement of lung compliance during postnatal adaptation correlates with airway sodium transport. Am J Respir Crit Care Med 2006;173(4):448–452.

[46] Yeh TF, Lilien LD, Barathi A, Pildes RS. Lung volume, dynamic lung compliance, and blood gases during the first 3 days of postnatal life in infants with meconium aspiration syndrome. Crit Care Med 1982;10(9):588–592.

[47] Szymankiewicz M, Gadzinowski J, Kowalska K. Pulmonary function after surfactant lung lavage followed by surfactant administration in infants with severe meconium aspiration syndrome. J Matern Fetal Neonatal Med 2004;16(2):125–130.

[48] Hintz SR, Van Meurs KP, Perritt R, Poole WK, Das A, Stevenson DK, et al. Neurodevelopmental outcomes of premature infants with severe respiratory failure enrolled in a randomized controlled trial of inhaled nitric oxide. J Pediatr 2007;151(1):16–22. 22.e11–13.

[49] Carlo WA, Finer NN, Walsh MC, Rich W, Gantz MG, SUPPORT Study Group of the Eunice Kennedy Shriver NICHD Neonatal Research Network. et al. Target ranges of oxygen saturation in extremely preterm infants. N Engl J Med 2010;362(21):1959–1969.

[50] Jobe AH. The new BPD. NeoReviews 2006;7(10):e531.

[51] Greenough A, Pahuja A. Updates on functional characterization of bronchopulmonary dysplasia: the contribution of lung function testing. Front Med 2015;2:35.

[52] Baraldi E, Filippone M, Trevisanuto D, Zanardo V, Zacchello F. Pulmonary function until two years of life in infants with bronchopulmonary dysplasia. Am J Respir Crit Care Med 1997;155(1):149–155.

[53] Mello RR, Silva KS, Costa AM, Ramos JR. Longitudinal assessment of the lung mechanics of very low birth weight preterm infants with and without bronchopulmonary dysplasia. Sao Paulo Med J 2015;133(5):401–407.

[54] Bhutani VK, Bowen FW, Sivieri EM. Postnatal changes in pulmonary mechanics and energetics of infants with respiratory distress syndrome following surfactant treatment. Biol Neonate 2005;87(4):323–331.

[55] May C, Kennedy C, Milner AD, Rafferty GF, Peacock JL, Greenough A. Lung function abnormalities in infants developing bronchopulmonary dysplasia. Arch Dis Child 2011;96(11):1014.

[56] Kavvadia V, Greenough A, Itakura Y, Dimitriou G. Neonatal lung function in very immature infants with and without RDS. J Perinat Med 1999;27(5):382–387.

[57] Fakhoury KF, Sellers C, Smith EO, Rama JA, Fan LL. Serial measurements of lung function in a cohort of young children with bronchopulmonary dysplasia. Pediatrics 2010;125(6):e1441.

[58] Robin B, Kim YJ, Huth J, Klocksieben J, Torres M, Tepper RS, et al. Pulmonary function in bronchopulmonary dysplasia. Pediatr Pulmonol 2004;37(3):236–242.

[59] Anand D, Stevenson CJ, West CR, Pharoah POD. Lung function and respiratory health in adolescents of very low birth weight. Arch Dis Child 2003;88(2):135.

[60] Thunqvist P, Gustafsson P, Norman M, Wickman M, Hallberg J. Lung function at 6 and 18 months after preterm birth in relation to severity of bronchopulmonary dysplasia. Pediatr Pulmonol 2015;50(10):978–986.

[61] Kotecha SJ, Edwards MO, Watkins WJ, Henderson AJ, Paranjothy S, Dunstan FD, et al. Effect of preterm birth on later FEV1: a systematic review and meta-analysis. Thorax 2013;68(8):760–766.

[62] Fanaroff AA, Fanaroff JM, Klaus MH. Klaus and Fanaroff's Care of the High-Risk Neonate. 6th ed. Philadelphia, PA: Elsevier/Saunders; 2013.

[63] Sivieri EM, Bhutani VK. Pulmonary mechanics. In: Sinha SK, Donn SM, editors. Manual of neonatal respiratory care. 2nd ed. Philadelphia, PA: Mosby; 2006. p. 50–60. [chapter 7].

Chapter | 7 |

Genesis of Lung Injury

Mitali Sahni, MD, Vineet Bhandari, MD, DM

CHAPTER POINTS

- The pathogenesis of "new" BPD is secondary to gene-environmental interactions; the latter includes pre- and/or post-natal factors
- The major environmental factors contributing to lung injury are invasive mechanical ventilation, hyperoxia, and sepsis (chorioamnionitis, local and systemic early- and late-onset neonatal sepsis)
- Avoiding intubation or early extubation, minimizing hyperoxia exposure, prevention of infection and adequate nutrition are ways to prevent/decrease lung injury

Introduction

Northway et al. first used the term "bronchopulmonary dysplasia" (BPD) to describe a chronic form of neonatal lung injury associated with barotrauma in preterm infants [1].

Although there has been significant advancement in this field over the last couple of decades including sophisticated, newer and gentler methods of mechanical ventilation (MV), surfactant replacement therapy, and so on, the prevalence of BPD remains quite high. Ventilator-associated lung injury is a recurring problem in neonatal intensive care units (NICUs) and continues to occur at an unacceptably high rate. Among the various factors leading to BPD, it has been well established that prolonged MV can injure the lungs, causing ventilator-induced lung injury (VILI). VILI is multifactorial and there are various forms of injury that contribute to the final common pathway causing BPD [2]. Barotrauma, or excessive pressure, may damage airway epithelium and disrupt alveoli. Volutrauma refers to the injury caused by overdistention of the lungs. Atelectotrauma is a term used to describe the injury due to repeated opening and closing of the smaller lung units/alveoli. Biotrauma is the lung injury caused or aggravated by the release of inflammatory mediators [3]. This chapter will focus on the factors involved in the pathogenesis of lung injury, including the various forms of VILI, in preterm neonates.

Old versus new BPD

Classical or old BPD, present in the presurfactant era, was a sequela of respiratory distress syndrome treated with high oxygen, barotrauma, and volutrauma. It involved an evolution of injury and repair that started with an exudative and early reparative stage and progressed through a subacute fibroproliferative stage to a chronic fibroproliferative stage [1]. By early 1990s, exogenous surfactant replacement had become a common practice and was followed by the use of antenatal steroids in preterm labor. These new practices combined with improved ventilation strategies and better nutrition, allowed survival of more very low birth weight (VLBW) infants with lungs in the late canalicular/early saccular stages [4]. Jobe coined the term "new BPD" in 1999 to refer to the chronic lung disease of preterm infants at that time [5]. This "new BPD" demonstrated much less alveolar septal fibrosis and airway damage when compared to its old counterpart, and was characterized by alveolar simplification and dysmorphic microvasculature [6]. Other findings reported include bronchial and bronchiolar smooth muscle hyperplasia as well as altered number of neuroendocrine cells [4]. Fig. 7.1 shows the differences in lung morphology in "old" and "new" BPD.

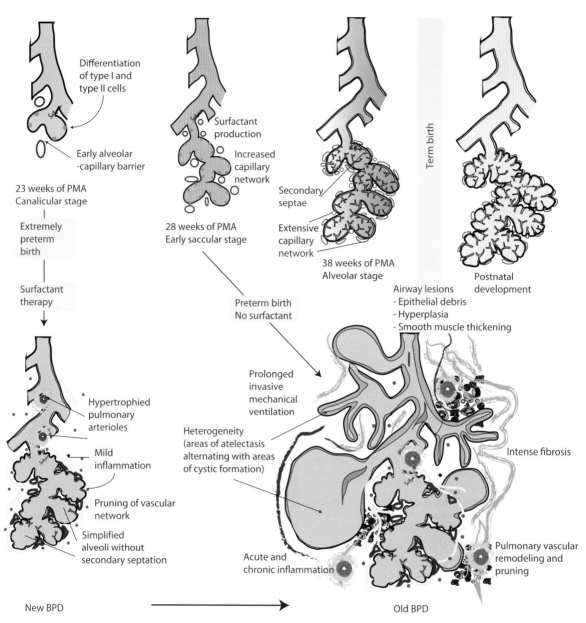

Fig. 7.1 Changes in Lung Morphology With Gestation and "Old" and "New" Bronchopulmonary Dysplasia (BPD). The normal fetal lung is in the canalicular stage between 16 and 27 weeks of PMA. This stage is characterized by differentiation of type I and type II cells and establishment of an early alveolar–capillary barrier. The fetal lung progresses into the saccular stage at 27–36 weeks of PMA and is associated with surfactant production and increased capillary network. Extreme preterm birth at 23–25 weeks of gestation during the canalicular stage requiring surfactant therapy, associated with mild inflammation, can lead to "new" BPD. "New" BPD is associated with simplified alveoli without secondary septation and pruning of vascular network. Preterm birth during early saccular stage followed by prolonged mechanical ventilation without surfactant leads to "old" BPD. "Old" BPD is associated with airway lesions associated with epithelial debris, intense fibrosis, and areas of atelectasis alternating with cyst formation. Copyright: Satyan Lakshminrusimha.

Factors involved in pathogenesis of lung injury

The pathogenesis of "new" BPD involves various genetic and environmental factors, which—when they act on the immature preterm lung—lead to persistent inflammation and lung remodeling. The factors involved in the evolution of "new" BPD are listed in Table 7.1. Multiple recent studies have focused on the role of inflammatory mediators and immune dysregulation in BPD. Increased levels of proinflammatory mediators present in amniotic fluid, tracheal aspirates, lung tissue, and serum of premature infants at risk for BPD support their role in the development of "new" BPD [7]. Fig. 7.2 demonstrates the pathogenesis of "new" BPD.

Table 7.1 Factors involved in the pathogenesis of lung injury in "new" BPD

Prenatal factors

- Pregnancy-induced hypertension
- Hypoxia
- Infection including chorioamnionitis
- Smoking
- Lack of antenatal steroids
- Genetic susceptibility
- Congenital anomalies causing pulmonary hypoplasia

Postnatal factors

- Lung immaturity
- Oxygen injury
- Mechanical ventilation
- Infection/Sepsis
- Corticosteroids
- Inadequate nutrition

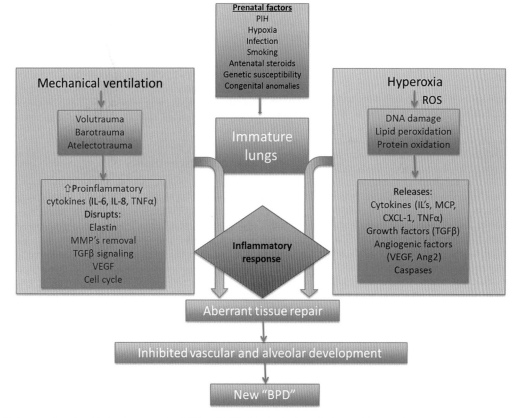

Fig. 7.2 Factors Involved in Pathogenesis of "New" BPD. Mechanical ventilation and hyperoxia act on premature lungs in the presence of prenatal factors predisposing to BPD, leading to exaggerated inflammatory response with aberrant tissue repair causing BPD. See text for details. *Ang 2*, Angiopoietin 2; *CXCL-1*, chemokine (C-X-C motif) ligand 1; *IL*, interleukin; *MCP*, monocyte chemoattractant protein; *MMP*, matrix metalloproteinase; *PIH*, pregnancy-induced hypertension; *ROS*, reactive oxygen species; *TGF*, transforming growth factor; *TNF*, tumor necrosis factor; *VEGF*, vascular endothelial growth factor.

Prenatal factors

Pregnancy-induced hypertension

Multiple studies have found preeclampsia (PE) or pregnancy-induced hypertension (PIH) to be associated with increased risk of BPD. In a large observational cohort study including 106,339 preterm infants, PE was the strongest risk factor for BPD (ajusted odds ratio [OR] 2.04, 95% confidence interval [CI]: 1.83–2.29) [8]. Another systematic review which included 15 studies also identified hypertensive disorders in pregnancy to be associated with increased risk of BPD (P = 0.01; OR = 1.59, 95% CI = 1.11–2.26) [9]. However, in another study, PE did not significantly affect the risk of BPD in extremely preterm (EP) or extremely LBW (ELBW) subjects [10], and hence this association is still considered controversial.

Hypoxia

In animal studies, mice exposed to prenatal hypoxia and postnatal hyperoxia developed intrauterine growth restriction due to prenatal hypoxia, which had an amplification effect on the lung pathology. This model is closer to the clinical events corresponding to the development of the so-called "new" BPD [11,12].

Infection

Chorioamnionitis (CA) is an inflammatory condition of the placenta that occurs in response to microbial invasion or pathological processes and causes subsequent induction of preterm labor. Increased concentrations of proinflammatory cytokines in human amniotic fluid and fetal cord blood have been shown to be independent risk factors for BPD [13]. A meta-analysis of 59 studies, involving 15,000 infants, confirmed an association between histologic CA and development of BPD [14]. However, the Alabama Preterm Birth Study found no association between BPD and CA, but in the same study, umbilical cord blood culture positive for *Ureaplasma* spp. was associated with increased risk for BPD [15]. A nested case control study found a protective effect of CA in the absence of postnatal sepsis and prolonged ventilation, but demonstrated an increased risk for BPD in infants exposed to histologic CA along with mechanical ventilation and postnatal sepsis [16]. Lastly, a cohort study involving preterm infants <32 weeks of gestation concluded that in these infants exposed to histologic CA there was a decreased response to surfactant replacement therapy and a need for prolonged ventilation which led to increased risk for BPD [17]. Hence, we can conclude that CA clearly increases risk for premature preterm birth, which in turn is one of the most important risk factors for the development of BPD. In addition, CA likely induces a chronic inflammatory process that predisposes the lung to postnatal injuries [13]. Fig. 7.3 demonstrates the relationship between CA and BPD.

Maternal smoking

A case control study investigating VLBW infants proposed intrauterine smoke exposure to be an independent risk factor for the development of BPD [18]. These findings were further confirmed in a multicenter study, which evaluated the influence of smoking and alcohol during pregnancy on the outcome of VLBW infants. They concluded that smoking during pregnancy results in a high rate of growth-restricted VLBW infants along with increased postnatal complications including BPD [19].

Antenatal steroids

Antenatal steroids are known to be associated with a decrease in severity of respiratory distress syndrome and neonatal mortality, and hence they were initially expected to decrease the risk of BPD [20]. In a Cochrane analysis that included 818 infants from 6 studies, the risk of BPD (defined as oxygen supplementation at 36 weeks of postmenstrual age or PMA) was not significantly different between infants who were exposed to antenatal steroids as compared to controls (relative risk [RR] 0.86, 95% CI: 0.61–1.22) [21]. Overall, these studies suggest that antenatal steroid exposure does not modify the risk of BPD; however, this may be due to an increase in survival of the more immature antenatal steroid-exposed infants [22].

Genetic susceptibility

Comparison studies among monozygotic and dizygotic premature twins have shown that genetic factors accounted for 53%–82% variance in liability for BPD [23,24]. Since the publication of these 2 studies, over 65 genetic associations have been implicated in candidate gene association studies [25]. Most of these genes are implicated in inflammation and antioxidant responses [25]. Genetic variations in SPOCK2, Toll-like receptors 4 and 5, interleukin-18 (IL-18), macrophage migration inhibitory factor (MIF), surfactant proteins, and vascular endothelial growth factor (VEGF), among others, have been suspected as playing a role in the development of BPD [25].

Congenital anomalies

Survival at birth is dependent on adequate development and maturation of the lung *in utero*. The disruption of alveolarization in preterm birth causes BPD. Abnormal bronchopulmonary development, resulting in congenital lung malformations, and inadequate development are thought to contribute to BPD [26].

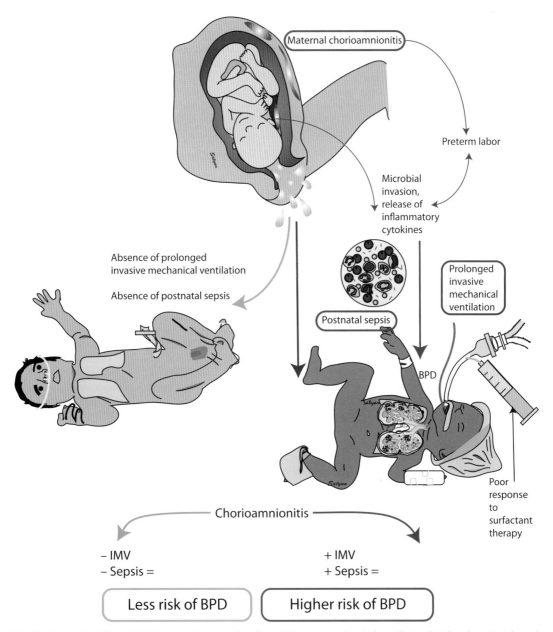

Fig. 7.3 Chorioamnionitis and BPD. In the absence of prolonged invasive mechanical ventilation (IMV) and postnatal sepsis, maternal chorioamnionitis is associated with less risk of BPD *(green arrows)*. In contrast, maternal chorioamnionitis associated with prolonged invasive mechanical ventilation and/or postnatal sepsis can lead to microbial invasion and release of inflammatory cytokines resulting in a higher risk of BPD *(red arrows)*. See text for details. Copyright: Satyan Lakshminrusimha.

Postnatal factors

Lung immaturity

Neonates predisposed to develop BPD are born premature and their lungs are either in the late canalicular (characterized by formation of primitive alveoli, differentiation of type I and type II pneumocytes, and formation of alveolar–capillary barrier) or in early saccular (initiation of surfactant production, enlargement of terminal airways, pulmonary vascularization) stages of development [27].

Alveolar sacs are formed by secondary septation of alveolar ducts. With preterm birth, this programed development is disrupted, and in the setting of inflammation, alveolarization is impaired leading to BPD [28]. Recent studies show that telomere length in circulating leukocytes or salivary cells in young adults born preterm is shorter than in young adults born at term [29,30]. This accelerated attrition of telomeres, which is one of the major causes of premature aging, may also be associated with the development and progression of chronic lung disease in preterm infants.

Hyperoxia/Oxygen-related injury

Acute pulmonary injury secondary to hyperoxia is characterized by an inflammatory response with destruction of the alveolar–capillary barrier, vascular leak, influx of inflammatory mediators, and pulmonary edema, ultimately followed by cell death [31]. In a neonatal mouse model of BPD, exposure to hyperoxia in the critical saccular stage of lung development replicates the changes seen in human BPD and these effects are dose-dependent on the fraction of inspired oxygen (FiO_2) concentration that was administered [32].

Based on animal studies, it has been postulated that when the preterm lung is exposed to hyperoxia, there is release of vascular mediators like VEGF and angiopoietin 2 (Ang2) that disrupt the alveolar–capillary membrane leading to pulmonary edema which contributes to lung injury [33,34]. VEGF is present in high amounts in lungs and promotes endothelial cell growth and remodeling [34]. Ang2 is an angiogenic growth factor that is known to destabilize blood vessels, enhance vascular leak, and induce vascular regression and endothelial cell apoptosis [33]. Other cytokines including IL-1, IL-6, IL-18, transforming factor beta (TGF-β), tumor necrosis factor alpha (TNFα), and VEGF are also released from lung cells that attract inflammatory cells to the lung [32]. These proinflammatory cytokines invoke significant damage to the capillary endothelium and the alveolar epithelium, resulting in hyaline membrane formation and leakage of protein-rich edema fluid into the alveoli [35].

Inflammatory cells as well as hyperoxia per se release reactive oxygen species (ROS). ROS is also known to be generated during normal mitochondrial respiration, the reperfusion of hypoxic tissue, and in association with inflammation and infection [36]. It is involved in many intracellular signaling pathways, including those important for normal cell growth and differentiation, as well as inflammatory responses during host defense. However, when the production of ROS exceeds the antioxidant capacity of the cell, oxidative stress follows, leading to cellular and tissue injury via lipid peroxidation, DNA damage, and protein oxidation [37]. These ROS further cause cell death by activation of key caspases and triggering surface

death receptors like Fas in the extrinsic pathway or via the mitochondrial cell death pathway in which Bax proteins interact with or form mitochondrial pores, release cytochrome *c*, activate caspase-9, and induce cell death [32]. This injurious process caused by hyperoxia, with a simultaneous attempt at repair, mediated via a variety of factors, results in lung pathology that culminates with the characteristic features of BPD in preterm infants.

Mechanical ventilation-related lung injury

In preterm infants, the need for intubation and MV is associated with ventilator-induced lung injuries and subsequent development of BPD. Lung injury from MV results due to volutrauma, barotrauma, or atelectotrauma [38]. The various elements involved in the genesis of lung injury in the setting of mechanical ventilation are described as follows:

1. *Susceptibility due to immature lungs*: Immature lungs are characterized by reduced amount of collagen and elastin as compared to mature lungs. Premature infants are most vulnerable to VILI in the period immediately following birth because their lungs are partially filled with fluid; they are not uniformly ventilated, and have reduced functional residual capacity (FRC) due to surfactant deficiency. As sacculi formation, mesenchymal thinning, and surfactant synthesis by type II cells occur late in pregnancy, any damage that occurs in the early stages of lung growth might affect those phenomena, resulting in long-lasting consequences [39].

2. *Barotrauma*: This is referred to the injury caused by high pressures used in ventilation. Exposure to pressure increases the risk of air leak syndromes, such as interstitial emphysema, pneumothorax, and pneumomediastinum, which in turn activate the inflammatory cascade [39]. In newborn infants, MV is usually time-cycled and pressure-limited, but the volume of gas supplied to the lungs is not controlled. However, some studies conducted with animals showed that lung injury is caused by changes in lung volume rather than by the pressure generated inside the airways [40].

3. *Volutrauma*: Volutrauma refers to the lung injury caused when the lungs are inflated to a volume larger than the total lung capacity during ventilation and resuscitation [39]. In premature infants, alveolar atelectasis and edema decrease the aerated lung capacity. The distribution of the underlying pathology is such that only a small portion of the lung is available for ventilation. If only a third of the lung is available for ventilation, then for a tidal volume of 10 mL/kg, the ventilated portion of the lung is stretched to an extent equivalent to 30 mL/kg in a healthy lung leading to regional overdistension [40]. Because of

the structural damage caused by stretching, there is migration of leukocytes to the lungs, increase in capillary permeability in the lungs, and interstitial and alveolar edema. On exposure to high-tidal volumes, overdistention of lungs leads to the production of proinflammatory cytokines, for example, IL-6, IL-8, and TNFα and reduced expression of anti-inflammatory cytokines such as IL-10 [38]. In a rat model of BPD, ventilation with high-tidal volume upregulated connective tissue growth factor (CTGF) expression (which inhibits branching morphogenesis), increased IL-6 mRNA, and upregulated the TGF-β signaling molecule [41].

Even ventilation with low-tidal volumes is also deleterious because stretch injury can occur with it by overdistention of partially collapsed lungs. In another study done on an 8-day-old neonatal rat model, high-, moderate-, and low-volume ventilation significantly elevated CXCL-2 and IL-6 mRNA levels. In the same study, high- and moderate-volume ventilation also increased IL-1β and CXCL-1 content [42]. Sustained lung inflation has been shown to increase levels of proinflammatory cytokines and cause BPD-like changes in the lungs of preterm lambs [43]. In newborn infants, an overdistention injury may occur even just after a few inflations with high-tidal volume and after periods as short as 30 min, which indicates the importance of performing resuscitation in the delivery room with appropriate positive end-expiratory pressure (PEEP) [44].

4. *Atelectotrauma*: In surfactant-deficient premature lungs, the alveolar units are prone to collapse, causing a cycle of recruitment and subsequent derecruitment of these units with each breath that causes lung injury [45]. This mechanism of injury explains the observation that recruitment of lung volumes to increase FRC protects against ventilator-induced lung injury and also reduces the need for high levels of inspired oxygen [46]. In premature lungs that have low FRC and are more prone to atelectasis, ventilation at low lung volumes causes release of cytokines along with accumulation and activation of peripheral leukocytes in the lungs [47].

5. *Biotrauma/Inflammation-related injury*: Biotrauma is a collective term used to describe the injurious effects of infection and inflammation (and oxidative stress) on the developing lung. Cytokines are small-secreted proteins that can act as inflammatory mediators, induce the release of other inflammatory mediators, recruit neutrophils, and increase vascular permeability. We have described above the inflammation caused secondary to volutrauma; however, there are other inflammatory mediators that are involved in the pathogenesis of BPD that are released due to a combination of different modes of lung injury. Studies

conducted in 2–6-day-old mice, which were ventilated for 8–24 h with room air or 40% O_2, revealed increased and dysregulated elastin assembly along with increase in lung cell apoptosis [48]. In an ovine model of BPD, lung tissue harvested from preterm lambs showed reduced expression of growth factors that regulate lung septation (VEGF-A and platelet-derived growth factor-A or PDGF-A and their receptors VEGF-R2 and PDGF-Rα) and increased lung expression of growth factors that regulate elastin production (TGF-α and TGF-β1) when compared to the lung protein levels in unventilated control lambs that were studied at the same postconceptional age [49].

In the preterm ventilated baboon model of BPD, alveolar hypoplasia and dysmorphic vasculature were noted to be similar to that seen in human BPD. This model also supported the role of inflammation by showing elevations of TNF-α, IL-6, IL-8 levels, but not of IL-1β and IL-10 [50]. In other studies on this model, increased matrix metalloproteinase-9 (MMP-9) levels were associated with lung inflammation and edema and alterations in VEGF were seen [51,52].

6. *Protective effect of noninvasive ventilation*: Previous studies using a chronically ventilated (3–4 weeks) preterm lamb model of BPD showed nonuniform inflation patterns and impaired alveolar formation with an abnormal abundance of elastin and inflammatory cells [53]. In the same model, reduced lung expression of growth factors that regulate alveolarization and differential alteration of matrix proteins that regulate elastin assembly were also demonstrated [49]. A noninvasive (nasal) ventilation approach preserved alveolar architecture [54] and had a positive effect on parathyroid hormone-related protein-peroxisome proliferator-activated receptor-gamma (PTHrP-PPARγ)-driven alveolar homeostatic epithelial–mesenchymal signaling in the preterm lamb model [55].

Similarly, in the 125-day-old baboon model, treatment with early nasal continuous positive airway pressure (NCPAP) for 28 days led to a pulmonary phenotype similar to 156 days of gestational control lungs, suggesting that this noninvasive approach could minimize lung injury [56]. In the same model, delayed extubation (till 5 days) versus early extubation to NCPAP at 24 h led to lower arterial to alveolar oxygen ratio, high $PaCO_2$, and worse respiratory function, likely secondary to poor respiratory drive that contributed to more reintubations and time on mechanical ventilation. The delayed NCPAP group also demonstrated increased cellular bronchiolitis and peribronchiolar alveolar wall thickening along with increased inflammatory mediators in the bronchoalveolar lavage [57].

Epidemiological studies have shown that replacing invasive MV with NCPAP was associated with the reduction in BPD [58]. However, no differences in the incidence of BPD or mortality were noted in the NCPAP group in the COIN study that randomized infants born at 25–28 weeks to receive either NCPAP or intubation with MV in the delivery room [59]. Other noninvasive ventilation options like nasal intermittent-positive pressure ventilation (NIPPV) have also been shown to reduce the need for intubation within the first 48–72 h of life and are associated with decreased mortality and/or BPD [60].

Infection/Sepsis

Immune dysregulation caused by infection in susceptible preterm infants has been implicated in the pathogenesis of BPD [38].

Corticosteroids

Corticosteroids are potent anti-inflammatory agents that have been used in VLBW infants to decrease the total number of days on mechanical ventilation and help in early extubation. Although postnatal use of steroids does not have any direct role in the pathogenesis of BPD, their use modulates the influence of inflammation in the pathogenesis of BPD. The 2010 Cochrane review and its revisions in 2014 and 2017 showed that early use of postnatal steroids facilitated extubation and decreased the risk of BPD, but did not have significant benefit in reducing neonatal or subsequent mortality [61].

Nutrition

Multiple studies have associated poor weight gain, small for gestational age status, and poor enteral nutrition as high risk factors for developing BPD [62,63]. Exclusive formula feeding has been shown to increase the risk for BPD [64]. High fluid intake has been associated with increased risk of cardiorespiratory morbidity and NEC [65]. A deficiency of vitamin A has been associated with decreased lung growth and repair.

How to minimize lung injury?

As discussed earlier, one of the most critical factors in the pathogenesis of BPD is exposure to hyperoxia. Hence it is important to avoid exposure to high concentrations of supplemental oxygen as early as possible given the immature antioxidant defenses of the preterm newborn [66]. Currently, the recommendation is to initiate resuscitation for preterm infants in the delivery room with a default setting of FiO_2 of 0.3–0.4 and titrate by

5%–10% upward or downward [67]. There is significant controversy regarding the precise SpO_2 target ranges recommended for preterm infants beyond the initial resuscitation in the delivery room. We recommend using a lower alarm limit of 88% and a higher alarm limit of 96% while attempting to target SpO_2 of 88%–94% for this population [68].

The next area to focus would be to minimize barotrauma and volutrauma due to mechanical ventilation. For this purpose, noninvasive ventilation should be the initial therapy of choice in preterm infants wherever feasible. A recent meta-analysis comparing prophylactic NCPAP with invasive mechanical ventilation demonstrated that the use of NCPAP resulted in a modest decrease in the risk of developing BPD (RR 0.89, 95% CI: 0.79–0.99, $P = 0.04$) [69]. If a preterm infant is intubated, attempts at extubation should be done as soon as possible. In a study examining 224 preterm infants born at <27 weeks, the age at first extubation attempt correlated directly with total number of days on mechanical ventilation and length of stay. They also reported that the earlier an extubation attempt, the lower the rate of BPD [70]. Extubation should be attempted when there is sufficient spontaneous respiratory effort, the level of mechanical ventilatory support (particularly the peak inspiratory pressures or PIP) has been weaned to reasonable levels (PIP ≤16 cmH_2O), and the patient is a suitable candidate for noninvasive mechanical support as a transitional therapy [68,71].

For infants at high risk of BPD, initial fluid intake should be limited to 80–100 mL/kg/day and progressive increase should aim for a maximum intake of 120–150 mL/kg/day by day 7 of life [72]. In a study evaluating effect of human milk use on chronic lung disease in VLBW infants, the incidence of BPD fell as the cumulative percentage of human milk use for enteral feedings increased. Specifically, by multivariate logistic regression, they demonstrated that each 10 mL/kg/day increase in human milk intake was associated with a 12% reduction in odds of BPD [73]. Therefore, maximizing early nutrition, preferably using breast milk should be a priority to prevent BPD.

Another nutritive factor that has shown some benefit in preventing BPD is vitamin A. National Institute of Child Health and Human Development (NICHD)-sponsored randomized controlled trials and a systematic review of other trials have shown that postnatal supplementation with intramuscular vitamin A (5000 IU) started within a few days of birth and given 3 times a day for 4 weeks reduces the risk of BPD in about 7% [74]. This translates into a number needed to treat of 14 infants to prevent one case of BPD [75].

Prevention of infection using meticulous infection control measures as well as good antibiotic stewardship should be the standard of care for preterm infants.

Fig. 7.4 demonstrates the summary of factors helping in prevention of BPD in preterm infants.

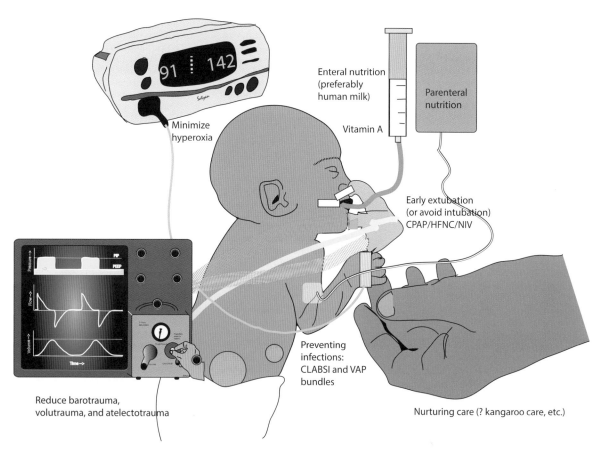

Fig. 7.4 Prevention of BPD in Preterm Infants. Reducing volutrauma, barotrauma, and atelectotrauma, early extubation (or avoiding intubation), minimizing hyperoxia, prevention of infections, enteral nutrition and vitamin A along with nurturing care may play a role in reducing rates of BPD in preterm infants. *CLABSI*, central line associated blood stream infection; *CPAP*, continuous positive airway pressure; *HFNC*, high flow nasal cannula; *NIV*, noninvasive ventilation; *VAP*, ventilator associated pneumonia. Copyright: Satyan Lakshminrusimha.

Conclusions

BPD remains a significant cause of mortality and morbidity in the NICUs all over the world despite use of newer and gentler means of ventilation. The pathogenesis of BPD involves a multifactorial pathway where lung injury due to hyperoxia and MV leads to dysregulated immune response and aberrant tissue repair in preterm infants. MV causes lung injury by various mechanisms that include barotrauma, volutrauma, atelectotrauma, and biotrauma. Use of noninvasive modes of MV and minimizing free radical injury due to hyperoxia have shown significant reduction in the rates of BPD in preterm neonates.

References

[1] Northway WH Jr, Rosan RC, Porter DY. Pulmonary disease following respirator therapy of hyaline-membrane disease. Bronchopulmonary dysplasia. N Engl J Med 1967;276(7):357–368.

[2] Kneyber MC, Zhang H, Slutsky AS. Ventilator-induced lung injury. Similarity and differences between children and adults. Am J Respir Crit Care Med 2014;190(3):258–265.

[3] Donn SM, Sinha SK. Minimising ventilator induced lung injury in preterm infants. Arch Dis Child Fetal Neonatal Ed 2006;91(3):F226–F230.

[4] De Paepe ME. Pathology of bronchopulmonary dysplasia. In: Bhandari V, editor. Bronchopulmonary dysplasia. Cham: Springer International Publishing; 2016. p. 149–164.

[5] Jobe AJ. The new BPD: an arrest of lung development. Pediatr Res 1999;46(6):641–643.

[6] Husain AN, Siddiqui NH, Stocker JT. Pathology of arrested acinar development in postsurfactant bronchopulmonary dysplasia. Hum Pathol 1998;29(7):710–717.

[7] Pryhuber GS. Postnatal infections and immunology affecting chronic lung disease of prematurity. Clin Perinatol 2015;42(4):697–718.

[8] Eriksson L, Haglund B, Odlind V, Altman M, Kieler H. Prenatal inflammatory risk factors for development of bronchopulmonary dysplasia. Pediatr Pulmonol 2014;49(7):665–672.

[9] Bi GL, Chen FL, Huang WM. The association between hypertensive disorders in pregnancy and bronchopulmonary dysplasia: a systematic review. World J Pediatr 2013;9(4):300–306.

[10] O'Shea JE, Davis PG, Doyle LW. Maternal preeclampsia and risk of bronchopulmonary dysplasia in preterm infants. Pediatr Res 2012;71(2):210–214.

[11] Schmiedl A, Roolfs T, Tutdibi E, Gortner L, Monz D. Influence of prenatal hypoxia and postnatal hyperoxia on morphologic lung maturation in mice. PLoS One 2017;12(4):e0175804.

[12] Gortner L, Monz D, Mildau C, et al. Bronchopulmonary dysplasia in a double-hit mouse model induced by intrauterine hypoxia and postnatal hyperoxia: closer to clinical features? Ann Anat 2013;195(4):351–358.

[13] Glaser K, Speer CP. Pre and postnatal inflammation in the pathogenesis of bronchopulmonary dysplasia. In: Bhandari V, editor. Bronchopulmonary dysplasia. Cham: Springer International Publishing; 2016. p. 55–77.

[14] Hartling L, Liang Y, Lacaze-Masmonteil T. Chorioamnionitis as a risk factor for bronchopulmonary dysplasia: a systematic review and meta-analysis. Arch Dis Child Fetal Neonatal Ed 2012;97(1):F8–F17.

[15] Goldenberg RL, Andrews WW, Goepfert AR, et al. The Alabama Preterm Birth Study: umbilical cord blood *Ureaplasma urealyticum* and *Mycoplasma hominis* cultures in very preterm newborn infants. Am J Obstet Gynecol 2008;198(1). 43.e41–45.e41.

[16] Van Marter LJ, Dammann O, Allred EN, et al. Chorioamnionitis, mechanical ventilation, and postnatal sepsis as modulators of chronic lung disease in preterm infants. J Pediatr 2002;140(2):171–176.

[17] Been JV, Rours IG, Kornelisse RF, Jonkers F, de Krijger RR, Zimmermann LJ. Chorioamnionitis alters the response to surfactant in preterm infants. J Pediatr 2010;156(1). 10.e11–15.e11.

[18] Antonucci R, Contu P, Porcella A, Atzeni C, Chiappe S. Intrauterine smoke exposure: a new risk factor for bronchopulmonary dysplasia? J Perinat Med 2004;32(3):272–277.

[19] Spiegler J, Jensen R, Segerer H, et al. Influence of smoking and alcohol during pregnancy on outcome of VLBW infants. Z Geburtshilfe Neonatol 2013;217(6):215–219.

[20] Van Marter LJ, Leviton A, Kuban KC, Pagano M, Allred EN. Maternal glucocorticoid therapy and reduced risk of bronchopulmonary dysplasia. Pediatrics 1990;86(3):331–336.

[21] Roberts D, Brown J, Medley N, Dalziel SR. Antenatal corticosteroids for accelerating fetal lung maturation for women at risk of preterm birth. Cochrane Database Syst Rev 2017;3:Cd004454.

[22] Trembath A, Laughon M. Predictors of bronchopulmonary dysplasia. Clin Perinatol 2012;39(3):585–601.

[23] Bhandari V, Gruen JR. The genetics of bronchopulmonary dysplasia. Semin Perinatol 2006;30(4):185–191.

[24] Lavoie PM, Pham C, Jang KL. Heritability of bronchopulmonary dysplasia, defined according to the consensus statement of the national institutes of health. Pediatrics 2008;122(3):479–485.

[25] Lavoie PM. Genetics of bronchopulmonary dysplasia. In: Bhandari V, editor. Bronchopulmonary dysplasia. Cham: Springer International Publishing; 2016. p. 109–127.

[26] Mullassery D, Smith NP. Lung development. Semin Pediatr Surg 2015;24(4):152–155.

[27] Joshi S, Kotecha S. Lung growth and development. Early Hum Dev 2007;83(12):789–794.

[28] Bhandari V. Postnatal inflammation in the pathogenesis of bronchopulmonary dysplasia. Birth Defects Res A Clin Mol Teratol 2014;100(3):189–201.

[29] Smeets CC, Codd V, Samani NJ, Hokken-Koelega AC. Leukocyte telomere length in young adults born preterm: support for accelerated biological ageing. PLoS One 2015;10(11):e0143951.

[30] Hadchouel A, Marchand-Martin L, Franco-Montoya ML, Peaudecerf L, Ancel PY, Delacourt C. Salivary telomere length and lung function in adolescents born very preterm: a prospective multicenter study. PLoS One 2015;10(9):e0136123.

[31] Warner BB, Stuart LA, Papes RA, Wispe JR. Functional and pathological effects of prolonged hyperoxia in neonatal mice. Am J Physiol 1998;275(1 Pt. 1):L110–L117.

[32] Bhandari V. Hyperoxia-derived lung damage in preterm infants. Semin Fetal Neonatal Med 2010;15(4):223–229.

[33] Bhandari V, Choo-Wing R, Lee CG, et al. Hyperoxia causes angiopoietin 2-mediated acute lung injury and necrotic cell death. Nat Med 2006;12(11):1286–1293.

[34] Bhandari V, Elias JA. Cytokines in tolerance to hyperoxia-induced injury in the developing and adult lung. Free Radic Biol Med 2006;41(1):4–18.

[35] Iliodromiti Z, Zygouris D, Sifakis S, et al. Acute lung injury in preterm fetuses and neonates: mechanisms and molecular pathways. J Matern Fetal Neonatal Med 2013;26(17):1696–1704.

[36] Wilborn AM, Evers LB, Canada AT. Oxygen toxicity to the developing lung of the mouse: role of reactive oxygen species. Pediatr Res 1996;40(2):225–232.

[37] Buczynski BW, Maduekwe ET, O'Reilly MA. The role of hyperoxia in the pathogenesis of experimental BPD. Semin Perinatol 2013;37(2):69–78.

[38] Balany J, Bhandari V. Understanding the impact of infection, inflammation, and their persistence in the pathogenesis of bronchopulmonary dysplasia. Front Med (Lausanne) 2015;2:90.

[39] Carvalho CG, Silveira RC, Procianoy RS. Ventilator-induced lung injury in preterm infants. Rev Bras Ter Intensiva 2013;25(4):319–326.

[40] Auten RL, Vozzelli M, Clark RH. Volutrauma. What is it, and how do we avoid it? Clin Perinatol 2001;28(3):505–515.

[41] Wu S, Capasso L, Lessa A, et al. High tidal volume ventilation activates Smad2 and upregulates expression of connective tissue growth factor in newborn rat lung. Pediatr Res 2008;63(3):245–250.

[42] Kroon AA, Wang J, Huang Z, Cao L, Kuliszewski M, Post M. Inflammatory response to oxygen and endotoxin in newborn rat lung ventilated with low tidal volume. Pediatr Res 2010;68(1):63–69.

[43] Hillman NH, Polglase GR, Pillow JJ, Saito M, Kallapur SG, Jobe AH. Inflammation and lung maturation from stretch injury in preterm fetal sheep. Am J Physiol Lung Cell Mol Physiol 2011;300(2):L232–L241.

[44] Stenson BJ, Boyle DW, Szyld EG. Initial ventilation strategies during newborn resuscitation. Clin Perinatol 2006;33(1):65–82.

[45] Muscedere JG, Mullen JB, Gan K, Slutsky AS. Tidal ventilation at low airway pressures can augment lung injury. Am J Respir Crit Care Med 1994;149(5):1327–1334.

[46] Clark RH, Gerstmann DR, Jobe AH, Moffitt ST, Slutsky AS, Yoder BA. Lung injury in neonates: causes, strategies for prevention, and long-term consequences. J Pediatr 2001;139(4):478–486.

[47] Jobe AH, Ikegami M. Mechanisms initiating lung injury in the preterm. Early Hum Dev 1998;53(1):81–94.

[48] Bland RD, Ertsey R, Mokres LM, et al. Mechanical ventilation uncouples synthesis and assembly of elastin and increases apoptosis in lungs of newborn mice. Prelude to defective alveolar septation during lung development? Am J Physiol Lung Cell Mol Physiol 2008;294(1):L3–L14.

[49] Bland RD, Xu L, Ertsey R, et al. Dysregulation of pulmonary elastin synthesis and assembly in preterm lambs with chronic lung disease. Am J Physiol Lung Cell Mol Physiol 2007;292(6):L1370–L1384.

[50] Coalson JJ, Winter VT, Siler-Khodr T, Yoder BA. Neonatal chronic lung disease in extremely immature baboons. Am J Respir Crit Care Med 1999;160(4):1333–1346.

[51] Tambunting F, Beharry KD, Hartleroad J, Waltzman J, Stavitsky Y, Modanlou HD. Increased lung matrix metalloproteinase-9 levels in extremely premature baboons with bronchopulmonary dysplasia. Pediatr Pulmonol 2005;39(1):5–14.

[52] Tambunting F, Beharry KD, Waltzman J, Modanlou HD. Impaired lung vascular endothelial growth factor in extremely premature baboons developing bronchopulmonary dysplasia/chronic lung disease. J Investig Med 2005;53(5):253–262.

[53] Albertine KH, Jones GP, Starcher BC, et al. Chronic lung injury in preterm lambs. Disordered respiratory tract development. Am J Respir Crit Care Med 1999;159(3):945–958.

[54] Reyburn B, Li M, Metcalfe DB, et al. Nasal ventilation alters mesenchymal cell turnover and improves alveolarization in preterm lambs. Am J Respir Crit Care Med 2008;178(4):407–418.

[55] Rehan VK, Fong J, Lee R, et al. Mechanism of reduced lung injury by high-frequency nasal ventilation in a preterm lamb model of neonatal chronic lung disease. Pediatr Res 2011;70(5):462–466.

[56] Thomson MA, Yoder BA, Winter VT, et al. Treatment of immature baboons for 28 days with early nasal continuous positive airway pressure. Am J Respir Crit Care Med 2004;169(9):1054–1062.

[57] Thomson MA, Yoder BA, Winter VT, Giavedoni L, Chang LY, Coalson JJ. Delayed extubation to nasal continuous positive airway pressure in the immature baboon model of bronchopulmonary dysplasia: lung clinical and pathological findings. Pediatrics 2006;118(5):2038–2050.

[58] Aly H, Milner JD, Patel K, El-Mohandes AA. Does the experience with the use of nasal continuous positive airway pressure improve over time in extremely low birth weight infants? Pediatrics 2004;114(3):697–702.

[59] Morley CJ, Davis PG, Doyle LW, Brion LP, Hascoet JM, Carlin JB. Nasal CPAP or intubation at birth for very preterm infants. N Engl J Med 2008;358(7):700–708.

[60] Bhandari V. The potential of non-invasive ventilation to decrease BPD. Semin Perinatol 2013;37(2):108–114.

[61] Doyle LW, Cheong JL, Ehrenkranz RA, Halliday HL. Early (<8 days) systemic postnatal corticosteroids for prevention of bronchopulmonary dysplasia in preterm infants. Cochrane Database Syst Rev 2017;10:Cd001146.

[62] Ehrenkranz RA, Dusick AM, Vohr BR, Wright LL, Wrage LA, Poole WK.

Growth in the neonatal intensive care unit influences neurodevelopmental and growth outcomes of extremely low birth weight infants. Pediatrics 2006;117(4):1253–1261.

[63] Wemhoner A, Ortner D, Tschirch E, Strasak A, Rudiger M. Nutrition of preterm infants in relation to bronchopulmonary dysplasia. BMC Pulm Med 2011;11:7.

[64] Spiegler J, Preuss M, Gebauer C, et al. Does breastmilk influence the development of bronchopulmonary dysplasia? J Pediatr 2016;169. 76.e74–80.e74.

[65] Van Marter LJ, Leviton A, Allred EN, Pagano M, Kuban KC. Hydration during the first days of life and the risk of bronchopulmonary dysplasia in low birth weight infants. J Pediatr 1990;116(6):942–949.

[66] Torres-Cuevas I, Cernada M, Nuñez A, Vento M. Oxygen modulation and bronchopulmonary dysplasia: delivery room and beyond. In: Bhandari V, editor. Bronchopulmonary dysplasia. Cham: Springer International Publishing; 2016. p. 183–198.

[67] Oei JL, Ghadge A, Coates E, et al. Clinicians in 25 countries prefer to use lower levels of oxygen to resuscitate preterm infants at birth. Acta Paediatr 2016;105(9):1061–1066.

[68] Nelin LD, Bhandari V. How to decrease bronchopulmonary dysplasia in your neonatal intensive care unit today and "tomorrow". F1000Res 2017;6:539.

[69] Subramaniam P, Ho JJ, Davis PG. Prophylactic nasal continuous positive airway pressure for preventing morbidity and mortality in very preterm infants. Cochrane Database Syst Rev 2016;6:Cd001243.

[70] Robbins M, Trittmann J, Martin E, Reber KM, Nelin L, Shepherd E. Early extubation attempts reduce length of stay in extremely preterm infants even if re-intubation is necessary. J Neonatal Perinatal Med 2015;8(2):91–97.

[71] Bhandari V. Nasal intermittent positive pressure ventilation in the newborn: review of literature and evidence-based guidelines. J Perinatol 2010;30(8):505–512.

[72] Ehrenkranz RA, Moya FR. Nutrition in bronchopulmonary dysplasia: in the NICU and beyond. In: Bhandari V, editor. Bronchopulmonary dysplasia. Cham: Springer International Publishing; 2016. p. 223–241.

[73] Patel AL, Johnson TJ, Robin B, et al. Influence of own mother's milk on

bronchopulmonary dysplasia and costs. Arch Dis Child Fetal Neonatal Ed 2017;102(3):F256–F261.

[74] Tyson JE, Wright LL, Oh W, et al. Vitamin A supplementation for extremely-low-birth-weight infants.

National Institute of Child Health and Human Development Neonatal Research Network. N Engl J Med 1999;340(25):1962–1968.

[75] Londhe VA, Nolen TL, Das A, et al. Vitamin A supplementation in

extremely low-birth-weight infants: subgroup analysis in small-for-gestational-age infants. Am J Perinatol 2013;30(9):771–780.

Chapter | 8 |

Hypoxic Respiratory Failure

Praveen Kumar, MBBS, DCH, MD, FAAP

CHAPTER POINTS

- Hypoxemic respiratory failure (HRF) in neonates is commonly due to hypoventilation, impaired diffusion and/or ventilation-perfusion mismatch and is often associated with persistent pulmonary hypertension of the newborn (PPHN) and right-to-left shunt.
- Severity of HRF is assessed by calculating Alveolar-arterial oxygen gradient (A-a DO$_2$), arterial to Alveolar oxygen ratio (a/A ratio), oxygenation index (OI), oxygen saturation index (OSI), respiratory severity score (RSS), PaO$_2$/FiO$_2$ (P/F) ratio and SpO$_2$/FiO$_2$ (S/F) ratio.
- Management of HRF includes gentle respiratory support with permissive hypercapnia, permissive hypoxemia (SpO$_2$ in low to mid-90s) and surfactant replacement in cases with parenchymal lung disease, inhaled nitric oxide in patients with PPHN and if intractable despite medical therapy, extracorporeal membrane oxygenation (ECMO).

Introduction

Hypoxemic respiratory failure (HRF) is frequently encountered in neonatal intensive care unit (NICU) and can occur in both term and preterm infants. Although the exact incidence of HRF is not known, it has been estimated that nearly 80,000 newborn infants require mechanical ventilation in the United States each year and nearly 11% of these infants die [1]. The annual cost of hospital care of these infants was estimated to be US$4.4 billion [1]. A diagnosis of HRF is characterized by presence of hypoxemia and/or hypercarbia on blood gases and is associated with significant morbidity and mortality in these critically ill infants. This failure to maintain normal PCO$_2$ and PaO$_2$ can either be secondary to pulmonary disorders such as hyaline membrane disease (HMD) in a preterm infant or meconium aspiration syndrome (MAS) in a term infant, or cardiac dysfunction such as persistent pulmonary hypertension in newborn (PPHN) or a large left-to-right shunt in an infant with patent ductus arteriosus (PDA). Often, it is a result of combination of both pulmonary and cardiac dysfunction in the same patient.

Pathophysiology of HRF

Maintenance of normal PCO$_2$ and PaO$_2$ depends on composition of air entering lungs, adequate blood flow to the lungs, mature gas-exchange surface, and an intact neuromuscular system. The pathophysiology of HRF can be attributed to one or more of the following mechanisms.

1. **Hypoventilation**: Hypoventilation is described as a condition in which the total air volume reaching alveolar space is inadequate to maintain gas exchange. Ventilation, usually reported as minute ventilation (VE), is the volume of air expired in 1 min. VE is calculated by multiplying respiratory rate (f) by tidal volume (V_t), which is a sum of alveolar ventilation (VA) and dead space ventilation (VD). Since only alveolar air participates in gas exchange, a decrease in VA will result in hypercarbia and hypoxemia (Fig. 8.1). Administration of oxygen alone may improve PaO$_2$ with no significant effect on PaCO$_2$. Correction of

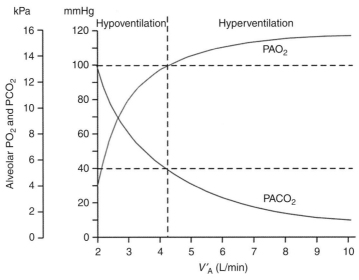

Fig. 8.1 The effects of hyper- and hypoventilation on the PAO_2 *(red)* and $PACO_2$ *(blue)* and, therefore, also on PaO_2 and $PaCO_2$ if no other V'_A/Q' mismatch is present. The *dashed lines* indicate normal values for V'_A, PAO_2 and $PACO_2$. The diagram is derived assuming unchanged cardiac output, O_2 consumption, and CO_2 production with mixed venous values changing with changes in PaO_2 and $PaCO_2$. With hypoventilation, PvO_2 and $PvCO_2$ are lower and higher than normal, respectively. Note that changes in V'_A correspond to changes in V'_A/Q' ratio, as blood flow (cardiac output) is held constant. Thus, decreased ventilation (low V'_A/Q' ratio) causes PAO_2 and $PACO_2$ to move toward the mixed venous values while hyperventilation shifts PAO_2 and $PACO_2$ toward their inspired values. Hypoventilation thus results in both hypoxemia and hypercapnia. An increase in FiO_2 results in an upward shift of the PO_2 curve while the PCO_2 curve remains fixed. In this situation, $PaCO_2$ might be high even in the absence of hypoxemia. Reproduced with permission from Petersson J, Glenny RW. Gas exchange and ventilation-perfusion relationships in the lung. Eur Respir J 2014;44(4):1023–1041 [2]. Copyright: ERS 2014.

$PaCO_2$ will require increase in VE. Common causes of hypoventilation leading to HRF are neuromuscular disorders, chest wall deformities, central nervous system depression (either due to a primary pathology or secondary to maternal or neonatal narcotics/sedation use), and airway obstruction.

2. **Impaired diffusion**: Gas exchange across alveolar–capillary membrane occurs by passive diffusion. Hypoxemia is a more prominent finding in conditions associated with impaired diffusion. Since CO_2 diffuses much more rapidly, about 20 times faster than oxygen, impaired diffusion by itself is an uncommon cause of hypercarbia [2,3]. Factors leading to impaired diffusion include thickness of alveolar–capillary junction, impaired alignment of alveoli and capillaries, reduced number of alveolar capillaries, and shorter RBC transit time through capillaries [3]. The examples of clinical conditions in a neonate in which impaired diffusion contributes to HRF are interstitial lung diseases (ILD), bronchopulmonary dysplasia (BPD), and alveolar capillary dysplasia (ACD).

3. **Ventilation–perfusion mismatch**: Ventilation–perfusion ratio (V/Q ratio) is described as the ratio of alveolar ventilation to alveolar perfusion. An

ideal V/Q ratio of 1 requires that all regions of lungs participate in gas exchange, all ventilated alveoli are adequately perfused, and all perfused alveoli are fully ventilated. Low V/Q ratio, ranging from 0 to 1, will occur in parts of lung with decreased or no ventilation but with adequate perfusion (Fig. 8.2). This is also described as intrapulmonary shunting as some deoxygenated blood passes through pulmonary circulation without participating in gas exchange. Effects of changes in V/Q mismatch on ventilation and oxygen are shown in Fig. 8.3. Patients with low V/Q ratio will present with hypercapnia and hypoxia (Fig. 8.3). In contrast, high V/Q ratio (ranging from more than 1 to infinity) occurs when ventilation is maintained in presence of decreased or absent perfusion. This will increase the dead space and reduce the overall gas exchange area of the lung. However, under normal condition in a healthy human adult in erect position, V/Q ratio is between 0.8 and 0.9 because of the effects of gravity on ventilation and perfusion in different regions of the lung. It has been known that the ventilation and perfusion of lungs is not uniform and vary in different areas of the lungs depending on the

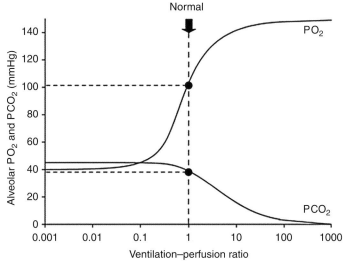

Fig. 8.2 Alveolar Oxygen and Carbon Dioxide Partial Pressures (PO_2 and PCO_2) in Homogeneous Regions With Different Alveolar Ventilation–Perfusion Ratio Indicated on the Abscissa. Reproduced with permission from Wagner PD. The physiological basis of pulmonary gas exchange: implications for clinical interpretation of arterial blood gases. Eur Respir J 2015;45(1):227–243 [3]. Copyright: ERS 2014.

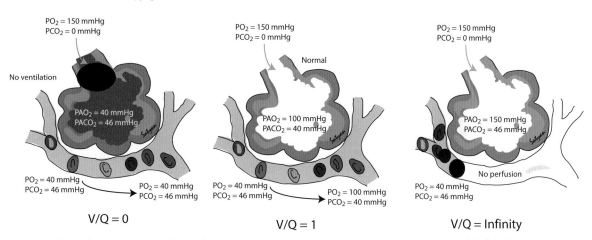

Fig. 8.3 Effect of Ventilation–Perfusion (V/Q) on Oxygenation in Lungs. Three-compartment model of the lung with V/Q equal to 1 in normal lungs (center figure), V/Q equal to infinity due to no perfusion, and V/Q equal to zero in airway obstruction with no ventilation. Copyright: Satyan Lakshminrusimha.

airway and hydrostatic pressures [4–7]. Based on the differences in V/Q, the lung has three distinct zones in an erect position (Fig. 8.4). Zone 1 (*upper zone* in Fig. 8.4) is described as part of the lung in which pulmonary arterial pressure is lower than the pulmonary alveolar pressure. As a result, capillaries in this part of the lung are either collapsed or poorly perfused, do not participate in gas exchange, and add to the dead space ventilation. Thus, the V/Q ratio is more than 1 in this part of the lung. This zone may be nonexistent in healthy adults but becomes important

in ventilated patients with high alveolar pressures and/or low pulmonary arterial pressures. Zone 2 (*middle zone* in Fig. 8.4) is the region of the lung few centimeters above the heart. The blood flow in this zone is pulsatile and pulmonary artery pressure is greater with the pulmonary venous pressure being lower than the alveolar pressure. The V/Q ratio in this region of lung is closest to 1. Both pulmonary artery and venous pressures are higher than the alveolar pressure in zone 3 (*lower zone* in Fig. 8.4) and the V/Q ratio is below 1 in this part of the lung.

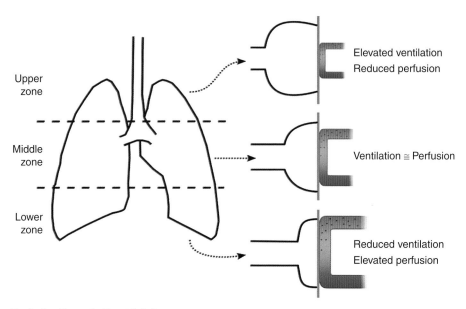

Fig. 8.4 **Lung Perfusion Zones in Erect Adult.**

Most patient with cardiopulmonary disorders has a variable combination of lung units with normal, low, and infinite V/Q ratios. This variation in V/Q mismatch is less in supine position because the vertical dimension of the lung is smaller. Although the effect of prone position on V/Q matching has been controversial, several animal and human studies have shown that clinically observed improvement in ventilation and oxygenation in mechanically ventilated patients in prone position is due to better V/Q match in prone position [6,7]. Minor reduction in overall V/Q mismatch is compensated by increase in VE till a point is reached when increase in ventilation is not sustainable either due to fatigue or degree of mismatch. V/Q mismatch is one of the primary underlying mechanisms in most patients with HRF.

4. **Right-to-left shunts**: In presence of right-to-left shunts, deoxygenated blood passes from right side to the left or oxygenated side of the circulation without participating in gas exchange in lungs. Due to the bronchial and thebesian (small cardiac veins) circulations, about 2%–3% of deoxygenated blood passes from right to the left side of the circulation in healthy adults. The amount of this physiologic right-to-left shunt is higher, about 5%–10%, in newborn infants because of presence of PFO and PDA in first few days of life and contributes to lower resting PaO_2 in healthy newborns. Right-to-left shunts can be either intracardiac or intrapulmonary and can lead to severe hypoxemia and respiratory failure. The severity of hypoxemia depends

on the size of right-to-left shunt (Fig. 8.5). In patients with a small right-to-left shunt ($\leq$10%–20% of cardiac output), the decrease in PaO_2 will be small and it will improve with increasing FiO_2. In contrast, in patients with a large right-to-left shunt (>30%–50% of cardiac output) PaO_2 will be significantly lower and will have minimal or no increase even with administration of 100% oxygen (Fig. 8.5). Changes in $PaCO_2$ are less striking. If VE remains unchanged, $PaCO_2$ will increase in nonlinear fashion with increase in the size of right-to-left shunt. However, $PaCO_2$ in patients with right-to-left shunt is usually either low or normal because of hypoxia-driven increase in VE.

Cardiac catheterization with the use of Fick principle is the gold standard to determine the size of shunt. However, several noninvasive methods, such as echocardiography, magnetic resonance study of the heart, and radionuclide scintigraphy have been developed and can provide good estimates of the size of shunt in these patients [8–12]. A rough estimate of right-to-left shunt can also be obtained by evaluating the effect of FiO_2 on SaO_2 as described earlier (Fig. 8.5). However, these techniques are helpful in patients with no pulmonary disease and V/Q mismatch. Based on the observation that increase in FiO_2 has minimal or no effect on PAO_2 or SaO_2 in patients with right-to-left shunt but will restore PAO_2 or SaO_2 to near normal in patients with V/Q mismatch alone, a simplified slide rule method has been proposed to evaluate the size of shunt in presence

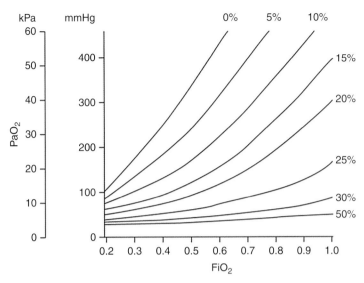

Fig. 8.5 The Iso-Shunt Diagram Illustrating the Relationship Between PaO$_2$ and FiO$_2$ in the Presence of a Shunt Corresponding to Different Percentages of Total Lung Blood Flow. Note the near linear relationship between PaO$_2$ and FiO$_2$ in the absence of shunt. With increasing shunt fractions, the change in PaO$_2$ with increasing FiO$_2$ is much more flat. Hence, a large increase in FiO$_2$ results in little change in PaO$_2$. For a shunt >30% of cardiac output, even a FiO$_2$ of 1.0 fails to result in a PaO$_2$ of 100 mmHg (13.3 kPa). Modeling is based on a hemoglobin concentration of 14 g/dL, PaCO$_2$ of 40 mmHg (5.3 kPa) and an arterial–mixed venous oxygen content difference (Ca – v̄O$_2$) of 5 mL/dL. Reproduced with permission from Petersson J, Glenny RW. Gas exchange and ventilation-perfusion relationships in the lung. Eur Respir J 2014;44(4):1023–1041 [2]. Copyright: ERS 2014.

of V/Q mismatch [13–16]. A online free version of the slide-rule calculator is available from http://www.noranaes.org/shuntcurves/. Using SaO$_2$ values at different FiO$_2$ and patient's hemoglobin, both the size of shunt and extent of V/Q mismatch can be calculated.

Some common causes of intrapulmonary right-to-left shunt in newborns include atelectasis, hyaline membrane disease, and pneumonia. Extrapulmonary right-to-left shunt is the cause of hypoxemia in neonates with cyanotic congenital heart disease.

5. **Low inspired oxygen pressure**: A low partial pressure of oxygen in alveoli (PAO$_2$) is an uncommon cause of hypoxemia in most clinical situations but can occur at high altitude (such as during air transport), by inhaling gas mixture with less than 21% oxygen or due to an increased alveolar amount of other gases such carbon monoxide and dioxide (Fig. 8.6).

6. **Low pulmonary arterial PO$_2$**: Another contributing mechanism of arterial hypoxemia is the presence of low PO$_2$ in the blood entering the pulmonary circulation. This could be due to low cardiac output, increased oxygen extraction by tissues, and presence of abnormal hemoglobin.

Etiology of HRF

A wide range of pulmonary and nonpulmonary disorders can cause HRF in newborns. It is important to note that most newborns with these conditions have mild to moderate clinical symptoms with minor alterations in PCO$_2$ and PaO$_2$ and only infants with severe disease may need mechanical ventilation. The disorders associated with HRF can present either at or after birth and can be divided into intra- and extrapulmonary disorders (Table 8.1).

Clinical features and assessment

A detailed history, including events in the antenatal period, can be helpful in identifying the likely etiology, the course of the disease, and the evaluation and management. The gestational age can help clinicians in narrowing down the differential diagnosis in a newborn with HRF. While HMD is more likely in a preterm infant with no maternal steroid treatment prior to delivery, MAS and PPHN are more likely to be a cause of HRF in a term or postterm infant. Other

of these infants. Chest X-ray can provide useful information about the cause of HRF and help in identifying complications of treatment and optimizing the ventilator support. Table 8.4 summarizes the typical chest X-ray findings in various disorders responsible for HRF in newborns (Figs. 8.7–8.19).

Blood gas estimation can provide crucial information about ventilation, degree of hypoxemia, and derangements in acid–base status. Normal ABG values for a newborn

Table 8.4	Chest X-ray findings in common disorders responsible for HRF in newborns
Disorder	**Typical chest X-ray findings**
HMD	Poor lung expansion, bilateral symmetric diffuse reticulogranular opacities, atelectasis, air bronchograms (Fig. 8.7)
MAS	Unilateral or bilateral fluffy infiltrates or coarse opacities, hyperexpanded lungs (Fig. 8.8)
Pneumonia	Variable ranging from patchy infiltrates or consolidation to being indistinguishable from X-ray of HMD (Fig. 8.9)
Air leak syndromes	Pneumothorax (Fig. 8.10), PIE (Fig. 8.11)
Pulmonary hypoplasia	Poor lung expansion with clear lung fields (Fig. 8.12)
PPHN	Primary PPHN—variable lung expansion with clear lung fields (Fig. 8.13) Secondary PPHN—consistent with underlying etiology
CDH	Absent diaphragm on the affected side with bowel gas in the chest presenting as cysts, poor lung expansion (Fig. 8.14)
CCAM	Pulmonary cysts localized to one lobe of the lung (Fig. 8.15)
Pleural effusion	Unilateral or bilateral opacities with shift of heart to contralateral side in unilateral effusion (Fig. 8.16)
Hydrops fetalis	Cardiomegaly with unilateral or bilateral pleural effusions, increased pulmonary vascular markings (Fig. 8.17)
BPD	Variable from increased interstitial markings to diffuse cystic changes, hyperexpansion (Fig. 8.18)
Skeletal dysplasias	Bell-shaped chest with findings of pulmonary hypoplasia, thin ribs, abnormal long bones (Fig. 8.19)

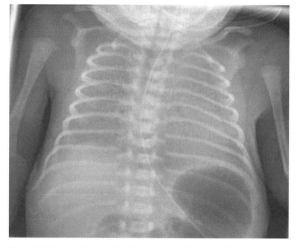

Fig. 8.7 Chest X-ray of a Newborn With Hyaline Membrane Disease (HMD).

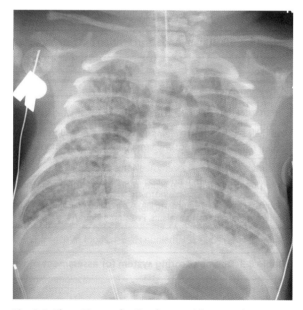

Fig. 8.8 Chest X-ray of a Newborn With Meconium Aspiration Syndrome (MAS).

breathing room air at sea level are shown in Table 8.5. Although the target PaO_2 in patients with HRF is between 60 and 80 mmHg, a PaO_2 between 40 and 60 mmHg can be accepted, in order to minimize adverse effects of increasing barotrauma, if there are no signs of end-organ hypoxia as assessed by serum lactic acid, blood pressure, and urine output. A PaO_2 value below 40 mmHg in absence of cyanotic congenital heart disease is always considered critical

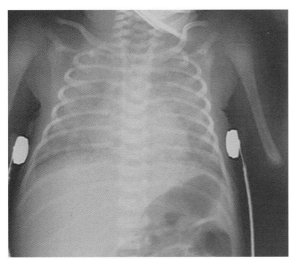

Fig. 8.9 **Chest X-ray of a Newborn With Pneumonia.**

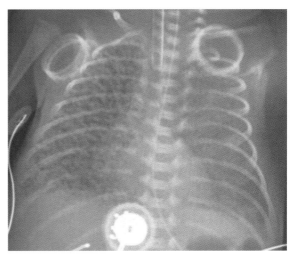

Fig. 8.11 **Chest X-ray of a Newborn With Pulmonary Interstitial Emphysema (PIE).**

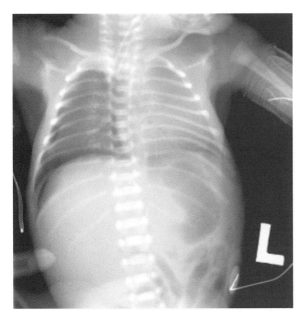

Fig. 8.10 **Chest X-ray of a Newborn With Right Pneumothorax.**

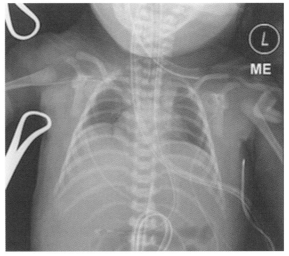

Fig. 8.12 **Chest X-ray of a Newborn With Pulmonary Hypoplasia.**

and is associated with significant increase in morbidity and mortality in patients with HRF. As oxygen is one of the most potent pulmonary vasodilators, it was believed that maintaining PaO_2 values higher than 80 mmHg could be beneficial in patients with pulmonary hypertension. However, the data from several animal studies have clearly shown that PaO_2 values above 80 mmHg provide no additional benefit

and may even be harmful due to increased production of the free-oxygen radicals and its harmful effects on surfactant and pulmonary vasculature.

In contrast to the interpretation of PaO_2, interpretation of $PaCO_2$ requires attention to pH and HCO_3^- values in the patient. An increase in $PaCO_2$ and/or decrease in HCO_3^- values will lower the pH while a decrease in $PaCO_2$ and/or increase in HCO_3^- values will have the opposite effect on pH. It is estimated that in patients with acute HRF every 10 mmHg change in $PaCO_2$ will change pH

89

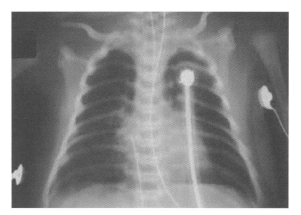

Fig. 8.13 **Chest X-ray of a Newborn With Primary Pulmonary Hypertension.**

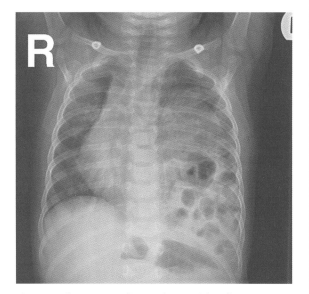

Fig. 8.14 **Chest X-ray of a Newborn With Left CDH.**

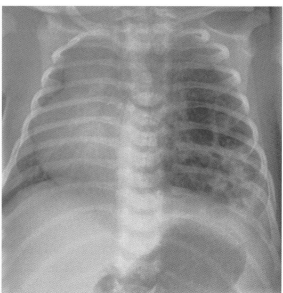

Fig. 8.15 **Chest X-ray of a Newborn With CCAM.**

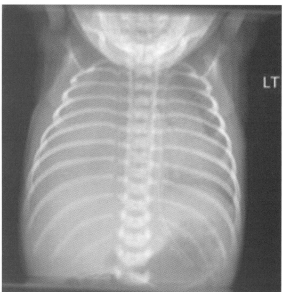

Fig. 8.16 **Chest X-ray of a Newborn With Right Pleural Effusion.**

by 0.07–0.08 units. The effect of change in $PaCO_2$ on pH in patients with long-standing respiratory failure is less marked. Table 8.6 summarizes the interpretation of different alterations in $PaCO_2$, pH, and HCO_3^- values. The most common abnormalities in an acute phase of HRF are respiratory and metabolic acidosis. Respiratory acidosis is a result of hypoventilation seen in patients with HRF. Metabolic acidosis in patients with HRF is frequently a sign of tissue hypoxia and hypoperfusion and is associated with increased serum lactic acid and anion gap. The common causes of metabolic acidosis with normal anion gap in newborns include renal bicarbonate loss, renal tubular

acidosis, and diarrhea. Respiratory alkalosis is a result of hyperventilation, which can be in response to hypoxemia or in some cases as a result of central hyperventilation with brain injury or hyperammonemia. The most common causes of metabolic alkalosis in newborns include diuretics and loss of excessive amounts of gastric contents.

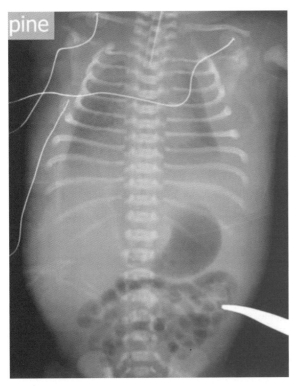

Fig. 8.17 **Chest X-ray of a Newborn With Hydrops Fetalis.**

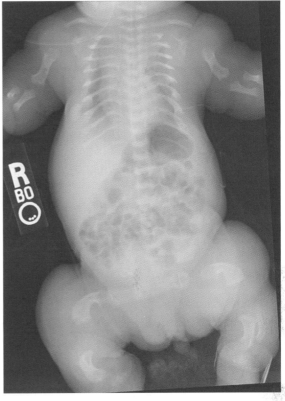

Fig. 8.19 **Chest X-ray of a Newborn With Skeletal Dysplasia.**

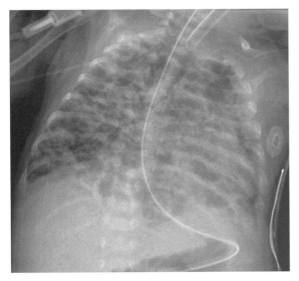

Fig. 8.18 **Chest X-ray of a Newborn With Bronchopulmonary Dysplasia (BPD).**

Table 8.5	Normal ABG values for a newborn breathing room air at sea level	
	Normal range
pH	7.35–7.45
$PaCO_2$	35–45 mmHg
PaO_2	60–80 mmHg
HCO_3	22–26 mEq/L
Base excess	±2–4 mEq/L
SaO_2	95%–98%
MetHb	<1%
COHb	<2%
CaO_2	16–22 mL O_2/dL

Table 8.6 Interpretation of alterations in $PaCO_2$, pH, and HCO_3^- values

Interpretation	pH	$PaCO_2$	HCO_3^-	BE
Uncompensated respiratory acidosis	↓	↑	N	N
Partially compensated respiratory acidosis	↓	↑	↑	↑
Compensated respiratory acidosis	N	↑	↑	↑
Uncompensated respiratory alkalosis	↑	↓	N	N
Partially compensated respiratory alkalosis	↑	↓	↓	↓
Compensated respiratory alkalosis	N	↓	↓	↓
Uncompensated metabolic acidosis	↓	N	↓	↓
Partially compensated metabolic acidosis	↓	↓	↓	↓
Compensated metabolic acidosis	N	↓	↓	↓
Uncompensated metabolic alkalosis	↑	N	↑	↑
Partially compensated metabolic alkalosis	↑	↑	↑	↑
Compensated metabolic alkalosis	N	↑	↑	↑
Mixed respiratory and metabolic acidosis	↓↓	↑	↓	↓
Mixed respiratory and metabolic alkalosis	↑↑	↓	↑	↑

↓, Decreased; ↑, increased; N, normal.

Although an arterial blood sample is ideal and provides most reliable information, both venous and capillary blood samples can be used in absence of arterial access but require appropriate interpretation based on the site of sampling. However, it is important to note that venous or capillary blood gases should only be used to assess the ventilation (based on $PaCO_2$) and the acid–base status (based on pH and bicarbonate values). PO_2 in either venous or capillary blood gas sample can provide some information on adequacy of tissue oxygenation but has no correlation with PaO_2. A blood gas analyzer provides actual pH, PCO_2, and PO_2, with calculated values of HCO_3 and base excess. In addition, most blood gas machines

also have a cooximeter which is required to measure Hb, carboxyhemoglobin (COHb), methemoglobin (MetHb), and SaO_2 and this data can be used to calculate the oxygen content in the blood (CaO_2). Proper interpretation of a blood gas result requires information on altitude and fraction of oxygen in inspired air (FiO_2) to determine partial inspiratory pressure of oxygen (PiO_2) by using the alveolar gas equation.

Alveolar gas equation
$$PiO_2 = FiO_2 \times Barometric\ pressure\ (PB)$$

Alveolar PO_2 (PAO_2) is directly related to partial pressure of inspired oxygen PiO_2 and inversely related to alveolar PCO_2. Since alveolar gas exchange occurs by simple diffusion, PaO_2 can never exceed PAO_2. This difference between PAO_2 and PaO_2 is called alveolar–arterial oxygen gradient or difference (A–aDO_2) and can be used as a marker of severity of the lung disease.

Erroneous blood gas results can occur if blood sample contains air bubbles, dilution from infusing fluids (especially TPN containing dextrose), and excessive heparin. Air bubbles can lead to overestimation of PaO_2 and underestimation of $PaCO_2$. Dilution of a blood gas sample with IV fluids will lead to spuriously low PaO_2 and $PaCO_2$ as both CO_2 and O_2 will diffuse from blood into the diluting fluid. However, due to the buffering capability of blood, pH may not change much. Excessive heparin can lower the pH of the sample. Another factor affecting the results of a blood gas sample is the body temperature. Blood gas machines analyze all samples at $37\,°C$. This means that a blood sample from a febrile patient gets cooled down and a sample from a hypothermic patient is warmed up during the analysis thus altering the values of PaO_2 and $PaCO_2$. As a result, measured PaO_2 and $PaCO_2$ are higher than in a hypothermic patient and lower in a febrile patients [17,18]. A change in temperature by each degree centigrade will change PaO_2 by about 5 mmHg and $PaCO_2$ by about 2 mmHg. Because of the effects of temperature on oxyhemoglobin dissociation curve and basal oxygen consumption, both SaO_2 and SvO_2 are affected by changes in the body temperature. A decrease in the body temperature shifts oxyhemoglobin dissociation curve to the left and lowers the tissue oxygen consumption. In contrast, any increase in body temperature has the opposite effect. As a result at any given PaO_2, both SaO_2 and SvO_2 will be higher in a hypothermic patient and lower in a febrile patient [17].

Noninvasive monitoring

Pulse oximetry

Use of pulse oximetry for continuous assessment of oxygen saturations has significantly improved care of critically ill patients of all ages and is the standard of care in all developed countries. In addition to being noninvasive, oxygen saturations using pulse oximetry (SpO_2) have been shown to correlate well with arterial oxygen saturations (SaO_2) measured by cooximeter on blood gas analyzers. However, there are differences between SpO_2 and SaO_2, which are important for all clinicians to know in order to make appropriate decisions about the patient care. SpO_2 is also referred to as functional oxygen saturations and is expressed as:

Functional oxygen saturations = Oxyhemoglobin/ (Oxyhemoglobin + Deoxyhemoglobin)

In contrast, SaO_2 is the oxygenated fraction of the total hemoglobin and is also called fractional oxygen saturations.

Fractional oxygen saturations = Oxyhemoglobin/ Total hemoglobin

The total hemoglobin in the above equation includes types of hemoglobin with limited or no capacity to bind with oxygen, such as COHb, MetHb, and others. Since levels of COHb and MetHb are low in most clinical situations, the correlation between SpO_2 and SaO_2 is fairly good with SaO_2 being 2%–3% lower than accurately measured SpO_2. However, under certain clinical conditions, a pulse oximeter can overestimate oxygen saturations by as much as 6% and the correlation between SpO_2 and SaO_2 is significantly lower when less than 80% of hemoglobin is oxygenated [19]. Other factors affecting the accuracy of SpO_2 include improper probe placement, motion artifact, electromagnetic and ambient light interference, irregular rhythm, loss of pulsatile circulation, and poor perfusion states [20]. These factors tend to cause erroneously low SpO_2 readings. The effect of skin color on SpO_2 has been evaluated in several studies [20–25]. Although pulse oximetry is considered accurate in presence of jaundice, some earlier studies observed that SpO_2 readings in dark infants may not be reliable especially when SaO_2 is less than 80% [22–24]. However, a recent study using current generation of pulse oximeters in infants with hypoxemia secondary to CCHD did not find any difference in SpO_2 based on skin pigment [25].

Simultaneous pre- and postductal SpO_2 measurement can provide significant clues to the etiology of HRF in infants with PDA. A lower postductal SpO_2 suggests right-to-left shunt at the level of PDA and is seen in infants with PPHN and many duct-dependent CCHD such as hypoplastic left heart and coarctation of aorta. As per current guidelines, a postductal SpO_2 lower by 4% or more is considered significant and an indication to obtain echocardiogram to exclude critical congenital heart disease [26]. A higher postductal SpO_2, sometimes referred to as "reverse differential cyanosis", is rare and seen in infants with complex critical congenital heart lesions such as dextrotransposition of the great arteries with persistent pulmonary hypertension or aortic interruption/coarctation.

Noninvasive PO_2 and PCO_2 monitoring

Transcutaneous PO_2 ($PtcO_2$) and transcutaneous PCO_2 ($PtcCO_2$) monitoring equipment are available but have significant limitations for widespread use. These systems require skin temperature to be 42–45°C to improve perfusion, which increases the risk of skin burns with prolonged use. Factors affecting the results include hypotension, shock, peripheral vasoconstriction, edema, patient movement, improper placement of the sensor and equipment calibration errors [27]. In a recent retrospective, cohort study from a large neonatal ICU, authors observed only a moderate correlation between $PtcCO_2$ and PCO_2 but reported reduction in the number of blood gases done in infants on $PtcCO_2$ monitors [28]. No difference in duration of mechanical ventilation and major morbidities was noted [28].

End-tidal CO_2 ($PetCO_2$) measurement, also called capnography, has been suggested as an alternative method of continuous, noninvasive monitoring of PCO_2 [29–35]. These devices can be either qualitative, also known as colorimetric detectors, detect the presence or absence of CO_2 in exhaled air, or quantitative which provide the exact value of PCO_2 in exhaled air. Use of these devices to confirm successful endotracheal intubation is strongly recommended and is becoming a routine practice in most units [36,37]. The continuous quantitative measurements of $PetCO_2$ correlate well with $PaCO_2$ in healthy adults but are somewhat less reliable in critically ill patients with high PCO_2 values. Higher respiratory rates and smaller tidal volumes in neonates have been cited as some of the reasons for poor correlation between $PetCO_2$ and $PaCO_2$ in neonates and young infants [29]. Although capnography has become a standard of care for intubated patients in operating rooms, its use in neonatal intensive care is variable.

Assessment of severity

Alveolar–arterial gradient and ($A-aDO_2$)

$A-aDO_2$, the difference between PAO_2 and PaO_2, reflects the degree of V/Q mismatch or diffusion impairment. Normal $A-aDO_2$ in healthy adults in room air is 5–15 mmHg but is usually between 25 and 30 mmHg in a newborn due to small amount of right-to-left shunt through PFO. Normal value for $A-aDO_2$ in healthy adults breathing 100% oxygen can be significantly higher in absence of any cardiopulmonary disease because high FiO_2 will lead to increase in both PAO_2 and PaO_2 but the increase in PAO_2 is higher than the increase in PaO_2. A–aDO_2 in healthy adults breathing 100% can be 80–120 depending on the age of the patient [38]. A–aDO_2 is calculated using the following formula:

$$A - aDO_2 = [(PB - PH_2O) \times FiO_2] - (PaCO_2 \div RQ) - PaO_2$$

PB = Atmospheric pressure (760 mmHg at sea level)
PH_2O = Partial vapor pressure (47 mmHg in inhaled air in alveoli at 37°C)
FiO_2 = Fraction of oxygen in inspired air
PaO_2 = Partial pressure of oxygen in arterial blood
$PaCO_2$ = Partial pressure of carbon dioxide in arterial blood
RQ = Respiratory quotient (1 with purely carbohydrate diet but 0.8 on a regular diet)

For all practical purposes, for an infant on 100% oxygen at sea level this equation can be simplified as

$$A - aDO_2 = 713 - PaO_2 - PaCO_2$$

Based on observations that A–aDO_2 higher than 600–620 mmHg for 8–12 consecutive hours is associated with 80%–100% mortality rate, an A–aDO_2 >605–620 mmHg for 4–12 h is recommended as one of the criteria for considering extracorporeal membrane oxygenation (ECMO) [39–42].

Arterial to alveolar (a–A) oxygen ratio

The a–A oxygen ratio is calculated by dividing the PaO_2 by PAO_2 and is another measure of oxygen transfer across the lung. The normal value of a–A oxygen ratio is greater than 0.9. In patients breathing higher FiO_2, a–A oxygen ratio is reported to be more reliable indicator of pulmonary gas exchange as compared to A–aDO_2 [43]. Arterial to alveolar (a–A) oxygen ratio of less than 0.22 has been used in several studies as a cutoff for administration of surfactant and ≤0.10 was considered as severe respiratory failure [44,45].

Oxygenation index

The oxygenation index (OI), a frequently used indicator of severity of lung disease in neonates with HRF, is calculated as follows:

$$OI = [MAP \times FiO_2 \div PaO_2] \times 100$$

The OI has been recommended to determine the need for rescue therapies such as ECMO, as well as to predict survival and outcome in conditions such as CDH. OI of more than 15–20 has been used as a cutoff for moderate

disease severity and initiation of iNO in several studies. The OI of ≥25 indicates severe hypoxemic respiratory failure and a value of >40 has been a long-standing criterion for consideration of ECMO in many centers. In a prospective study of pediatric HRF, peak OI was an independent predictor of outcome and a steadily increasing risk of death was observed with increasing OI [46]. A recent retrospective, multicenter study of infants born with CDH reported that best OI on first day of life is one of the best prognostic factors for survival in these infants [47].

Oxygen saturation index

Oxygen saturation index (OSI) is similar to OI but substitutes SpO_2 for PaO_2.

$$OSI = [100 \times MAP \times FiO_2] \div SpO_2$$

Correlation between OSI and OI and utility of OSI in newborns and children with HRF has been evaluated in several studies [48,49]. Based on the data from 255 children with ALI/ARDS, investigators estimated that an OSI of 6.5 would be equivalent to an OI of 5.3 and PaO_2/FiO_2 ratio of 300 (well accepted criteria for the diagnosis of ALI in children), and an OSI of 7.8 would equal PaO_2/FiO_2 ratio of 200 (criteria for the diagnosis of ARDS) and an OI of 8.1 [48].

Respiratory severity score

The respiratory severity score (RSS) is calculated using the following formula:

$$RSS = MAP \times FiO_2$$

An advantage of RSS is that it can be calculated in patients with no arterial access and PaO_2. RSS was used in a large multicenter trial in which preterm infants undergoing mechanical ventilation were treated with a SpO_2 goal of 88%–94% and were expected to have a PaO_2 range of 40–70 mmHg. Based on these assumptions, a severity score of 3.5 was considered equivalent to an oxygenation index between 5 and 9 [50]. Other investigators have reported a strong association between RSS and OI in infants with oxygen saturation (SaO_2) between 88% and 94% ($R^2 = 0.982$, $n = 101$; $P < 0.001$) [51]. With SpO_2 between 88% and 94%, RSS of ≥3 correlated with an OI of ≥4.9 (95% CI, 3.4–6.5) and RSS of ≥10 was consistent with an OI of ≥14.1 (12.5–15.8) [51]. A correlation outside these SpO_2 range has not been evaluated.

PaO_2/FiO_2 ratio

The PaO_2/FiO_2 ratio, also called P/F ratio, is another common measure of oxygenation and is most often employed in ventilated patients. A normal PaO_2/FiO_2 ratio is

300–500 mmHg, with values less than 300 mmHg indicating abnormal gas exchange and values less than 200 mmHg indicating severe hypoxemia. A P/F ratio ≤ 300 and ≤ 200, respectively, have been used to define ALI and ARDS [52].

SpO$_2$/FiO$_2$ ratio

SpO$_2$/FiO$_2$ (S/F) ratios provide information like P/F ratio but have the advantage of being calculated in patients with no arterial access and PaO$_2$. However, it can only be used in patients with saturations in 80%–97% range since the oxyhemoglobin dissociation curve is nearly linear with SpO$_2$ in this range. In a large ARDS network trial of 672 patients, S/F ratios correlated well with P/F ratios [52]. It was estimated that an S/F ratio of 235 correlates with a P/F ratio of 200 and an S/F ratio of 315 correlates with P/F ratio 300 in a cohort of patients with ALI and ARDS [52]. These findings have been validated by several subsequent studies in children with ALI or ARDS [53–56].

Use of P/F and S/F ratio has not been validated in neonatal HRF yet.

Different studies have used different indices of severity of HRF, but it is important to note that each scoring system provides somewhat different information, and these are not completely interchangeable. Of these indices, OI, A–aDO$_2$, and a/A ratio are used most frequently in newborns. In a study of 155 preterm infants below 34 weeks of gestation, investigators compared ability of these three indices to predict respiratory outcome [57]. All three parameters, OI, A–aDO$_2$, and a/A ratio, were similar in their ability to predict the combined outcome of CLD/death. However, none of these indices were superior to birth weight or gestational alone in predicting this outcome [57]. In a similar study in late preterm infants (gestational age 34 0/7–36 6/7), the ability of the maximum A–aDO$_2$ (AUC 0.97), minimum a/A ratio (AUC 0.95), and minimum PaO$_2$/FiO$_2$ (AUC 0.95) to predict need for mechanical ventilation were similar [58]. The cutoff values with highest predictive ability were reported to be >200 mmHg for A–aDO$_2$, <180 mmHg for PaO$_2$/FiO$_2$, and <0.3 for a/A ratio [58].

Management

The initial steps in management of an infant with HRF include stabilizing and securing the airway, and attention to breathing and circulation. Supplemental oxygen and appropriate ventilator support should be provided, and vascular access should be established. Appropriate treatment of underlying condition responsible for HRF such as HMD, pneumonia must be initiated without delay. Other goals of care include prevention of iatrogenic lung injury while maintaining adequate perfusion and oxygenation to avoid organ injury. The clinical management of underlying conditions such as HMD or PPHN is discussed in individual chapters on these topics. However, certain basic principles guiding care of neonates with HRF are briefly discussed here.

Respiratory support

Adequate and optimum respiratory support is the key to the management of neonates with HRF. Patients in initial stages of HRF can be managed effectively with different modes of respiratory support, such as low/high flow nasal cannulas, CPAP, noninvasive mechanical ventilation, and supplemental oxygenation [59–63]. However, most cases with severe and advanced HRF will require intubation and mechanical ventilation. Different ventilation modalities such as pressure-limited ventilation, volume-targeted ventilation and high frequency ventilation among others have been studied in neonates. However, there is limited evidence to support if any one modality is superior to others [59,63–67]. Some recent studies have shown that volume-targeted ventilation may be better than pressure-limited ventilation in preterm infants [68,69]. Irrespective of the ventilation modality used, adequate lung expansion and synchronization between patient and ventilator are necessary to obtain good gas exchange. Optimum continuous airway distending pressure is the key to adequate lung expansion. The goal is to use the minimum airway distending pressure necessary to achieve lung expansion up to 9–10 ribs on chest X-ray. A prudent use of sedatives and analgesics may help in reducing pain, decreasing oxygen utilization, and improve ventilation by improving synchronization and compliance. Use of permissive hypercapnia and permissive hypoxia has also been suggested in order to minimize iatrogenic lung injury in these patients.

Permissive hypercapnia

Permissive hypercapnia is a frequently used lung protective strategy in mechanically ventilated patients. The underlying concept is that accepting higher than normal PCO$_2$ will reduce the barotrauma and thus decrease the likelihood of ventilator-induced lung injury and chronic lung disease. Mild to moderate hypercapnia in animal models has been shown to increase lung compliance, improve V/Q match, but has variable effects on airway resistance and diaphragmatic function [70]. Hemodynamic effects of hypercapnia include increased cardiac output, cerebral vasodilatation with increased cerebral blood flow, and reduced microvascular permeability [70]. Effects of mild to moderate hypercapnia in the setting of pulmonary hypertension and sepsis are less clear.

Although this strategy has been used in patients of all ages, its use in neonates gained acceptance in late 1990s and continues to be widely practiced despite the lack of evidence to support its use in neonates [71,72]. There is a lack of consensus on what level of PCO_2 is safe and acceptable in newborns, and different studies have used different cutoffs to describe permissive hypercapnia. One of the earliest studies focused on short-term outcomes of infants with permissive hypercapnia ($PaCO_2$ in 45–55 mmHg range) compared to infants with normal $PaCO_2$ (35–45 mmHg) in the first 96 h of life and reported that permissive hypercapnia allowed faster weaning from the ventilator [73]. Two subsequent randomized studies with higher $PaCO_2$ targets in permissive hypercapnia groups reported no reduction in the incidence of death or BPD [74,75]. However, a significantly increased combined outcome of mental impairment or death ($P < 0.05$) was reported in the permissive hypercapnia group (target $PaCO_2$ between 55 and 65 mmHg for the first 7 days of life) in one of these studies [75]. Two other studies also reported that hypercapnia in first few days of life was associated with severe intraventricular hemorrhage and adverse neurodevelopmental outcome in preterm infants [76,77].

In a randomized controlled multicenter trial from Germany entitled permissive hypercapnia in extremely low birth weight infants (PHELBI), 362 ELBW infant were enrolled and randomly assigned to either a high target or control group [78]. Target PCO_2 values in permissive hypercapnia group were 55–65 mmHg for first 3 postnatal days, 60–70 mmHg from days 4 to 6, and 65–75 mmHg on days 7–14, the target PCO_2 in the control group was 40–50 mmHg, 45–55 mmHg, and 50–60 mmHg for the corresponding three periods. There were no significant differences in important neonatal outcomes, such as rates of BPD or death, mortality, intraventricular hemorrhage, and retinopathy of prematurity in the two groups [78]. No differences were found on neurodevelopmental assessment at 2 years ± 3 months corrected age either [79]. A recently published meta-analysis of these studies concluded that permissive hypercapnia is of no benefit in extremely low birth weight infants and does not reduce the rates of BPD, mortality, IVH, PVL, NEC, ROP, and had no impact on neurodevelopmental outcomes of these infants [72]. The risks and benefits of PH in term infants with HRF have not been studied systematically. However, several studies have reported it to be well tolerated and to improve survival in patients with congenital diaphragmatic hernia [80–82].

Permissive hypoxia

Although supplemental oxygen is necessary for management of newborns with HRF, controversy exists on ideal oxygen saturation targets in infants requiring supplemental oxygen especially in preterm infants. A better understanding of harmful effects of free-oxygen radicals and reports of associations between liberal oxygen use and adverse outcomes such as retinopathy of prematurity and lung injury promoted the practice of accepting relatively low oxygen saturations in infants with HRF [83–93]. On the other hand, there are concerns that too restrictive use of oxygen can lead to tissue hypoxia, adverse neurodevelopmental outcomes, and even increased mortality. The ideal range of oxygen saturation in these infants remains unclear. To answer this important question, several large double-blind, randomized, multicenter studies have been completed [94–98]. Although there were some minor differences in the protocol design of these studies, all studies compared short- and long-term outcome of ELBW infants managed with low oxygen saturation (high 80's) compared to higher oxygen saturation target (low 90's). Some of the concerns cited about these studies include significant overlap in SpO_2 between the two groups, accuracy of SpO_2 monitors, and oxygen-saturation calibration problem requiring update to the SpO_2 monitor in two of these studies. Two meta-analyses of these studies have been published [99–100]. The first meta-analysis, neonatal oxygenation prospective meta-analysis (NEOPROM), concluded that relative risks for mortality (1.41, CI 1.14–1.74) and NEC (1.25, CI 1.05–1.49) are significantly increased in low compared to high oxygen saturation target infants [99]. The RR for severe retinopathy of prematurity was significantly reduced to low as compared with high oxygen saturation target infants, and there were no differences in rates of BPD and brain injury between the two groups [99]. Although the second meta-analysis also observed a significant increase in mortality and NEC in low oxygen saturation group, the authors cautioned that the quality of evidence for these outcomes was moderate to low and uncertainty remains about the optimal target range for SpO_2 in ELBW infants [100]. Follow-up at 18–24 months corrected age has been published for these studies and no significant differences in the primary outcome of death or major disability between the low and high oxygen saturation target groups were seen [97,101,102]. A recently published Cochrane review concluded that targeting lower (85%–89%) SpO_2 increased the average risk of mortality by 28 per 1000 infants but had no significant effect on the composite outcome of death or major disability or on major disability alone [103]. In a clinical report on this topic, the AAP Committee on Fetus and Newborn concluded that the ideal oxygen saturation range is likely to be patient-specific and will vary based on several factors, such as gestational age at birth, postnatal age, and presence or absence of different complications of prematurity [104]. Although there are no evidence-based recommendations for SpO_2 targets in late preterm and term infants, it is prudent to keep SpO_2 levels in the range of 90%–95% in all newborns with HRF.

Surfactant replacement therapy

Surfactant deficiency is one of the most common causes of HRF in premature infants. Exogenous administration of surfactant in these infants has been shown to reduce mortality and morbidity [105–108]. Although multiple randomized trials and meta-analyses have shown surfactant therapy to be beneficial in preterm infants with HRF, the optimal dose and timing of administration have not been clearly defined [105–108]. Current evidence supports an individualized approach and the decision to administer surfactant should be based on the severity of lung disease and the degree of respiratory support to maintain ventilation and oxygenation [105]. Although a detailed discussion on this topic is provided in chapter on surfactant (Chapter 24: Respiratory Distress Syndrome and Surfactant Therapy) of this book, some key principles are:

- Currently available natural and synthetic surfactants are equally effective. However, clinical trials are on the way to produce improved synthetic surfactants.
- A phospholipid dose of at least 100 mg/kg is required for good clinical response but an initial dose of 200 mg/kg may be superior.
- Although routine prophylactic administration is not recommended at any gestational age, it should be administered early in the course of the disease.
- Surfactant replacement in infants with MAS improves oxygenation and reduces the need for ECMO.
- Role of surfactant replacement in patients with conditions associated with possible surfactant inactivation such as in patients with neonatal pneumonia, pulmonary hemorrhage, and others is less well established and requires further study.

- Routine use of surfactant in term infants with CDH has not been shown to improve clinical course or outcome.

Extracorporeal membrane oxygenation (ECMO)

ECMO, a form of cardiopulmonary bypass, has been shown to be a lifesaving intervention in newborns with HRF unresponsive to maximal medical management. A multicenter, randomized trial from the United Kingdom demonstrated that the use of ECMO in critically ill neonates reduced mortality nearly by half (59% without use of ECMO and 39% with ECMO) [109]. The improvement in survival was noted irrespective of the underlying pathology. Use of inhaled nitric oxide and other vasodilator therapies in addition to improved ventilation strategies have led to a significant reduction in the number of infants requiring ECMO over the last 2 decades. An important limiting factor is the gestational age of the infant. The need for systemic heparinization and technical difficulties of cannulating infants below 2000 g birth weight preclude its use in newborns born at less than 34 weeks of gestation at birth. Other common exclusion criteria include presence of major IVH, significant coagulopathy, lethal congenital malformation, irreversible brain injury or pulmonary pathology. Currently, ECMO is only used as a rescue therapy for late preterm and term newborns with a very high risk of death with standard treatment. Further research is necessary to evaluate if it can be beneficial in infants with less severe disease. A detailed discussion of different types of ECMO, inclusion criteria, complications, and outcome is provided in chapter on ECMO (Chapter 22: Extracorporeal Membrane Oxygenation for Refractory Respiratory Failure) of this book.

References

[1] Angus DC, Linde-Zwirble WT, Clermont G, Griffin MF, Clark RH. Epidemiology of neonatal respiratory failure in the United States. Am J Respir Crit Care Med 2001;164:1154–1160.

[2] Petersson J, Glenny RW. Gas exchange and ventilation-perfusion relationships in the lung. Eur Respir J 2014;44(4):1023–1041.

[3] Wagner PD. The physiological basis of pulmonary gas exchange: implications for clinical interpretation of arterial blood gases. Eur Respir J 2015;45(1):227–243.

[4] West JB. Ventilation-perfusion inequality and overall gas exchange in computer models of the lung. Respir Physiol 1969;7:88–110.

[5] West Jb, Dollery CT, Naimark A. Distribution of blood flow in isolated lung; relation to vascular and alveolar pressures. J Appl Physiol 1964;19:713–724.

[6] Galvin I, Drummond GB, Nirmalan M. Distribution of blood flow and ventilation in the lung: gravity is not the only factor. Br J Anaesth 2007;98(4):420–428.

[7] Richard JC, Bregeon F, Costes N, Bars DL, Tourvieille C, Lavenne F, et al. Effects of prone position and positive end-expiratory pressure on lung perfusion and ventilation. Crit Care Med 2008;36(8):2373–2380.

[8] Marx GR, Allen HD, Goldberg SJ, Flinn CJ. Transatrial septal velocity measurement by Doppler echocardiography in atrial septal defect: correlation with Qp:Qs ratio. Am J Cardiol 1985;55(9): 1162–1167.

[9] Morimoto K, Matsuzaki M, Tohma Y, Ono S, Tanaka N, Michishige H, et al. Diagnosis and quantitative evaluation of secundum-type atrial septal defect by transesophageal Doppler echocardiography. Am J Cardiol 1990;66(1):85–91.

[10] Cloez JL, Schmidt KG, Birk E, Silverman NH. Determination of pulmonary to systemic blood flow ratio in children by a simplified Doppler echocardiographic method. J Am Coll Cardiol 1988;11(4):825–830.

[11] Wang ZJ, Reddy GP, Gotway MB, Yeh BM, Higgins CB. Cardiovascular shunts: MR imaging evaluation. RadioGraphics 2003;23(Suppl. 1):S181–S194.

[12] Parker JA, Treves S. Radionuclide detection, localization, and quantitation of intracardiac shunts

and shunts between the great arteries. Prog Cardiovasc Dis 1977;20:121–150.

[13] Smith HL, Jones JG. Non-invasive assessment of shunt and ventilation/perfusion ratio in neonates with pulmonary failure. Arch Dis Child Fetal Neonatal Ed 2001;85:F127–F132.

[14] Rowe L, Jones JG, Quine D, Bhushan SS, Stenson BJ. A simplified method for deriving shunt and reduced VA/Q in infants. Arch Dis Child Fetal Neonatal Ed 2010;95(1):F47–F52.

[15] Quine D, Wong CM, Boyle EM, Jones JG, Stenson BJ. Non-invasive measurement of reduced ventilation:perfusion ratio and shunt in infants with bronchopulmonary dysplasia: a physiological definition of the disease. Arch Dis Child Fetal Neonatal Ed 2006;91(6):F409–F414.

[16] Dassios T, Curley A, Morley C, Ross-Russell R. Using measurements of shunt and ventilation-to-perfusion ratio to quantify the severity of bronchopulmonary dysplasia. Neonatology 2015;107(4):283–288.

[17] Bacher A. Effects of body temperature on blood gases. Intensive Care Med 2005;31(1):24–27.

[18] Alston TA. Blood gases and pH during hypothermia: the "-stats". Int Anesthesiol Clin 2004;42(4):73–80.

[19] Shiao SY, Ou CN. Validation of oxygen saturation monitoring in neonates. Am J Crit Care 2007;16(2):168–178.

[20] Fouzas S, Priftis KN, Anthracopoulos MB. Pulse oximetry in pediatric practice. Pediatrics 2011;128(4):740–752.

[21] Nitzan M, Romem A, Koppel R. Pulse oximetry: fundamentals and technology update. Med Devices (Auckl) 2014;7:231–239.

[22] Callahan JM. Pulse oximetry in emergency medicine. Emerg Med Clin North Am 2008;26(4):869–879.

[23] Feiner JR, Severinghaus JW, Bickler PE. Dark skin decreases the accuracy of pulse oximeters at low oxygen saturation: the effects of oximeter probe type and gender. Anesth Analg 2007;105(Suppl. 6):S18–S23.

[24] Bickler PE, Feiner JR, Severinghaus JW. Effects of skin pigmentation on pulse oximeter accuracy at low saturation. Anesthesiology 2005;102(4):715–719.

[25] Foglia EE, Whyte RK, Chaudhary A, Mott A, Chen J, Propert KJ, et al. The effect of skin pigmentation on the accuracy of pulse oximetry in infants with hypoxemia. J Pediatr 2017;182:375–377.

[26] Kemper AR, Mahle WT, Martin GR, Cooley WC, Kumar P, Morrow WR, et al. Strategies for implementing screening for critical congenital heart disease. Pediatrics 2011;128(5):e1259–e1267.

[27] Restrepo RD, Hirst KR, Wittnebel L, Wettstein R. AARC clinical practice guideline: transcutaneous monitoring of carbon dioxide and oxygen: 2012. Respir Care 2012;57(11):1955–1962.

[28] Mukhopadhyay S, Maurer R, Puopolo KM. Neonatal transcutaneous carbon dioxide monitoring—effect on clinical management and outcomes. Respir Care 2016;61(1):90–97.

[29] Molloy EJ, Deakins K. Are carbon dioxide detectors useful in neonates? Arch Dis Child Fetal Neonatal Ed 2006;91(4):F295–F298.

[30] Saunders R, Struys MMRF, Pollock RF, Mestek M, Lightdale JR. Patient safety during procedural sedation using capnography monitoring: a systematic review and meta-analysis. BMJ Open 2017;7(6):e013402.

[31] Wall BF, Magee K, Campbell SG, Zed PJ. Capnography versus standard monitoring for emergency department procedural sedation and analgesia. Cochrane Database Syst Rev 2017;3:CD010698.

[32] Leone TA, Lange A, Rich W, Finer NN. Disposable colorimetric carbon dioxide detector use as an indicator of a patent airway during noninvasive mask ventilation. Pediatrics 2006;118(1):e202–e204.

[33] Ornato JP, Shipley JB, Racht EM, Slovis CM, Wrenn KD, Pepe PE, et al. Multicenter study of a portable, hand-size, colorimetric end-tidal carbon dioxide detection device. Ann Emerg Med 1992;21(5):518–523.

[34] Garey DM, Ward R, Rich W, Heldt G, Leone T, Finer NN. Tidal volume threshold for colorimetric carbon dioxide detectors available for use in neonates. Pediatrics 2008;121(6):e1524–e1527.

[35] Bhende MS, Thompson AE, Cook DR, Saville AL. Validity of a disposable end-tidal CO_2 detector in verifying endotracheal tube placement in infants and children. Ann Emerg Med 1992;21(2):142–145.

[36] Hawkes GA, Kelleher J, Ryan CA, Dempsey EM. A review of carbon dioxide monitoring in preterm newborns in the delivery room. Resuscitation 2014;85(10):1315–1319.

[37] Blank D, Rich W, Leone T, Garey D, Finer N. Pedi-cap color change precedes a significant increase in heart rate during neonatal resuscitation. Resuscitation 2014;85(11):1568–1572.

[38] Kanber GJ, King FW, Eshchar YR, Sharp JT. The alveolar-arterial oxygen gradient in young and elderly men during air and oxygen breathing. Am Rev Respir Dis 1968;97(3):376–381.

[39] Krummel TM, Greenfield LJ, Kirkpatrick BV, Mueller DG, Kerkering KW, Ormazabal M, et al. Alveolar-arterial oxygen gradients versus the Neonatal Pulmonary Insufficiency Index for prediction of mortality in ECMO candidates. J Pediatr Surg 1984;19(4):380–384.

[40] Beck R, Anderson KD, Pearson GD, Cronin J, Miller MK, Short BL. Criteria for extracorporeal membrane oxygenation in a population of infants with persistent pulmonary hypertension of the newborn. J Pediatr Surg 1986;21(4):297–302.

[41] Fakioglu H, Totapally BR, Torbati D, Raszynski A, Sussmane JB, Wolfsdorf J. Hypoxic respiratory failure in term newborns: clinical indicators for inhaled nitric oxide and extracorporeal membrane oxygenation therapy. J Crit Care 2005;20(3):288–293.

[42] Suttner DM, Short BL. Neonatal respiratory ECLS. In: Annich GM, Lynch WR, MacLaren G, Wilson JM, Bartlett RH, editors. Extracorporeal cardiopulmonary support in critical care. 4th ed. Ann Arbor, MI: Extracorporeal Life Support Organization; 2012. p. 225–250.

[43] Doyle DJ. Arterial/alveolar oxygen tension ratio: a critical appraisal. Can Anaesth Soc J 1986;33(4):471–474.

[44] Berry DD, Pramanik AK, Philips JB 3rd, Buchter DS, Kanarek KS, Easa D, et al. Comparison of the effect of three doses of a synthetic surfactant on the alveolar-arterial oxygen gradient in infants weighing > or = 1250 grams with respiratory distress syndrome. American Exosurf Neonatal Study Group II. J Pediatr 1994;124(2):294–301.

[45] Hudak ML, Farrell EE, Rosenberg AA, Jung AL, Auten RL, Durand DJ, et al. A multicenter randomized, masked comparison trial of natural versus synthetic surfactant for the treatment of respiratory distress syndrome. J Pediatr 1996;128(3):396–406.

[46] Trachsel D, McCrindle BW, Nakagawa S, Bohn D. Oxygenation index predicts outcome in children with acute hypoxemic respiratory failure. Am J Respir Crit Care Med 2005;172(2):206–211.

[47] Ruttenstock E, Wright N, Barrena S, Krickhahn A, Castellani C, Desai AP, et al. Best oxygenation index on day 1: a reliable marker for outcome and survival in infants with congenital diaphragmatic hernia. Eur J Pediatr Surg 2015;25(1):3–8.

[48] Thomas NJ, Shaffer ML, Willson DF, Shih MC, Curley MA. Defining acute lung disease in children with the oxygenation saturation index. Pediatr Crit Care Med 2010;11(1):12–17.

[49] Rawat M, Chandrasekharan PK, Williams A, Gugino S, Koenigsknecht C, Swartz D, et al. Oxygen saturation index and severity of hypoxic respiratory failure. Neonatology 2015;107(3):161–166.

[50] Ballard RA, Truog WE, Cnaan A, Martin RJ, Ballard PL, Merrill JD, et al. NO CLD Study Group. Inhaled nitric oxide in preterm infants undergoing mechanical ventilation. N Engl J Med 2006;355(4):343–353.

[51] Iyer NP, Mhanna MJ. Non-invasively derived respiratory severity score and oxygenation index in ventilated newborn infants. Pediatr Pulmonol 2013;48(4):364–369.

[52] Rice TW, Wheeler AP, Bernard GR, Hayden DL, Schoenfeld DA, Ware LB. National Institutes of Health, National Heart, Lung, and Blood Institute ARDS Network. Comparison of the SpO_2/FiO_2 ratio and the PaO_2/FiO_2 ratio in patients with acute lung injury or ARDS. Chest 2007;132(2):410–417.

[53] Khemani RG, Patel NR, Bart RD 3rd, Newth CJL. Comparison of the pulse oximetric saturation/fraction of inspired oxygen ratio and the PaO_2/fraction of inspired oxygen ratio in children. Chest 2009;135(3):662–668.

[54] Khemani RG, Thomas NJ, Venkatachalam V, Scimeme JP, Berutti T, Schneider JB, et al. Pediatric Acute Lung Injury and Sepsis Network Investigators (PALISI). Comparison of SpO_2 to PaO_2 based markers of lung disease severity for children with acute lung injury. Crit Care Med 2012;40(4):1309–1316.

[55] Bilan N, Dastranji A, Ghalehgolab Behbahani A. Comparison of the SpO_2/FiO_2 ratio and the PaO_2/FiO_2 ratio in patients with acute lung injury or acute respiratory distress syndrome.

J Cardiovasc Thorac Res 2015;7(1):28–31.

[56] Chen W, Janz DR, Shaver CM, Bernard GR, Bastarache JA, Ware LB. Clinical characteristics and outcomes are similar in ARDS diagnosed by oxygen saturation/FiO_2 ratio compared with PaO_2/FiO_2 ratio. Chest 2015;148(6):1477–1483.

[57] Subhedar NV, Tan AT, Sweeney EM, Shaw NJ. A comparison of indices of respiratory failure in ventilated preterm infants. Arch Dis Child Fetal Neonatal Ed 2000;83(2):F97–F100.

[58] Dimitriou G, Fouzas S, Giannakopoulos I, Papadopoulos VG, Decavalas G, Mantagos S. Prediction of respiratory failure in late-preterm infants with respiratory distress at birth. Eur J Pediatr 2011;170(1):45–50.

[59] Dunn MS, Kaempf J, de Klerk A, de Klerk R, Reilly M, Howard D, et al. Vermont Oxford Network DRM Study Group. Randomized trial comparing 3 approaches to the initial respiratory management of preterm neonates. Pediatrics 2011;128:e1069–e1076.

[60] Morley CJ, Davis PG, Doyle LW, Brion LP, Hascoet JM, Carlin JB. COIN Trial Investigators. Nasal CPAP or intubation at birth for very preterm infants. N Engl J Med 2008;358:700–708.

[61] Finer NN, Carlo WA, Walsh MC, Rich W, Gantz MG, Laptook AR, et al. SUPPORT Study Group of the Eunice Kennedy Shriver NICHD Neonatal Research Network. Early CPAP versus surfactant in extremely preterm infants. N Engl J Med 2010;362:1970–1979.

[62] Finer NN, Carlo WA, Duara S, Fanaroff AA, Donovan EF, Wright LL, et al. National Institute of Child Health and Human Development Neonatal Research Network. Delivery room continuous positive airway pressure/positive end-expiratory pressure in extremely low birth weight infants: a feasibility trial. Pediatrics 2004;114:651–657.

[63] Kirpalani H, Millar D, Lemyre B, et al. A trial comparing noninvasive ventilation strategies in preterm infants. N Engl J Med 2013;369:611–620.

[64] Rojas-Reyes MX, Orrego-Rojas PA. Rescue high-frequency jet ventilation versus conventional ventilation for severe pulmonary dysfunction in preterm infants. Cochrane Database Syst Rev 2015;10:CD000437.

[65] Cools F, Offringa M, Askie LM. Elective high frequency oscillatory ventilation versus conventional ventilation for acute pulmonary dysfunction in preterm infants. Cochrane Database Syst Rev 2015;3:CD000104.

[66] Cools F, Askie LM, Offringa M, Asselin JM, Calvert SA, Courtney SE, et al. PreVILIG collaboration. Elective high-frequency oscillatory ventilation versus conventional ventilation in preterm infants: a systematic review and meta-analysis of individual patients' data. Lancet 2010;375(9731):2082–2091.

[67] Tapia JL, Urzua S, Bancalari A, Meritano J, Torres G, Fabres J, et al. South American Neocosur Network. Randomized trial of early bubble continuous positive airway pressure for very low birth weight infants. J Pediatr 2012;161(1). 75.e1–80.e1.

[68] Klingenberg C, Wheeler KI, McCallion N, Morley CJ, Davis PG. Volume-targeted versus pressure-limited ventilation in neonates. Cochrane Database Syst Rev 2017;10:CD003666.

[69] Peng W, Zhu H, Shi H, Liu E. Volume-targeted ventilation is more suitable than pressure-limited ventilation for preterm infants: a systematic review and meta-analysis. Arch Dis Child Fetal Neonatal Ed 2014;99(2):F158–F165.

[70] Contreras M, Masterson C, Laffey JG. Permissive hypercapnia: what to remember. Curr Opin Anaesthesiol 2015;28(1):26–37.

[71] Woodgate PG, Davies MW. Permissive hypercapnia for the prevention of morbidity and mortality in mechanically ventilated newborn infants. Cochrane Database Syst Rev 2001;2:CD002061.

[72] Ma J, Ye H. Effects of permissive hypercapnia on pulmonary and neurodevelopmental sequelae in extremely low birth weight infants: a meta-analysis. Springerplus 2016;5(1):764.

[73] Mariani G, Cifuentes J, Carlo WA. Randomized trial of permissive hypercapnia in preterm infants. Pediatrics 1999;104(5 Pt. 1):1082–1088.

[74] Carlo WA, Stark AR, Wright LL, Tyson JE, Papile LA, Shankaran S, et al. Minimal ventilation to prevent bronchopulmonary dysplasia in extremely-low-birth-weight infants. J Pediatr 2002;141(3):370–374.

[75] Thome UH, Carroll W, Wu TJ, Johnson RB, Roane C, Young D, et al. Outcome of extremely preterm infants randomized at birth to

different PaCO$_2$ targets during the first seven days of life. Biol Neonate 2006;90(4):218–225.

[76] McKee LA, Fabres J, Howard G, Peralta-Carcelen M, Carlo WA, Ambalavanan N. PaCO$_2$ and neurodevelopment in extremely low birth weight infants. J Pediatr 2009;155(2). 217.e1–221.e1.

[77] Kaiser JR, Gauss CH, Pont MM, Williams DK. Hypercapnia during the first 3 days of life is associated with severe intraventricular hemorrhage in very low birth weight infants. J Perinatol 2006;26(5):279–285.

[78] Thome UH, Genzel-Boroviczeny O, Bohnhorst B, Schmid M, Fuchs H, Rohde O, et al. PHELBI Study Group. Permissive hypercapnia in extremely low birthweight infants (PHELBI): a randomised controlled multicentre trial. Lancet Respir Med 2015;3(7):534–543.

[79] Thome UH, Genzel-Boroviczeny O, Bohnhorst B, Schmid M, Fuchs H, Rohde O, et al. Neurodevelopmental outcomes of extremely low birthweight infants randomised to different PCO$_2$ targets: the PHELBI follow-up study. Arch Dis Child Fetal Neonatal Ed 2017;102(5):F376–F382.

[80] Boloker J, Bateman DA, Wung JT, Stolar CJ. Congenital diaphragmatic hernia in 120 infants treated consecutively with permissive hypercapnea/spontaneous respiration/elective repair. J Pediatr Surg 2002;37(3):357–366.

[81] Guidry CA, Hranjec T, Rodgers BM, Kane B, McGahren ED. Permissive hypercapnia in the management of congenital diaphragmatic hernia: our institutional experience. J Am Coll Surg 2012;214(4). 640–645, 647.

[82] Puligandla PS, Grabowski J, Austin M, Hedrick H, Renaud E, Arnold M, et al. Management of congenital diaphragmatic hernia: a systematic review from the APSA outcomes and evidence based practice committee. J Pediatr Surg 2015;50(11):1958–1970.

[83] Flynn JT, Bancalari E, Snyder ES, Goldberg RN, Feuer W, Cassady J. A cohort study of transcutaneous oxygen tension and the incidence and severity of retinopathy of prematurity. N Engl J Med 1992;326:1050–1054.

[84] Tin W, Milligan DW, Pennefather P, Hey E. Pulse oximetry, severe retinopathy, and outcome at one year in babies of less than 28 weeks gestation. Arch Dis Child Fetal Neonatal Ed 2001;84:F106–F110.

[85] Sun SC. Relation of target SpO$_2$ levels and clinical outcome in ELBW infants on supplementary oxygen (abstract). Pediatr Res 2002;51:350A.

[86] Anderson CG, Benitz WE, Madan A. Retinopathy of prematurity and pulse oximetry: a national survey of recent practices. J Perinatol 2004;24:164–168.

[87] Wright KW, Sami D, Thompson L, Ramanathan R, Joseph R, Farzavandi S. A physiologic reduced oxygen protocol decreases the incidence of threshold retinopathy of prematurity. Trans Am Ophthalmol Soc 2006;104:78–84.

[88] Vanderveen DK, Mansfield TA, Eichenwald EC. Lower oxygen saturation alarm limits decrease the severity of retinopathy of prematurity. J AAPOS 2006;10: 445–448.

[89] Deulofeut R, Critz A, Adams-Chapman I, Sola A. Avoiding hyperoxia in infants < or = 1,250 g is associated with improved short- and long-term outcomes. J Perinatol 2006;26:700–705.

[90] Wallace DK, Veness-Meehan KA, Miller WC. Incidence of severe retinopathy of prematurity before and after a modest reduction in target oxygen saturation levels. J AAPOS 2007;11:170–174.

[91] Noori S, Patel D, Friedlich P, Siassi B, Seri I, Ramanathan R. Effects of low oxygen saturation limits on the ductus arteriosus in extremely low birth weight infants. J Perinatol 2009;29:553–557.

[92] Saugstad OD, Aune D. In search of the optimal oxygen saturation for extremely low birth weight infants: a systematic review and meta-analysis. Neonatology 2011;100:1–8.

[93] Askie LM, Henderson-Smart DJ, Ko H. Restricted versus liberal oxygen exposure for preventing morbidity and mortality in preterm or low birth weight infants. Cochrane Database Syst Rev 2009;1:CD001077.

[94] Carlo WA, Finer NN, Walsh MC, Rich W, Gantz MG, Laptook AR, et al. SUPPORT Study Group of the Eunice Kennedy Shriver NICHD Neonatal Research Network. Target ranges of oxygen saturation in extremely preterm infants. N Engl J Med 2010;362: 1959–1969.

[95] Stenson B, Brocklehurst P, Tarnow-Mordi W. UK BOOST II Trial, Australian BOOST II Trial, New Zealand BOOST II Trial. Increased 36-week survival with high oxygen saturation target in extremely preterm infants. N Engl J Med 2011;364:1680–1682.

[96] Stenson BJ, Tarnow-Mordi WO, Darlow BA, Simes J, Juszczak E, Askie L, et al. BOOST II United Kingdom Collaborative Group, BOOST II Australia Collaborative Group, BOOST II New Zealand Collaborative Group. Oxygen saturation and outcomes in preterm infants. N Engl J Med 2013;368:2094–2104.

[97] Schmidt B, Whyte RK, Asztalos EV, Moddemann D, Poets C, Rabi Y, et al. Canadian Oxygen Trial (COT) Group. Effects of targeting higher vs lower arterial oxygen saturations on death or disability in extremely preterm infants: a randomized clinical trial. JAMA 2013;309:2111–2120.

[98] Johnston ED, Boyle B, Juszczak E, King A, Brocklehurst P, Stenson BJ. Oxygen targeting in preterm infants using the Masimo SET Radical pulse oximeter. Arch Dis Child Fetal Neonatal Ed 2011;96(6):F429–F433.

[99] Saugstad OD, Aune D. Optimal oxygenation of extremely low birth weight infants: a meta-analysis and systematic review of the oxygen saturation target studies. Neonatology 2014;105(1):55–63.

[100] Manja V, Lakshminrusimha S, Cook DJ. Oxygen saturation target range for extremely preterm infants: a systematic review and meta-analysis. JAMA Pediatr 2015;169(4):332–340.

[101] Vaucher YE, Peralta-Carcelen M, Finer NN, et al. SUPPORT Study Group of the Eunice Kennedy Shriver NICHD Neonatal Research Network. Neurodevelopmental outcomes in the early CPAP and pulse oximetry trial. N Engl J Med 2012;367(26):2495–2504.

[102] Darlow BA, Marschner SL, Donoghoe M, et al. Benefits of Oxygen Saturation Targeting-New Zealand (BOOST-NZ) Collaborative Group. Randomized controlled trial of oxygen saturation targets in very preterm infants: two year outcomes. J Pediatr 2014;165(1):30–35.

[103] Askie LM, Darlow BA, Davis PG, Finer N, Stenson B, Vento M, et al. Effects of targeting lower versus higher arterial oxygen saturations on death or disability in preterm infants. Cochrane Database Syst Rev 2017;4:CD011190.

[104] Cummings JJ, Polin RA. Committee on Fetus and Newborn. Oxygen targeting in extremely low birth weight infants. Pediatrics 2016;138(2). pii: e20161576.

[105] Polin RA, Carlo WA. Committee on Fetus and Newborn. Surfactant replacement therapy for preterm and term neonates with respiratory distress. Pediatrics 2014;133(1):156–163.

[106] Lopez E, Gascoin G, Flamant C, Merhi M, Tourneux P, Baud O. French Young Neonatologist Club. Exogenous surfactant therapy in 2013: what is next? Who, when and how should we treat newborn infants in the future? BMC Pediatr 2013;13:165.

[107] Speer CP, Sweet DG, Halliday HL. Surfactant therapy: past, present and future. Early Hum Dev 2013;89(Suppl. 1):S22–S24.

[108] Sardesai S, Biniwale M, Wertheimer F, Garingo A, Ramanathan R. Evolution of surfactant therapy for respiratory distress syndrome: past, present, and future. Pediatr Res 2017;81(1–2):240–248.

[109] UK collaborative randomised trial of neonatal extracorporeal membrane oxygenation. UK Collaborative ECMO Trail Group. Lancet 1996;348(9020):75–82.

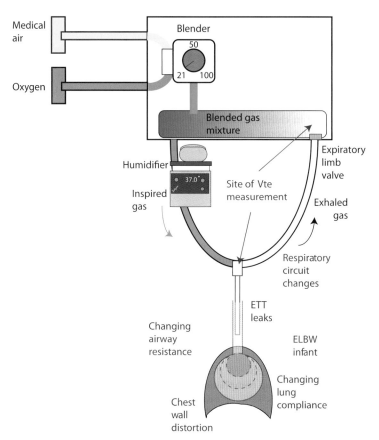

Fig. 9A.1 Basic ventilator design and factors contributing to discrepancies *(red font)* between set and measured values. Copyright: Satyan Lakshminrusimha.

pressure across a fixed resistance type. The Avea, SLE, and VIP Bird all measured airway pressure at the patient connection, while the Dräger ventilators use internal inspiratory and expiratory pressure sensors to compute airway pressure based on the known pressure drop in the patient circuit. And again, a unique circuit is supplied by the manufacturer in some cases (i.e., SLE) but not in others.

During real ventilation of infants, which involves all the variables mentioned, the differences between values set on the ventilators and the delivered ones may at times be even larger than those identified and published in bench studies. These are reasons why it is objectively challenging to make truly meaningful comparisons in clinical ventilatory care. Clinicians that utilize these ventilator parameters should understand the limitations of these measures.

An important significant discrepancy exists between V_{te} measured at a ventilator and that measured with a pneumotachometer sensing at the endotracheal tube in infants. Therefore, in ventilated infants, V_{te} should be determined

with a pneumotachometer or sensor placed at the proximal airway. The Siemens ventilator, the flow sensor measures flow at the distal end of the expiratory tubing.

All ventilators in all bench studies underread the true value in normal simulated lungs by about 2%–8%, reaching a peak of -9% to -11% bias. In contrast, they can overestimate V_{te} for simulated sick lungs (+4% to 10%).

The Avea had the least bias and tighter confidence limits, and remained at a constant mean bias of about -2.0% across various simulated lung conditions. The Dräger Babylog consistently underestimated V_{te} across all three simulated lung conditions at between -8 and -11%.

Bias in the compliance measurements

Some respirators (Avea, VIP Bird, SLE, and others) basically compute compliance as the ratio of V_{te} to peak airway pressure minus PEEP. This would result in underestimation of compliance, as peak airway pressure usually includes a

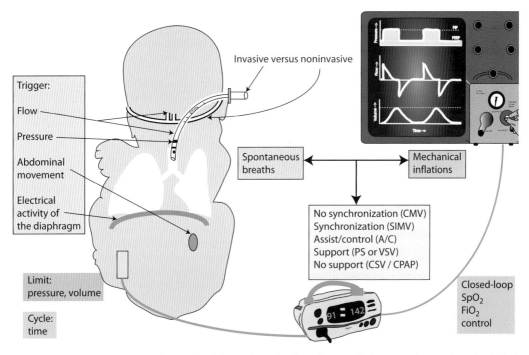

Fig. 9A.2 Modes of Ventilation. The basic factors that define each mode of ventilation include invasive (e.g., endotracheal tube) versus noninvasive (e.g., nasal cannula), synchrony of spontaneous breaths with ventilator inflations, trigger (initiation), limit (maintenance), and cycling (termination of inflation). Closed-loop SpO_2–FiO_2 control is a new feature available with some ventilators. Copyright: Satyan Lakshminrusimha.

resistive element. The Dräger Evita in one study underestimated compliance for all three simulated abnormal lung conditions but overestimated compliance in the simulated normal lung condition (+17% bias).

As another finding from studies, the Avea and SLE both increased in progressing from simulated normal lung condition (−18 and −19%, respectively) to simulated severely ill lung condition (−26% for Avea and −40% for SLE), whereas bias in compliance measurements for the Dräger Babylog remained within the range of −8% to −16% in progressing from normal to severe simulated lung conditions. The observed accuracy differences likely reflect inconsistent methodologies and algorithms used by the manufacturers to compute compliance.

Likewise, inconsistent computation algorithms may account for the wide range in resistance.

Bias in the resistance measurements

There are also difficulties with the measurement of resistance, where the bias could be as low as 1.5–2.0 (Dräger) or 5–7 times worse in other respirators. The Avea does not display resistance values > 100 $cmH_2O/L/s$ by manufacturer design.

Assessment of accuracy and precision of measurements

In an actual lung, changes in PEEP and PIP level may both alter the functional residual capacity and shift V_t excursions along the sigmoidal pressure–volume response of the lung with concomitant changes in compliance and resistance. But for testing and comparison purposes, it is desirable to keep compliance and resistance constant, as is the case with the single or multicompartment linear lung model.

According to the International Standards Organization for testing ventilators, all of the ventilator manufacturers stated a range of accuracy of ±8% to ±10% for pulmonary function measures. Most of the tested ventilators generally conform to this with normal lung mechanics when V_t are largest. However, in preterm sick infants and in simulated severe lung mechanics V_t are smallest. We and others have shown inaccuracies in the measurements of neonatal ventilators. Accuracy of the V_t measurements also demonstrates some dependency on the level of PIP and PEEP and the degree of bias or errors in measurements in all machines studied varied by the severity of simulated lung condition. Such variability limits clinical use of these measurements. As we first demonstrated that V_{te} as measured by three then commonly used ventilators and two freestanding PMM, differed markedly and that in clinical neonatology no "gold standards" for V_{te} or other respiratory parameters existed, we and others concluded that V_t readings are inaccurate and vary widely between different ventilators and freestanding PMM.

Additionally, and probably as important, the shape of the V_t delivery over time may also influence pathology. Only further studies can delineate the underlying causes for the discrepancies, errors, and impact on pathology, perhaps using a multicompartment nonlinear lung model.

Ventilator mode classification

In the past several years, automatization of neonatal ventilators has progressively increased with advances on sensor technology and microprocessors. The different modes of neonatal ventilation have expanded tremendously with this automatization. It is really amazing that modern infant ventilators have 15 and up to 25 modes possibilities. This is not simple for clinicians at the bedside!

With the aim of easing comprehension and simplifying the approach to neonatal ventilation, one tactic is to first identify and describe three main points (Table 9A.2). First, is the ventilation invasive (endotracheal tube) or noninvasive (nasal/facial interphase)? Second, how are the infant's breaths? Is she or he breathing spontaneously all the time? When all breaths are spontaneous, we speak of continuous spontaneous ventilation (CSV) as it happens with CPAP and cannula. IMV is when spontaneous breaths are possible between mandatory breaths controlled by the ventilator. The spontaneous respirations may or may not be supported with pressure support (PS), which by definition occurs only in spontaneous breaths. Continuous mandatory ventilation (CMV) is where all breaths are mandatory without spontaneous breathing or triggering (like in apnea of any cause and with high frequency). When some of the spontaneous breaths trigger ventilator breaths, synchronized intermittent ventilation (SIMV) occurs. If the infant triggers all ventilator breaths, the mode is called assist/control (A/C).

Finally, in this initial approach, the modes can be classified according to which is the controlling variable, the pressure, or the volume.

There are many variables that may trigger, limit, and/or end the inspiratory phase and others that influence the expiratory phase and baseline pressure. The more frequently used neonatal ventilators, described later in Table 9A.3, can provide one or more of the different modalities listed in Table 9A.2, where accepted abbreviations are also listed.

Newer ventilatory modes such as VAPS and MMV may prove very beneficial for weaning but have limited clinical experience in the newborn at present. Nasal (noninvasive) HFOV modes have potential, but the problem of insufficient data still persists.

Table 9A.2 Modes of ventilation

Invasive ventilation (synchronized or not)
Noninvasive (nasal) (synchronized or not)
Breathing spontaneously (CPAP; pressure support)
Triggering assisted breaths (SIMV vs. A/C)
No triggering (IMV; HFV; apneic)
Intermittent mandatory ventilation—IMV (spontaneous breaths are possible between mandatory breaths)
Continuous mandatory ventilation—CMV (all breaths are mandatory)
Continuous spontaneous ventilation—CSV (all breaths are spontaneous)
Volume control—VC or pressure control—PC
Time cycled/pressure limited —TCPL (or PC-IMV)
Flow cycled/pressure limited—FCPL
Synchronized intermittent mandatory ventilation—SIMV
Assist/control ventilation—A/C
Inspiratory time termination—ITT
Pressure control ventilation—PCV
Pressure-regulated volume control—PRVC
Pressure support ventilation—PSV
Volume support ventilation—VSV
Volume-targeted ventilation—VTV
Volume guarantee ventilation—VG
Targeted tidal volume plus—TTV^{plus}
Volume assured pressure support—VAPS
Volume target pressure control—VTPC
Volume target pressure support—VTPS
Proportional assist ventilation—PAV
Neurally adjusted ventilatory assist—NAVA *(EAdi: monitoring the electrical activity of the diaphragm)*
High-frequency jet ventilation—HFJV
High-frequency oscillatory ventilation—HFOV
High-frequency "hybrid" ventilation
Noninvasive ventilation (NIV); synchronized (NISIMV)
Nasal intermittent positive ventilation (NIPPV); synchronized (sNIPPV)
Mandatory minute ventilation—MMV
Airway pressure release ventilation—APRV
Auto-FiO$_2$: Closed-loop automatic oxygen control

Commonly used ventilators and ventilator performance comparison

The following tables show salient comparison points for "conventional" ventilators (Table 9A.3) and high-frequency ventilators (HFV) (Table 9A.4).

Based on factors discussed previously, it is difficult, if not impossible, to have a true in vivo performance analysis and comparison. The controlled and rigid conditions that exist

Table 9A.3 Commonly used ventilators in 2017 (alphabetic order)

Respirator	Control variable: volume	Control variable: pressure	Other modes available	Sensor	Other
Avea	A/C (with demand flow); SIMV (demand flow and artificial airway compensation)	A/C; SIMV; TCPL; VG; pressure-regulated volume control	CPAP + PS with volume limit; nasal IMV; airway pressure release; biphasic ventilation	Proximal flow	Flow cycle, demand flow, artificial airway compensation, port for Heliox Closed-loop FiO_2–SpO_2 controls
Bird VIP Gold series^	A/C; SIMV	A/C; SIMV; TCPL; volume target; PS	CPAP + PS		Not manufactured any longer
Bourns/Bear Cub 750^	No	A/C; SIMV		Proximal flow	Not manufactured any longer
Dräger Babylog VN500	No	A/C; SIMV; VG; MMV	APRV; nasal CPAP, noninvasive IMV	Proximal hot wire anemometer	HFOV optional
Dräger Evita XL-neo; Infinity V500 (Various)	A/C; MMV	A/C; SIMV; VG; PS	APRV; CPAP +PS; noninvasive	Flow trigger	Variable PS
Dräger Babylog 8000	No	VG			Not manufactured any longer
Fabian	No	A/S; SIMV;VG; volume limit	Noninvasive; nasal CPAP; PS	Volume trigger; flow trigger	Closed-loop FiO_2–SpO_2 controls; HFOV
Leoni Plus	No	SIMV (+ PS) (+ VG and limitation)	NIV; nasal CPAP		Auto-FiO_2; HFOV
Newport e360 and WAVE	No	A/C; SIMV	VTPC and VTPS; biphasic pressure release	Flow or pressure trigger	Cycling-off timing, breath by breath
HT70 Plus		A/C; SIMV	Noninvasive		Transport
Puritan Bennett 840; 980*	A/C; SIMV (+ PS) volume support	A/C; SIMV (+ PS)	Bilevel (+ PS); synchronized noninvasive		Leak compensation; volume control plus; PAV
Servo-I; NAVA	SIMV; volume control with flow adaptation automode	PRVC; SIMV; Bi-vent; automode	Nasal CPAP; PS; NAVA; volume support; noninvasive	Differential pressure and EAdi	CO_2 monitor; port for Heliox; active exhalation valve
SLE 4000 and 5000	No	SIMV (TCPL and FCPL)	PS; TTV	Differential pressure and flow triggering	HFOV in 5000 model Valveless TTV^plus
Siemens Servo 300A	SIMV; PS	SIMV; PS	PRVC and volume support	Expiratory flow and pressure transducer	
Stephanie (Stephan)	A/C; IMV; SIMV (flow controlled; pressure limit)	A/C; SIMV (pressure controlled; volume limitation)	PS; PAV; NIV (apc*); CPAP: HFV	Flow; pressure (proximal) and apc*	Auto-FiO_2 (Nova) HFOV
Sophie (Stephan)	No	A/C; SIMV; VG (volume target with volume limit; with ITT or not)	PS; NIV; CPAP	Flow (proximal) and apc*	Auto-FiO_2 (Masimo) Optional HFOV

The abbreviations used in this table are summarized in Table 9A.2.
*apc: abdominal pressure capsule

Table 9A.4 High-frequency ventilators

Respirator	Principle for operation	Rate (Hz)	M-MAP (cmH₂O)	Amplitude (cmH₂O)	VTV	Exhalation	Other
Bunnell Life Pulse Jet ventilator	Microprocessor controlled, time cycled, pressure controlled	4–11	Adjusting PEEP	Indirectly by setting PIP and PEEP	No	Passive, unimpeded	Unique mechanism
Sensormedics	Valve oscillator	3–15	45	90	No	Active valve	Electromagnetic flow generator
Twinstream	Electric-driven microprocessor-controlled jet ventilator	1–25	PIP <35	Variable	No	Venturi assisted	Two different jet streams (Pulsatile BiLevel ventilation); Pulsatile CPAP
Dräeger VN500	Venturi assisted expiration (hybrid)	5–20	40	90	Yes	Active valve. Ejector integrated in the valve	Volume guarantee available (VTV)
BabyLog 8000+				% Maximum	NO		*No longer sold*
SLE 5000	Bidirectional jets + CMV	3–20	45	180	No	Valveless	Significant O₂ consumption
Stephanie/ Sophie	Valve oscillator	5–20	30	% Maximum	Yes	Active valve	Differential pressure
Leoni +	Membrane-integrated diaphragms	5–20	40	100	Yes	Active	VTV
Fabian	Voice coil generator	5–20		80	Yes	Active	VTV

M-MAP, Maximum mean airway pressure; *VTV*, volume-targeted ventilation mode. MAP is the "average" pressure delivered to the lung throughout the respiratory cycle.

in simulation models (under which studies have been performed) do not exist in clinical practice.

Table 9A.3 summarizes salient features of commonly used ventilators in 2017, and provides a comparison between them, including the two control variables (volume and/or pressure), the various ventilator modes available, and other issues. As mentioned previously, there are differences in accuracy and precision in V_{te}. It is beyond the scope of this chapter to describe each and every aspect and feature of every single ventilator currently used. Other variables, including sensors used, are briefly described later.

Summary of various factors in neonatal ventilators

Historically, infant ventilators were designed to deliver pressure-limited breaths by diverting a preset constant flow through a pressure pop-off valve. This is referred to as the "time-cycled and pressure-limited" mode. Some modern ventilators like AVEA (CareFusion) still offer this modality.

There are differences in available features in the different respirators and also on the specific terminology each may be using. To stress the importance of knowing completely the ventilator a clinician decides to use for the baby in NICU, I will describe below a few points and examples that show how complex and variable things could be.

Inspiratory flow

This is variable in different ventilators. In volume control modes, it is directly set. The higher the flow for a given V_t, the shorter the T_i. Inspiratory flow is indirectly set during pressure control modes and is a function of the set ΔP and the pressure rise time, for a given value of respiratory system time constant. Peak inspiratory flow decreases as respiratory system resistance increases or the pressure rise time increases. Some ventilators adjust flow according to infant needs.

Flow triggering involves less patient effort and is more commonly used in neonatal/infant ventilators. It has become clear that proximal flow sensors are the best to provide flow-triggered synchronization of ventilator breaths as well as proximal volume measurements. All ventilators except one are that way. However, validity and comparison studies on the wide range of flow sensors clinically in use are very necessary.

Sensors

1. Heated wire anemometer: It measures the amount of current required to keep a heated wire at a constant temperature as gas flows past the wire and heat is convected. This current can be converted to a flow measurement, and integrated to determine volume.
2. Differential pressure pneumotachometer: As gas flows through the sensor across an element, a differential pressure is created between the upstream and downstream sensing ports. The change in pressure across the element is proportional to flow.
3. Abdominal pressure capsule (apc): It is placed over the abdomen "under" the diaphragm. It senses initiation of diaphragmatic excursion. Such capsule (Graseby capsule) was previously used for invasive SIMV ventilation by a ventilator no longer in the market. Currently, one ventilator has it for noninvasive ventilation (Table 9A.3).
4. Neurally adjusted ventilatory assist (NAVA) triggers a ventilator breath with a diaphragmatic neural sensor, by monitoring electrical activity from the diaphragm (EAdi). This technique uses a modified feeding tube containing a number of electrode sensors for the measurement of diaphragmatic EMG (Table 9A.3).

It is known that differing pressure and flow patterns may play a role in observed compliance and resistance discrepancies and have been related to significant variability in the performance of neonatal ventilators.

Pressure triggering

It is sometimes difficult for the VLBW infant to consistently trigger PS with this mode of triggering as compared with flow triggering.

Differences in setting pressure support

In SIMV + PSV mode, the PS level for spontaneous breaths is set (and read) differently in different ventilators. PS is a pressure in cmH_2O above PEEP during spontaneous breaths. In some ventilators, it is set (and read) directly in cmH_2O as such (i.e., 5 cmH_2O). In others, it is read as the pressure above atmospheric pressure (adding PEEP + PS). So, for example, if PEEP were 6 cmH_2O and PS 8 cmH_2O, the pressure above atmospheric pressure will be 14 cmH_2O. In other ventilator, PS is set as % of the delta pressure (PIP–PEEP) used for the mandatory breaths. In such cases, if mandatory breaths were set at PIP 18 cmH_2O and PEEP 6 cmH_2O, the delta pressure will be 12 cmH_2O. If PSV PS is set at 50%, then the PS level during spontaneous breaths will be 0.5 × 12, which would of course be 6 cmH_2O above PEEP. Obviously, pressure above atmospheric pressure during PS spontaneous inflations will be then 6 + 6 = 12 cmH_2O.

Leak compensation

Some ventilators have artificial airway compensation and calculate the drop in pressure through the endotracheal tube and add that amount of pressure to the system. When there is leak compensation, the flow control valve and the exhalation valve work together to compensate for baseline leaks. Leak compensation in invasive and noninvasive modes has wide variations between ventilators. It is not clear if these variations have clinical importance but they can affect synchronization; additionally, leak has been shown to be a major factor leading to autotriggering. A recent study found that the median asynchrony index was up to 29% in invasive ventilation, and 48% in NIV. In view of the fact that an asynchrony index >10% has been considered severe asynchrony in previous studies, the appropriateness of premature/neonatal patient-triggered modes on many ICU ventilators must be questioned.

I will end this section with a few more examples of some terminology and features. The Puritan Bennet respirator has variable features depending on the manufacture date (before 2005 or from later) and the availability of the NeoMode option. Trigger could be chosen to be by flow (preferred) or pressure. PEEP can be predefined. There is a "bilevel" mode which has not been well studied in neonates. This ventilator uses a terminology for pressures which include "Ppeak" which in some way is the limit for the maximum pressure in the circuit. The high alarm will be 2 cmH_2O above maximum pressure. The peak pressure delivered to the baby is called P_i (inspiratory pressure) in this respirator. This P_i is pressure *above* PEEP, and it is the pressure delivered to the lungs during each ventilator breath. If PEEP were 6 cmH_2O and P_i 18, the ventilator will deliver 24 cmH_2O. In order to increase P_i, it is necessary to ensure that the high alarm limit of Ppeak is increased. If not, the chosen P_i will not be delivered. This ventilator also has an algorithm that does not allow to decrease inspiratory pressure to less than PEEP + 5 cmH_2O. Therefore, if PEEP were 6 cmH_2O inspiratory pressure cannot be less than 11 cmH_2O. When the volume mode is used, P_i is usually the same as Ppeak.

Proportional assist ventilation (PAV) is available in some ventilators (Table 9A.3). Elastic and resistive unloading may be used to support the infant's own respiratory effort. Adjusting the degree of elastic and resistive unloading is possible according to the patient's individual needs. This allows compensation for decreased compliance (i.e., increased elastance) and increased resistance of the respiratory system, allowing the patient to use his/her own respiratory control mechanisms.

Close loop or automated FiO$_2$-control (auto-FiO$_2$) is available in a few modern respirators (Table 9A.3). This is not in use in the United States as it has not been approved by the FDA.

Other: The vast majority of current ventilators have low and high alarms, a wide range of pressures and V_t that can be delivered, and "nice graphics," but these are not included in Table 9A.3. Some ventilators allow for Heliox and nitric oxide delivery and most have internal battery and compressor.

High-frequency ventilators

Different HFV are compared in Table 9A.4.

HFV uses lower transpulmonary pressure and V_t than any other modality of assisted ventilation. It can be defined by the type and method of pressure and flow wave measured at the proximal endotracheal tube. These can be considered as square or sine (sinusoidal; triangular) waves. The wave form of most of the HFV is sinusoidal, except for Sensormedics and SLE5000 which have a square waveform. At an alveolar level, all devices deliver some form of a sine wave.

The Bunnell Jet is FDA-approved in the United States. The Sensormedics 3100A and 3100B are the only dedicated HFO ventilators; most other devices are hybrid devices offering conventional and high-frequency ventilation options. Table 9A.4 shows the most significant points comparing HFV.

Amplitude: In HFV, it is the principal determinant of V_t. It is the difference between peak inspiratory pressure (PIP) and positive end-expiratory pressure (PEEP), or "height" of the wave or "delta" pressure (ΔP). Most ventilators display ΔP in cmH$_2$O. The Leoni plus compensates for any leak or change in compliance. Sensor Medics 3100A has lower V_t output at higher frequencies. This can be compensated by increasing the power setting or amplitude.

% Maximum amplitude: Two respirators (Dräger Baby-Log 8000+ and Sophie) display amplitude as a percentage of the maximum delta pressure that the ventilator can generate in that individual infant at the preset frequency, I:E ratio, endotracheal tube, and mean airway pressure (MAP). Therefore, amplitude delivery cannot be assumed to be exchangeable from different ventilators, between infants, or even in the same infant with variable settings. As one example of variability, maximum reported amplitude in vivo settings for Sophie is 80 cmH$_2$O and for Dräger Baby-Log 8000+ is 35 cmH$_2$O.

Inspiratory:expiratory (*I:E*) ratio is usually 1:1–1:3 in most HFV, but the Babylog 8000+ has up to 1:5. V_t is higher with a 1:1 ratio, but expiratory time is shorter.

Diffusion coefficient of CO$_2$ and V_t monitoring: All of the listed ventilators in Table 9A.4, except Sensormedics, Bunnell Jet, and Twinstream, have this capability.

Clinicians should be aware that modern high-frequency oscillators exhibit important differences in the delivered ΔP and V_t. Ventilator-displayed settings are not directly transferable between devices due to differences in oscillator performance. Understanding the behavior of each ventilator remains paramount to its optimal use and application, especially given the wide range of oscillators available. The traditional definition of high-frequency devices as oscillators, jet, or flow-interrupters, with or without active expiratory mechanisms, is no longer appropriate. The characteristics of the generated pressure and flow waveforms vary between devices, and classifying devices as square wave (complex waveform harmonics) or sine wave (simple harmonics) devices is more appropriate. In all published studies, the pattern of attenuation of the pressure wave through the circuit and test lung, and thus delivered V_t, is not consistent for the various oscillators. Additionally, humidification provides a variable that is difficult to standardize. Gas compressive effects of the chamber and the circuits used influence the fidelity of the pressure and flow measurements. Some ventilators (Sophie, Fabian, and Leoni Plus) have dedicated circuits; others do not.

With larger inner diameter of endotracheal tubes (3.5 mm) and low-frequency conditions and I:E ratio 1:1, many devices could generate V_t that would potentially be greater than dead space. At frequencies of 5 and 10 Hz, all ventilators, except Babylog 8000, generated airway pressure amplitudes greater than 28.6 cmH$_2$O and V_t greater than 6 mL at the airway opening. By contrast, at 15 Hz some HFV were unable to produce V_t >3.0 mL at maximum ΔP (i.e., Leoni Plus, Dräger VN500, and BabyLog 8000).

The wide range of flow sensors is also a confounding factor for HFV, especially as more devices offer "volume guarantee" during HFOV.

Similar to conventional ventilators, HFV parameters are not perfect and there are errors and differences in ΔP, T_i, and I:E ratio. MAP may show drifting over time. This may affect CO$_2$ elimination if alveolar ventilation suffers. Insufficient MAP, with inadequate lung volume, can lead to elevated PaCO$_2$, similar to insufficient CPAP and PEEP in conventional modes. Excessive MAP can lead to air trapping and also produce hypercarbia due to "airway obstruction."

Regarding V_t measurements and the mode of VG on HF ventilation, it sounds "attractive," but much more is still needed to determine its accuracy and reliability and whether it has any impact on neonatal outcomes.

Discussion and final comments

The ability to evaluate respiratory mechanics in response to ventilator settings and clinical interventions was difficult or impossible to accomplish in the NICU. Automatization of neonatal ventilation has brought significant advantages, but unfortunately many of them are still not fully understood or used to their full capacity by bedside care providers.

In the past, the clinician had to choose all parameters delivered by the ventilator, and the possibility to track disease progress by measuring pulmonary mechanics and respiratory physiology was nonexistent. Currently, we can evaluate graphics and waves, but setting online continuous estimates of respiratory function is far from perfect in accuracy and reliability; even in preset values of neonatal test lungs there are systematic deviations from true values. Limitations in pulmonary mechanics monitoring exist, and should be considered in the interpretation of data used to guide clinical management. Comparison of V_{te} and other pulmonary mechanics measures between babies in the same unit or between centers may be very inaccurate. Pulmonary mechanics monitoring should never replace the expertise of skilled caregivers, as the use of flawed information for clinical decision-making may be more detrimental than no information at all.

In several available modes, the newborn baby is the one who chooses parameters. In some circumstances, this has proven not to be the best or ideal for that particular baby. Drawing an analogy with teenagers, the babies may ask for things that are not good for them at a time they are not fully mature or capable to make that decision and understand the potential ramifications or adverse consequences.

There are many dimensions necessary for adequacy of mechanical ventilation of a newborn infant. Five or six of them should never be forgotten in clinical care:

1. Knowing the infant, his/her clinical condition, and changing status over minutes, hours, or days.
2. Individualized care.
3. Pulmonary and cardiovascular physiology.

4. Do not overexpand alveoli in inspiration—that is, do not tolerate chest excursions during manual or mechanical ventilation. It is sufficient to auscultate good air entry and see improvements in clinical condition (SpO$_2$, CO$_2$, and other).
5. Understand completely the ventilator you are using.

Many people ask which is the best respirator. Or, which is the best mode to use? I have heard various and discrepant answers to these two questions. Individual studies, some with significant biases and methodological issues, try to provide us with answers. However, network meta-analysis does not provide a clear answer and it is very unlikely that one mode of ventilation will be found to be "the best" for all babies in all NICUs. Some reply "A/C + VG," others "SIMV + PS + VG," and so on. The former can pose significant difficulties for some infants. A recent meta-analysis in Cochrane mentions that infants ventilated using VTV modes had reduced death and chronic lung disease compared with infants ventilated using pressure-limited modes, but comment on the further needs to compare and refine VTV strategies. I would like to emphasize that each individual baby and the dimensions mentioned above (and others) should be considered to guide individualized clinical care.

With over 43 years of ventilating newborn infants, I would like to share that I learnt almost all I know today about respiratory physiology and neonatal ventilation starting in medical school in Argentina (Physiology) and then pediatric residency and neonatal fellowship in the United States (1974–79). During those times many babies survived well, with no sequelae, using a good and reliable pressure-limited and time-cycled neonatal ventilation (Baby Bird). Other infants, no doubts, could have benefited from what is available today. The caveats today are not to rely solely and completely on a machine nor to trust baby's "wishes." To continue to improve outcomes, the best ventilation strategy, still today, necessitates physiology, detailed clinical evaluation, and unswerving dedication by the bedside. It is likely that using them as the basis, the potentially optimal ventilation strategy is one that uses the lowest possible V_t with FiO$_2$-guided higher PEEP and prone positioning, regardless of the mode chosen.

Further reading

[1] Abbasi S, Sivieri E, Roberts R, Kirpalani H. Accuracy of tidal volume, compliance, and resistance measurements on neonatal ventilator displays: an in vitro assessment. Pediatr Crit Care Med 2012;13:e262–e268.

[2] Baldoli I, Tognarelli S, Scaramuzzo S, et al. Comparative performances analysis of neonatal ventilators. Ital J Pediatr 2015;41:9.

[3] Chow L, Vanderhal A, Raber J, Sola A. Are tidal volume measurements in neonatal pressure-controlled ventilation accurate? Pediatr Pulmonol 2002;34(3):196–202.

[4] Gerhardt TO. Limitations and pitfalls of pulmonary function testing and pulmonary graphics in the clinical setting. In: Donn SM, editor. Neonatal and pediatric pulmonary graphics: principles and clinical applications.

New York: Futura Publishing Co; 1998. p. 129–153.

[5] Grazioli S, Karam O, Rimensberger PC. New generation neonatal high frequency ventilators: effect of oscillatory frequency and working principles on performance. Respir Care 2015;60:363–370.

[6] Harcourt ER, John J, Dargaville PA, Zannin E, Davis PG, Tingay DG. Pressure and flow waveform

characteristics of eight high-frequency oscillators. Pediatr Crit Care Med 2014;15:e234–e240.

[7] Heulitt MJ, Thurman TL, Holt SJ, Jo CH, Simpson P. Reliability of displayed tidal volume in infants and children during dual-controlled ventilation. Pediatr Crit Care Med 2009;10(6):661–667.

[8] Hokenson M, Shepherd EG. Neonatal pressure support ventilation: are we doing what we think we are doing? Respir Care 2014;59(10):1606.

[9] Isayama T, Iwami H, McDonald S, Beyene J. Association of noninvasive ventilation strategies with mortality and bronchopulmonary dysplasia among preterm infants: a systematic review and meta-analysis. JAMA 2016;316(6):611–624.

[10] Itagaki T, Bennett DJ, Chenelle CT, Fisher DF, Kacmarek RM. Performance of leak compensation in all-age ICU ventilators during volume-targeted neonatal ventilation: a lung model study. Respir Care 2017;62(1):10–21.

[11] Itagaki T, Bennett DJ, Chenelle CT, Fisher DF, Kacmarek RM. Effects of leak compensation on patient-ventilator synchrony during premature/neonatal invasive and noninvasive ventilation: a lung model study. Respir Care 2017;62:22–33.

[12] Iyer NP, Chatburn R. Evaluation of a nasal cannula in noninvasive ventilation using a lung simulator. Respir Care 2015;60(4):508–512.

[13] Kavvadia V, Greenough A, Itakura Y, Dimitriou G. Neonatal lung function in very immature infants with and without RDS. J Perinat Med 1999;27:382–387.

[14] Keszler M. Volume-targeted ventilation. Early Hum Dev 2006;82(12):811–818.

[15] Kim P, Salazar A, Ross PA, et al. Comparison of tidal volumes at the endotracheal tube and at the ventilator. Pediatr Crit Care Med 2015;16(9):e324–e331.

[16] Klingenberg C, Wheeler K, McCallion N, Morley CJ, Davis PG. Volume-targeted versus pressure-limited ventilation in the neonate. Cochrane Database Syst Rev 2017;10.CD003666.

[17] Mahmoud RA, Proquitté H, Fawzy N, Bührer C, Schmalisch G. Tracheal tube airleak in clinical practice and impact on tidal volume measurement in ventilated neonates. Pediatr Crit Care Med 2011;12(2):197–202.

[18] Oto J, Chenelle CT, Marchese AD, Kacmarek RM. A comparison of leak compensation in acute care ventilators during non-invasive and invasive ventilation: a lung model study. Respir Care 2013;58(12):2027–2037.

[19] Oto J, Chenelle CT, Marchese AD, Kacmarek RM. A comparison of leak compensation during pediatric noninvasive ventilation: a lung model study. Respir Care 2014;59(2):241–251.

[20] Pisani L, Carlucci A, Nava S. Interfaces for noninvasive mechanical ventilation: technical aspects and efficiency. Minerva Anestesiol 2012;78(10):1154–1161.

[21] Sinha SK, Donn SM, Gavey J, McCarty M. Randomised trial of volume controlled versus time cycled, pressure limited ventilation in preterm infants with respiratory distress syndrome. Arch Dis Child 1997;77:202–205.

[22] Sivieri EM, Gerdes JS, Abbasi S. Effect of HFNC flow rate, cannula size, and nares diameter on generated airway pressures: an in vitro study. Pediatr Pulmonol 2013;48(5):506–514.

[23] Sola A. Oxygen management: concerns about both hyperoxia and hypoxia in neonates during critical care and intraoperatively. Section 1, Chapter 7: essentials of anesthesia for infants and neonates. In: McCan ME, Greco C, Matthes K, editors. Cambridge University Press. ISBN 978-1-107-06977-0.

[24] Sola A. Oxygen saturation in the newborn and the importance of avoiding hyperoxia-induced damage. NeoReviews 2015;16(7):e393.

[25] Sola A. Oxygen management in essentials of anesthesia for infants and neonates. In: McCan ME, Greco C, Matthes K, editors. Cambridge University Press. ISBN 978-1-107-06977-0.

[26] Sola A, Golombek S. Oxygen Saturation monitoring in neonatal period. In: Buonocore G, editor. Neonatology. Switzerland: Springer International Publishing; 2016.

[27] Sola A, Golombek S (Spanish language). Chapters in Sola, A and Golombek SG. *Cuidando al recién nacido a la manera de SIBEN. Tomo I. 2017 EDISIBEN, ISBN 978-1-5323-3453-5* (Gráfica IMPRIMAX, Santa Cruz, Bolivia, September 2017): Respiradores neonatales p:355-364; Diferentes modos ventilatorios p:364-383; Automatización de los respiradores p 396-401.

[28] Sola A, Golombek S, Gregory GA (Spanish language). Fisiología respiratoria y medición de la función y mecánica pulmonary. p:245-252 in Sola, A and Golombek SG. *Cuidando al recién nacido a la manera de SIBEN. Tomo I. 2017 EDISIBEN, ISBN 978-1-5323-3453-5* (Gráfica IMPRIMAX, Santa Cruz, Bolivia, September 2017).

[29] Stocks J. Lung function testing in infants. Pediatr Pulmonol Suppl 1999;18:14–20.

[30] Stocks J. Respiratory function testing in early childhood: where have we come from and where are we going? Pediatr Pulmonol Suppl 1999;18:24–28.

[31] Thille AW, Rodriguez P, Cabello B, Lellouche F, Brochard L. Patient-ventilator asynchrony during assisted mechanical ventilation. Intensive Care Med 2006;32(10):1515–1522.

[32] Tingay DG, Jubal J, Harcourt ER, Dargaville PA, et al. Are all oscillators created equal? In vitro performance characteristics of eight high-frequency oscillatory ventilators. Neonatology 2015;108:220–228.

[33] Tingay DG, Mills JF, Morley CJ, Pellicano A, Dargaville PA. Indicators of optimal lung volume during high-frequency oscillatory ventilation in infants. Crit Care Med 2013;41:237–244.

[34] Vignaux L, Grazioli S, Piquilloud L, Bochaton N, Karam O, Jaecklin T, et al. Optimizing patient-ventilator synchrony during invasive ventilator assist in children and infants remains a difficult task. Pediatr Crit Care Med 2013;14(7):e316–e325.

[35] Vignaux L, Grazioli S, Piquilloud L, Bochaton N, Karam O, Levy-Jamet Y, et al. Patient-ventilator asynchrony during noninvasive pressure support ventilation and neurally adjusted ventilatory assist in infants and children. Pediatr Crit Care Med 2013;14(8):e357–e364.

[36] Wang C, Wang X, Chi C, Guo L, Guo L, Zhao N, et al. Lung ventilation strategies for acute respiratory distress syndrome: a systematic review and network meta-analysis. Sci Rep 2016;6:22855.

[37] Wheeler KI, Klingenberg C, Morley CJ, Davis PG. Volume-targeted versus pressure-limited ventilation for preterm infants: a systematic review and meta-analysis. Neonatology 2011;100(3):219–227.

Also: Manuals prepared by manufactures of all different ventilators presented were used as informational sources.

Chapter | **9B** |

The Importance of Heating and Humidifying the Inspired Gases During Mechanical Ventilation: Identifying the Ideal Settings and Circuit Configuration During Ventilation

David A. Todd, FIMLS, MSc, PhD, MBBS, K.Y. Ashok Murthy, P.K. Rajiv, DCH, MD

CHAPTER POINTS

- During intubation and mechanical ventilation it is essential that the inspired gases are optimally heated and humidified
- Failure to achieve optimum heat and humidification of inspired gases will result in acute and potential long term damage to the upper and peripheral airways
- In this chapter we will explore the natural processes that heat and humidity the inspired gases and the devices that are commonly used to artificially attain these natural processes.
- We will then state our recommendations and our "do's and don'ts" during ventilation to achieve the least damage to the airways

Normal gas conditioning in the respiratory tract

When intubated, the upper airway (UAW), which heats and humidifies inspired air to core body temperature and 100% relative humidity (RH), is bypassed [1]. The UAW promotes viable pulmonary function by regulating the heat and humidity of inspired and expired gases. During inspiration, the UAW progressively adds heat and humidity from the mucosa to the inspired gases in the nasopharynx and trachea. Heat and humidity is transferred back, during expiration, from the moist and warm alveolar gases to the mucosa, thereby preparing it for use in the next cycle. Unlike in the adult population, where thermal mapping of the respiratory tree has yielded clear data about the heat and moisture exchange in the UAW, there is very little data for neonates [2–10]. The typical values of heat and humidity along the respiratory tract for the adult are shown in Table 9B.1 [3].

Moisture and heat are added or removed from the inspiratory and expiratory gases by evaporation, condensation, and convection, and are a continuum with the inspired gas humidity (IH) at the lower trachea/main bronchi measured at 44 mgH$_2$O/L absolute humidity (AH), equivalent to core body temperature (37°C) and 100% RH (Table 9B.1, Fig. 9B.1) [1–3,11,12].

However, the minimum standards for IH during mechanical ventilation are recommended to be an AH of 33 mgH$_2$O/L in the United Kingdom [13] and 30 mgH$_2$O/L in the United States [14].

Table 9B.1 Change of temperature and humidity during inspiration and expiration in the adult			
Position	Inspired temperature (°C)	Relative humidity (%)	Absolute humidity (mgH$_2$O/L)
Change of temperature and humidity during inspiration in the adult			
Nares	22	51	10
Larynx	31–33	81–89	26–32
Mid Trachea	34–35	90–96	34–38
Main Bronchi	37	100	44
Change of temperature and humidity during expiration in the adult			
Nares	32–34	86–90	27–34
Larynx	36	96	40

Extracted and modified from McFadden ER, Pachinko B, Bowman H, et al. Thermal mapping of the airways in humans. J Appl Physiol 1985;58:564–570 [3].

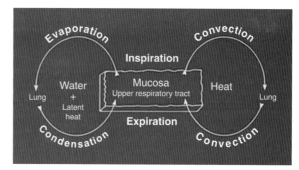

Fig. 9B.1 Heat and Moisture Changes in the Upper Airway. Modified from Walker JEC, Wells RE, Merrill EW. Heat and Moister exchange in the respiratory tract. Am J Med 1961;2:259–267 [11].

Essential terminologies and definitions

AH, expressed in mgH$_2$O/L, is defined as the amount of water vapor (mg) per unit volume (L) of gas.

RH, expressed in %, is the ratio of the actual water vapor content of a gas to the amount required to saturate the same gas volume at the same temperature. There is a fixed relationship between AH, RH, and temperature.

Suboptimal conditioning of inspired gases to the AW

During both conventional and high-frequency ventilation, the gases entering the ventilators are at extremely low temperature and humidity (15°C, 0.3 mgH$_2$O/L) and must be heated and humidified prior to entering the AW [1,4–16]. The longer the respiratory system is exposed to suboptimal heat and humidity, the more likelihood that there will be acute and potentially long-term damage. This will affect mucociliary transport velocity (MTV) which normally runs at 19.2 ± 1.6 mm/min due to the ciliary beat frequency (CBF) of around 17–25 beats/s when at the body temperature (37°C), atmospheric pressure and saturated with water vapor (BTPS: 37 mmHg or 6.2 kPa) (Fig. 9B.2) [1]. The longer the exposure to the suboptimal heat and humidity, the higher the likelihood of reducing the delicate balance between the pericellular fluid (aqueous sol) depth, CBF, and MTV (Figs. 9B.2–9B.5).

In the preterm baby (PB), this is especially important as the AW is immature both in respect to UAW and peripheral AW (PAW), where the alveoli may not be fully matured in the both the type I and type II cells. In the PB, the damage to the AW from suboptimal heat and humidification of the inspiratory gases may be more rapid and with greater long-term consequences such as bronchopulmonary dysplasia (BPD) [17]. Exposure to suboptimal heat and humidity beyond the endotracheal tube (ETT) leads to increased lung damage [1,4–8].

Low heat and humidity delivered to the UAW and respiratory tract leads to flattening of normal tracheal mucosa, replacement of epithelial cells by nonciliated epidermoid squamous metaplastic cells, and exposed openings of the submucosal glands—indicative of erosion similar to PBs with BPD (Figs. 9B.3 and 9B.6) [4–7].

Excess heat and humidity results in condensation of water. This may cause thermal damage, decreased mucous viscosity resulting in reduced effective mucociliary transport, dilution of surfactant, hypotonic challenge, and injury causing cell damage with interstitial edema, especially in the PAW (Figs. 9B.3 and 9B.6) [1,4,8,9,15].

In addition, the ETT, through mechanical irritation, has a significant effect on the integrity of the UAW and can precipitate damage to the vocal cords, tracheal rings, beyond the ETT and at the carina (Fig. 9B.4).

Structure and function of the AW lining

The respiratory tract is lined with ciliated epithelial cells (Fig. 9B.5) [1]. Each cell carries about 200 cilia at its apex. The mature cilia are 5–6 μm in length and carry a crown of short claws at their tip. The cilia support and push an aqueous layer of mucus upward so that it can be expectorated. This is known as the mucociliary escalator.

Mucus is secreted by goblet cells and submucosal mucous glands as globules of 1–2 mm in diameter. They absorb

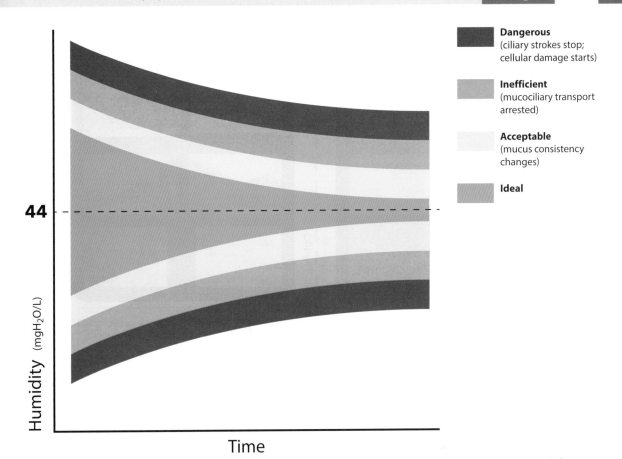

Fig. 9B.2 Diagrammatic representation of mucosal function during changes over time in heat and humidity levels from optimum to suboptimum levels. This ranges is from "ideal" mucus transport velocity (MTV) at optimum heat and humidity levels to negligible MTV and cell damage at suboptimum levels of heat and humidity. Modified from Williams R, Rankin N, Smith T, et al. Relationship between the humidity and temperature of inspired gas and the function of airway mucosa. Crit Care Med 1996;24:1920–1929 [1].

water from the aqueous layer and subsequently swell rapidly. Mucus consists of glycoproteins, proteoglycans, lipids, and 95% water. It forms small flakes, larger plaques, or blanket-like covers that float on the luminal surface and trap inhaled particles and other compounds, such as bacteria, macrophages, and cell debris. Experimental evidence exists that mucus secretion is stimulated when particles come into contact with the ciliated surface. Such particles are subsequently encapsulated by mucus and carried away by the mucociliary escalator.

Achieving the optimum heat and humidity

Circuit configuration

Situations of low or inadequate heat and humidity delivered to the respiratory tract may arise whenever assisted ventilation (invasive or noninvasive) is initiated. This may occur at birth in the delivery suite to the neonatal intensive care unit, for example, during resuscitation, stabilization, or transport of a neonate.

Low levels of humidity contribute to a fall in compliance, with decreased surfactant activity, and a rise in AW resistance, alveolar gas trapping, thereby increasing the risk of hypoventilation [1,12]. Systemic moisture loss could also result [1,12]. It is our suggestion that the optimum heat and humidity targets for PBs be at or close to a temperature of $37\,^{\circ}$C and AH of 44 mgH$_2$O/L in the inspired gas as it passes beyond the ETT and into the respiratory tract. This is higher than the recommended UK and US minimum standards [13,14].

High humidity levels, on the other hand, will lead to inflammatory responses, thermal injury, and low-viscosity secretions (Fig. 9B.3) [10,15,16]. Mucociliary transport is impacted adversely. Prolonged exposure exacerbates these effects. When the exposure to suboptimal humidification

115

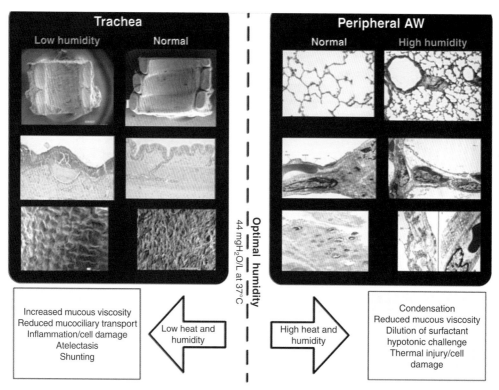

Fig. 9B.3 The UAW and PAW Changes During Low and High Heat and Humidity of Inspired Gases. Middle: Photomicrographs of UAW and PAW of normal trachea by scanning electron microscopy (SEM) and normal alveoli by light microscopy (LM) and transmission electron microscopy (TEM). UAW showing the folding and a predominance of ciliated columnar epithelial cells on the crests and a predominance of goblet cells in the furrows with the "wheatfield"-like appearance of the cilia on the crests of the mucosal folds. PAW showing normal appearance of alveoli, thin epithelium (EPI), and endothelium (END) of the type I and endothelial cells and type II cells. Left: Photomicrograph showing UAW during low heat and humidity conditions and showing abnormal trachea loss of the folding and complete loss of ciliated columnar epithelial cells and goblet cells in the furrows by LM. Photomicrographs showing abnormal tracheal epithelium SEM × 12.5, bar = 1 mm, showing dried mucous of tracheal epithelium and complete loss of ciliated epithelium; SEM × 750, bar = 10 μm, loss of the "wheatfield"-like appearance and replaced by dried mucous layer. Right: Photomicrograph showing PAW during high heat and humidity conditions by LM and TEM showing interstitial edema and breakdown of the cellular integrity with vesicles (V) in the type I cell epithelium. Todd collected photomicrographs.

crosses 20–30 min, shearing of the PAW due to surfactant deficiency results in the greatest damage. With continued excess humidity and water of condensation, this could potentially lead to ventilator-associated pneumonia (VAP).

Excess heat and humidity may occur during ventilation of the newborn, but the common scenario is low heat but high humidity. Thermal energy is trapped in water at high temperatures as moist gases (steam) and will cause severely more damage than dry gas at the same high temperature. High humidity with low temperatures will affect the mucociliary transport of the ciliated epithelium within the trachea and UAW and will cause disruption of the type I and type II cells in the PAW. In the PAW, this will lead to interstitial edema and may lead to fibrosis and potentially BPD in the PB (Figs. 9B.3 and 9B.6) [10,15–17].

Humidifiers add water vapor to the inspired gases by heating water in a chamber. The humidification device does not measure humidity in the system, but it relies on a measurement of temperature, which is performed by the proximal airway temperature probe (ATP) in a dual TP system (Fig. 9B.7).

The two configurations of ATP placement are shown in Fig. 9B.7. In configuration Fig. 9B.7.1, the proximal ATP (pATP) is placed at the outlet of the humidifier chamber (position A). This is often combined with the heater hose adapter for ease of assembly. The other measurement of temperature is performed by placing the distal ATP (dATP) as position B at the end of the heated inspiratory limb close to the ETT (Fig. 9B.7.1). The inspiratory limb between these two ATP positions is heated by a heater wire in the inspiratory

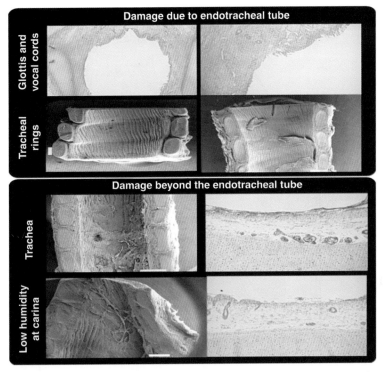

Fig. 9B.4 Damage to the Vocal Cords and Trachea From the ETT and Beyond the Carina, and Erosion and Deciliation of the Epithelial Cells With Mucous Strands.

limb either within the inspiratory limb or incorporated into the tubing and surrounding the inspired gases. In configuration Fig. 9B.7.2, there is a small unheated extension tube after the dATP, at position C. To achieve optimum heat and humidification to the PB and term neonate, this extension should not be used as this will cause a drop in inspired temperature and rain out of water leading to potential lung damage (Table 9B.2) [5,10,15,16].

Temperature and humidity (offset) settings

To achieve a target of 37°C and 44 mgH$_2$O/L beyond the ETT in the trachea, it is common to set 37°C as the target temperature at the humidifier chamber outlet (pATP). This will condition the gas exiting the humidifier to 37°C and an AH of 44 mgH$_2$O/L of water vapor. The inspiratory limb will heat the gas as it progresses to the patient, using the heater hose wires. At the end of the heated section, the temperature should have been elevated by 3°C from 37°C to 40°C (thus the humidifier is set at 40-3 [offset]). The water vapor should remain 44 mgH$_2$O/L, but this may be affected by humidicrib and environmental temperature [4]. As the gas now traverses past the

pneumotach (or hotwire anemometer [Table 9B.2]), ETT, and its adapter, there will be a temperature drop due to this section being unheated. The fall should be the 2–3°C depending on the temperature of the humidicrib, circuit setup, and position of the pATP and dATP, and may be up to 4.5°C (Table 9B.2). This should result in the desired target of 37°C and 44 mgH$_2$O/L being achieved in the trachea (Fig. 9B.8).

Clinical situations with suboptimum conditions

There are other factors that may interfere with the achievement of the target temperature and moisture gas conditioning and should be managed appropriately. These factors include:

1. **Ambient air conditions:** In high ambient air temperature conditions, the environment will also provide heat to the humidifier chamber and inspiratory limb. The humidifier chamber will add less heat energy to the inspiratory gas, as it is easier to attain the target temperature. This will reduce the water vapor content added to the inspired gas, as the water in the chamber will not evaporate as much due to it being cold. During

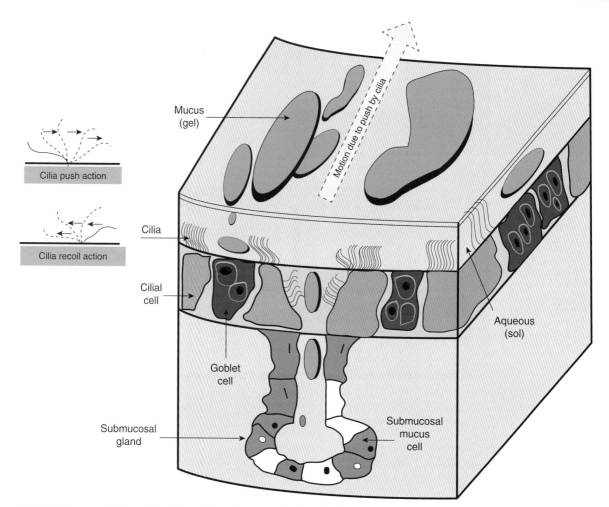

Fig. 9B.5 Representation of the Mucociliary Transport Escalator in the Upper Airways (UAW). This depicts (1) the submucosal gland producing the more thicker mucus gel (mucus flakes) that trap microparticles in the UAW, (2) the goblet cells that produce the aqueous sol that baths the cilia of the ciliated epithelial cell, and (3) the movement of the mucus flakes toward the glottis. Modified from Williams R, Rankin N, Smith T, et al. Relationship between the humidity and temperature of inspired gas and the function of airway mucosa. Crit Care Med 1996;24:1920–1929 [1].

therapeutic hypothermia, excessive humidity and rainout of water may occur due to the low ambient temperature [18].

2. **Location of dATP in a heated field:** In conditions where the baby is nursed with a radiant warmer, if the distal ATP is placed in the radiant field it may falsely register a higher temperature than that of the inspired gas. The humidifier will respond by reducing the heat added, causing a fall in the water vapor to suboptimal levels. We recommend a small foil reflector disc placed over the dATP to prevent this. A similar situation may arise if the dATP is located within a hot incubator that may cause the same suboptimal humidity delivered

to the patient. Less mature neonates with low birth weight (who have higher incubator temperatures) require close attention to this factor. Colder inspired gases where condensation of water may occur could lead to more instances of VAP, chronic lung disease, especially in very PBs [15–17]. Potentially altered pressure and changing alarm may also occur with rainout of water [19].

3. **During resuscitation, transport, changing ventilator circuits, and setting up of the ventilator equipment and circuit:** It is essential that during resuscitation, transport, and changing ventilator circuits, a heated and humidified respiratory circuit be used to prevent

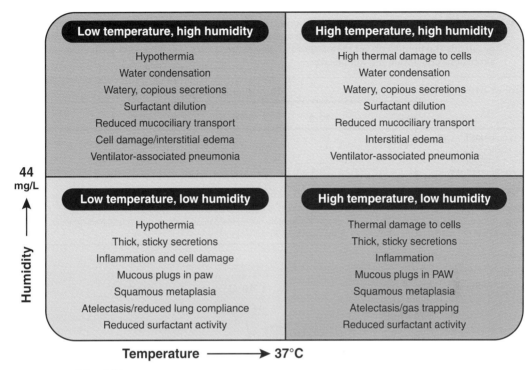

Fig. 9B.6 **Heat Humidity Grid.**

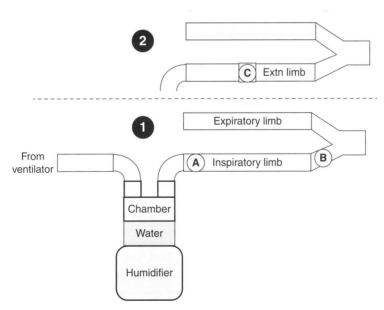

Fig. 9B.7 **Common Humidifier Configurations.** (1) The airway temperature probes are placed at position A—the outlet of the humidifier chamber (pATP) and position B—patient proximal or distal to the heated inspiratory tube (dATP). (2) The dATP is placed at position C—between the heated inspiratory tube and an unheated extension limb that is patient proximal.

Table 9B.2 Inspired gas temperature at different humidicrib temperatures with the distal airway temperature probe (dATP) either inside the humidicrib with the set temperature at 36.5°C (position B, Fig. 9B.7.1) or outside the humidicrib set temperature at 39.0°C (position C, Fig. 9B.7.2) with the unheated extension tube within the humidicrib

Position of ATP	Humidicrib temperature (°C)				
	30.8	32.9	35.2	36.2	37.2
Inspired temperature with dATP at position B (°C)	36.4 ± 0.1	36.4 ± 0.1	36.4 ± 0.1	36.4 ± 0.1	36.4 ± 0.1
Inspired temperature with dATP at position C (°C)	34.7 ± 0.2	35.5 ± 0.3	36.6 ± 0.1	36.8 ± 0.1	37.7 ± 0.1

All inspired temperatures were measured proximal to the pneumotach or hotwire anemometer to avoid increases in reading.
Modified from Todd DA, Boyd J, Lloyd J, John E. Inspired gas temperature during mechanical ventilation: effects of environmental temperature and airway temperature probe position. J Paediatr Child Health 2001;37:495–500 [5].

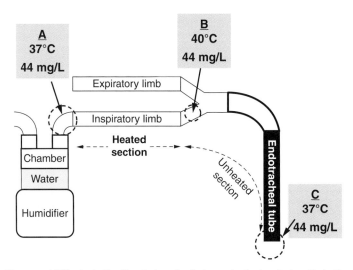

Fig. 9B.8 Humidifier Settings and Effects. In the "heated section" shown in the inspiratory limb, the gas exiting the humidifier chamber is heated to attain 2 or 3°C elevation at the patient proximal end. The amount of water vapor remains the same. In the "unheated section," consisting of the extension piece/adapter and endotracheal (or tracheostomy) tube, there will be a corresponding temperature drop.

damage to the lungs (Figs. 9B.3 and 9B.4). In addition, it has been shown that heating and humidifying the inspired gases during resuscitation prevents hypothermia in PBs <32-week GA, and this may also be the case while using mask ventilation during resuscitation [20,21]. The clinical situations below are examples where there may be suboptimum heat and humidity delivered to the baby:

a. During resuscitation and transport of the PB or even term infants, it is essential that the inspired gases are heated and humidified. Because PBs are more prone to rapid heat losses, they have an even greater need for such protective measures.

b. During ventilator circuit changes that should be performed weekly, it is usual to bag/hand ventilate the babies. It is essential that the bagging circuit is attached to a heat and humidifier system.

Ventilators/ventilation: types, modes, and circuitry

In this chapter we will consider heat and humidifying the respiratory circuit during different types of ventilation, including conventional ventilation (CV), high-frequency

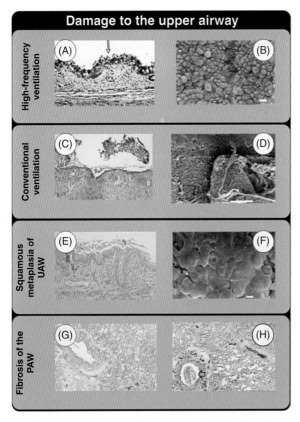

Damage to the upper airway

(A) High-frequency ventilation
(B)
(C) Conventional ventilation
(D)
(E) Squamous metaplasia of UAW
(F)
(G) Fibrosis of the PAW
(H)

Fig. 9B.9 Various Types of Damage to UAW. Differing type of damage to upper AW at low humidity and temperature caused by high frequency (A and B) versus conventional ventilation (C and D); chronic changes that occur in BPD from either type of initial damage (A–D) with squamous metaplasia of the UAW (E and F) and fibrosis of the PAW with mucous plugging of the UAW (G and H). Modified from Todd DA, John E, Osborn R. Tracheal damage following conventional and high frequency ventilation at low and high humidity. Crit Care Med. 1991;19:1310–1316 [8]. Todd collected photomicrographs.

ventilation (HFV), continuous positive airway pressure (CPAP), high-flow nasal cannula (HFNC), and low-flow nasal cannula (LFNC).

There are different types of ventilators and ventilation devices on the market, and these have varying modes of ventilation, but the most important difference for the invasive ventilation is the difference between CV and HFV. Due to the mechanism of flow and tidal volume differences between CV and HFV, there is a difference in the type of damage seen with low inspired gas temperature and humidity (Fig. 9B.9A–D), and thus it is vitally important to adequately heat and humidify the inspired gases with the correct ventilator circuit setup. If this damage continues in prolonged ventilation, regardless of the initial cause of the damage, then

metaplasia of the UAW (Fig. 9B.9E and F) and fibrosis of the PAW may be the outcome (Fig. 9B.9G and H) that is essentially BPD. Several mechanisms are in place during HFV including the type of high-frequency generator (flow interrupter, jet and oscillator [High Frequency Oscillatory Ventilation {HFOV}]) as well as inspiratory flow; increased inspiratory flow will produce increased inspired temperature but decreased humidity delivered [22–25]. As well, amplitude has an effect on inspired humidity—the higher the amplitude, the lower the inspired humidity [25]—while oscillation frequency has less effect on inspired humidity [25].

The necessity of additive heat and humidification remains essential in noninvasive modes, even though the nares and UAW are not bypassed. Medical gases that are cold and dry (15°C, 0.3 mgH$_2$O/L) drive CPAP, HFNC, and LFNC systems and will lead to drying of mucosal secretions and hypothermia if not conditioned adequately (heated and humidified). More CPAP is now being used in the PBs as the delivery of surfactant either by the INSURE method (intubation, surfactant, extubation) or MIST (minimally invasive surfactant therapy) has gained popularity, similarly for HFNC as this mode of noninvasive ventilation is becoming more popular [26]. The inspired gases from both CPAP and HFNC must be passed through a heated humidification system prior to entering the patient. Some HFNC systems base their heat and humidification on using vapor transfer cartridges to enrich the gas stream with water vapor. For LFNC, the gases must be passed through a water bubbler system prior to entering the nares.

Types of heat and humidifiers

1. External: to ventilator
   a. F&P
   b. Wilhamed
2. Internal: to the ventilator
   a. Stephanie
   b. Sophie

External heat and humidifiers

In external heat and humidifiers, the basic principles are similar. Cold gases with low humidity (15°C, 0.3 mgH$_2$O/L) are directed from the ventilator to the heated humidifier chamber where the gases pass through the humid gas above the heated water. The water in the humidifier chamber is heated via a "hot plate" below the humidifier chamber. During the passage over the heated water, the dry gas will obtain heat and moisture from the moist air and pass into the heated inspiratory limb with a temperature of 37°C containing 44 mgH$_2$O/L gas. In the heated inspiratory limb, the gas is then warmed to 40°C (may be variable depending on the type and manufacturer of humidifier base) and thus maintains the AH of 44 mgH$_2$O/L. Prior to entering the ETT, the gas will drop in temperature, but this will depend mainly on the ventilator type, humidicrib temperature, position of the dATP, and ventilator circuit setup [4,5,22,25].

Internal or inbuilt heat and humidifiers with ventilator such as Stephanie/Sophie

When ventilating infants with ventilators that have inbuilt heating and humidification systems, it is important to position the humidification system correctly within the circuit together with optimizing the system. With the Stephanie/Sophie ventilator, the inbuilt heating and humidification system is essentially a heater block immersed in a chamber ½ to ¾ filled with water. The inspiratory gases flow into the chamber and pass over the heated moist air above the water increasing in heat and humidity. They exit of the heater and humidifier block to the proximal ATP (pATP) and distal ATP (dATP) that are within the inspiratory limb away from the heater block (Fig. 9B.10) [22,25]. This is dissimilar to the external heat and humidifiers (Figs. 9B.7 and 9B.8), where the pATP is at the exit of the heat and humidifier chamber and it is essential in the Stephanie and Sophie ventilators to insulate the inspiratory limb to reduce rainout of water and reduction of inspired temperature and humidity [22,25].

We recommend the following settings:

1. Stephanie ventilator: "39-2°C," that is, 39°C at the dATP, and 37°C at the exit from the humidifier. This differs from the manufacturer's specification of "37-2°C" [22].
2. Sophie ventilator: "40-3°C" as the Sophie ventilator has a higher setting. We also recommend using the long circuit rather than the short circuit supplied with these ventilators as this improves the AH of the inspired gases [25].

Achieving optimum humidity

Recommendations for inspired gases during intubation and ventilation are as follows:
- **Humidity**
  - UK recommendation >34 mgH$_2$O/L gas
  - US recommendation >30 mgH$_2$O/L gas
  - Our recommendation: 44 mgH$_2$O/L gas (or as close to this)
- **Temperature**
  - Our recommendation: 37°C at the distal ATP (or as close to this)
- Optimal heat and humidification of inspired gases is essential during intubation and ventilation. Many factors contribute to the conditioning of inspired gases, including
  - Ventilator type (CV/HFV)
  - Ventilator mode (CV/HFV)
  - Ventilator settings
  - Humidifier type (external and type of external/inbuilt with ventilator)
  - Humidifier settings (proximal and distal ATP)
- Thus, it is imperative to optimize and therefore adjusts the setting of the heat and humidifier system accordingly

Dos and Don'ts

1. The ventilator circuit must be changed at least once per week.
2. The humidifier system must be inspected at least once a shift (3 times/day) for correct temperature

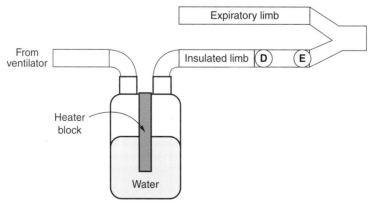

Fig. 9B.10 Respiratory Circuit for Stephanie and Sophie Ventilators Showing the Heater Block Immersed in Water and Temperature Probes in Distal Inspiratory Limb. There are two temperature probes (D and E) that follow an insulated inspiratory limb.

probe positioning, signs of any damage to any of the accessories, the adequacy of water level in the chamber, the presence of condensate in the circuit, and any other manufacturer's recommended guidelines. Overheating (although less common) can lead to a cascade of effects beginning with mucosal heating. Overhumidification can lead to increased secretions and hypoxemia. Excess condensate in the circuit indicates an inappropriate humidifier setting. Unlike the vapor associated with the delivery of heat and

humidity into the AWs, the condensate may be contaminated by bacterial colonization and may lead to VAP.

3. The humidifier chamber and circuits must always be below the ETT height. This will prevent any condensate from inadvertently flowing into the airways, which can be catastrophic.

4. If the condensate is difficult to manage, the use of water traps in the inspiratory and expiratory limbs may be considered.

References

[1] Williams R, Rankin N, Smith T, et al. Relationship between the humidity and temperature of inspired gas and the function of airway mucosa. Crit Care Med 1996;24: 1920–1929.

[2] Schiffmann H. Humidification of respired gases in neonates and infants. Respir Care Clin N Am 2006;12:321–336.

[3] McFadden ER, Pachinko B, Bowman H, et al. Thermal mapping of the airways in humans. J Appl Physiol 1985;58:564–570.

[4] Todd DA, Boyd J, Lloyd J, et al. Inspired gas humidity during mechanical ventilation: effects of humidification chamber, airway temperature probe position and environmental conditions. J Paediatr Child Health 2001;37:489–494.

[5] Todd DA, Boyd J, Lloyd J, John E. Inspired gas temperature during mechanical ventilation: effects of environmental temperature and airway temperature probe position. J Paediatr Child Health 2001;37:495–500.

[6] Davies MW, Dunster KR, Cartwright DW. Inspired gas temperature in ventilated neonates. Pediatr Pulmonol 2004;38:50–54.

[7] Todd DA, John E, Osborn R. Epithelial damage beyond the tip of the endotracheal tube. Early Hum Dev 1990;24:187–200.

[8] Todd DA, John E, Osborn R. Tracheal damage following conventional and high frequency ventilation at low and high humidity. Crit Care Med 1991;19:1310–1316.

[9] Todd DA, John E, Osborn R. Recovery of tracheal epithelium following high frequency ventilation at low inspired humidity. Early Hum Dev 1992;31:53–66.

[10] Williams R. The effects of excessive humidity. Respir Care Clin N Am 1998;4:215–228.

[11] Walker JEC, Wells RE, Merrill EW. Heat and Moister exchange in the respiratory tract. Am J Med 1961;2:259–267.

[12] Chatburn R. Physiologic and methodologic issues regarding humidity therapy. J Pediatr 1989;114:416–420.

[13] British Standards Institution. Specifications for humidifiers for use with breathing machines (PuBLVication no. BS 4494). London: The Institution; 1970.

[14] American National Standards Institute. American National Standard for Humidifiers and Nebulizers for Medical Use (PuBLVication no. ANSI Z79.9-179). New York: The Institute; 1979.

[15] Todd DA, John E. Lung injury and repair in rabbits from ventilation with most air. Br J Exp Pathol 1989;17:637–645.

[16] John E, Ermocilla R, Golden J, Cash R, McDevitt M, Cassady G. Effects of gas temperature and particulate water on rabbit lungs during ventilation. Pediatr Res 1980;14:1186–1191.

[17] Todd DA, Jana A, John E. Chronic oxygen dependency in infants at 24 to 32 weeks gestation: the role of antenatal and neonatal factors. J Paediatr Child Health 1997;33:402–407.

[18] Tanaka S, Iwata S, Kinoshita M, Tsuda K, Sakai S, Saikusa M, et al. Use of normothermic default humidifier settings causes excessive humidification of respiratory gases during therapeutic hypothermia. Ther Hypothermia Temp Manag 2016;6:180–188.

[19] Hinder M, Perdomo A, Tracy M. Dangerous pressurization and inappropriate alarms during water

occlusion of the expiratory circuit of commonly used infant ventilators. PLoS One 2016;11. e0154034.

[20] Meter MP, Hou D, Ishrar NN, Dito I, te Pas AB. Initial respiratory support with cold, dry gas versus heated humidified gas and the admission temperature of preterm infants. J Pediatr 2015;116:245–250.

[21] Owen LS, Dawson JA, Middleburgh R, Buttner S, McGrory L, Davis PG. Feasibility and practical considerations for heating and humidifying gases during newborn stabilisation: an in vitro model. Neonatology 2014;106:156–162.

[22] Preo B, Shadbolt B, Todd DA. Inspired gas humidity and temperature during mechanical ventilation with the Stephanie ventilator. Pediatr Anesth 2013;23:1062–1068.

[23] Nagaya K, Okamoto T, Nakamura E, Hayashi T, Fujieda K. Airway humidification with the heated wire humidifier during high frequency ventilation using the Babylog 8000 Plus in neonates. Pediatr Pulmonol 2009;44:260–266.

[24] Chikata Y, Imanaka H, Onishi Y, Ueta M, Nishimura M. Humidification during high-frequency osilation ventilation is affected by ventilator circuit and ventilator settings. Pediatr Anesth 2009;19:779–783.

[25] Deloit V, Shadbolt B, Todd DA. Inspired humidity using during high frequency ventilation. Annual Perinatal Society of Australia and New Zealand meeting: Hobart, Tasmania 2011 and Pediatric Anesthesia; 2018 submitted for publication.

[26] Heath-Jeffery RA, Todd DA. Heated humidified high-flow nasal cannula: impact on neonatal outcomes. Respir Care 2016;61:1428–1429.

Chapter 10

Ventilator Graphics

Manoj Biniwale, MBBS, MD, MRCP, MRCPCH, FAAP, Rangasamy Ramanathan, MBBS, MD, FAAP, Mark C. Mammel, MD, FAAP

CHAPTER POINTS

Real-time ventilator graphics are an integral part of understanding the pathophysiology of mechanically ventilated infants. Breath to breath patient ventilator interactions give insight to underlying lung function through evaluations of waves and loops. Responses of individual patient as reflected by displays showing pressure, volume, and flow waveforms, pressure–volume and flow–volume loops, and trend screens, helps clinicians to enhance understanding of underlying lung pathophysiology leading to optimizing ventilator management. Knowledge of graphics further aides in early troubleshooting while adjusting ventilator parameters and preventing potentially detrimental complications.

Introduction

Real-time ventilatory graphics are the display of measured and derived values captured when a patient is treated with mechanical ventilation. Physicians, nurses, and respiratory therapists working with critically ill newborns should recognize these visual representations in order to understand adequacy of the ventilation support used and response of the infant.

Most of today's ventilators, including high-frequency machines, capture many ventilator parameters and can generate multiple graphic displays. Sadly, most often clinicians fail to understand or ignore the potentially valuable information provided by these displays.

Historical timeline

As early as the 1929, pressure–volume (P–V) relationships were studied by Von Neergaard and Wirtz in isolated liquid- and air-filled cat lungs. They observed a difference in the inspiratory and expiratory P–V relationship in the air-filled but not with water-filled lungs. They concluded the existence of a surface-acting material, which produced the different mechanical actions [1].

In 1960s, there was tremendous advancement in neonatal respiratory support as neonatal ventilation was considered as a viable therapy. Gregory et al. published their seminal work in 1971 showing that the application of continuous positive airway pressure (CPAP) in newborns with respiratory distress syndrome reduced mortality [2]. Continuous real-time display of ventilator parameters became possible in the 1980s after introduction of the portable computer. Bhutani et al. in 1988 described a stand-alone device to evaluate the respiratory status of sick neonates with bedside analysis of pulmonary mechanics, providing graphical information, and quantitative data for day-to-day pulmonary management [3]. By the 1990s, the manufacturers of neonatal respirators started displaying various types of graphics, from simple to complex. Over last 20 years there has been tremendous progress with sophisticated computer-generated models calculating a number of parameters from various modes of respiratory support provided to the infants.

Role of ventilator waveforms

- Identify pathophysiologic processes
- Recognize patient's response to therapy and monitor patient's disease status
- Calculate respiratory mechanics
- Optimize ventilator settings and treatment
- Determine effectiveness of ventilator settings
- Detect adverse effects of mechanical ventilation
- Minimize risk of ventilator-induced complications— allow user to interpret, evaluate, and troubleshoot ventilator and patients' response to ventilator

Ventilator graphic classification

Basic waveforms (scalar graphic)—any single variable (e.g., flow, pressure, volume) plotted against time.
- Pressure versus time scalar
- Flow versus time scalar
- Volume versus time scalar
Loops—the two-dimensional graphic display of two scalars.
- P–V loop
- Flow–volume loop

Basic waveforms

The three basic plots of airway pressure, gas flow change, and volume change are referred as scalar tracings. Most

systems display these settings simultaneously in real time during respiratory support. Basically, the information provided shows the pressure and flow needed to produce the resulting tidal volume on a breath-to-breath basis. Most ventilators define a volume target for each patient and that can be seen on the display. Additionally, the ventilators show two loops which combine these measured values, and which change their shape according to the different conditions affecting the infant. The P–V loop essentially shows the relationship of change in volume with change in pressure, whereas the flow–volume loop informs about flow dynamics and the effects on volume (Fig. 10.1).

Pressure waveform

Pressure waveforms contain both inspiratory and expiratory components. Inspiratory waveforms demonstrate several components. Peak inspiratory pressure (PIP) is the maximum pressure generated in the system. Resistance pressure is the pressure produced secondary to resistance of the whole circuit including hoses, endotracheal tube, and bronchi. It is related to dynamic compliance of the chest and present only with movement of air. Plateau pressure is alveolar compliance pressure generated by delivered volume. It is related to static compliance of the lung. Expiratory pressure waveform shows the pressure returning to baseline positive end-expiratory pressure (PEEP) level. Mean airway pressure is defined by the area under curve for a single inspiratory and expiratory cycle. PEEP remains at the preset level above atmospheric pressure in between breaths. Decrease in pressure below that level indicates patient effort, artifact, or circuit leaks [4]. This pressure waveform typically seen in adults is not as conspicuous in newborns. Neonatal ventilators typically do not show the PIP peak and a lower pressure plateau (Fig. 10.2).

Flow waveform

Flow waveform also has inspiratory and expiratory components. Both inspiratory and expiratory waveforms consist of accelerating and decelerating flow. Inspiratory flow denotes a positive wave, whereas expiratory flow is shown as a negative wave below the baseline zero. Maximum flow is the flow generated during the inspiratory phase. In volume control mode, machine delivers a steady flow of gas while target volume is reached and the inspiratory waveform thus becomes rectangular [5]. As against in pressure

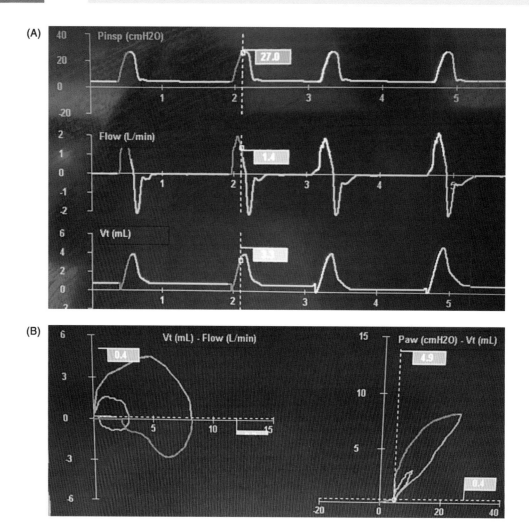

Fig. 10.1 (A and B) Basic waveforms and loops displayed on ventilator. In frame (A), the scalar tracings from top to bottom are pressure, flow, and volume; in frame (B), the flow–volume loop is on the left, and the pressure–volume loop is on the right.

control mode, the machine delivers just enough flow to produce the pressure desired and inspiratory waveform is decelerating [6]. Expiratory flow wave has an acceleration phase in the beginning which ends in peak value and this is usually followed by slow phase retuning back to baseline (Figs. 10.3 and 10.4).

Volume waveform

Pressure and flow impact is summarized and shown on the volume waveform. Most clinicians rely on the displayed

number rather than the wave to determine delivered volume. However, the displayed volume number often reflects an average value, and during SIMV, where both spontaneous and mechanically generated breaths occur, this average may reflect neither volume correctly. The volume waveform, on the other hand, shows comparative size of spontaneous and ventilator-generated volumes. Tidal volume may be more accurately determined by inspecting this waveform. The volume waveform is useful also in assessing the presence of air leak, adequacy of volume delivery, impact of changing ventilator settings, and to evaluate whether patient is generating enough volumes (Fig. 10.5).

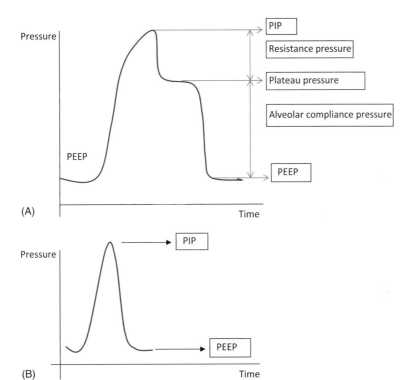

Fig. 10.2 (A) Pressure waveform in adults. (B) Pressure waveform in newborn.

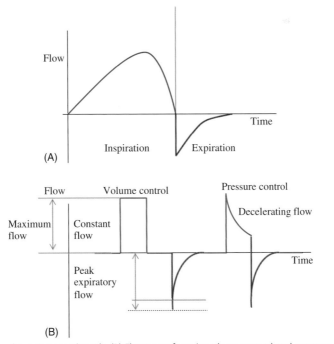

Fig. 10.3 (A) Flow waveform of spontaneous breath. (B) Flow waveform in volume control and pressure control ventilation.

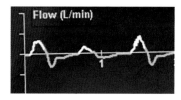

Fig. 10.4 Spontaneous and Ventilated Flow Waveforms.

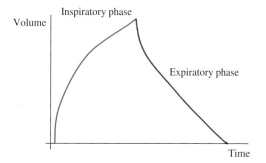

Fig. 10.5 Volume Waveform.

Pulmonary mechanics and loops

Assessment of pulmonary mechanics can be done by graphing changes in pressure or flow with volume over time.

Pressure–volume loop

Lungs change shape according to force applied and the lung behaves differently during inspiration and expiration. This defines hysteresis. After release of inspiratory force, the recoil in elastic components brings the lungs back to their original state. Plotted against volume, the pressure changes required to inflate and deflate form a P–V loop. The different appearance of the inspiratory and expiratory limbs of the P–V loop is a display of hysteresis [7]. This loop shows change in compliance with change in volume. Over last several years this assessment has played important part in developing protective lung strategies for the support of patients with respiratory distress syndrome [8].

In spontaneously breathing patients, inspiration creates a negative pressure that produces filling of the lungs to the tidal volume. Positive pressure is created at the expiration due to elastic recoil and it decreases to zero at the end of expiration. In a spontaneously breathing patient, the volume added to the circuit leads to decrease in circuit pressure, hence the tracing of the loop proceeds in a clockwise fashion. The whole loop shifts to right with application of CPAP or PEEP (Fig. 10.6A–B).

In a ventilated patient, the loop begins not at zero pressure, but at the set PEEP. With increasing pressure from the PEEP baseline, there is gas volume delivery to the lungs, producing the inspiratory portion of the loop. Inspiration ends based on how ventilation is set to be delivered: in time cycled modes when the preset inspiratory time has passed; in flow triggered modes when inspiratory flow has fallen to a set percentage; and in volume-triggered modes when a set tidal volume has been achieved. Pressure and volume fall as the lung deflates. Opening pressure reflects the minimum pressure required to recruit alveoli. Initial rapid rise corresponds to alveolar recruitment. Maximum pressure is the pressure above which there is very little increase in volume with increase in pressure at which point the beaking occurs. Closing pressure is the pressure on expiratory limb at which point volume steeply drops. It reflects elastic recoil of the lung and chest wall. The pressure and volume values recorded at the highest value of the loop correspond to PIP and tidal volume, respectively. However, PEEP lies somewhere in between opening and closing pressures (Fig. 10.6C).

As there is no significant circuit flow at the beginning and end of inspiration, the change in pressure required is that needed to distend the lung. If a line is drawn in the P–V loop from beginning to end inspiration, essentially bisecting the loop, its slope is change in volume over change in pressure–dynamic respiratory system compliance.

P–V loops can show changes in mechanical properties of the lungs, air leaks, evidence of overdistension, adequacy of applied PEEP, and circuit problems (Fig. 10.7).

Patient-triggered pressure–volume loop

Efforts by the patient while on ventilator may show trigger on the P–V [9]. This patient ventilator dyssynchrony is reflected on lower left quadrant. This area can increase or decrease based on adjusting trigger sensitivity on the ventilator (Fig. 10.8).

Increased resistance

With an increase in airway or circuit resistances or both, the loop flattens out away from the dynamic compliance line indicating that relatively higher pressure is required to overcome the resistance and reach targeted volume. In this scenario the dynamic compliance decreases. Increased bowing of the P–V loop should alert the clinician to investigate

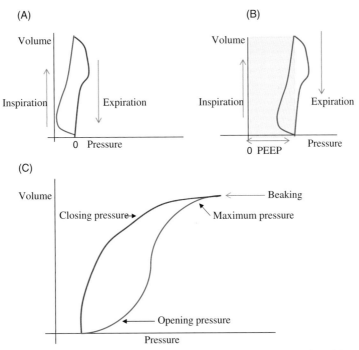

Fig. 10.6 (A) Pressure–volume loop in spontaneously breathing patient and (B) a spontaneous breath in a patient on CPAP or PEEP. (C) Opening, maximum, and closing pressures on a pressure–volume loop.

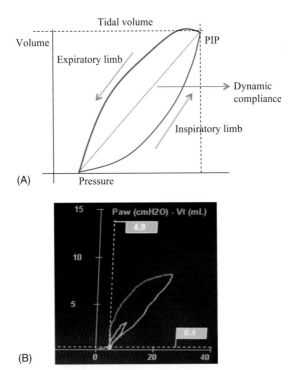

Fig. 10.7 Pressure–Volume Loop in Ventilated Patient. (A) Representation of pressure volume loop in ventilated patient. (B) Pressure volume loop as viewed on ventilator screen.

129

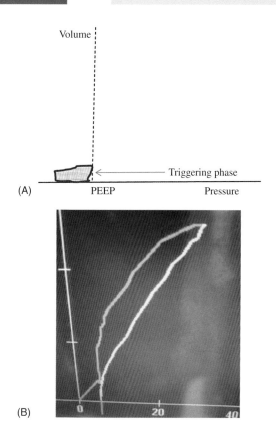

Fig. 10.8 Patient-Triggered Pressure–Volume Loop.
(A) representation of triggering phase (B) Patient triggering on ventilator screen.

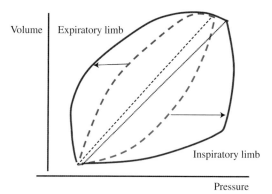

Fig. 10.9 Pressure–Volume Loop With Increased Resistance.

whether the endotracheal tube is kinked or obstructed, whether suctioning is needed or bronchodilator administration is necessary for airway narrowing (Fig. 10.9).

Compliance changes

The shape and position of P–V loop can be altered by change in compliance. Decreases in compliance reflect the need for greater pressure application to cause a fixed volume change. This will cause the P–V loop to rotate toward the x-axis. On the other hand, if compliance increases, with less pressure required for a given change in volume, the loop then rotates toward the y-axis. Slopes of dynamic compliance are significantly altered with these changes (Fig. 10.10).

Alveolar overdistension

Larger tidal volumes in some patients can lead to alveolar overdistension which would then appear on P–V loop as "beaking." It is appreciated at the terminal portion of

the inspiratory limb [10]. Beaking denotes that any further increase in pressure would lead to minimal change in tidal volume. Clinician in this scenario should be cautious managing infant on the ventilator because at this point alveoli are likely to have near-maximal expansion. Active weaning of pressure is recommended until beaking is no longer seen (Fig. 10.11).

Volutrauma and atelectotrauma

P–V loops can greatly influence outcomes related to the ventilator-induced lung injury by helping the clinician to optimizing ventilator settings [11]. Pulmonary compliance increases at pressures above the lower inflection point. This is the point at which alveoli begin to open. Repeated alveolar opening and collapse can lead to atelectotrauma. Minimizing pulmonary damage secondary to atelectasis can be achieved by optimizing the PEEP to a value near or above the lower inflection point. On the other hand, pulmonary compliance decreases at the upper inflection point, at which alveolar overdistension occurs. This in turn may put the infant at risk for volutrauma [12]. Keeping PIP below the maximum pressure may decrease this risk (Fig. 10.12).

Circuit leak

The P–V loop makes identifying a leak in the ventilator circuit easy. The expiratory limb of the loop will not return to zero volume. The ventilator display may also show a % leak value; the loops will quickly provide visual confirmation (Fig. 10.13).

Air hunger

If the infant is not getting adequate flow, the P–V loop may assume the shape of figure of 8. That usually would

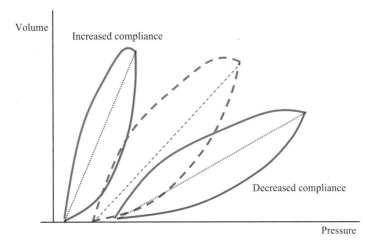

Fig. 10.10 **Pressure–Volume Loop With Change in Compliance.**

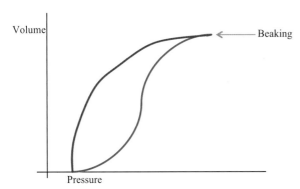

Fig. 10.11 **Beaking of Pressure–Volume Loop Secondary to Alveolar Overdistension.**

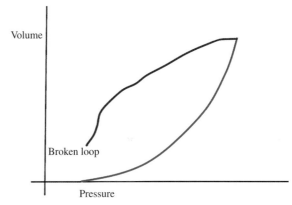

Fig. 10.13 **Circuit Leak on Pressure–Volume Loop.**

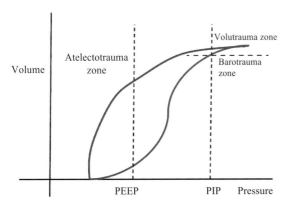

Fig. 10.12 **Zones of Barotrauma and Atelectotrauma on Pressure–Volume Loop.**

indicate inadequate hysteresis. This may also reflect the unstable chest wall of the neonate. This can be corrected by increasing flow or rise time (Fig. 10.14).

Flow–volume loop

The flow–volume loop describes the airflow during tidal breathing. Volume is shown on the x-axis and flow is on the y-axis. Flow–volume loops are particularly important in the assessment of excessive airway resistance and in alerting for the presence of copious airway secretions or circuit leaks. Neonatal ventilators show the flow–volume loop with the inspiratory limb above the x-axis and expiratory limb below the x-axis. The loop moves clockwise

131

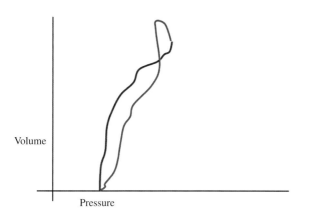

Fig. 10.14 **Air Hunger on Pressure–Volume Loop.**

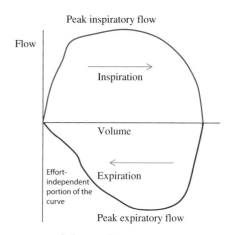

Fig. 10.15 **Normal Flow–Volume Loop.**

with inspiration proceeding up and to the right, while expiration begins when flow drops to zero, then continues below the x-axis, and returns back to zero flow at the end of expiration. The loop shows the rapid rise in flow in early inspiration, with constant flow as volume is delivered, and a rapid fall in flow back to zero as volume delivery ceases. In the expiratory limb, peak expiratory flow occurs early in exhalation depending on patient's efforts. After peak flow is achieved, the expiratory limb tracing progresses to the effort-independent portion of the curve. This area is of particular interest when assessing airway resistance (Fig. 10.15).

Variable extrathoracic obstruction

Increase in inspiratory resistance, suggesting an extrathoracic obstruction, is demonstrated on flow–volume loop with flattening of only inspiratory portion of the loop (Fig. 10.16).

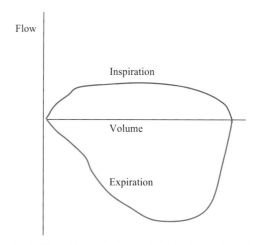

Fig. 10.16 **Flow–Volume Loop in Variable Extrathoracic Obstruction.**

Variable intrathoracic obstruction

Intrathoracic obstruction such as in obstructive airway disease preferentially flattens expiratory portion of the flow–volume loop (Fig. 10.17).

Fixed airway obstruction

Airway obstruction such as in airway anomalies (e.g., tracheal stenosis) or related to endotracheal tube block or kink produces variable changes in both inspiratory and expiratory positions, either flattening both inspiratory and expiratory components (Fig. 10.18A and B) or scooping out of expiratory limb (Fig. 10.18C). Excessive tracheal

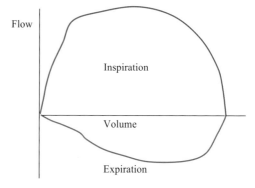

Fig. 10.17 **Flow–Volume Loop in Variable Intrathoracic Obstruction.**

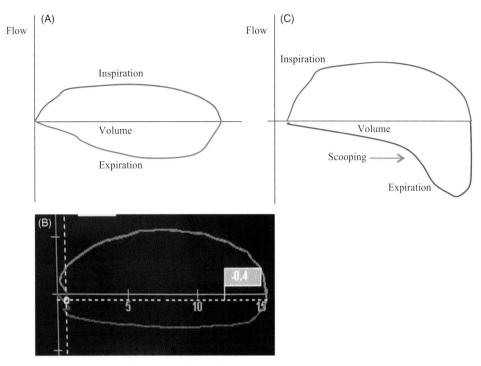

Fig. 10.18 (A–C) Flow–volume loop in fixed airway obstruction.

secretions on the other hand often produce a sawtooth appearance to the expiratory limb of the flow–volume loop which is generally considered a reliable indicator that tracheal suctioning is required.

Turbulence

The circuit airway flow is set too high, or if there are secretions in the airway, sensor, or circuit that interfere with the flow, the flow–volume loop may create a noisy signal. This can be seen on both inspiratory and expiratory components of flow–volume loop as having waveform with serrated edges. Careful inspection for secretions or condensation as well as consideration for endotracheal tube suctioning should be undertaken when the loop produces such sawtooth appearance (Fig. 10.19).

Airway leak

Similar to the P–V loop, an airway leak is seen in the flow–volume loop when the expiratory limb returns to zero without a return to the zero volume point. This is due to the fact that the inspiratory volume is greater than the expiratory volume because of an airway leak (Fig. 10.20).

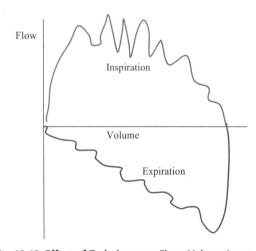

Fig. 10.19 **Effect of Turbulence on Flow–Volume Loop.**

Extubation

If a patient is accidentally extubated, then the flow–volume loop shows flow going in the inspiratory loop but not returning to zero at the end of expiration. The expiratory loop on the other hand is missing as the machine does not

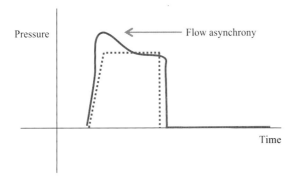

Fig. 10.26 **Flow Asynchrony on Pressure Waveform.**

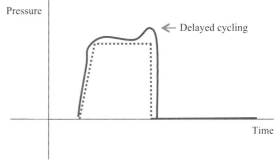

Fig. 10.28 **Delayed Cycling on Pressure Waveform.**

the airway pressure waveform. Adjusting rise time is needed in this setting until the pressure waveforms appear square, have no plateau concavity, and have no evidence of overshoot (Fig. 10.26).

Termination asynchrony

Termination asynchrony or cycling asynchrony involves inspiration being terminated too early (premature cycling) or too late (delayed cycling).

In premature cycling, the patient is continuing to make inspiratory efforts at the time the ventilator cycles off. It may be a feature of unsynchronized ventilation. On the ventilator flow waveforms, premature cycling may be detected by noticing an abrupt initial reversal in the expiratory flow waveform. Synchronizing ventilator may be able to fix this issue (Fig. 10.27).

In delayed cycling, the patient initiates active expiratory efforts while the ventilator is continuing to deliver inspiratory flow. Pressure spike on the pressure waveform during middle-to-late inspiration can be seen. On the flow waveform, it is seen as an abrupt, rapid decline in inspiratory flow near end inspiration. It can be fixed by reducing inspiratory time or tidal volumes (Fig. 10.28).

Expiratory asynchrony

Expiratory asynchrony typically manifests as auto-PEEP with increased peek airway pressure leading to gas trapping. If auto-PEEP is detected, one of the maneuvers to prolong expiratory time (i.e., trigger sensitivity, peak flow, flow pattern, rise time, inspiratory time, cycle threshold, I:E ratio, and respiratory rate) is usually needed [18]. With auto-PEEP increasing, the patient may have difficulty in reaching the triggering threshold. Increasing PEEP may lead to improvement in triggering sensitivity and efficacy. Now that rapid rates are no longer used in favor of fully synchronized modes, this is rarely, if ever, seen in newborns. Auto-PEEP is a result of violating the expiratory time constant (Fig. 10.29).

Pulmonary mechanics and graphics

Using the pulmonary graphics, various pulmonary measurements can be calculated which may be useful diagnostically as well as prognostically.

Compliance

Compliance is a measure of the lung's ability to stretch and expand between inflation and deflation (distensibility of elastic tissue). In clinical practice it consists of two different measurements, static compliance and dynamic compliance. Compliance is measured by P–V loop through ratio of change in volume for change in pressure. The relationship is linear starting at functional residual capacity. As the lung compliance decreases such as in respiratory distress syndrome, pneumonia, and atelectasis, the P–V loop becomes more flat. Healthy newborns have lung compliance between 1.5 and 2 mL/cmH$_2$O. In preterm infant, compliance varies with gestational age

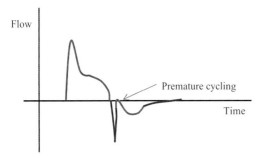

Fig. 10.27 **Premature Cycling on Flow Waveform.**

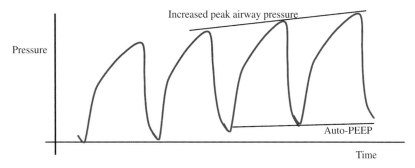

Fig. 10.29 **Expiratory Asynchrony With Generation of Auto-PEEP.**

and weight [19] (Table 10.1). Also, it improves as preterm infants mature. Static compliance is the compliance without any gas flow through the lungs, whereas dynamic compliance is determined by tidal volume for change in driving pressure. Dynamic compliance measurement is useful to estimate change in volume for every pressure change on ventilator.

$$Dynamic\ compliance = Tidal\ volume / PIP - PEEP$$

Resistance

Resistance is any opposition to airflow throughout the respiratory system. It consists of frictional resistance to airflow (80%), tissue resistance (19%), and inertial forces (1%). Resistance is calculated by driving pressure divided by airflow volume. Normal airway resistance in term newborn is 20–40 $cmH_2O/L/s$. Hysteresis of P–V loop represents resistive work of breathing. Resistance decreases with increase in gestational age. Patients with BPD have high airway resistance due to associate barotrauma and therefore increased resistive work of breathing.

Role of pulmonary graphics in bedside ventilator management

Optimizing PIP

PIP can be adjusted for infants managed on pressure-limited ventilator by viewing tidal volume for chosen PIP value with goal of providing volume of 5–6 mL/kg.

Optimizing PEEP (Fig. 10.30)

PEEP can be adjusted to provide adequate tidal volume and viewing favorable P–V relationship on loops avoiding over-distention and underinflation.

Optimizing airflow

Flow–volume loops may aide in adjusting flow. Excessive circuit flow may lead to overdistention and excessive PEEP. This in turn can lead to hypoventilation with wider hysteresis and turbulence.

Table 10.1 Variation in compliance and resistance at different gestational ages

Gestational age	≤26 weeks	27–28 weeks	29–30 weeks	≥31 weeks
Tidal volume, mL/kg	6.1 ± 1.7	5.7 ± 1.5	5.1 ± 1.2	5.2 ± 0.8
Pulmonary compliance, mL/cmH$_2$O/kg	0.27 ± 0.18	0.35 ± 0.22	0.40 ± 0.23	0.77 ± 0.75
Pulmonary resistance, cmH$_2$O/L/s	194 ± 161	139 ± 117	101 ± 64	87 ± 76
Flow-resistive work, g.cm/kg	38 ± 29	28 ± 17	21 ± 14	15 ± 1.2
Change in compliance per week, mL/cmH$_2$O/week	0.16	0.19	0.19	0.24

Adapted from Bhutani VK, Bowen FW, Sivieri EM. Postnatal changes in pulmonary mechanics and energetics of infants with respiratory distress syndrome following surfactant treatment. Biol Neonate 2005;87:323–331 [19].

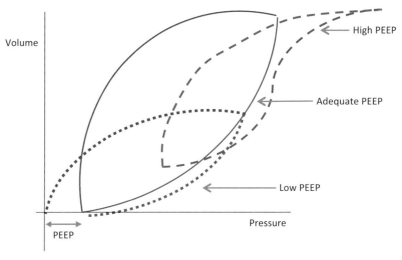

Fig. 10.30 Effect of PEEP on pressure–volume curve with *bold line* showing adequate PEEP, *dotted line* showing low PEEP, and *dashed line* showing excessive PEEP.

Optimizing inspiratory time

Effects on tidal volume, hysteresis, P–V and flow–volume relationships can be assessed by changing inspiratory time. Higher inspiratory time may lead to excessive pressures, decrease in expiratory time, and inadvertent PEEP.

Optimizing synchrony

Real-time evaluation is helpful for team to visualize synchrony on displays. Patient discomfort can be predicted earlier with these displays showing discomfort.

Optimizing tidal volume

Optimal functional residual capacity (FRC) can be predicted by adequate tidal volume and shape of P–V loops. Changes in volume noted on displays can be troubleshooted for various conditions.

Troubleshooting for ventilator graphics

Air trapping (auto-PEEP)

Causes

- Increased expiratory resistance (either in the airways or in the circuit)—thick secretions, bronchospasm

- Insufficient expiratory time
- Early collapse of unstable alveoli/airways during exhalation

How to identify it on the graphics

- Pressure–time: While performing an expiratory hold, the waveform rises above baseline
- Flow–time: The expiratory flow does not return to baseline before the next breath begins
- Volume–time: The expiratory portion does not return to baseline
- Flow–volume loop: The loop does not meet at the baseline
- P–V loop: The loop does not meet at the baseline

How to fix

- Identify the cause and resolve
- Give a treatment or suction
- Decrease inspiratory time
- Increase flow
- Add PEEP

Increased resistance

Causes

- Bronchospasm
- Damp or blocked expiratory valve/filter
- Endotracheal tube problems (too small, kinked, obstructed)

- High flow
- Secretion buildup
- Water in the circuit

How to identify

- Pressure–time: The PIP increases, but the plateau stays the same
- Volume–time: It takes longer for the expiratory curve to reach the baseline
- Flow–time: It takes longer for the expiratory curve to reach baseline and the expiratory flow rate is reduced
- Flow–volume loop: Decreased expiratory flow with a scoop in the expiratory curve
- P–V loop: The loop will be fatter, bulges to the right with inspiratory resistance and to the left with expiratory resistance

How to fix

- Identify cause and fix it
- Bronchodilator treatment
- Suction
- Drain water
- Change circuit
- Change endotracheal tube
- Decrease PF rate
- Change expiratory filter

Decreased compliance

Causes

- ARDS
- Atelectasis
- Abdominal distension
- Congestive heart failure
- Consolidation
- Fibrosis
- Hyperinflation
- Pneumothorax
- Pleural effusion

How to identify it

- Pressure–time: The PIP and plateau both increase
- P–V loop: Lays more horizontal

How to fix

- Treat the cause
- Increase PEEP

Increased compliance

Causes

- Surfactant therapy
- Natural resolution of RDS/pneumonia
- Intercostal drain for pneumothorax

How to identify it

- Pressure–time: PIP and plateau both decrease
- P–V loop: Stands more vertical (upright)

How to fix

- Aggressive weaning of pressures

Active exhalation

Causes

- Patient is exhaling below FRC due to air trapping (volume dumping)
- Pain
- Positional change
- Equipment calibration problem

How to identify it

- Volume–time: Expiratory waveform goes below the baseline
- P–V loop: Expiratory loop goes past the zero point
- Flow–volume loop: Expiratory part goes past the zero point

How to fix

- Reduce air trapping
- Calibrate equipment
- Relieve pain

Partial obstruction

Causes

- Suction catheter left in ETT
- Tissue flap
- Mucus plug
- Water/secretions in the circuit or airway

How to identify

- Flow–volume: Flow is not steady and constant, but varies as the obstruction moves around
- P–V loop: Jagged instead of smooth
- Flow–volume loop: Jagged with fluctuating flow

How to fix it

- Pull catheter out of ETT
- Suction
- Drain water
- Change circuit
- Move the endotracheal tube

Overdistension

Causes

- Tidal volume set too high (volume ventilation)
- Pressure set too high (pressure ventilator)
- Could occur in pressure ventilator with compliance or airway resistance changes

How to identify it

- P–V loop: Bird beak at the top of the loop

How to fix it

- Reduce tidal volume (volume ventilation)
- Reduce pressure (pressure ventilation)

Leak

Causes

- Expiratory leak: Air leak through a chest tube, BP fistula, ETT cuff leak, NG tube in trachea
- Inspiratory leak: Loose connections, ventilator malfunction, faulty flow sensor

How to identify

- Pressure–time: Decreased PIP
- Volume–time: Decreased tidal volume, in expiratory leaks keep tidal volume returning to baseline
- Flow–time: Peak expiratory flow decreases
- P–V loop: Expiratory side does not return to the baseline
- Flow–volume loop: Expiratory part does not return to baseline

How to fix it

- Identify source of leak and fix it
- Do a leak test and make sure all connections are tight

Ventilator graphics in special situations

Surfactant administration

The administration of exogenous surfactant to an infant with RDS typically lowers alveolar surface tension and improves pulmonary compliance. It happens rapidly, and one must monitor loops as both flow–volume and P–V loops will show significantly higher volume administered. There is a risk of overdistension of the lung if pressure is not reduced rapidly enough to reduce volume.

Bronchopulmonary dysplasia

Infants with bronchopumonary dysplasia (BPD) can demonstrate combination of restrictive and obstructive patterns based on the severity. Flow–volume loop may demonstrate flattening of both components of loops, demonstrating diminished inspiratory as well as expiratory flow rates. Infants with BPD may at times manifest with abnormal central airway collapse causing BPD spell where wheezing becomes prominent with increased expiratory effort, and infant may become cyanotic. Infants on ventilator may show lack of air movement or acute obstructive pattern with near-zero volume on inspiratory as well as expiratory components (Fig. 10.31). Bronchodilator effects can also be demonstrated in patients with BPD with loops. Effective treatment would show significant improvement in both the inspiratory and expiratory flows. The loop would be opened with improved tidal volume delivery.

Pneumothorax

Pneumothorax is suspected when autocycling occurs with sudden increase in respiratory rate without any patient input associated with sudden decrease in the exhaled tidal volume and minute ventilation. It may occur because of a leak anywhere in the system starting from the ventilator right up to the patient's lungs. The exhaled tidal volume

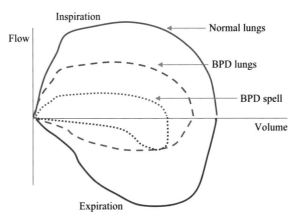

Fig. 10.31 Flow–volume loop comparing normal lungs (bold line), BPD lungs (dashed line), and BPD while having a spell (dotted line).

will be lower than the set parameters, and this may set off a ventilator alarm for low exhaled tidal volume, low minute ventilation, circuit disconnect, or rapid respiratory rate. The lung compliance may acutely decrease with atelectasis of the affected lung.

Waveforms with high-frequency ventilators (Fig. 10.32)

Unlike conventional ventilation, HFOV is reliant on the waveforms generated to achieve gas exchange at much smaller tidal volumes. The waveforms generated by modern oscillators have unique shape, frequency characteristics, and resultant amplitudes at comparable settings. Oscillators generate either a square or sine wave pattern with varying frequencies. The Fabian, Leonie+, and BL8000 mainly show sine waves, whereas VN500 pressure waveform is a sine wave with steep expiratory slope. The SensorMedic 3100B waveforms at 1:2 I:E ratio and SM3100A at both I:E settings show square waves. At 1:2 ratio, the SM3100B waveforms produce an initial inspiratory pulse followed by a notch, then stepwise reductions in pressure and flow preceding peaks. The SLE5000 exhibits a square wave comparable to SM3100A and B at 1:1 ratios. It is hard to determine whether the marked differences in delivered waveforms are likely to translate into clinical differences in oscillatory performance or lung protection [20].

Limitations of ventilator graphics

With increasing use of noninvasive ventilation, there has been decrease in trend in following waveforms on the ventilator. Both pressures and volumes are reliable when infants are intubated. The current ventilators providing noninvasive support cannot optimally measure both these parameters partly due the fact that nasal interface does not block nostrils. Additionally, pressures and volume generated at the nasal interface cannot reliably measure the same parameters at the laryngeal opening as both pressures and volumes are lost in variable proportions to esophagus. Also, with uncuffed endotracheal tubes used in newborns measured volumes and pressures could be different depending on the leak. With use of new sophisticated ventilators, clinicians try to focus on the numbers and pay less attention to the waveforms. Unfortunately, in this day and age less and less clinicians have knowledge of how the ventilator works and how to troubleshoot them.

Summary

- Ventilator graphics analyze breath-to-breath performance of the infant on the ventilator which is then displayed as waveforms, loops, and trends.

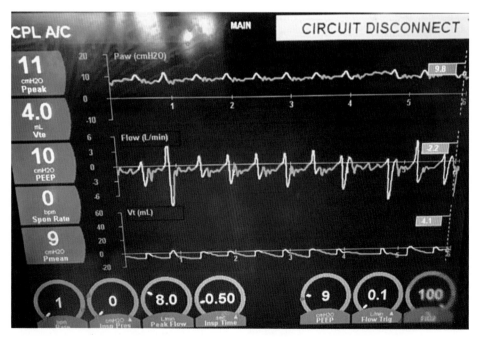

Fig. 10.32 Scalar Waveforms With High-Frequency Jet Ventilator Connected to AVEA® Ventilator.

- Respiratory physiology can be easily understood by reviewing the ventilator graphics.
- Some of the complications including hyperinflation, extubation, auto-PEEP, and so on may be evident from graphics before they are clinically apparent.

- Continuous monitoring can help decrease the frequency of blood gas analysis and radiography, reducing the cost of care as well as increasing the comfort of the patient.

References

[1] Von Neergaard K, Wirtz K. Neue Auffassungen über einen Grudbegriff der Atemmechanik: Die Retraktionskraft der Lunger, abh€angig von der Oberfl€achenspannug in den Alveolen. Zeitschr Gesamte Exp Med 1929;66:373–394.

[2] Gregory GA, Kitterman JA, Phibbs RH, Tooley WH, Hamilton WK. Treatment of the idiopathic respiratory-distress syndrome with continuous airway pressure. N Engl J M ed 1971;284:1333–1340.

[3] Bhutani VK, Sivieri EM, Abbasi S, Shaffer TH. Evaluation of neonatal pulmonary mechanics and energetics: a two factor least mean square analysis. Pediatr Pulmonol 1988;4:150–158.

[4] Vignaux L, Vargas F, et al. Patient-ventilator asynchrony during non-invasive ventilation for acute respiratory failure: a multicenter study. Intensive Care Med 2009;35:840–846.

[5] Koh SO. Mode of mechanical ventilation: volume controlled mode. Crit Care Clin 2007;23:161–167.

[6] Singer BD, Corbridge TC. Pressure modes of invasive mechanical ventilation. South Med J 2011;104:701–709.

[7] Brusasco V, Pellegrino R. Hysteresis of airways and lung parenchyma. Respir Med 1995;89:311–322.

[8] Terragni PP, Rosboch GL, Lisi A, Viale AG, Ranieri VM. How respiratory system mechanics may help in minimising ventilator-induced lung injury in ARDS patients. Eur Respir J Suppl 2003;42:15s–21s.

[9] Waugh JB, Deshpande VM, Harwood RJ. Pressure-volume and flow-volume loops. Rapid interpretation of ventilator waveforms. Upper Saddle River, NJ: Pearson Education, Inc; 2007. 23–52.

[10] Fisher JB, Mammel MC, Coleman JM, Bing D, Boros SJ. Identifying lung overdistention during mechanical ventilation by using volume-pressure loops. Pediatr Pulmonol 1988;5:10–14.

[11] Muscedere JG, Mullen JB, Gan K, Slutsky AS. Tidal ventilation at low airway pressures can augment lung injury. Am J Respir Crit Care Med 1994;149:1327–1334.

[12] Dreyfuss D, Soler P, Basset G, Saumon G. High inflation pressure pulmonary edema. Respective effects of high airway pressure, high tidal volume, and positive end-expiratory pressure. Am Rev Respir Dis 1988;137:1159–1164.

[13] Donn SM, Nicks JJ, Becker MA. Flow-synchronized ventilation of preterm infants with respiratory distress syndrome. J Perinatol 1994;14:90–94.

[14] Perlman JM, McMenanim JB, Volpe JJ. Fluctuating cerebral blood flow velocity in respiratory distress syndrome: relationship to subsequent development of intraventricular hemorrhage. N Engl J Med 1983;309:204–209.

[15] de Wit M. Monitoring of patient-ventilator interaction at the bedside. Respir Care 2011;56:61–72.

[16] Thille AW, Rodriguez P, Cabello B, Lellouche F, Brochard L. Patient-ventilator asynchrony during assisted mechanical ventilation. Intensive Care Med 2006;32:1515–1522.

[17] Thille AW, Cabello B, Galia F, Lyazidi A, Brochard L. Reduction of patient-ventilator asynchrony by reducing tidal volume during pressure-support ventilation. Intensive Care Med 2008;34:1477–1486.

[18] Laghi F, Goyal A. Auto-PEEP in respiratory failure. Minerva Anesthesiol 2012;78:201–221.

[19] Bhutani VK, Bowen FW, Sivieri EM. Postnatal changes in pulmonary mechanics and energetics of infants with respiratory distress syndrome following surfactant treatment. Biol Neonate 2005;87:323–331.

[20] Harcourt ER, John J, Dargaville PA, Zannin E, Davis PG, Tingay DG. Pressure and flow waveform characteristics of eight high-frequency oscillators. Pediatr Crit Care Med 2014;15:e234–e240.

Chapter | 11A |

Initiation of Mechanical Ventilation

Dushyant Batra, MRCPCH, Craig Smith, MRCPCH, Bernard Schoonakker, MRCPCH

CHAPTER POINTS

- Mechanical ventilation may be associated with harm.
- A structured algorithm for initiation and weaning is suggested.

Introduction

Despite advances in antenatal and neonatal care, many preterm as well as term newborn babies need mechanical ventilation to ensure survival and reduce suboptimal outcomes. However, mechanical ventilation may contribute to mortality as well as morbidities. Strategies aimed at avoiding mechanical ventilation have shown a significant impact on the incidence of bronchopulmonary dysplasia (BPD) in preterm infants [1]. Even term babies requiring ventilatory support may suffer from significant morbidity and mortality [2,3]. In spontaneously breathing preterm infants, continuous positive airway pressure (CPAP) [4] or nasal intermittent positive pressure ventilation (NIPPV) [5] from birth is recommended with intubation reserved for babies not responding to noninvasive respiratory support [4]. The use of minimally invasive surfactant therapy in spontaneously breathing preterm infants is becoming more common [6] and has been shown to reduce the need for ventilation [7].

New advances in ventilation technology and patient monitoring, including pulmonary graphics, can help optimize the management of preterm as well as term babies needing respiratory support. This section provides practical guidance for the initiation and early optimization of ventilation for critically unwell babies.

Indications for mechanical ventilation

Newborn babies may require mechanical ventilation for respiratory and nonrespiratory reasons within either an urgent or elective time frame. Attending clinicians must always ask: *Do I need to intubate and ventilate this baby or can I manage them with less invasive support?*

The common indications for mechanical ventilation include:

- Respiratory
  - Anticipated significant surfactant deficiency or apnea at birth
  - Early and significant respiratory distress syndrome (RDS) not responding to noninvasive respiratory support (including less invasive surfactant therapy administration)
  - Worsening respiratory failure on noninvasive support
  - Inadequate respiratory drive/strength
- Nonrespiratory
  - Inability to maintain safe airway
  - Systemically unwell, for example, hypotension requiring intervention or severe sepsis
  - Certain surgical conditions directly or indirectly affecting airway or respiratory status, for example,

congenital diaphragmatic hernia, necrotizing enterocolitis
- Surgery (perioperative period)

The decision to ventilate may not be simple and may require a risk to benefit assessment by senior team members, reviewing key information such as:
- Indication for mechanical ventilation
- Gestational age and weight
- Antenatal history (e.g., antenatal steroids, prolonged rupture of membranes)
- Current respiratory status including chest X-ray (CXR)
- Recent and anticipated respiratory course
- Current systemic status, for example, hypotension, NEC, HIE
- Imminent transport

Equipment

A number of modern neonatal ventilators are available. They offer advances in patient safety but are complex, and this complexity may increase the risk of human error. Further, the use of different nomenclature can be confusing. Each service needs to be very familiar with its ventilator of choice and be clear as to how it complements their respiratory support strategy.

An ideal modern ventilator should have the following properties:
- Offer a variety of modes of ventilation including high frequency ventilation (HFOV)
- Easy transition to HFOV
- User friendly interface and simple controls
- Reliable performance
- Accuracy with ability to make small changes in parameters
- Circuits with low compliance
- Facility for efficient and accurate volume targeting
- Reliable pulmonary graphics to guide changes
- Informative alarm system
- Ability to work with other equipment, for example, nitric oxide delivery, end-tidal CO_2 monitoring

Goals of mechanical ventilation

Generic goals of intubation and ventilation include [8]:
- Secure airway
- Support baby's own respiratory efforts when feasible
- Optimal oxygenation with acceptable CO_2 clearance
- Minimal adverse effects, for example, ventilator-associated lung injury (VALI)

- Prepare for safe surgery or transport
- Add to stabilization of the critically unwell baby

Initiation of mechanical ventilation

Algorithm 11A.1 provides a framework for the initiation of mechanical ventilation [8]. Recently, a greater proportion of babies have been managed without intubation, using alternative approaches alongside improved antenatal care. Each service needs to be clear about indications for ventilation and ventilation avoidance. Some services will direct staff to manage extreme prematurity with intubation based on factors, such as gestational age; whereas others will aim to avoid intubation and manage respiratory care with alternative methods until intubation is required as a rescue strategy. Once intubation has been deemed necessary, most clinicians will opt for a version of conventional mechanical ventilation. Some services choose HFOV as the default modality to start ventilation.

After setting up the ventilator for safe use, key initial ventilation settings need to be chosen, including peak inspiratory pressure (PIP), peak-end expiratory pressure (PEEP), inhaled oxygen concentration (FiO_2), inspiratory time (T_i), and respiratory rate (RR). Knowledge of antenatal factors as well as use of premedication and surfactant is important. Settings used in stabilization can guide these but typical initial settings for most preterm babies would be within the following ranges:
- PIP: 16–20 cmH_2O
- PEEP: 4–6 cmH_2O
- Ti: 0.3–0.35 sec
- Rate: 40–60 bpm

A new 25-week gestation baby, who received surfactant in the delivery room, may be started on 18/5, T_i 0.3 s and RR of 40 bpm. Early observation of minute ventilation, tidal volume, and saturation, combined with chest examination can be used to guide minor changes as lung volumes stabilize and synchrony improves. Alternatively, a baby receiving surfactant later, for respiratory distress and rising FiO_2, after a trial of CPAP, may require a higher PIP (>20 cmH_2O) to ensure adequate recruitment. A higher PEEP of 5–6 cmH_2O will reduce atelectasis. When initiating ventilation in babies with abdominal distension, significant atelectasis or pulmonary hemorrhage, a PEEP of 6–8 cmH_2O should be used. Again observation of tidal volumes and minute ventilation will help. Determining optimum T_i and rate requires knowledge of the lung disease and observation of pulmonary graphic waveforms. In low compliance lung disease, a shorter T_i of 0.2–0.3 s and a higher rate of 50–60 bpm will allow you to achieve a target minute ventilation of 200–300 mL/kg/min.

If the severity of lung disease is unclear or breathing is reduced, we recommend initiating ventilation with synchronized intermittent mandatory ventilation (SIMV) mode. The clinician should stay with the patient to assess synchrony

ALGORITHM 11A.1 INITIATION OF VENTILATION.

Setup Ventilator

1. Set appropriate PIP, PEEP, T_i, and FiO_2 (see guidance on starting values above)
2. Choose SIMV mode
3. Set pressure-rise time (time from PEEP to PIP) at 0.1–0.16 s

↓

Connect the intubated baby to the ventilator

↓

Initiate ventilation

1. Observe immediate ventilation responses: chest movement, air entry, V_{te} and minute ventilation, saturation, and FiO_2
2. Be aware of ETT leak and hemodynamic status
3. Consider volume guided ventilation when the above parameters, for example, V_{te} and FiO_2 are stable and the leak is <40%
4. Blood gas (arterial or capillary) after 20–30 min
5. Consider assist-control (AC) mode if the respiratory drive is sufficient

↓

Reassess and review
Is the patient likely to remain ventilated for >12 h?

Yes	No
Follow Algorithm 11.2	Follow Algorithm 11.3

and response. As parameters stabilize, the use of volume targeting and a better trigger mode should be considered.

The anticipated duration of ventilation will vary according to the underlying diagnosis and predicted natural history. If the duration of ventilation is anticipated to be short, for example, a 30-week gestation baby showing a good response to early surfactant, then initiation of a weaning process (see later) including adjunctive therapy, for example, caffeine citrate should be considered early. Alternatively, babies expected to be on the ventilator for longer periods, for example, a 23-week gestation baby in poor condition, the focus should be on early optimal ventilation aimed at minimizing VALI, with a package of good intensive care support including sedation. For babies with good respiratory drive, assist-control (AC) ventilation mode in combination with volume targeting (see below) provides uniform tidal volumes and a lower work of breathing [9]. A lower backup rate should increase the number of triggered breaths, ventilator synchrony [10], and reduce the work of breathing [11,12]. When entering the weaning phase, volume targeted pressure support ventilation (PSV) mode can allow babies to determine their own respiratory pattern with better synchrony and at a lower MAP [13]. Most babies will usually require a brief period of SIMV followed by either AC or PSV.

Neurally adjusted ventilatory assist (NAVA) mode can aid ventilator synchrony by unloading respiratory muscles [14].

Ventilation strategies and choosing the right mode

A practical approach (Algorithm 11A.2) to achieve optimal ventilation for each individual patient can be achieved by

ALGORITHM 11A.2 VENTILATION STRATEGY.

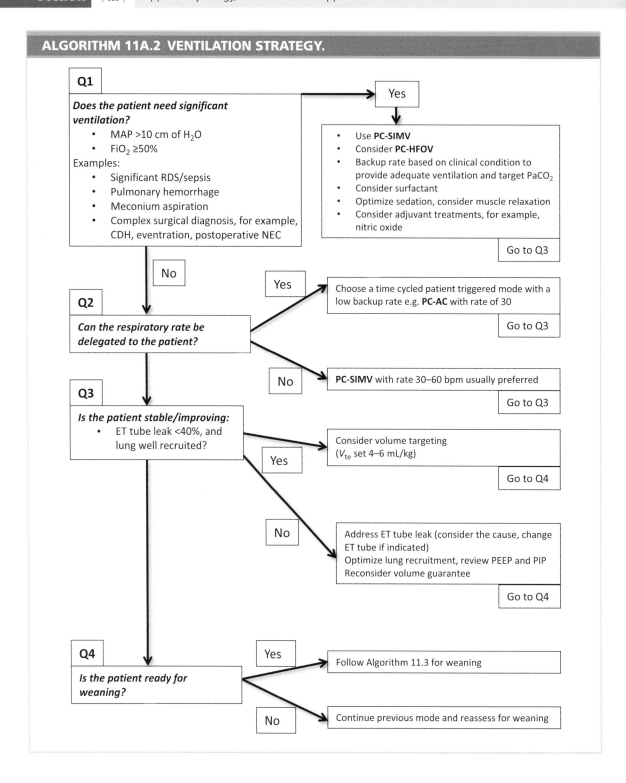

Q1

Does the patient need significant ventilation?
- MAP >10 cm of H_2O
- FiO_2 ≥50%

Examples:
- Significant RDS/sepsis
- Pulmonary hemorrhage
- Meconium aspiration
- Complex surgical diagnosis, for example, CDH, eventration, postoperative NEC

Yes

- Use **PC-SIMV**
- Consider **PC-HFOV**
- Backup rate based on clinical condition to provide adequate ventilation and target $PaCO_2$
- Consider surfactant
- Optimize sedation, consider muscle relaxation
- Consider adjuvant treatments, for example, nitric oxide

Go to Q3

No

Q2

Can the respiratory rate be delegated to the patient?

Yes

Choose a time cycled patient triggered mode with a low backup rate e.g. **PC-AC** with rate of 30

Go to Q3

No

PC-SIMV with rate 30–60 bpm usually preferred

Go to Q3

Q3

Is the patient stable/improving:
- ET tube leak <40%, and lung well recruited?

Yes

Consider volume targeting (V_{te} set 4–6 mL/kg)

Go to Q4

No

Address ET tube leak (consider the cause, change ET tube if indicated)
Optimize lung recruitment, review PEEP and PIP
Reconsider volume guarantee

Go to Q4

Q4

Is the patient ready for weaning?

Yes

Follow Algorithm 11.3 for weaning

No

Continue previous mode and reassess for weaning

asking four questions [8]. These questions may need to be revisited with changes in the clinical course.

1. *Does the baby require significant ventilation, for example, MAP > 10 cmH₂O?*
   Clinical scenarios include those with very low compliance, such as significant surfactant deficiency, pulmonary hemorrhage, meconium aspiration syndrome, and patients with pulmonary hypoplasia. Typically, the baby will require support with a high-mean airway pressure (> 10 cmH₂O), high-inspired oxygen requirement (> 50%), and high respiratory rate, typically 50–60 bpm.
   If the answer is yes, then the clinician must strive to optimize the patient–ventilator interaction, at these higher settings. Effective early sedation and the occasional brief use of muscle relaxants can help stabilize the clinical situation, achieve an open lung, and reduce the risk of air leak. PEEP values between 5 and 8 cmH₂O will maintain lung recruitment. Occasionally, higher PEEP values of 9–10 cmH₂O are used as part of a recruitment maneuver [15]. Observing trends in expiratory tidal volume (V_{te}) (4–6 mL/kg) and minute ventilation is a useful guide to stable ventilation.
   Oxygenation index values above 25 indicate severe ventilation–perfusion imbalance [16] and worsening values may need consideration of HFOV and adjuvant treatments, such as surfactant and nitric oxide.
   If the answer is no, then move on to the second question.

2. *Can the respiratory rate be delegated to the patient?*
   This explores how good the patient's respiratory drive is.
   If the answer is yes, then the patient can be put on a time cycled patient triggered mode, for example. AC with a low backup rate [11], that is, set typically at 30 bpm.
   If the answer is no, and you anticipate the baby won't trigger many breaths then use SIMV.

3. *Are the patient's lungs adequately recruited and is the ET leak <40%?*
   If the answer is yes, then the patient would benefit from using volume targeting. Adequate recruitment at this stage can be confirmed with clinical signs and CXR. V_{te} is usually set at 4–6 mL/kg.
   If the answer is no, then review the patient to see what could be optimized. If the leak is >40%, consider the cause and change ET tube if indicated. If the lungs are underrecruited then consider a recruitment maneuver. Reconsider volume guarantee after performing these steps.
   The final question is

4. *Is the patient ready for weaning?* Typically, this will be true once the oxygen requirement and MAP have

stabilized and are at acceptable levels, for example, <40% and 8–10 cmH₂O, respectively. The mean airway pressure prior to successful extubation will vary with the underlying lung disease and other patient factors. The relationship between MAP, weaning, and extubation is unclear [17]. The patient should be hemodynamically stable with no contraindications to extubation.

If the answer is yes, AC mode with a low backup rate (typically 30 bpm) and a set volume target (typically 4–6 mL/kg) will allow the MAP to fall as the lung mechanics improve (Algorithm 11A.3) [8]. Ensure that the sedation is appropriately weaned and the patient

---

ALGORITHM 11A.3 WEANING VENTILATION.

Is the patient ready for weaning?
- Stable and acceptable FiO₂
- Acceptable MAP (generally 8–10 cm H₂O)
- Hemodynamic stability (stable BP off inotropes or on low dose inotropes)
- No contraindications to extubation (e.g., continued muscle relaxation, surgical plan to continue ventilation after major surgery)

↓

Review the mode of ventilation
- Weaning with PC-AC or PC-PSV usually preferred
- Backup rate typically 30 bpm
- Monitor MAP, it should wean itself on volume targeted ventilation as lung mechanics improve
- Wean sedation as appropriate and ensure good respiratory drive
- Consider caffeine

↓

Readiness for extubation assessment
- Improving or stable blood gas (arterial or capillary)
- Improving or stable respiratory diagnosis
- Good respiratory drive
- Non–invasive respiratory support is available (if indicated)

↓

Postextubation care
- Good positioning and minimize handling as appropriate
- Repeat blood gas (arterial/capillary) after 30–60 min

has been given caffeine, if indicated. To improve synchrony, switch to the flow-cycled mode PSV [18]. Continue with a low backup rate (typically 30 bpm). Monitor the T_i as values consistently below 0.2 s may lead to progressive atelectasis [19].

HFOV as the initial mode

Some services have become skilled with HFOV as the initial mode of respiratory support. Compared to services choosing conventional modes, these services have a high number of medical and nursing staff who are familiar with the theory, effective use, and problem-solving associated with HFOV. Although not consistently proven, HFOV may offer some advantages to some patient groups requiring ongoing ventilation [20]. However, HFOV is usually reserved as a rescue mode.

References

[1] Fischer H, Buhrer C. Avoiding endotracheal ventilation to prevent bronchopulmonary dysplasia: a meta-analysis. Pediatrics 2013;132:e1351–e1360.

[2] Ramadan G, Paul N, Morton M, Peacock J, Greenough A. Outcome of ventilated term infants born at term without major congenital abnormalities. Eur J Pediatr 2012;171(171):331–336.

[3] Clark R. The epidemiology of respiratory failure in neonates born at an estimated gestational age of 34 weeks of more. J Perinatol 2005;25:251–257.

[4] Sweet DG, Carnielli V, Greisen G, Hallman M, Ozek E, Plavka R, et al. Consensus Guidelines European Consensus Guidelines on the Management of Neonatal Respiratory Distress Syndrome in Preterm Infants—2013 Update. Neonatology 2013; 103103.

[5] Lemyre B, Laughon M, Bose C, Davis PG. Early nasal intermittent positive pressure ventilation (NIPPV) versus early nasal continuous positive airway pressure (NCPAP) for preterm infants. In: Lemyre B, editor. Cochrane database of systematic reviews. Chichester, UK: John Wiley & Sons, Ltd; 2016.

[6] Klotz D, Porcaro U, Fleck T, Fuchs H. European perspective on less invasive surfactant administration—a survey. Eur J Pediatr 2017;176(2):147–154.

[7] Oncel MY, Arayici S, Uras N, Alyamac-Dizdar E, Sari FN, Karahan S, et al. Nasal continuous positive airway pressure versus nasal intermittent positive-pressure ventilation within the minimally invasive surfactant therapy approach in preterm infants: a randomised controlled trial. Arch Dis Child Fetal Neonatal Ed 2016;101(4):F323–F328.

[8] Batra D, Schoonakker B, Smith C. Mechanical ventilation in neonates. Nottingham neonatal service—clinical guidelines. Nottingham: Nottingham Neonatal Service; 2017. p. 1–26.

[9] Keszler M. State of art in conventional mechanical ventilation. J Perinatol 2009;29:262–275.

[10] Banacalari E, Claure N. Chapter 17: patient-ventilator interaction. In: Polin RA, editor. The newborn lung: neonatology questions and controversies. 2nd ed. Philadelphia: Elsevier; 2012. 339–354.

[11] Wheeler KI, Morley CJ, Hooper SB, Davis PG. Lower back-up rates improve ventilator triggering during assist-control ventilation: a randomized crossover trial. J Perinatol 2012;32(2):111–116.

[12] Carlucci A, Pisani L, Ceriana P, Malovini A, Nava S. Patient-ventilator asynchronies: may the respiratory mechanics play a role? Crit Care 2013;17(2):R54.

[13] Abubakar KM, Keszler M. Patient-ventilator interactions in newer modes of patient triggered ventilation. Pediatr Pulmonol 2001;32:71–75.

[14] Stein H, Firestone K, Rimensberger PC. Synchronized mechanical ventilation using electrical activity of the diaphragm in neonates. Clin Perinatol 2012;39(3):525–542.

[15] Keszler M, Sant'Anna G. Mechanical ventilation and bronchopulmonary dysplasia. Clin Perinatol 2015;42(4):781–796.

[16] Donn SM, Sinha SK. Pulmonary diagnostics. Semin Fetal Neonatal Med 2017;22(4):200–205.

[17] Wang HW, Jyun-You L, Chien-Yi C, Chou H-C, Hsieh W-S, Tsao P-N. Risk factors for extubation failure in extremely low birth weight infants. Pediatr Neonatol 2017;58:145–150.

[18] Keszler M. Mechanical ventilation strategies. Semin Fetal Neonatal Med 2017;22:267–274.

[19] Klingenberg C, Wheeler KI, Davis PG, Morley CJ. A practical guide to neonatal volume guarantee ventilation. J Perinatol 2011;31(9):575–585.

[20] Cools F, Offringa M, Askie LM. Elective high frequency oscillatory ventilation versus conventional ventilation for acute pulmonary dysfunction in preterm infants. In: Cools F, editor. Cochrane database of systematic reviews. Chichester, UK: John Wiley & Sons, Ltd; 2015.

Chapter | 11B |

Deterioration on the Ventilator

Craig Smith, MRCPCH, Dushyant Batra, MRCPCH, Bernard Schoonakker, MRCPCH

CHAPTER POINTS

- Modern intensive care should aim to predict and prepare for deterioration events.

Approach to deterioration on a ventilator

Intensive care is associated with adverse outcomes independent of the underlying disease [1]. The origin of these may be "silent," for example, hypocapnia and hyperoxia during excess ventilatory support or be directly associated with deterioration events while on the ventilator, for example, hypoxia secondary to a blocked endotracheal tube (ETT). Deterioration events are common [2] and can be anticipated in certain situations, for example, air leak in pulmonary hypoplasia. Services should target these events as a part of their quality improvement strategy. Exposure to approved guidance and simulation training [3] can enhance the recognition and management of these episodes by key decision makers and the intensive care team.

Deterioration awareness strategy

- Anticipation
- Rapid information synthesis
- Assessment maneuvers, analysis, and diagnosis

Anticipation of potential deterioration events should be a part of the narrative of daily assessments and decision-making. Once the underlying disease has been diagnosed and assessed, the natural history on the ventilator should be discussed by the team. This should include duration of ventilation, need for other organ support, and the anticipation of likely complications and when they may occur.

Modern intensive care collects and presents important diagnostic information at very frequent intervals, for example SaO_2 trends, pulmonary graphic data, and blood gases. Recognizable patterns in these information flows can be used to warn of impending deterioration to prepared decision-makers and team members, for example, trend data on minute ventilation, tidal volume, and resistance may herald a blocked ETT before profound desaturation and bradycardia. Information immediately available to the team includes clinical examination, ventilation parameters, pulmonary graphics, monitoring data, nursing feedback, as well as recent blood gases and X-rays (Table 11B.1).

The rapid collection, synthesis, and analysis of these data into recognizable patterns based on common problems are the key to correct timely intervention to minimize risk of sudden death or long-term morbidity (Algorithm 11B.1).

The majority of the deterioration events are either respiratory or cardiorespiratory in nature and present as a desaturation episode, usually accompanied by bradycardia. Less

Table 11B.1 BOLDPEEP approach to deterioration on a ventilator

	B Bad or worsening lung disease	O Obstructed ETT	L Long ETT	D Displaced ETT	P Pneumothorax	E Equipment failure	EP Equipment-patient asynchrony
History	No antenatal steroids, PPROM, high FiO_2, weaned too quickly, blood up ETT	Secretions, sepsis, blood up ETT, variable FiO_2	Never settled on ventilator, long ETT on X-ray, dental rolls in use	Sudden desaturation, no response to T-piece ventilation or increasing FiO_2 and PIP	No antenatal steroids, moderate to severe RDS or hypoplasia, delayed or poor early care including late surfactant, high PIP, drop in BP	Frequent alarms, frequent water in circuits, ventilator cutting out, unexplained hypotension or hypoglycemia (lines)	Old BPD baby, bad lung disease, long ETT, recently reduced or stopped morphine or atracurium, hyperinflation
Exam	Poor chest movement, reduced air entry bilaterally, negative cold light	Variable chest movement, reduced air entry, crepitations and wheeze	Poor chest movement and air entry, often worse on left. Air entry improves with pulling ETT back	No chest movement or air entry, audible leak, no colour change with $ETCO_2$ sensor	Asymmetry of chest shape, movement and air entry. Positive transillumination	Poor chest movement and air entry, improves with T-piece on same settings	Active baby, variable chest movement, chest splinting, hyperinflation
Charts	Rising FiO_2, desaturations, poor handling	Rising FiO_2, desaturations, poor handling, frequent suction	Rising FiO_2, desaturations, poor handling	Previously stable, recent handling, poorly sedated, very active	Sudden change or deterioration	Nurse may indicate concern over the ventilator	Desaturations, pain score, high HR/BP, rising/high FiO_2
Blood gas	Respiratory acidosis	Respiratory acidosis, mixed acidosis in pulmonary hemorrhage	Respiratory acidosis	Previously stable	Worsening respiratory acidosis	Previously stable	Variable

Pulmonary graphics	Low compliance, high resistance, blunted flows, flat VP loops, low MV/VTE, possible leak	Variable resistance and compliance, variable flows, often blunted	High resistance, blunted flows	No expiratory flow, incomplete loops, MV and TV alarms	Look for leak on V/P loop and VT waveform, high percentage leak, leak may be minimal or variable with stiff lungs	Obstructive pattern if water in the circuit, Interference in time flow waveform	Normal to high resistance, periods of no flow with splinting, "Beaking" on V/P loop
X-ray	Bad RDS, low volume lungs, consolidation	Variable or non-specific	Long ETT, asymmetry, right-side hyperinflation, right upper lobe collapse	ETT seen to right of trachea or left of NGT	Pneumothorax, tension pneumothorax	Not necessary for minor ventilator problem but always check central lines are not in the heart or misplaced	Significant BPD. Recent worsening, hyperinflation, "squeezed heart"
Actions	Responds to increasing PIP/MAP, surfactant, pulmonary hemorrhage treatment	Improves on suction. May require new ETT if completely blocked. Increasing PIP briefly may overcome secretions at tip of ETT	Pull back ETT and observe response (may need to increase PIP to inflate left side). Plan reintubation after pulling ETT back and recruiting deflated areas	Consider blocked ETT; Try ↑FiO$_2$, PIP, T-piece ventilation, and suction; remove ETT and replace	Transillumination, needle if unstable or tension identified, place ICD	Look for leaks or obstructions in circuit. Review alarm settings. Clear water from circuit. Ensure flow sensor is vertical and not soiled. Manage line position	Confirm tube patency and length. Optimize Mode/trigger. Consider paralysis/Chloral hydrate or extubation if otherwise stable. Normalize lung volume

ETT, Endotracheal tube; *ICD*, Intercostal drain; *NGT*, Nasogastric tube; *PROM*, Prolonged premature rupture of membranes.

ALGORITHM 11B.1 SUGGESTED ALGORITHM FOR DETERIORATION ON VENTILATOR

```
                              ┌──────────────────────────┐
                              │    Stable on ventilator   │◄──────────────────────┐
                              │     Know history and      │                        │
                              │  anticipate complications │                        │
                              └──────────────────────────┘                        │
                                          │                                        │
                                          ▼                                        │
                              ┌──────────────────────────┐                        │
                              │  Acute desaturation and   │                        │
                              │       bradycardia         │                        │
                              └──────────────────────────┘                        │
                                          │                                        │
┌──────────────────────────────┐         ▼                                        │
│ Local governance and training │  ┌──────────────────────────┐                   │
│          strategies           │  │    Bedside assessment     │                   │
│ • National resuscitation      │  │  History from bedside     │                   │
│   guidance                    │  │          team             │                   │
│ • National and local advanced │  │       Examination         │                   │
│   resuscitation guidance      │  │  Trend data on monitor    │                   │
│ • Local teamwork training     │  │   Pulmonary graphics      │                   │
│ • Local equipment training    │  │      Blood gases          │                   │
│ • Advanced ventilator use     │  │       CXR review          │                   │
│   training                    │  └──────────────────────────┘                   │
│ • Local regular scenario      │            │                                     │
│   simulation training         │            ▼                                     │
└──────────────────────────────┘  ┌──────────────────────────┐                    │
                                   │         BOLDPEEP          │                    │
                                   └──────────────────────────┘                    │
                                             │                                      │
                                             ▼                                      │
                              ┌──────────────────────────┐   ┌──────────────────────────────┐
                              │     Bedside actions       │   │ Diagnose and manage specific   │
                              │      Suction ETT          │   │      respiratory event         │
                              │      Adjust ETT           │──▶│       Open airway              │
                              │     Increase PIP          │   │   Adjust or replace ETT        │
                              │   Transillumination       │   │        Open lungs              │
                              │    New blood gas          │   │     Normalize PaCO2            │
                              │       New CXR             │   └──────────────────────────────┘
                              └──────────────────────────┘                    │
                                          │                                    │
                                          ▼                                    │
                              ┌──────────────────────────┐                    │
                              │ Acute nonrespiratory events│                   │
                              │         Sepsis            │                    │
                              │       Hypotension         │                    │
                              │  Acute anemia/blood loss  │                    │
                              │ Profound metabolic acidosis│   ┌──────────────────────────────┐
                              │      Acute abdomen        │   │ Manage specific nonrespiratory │
                              │        Seizure            │   │          event                 │
                              └──────────────────────────┘   │         Volume                 │
                                          │                   │       Transfusion              │
                                          ▼                   │       Antibiotics              │
                              ┌──────────────────────────┐   └──────────────────────────────┘
                              │ AXR, cranial U/S, ECHO    │                    ▲
                              │ Septic screen, lactate, FBC,│──────────────────┘
                              │      clotting, aEEG       │
                              └──────────────────────────┘
```

commonly, the presenting feature needing timely review is pallor, hypotension, bradycardia, or seizure.

Importantly, acronyms can be used as aide-memoires in stressful situations and can be enabling in simulation training. The acronym BOLDPEEP is useful in this setting to prompt the memory and pattern recognition [4] (Table 11B.1) of the common causes for acute desaturation events.

Bad lung disease

This refers to a gradual or sudden deterioration in the lung disease. This includes severe RDS and development of PIE, bilateral atelectasis, or pulmonary hemorrhage. A mismatch between the level of ventilator support and the evolving lung disease may contribute, that is, insufficient MAP or minute ventilation for the severity of disease. Trend data may herald this event, which if left unattended will present with a rising oxygen requirement, desaturations, and bradycardia, as respiratory acidosis worsens. The chest X-ray, the nursing history, and the recent changes to respiratory support, for example, excessive weaning, will enhance rapid assessment. An acute pulmonary hemorrhage usually presents as a sudden event with signs of obstruction to ventilation associated with pallor secondary to blood loss and acidosis. Suction to the ETT revealing fresh blood allows immediate confirmation of the diagnosis.

Obstructed, Long, or Displaced ETT

These are common problems in neonatal intensive care. The advent of pulmonary graphics in combination with good bedside medical and nursing assessment should allow prompt diagnosis and management (Table 11B.1).

Pneumothorax

Pneumothorax is more likely in certain settings, for example, pulmonary hypoplasia, ventilation with high pressure or high volume in RDS, late use of CPAP in established RDS without surfactant.

Pneumothorax may present with the clinical signs of chest-size asymmetry, asymmetrical breath sounds, desaturation, and hypotension. Pulmonary graphics may reveal a new leak on the volume–time waveform and pressure–volume graph. Careful thoracic transillumination in an adequately darkened room is usually diagnostic in extreme prematurity [5,6].

Equipment

Occasionally, ventilator malfunction causes deterioration. Excess water in the circuit or a disconnected circuit are usually quickly identified and managed. However, it is also always important to consider the abnormal position of central lines [7]. An umbilical venous line can enter the peritoneal cavity, but appears to be in a good central position on AP film. The baby may then present with refractive hypoglycemia or hypotension. Ultrasound or lateral X-ray may be required to confirm the abnormal position. Cardiac tamponade following line damage to the heart is well recognized and may present with sudden refractive bradycardia despite adequate ventilation [8]. Careful regular inspection of line positions is essential to limit these complications and highlight them to new members of the team. Further, unexplained hypotension in a baby established on inotropes may simply be due to accidental clamping of central lines, infusion changes, or leakage.

Equipment–Patient asynchrony

Asynchrony between the patient and ventilator increases the risk of air leaks [9,10] and intraventricular hemorrhage [11]. Older babies with chronic lung disease complicated by new infection may require reventilation and quickly develop a difficult course characterized by secretions and areas of hyperinflation and atelectasis, leading to higher FiO_2 and frequent desaturations and bradycardias. These babies may require increased sedation or temporary muscle relaxation tailored with effective triggered ventilation during the period when they are most unstable. Further, if spontaneously breathing, setting a low backup rate can reduce asynchrony. However, once stabilized with open lungs, early extubation should be pursued. Occasionally. a baby with overwhelming sepsis, for example, Group B streptococcus (GBS) may present with acidosis and pulmonary hypertension leading to high FiO_2. Inadvertently, increasing the ventilatory support can lead to hyperinflation, air trapping, poor venous return, and ventilation–perfusion mismatch. The lung fields may be relatively clear. An urgent chest X-ray can reveal the need to reduce lung volumes quickly. This is similar to what happens with air trapping in meconium and blood aspiration syndromes.

Nonrespiratory causes of deterioration on the ventilator

Acute nonrespiratory deterioration on the ventilator may be due to acute anemia (large IVH, subgaleal hemorrhage, GI bleed, umbilical cord, and arterial line events), profound acidosis (sepsis, metabolic acidosis), or an acute abdomen (NEC, perforation, volvulus). Hypotension is common to many of these events. Careful systematic review with appropriate urgent investigations will help elicit the cause.

Approach to ventilator alarms

Ventilator alarms are designed to alert the health care professionals to unexpected changes in the ventilator-baby unit which may have a significant impact on the baby, for example, disconnection or a dislodged tube. Color and sound coding of alarms highlights their relative urgency. The service should agree to set up alarm parameters for safe use, for example, never set the lower limit of minute ventilation to zero.

Table 11B.2 provides information about responding to common ventilator alarms. A pragmatic approach should include:

1. Review the patient with the nurse and ask for help if required.
2. Check for chest movement and air entry.
3. Review bedside monitoring including saturations, heart rate, etc.
4. Does the baby need resuscitation?
5. Review the ventilator current trend data and blood gases for key parameters and pattern recognition.

Table 12.1 Checklist for extubation readiness

Checklist question	Items to check	Pre- and postextubation plan activities
What is the respiratory history and extubation history?	Antenatal history, for example, steroids, PROM, or previous immediate extubation failure	Address previous cause of failure
Did the baby receive surfactant?	Timing, dose, and response to surfactant	Optimize total dose of surfactant, for example, 200 mg/kg Curosurf [6], Survanta 100 mg/kg [7]
Is there evidence of improving or stable lung disease?	Trends in markers of compliance, for example, MAP, PIP, MV, V_{te}, and FiO_2	Identify MAP to target postextubation PEEP
Is there evidence of open lungs, that is, good lung volumes?	Recent chest X-ray and pulmonary graphics	Optimize PEEP and ETT position
Is there evidence of secretions or airway edema or airway narrowing?	Recent burden of secretions, respiratory pathogens, intubation history, and extubation history	Consider antibiotics and steroids. Optimize positioning, physiotherapy, and suction prior to extubation
Is there evidence of metabolic compensation to hypercapnia?	Chloride, pH, and $PaCO_2$	Agree a pH lower limit, for example, 7.20 Review chloride intake
Is there evidence of good respiratory drive?	Baby is breathing above backup rate without significant recession	Consider a short trial of ET CPAP (SBT) or low backup rate in patient triggered modes
Has sedation or analgesia been minimized or stopped?	History of medication and responses	Consider need for ongoing sedation or analgesia after extubation, for example, tolerance of CPAP in an older baby
Would the baby benefit from caffeine?	Local guidance on Caffeine use	Give 24 h before extubation [8] Consider need for exceptional use, for example, apneas with sepsis
Will the lung disease or respiratory drive benefit from CPAP?	Consider gestational age and severity of current lung disease	Identify MAP required to keep lungs open
Are there abdominal contraindications to CPAP?	Abdominal assessment	Await evidence of abdominal stability, for example, peristalsis
Is there an NGT in place?	Last CXR assessing recent NGT position	Deflate stomach via NGT
Is there evidence of systemic stability, for example, off inotropes or resolving sepsis?	Cardiac status and recent history of sepsis with evidence of resolution, for example, improving lactate and sepsis markers	Observe period of stability on stopping inotropes
Is there a hemodynamically significant PDA?	Cardiac status	Clinical and echocardiography assessment
Is the hemoglobin (Hb) optimal?	Hb in context of age, clinical status, and degree of ventilatory support	Consider red cell transfusion [9] if Hb ≤10 g/dL and MAP >8 cmH_2O and or FiO_2 >0.4
Is there evidence of excess tissue fluid?	Recent renal function, weight changes, and nutritional status	Consider short course of diuretics to improve lung compliance
Are the parents aware of the plan?	Aware of risk of reintubation or complications	Ensure good and consistent communication
Is a very experienced nurse available when extubation success is deemed less likely?	Skill mix check	Optimize position and device interface Experienced tolerance of initial postextubation instability
Who should be present at the extubation?	Check personnel skill mix and numbers	Consider time of day and service workload
What are the reintubation thresholds?	Patient course and physiological markers	Individualize threshold parameters for reintubation

Table 12.2 Clinical and ventilator parameters for extubation

Parameter	Typical extubation settings	Comments
Bedside clinical parameters		
Heart rate (HR)	Stable within normal range [17], variability-normal [18], no bradycardias	Reduced HR variability is associated with extubation failure [18]
Respiratory rate (RR)	Good respiratory drive with RR above backup rate	Load with Caffeine as appropriate
Blood pressure	Stable, usually off inotropes [17]	Consider echocardiogram if concerned about impact of a PDA
O_2 saturations	Stable within target limits—91%–95% [19]	
Ventilator parameters		
Mode of ventilation	PC-AC or PC-PSV [20]	Additional parameters measuring respiratory variability like T_i, T_e, mean inspiratory flow during SBT can aid in assessing readiness for extubation [14]
FiO_2	Stable oxygenation at FiO_2 ≤0.4 [4,16,21,22]	In infants with established lung disease, extubation may be appropriate from a higher FiO_2
MAP	Consistently ≤7–9 cmH_2O [3,17]	May be higher in babies with established lung disease
Backup rate	Below the spontaneous RR, typically 20–30 [23]	Optimize respiratory drive, consider Caffeine
Blood gas parameters		
pH	≥7.20 [3]	Care should be given to manage respiratory as well as metabolic component of acidosis
$PaCO_2$	First 3–4 days: 4–6 kPa; subsequently more permissive hypercapnia tolerated [3]	After first 3–4 days, babies tolerate higher $PaCO_2$ and extubation decision should be based on clinical status, $PaCO_2$ trend and pH
Lactate	≤2.5 mmol/L	If higher consider the cause and manage as appropriate
Hemoglobin	>10 g/dL with hematocrit >30% [9]	Consider aiming for higher threshold if higher MAP or need of inotropes

birth weight babies [5,13–15]. It involves assessing the baby's ability to breathe while receiving minimal or no respiratory support [16], typically with endotracheal CPAP over 3–5 min [13–15]; while observing key parameters, for example, FiO_2, saturations, heart rate, blood pressure, and respiratory rate. A drop in heart rate below 100 bpm lasting more than 15 s or a drop in oxygen saturation to below 85% despite a 15% increase in FiO_2 or apnea suggests the baby is not ready for extubation [14].

Patient groups

26–31 weeks of gestation

Many preterm babies will have received surfactant, have minimal lung disease, and no significant systemic concerns.

They will routinely receive caffeine and, provided CPAP is applied correctly, will extubate successfully. In this cohort, MAP <10 cmH_2O and an FiO_2 less than 0.3 will normally suggest sufficiently improved lung compliance. However, occasionally these values are achieved with moderate RDS during active weaning and a review of the CXR and history, for example, use of antenatal steroids or associated sepsis in conjunction with a short SBT, may help identify the small group whose lung disease will predict extubation failure.

23–25 weeks of gestation

Early on this group may require ongoing ventilation for a combination of lung disease, respiratory muscle fatigue, poor drive, sepsis, poor tolerance of hypercapnia, and acidosis. A hyperchloremic acidosis compromises

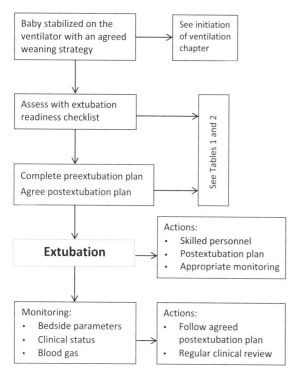

Fig. 12.1 **Extubation Algorithm.**

the ability to tolerate permissive hypercapnia in these patients. Careful assessment includes anticipating problems with tolerance of CPAP and the patient interface; with particular attention to birth weight (especially <500 g), condition at birth skin integrity. BiPAP may be especially useful for this group to reduce the risk of extubation failure [24]. A suggested algorithm for extubation is shown in Fig. 12.1.

Evolving severe BPD

Babies with more significant lung disease or with previous failed extubation attempts benefit from more detailed planning to ensure success. Tolerance of higher MAP, FiO_2, and $PaCO_2$ is necessary provided the baby is systemically well with open lungs at the time of extubation. This is particularly true in the presence of episodes of patient-ventilator asynchrony, copious secretions, blocked ETTs, and displaced ETTs. This patient group, whose ventilatory requirements are higher at the time of extubation require expert nursing care in the first 12 h to ensure stabilization on noninvasive respiratory support, for example, CPAP/BiPAP (see later).

Recurrent air leaks

Respiratory function and stability can deteriorate quickly with PIE and pneumothoraces. Ongoing ventilation can make these worse and contribute to a trajectory of severe BPD. A more aggressive approach to extubation is required with assessment of the underlying lung disease (CXR, MAP, and FiO_2), tailored volume ventilation, and ensuring correctly placed intercostal drains (ICD) and ETT. If air leaks are recurrent as in persistent pleural hole or bronchopleural fistula, removing positive pressure ventilation with the ICD still in situ should be considered, provided the underlying lung disease is stable and the lungs are well recruited.

Surgical

The timing of extubation in surgical conditions is often influenced by nonrespiratory factors such as the nature of the abdominal pathology. A tight esophageal atresia repair or pneumotosis in NEC may dictate a delay in extubation.

Postextubation noninvasive respiratory support

Many babies <28 weeks or <1 kg benefit from noninvasive respiratory support, for example, CPAP, BiPAP, or high-flow nasal cannula (HFNC). CPAP should be applied before or at extubation to avoid atelectasis. The use of nasal CPAP increases the likelihood of maintaining a successful extubation [25]. Caution is needed while using CPAP in babies with necrotizing enterocolitis and abdominal pathology. To augment the tidal volume during noninvasive respiratory support, further inspiratory pressure can supplement the continuous distending pressure of CPAP as synchronized (SIPAP) or asynchronized with low (BIPAP) or high (NIPPV) pressures [26]. In a study in preterm infants below 30 weeks receiving CPAP or NIPPV, NIPPV was associated with reduction in reintubation and duration of mechanical ventilation [27]. A meta-analysis comparing nasal CPAP to various forms of NIPPV showed latter to be better to reduce extubation failure, but showed no difference in the incidence of chronic lung disease or mortality [24]. Reassuringly, there was no increase in gastrointestinal adverse effects [24].

Recurrent failure of extubation

Failure to maintain extubation is usually explained by poor equipment seal, loss of lung volume, excessive secretions, poor respiratory drive, or occasionally airway narrowing. These should be predicted with the checklist and addressed. However, if failure to extubate is recurrent, consider the causes listed in Table 12.3.

Table 12.3 Causes of recurrent failure to extubate

Airway/lung problem	Decreased respiratory drive	Muscular dysfunction	Neuromuscular	Cardiac
Mucus plugs and secretions	Excessive sedation	Muscle weakness	Diaphragmatic dysfunction	Hemodynamically significant PDA
Consolidation	Need for caffeine	Severe electrolyte disturbances	Prolonged neuromuscular blockade	Cor pulmonale
Severe cystic BPD	Infection		Myotonic dystrophy	
Nasal obstruction	CNS abnormality		Spinal muscular atrophy	
Postextubation stridor (laryngeal edema, subglottic stenosis)	Hypocapnia		Brain anomaly	
Large airway anomalies, for example, tracheomalacia			Cervical spinal injury	
Congenital lung anomalies, for example, CLE				

References

[1] Manley BJ, Davis PG. Solving the extubation equation: successfully weaning infants born extremely preterm from mechanical ventilation. J Pediatr 2017;189:17–18.

[2] Venkatesh V, Ponnusamy V, Anandaraj J, Chaudhary R, Malviya M, Clarke P, et al. Endotracheal intubation in a neonatal population remains associated with a high risk of adverse events. Eur J Pediatr 2011;170:223–227.

[3] Shalish W, Sant'Anna GM, Natarajan G, Chawla S. When and how to extubate premature infants from mechanical ventilation. Curr Pediatr Rep 2014;2(1):18–25.

[4] Chawla S, Natarajan G, Shankaran S, Carper B, Brion LP, Keszler M, et al. Markers of successful extubation in extremely preterm infants, and morbidity after failed extubation. J Pediatr 2017;189:113–119.e2.

[5] Manley BJ, Doyle LW, Owen LS, Davies PG. Extubating extremely preterm infants: predictors of success and outcomes following failure. J Pediatr 2016;173:45–49.

[6] Cloete E, Lo C, Buksh MJ. Respiratory outcomes following 100 mg/kg v. 200 mg/kg of poractant alpha: a retrospective review. South African J Child Health 2013;7(4):148.

[7] Singh N, Halliday HL, Stevens TP, Suresh G, Soll R, Rojas-Reyes MX. Comparison of animal-derived surfactants for the prevention and treatment of respiratory distress syndrome in preterm infants. In: Singh N, editor. Cochrane database of systematic reviews. Chichester, UK: John Wiley & Sons, Ltd; 2015. p. 1–69.

[8] Dobson NR, Hunt CE. Pharmacology review: caffeine use in neonates: indications, pharmacokinetics, clinical effects, outcomes. NeoReviews 2013;14(11):e540–e550.

[9] Bishara N, Ohls RK. Current Controversies in the management of the anemia of prematurity. Semin Perinatol 2009;33:29–34.

[10] Keszler M, Sant'Anna G. Mechanical ventilation and bronchopulmonary dysplasia. Clin Perinatol 2015;42(4):781–796.

[11] Newth CJL, Venkataraman S, Willson DF, Meert KL, Harrison R, Dean JM, et al. Weaning and extubation readiness in pediatric patients. Pediatr Crit Care Med 2009;10(1):1–11.

[12] Mhanna MJ, Iyer NP, Piraino S, Jain M, Bauer K, Caughey AB, et al. Respiratory severity score and extubation readiness in very low birth weight infants. Pediatr Neonatol. 2017;16:968–973.

[13] Chawla S, Natarajan G, Gelmini M, Nadya S, Kazzi J. Role of spontaneous breathing trial in predicting successful extubation in premature infants. Pediatr Pulmonol 2013;48(5):443–448.

[14] Kaczmarek J, Kamlin COF, Morley CJ, Davis PG, Sant'Anna GM. Variability of respiratory parameters and extubation readiness in ventilated neonates. Arch Dis Child Fetal Neonatal Ed 2013;98(1):F70–F73.

[15] Kamlin COF, Davis PG, Morley CJ. Predicting successful extubation of very low birthweight infants. Arch Dis Child Fetal Neonatal Ed 2006;91(3):F180–F183.

[16] Biban P, Gaffuri M, Spaggiari S, Silvagni D, Zaglia F, Santuz P. Weaning newborn infants from mechanical ventilation. J Pediatr Neonatal Individ Med 2013;22(22):1–7.

[17] Batra D, Schoonakker B, Smith C. Mechanical ventilation in neonates. Nottingham neonatal service—clinical guidlines. Nottingham: Nottingham Neonatal Service; 2017. p. 1–26.

[18] Kaczmarek J, Chawla S, Marchica C, Dwaihy M, Grundy L, Sant'Anna GM. Heart rate variability and extubation readiness in extremely preterm infants. Neonatology 2013;104:42–48.

[19] The BOOST II United Kingdom Australia and New Zealand Collaborative Groups. Oxygen saturation and outcomes in preterm infants. N Engl J Med 2013;368(22):2094–2104.

[20] Banacalari E, Claure N. Patient-ventilator interaction. In: Polin RA, editor. The newborn lung: neonatology questions and controversies. 2nd ed. Philadelphia, PA: Elsevier; 2012. p. 339–354.

[21] Wang HW, Jyun-You L, Chien-Yi C, Chou H-C, Hsieh W-S, Tsao P-N. Risk factors for extubation failure in extremely low birth weight infants. Pediatr Neonatol 2017;58:145–150.

[22] El-Beleidy ASE-D, Khattab AAE-H, El-Sherbini SA, Al-Gebaly HF. Automatic tube compensation versus pressure support ventilation and extubation outcome in children: a randomized controlled study. ISRN Pediatr 2013;2013:871376.

[23] Wheeler KI, Morley CJ, Hooper SB, Davis PG. Lower back-up rates improve ventilator triggering during assist-control ventilation: a randomized crossover trial. J Perinatol 2012;32(2):111–116.

[24] Lemyre B, Davis PG, De Paoli AG, Kirpalani H. Nasal intermittent positive pressure ventilation (NIPPV) versus nasal continuous positive airway pressure (NCPAP) for preterm neonates after extubation. In: Lemyre B, editor. Cochrane database of systematic reviews. Chichester, UK: John Wiley & Sons, Ltd; 2017.

[25] Davis PG, Henderson-Smart DJ. Nasal continuous positive airway pressure immediately after extubation for preventing morbidity in preterm infants. In: Davis PG, editor. Cochrane database of systematic reviews. Chichester, UK: John Wiley & Sons, Ltd; 2003.

[26] Garg S, Sinha S. Non-invasive ventilation in premature infants: based on evidence or habit. J Clin Neonatol 2013;2(4):155–159.

[27] Ramanathan R, Sekar KC, Rasmussen M, Bhatia J, Soll RF. Nasal intermittent positive pressure ventilation after surfactant treatment for respiratory distress syndrome in preterm infants <30 weeks' gestation: a randomized, controlled trial. J Perinatol 2012;32(5):336–343.

Chapter |13A|

Complications of Mechanical Ventilation

Srinivas Murki, MD, DM, Sai Sunil Kishore, MD, DM, Sreeram Subramanian, MD, DM

CHAPTER POINTS

- Barotrauma, volutrauma, alelectotrauma and biotrauma are essential components of Ventilator Induced Lung Injury (VILI)
- Incidence of ventilation associated pneumonia is a quality indicator of neonatal ventilation

Mechanical ventilation (MV) is a nonphysiological process as the gas is driven into the lungs with positive pressure in contrast to negative pressure breathing (air passively flows into lungs) in spontaneous natural breathing process. Hence it is prone for complications. Health care professional should not only be aware of these complications but also be able to prevent, anticipate, identify, and circumvent it at the earliest. In MV, as the gases containing high oxygen concentration are driven into the lungs with certain pressure and volume, lung experiences special (artificial) trauma, commonly named as ventilator-induced lung

injury (VILI) [1]. The predominant modes of VILI are as follows:

1. Barotrauma—use of high pressure
2. Volutrauma—use of high tidal volume
3. Oxytrauma—use of high oxygen concentration
4. Atelectotrauma—repeated closing and opening of alveoli often due to inadequate positive end-expiratory pressure (PEEP)
5. Biotrauma—inflammatory response-related injury
6. Injury related to endotracheal tube
7. Ventilator asynchrony
8. Lack of warmidification (inappropriate temperature and relative humidity of gases)

These types of VILI injure the fragile alveoli, causing leakage of capillaries in the interstitium and also into the alveolar lumen. The mechanical injury activates the inflammatory system of the lungs, causing more leakage. Microbial colonization adds fuel to the fire. This cascade of events worsens the primary pathology for which the ventilation was instituted. All these events prolong the duration of MV, exacerbate extubation failures, and pave the way for chronic lung disease which has enormous short- and long-term adverse respiratory and neurological implications [2,3].

Barotrauma

High inflation pressures may cause shear stress, creating microtears in the alveolar walls. Intrathoracic pressures can rise due to overdistention of the lungs [4]. Air leaks, decreased venous return to the heart, and intraventricular hemorrhages in preterm neonates are known consequences. Excessive flow of gas can also result in barotrauma due to increase in mean airway pressure (sine wave to square wave form).

How to recognize it

- Clinical—excessive chest rise; increased anteroposterior diameter of the chest (Fig. 13A.1); poor capillary refill time; and decreased urine output. Differential air entry, sudden desaturations, and a positive transillumination test are signs of air leaks. Arterial blood gas may reflect retention of carbon dioxide.
- Chest X-ray—hyperinflated lungs with flattened domes of diaphragm and more than eight rib spaces on the AP view (Fig. 13A.2). Pulmonary interstitial emphysema or small air leaks into mediastinum or near the apical regions of the lungs should serve as warning signs (Fig. 13A.3A–B).

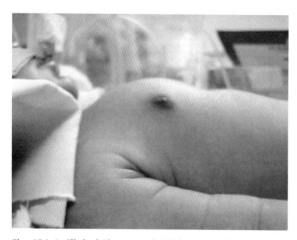

Fig. 13A.1 **Clinical Photograph With Hyperinflated Chest.**

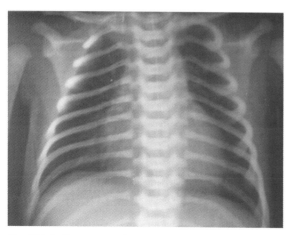

Fig. 13A.2 **Chest X-ray Showing Hyperinflated Lung Fields.**

- Pulmonary graphics—beaking can be seen in the pressure–volume loops (Fig. 13A.4).

Remedial measures

PIP or PEEP should be kept optimal. Keep flow of gas between 5 and 8 L/min.

Volutrauma

Volutrauma is considered to be the predominant reason for VILI. High tidal volumes (>8 mL/kg) and low tidal volumes (<4 mL/kg) can initiate VILI [2]. Tidal volume in a pressure-controlled ventilation is dependent upon the driving pressure (delta P = PIP – PEEP). Thus, increasing PIP and decreasing PEEP result in more tidal volumes. In volume-controlled ventilation, tidal volume is determined by operator. Physiological tidal volumes between 5 and 8 mL/kg have been shown to minimize lung injury. High tidal volumes especially with short expiratory times result in overdistention, gradually increasing the intrathoracic pressure called as auto-PEEP. The consequences are similar to barotrauma, but are more profound.

Excessive tidal volumes can result in low $PaCO_2$; persistent low values ($PaCO_2$ <30 mmHg) can cause cerebral ischemia, especially the periventricular white matter culminating in periventricular leukomalacia (PVL). Permissive hypercapnea (PCO_2: 55–60 mmHg and pH >7.25) is used as a strategy to restrict tidal volumes and minimize VILI [5].

Volume-targeted ventilation is a proven strategy to reduce the duration of ventilation, the need for oxygen for 36 weeks, incidence of hypocarbia, incidence of IVH, and PVL in preterm neonates in comparison to pressure-limited ventilation [6].

How to identify

- Clinical—excessive tidal volumes result in excessive/increased chest rise, harsh breath sounds, and low $PaCO_2$ on the arterial blood gas. The spontaneous respiratory efforts of the baby may be lost and it may stop triggering the breaths in a synchronized mode of ventilation with fixed rates (SIMV or A/C).
- Hyperinflation can be seen on chest X-ray.
- Pulmonary graphics can pick up early—prolonged expiratory pattern in flow–time graph, and termination of expiratory limb of flow–volume loop on the y-axis below the point of origin of the loop (Fig. 13A.5).

Remedial measures

- In volume controlled or targeted ventilation - use tidal volumes between 5 to 8 mL/kg.

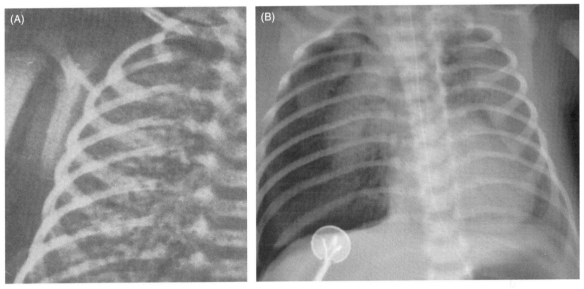

Fig. 13A.3 (A) Pulmonary interstitial emphysema. (B) Subtle pneumothorax on right side.

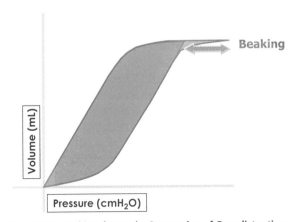

Fig. 13A.4 Beaking (Arrow)—Suggestive of Overdistention.

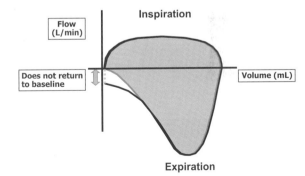

Fig. 13A.5 Air Trapping Seen (Green Arrow) in Flow–Volume Loop.

- In pressure-controlled ventilation—monitoring the tidal volumes and keeping the driving pressure optimal to achieve the normal tidal volumes.

Oxytrauma

Exposure of high concentration of oxygen in the inspired gas (FiO_2) to the respiratory tract is Oxytrauma. Oxygen,

being a potent free radical, can not only potentiate VILI but also induce free radical injury in other vital organs like brain, retina and intestines. Limiting FiO_2 to keep saturations with in target range reduces exposure to excessive oxygen (91%–95% in preterm infants). Targeting saturations below 90% was associated with increased mortality but lower risk of retinopathy of prematurity (ROP). There was no effect on need for oxygen at 36 weeks [7]. Higher saturation targets (>95 %) are not indicated even in babies with severe pulmonary hypertension in term neonates.

How to identify

- Flushed and pink extremities—persistent SpO_2 values greater than 95% is an indication of hyperoxia.
- Arterial blood gas with PaO_2 >80 mmHg.

Remedial measures

Modify the FiO_2 to target SpO_2 between 91% and 95%. Optimize the mean airway pressure to achieve the ideal functional residual capacity and reduce the need for high oxygen. Use of surfactant and HFOV may be useful options to reduce the airway and lung exposure to high oxygen.

Atelectotrauma

Suboptimal pressures can result in lung injury. Suboptimal PEEP results in under-recruitment of alveoli in alveolar diseases (HMD, pneumonia, pulmonary hemorrhage). Low functional residual capacity (FRC) results in persistence of V/Q mismatch, negating the purpose of MV and prolonging the duration of ventilation [1,8].

How to identify

- Poor chest rise (inadequate PIP), persistent intercostals and subcostal retractions (inadequate PEEP), reduced air entry, disproportionate need for oxygen in relation to pressure requirements are signs of atelectasis. High and worsening Silverman Anderson score are objective signs of poor functional residual capacity and alveolar atelectasis.
- Low volume lungs on chest X-ray (Fig. 13A.6).

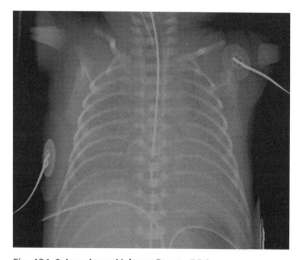

Fig. 13A.6 **Low Lung Volume Due to RDS.**

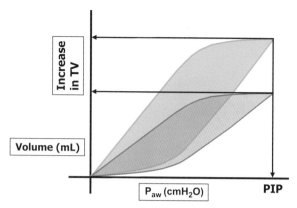

Fig. 13A.7 **Low Compliance** *(Pink)* **and Normal Compliance** *(Green)* **on Pressure–Volume Loop.**

- Tidal volume will be lower than normal. Pulmonary graphics can show low compliance pattern in pressure–volume loops (Fig. 13A.7). The lower inflection on the pressure–volume loop is displaced to the right.

Remedial measures

Optimal PEEP to keep the lungs at FRC (minimal chest recessions, SAS score ≤3 and 6–8 rib spaces on the chest X-ray). Increase PEEP till the lower inflection point on the PV loop is close to the left. In open lung concept (alveolar recruitment maneuver) one can increase PEEP keeping the ΔP constant (PIP–PEEP difference) till a drop in FiO_2 is noticed.

Biotrauma

All of the above factors will cause an increase in alveolar–capillary permeability with leakage of fluids and proteins into the alveolar space, surfactant inactivation, and an inflammatory response [1,3].

Injury related to endotracheal tube

This is due to the presence of endotracheal tube, a foreign body in the trachea. It initiates inflammation, and favors microbial colonization. Improper unsterile suctioning technique can cause tracheal mucosal injury and enhance microbial colonization. Tube blocks can occur due to inadequate humidification, improper suctioning, excessive secretions, or blood clots. This results in under-ventilation and worsening of the primary pathology [2].

The position of endotracheal tube can also lead to mechanical complications. The optimal position is 1 cm

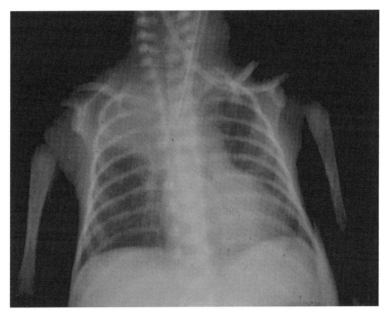

Fig. 13A.8 Right Upper Lobe Collapse Due to Right Bronchial Intubation.

above the carina, radiologically corresponding to lower border of T2 vertebra. Right bronchial intubation results in under-ventilation of left lung and right upper lobe, causing collapse (Fig. 13A.8). As a result the right lung can become hyperinflated. High position of the tube causes excessive air leak resulting in under-ventilation of the lungs and distension of stomach negating the primary reason for ventilation.

Improper ET size: ET size cannot be judged by looking at the vocal cords as the narrowest part in neonates is subglottic area. Larger ET size can result in extubation failures due to subglottic edema. Small ET can result in increased resistance and more work of breathing.

How to identify

- Clinical—proper position and patency of endotracheal tube can be confirmed by equal air entry in bilateral lung fields, good chest rise, mist formation in the ET, and absence of air entry in the stomach. In difficult situations, endotracheal tube placement in the esophagus may be confirmed by placing the end of the orogastric tube in a bowl of water and looking for bubbling. Auscultation on the carina may identify the peritubal leaks.
- Chest X-ray can confirm the position. Bedside ultrasound is increasingly being used to identify the tube position in children and in newborn.
- ET CO_2 monitors are not widely used in neonates as they tend to increase the dead space.

- Excessive ET leak can be identified using pulmonary graphics (pressure–volume loop, flow–volume loop) (Fig. 13A.9).

Remedial measures

Aseptic precautions during intubation, choosing the right ET size, intubating till the vocal cord guide, avoiding blind intubation, proper fixation, ensuring utmost sterility during endotracheal suctioning, and early extubation are some of the strategies to minimize complications.

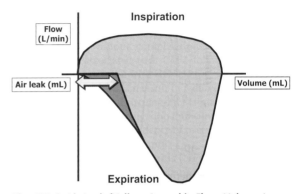

Fig. 13A.9 Air Leak (Yellow Arrow) in Flow–Volume Loop.

165

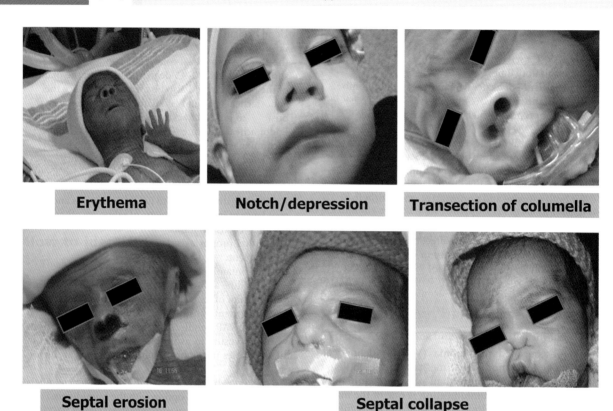

Fig. 13A.11 **Progression of Nasal Septal Injury.**

increases the risk of NTB. This complication has to be suspected if neonate develops acute hypercapnia and reduced chest wall movement that does not improve with endotracheal suctioning.

- **Air leaks**: This complication can occur when HFV is used as rescue therapy in failed CMV.
- **Intraventricular hemorrhage and PVL**: These have been reported as complications of HFV in some studies, but most recent studies using the optimal volume strategy have not shown any difference in the incidence of these complications between babies on conventional and HFV.

Complications associated with interface in NIMV

All the interface devices used for NIMV are associated with local complications, though the spectrum and severity vary. The spectrum of complications with short binasal prongs include nasal irritation, reddening, damage to the septal mucosa, columellar transection, septal erosion, and septal collapse (Fig. 13A.11). Nasal masks are associated with contusion of the nasal bridge.

How to prevent interface-related nasal injuries

Nasal care

- Assess for any discoloration, blanching is the earliest sign.
- Moisturize the nares with saline drops, do gentle suction.
- Use correct prong size.
- Maintain a small gap (2–3 mm) between base of the prong and nasal septum.
- For binasal prong—use transparent semipermeable film, cotton plug at nasal septum.
- Prevent upward traction on the ala nasi.
- Use normal saline as a lubricant when inserting the prongs.
- For nasal mask: use skin barriers (e.g. Tegaderm, Cannulaide) over bridge of nose and pressure points.

Extrapulmonary complications

Retinopathy of prematurity: The risk of severe ROP is lesser with lower oxygen saturation targets (85%–89%) as opposed to higher targets (91%–95%) [RR 0.52, 0.37–0.73) but at the cost of increased mortality (19.9% vs.

16.2%). From available evidence, it is clear that targeting higher oxygen saturations in the initial weeks of birth result in an increased rate of severe ROP needing treatment. A meticulous analysis of oxygenation patterns with a closed loop system oxygen analyzer may be the way forward in this regard [7].

Intraventricular hemorrhage/PVL: The risk factors for IVH include ventilator asynchrony, use of excessive pressures, air leaks, and sudden fluctuations in $PaCO_2$ (partial

pressure of carbon dioxide). More prolonged exposure to hypocapnoea increases risk of PVL by nearly 5 times (7.4% vs. 1.4%). As in prevention of BPD, the importance of gentle ventilation with optimal tidal volumes and prevention of hypocapnoea is essential. The use of volume-targeted ventilation has been found to reduce IVH (RR 0.65, 95% CI 0.42–0.99) and PVL (RR 0.33, 95% CI 0.15–0.72) as compared to pressure-controlled ventilation [6].

References

[1] Attar MA, Donn SM. Mechanisms of ventilator-induced lung injury in premature infants. Semin Neonatol 2002;7(5):353–360.

[2] Miller JD, Carlo WA. Pulmonary complications of mechanical ventilation in neonates. Clin Perinatol 2008;35(1):273–281.

[3] Van Kaam A. Lung-protective ventilation in neonatology. Neonatology 2011;99(4):338–341.

[4] Slutsky AS. Ventilator-induced lung injury: from barotrauma to biotrauma. Respir Care 2005;50(5):646.

[5] Ambalavanan N, Carlo WA. Ventilatory strategies in the prevention and management of bronchopulmonary dysplasia. Semin Perinatol 2006;30(4):192–199.

[6] Klingenberg C, Wheeler KI, McCallion N, Morley CJ, Davis PG. Volume-targeted versus pressure-limited ventilation in neonates. Cochrane Database Syst Rev 2017;10:CD003666.

[7] Stenson BJ. Oxygen saturation targets for extremely preterm infants after the NeOProM trials. Neonatology 2016;109(4):352–358.

[8] Muscedere JG, Mullen JB, Gan K, Slutsky AS. Tidal ventilation at low airway pressures can augment lung injury. Am J Respir Crit Care Med 1994;149(5):1327–1334.

[9] Greenough A, Rossor TE, Sundaresan A, Murthy V, Milner AD. Synchronized mechanical ventilation for respiratory support in newborn

infants. Cochrane Database Syst Rev 2016;9:CD000456.

[10] Cernada M, Brugada M, Golombek S, Vento M. Ventilator-associated pneumonia in neonatal patients: an update. Neonatology 2014;105(2):98–107.

[11] Garland JS. Strategies to prevent ventilator-associated pneumonia in neonates. Clin Perinatol 2010;37(3):629–643.

[12] Mammel MC, Courtney SE. High-frequency ventilation A2. In: Goldsmith JP, Karotkin EH, Keszler M, Suresh GK, editors. Assisted ventilation of the neonate. 6th ed. Philadelphia, PA: Elsevier; 2017. p. 211–228.

Chapter | **13B**

Pulmonary Air Leaks

Nalinikant Panigrahy, MD, DNB (Neonatology), Dinesh Kumar Chirla, MD, DM, MRCPCH, CCST, P.K. Rajiv, MBBS, DCH, MD

CHAPTER POINTS

- Risk factors for different air leaks
- Ventilatory strategies to prevent air leaks
- Identification and optimum management of air leaks

Pulmonary air leak refers to accumulation of air outside the pulmonary space. It is a well-recognized complication of neonates with lung disease, particularly those who need mechanical ventilation, and can increase morbidity and mortality in preterm infants. Pulmonary interstitial emphysema (PIE) and pneumothorax are the most common forms of air leak, followed by pneumomediastinum and pneumopericardium.

All clinical air leak conditions are caused by high intra-alveolar pressure leading to alveolar overdistension which, in turn, causes the alveoli to rupture.

Thoracic air leaks (Figs. 13B.1 and 13B.2)

Pneumothorax

Pneumothorax is the commonest air leak condition, and results from accumulation of air in between visceral and parietal pleural surface. It is relatively common in neonatal period (Fig. 13B.3A–B).

Etiology

The majority of pneumothoraces occur in neonates who receive positive pressure ventilation such as bag and mask ventilation at delivery room, or later require respiratory support in the neonatal ICU. Spontaneous pneumothorax also may occur in immediate perinatal period in a nonventilated neonate, and may result from high transpulmonary pressure generated by the infant's first breath. In infants who receive respiratory support (mechanical ventilation, continuous positive airway pressure [CPAP]) alveolar hyperinflation causes alveoli to rupture. Poor compliance of the lungs may result into unequal ventilation which may cause overdistension of some alveoli. The overinflated alveoli may rupture and air may reach to pleural space through perivascular bundle and root of lungs causing pneumothorax. Pneumothoraces (70%–80%) are unilateral and two-third of those occur on the right side [1].

Risk factors for pneumothorax

The incidence of air leak is influenced by gestational age, birth weight, and the underlying disease for which respiratory care was initiated. Therefore, the incidence varies in different study populations, and is reported to be 1%–2% in term infants [2] and 5%–14% in preterm infants [3,4], although the incidence has decreased with use of antenatal steroids (ANSs) and surfactant. The incidence of pneumothorax is inversely proportional to *birth weight and gestation age at birth* (Table 13B.1).

EuroNeoNet data cohort from 80 neonatal units showed 4% incidence with variation of 0.5%–15.8% within units.

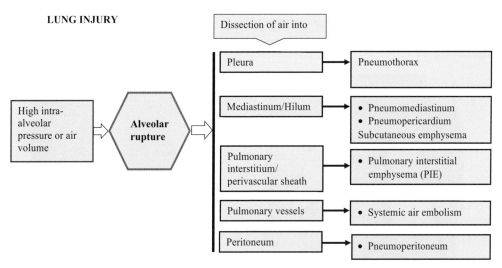

Figure 13B.1 **Classification of Thoracic Air Leaks.**

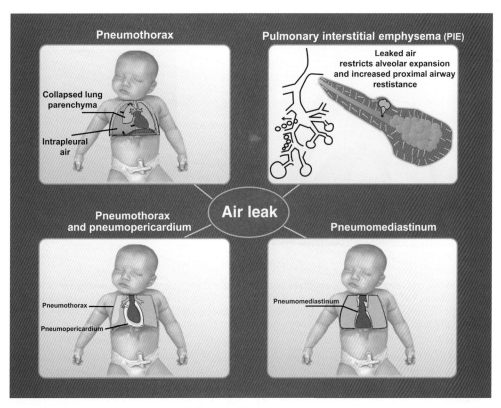

Figure 13B.2 **Cartoon Describes Various Forms of Air Leaks.**

(A)
Chest X-ray—diagrammatic representation of thoracic structures

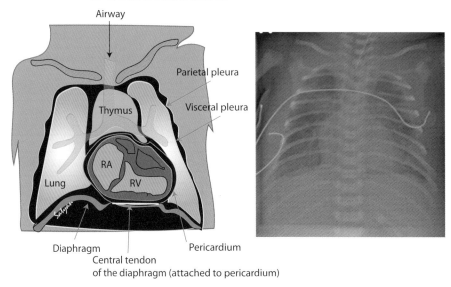

(B)
Pneumothorax

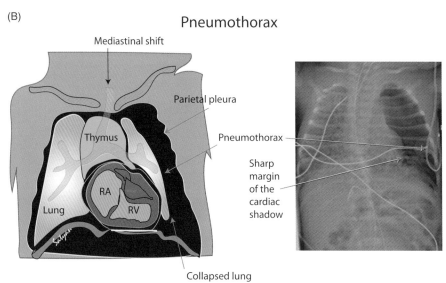

Figure 13B.3 (A) Normal orientation of thoracic structures associated with a chest X-ray without any evidence of air leak. (B) Chest X-ray in left pneumothorax. Part A: Adapted from Satyan's illustrative neonatology by Drs. Chandrasekharan and Rawat at https://itunes. apple.com/us/app/illustrative-neonatology/id1220324936?mt=8 and https://play.google.com/store/apps/details?id=com.pediatrics. droid&hl=en. Part B: Adapted from Satyan's illustrative neonatology by Drs. Chandrasekharan and Rawat.

The incidence was 9% in very low birth weight (VLBW) infants and 11% in extremely low birth weight (ELBW) infants [5]. A review of the Vermont Oxford network (VON) database demonstrates a pneumothorax rate of 5%–7% in infants with birth weight less than 1500 g [6]. Australia and New Zealand Neonatal Network database (ANZNN 2015) shows an overall incidence of 4% with an incidence as high as 15% in extremely preterm neonates [7] (Fig. 13B.4).

Table 13B.1 List of various risk factors for pneumothorax in newborn

Prematurity
Very low birth weight
Oligohydramnios
IUGR and SGA neonate
Resuscitation at birth—bag and mask ventilation
Respiratory disease (HMD, MAS, pneumonia), requiring CPAP, mechanical ventilation
Ventilation with high positive inspiratory pressure (PIP), tidal volume (V_t), and inspiratory time (T_i)
Patient ventilator asynchrony, ET suction

CPAP, Continuous positive airway pressure; *IUGR*, intrauterine growth restriction; *HMD*, hyaline membrane disease; *MAS*, meconium aspiration syndrome; *SGA*, small for gestation age.

Pneumothorax risk increases in babies receiving *respiratory support* for respiratory distress syndrome (RDS), meconium aspiration syndrome (MAS), pneumonia, congenital bullous lesion, and pulmonary hypoplasia. The incidence of pneumothorax is 10%–30% in newborn with MAS and 5%–20% in preterm infants with hyaline membrane disease [8], but decreasing with increased surfactant use.

The incidence of air leak was reported to relate to the *level of respiratory support* used, being 34% in those received mechanical ventilation in presurfactant era which reduced now to 5%, 16% in infants on CPAP, and 4% in infants

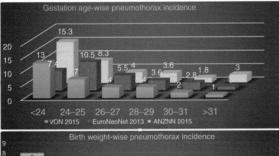

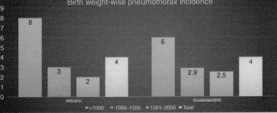

Figure 13B.4 Graph Depicts Incidence of Pneumothorax Across Different Gestation Age and Birth Weight From Different International Neonatal Database.

receiving oxygen only [9,10]. Preterm infants who need CPAP for respiratory distress are 2.64 (1.39–5.04) times more prone for pneumothorax in comparison to newborn without any respiratory support [11], but have similar incidence in comparison to intubation and surfactant group as noted in SUPPORT trial (6.8% Vs7.4%) among infants born less than 28 weeks of gestational age [12].

Ventilator settings like mean airway pressure (MAP) of more than 12 cmH$_2$O which overdistend alveoli, prolonged inspiratory time (*I:E* ratio ≥1:1), which may provoke active expiration, may increase pneumothorax rate [13,14]. Poor ventilator and patient synchrony, low inspired gas temperature (<36.5°C) especially in VLBW infants, direct injury during intubation with an introducer or during ET suction also increase incidences of pneumothorax.

Preventive strategies

1. **ANS**: A few published studies report ANS may decrease pneumothorax, but recently a Cochrane systematic review and meta-analysis found no significant reduction in incidence, RR, 0.76 (0.32–1.80) [15].
2. **Surfactant use**: Surfactant administration has been shown to significantly reduce the incidence of pneumothorax (OR, 0.35, 95% CI, 0.26–0.49) [16].

a.	Early surfactant versus delayed surfactant	RR, **0.69** (95% CI, 0.59–0.82) [17]
b.	Multiple doses versus single dose	RR, **0.51** (95% CI, 0.30–0.88)
c.	Early surfactant with brief ventilation versus surfactant and continued ventilation	RR, **0.52** (95% CI, 0.28–0.84)

However, the rate pneumothorax in the recent CURPAP study trial was found to be higher (6.7% versus 1%) among the preterm neonates who received prophylactic surfactant within 30 min of birth in comparison to neonates who received surfactant later with a median time of administration 4 hours of life, after initial stabilization with delivery room CPAP [18].

3. **Ventilation strategies**: Optimization of mechanical ventilation can reduce risk of pneumothorax.
    a. Meta-analysis of three RCTs comparing *high RR* (>60/min, HFPPV) versus lower RR with conventional ventilation showed decrease in air leak in high RR group (RR, 0.69, 95% CI, 0.51–0.93) [19]. Meta-analysis of five RCTs showed *long Ti* (>0.5 s) was associated with increased risk of pneumothorax (RR, 1.56, 95% CI, 1.24-1.97) [20]. However, many of those studies were done

in presurfactant era and before the introduction of antenatal steroids.

b. *Patient triggered ventilation* (PTV): Patient triggered ventilation like assist control (AC) and synchronized intermittent mandatory ventilation with or without pressure support (SIMV ± PS) did not show any reduction in incidence of pneumothorax when compared with continuous mandatory ventilation (CMV) mode (RR, 1.03, 95% CI, 0.80–1.34) [19].

c. Elective *high-frequency ventilation* (HFOV or jet ventilation) compared with conventional ventilation has not shown any advantage in preventing pneumothorax, instead showed increased incidence of pneumothorax in HFOV group (RR, 1.23, 95% CI, 1.06–1.44). The HFO group had significantly lower incidence of new air leak (RR, 0.73, 95% CI, 0.55–0.96) when used as rescue in newborn with pneumothorax [21].

d. Routine use of *sedation and analgesia* has not been shown any advantage over synchronized ventilation in decreasing pneumothorax, but may be it seems prudent to use sedation or analgesia in an infant with air leak who is on mechanical ventilation. A meta-analysis showed muscle relaxants use during mechanical ventilation may decrease air leaks, but their use after air leak has occurred is not well studied.

e. A meta-analysis of 16 RCTs (977 infants) showed moderate quality evidence that use of *volume-targeted ventilation* (VTV with time cycled pressure limited mode) resulted in significant reduction in rates of pneumothorax in comparison to pressure limited mode of ventilation (RR, 0.52, 95% CI, 0.31–0.87, NNT for benefit-20) [22].

f. In a recent quality initiative (QI) study, bundle of interventions such as close monitoring of tidal volume (V_t) and PIP depending on ventilator mode, with a V_t goal of 4–6 mL/kg body weight of infant, and prompt feedback of bedside nursing staff to clinical care provider whenever sustained elevations of these parameters helped in reducing incidence of pneumothorax from 10.45% to 2.6% in VLBW infants [23].

g. Among VLBW infant population, maintaining inspired gas >36.5 °C was associated with a reduction in pneumothorax incidence by 2/3 [24].

Practical respiratory strategies that can reduce potential air leaks are described as follows (Table 13B.2).

Diagnosis

A high index of suspicion is needed to diagnose pneumothorax. In a ventilated baby any sudden unexplained deterioration should always raise a suspicion for pneumothorax, as a part of displacement, obstruction, pneumothorax and equipment (DOPE) failure evaluation. Diagnosis is usually made by the presence of clinical signs, physical examination, transillumination, and chest X-ray or chest ultrasound.

Table 13B.2 Proposed respiratory management strategies to reduce air leaks

Initial ventilator settings—at admission				
Early use of surfactant whenever indicated	1. Volume targeted ventilation V_t 4–6 mL/kg 2. If TCPL mode V_t to be achieved 4–6 mL/kg 3. Careful monitoring, specially postsurfactant administration	1. PIP = 14–16 cm in preterm and 16–20 cmH$_2$O in term infants 2. To avoid PIP >24 cmH$_2$O 3. MAP >12 cmH$_2$O, careful monitoring—consider HFOV	PEEP = 5 cmH$_2$O Aggressive weaning to CPAP	1. Respiratory rate at 40–60/min 2. Inspiratory time (T_i) = 0.3–0.4 s, avoid T_i > 0.5 s	1. Inspiratory gas temperature between 36.5–37.5°C 2. Adequate analgesia to facilitate patient ventilator synchrony 3. ET care protocol to avoid direct airway injury
Ideal blood gas and oxygenation target				
pH = 7.25–7.35	PCO$_2$ = 40–50 mmHg, accepting 60 mmHg, if pH >7.25	PaO2 = 50–60 mmHg, accepting >40 mmHg in small preemies.	SpO$_2$ = 90%–95%	

HFOV, High-frequency oscillation ventilation; *MAP*, mean airway pressure; *TCPL*, time cycled pressure limited.

Clinical presentations

1. Asymptomatic: Mild air leaks or anterior pneumothorax without lung collapse may be asymptomatic and sometimes detected during chest X-ray, but usually pneumothorax presents as an acute clinical deterioration of baby's condition.
2. In ventilated babies there may be sudden deterioration of infants' clinical condition with agitation, desaturations, or increase need in oxygenation; ventilator requirements may increase or may present with sudden change in cardiovascular status of the baby.
3. Large/Tension pneumothorax may present with:
   a. increased work of breathing
   b. signs of respiratory distress such as tachypnea, grunting, and cyanosis
   c. sign of mediastinal shift
   d. diminished air entry in pneumothorax side
   e. weak peripheral pulse and pallor
4. Advanced tension pneumothorax—a large tension pneumothorax increases intrathoracic pressure, which may cause increased central venous pressure and decreased venous return which may present with hypotension and narrow pulse pressure, bradycardia, and hypoxemia. Arterial blood gas shows respiratory or mixed acidosis and hypoxemia.

Sudden decrease in voltage of QRS complex on cardiac ECG tracing may be one of the earliest signs of pneumothorax. Pulse oximetry "pseudobradycardia" sign may be another characteristic finding in pneumothorax where pulse oximeter displays low pulse rate and desaturations when auscultation heart rate will be in normal range. This finding can be explained by the fact that pulse oximeter missing out the low amplitude pulse wave signals results in the "pseudobradycardia" [25]. Pulsus paradoxus, a clinical sign with diagnostic and prognostic significance in pericardial diseases, also can be seen in tension pneumothorax. This is an exaggeration of normal decrease in systolic blood pressure during inspiration and increase in expiration. The "pararadox" refers to the fact that heart sounds may be heard over the precordium when the radial pulse is not felt. The clinical method of assessment of this "pulse" is by measurement of the "systolic blood pressure." In ICU care settings, where the arterial waveform is available, pulsus paradoxus can be diagnosed by visualizing changes in the systolic blood pressure tracing during the inspiratory and expiratory phases of respiration. Pulse oximetry waveform analysis has been found useful in the neonates with cardiac tamponade, and it is a useful adjunct for continually assessing pulsus paradoxus and air trapping severity.

Cyanosis of the head with pallor of the trunk may occur in tension pneumothorax with or without pneumopericardium.

On examination the side of the pneumothorax may be prominent compared with the other side. Abdominal distension may also be observed as a result of the pressure of the pneumothorax on the diaphragm. *Paradoxical symmetry of the chest* has been described as a clinical sign of unilateral pneumothorax [26]. In health, rotation of the neck causes the hemithorax on the side to which the head is turned to be less prominent than on the other side. In the presence of a unilateral pneumothorax, in contrast, the hemithorax on the side to which the head is turned is as prominent as the contralateral side.

Transillumination

Transillumination of the chest with a high-intensity fiber optic probe in a darkened room is a very useful beside tool, allowing a very rapid diagnosis in a preterm infant with sudden deterioration. When placed against the chest wall, it illuminates whole hemithorax on the affected side. This technique is useful in the emergency treatment of the pneumothorax without waiting for the radiograph in a rapidly deteriorating infant. Reported sensitivity is 87%–100% with false positive in the presence of PIE and pneumomediastinum, *specificity* is 95%–100% with false negative results in edematous infants, and small pneumothorax in term infants [27] (Fig. 13B.5).

Chest X-ray

Chest X-ray is gold standard in diagnosing pneumothorax in an infant. In a large pneumothorax under tension, air may be seen in the pleural space outlining visceral pleura appears hyperlucent with the absence of lung markings, flattening of the diaphragm, and displacement of the mediastinum. The collapsed lung edge is clearly visible. Small pneumothoraces on chest X-ray obtained in the supine position may also be detected only by a difference of radiolucency in one lung which appears to be "clearer" despite the presence of lung parenchyma. An anteroposterior chest X-ray with horizontal beam taken with the infant kept in lateral decubitus with affected side up may improve the detection of small pneumothoraces and a lateral radiograph with horizontal beam while the infant is in the supine position, which helps in detecting anterior pneumothorax. Shadows of skin folds, the latissimus dorsi, and bed clothes mimicking a lung edge may all cause diagnostic dilemmas. The sources of these extraneous (extrathoracic) findings can be identified by following the shadows which may extend beyond lungs field. Diagnostic accuracy of chest X-ray is reported as *sensitivity* of 87%–96% and *specificity* of 96%–99% [28] (Fig. 13B.6).

Lungs ultrasound

Lungs ultrasound (LUS) may be a useful point of care tool for diagnosing pneumothorax in neonates. Ultrasound of

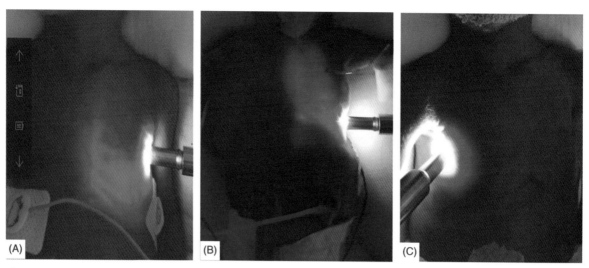

Figure 13B.5 High-intensity fiber optic light demonstrating increased transillumination on left half of chest suggestive of left side pneumothorax (A–B) compared to normal right chest (C).

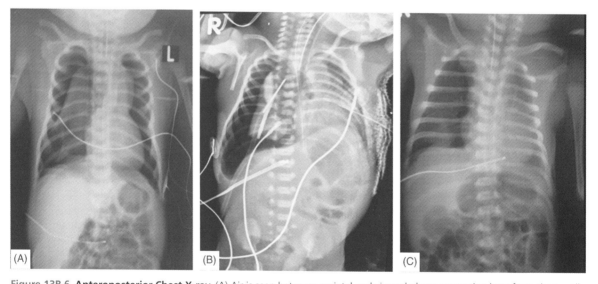

Figure 13B.6 Anteroposterior Chest X-ray. (A) Air is seen between parietal and visceral pleura separating lung from chest wall and collapsing the ipsilateral lung and with shift of mediastinum to other side. (B) Bilateral pneumothorax with ICD in left-side chest. (C) Free air is seen anteriorly suggestive of anterior pneumothorax with out collapse of lungs.

the healthy lung reveals "lung sliding" and "seashore sign" on B- and M-mode imaging, respectively. Using B-mode, in a normal lung you should be able to see the pleura, visible as a hyperechoic line beneath subcutaneous tissue, sliding up and down. In cases of pneumothorax, however, the presence of air between visceral and parietal pleura abolishes lung sliding on the B-mode imaging. Infant should be kept in a reclining position for letting air collection within the anterior nondependent portions of the pleural space and place the transducer anteriorly (midclavicular line, fifth to eighth intercostal space). It is possible to identify the edge of the collection of air with ultrasound (the lung point) where the pleura stop sliding. Other USG findings suggestive of pneumothorax are double lung point, the absence of B lines, and the absence of lung pulse. Using M-mode, the normal lung is seen beneath pleura (the waves), as a

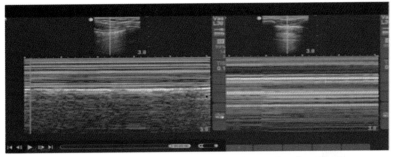

Sand and sea/seashore sign   Sea only/stratosphere/barcode sign

Figure 13B.7 Chest USG Using M-Mode. *Left side* shows normal lung with sand and seashore pattern and *right side* with pneumothorax shows "barcode" pattern. Image modified from Kurepa D, Zaghloul N, Watkins L and Liu J. Neonatal lung ultrasound exam guidelines. J Perinatol 2018;38:11–22 [29].

granular pattern (the gravelly beach), and as a seashore. In pneumothorax, the pattern is replaced by the "stratosphere" or "barcode" sign where lung sliding disappears, lung no longer visible, but instead artifacts (A-line) is visible [29] (Fig. 13B.7).

Cattarossi et al. in a recent study reported that the sensitivity and the specificity in diagnosing pneumothorax were 100% for LUS, 96% and 100% for CXR, and 87% and 96% for transillumination [28]. Another recent study by Liu et al., observed accuracy and reliability of the LUS signs of lung sliding disappearance as well as the existence of the pleural line and the A-line in diagnosing pneumothorax were as follows: 100% sensitivity, 100% specificity, 100% PPV, and 100% NPV [30]. Studies in the adult population have shown a high sensitivity (95%), specificity (100%), and diagnostic effectiveness (98%) of LUS in comparison to CT scan as gold standard.

Management

There is paucity of evidence-based recommendations for the management of pneumothorax in newborns. There are different strategies available in various clinical situations.

If pneumothorax detected in spontaneous breathing baby or with respiratory support oxygen supplementation should be provided to maintain adequate oxygen saturation. Increasing the inspired concentration of oxygen to 50%–100% may help in the resorption of air from the pleural spaces by nitrogen washout, but this practice is not supported by any high-quality evidence and with a risk of hyperoxia it may be dangerous in preterm infants. In mechanical ventilated infants, ventilator settings should be adjusted to minimize MAP by reducing PIP, PEEP, and inspiratory time (T_i). Treatment options for pneumothorax include expectant management, needle aspiration, and chest tube drainage (intercostal chest drain [ICD]).There is little consensus about methods of treatment in neonatal pneumothorax.

Expectant management with careful monitoring: This may be useful for infants with small and medium pneumothoraces, who are asymptomatic or stable and on minimal respiratory support. In a retrospective cohort study of 136 ventilated infants who developed pneumothorax, 26% infants managed without need of an intercostal catheter [31].

Needle thoracocentesis: This emergency management is warranted when rapid deterioration in gas exchange or cardiovascular status occurs, usually in tension pneumothorax. In a recent randomized clinical trial, needle aspiration reduced rate of ICD insertion by 30%, relative risk (0.70; 95% CI, 0.56–0.87) in newborn with symptomatic pneumothoraces [32]. Needle thoracocentesis when required should not be delayed pending a chest X-ray. This can be used both as therapeutic or diagnostic method. Site of aspiration should be in the second intercostal space on the affected side and in the midclavicular line just above the lower rib. Aspiration can be done by 10 mL syringe attached to intravenous cannula or butterfly with a three-way tap or connecting to underwater seal. Once the baby is stabilized with needle aspiration, a chest drain should be inserted.

Intercostal chest tube drainage: A chest drain should be inserted as the primary treatment for a significant pneumothorax that is not under tension, or following needle drainage for a tension pneumothorax.

1. *Site of tube insertion* is usually safe and effective in the fourth or fifth intercostal space in the mid- or anterior axillary line in the anatomical safe triangle and it should be away from nipple line. In an anterior pneumothorax this lateral approach may fail to drain the air, in which case the chest tube may have to be inserted in a more anterior position such as the second intercostal space on anterior axillary line can be used.

2. The *sizes of chest drains* used in newborns usually varies according to gestation and birth weight of infants. Trochar chest drain (polyvinyl) size 8,10, and 10–12 Fr are appropriate for infants with birth weight of <1,

1–1.5, and >1.5 kg, respectively. Similarly, 6 Fr (8 cm), 6 Fr (15 cm), and 8.5 Fr (15 cm) are recommended for <1, 1–1.5, and >1.5 kg birth weight group, respectively [33,34].

Large-bore, stiff chest drains have been used traditionally to drain pleural collections which require blunt dissection of the chest wall. Small-bore, flexible pigtail catheters inserted via the Seldinger technique or directly over an introducer are now found to be equally effective and safe and considered as primary choice of intercostal catheter in infants. These new soft, polyurethane pigtail catheters are easy to introduce with shorter time by 10 min, less painful during insertion and during ongoing care, and post procedure scars are also less in comparison to stiff large bore tubes and trocars. Studies showed complications like lung perforation and other viscera injuries are lesser (1% vs. 3%–6%), but the rate of tube dislodgement or dysfunction (blockage, kinking, or failure to drain) was slightly higher in pigtail group [35].

3. Indications for ICD removal: The aim is to remove the drain(s) with minimal risk of air entrapment or recurrence of pneumothorax. If there are two drains to be removed, remove the lower or dependent position drain first followed by the higher drain. Removal of ICD may be considered after stopping negative suction if used and when the following criteria are met [33]:
   a. Clinical and radiological signs of lung reexpansion with decreased work of breathing
   b. No signs of new air leak
   c. Air bubbling in chest tube drainage bottle or fluttering of Heimlich valve has subsided for more than 24 h

There is no consensus on routine use of negative suction to underwater seal chest drains in neonatal pneumothorax, but suction may be applied if chest drain fails to help in expansion collapsed alveoli or residual free air still present after ICD placement and appropriate positioning. In adult population, −10 or −20 cm of water negative suction was used effectively with reasonable safety both in spontaneous or postsurgical air leaks. Effectiveness of suction depends on height of water column which should be maintained at least 10–15 cm, once underwater seal connected to wall-mounted negative suction it should be switched on otherwise it will create a closed circuit which may increase pneumothorax [36]. In preterm neonates close monitoring of negative suction should be done as it may lead to other pulmonary complications. Stop negative suction if ICD clamping planned before removal of intercostal chest drain.

Whether to clamp an ICD before removal or not is a matter of controversy. A consensus statement from the American College of Chest Physicians (ACCP) showed that 60% physicians would clamp before removal [37] but cur-

rent BTS guidelines do not favor clamping, though both guidelines are from adult populations. There are many supporters for clamping considering lethal complications associated with premature removal of ICD without a clamp trial. In a recent study (2015) published in *European Respiratory Journal*, comparison between clamping for 6 versus 24 h duration found no difference in recurrence of air leaks within 7 days of chest drain removal [38]. Therefore, it may be appropriate to clamp ICD for 6–12 h duration and can be removed if air does not accumulate in the pleura, which can be found out with clinical and radiological assessment (Fig. 13B.8).

Bronchopulmonary fistula

Bronchopleural fistula (BPF) is the abnormal connection between the pleural space and the bronchial tree. It is both an indication for and a dreaded complication of chest tube placement. BPF exists if the bubbling continues for 24 h or more in chest tube and indicative of a persistent air leak into the pleural space. Volutrauma during ventilation is probably the major factor in the development of a BPF, but a large transpulmonary pressure gradient (i.e., the difference in the airway and pleural pressures) may also play a role.

Loss of tidal volume, gas exchange abnormalities, and the appearance of ventilator autocycling are initial diagnostic clues in a ventilated baby. The severity of the air leak can be categorized as bubbling during inspiration only, bubbling during both inspiration and expiration, or bubbling during both inspiration and expiration with a detectable difference in the inspired and expired tidal volumes. BPFs that fall into the last category can have physiological effects (e.g., tachypnea, hypercapnia, hypoxemia). The main problems with a large fistula in a ventilated patient are the loss of delivered tidal volume, inability to apply PEEP, persistent lung collapse, and delayed weaning from assisted ventilation. Diagnosis can be confirmed via bronchoscopy, bronchography, or computed tomography (CT) with 3D reconstruction, but bronchoscopy remains gold standard for diagnosis and evaluation [39].

Management strategies include general conservative measures such as large bore chest drains (multiple if necessary) and the use of drainage system with adequate capabilities. In mechanically ventilated patients, the goal is to maintain adequate ventilation and oxygenation while reducing the fistula flow to allow the leak to heal. Suggested ventilation strategies include reducing PIP, V_t, respiratory rate, PEEP, and inspiratory times, allowing more spontaneous breathing and accepting permissive hypercapnia and lower oxygen saturations. The decision to reduce PEEP is very critical in the acute phase of lung disease, and should not be undertaken casually. Most air leaks will settle spontaneously over a few days if the patient can be weaned

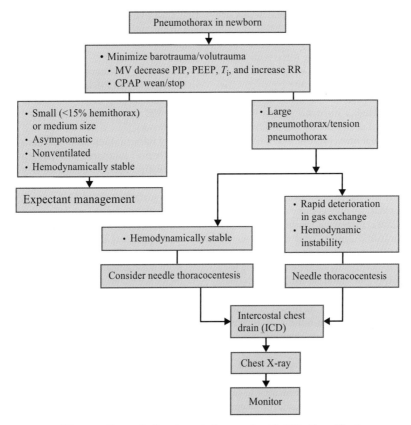

Figure 13B.8 Management of Pneumothorax in Newborn is Summarized in This Flow Chart.

onto spontaneous respiration without high levels of PEEP. Avoidance of negative pressure suction to ICD tube or underwater seal bottle will help in healing of BPF. The use of other modes of ventilation including high-frequency ventilation, oscillation, and differential lung ventilation through double-lumen tubes has been reported. For proximal leaks, fiber optic bronchoscopy and direct application of sealants (e.g., cyanoacrylate, fibrin agents, gelfoam) have been tried in pediatric population with limited success. Thoracotomy is definite therapy for selected infants requiring ventilator support who demonstrate a large air leak, persistent pneumothorax, and progressive hypoxia which is unresponsive to chest tube insertion. Refractory cases need surgical repair of the air leak by thoracoplasty, lung resection/stapling, pleural abrasion/decortication, or other techniques. Although rare, acute BPF is difficult to manage and is associated with high morbidity, prolonged hospital stay, high resource utilization, and mortality.

Pneumothorax prognosis: Pneumothorax in prematurely born infants with RDS increases mortality from 12% to 31% in VLBW infants [40]. Mortality is higher in infants who developed pneumothorax on day 1 or 4th day after

birth [41]. Air leaks are also associated with intraventricular hemorrhage, and there is higher chance of developing bronchopulmonary dysplasia (BPD) in preterm neonates (adjusted OR, -9.4, 95% CI, 3.6–24.8) with pneumothorax. About 15% term and late preterm newborns developed persistent pulmonary hypertension (PPHN) in a large cohort of symptomatic pneumothorax [42].

Pulmonary interstitial emphysema

PIE, most common form of air leak in preterm infants, occurs most often but not exclusively in the presence of clinical triad prematurity, RDS, and mechanical ventilation. The incidence, inversely proportional to gestation age at birth and birth weight, usually presents in the first 96 h of life. The incidence of PIE in the presurfactant era in mechanically ventilated babies under 1500 g was approximately 20% [43]. Recent studies showed incidence of PIE in 2%–3% of NICU admission and 25% in ELBW infants [44,45].

The highest incidence of PIE in preterm infants has been observed when intrauterine infection (chorioamnionitis) complicates the RDS [46]. MAS, resuscitation at birth, subsequent need of ventilation, and postnatal sepsis are other known risk factors for PIE.

PIE is a consequence of alveolar rupture into the peribronchial space with a positive driving force with subsequent spreading of air resulting in an endolymphatic air distribution and diffusion of air inside the connective tissue of the peribronchovascular sheets, interlobular septa, and the visceral pleura. Higher incidence found in ELBW preterm infants because of poor development of basement membrane layer of terminal bronchiole adjacent to alveoli, less compliant alveolus, incomplete development of peribronchial connective tissue till distal end, and increased need of mechanical ventilation in this population. The presence of interstitial air trapping causes alveolar compression, tissue inflammation, alters pulmonary mechanics by decreasing compliance, increasing residual volume and dead space which impair diffusion, and compresses the capillaries and hilum causing decreased venous return, contributing to ventilation–perfusion (V/Q) mismatching [47].

PIE commonly evolves and manifests during mechanical ventilation or CPAP use in preterm infants. PIE may present as a slowly progressive disease with increased ventilation requirement or with frequent desaturations or increased need of oxygen. PIE may present with agitation, frequent apneic episodes, or bradycardia. It may lead to hypercapnia, with profound hypoxemia and metabolic acidosis.

Diagnosis usually confirmed by chest radiograph (CXR) reveals hyperinflation with linear radiolucencies and small cysts, either localized or diffuse. The linear radiolucencies vary in width, coarse in nature, nonconfluent, they do not branch, seen in peripherals as well as medial lung fields. This may create a "salt and pepper" or "shattered glass" appearance in chest X-ray [48]. It must be distinguished from air bronchogram in which branching radiolucencies follow the normal anatomic distribution of the bronchial tree. Cyst-like radiolucencies of 0.5–4 mm may also present in the pulmonary parenchyma or in interlobular and subpleural connective tissue or in perivascular lymphatics (Fig. 13B.9).

No specific treatment is available for PIE, but main goal in management of PIE is focused on reducing or preventing further barotrauma or volutrauma to the lungs. Summary of different practices, which may influence PIE incidence, is as follows:

1. Early surfactant replacement therapy with brief ventilation compared with late surfactant and ventilation suggests decreased trend of air leak syndromes including PIE in premature infants in the early surfactant group [17].
2. Different modes of ventilation such as PTV, VTV, and early or rescue high-frequency ventilation have not much influence on the incidence of PIE [19].
3. Early CPAP, gentle ventilation, and early extubation from mechanical ventilation might influence PIE incidence. A recent study showed that the rate of PIE was significantly less while delivering nasal CPAP by mask as compared with prongs (4.9% vs. 17.5%; RR, 0.28, 95% CI, 0.08–0.96) [49].

Conventional ventilation strategy should include the following:

1. Decrease in PIP or tidal volume to achieve acceptable arterial blood gases (PaO_2, 45–50 mmHg or 6–6.7 kPa; PCO_2, <60 mmHg or 8 kPa with a pH >7.25) [50].
2. Decreasing PEEP to avoid hyperinflation *without compromising lung recruitment* should also be considered as hyperinflation in PIE is mainly extraalveolar in nature and too low PEEP may tilt the ventilation balance. This critical decision to reduce PEEP should not be casual.
3. Higher ventilator rate with short T_i (<0.3 s) may be beneficial to resolve PIE [51].

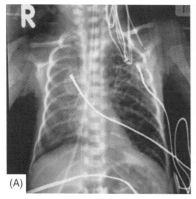 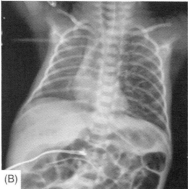 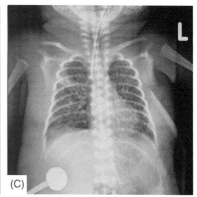

Figure 13B.9 (A–B) Localized PIE—coarse, nonbranching, radiolucencies that project toward the periphery of the lung in a disorganized fashion (left side). (C) Generalized PIE—coarse, nonbranching, radiolucencies that project toward the periphery of the lung in a disorganized fashion on both sides.

If conventional ventilation fails, high-frequency jet ventilation (HFJV) or high-frequency oscillation ventilation (HFOV) may improve oxygenation in infants with severe respiratory failure due to PIE in infants. Treatment with HFJV resulted in improved ventilation at lower peak and MAPs with more rapid radiological improvement of the PIE, but survival, the incidences of chronic lung disease, IVH, patent ductus arteriosus, airway obstruction, and new air leak did not differ significantly between infants supported on HFJV or CMV [52]. Although HFJV may be most effective in resolution of PIE (within 24–48 h), different studies showed only short-term benefits in improving ventilation.

HFJV strategy for PIE: Low MAP with relatively low PEEP on HFJV with its smaller tidal volume and lower intrapulmonary pressure amplitude facilitates healing.

Goals should be

1. Permissive hypercarbia—choose PIP 2 cmH$_2$O less than CMV, decrease delta P, and tolerate higher PCO$_2$ 55–65 mmHg with pH >7.25.
2. Minimize number and intensity of IMV (sigh breaths) by choosing IMV rate 0–3.
3. Decrease high MAP by decreasing PIP and PEEP, in this process if required achieve optimum oxygenation by transient increase in FiO$_2$.
4. Decrease rate—as inspiratory time is fixed (0.02 s), choosing 4 Hz (240 bpm; *I:E*, 1:12) to 6 Hz (360 bpm, I:E, 1:7) with adequate expiratory time can minimize air trapping.

HFOV strategy for PIE: HFOV is used more commonly worldwide as a rescue ventilation for air leaks. Although evidence-based recommendations of HFOV for PIE management are lacking, here we summarize some HFOV strategies for PIE when conventional ventilation fails. Weaning from HFOV to CMV considered 24–48 h after PIE resolves [53]. MAP is critical in management of PIE; aggressive lungs recruitment should be avoided and maintained at a pressure sufficient to stent small airways open which may help in maintaining oxygenation and reducing progression of the air leak (Table 13B.3).

There have been few descriptions of the utility of systemic corticosteroids in PIE. In 1987, Mosini et al. showed a dramatic effect in three neonates treated with 5–7 days of dexamethasone (0.5 mg/kg/day) [55]. Fitzgerald et al. reported a retrospective case review of the efficacy of a 3-day course of dexamethasone at the same dose in 10 infants with severe PIE, with a 78% resolution rate [56]. In both series steroid used after first week of life who requires high ventilator setting and hypoxemia with development of PIE. Recently, rapid resolution of a refractory unilateral PIE was reported with the use of a single dose of intravenous hydrocortisone (2 mg/kg) on day 18 of life followed by 1 mg/kg every 12 h for next 48 h [57]. Short steroid courses though look promising in resolution of PIE, it should be used with all caution as it may not be quite safe in those small preemies.

Treatment of localized PIE may need few alternative approaches.

1. Ventilation with very short T_i such as 0.15 s which will facilitate preferential volume delivery to normal time constant lung and simultaneously will avoid overdistension of longer time constant PIE lung [58]. This method may not be tolerated for longer period.

Table 13B.3 HFOV strategies in newborn with PIE

	Pathology	HFOV strategies
Group 1	1. Diffuse alveolar collapse with dilated distal bronchioles 2. CXR—small focal bubbles surrounded by opacities representing atelectasis and low lung volume	Goal Lung recruitment and avoid lung overinflation Settings of HFOV 1. MAP 1 or 2 cm higher than that used during CMV 2. Wean FiO$_2$ to 60% keeping optimal lung inflation, then weaning of MAP 3. Amplitude (delta P) for adequate wiggle 4. Rate (Hz)—start with 10–15 Hz keeping T_i 0.33, then further adjustment
Group 2	1. Interstitial collection of gas, focal, or diffuse, progressive compression may behave like tension pneumothorax 2. CXR—large tortuous cysts, focal, or diffuse with patchy hyperinflation	Goal Lowest possible ventilator setting Accept low PO$_2$ (45–50) and high PCO$_2$ (55–65, pH >7.25) Settings of HFOV 1. MAP equal or less than that used during CMV. Weaning MAP preferred over FiO$_2$ 2. Low oscillatory amplitude (delta P)—less than PIP in CMV 3. Rate (Hz)—10–12 in early PIE and 6–8 in established PIE [54]

2. *Independent lung ventilation* (ILV) strategy has been described in infants and children with unilateral lung disease but rarely used in preterm infants. Reports of ILV in neonates have been described with simultaneous intubation of with two separate ET tubes, one in trachea, providing ventilation to left lung, and other in right main bronchus, providing ventilation to right lung [59]. Alternatively, dual lumen single tube also has been used in bigger babies. Ventilation strategy such as "master and slave" method has been used in this procedure with independent lower ventilator setting for the PIE lungs.

3. *Selective bronchial intubation* (SBI) of contralateral lung can decompress PIE lung. Unilateral intubation can be facilitated by turning head of infant to opposite side [60].
   Ventilation of unilateral lung can also be obtained by a Swan–Ganz catheter by occlusion of a mainstem bronchus [61]. Duration of selective intubation is controversial—some suggest decompression happens with 48 h of intubation, and others advocate to continue till 5 days to prevent recurrence of PIE. Selective intubation should be accompanied by HFOV for better ventilation.

4. Placing the infant in the *lateral decubitus position* with the affected side down, minimal chest physiotherapy, and endotracheal suctioning facilitates gas exchange of unaffected lung and reduce aeration of lung with PIE. Lateral decubitus positioning for 3 days was associated with radiological resolution of tension PIE.

5. Refractory localized PIE which may be expanding and poorly responding to all treatment may require surgical resection.

Prognosis

PIE contributes for significant morbidity and mortality in preterm infants [62]:
- Respiratory failure, associated with other air leaks— prolonged ventilation.
- Chronic lung disease (CLD/BPD), IVH (twice as common preterm infants in the presence of PIE), and periventricular leukomalacia.
- Mortality increases significantly in the presence of PIE (OR, 14.4; 95% CI, 1–208; $P = 0.05$).

Pneumopericardium

Pneumopericardium is the severe form of air leak and results when air from the pleural space or mediastinum enters the pericardial sac through a defect that is often located at the reflection near the ostia of the pulmonary veins. It may occur in 2% of VLBW infants and 3.5% of ventilated neonates, usually reported with coexisting other form of air leaks [63]. The majority of reported cases are of preterm newborns with RDS who required PPV at birth and/or subsequent respiratory support, whether in the form of mechanical ventilation or CPAP. Ventilation parameters such as high PIP (>32 cmH$_2$O), high MAP (>17 cmH$_2$O), and long T_i (>0.7 s) are known risk factors for pneumopericardium, though these practices are not common now a days [64].

Pneumopericardium is usually symptomatic and should be suspected in infants with air leak and sudden cardiovascular deterioration. Clinically, it may present with worsening respiratory distress, hypotension with narrow pulse pressure, bradycardia, pallor, or cyanosis. Cyanosis of the head with pallor of the trunk may occur in pneumopericardium. On auscultation heart sounds are muffled and pericardial rub is rarely audible. Low voltage QRS complexes are also seen.

The diagnosis is confirmed by chest radiograph. The diagnosis is based on radiographs showing air surrounding the heart including the inferior surface and outlining the great vessels. The presence of air inferior to the diaphragmatic surface of the heart differentiates it from a pneumomediastinum in which the mediastinal gas is limited inferiorly by the attachment of the mediastinal pleura to the central tendon of the diaphragm (Figs. 13B.10 and 13B.11). Illumination of the substernal region that may flicker with the heart rate may be good clue for pneumopericardium in transillumination test. Ultrasound detection of air in pericardial sac can be life saving.

Conservative approach is reserved for asymptomatic infants. As with any air leak in an infant receiving mechanical ventilation, ventilator pressures should be minimized. Pneumopericardium whenever associated with pneumothorax, draining pneumothorax by placing a chest drain may decompress it. Drainage by direct pericardial tap via the subxiphoid route under USG guidance should be considered in rapid deteriorating pneumopericardium with or without a tamponade effect. The blood pressure should be monitored continuously and the tap repeated if bradycardia or hypotension recurs. Catheter drainage has been recommended only if there is persistent or recurrence pneumopericardium present. High mortality such as 60%–70% reported in different studies in symptomatic neonatal pneumopericardium cases [63].

Pneumomediastinum

Pneumomediastinum results from leakage of air into the mediastinal space. The most common reported causes of pneumomediastinum in the neonates are exposure to positive pressure ventilation, MAS, pneumonia, or RDS. It occurs in about 0.1%–0.2% of newborns, though this is an underestimate as majority isolated cases are asymptomatic.

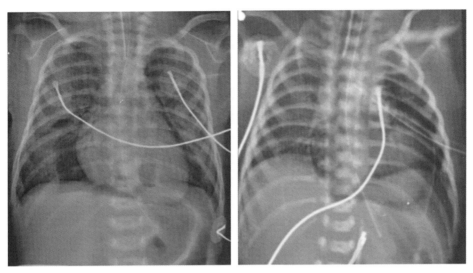

Figure 13B.10 **Pneumopericardium—Free Air Surrounding the Heart but Not Extending Beyond the Great Vessels and Extending to Inferior Border of Heart.**

Pneumopericardium

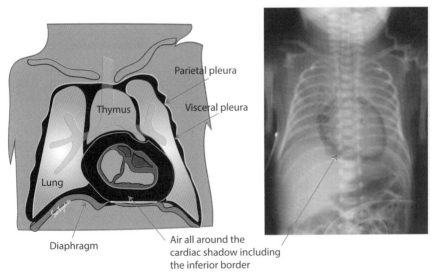

Parietal pleura

Thymus

Visceral pleura

Lung

Diaphragm

Air all around the cardiac shadow including the inferior border

Figure 13B.11 **Diagrammatic Representation of Pneumopericardium Showing a "Ring" of Air Surrounding the Cardiac Silhouette.** Adapted from Satyan's illustrative neonatology by Drs. Chandrasekharan and Rawat.

Pneumomediastinum may present with respiratory distress, a bowed sternum, and muffled heart sound. On radiograph, a pneumomediastinum is most commonly seen as air surrounding the thymus above the cardiac shadow. When large, it appears as a halo around the heart on AP view and as a retrosternal or superior mediastinal lucency on the lateral view. The mediastinal air can elevate the thymus away from the pericardium, resulting in a "spinnaker sail" or "Angel wing" appearance, which is best appreciated on a left anterior oblique view (Fig. 13B.12).

An isolated pneumomediastinum often resolves spontaneously and in general requires no treatment. It is very

183

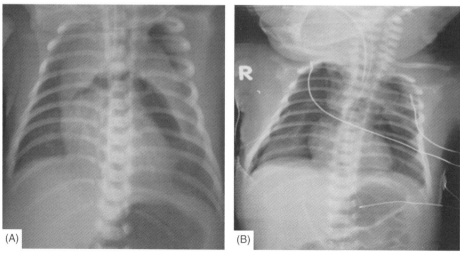

Figure 13B.12 (A) Isolated pneumomediastinum. (B) Pneumomediastinum associated with right-sided pneumothorax.

difficult to drain a symptomatic pneumomediastinum, as the gas is collected in multiple independent lobules but if under tension ultrasound-guided percutaneous drainage can be tried [65]. However, we have observed resolution of many pneumomediastinum cases, once coexisting pneumothorax was drained with the placement of chest drain (ICD) (Fig. 13B.13).

Pneumoperitonium

Pneumoperitoneum usually results from perforation of intestine or other abdominal viscera, so primarily surgical causes should be ruled out. A pneumoperitoneum may rarely be associated with an intrathoracic air leak due; it should be suspected whenever a ventilated newborn develops pneumoperitoneum simultaneously or shortly after pulmonary air leaks (pneumothorax, pneomomediastinum, etc.). It usually resolves with adequate management of the lung pathology and intrathoracic air leaks.

High and prolonged positive airway pressure or large tidal volume during mechanical ventilation may produce lung injury which may cause pneumoperitoneum through different routes.

1. Various thoracic air leaks may result air in mediastinum, from there air may leak around aorta and esophagus and dissects down into retroperitoneum and with rupture of parietal peritoneum may cause pneumoperitoneum.
2. Air after entering into pulmonary lymphatics may pass through retrograde path with positive pressure drive and can cause pneumoperitoneum.

3. Pleural air from pneumothorax or surgical emphysema air can traverse through pleuroperitoneal fistula into peritoneum.

A horizontal beam lateral or right lateral radiograph will demonstrate even a small pneumoperitoneum, abdominal X-ray along with chest may identify cause of pneumoperitoneum. High-intensity transillumination light can also identify free peritoneal air, though false positive is possible in the presence of very large dilated loops in small preterm infants (Fig. 13B.14).

Pulmonary air leak once drained usually coexisting free peritoneal air resolve [66] but rarely massive pneumoperitoneum causes respiratory embarrassment or may compress the portal, inferior vena cava and resulting decreased blood return to the heart resulting into poor perfusion, hypotension and metabolic acidosis. This large pneumoperitoneum may need needle drainage or the placement of a catheter for drainage (Fig. 13B.15).

Practice points

1. Pneumothorax and PIE are commonest air leaks in neonates, usually occurs in mechanical ventilated babies with high pressure or volume.
2. Early use of surfactant, volume-targeted ventilation, and early extubation may significantly reduce air leaks in preterm newborn.
3. Avoidance of high PIP, MAP, long T_i, monitoring of tidal volume, and choosing an appropriate PEEP are key ventilation practices which prevent air leaks.

4. Pneumothorax usually presents with acute deterioration, but PIE presents with slow deterioration in a ventilated preterm.
5. Tension pneumothorax should be suspected clinically and it should be managed as an emergency.
6. Asymptomatic air leaks can be managed with expectant management by monitoring and needle aspiration

can reduce one-third chest drain placement even in symptomatic pneumothoraces.
7. Small-bore, flexible pigtail catheters are preferred for chest drain when where needed in newborn with large symptomatic or tension pneumothorax.

(A)
Pneumomediastinum

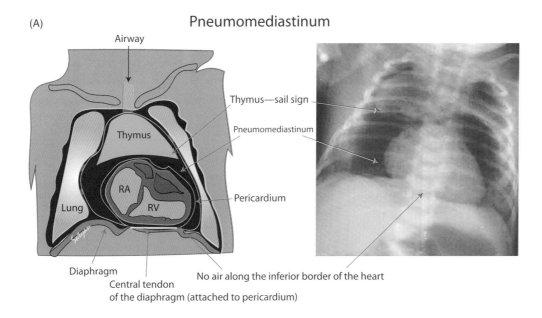

(B)
Pneumomediastinum—lateral view

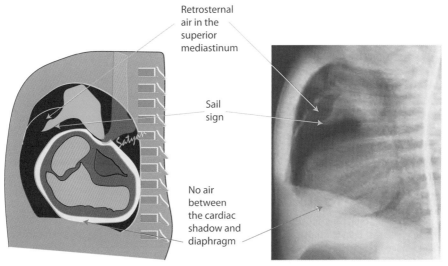

Figure 13B.13 (A) Diagrammatic representation of anteroposterior view of a pneumomediastinum. (B) Diagrammatic representation of a lateral view of a pneumomediastinum. Part A–B: Adapted from Satyan's illustrative neonatology by Drs. Chandrasekharan and Rawat.

185

Case 2

Air leak difficult case scenario

Baby S is a preterm (29 weeks of gestational age) baby boy, birth weight 1.1 kg, delivered to 22 years old primigravida mother by spontaneous vaginal delivery. This baby was a result of a spontaneous conception and mother had regular antenatal checkups with uneventful antenatal period. Antenatal scans were reported normal and Doppler study was also normal. She had preterm premature rupture of membrane (PPROM) for 20 days for which she received IV antibiotics. There was no clinical or biochemical evidence of chorioamnionitis. She received 2 doses of antenatal steroids 1 week prior to delivery.

Delivery room

Baby cried immediately after birth. Apgar scores were 7 and 8 at 1 and 5 min, respectively. Baby developed grunting and subcostal and intercostal retraction soon after birth for which CPAP started in delivery room (PEEP of 6 cmH$_2$O and maximum FiO$_2$ of 0.3) and shifted to NICU.

Course in NICU

Baby was continued on CPAP support with PEEP 6 cmH$_2$O and FiO$_2$ 0.3. IV Antibiotics were started after sending blood culture in view of history of PPROM and respiratory distress. Initial CXR was suggestive of mild RDS (Fig. 4). The first blood gas showed mild respiratory acidosis (pH 7.26, PCO$_2$ 53 mmHg, PO$_2$ 48 mmHg, BE 3 mEq/L).

Over next few hours baby had increase in retractions for which CPAP support was increased to 7 cmH$_2$O. Baby continued to have >40% oxygen requirement, so baby was intubated, one dose surfactant was given and continued on mechanical ventilator (Fig. 5).

Baby was continued on assist control (AC mode) (PIP 20, PEEP 6, T_i 0.30, RR 50, and FiO$_2$ 40%). After 2 h of ventilation baby had sudden increase in FiO$_2$ requirement with increased distress. Baby was hemodynamically stable during evaluation.

What could be the reason for sudden deterioration? Remember mnemonic: DOPED

- Tube displacement and obstruction
- Air leak (pneumothorax)
- Ventilation (equipment) failure
- Deterioration of RDS and lung derecruitment

Bedside immediate chest transillumination was suggestive of right-side pneumothorax which was confirmed by CXR.

What are the risk factors for pneumothorax?

- Preterm RDS
- PPROM with possible lung hypoplasia
- Increase in compliance post surfactant

How could we prevent this complication?

- Volume guarantee mode
- Continuous monitoring of tidal volumes postsurfactant and weaning of pressures

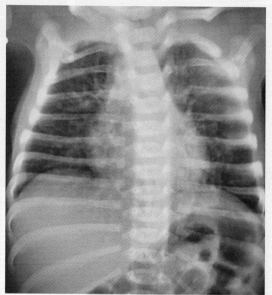
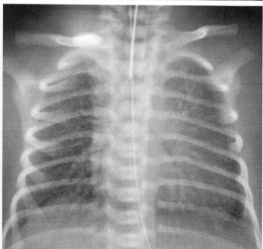

Fig. 4 Preterm RDS. Pre- and postsurfactant anteroposterior chest X-ray.

As baby was stable hemodynamically chest drain was planned without needle aspiration. Post-ICD baby improved with improvement in oxygenation (Fig. 5).

Ventilation strategy postpneumothorax?

- Patient trigger ventilation (AC, SIMV, PSV) or rescue HFOV
- High RR
- Keep PIP minimal to prevent further volutrauma and barotrauma
- PEEP to maintain adequate lung expansion
- Permissive hypercapnia

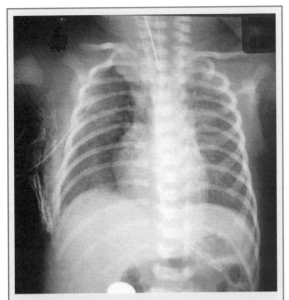

Fig. 5 **Right-Side Pneumothorax With ICD.**

Again after 2 h ventilator pressure and oxygen requirement increased. Repeat CXR done showed persistent
anterior pneumothorax with first ICD in proper position
(Fig. 6). As baby continued to have high pressure and oxygen requirement, second ICD was placed anteriorly to drain
pneumothorax, some time reposition of ICD helps but here
it did not drain pneumothorax. Requirement of multiple ICD
though rare nowadays with early surfactant use and gentle
ventilation but subsequent opposite side pneumothorax or
recurrent pneumothorax may occur during mechanical ventilation for which careful monitoring is required.

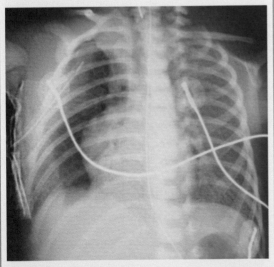

Fig. 6 **Persistent Pneumothorax Even After 1st ICD.**

Baby was switched over to high-frequency ventilator
with setting of MAP 10, frequency 10, amplitude 20 which
produced adequate chest wiggle (VN500, Draeger). FiO₂
requirement slowly came down to 30% after 4 h of HFOV.
Recurrence of pneumothorax observed in right side when
weaned to conventional patient-triggered ventilation. Next
48 h again managed by HFOV with MAP 8, frequency 12,
and amplitude as per need. (Fig. 7).

Next question to remove ICD first or extubate first

Considering recurrence of air leak, we continued HFOV for
next 3 days, one of ICDs removed. Once baby stable with
low settings extubated to CPAP of 5 cm and next 48 h baby
was on room air and 4 CPAP. CPAP was discontinued at
31 weeks, 3 days PMA. Baby discharged home at 36 weeks
PMA with 1.7 kg weight.

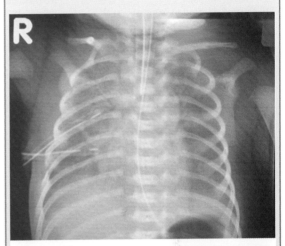

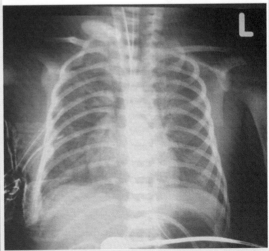

Fig. 7 **Resolution of Right-Sided Pneumothorax After
2nd ICD.**

Acknowledgments

We thank Dr Gautham Suresh MD, DM, MS, FAAP, Professor of Pediatrics, Baylor College of Medicine and Section Head and Service Chief of Neonatology, Texas Children's Hospital for reviewing this chapter and giving thoughtful comments and suggestions.

References

[1] Greenough A. Air leaks. In: Greenough A, Milner AD, editors. Neonatal respiratory disorders. 2nd ed. Arnold; London; 2003. p. 311–333.

[2] Chernick V, Avery ME. Spontaneous alveolar rupture at birth. Pediatrics 1963;32:816–824.

[3] Fanaroff AA, Stoll BJ, Wright LL, et al. Trends in neonatal morbidity and mortality for low birth weight infants. Am J Obstet Gynecol 2007;147:e1–e8.

[4] Horbar JD, Badger GJ, Carpenter JH, Fanaroff AA, Kilpatrick S, LaCorte M, et al. Trends in mortality and morbidity for very low birth weight infants, 1991–1999. Pediatrics 2002;110:143–151.

[5] Valls-I Soler A, Pijoan J, Cuttini M, Cruz J, Pallas C, et al. on behalf of the EuroNeoStat Consortium. Very low birthweight and gestational age babies in Europe: EuroNeoStat. In: Zeitlin J, Ashna M, editors. European Perinatal Health Report, 2008. EuroPeriStat Project; Spain; 2012. p. 183–194.

[6] Horbar JD, Soll RF, Edwards WH. The Vermont Oxford Network: a community of practice. Clin Perinatol 2010;37:29–47.

[7] Chow SSW, Le Marsney R, Creighton P, Kander V, Haslam R, Lui K. Report of the Australian and New Zealand Neonatal Network 2015. Sydney: ANZNN; 2017.

[8] Aly H, Massaro A, Acun C, Ozen M. Pneumothorax in the newborn: clinical presentation, risk factors and outcomes. J Matern Fetal Neonatal Med 2014;27(4):402–406.

[9] Madansky DL, Lawson EE, Chernick V, Taeusch HW. Pneumothorax and other forms of pulmonary air leak in newborns. Am Rew Resp Dis 1979;120:729–737.

[10] Goldeberg RN, Abdenour GE. Air leak syndrome. In: Spitzer AR, editor. Intensive care of the fetus and neonate. St. Louis, MO: Mosby; 1996. p. 629–640.

[11] Ho JJ, Subramaniam P, Davis PG. Continuous distending pressure for respiratory distress in preterm infants. Cochrane Database Syst Rev 2015;9:CD002271.

[12] Finer NN, Carlo WA, Walsh MC, Rich W, Gantz MG, Laptook AR, et al. Early CPAP versus surfactant in extremely preterm infants. N Engl J Med 2010;362:1970–1979.

[13] Greenough A, Dixon AK, Roberton NR. Pulmonary interstitial emphysema. Arch Dis Child 1984;59:1046–1051.

[14] Tarnow-Mordi WO, Narang A, Wilkinson AR. Lack of association between barotrauma and air leak in hyaline membrane disease. Arch Dis Child 1985;60:555–559.

[15] Roberts D, Brown J, Medley N, Dalziel SR. Antenatal corticosteroids for accelerating fetal lung maturation for women at risk of preterm birth. Cochrane Database Syst Rev 2017;3:CD004454.

[16] Soll RF. Prophylactic synthetic surfactant for preventing morbidity and mortality in preterm infants. Cochrane Database Syst Rev 1998;2:CD001079.

[17] Bahadue FL, Soll R. Early versus delayed selective surfactant treatment for neonatal respiratory distress syndrome. Cochrane Database Syst Rev 2012;11:CD001456.

[18] Sandri F, Plavka R, Ancora G, Simeoni U, Stranak Z, Martinelli S, et al. Prophylactic or early selective surfactant combined with nCPAP in very preterm infants. Pediatrics 2010;125:e1402–e1409.

[19] Greenough A, Rossor TE, Sundaresan A, Murthy V, Milner AD. Synchronized mechanical ventilation for respiratory support in newborn infants. Cochrane Database Syst Rev 2016;9:CD000456.

[20] Kamlin COF, Davis PG. Long versus short inspiratory times in neonates receiving mechanical ventilation. Cochrane Database Syst Rev 2003;4:CD004503.

[21] Cools F, Offringa M, Askie LM. Elective high frequency oscillatory ventilation versus conventional ventilation for acute pulmonary dysfunction in preterm infants. Cochrane Database Syst Rev 2015;3:CD000104.

[22] Klingenberg C, Wheeler KI, McCallion N, Morley CJ, Davis PG. Volume-targeted versus pressure-limited ventilation in neonates. Cochrane Database Syst Rev 2017;10:CD003666.

[23] Walker MW, Shoemaker M, Riddle K, Crane MM, Clark R. Clinical process improvement: reduction of pneumothorax and mortality in high-risk preterm infants. J Perinatol 2002;22:641–645.

[24] Tarnow-Mordi WO, Reid E, Griffiths P, Wilkinson AR. Low inspired gas temperature and respiratory complications in very low birth weight infants. J Pediatr 1989;114:438–442.

[25] Karthikeyan G, Narang A. Pulseoximetric pseudobradycardia in ventilated newborns with pneumothorax. Indian Pediatr 1999;36(8):841.

[26] Delport SA. Paradoxical symmetry of the chest in neonates—a new clinical sign in the diagnosis of a unilateral pneumothorax. South African Med J 1996;86:1465–1466.

[27] Wyman ML, Kuhns LR. Accuracy of transillumination in the recognition of pneumothorax and pneumomediastinum in the neonate. Clin Pediatr (Phila) 1977;16:323–324.

[28] Cattarossi L, Copetti R, Brusa G, Pintaldi S. Lung ultrasound diagnostic accuracy in neonatal pneumothorax. Can Respir J 2016;2016:6515069.

[29] Kurepa D, Zaghloul N, Watkins L, Liu J. Neonatal lung ultrasound exam guidelines. J Perinatol 2018;38:11–22.

[30] Liu J. Lung ultrasonography for the diagnosis of neonatal lung disease. J Matern Fetal Neonatal Med 2014;27(8):856–861.

[31] Litmanovitz I, Carlo WA. Expectant management of pneumothorax in ventilated neonates. Pediatrics 2008;122:e975–e979.

[32] Murphy MC, Heiring C, Doglioni N, Trevisanuto D, O'Donnell CPF, et al. Effect of needle aspiration of pneumothorax on subsequent chest drain insertion in newborns: a randomized clinical trial. JAMA Pediatr 2018;172:664–669.

[33] Wood B, Dubik M. A new device for pleural drainage in newborn infants. Pediatrics 1995;96:955–956.

[34] Otunla T, Thomas S. Pneumothorax-drainage guideline, neonatal intensive care unit clinical guideline. Ashford and St Peter Hospital, NHS Foundation. Available from: www.asph.mobi/Guidelines_Neonatal/Pneumothorax%20Nov%202014.pdf.

[35] Wei YH, Lee CH, Cheng HN, Tsao LT, Hsiao CC. Pigtail catheters versus traditional chest tubes for pneumothoraces in premature infants treated in a neonatal intensive care unit. Pediatr Neonatol 2014;55:376–380.

[36] Zisis C, Tsirgogianni K, Lazaridis G, Lampaki S, Baka S, Mpoukovinas I, et al. Chest drainage systems in use. Ann Transl Med 2015;3(3):43.

[37] Baumann MH, Strange C, Heffner JE, Light R, Kirby TJ, Klein J, et al. AACP Pneumothorax Consensus Group. Management of spontaneous pneumothorax: an American College of Chest Physicians Delphi consensus statement. Chest 2001;119(2):590–602.

[38] Kouritas V, Zissis C, Io B. Is clamping of chest tubes for air leak necessary? Eur Respir J 2013;42:202.

[39] Lois M, Noppen M. Bronchopleural fistulas: an overview of the problem with special focus on endoscopic management. Chest 2005;128:3955–3965.

[40] Silva IS, Flôr-de-Lima F, Rocha G, Alves I, Guimarães H. Pneumothorax in neonates: a level III neonatal intensive care unit experience. J Pediatr Neonatal Individualized Med 2016;5(2):e050220.

[41] Powers WF, Clemens JD. Prognostic implications of age at detection of air leak in very low birth weight infants requiring ventilatory support. J Pediatr 1993;123:611–617.

[42] Smith J, Schumacher RE, Donn SM, Sarkar S. Clinical course of symptomatic spontaneous pneumothorax in term and late preterm newborns: report from a large cohort. Am J Perinatol 2011;28(2):163–168.

[43] Yu VY, Wong PY, Bajuk B, Szymonowicz W. Pulmonary air leak in extremely low birthweight infants. Arch Dis Child 1986;61:239–241.

[44] Verma RP, Chandra S, Niwas R, Komaroff E. Risk factors and clinical outcomes of pulmonary interstitial emphysema in extremely low birth weight infants. J Perinatol 2006;26(3):197–200.

[45] Morley CJ, Davis PG, Doyle LW, Brion LP, Hascoet JM, Carlin JB. COIN Trial Investigators. Nasal CPAP or intubation at birth for very preterm infants. N Engl J Med 2008;358(7):700–708.

[46] Toledo Del Castillo B, Gordillo I, et al. Diffuse persistent pulmonary interstitial emphysema secondary to mechanical ventilation in bronchiolitis. BMC Pulm Med 2016;16(1):139.

[47] Stocker JT, Madewell JE. Persistent interstitial pulmonary emphysema: another complication of the respiratory distress syndrome. Pediatrics 1977;59(6):847–857.

[48] Sivit CJ. Diagnostic imaging. In: Martin RJ, Fanaroff AA, Walsh MC, editors. Neonatal-perinatal medicine. Philadelphia, PA: Elsevier/Mosby; 2006. p. 713–731.

[49] Goel S, Mondkar J, Panchal H, Hegde D, Utture A, Manerkar S. Nasal mask versus nasal prongs for delivering nasal continuous positive airway pressure in preterm infants with respiratory distress: a randomized controlled trial. Indian Pediatr 2015;52(12):1035–1040.

[50] Bermick JR, Donn SM. Thoracic air leaks. In: Donn SM, Sinha SK, editors, 4 edition. Manual of neonatal respiratory care. Springer; Switzerland; 2017. p. 665–672.

[51] Swingle HM, Eggert LD, Bucciarelli RL. New approach to management of unilateral tension pulmonary interstitial emphysema in premature infants. Pediatrics 1984;74:354–357.

[52] Keszler M, Donn SM, Bucciarelli RL, et al. Multicenter controlled trial comparing high-frequency jet ventilation and conventional mechanical ventilation in newborn infants with pulmonary interstitial emphysema. J Pediatr 1991;119:85–93.

[53] Clark RH, Null DM. High frequency oscillatory ventilation: clinical management strategies: critical care review current applications and economics. Available from: http://pages.carefusion.com/rs/565-YXD-236/images/RC_HFOV-Management-Strategies_WP_EN.pdf.

[54] Squires KA, De Paoli AG, Williams C, Dargaville PA. High frequency oscillatory ventilation with low oscillatory frequency in pulmonary interstitial emphysema. Neonatology 2013;104(4):243–249.

[55] Mohsini K, Reid D, Tanswell K. Resolution of acquired lobar emphysema with dexamethasone therapy. J Pediatr 1987;111:901–904.

[56] Fitzgerald D, Willis D, Usher R, Outerbridge E, Davis GM. Dexamethasone for pulmonary interstitial emphysema in preterm infants. Biol Neonate 1998;73(1):34–39.

[57] Mahapatra S, Scottoline B. Steroid-induced resolution of refractory pulmonary interstitial emphysema. J Matern Fetal Neonatal Med 2016;29(24):4092–4095.

[58] Meadow WL, Cheromcha D. Successful therapy of unilateral pulmonary emphysema: mechanical ventilation with extremely short inspiratory time. Am J Perinatol 1985;2:194–197.

[59] Nardo MD, Perrotta D, Stoppa F, Cecchetti C, Marano M, Pirozzi N. Independent lung ventilation in a newborn with asymmetric acute lung injury due to respiratory syncytial virus: a case report. J Med Case Rep 2008;2:212–216.

[60] Brooks JG, Bustamante SA, Koops BL, et al. Selective bronchial intubation for the treatment of severe localized pulmonary interstitial emphysema in newborn infants. J Pediatr 1977;91(4):648–652.

[61] Chalak LF, Kaiser JR, Arrington RW. Resolution of pulmonary interstitial emphysema following selective left main stem intubation in a premature newborn: an old procedure revisited. Paediatr Anaesth 2007;17(2):183–186.

[62] Verma RP, Chandra S, Niwas R, Komaroff E. Risk factors and clinical outcomes of pulmonary interstitial emphysema in extremely low birth weight infants. J Perinatol 2006;26(3):197–200.

[63] Hook B, Hack M, Morrison S, Borawski-Clark E, Newman NS, Fanaroff A. Pneumopericardium

in very low birth weight infants. J Perinatol 1995;15:27–31.

[64] Glenski JA, Hall RT. Neonatal pneumopericardium: analysis of ventilatory variables. Crit Care Med 1984;12:439–442.

[65] Mohamed IS, Lee YH, Yamout SZ, Fakir S, Reyonolds AM. Ultrasound guided percutaneous relief of tension pneumomediastinum in a 1-day-old newborn. Arch Dis Child Fetal Neonatal Ed 2007;92(6):F458.

[66] Bakal U, Aydin M, Orman A, Taskin E, Kazez A. A non-surgical condition of neonatal neumoperitoneum: retroperitoneal free air secondary to massive tension pneumothorax. J Med Cases 2016;7(1):13–14.

Chapter | **13C** |

Pulmonary Edema and Pulmonary Hemorrhage

Srinivas Murki, MD, DM, Sreeram Subramanian, MD, DM

CHAPTER POINTS

- Pulmonary Edema and Pulmonary Hemorrhage are rare but life threatening emergency in the newborn
- Timely diagnosis, systematic evaluation, use of optimal CPAP/PEEP during invasive and non invasive ventilation, general supportive care and management of underlying etiology are key to successful management

Pulmonary edema occurs due to accumulation of fluid in the interstitium and/or in the alveoli. The major mechanisms [1] involved are

1. Increase in transpulmonary pressure
2. Leakage of fluid due to increase in capillary permeability

Pulmonary edema occurs when the fluid transit into the lungs exceeds airway fluid clearance, which is a protective mechanism. Na,K-ATP channels play an important role in airway fluid clearance [2]. The development of these channels is gestation-dependent. Studies have shown that these channels are upregulated by antenatal corticosteroids.

Increase in transpulmonary pressures occurs in left atrial hypertension of any cause. Patent Ductus Arteriosus (PDA) with left to right shunt is a common condition in neonates responsible for pulmonary edema. Left Ventricular (LV) dysfunction due to asphyxia, sepsis, metabolic, or congenital conditions can result in pulmonary edema. Pulmonary edema due to increase in capillary permeability occurs in lung injury. Ventilator-induced lung injury, sepsis, asphyxia are the usual reasons. Combination of the above two processes albeit could be the common reason as is evident from the overlapping etiologies. Re-expansion pulmonary edema is a specific entity seen when lung expands after a prolonged period of collapse. The negative pressure generated during reexapansion of the lung is the probable mechanism [1].

Clinical features and diagnosis

Fluid in the interstitium or alveoli results in hypoxia. Respiratory distress, hypoxemia, pale skin are the usual manifestations. Intercoastal and subcoastal retractions are usually seen. Fine rales may be heard on auscultation of both lung fields. Hepatomegaly, gallop rhythm, and cardiac murmur are the clues for cardiac origin of pulmonary edema. Systemic examination of the neonate may provide clues for multiorgan involvement and generalized disease process (sepsis or asphyxia).

Chest X-ray: Cardiomegaly, diffuse fluffy infiltrates radiating from the hilum toward the periphery, hyperexpanded lung fields (interstitial pulmonary edema) are the signs of pulmonary edema on the chest X-ray. Cardiogenic causes will be identified on echocardiography.

Remedial measures

Diuretics, inotropic support, and supplemental oxygen may suffice in milder variants. Non-invasive and subsequently invasive ventilation support could be escalated for the management of moderate to severe pulmonary oedema. Neonates can be started on incremental PEEP titrating to retractions and saturations, keeping FiO_2 minimal. PEEP can be gradually increased from 5 to 8 cm. In case of noncardiogenic pulmonary edema (ARDS), PEEP can be increased gradually and cautiously to 10–12 cm optimizing lung expansion using chest X-ray and clinical monitoring of anteroposterior diameter of chest.

Pressure–volume (P–V) loop in pulmonary graphics may aid in determining optimum PEEP based on the lower inflection point. PEEP increments can be done till flat lower inspiratory portion of the P–V loop becomes vertical. The aim of ventilation is to minimize retractions, correct hypoxemia with optimal PEEP and lowest possible FiO_2.

Specific management must be tailored to the etiological process (e.g., PDA, sepsis, asphyxia, cardiac malformations) to prevent recurrence.

Pulmonary hemorrhage

Pulmonary hemorrhage can occur due to varied reasons. The origin can be cardiac or noncardiac. Cardiac causes include elevated left atrial pressures due to left ventricular dysfunction (asphyxia, sepsis), or volume overload (PDA), or valvular pathology (mitral stenosis—rare in neonates). Noncardiac causes include systemic disorders like sepsis, coagulation abnormalities, platelet dysfunction, or severe thrombocytopenia. Other factors, which may have independent association with pulmonary hemorrhage include intrauterine growth restriction, polycythemia, mechanical ventilation, and prematurity [3].

A well-recognized (albeit rare) scenario is pulmonary hemorrhage due to a rapid fall in pulmonary vascular resistance increasing the left to right shunt across PDA resulting in volume overload of the pulmonary capillaries following surfactant administration in preterm neonates. Cochrane review has shown an increased risk of pulmonary hemorrhage with protein-free synthetic surfactant especially when administered prophylactically [4]. Rescue surfactant therapy with natural surfactant is not associated with significant pulmonary hemorrhage.

Clinical features and diagnosis

Neonate on mechanical ventilation may have acute desaturation, increasing oxygen requirements, and poor chest rise. Endotracheal suction may reveal pink-colored hemorrhagic fluid (hematocrit of the fluid is less than the blood indicating admixture with edema fluid) [5]. Care must be taken to avoid deep suction of endotracheal tube as bleed from local trauma of the trachea can be misinterpreted as pulmonary hemorrhage. Tachycardia is usually noted. Bag and tube ventilation may reveal stiff lungs. In case of massive hemorrhage, neonate can become pale, apneic, and hypotensive.

Chest X-ray may show varied findings; many have bilateral fluffly opacities radiating from hilum toward peripheries. In severe cases, white out of the lungs can be seen.

Pulmonary graphics—loss of lung compliance in the PV loop.

Arterial blood gas may show hypoxia, hypercarbia, and mixed acidosis.

Remedial measures

Endotracheal suction is done to prevent clogging of endotracheal tube with blood clots. Increasing PEEP is an important strategy to reduce hemorrhage. Careful increments of PEEP (from 5 to 8 cm) aiming to reduce intercostal recessions, optimize lung volume on the chest X-ray, are useful in recruiting fluid-filled alveoli. This compresses the oozing capillaries, controlling or arresting the hemorrhage. PIP must be titrated to optimize chest rise. T_i can be prolonged to have good inflation time (0.4–0.5 s).

If conventional ventilation fails, high frequency ventilation can be employed as a tool to reduce pulmonary hemorrhage. MAP can be increased till adequate FRC is attained and oxygenation is maintained. High frequency ventilation can paradoxically increase the secretions, thereby increase the need for frequent suctioning and this can interfere with adequate and consistent delivery of MAP.

Surfactant paradoxically has been tried in severe pulmonary hemorrhage to restore the lost surfactant pool due to inactivation by blood with some benefit, but lack of well-designed trials preclude recommendation for routine use [6]. Endotracheal adrenaline (1:10000 dilution, 0.1 mL/kg) being a potent vasoconstrictor has been tried to decrease the bleed in small trials, but cannot be recommended as a standard of care. Similarly, endotracheal hemocoagulase—a purified enzyme extracted from South American Viper—has also been tried with some benefit, but cannot be recommended due to lack of robust evidence [7] (Algorithm 13C.1).

ALGORITHM 13C.1 MANAGEMENT OF PULMONARY HEMORRHAGE

Confirm pulmonary hemorrhage

    Blood in the endotracheal tube

    Increase in oxygen requirement, fall in PCV

    Suggestive CXR findings

Evaluate etiology

    PDA: Bounding pulses, wide pulse pressures, tachycardia, murmur, precordial activity, cardiomegaly

    Sepsis with coagulopathy: Off color, decreased activity, cold peripheries, temperature instability, GI bleeds, petechiae, sclerema

    IUGR: Sever IUGR—oligohydramnios, decreased fetal movements, doppler abnormalities, sudden onset, thrombocytopenia

    Asphyxia: Reduced fetal movements, poor Apgars, need for resuscitation at birth, seizures, encephalopathy, multiorgan dysfunction, coagulopathy

Steps of management

- Early ventilation (SIMV or assist control)

  - Increase PEEP in steps of 1 cm every 10–15 min to achieve fall in FiO_2 and keep delta P (PIP–PEEP) constant to obtain good chest rise or optimal tidal volume. Avoid frequent and deep suctioning (inline suctioning may be preferred)

- Supportive care

  - Correct hypothermia, hyperthermia, polycythemia, hypoglycemia and acidosis
  - Correct hypovolemia (normal saline or blood)
  - Correct shock or hypotension (inotropes or vasopressors)
  - Correct anemia (packed cells)

- Rescue HFO

  - HFO if the pressure required is high (PEEP >8 cm of Hg and PIP >24 cm of Hg). Increase MAP to achieve optimum oxygenation. Optimize humidification to deliver gases at 37°C and at 100% RH at the airway. Ensure endotracheal tube tip position at the correct place

- Adjuvant therapy

  - Surfactant if CXR suggestive of bilateral infiltrates and low volume lungs (high dose (200 mg/kg) may be needed as surfactant is deactivated by the blood in the alveoli)

- Endotracheal adrenaline: Rapid and repeated injections/instillations of 0.5 mL of epinephrine (1:10,000 dilution) may help in resolution of pulmonary hemorrhage
- Recombinant factor VIII: A dose of 80 µg/kg rFVIIa can normalize a prolonged prothrombin time. This drug has also been used with success in isolated cases of neonatal pulmonary hemorrhage at doses of 50 µg/kg/dose, repeated every 3 h for 2–3 days

- Specific therapies

  - PDA: Fluid restriction, Diuretics, Paracetamol, Ibuprofen, or Indomethacin as clinically indicated
  - Coagulopathy: Fresh frozen plasma or cryoprecipitate in aliquots of 15 mL/kg till PT and APTT normalizes
  - Thrombocytopenia: Platelet-rich plasma or single room platelets till platelets are greater than $50,000/mm^3$
  - Sepsis: Good supportive care and antibiotics to cover Gram-positive, Gram-negative, and fungal infections as appropriate
  - Asphyxia: Good supportive care

- Prevention

  - Antenatal steroids for all preterm deliveries
  - Gentle care in the delivery room. Avoid hyperoxia and hypoxia and also hypothermia and hyperthermia. Optimize transport to the NICU
  - Prevent PDA by appropriate fluid management and early treatment
  - Prefer natural surfactant over exogenous surfactant

References

[1] O'Brodovich H. Pulmonary edema in infants and children. Curr Opin Pediatr 2005;17(3):381–384.
[2] Verghese GM, Ware LB, Matthay BA, Matthay MA. Alveolar epithelial fluid transport and the resolution of clinically severe hydrostatic pulmonary edema. J Appl Physiol 1999;87: 1301–1312.
[3] Bendapudi P, Narasimhan R, Papworth S. Causes and management of pulmonary haemorrhage in the neonate. Paediatr Child Health 2012;22(12):528–531.
[4] Soll R, Ozek E. Prophylactic protein free synthetic surfactant for preventing morbidity and mortality in preterm infants. Cochrane Database Syst Rev 2010;1:CD001079.
[5] Zahr RA, Ashfaq A, Marron-Corwin M. Neonatal pulmonary hemorrhage. NeoReviews 2012;13(5):e302–e306.
[6] Aziz A, Ohlsson A. Surfactant for pulmonary hemorrhage in neonates. Cochrane Database Syst Rev 2008;2:CD005254.
[7] Shi Y, Zhao J, Tang S, et al. Effect of hemocoagulase for prevention of pulmonary hemorrhage in critical newborns on mechanical ventilation: a randomized controlled trial. Indian Pediatr 2008;45(3):199–202.

Chapter | **13D**

Neonatal Necrotizing Tracheobronchitis

Arun Nair, MD, FRCPCH, FRACP, P.K. Rajiv, DCH, MD, Aiman Rahmani, FAAP

CHAPTER POINTS

- This is a rare clinical entity in ventilator management
- The aetiology is possibly linked to inadequate humidification and hence imminently preventable
- High index of suspicion when encountering acute hypercarbia and hypoxemia especially on HFOV
- Judicious step by step increment in PEEP /MAP and Tidal volume to effect improvement in saturations

Necrotizing tracheobronchitis (NTB) is an inflammatory lesion of the upper airway seen in mechanically ventilated neonates. In its severe form, it causes necrosis and sloughing of the epithelium in the trachea and main stem bronchi with resultant acute obstruction of the airway. Neonates with NTB present a diverse clinical spectrum from asymptomatic disease to severe airway obstruction.

The term necrotizing tracheobronchitis was coined by Metlay et al. from Strong Memorial Hospital in Rochester and MacPherson and coworkers from Maggie Women's Hospital in Pittsburgh, USA in 1983. They jointly published a study of a series of cases, which had undergone assisted ventilator therapy and died of obstructive ventilator events; the autopsy findings of these babies' trachea were filled with friable red black debris [1]. There was no evidence of any viral, fungal, or bacterial infection. They found no such findings in babies who were still born or who were ventilated for less than 3 h. They therefore concluded that NTB is related to assisted ventilation and length of survival. In addition to trachea they found similar changes in both left and right main stem bronchi prompting them to rule out the mechanical injury of intubation to be a cause for these findings.

Several case reports were subsequently published in the 80s and with decreasing frequency in the 90s and beyond outlining the clinical and bronchoscopy findings [2–9]. With increasing survival of high-risk infants especially small preterm babies and the advent of high frequency ventilation especially jet ventilation, people started seeing and reporting increasing number of this rather rare disease process. Many authors have reported the role of high-frequency jet-ventilation (HJV) as the main modality to cause this lesion, but it has been reported in babies on other modes of ventilation including conventional ventilation [10–12]. It has now become clear that this is definitely an iatrogenic disease process seen in ventilated newborn babies, mostly in those born prematurely.

Pathogenesis

The pathogenesis is not well understood, many factors may be involved like mode and duration of ventilation, high pressure to which the airways are exposed during ventilation, ischemic injury in hemodynamic unstable babies, and so on [5,6]. The role of humidification or rather lack of it has been consistently shown in studies in human beings and in animal experiments specially using high frequency ventilation [13–16].

Clinical diagnosis

NTB should be suspected in the mechanically ventilated newborn with an acute onset of hypercarbia and respiratory acidosis, decreased chest excursions without obvious deterioration of the pulmonary parenchymal disease on chest X-ray when other causes like accidental displacement of ET tube, pneumothorax, or obstruction of the ET tube is ruled out. It is important to be aware of the possibility of NTB as one of the causes for increasing $PaCO_2$ in a baby well established on ventilator so that early intervention can be instituted to prevent it from escalating into a severe form (Fig.13D.1).

Investigations

Bronchoscopy is the main investigative tool. The typical appearance on bronchoscopy would show the necrotic plug and exfoliatiation of the tracheal mucosa as depicted in Fig. 13D.2.

On microscopy this debris would consist of thick homogenous basophilic material lined on the luminal aspect of the necrotic epithelium. The material has the appearance of detached necrotic mucosa admixed with mucous. The remaining mucosal tissue would usually be fibrotic with regenerating glands and minimal inflammation.

CT scan of the chest to look at the airways may be required in long standing cases to outline the degree of narrowing of the airways.

Prevention

Being an iatrogenic disease entity with high mortality and morbidity, every effort should be made to prevent it. Use of gentle ventilation, adequate humidification (with inspired gases at temperatures 37–37.5°C), and careful attention toward monitoring of blood gases have essentially seen a reduction in the frequency of occurrence as well as reporting of NTB in the last 2 decades. One other factor that may have played a role in decreasing rates of this dreaded

disease process is the increasing use of noninvasive modalities of respiratory support in smaller and smaller babies in recent times.

Treatment

In those babies where the NTB has just been diagnosed, there are very few treatment options. Ventilatory flow tracing, if available on the ventilator, it could help in picking up early signs of obstruction. Typically, the tracing would indicate air trapping, expiratory waveforms do not return to base line with no zero-flow state at the end of expiration (Fig. 13D.3).

The following adjustments may help to mitigate the following situations [17]:
1. Decrease the rate
2. Increase the expiratory time
3. Decrease the flow
4. Consider increasing the PEEP

As pointed out, the disease is a direct consequence of an artificial invasive respiratory care; one could try to reduce the ventilator settings if possible and aim to extubate under cover of steroids, if there are no contra indications. Try decreasing the ventilator setting while maintaining and titrating adequate PEEP on conventional ventilation or by increasing the MAP on HFV in steps about a cmH_2O to gain reductions in $PaCO_2$.

In those where the disease process is well established, two types of treatment are described: repeated bronchoscopies with membrane extraction [2,3] and extracorporeal membrane oxygenation [18,19]. In long standing cases with narrowing of the airways with stenosis following healing, there is no other option but for surgical attempts to increase the caliber of the airways.

Prognosis

There is a high mortality rate approaching 45%–100% [6]. Those who survive tend to have high morbidity related to stenosis of the upper airways. Long-term prognosis in those babies who survive will depend on the degree of airway narrowing and other comorbidities that go with the surviving high-risk newborn infant. In view of the rarity of the disease process, there is very little long-term data available to predict a population-based outcome.

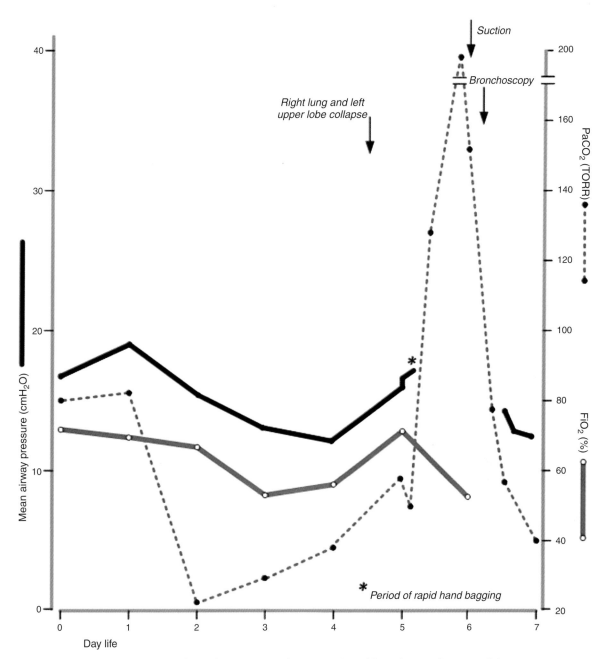

Fig. 13D.1 The Typical Sequence of Ventilatory Events That Occurs in Babies Who Develop Necrotizing Tracheobronchitis (NTB). Adapted from Kirpalani H, Higa T, Perlman M, Friedberg J, Cutz E. Diagnosis and therapy of necrotizing tracheobronchitis in ventilated neonates. Crit Care Med 1985;13:792–797 [2].

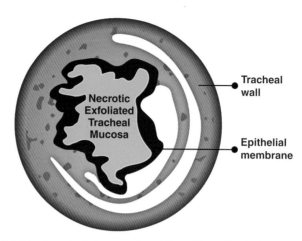

Fig. 13D.2 Cross section of distal trachea, just above carina. Adapted from Kirpalani H, Higa T, Perlman M, Friedberg J, Cutz E. Diagnosis and therapy of necrotizing tracheobronchitis in ventilated neonates. Crit Care Med 1985; 13:792-797 [2].

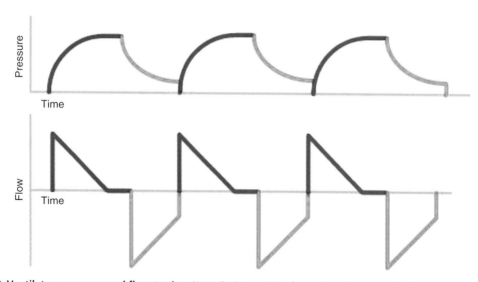

Fig. 13D.3 Ventilatory pressure and flow tracing. Note: Expiratory Waveforms do not return to baseline

References

[1] Metlay LA, MacPherson TA, Doshi N, et al. A new iatrogenic lesion in newborn requiring assisted ventilation (letter) N. Engl J Med 1983;309: 111–112.

[2] Kirpalani H, Higa T, Perlman M, Friedberg J, Cutz E. Diagnosis and therapy of necrotizing

tracheobronchitis in ventilated neonates. Crit Care Med 1985;13:792–797.

[3] Wilson KS, Carley RB, Mammel MC, Ophoven JP, et al. Necrotizing tracheobronchitis: a newly recognized cause of acute obstruction in mechanically ventilated neonates. Laryngoscope 1987;97:1017–1019.

[4] Pietsch JB, Nagaraj HS, Groff DB, Yacoub UA, Roberts JL. Necrotizing tracheobronchitis: a new indication for emergency bronchoscopy in the neonate. J Pediatr Surg 1988;23:798–801.

[5] Metlay LA, McPherson TA, Doshi N, Milley JR. Necrotizing tracheobronchitis in intubated

newborns: a complication of assisted ventilation. Pediatr Pathol 1987;7:575–584.

[6] Gaugler C, Astruc D, Donato L, Rivera S, Langlet C, Messer J. Neonatal necrotizing tracheobronchitis: three case reports. J Perinatol 2004;24:259–260.

[7] Bua J, Grasso D, Schleef J, Zennaro F, et al. Neonatal necrotizing tracheobronchitis. J Pediatr 2011;159:699.

[8] Mimouni F, Ballard Jl, Ballard ET, et al. Necrotising tracheobronchitis: case report. Pediatrics 1986;77:366–368.

[9] Pietsch JB, Nagarag HS, Groff DB, et al. Necrotizing tracheobronchitis: a new indication for emergency bronchoscopy in the neonate. J Pediatr Surg 1985;20:391–393.

[10] Ophoven JP, Mammel MC, Gordon MJ, et al. Histopathology associated with high-frequency jet ventilation. Crit Care Med 1984;12:829–832.

[11] Harris TR, Gouch WIII, Wilson JF, et al. Necrotizing tracheobronchitis associated with high-frequency jet ventilation. Clin Res 1984;32:132A.

[12] Fuksman R, Prudent L, Larguia M, et al. Necrotising tracheobronchitis (NTB) following conventional mechanical ventilation in newborn infants. Pediatr Res 1984;20:429.

[13] Circeo LF, Heard SO, Griffiths E, Nash G. Overwhelming necrotizing tracheobronchitis due to inadequate humidification during high-frequency jet ventilation. Chest 1991;100:268–269.

[14] Dalhamn T. Mucous flow and ciliary activity in the trachea of healthy rats and rats exposed to irritant gases. Acta Physiol Scand 1956;36(Suppl. 123):1.

[15] Chalon J, Loew D, Malbranche J. Effects of dry anaesthetic gases on tracheobronchial ciliated epithelium. Anaesthesiology 1972;37:338.

[16] Ophoven JP, Mammel MC, Gordon MJ, et al. Tracheobronchial histopathology associated with high frequency jet ventilation. Crit Care Med 1984;12:829.

[17] Donn SM. University of Michigan Health System. Available from: www.michiganrc.org/docs/Neonatal_Pulmonary_Graphics_-_S._Donn.pdf.

[18] Michael EJ, Zwillenberg D, Furnari A, et al. Treatment of neonatal necrotizing tracheobronchitis with extracorporeal membrane oxygenation and bronchoscopy. J Pediatr Surg 1988;23:798–801. 1984.

[19] Nicklaus PJ. Airway complications of jet ventilation in neonates. Ann Oto Rhinol Laryngol 1995;104:24–30.

Section | IV |

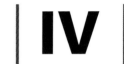

Bedside Application Principles of Assisted Ventilation Devices

Chapter | **14** |

Various Modes of Mechanical Ventilation

Gianluca Lista, PhD, Ilia Bresesti, MD

CHAPTER POINTS

- Mechanical ventilation can damage the lung by several mechanisms – volutrauma, barotrauma, atelectotrauma, biotrauma (inflammation) and rheotrauma (induced by flow) resulting in ventilator-induced lung injury (VILI).
- Conventional ventilation is characterized by factors dictating the initiation of breath (trigger – flow or pressure), control of gas flow during respiratory support (limit or control – pressure or volume) and termination of respiratory support (cycle – time or flow).
- Uncontrolled delivery of volume is the main determinant of VILI. Volume-targeted ventilation with synchronization reduces mortality and risk of BPD compared to non-synchronized pressure-limited ventilation.
- The types of patient triggered ventilation include synchronized intermittent mandatory ventilation (SIMV – often with pressure support), assist control, and pressure support ventilation (flow-cycled).

Introduction

The last decades have seen significant improvements in the care of premature infants. In particular, the introduction of new ventilation techniques, the use of antenatal steroids, and the administration of surfactant have led to a decrease in early mortality and to a reduction in long-term sequelae [1].

However, nowadays one of the most relevant causes of mortality in preterm infants remains respiratory failure.

Respiratory distress syndrome (RDS) affects a great proportion of these premature neonates and it is a multifactorial disease, mainly caused by the lack of surfactant production and the inefficiency of breathing effort at birth and in the following hours. However, while surfactant can now be replaced and administered in its exogenous form, respiratory work has to be supported by ventilators.

The introduction of mechanical ventilation (MV) in the neonatal field dates back to the early 1970s, when assistance started to be provided at an early stage of the disease, and no longer as a desperate final attempt to avoid death, using devices that were specifically designed according to infants' needs.

Initially, mortality and air leak were quite common, but over time, techniques of invasive ventilation have evolved. Although these new approaches have consistently improved neonatal survival and have led to the development of new techniques, bronchopulmonary dysplasia (BPD) is still a serious consequence following MV. This is the reason why great commitment has been devoted to the search for alternative, less invasive ventilation techniques, which would be able to provide the gentlest and most effective respiratory support. There is, in fact, wide consensus among neonatologists about the reduced lung damage using less invasive respiratory assistance compared to MV.

There are several types of damage that can occur in the lung during ventilation, and they are named according to the cause leading to them. These are (Fig. 14.1) as follows:

- volutrauma, which is caused by overdistension and excessive stretch of tissues
- barotrauma, when excessive pressure is delivered to the lung parenchyma
- atelectotrauma, when tidal ventilation is given in presence of atelectasis

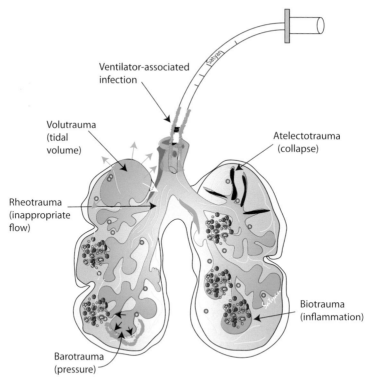

Fig. 14.1 Contributors to Ventilation-Induced Lung Injury (VILI)—Volutrauma, Barotrauma, Rheotrauma, Atelectotrauma, Biotrauma, and Ventilator-Associated Infections Play a Role in the Pathogenesis of VILI. Copyright: Satyan Lakshminrusimha.

- biotrauma, when MV of any form triggers a cascade of inflammatory mediators and cells causing biochemical and biophysical injury
- rheotrauma, when inappropriate flow is delivered, either excessive or inadequate

All of these injuries are covered by the definition of "ventilator-induced lung injury" (VILI).

Hence, nowadays the main goal for the neonatologist is to minimize VILI by reducing the duration of ventilation and optimizing the use of ventilators.

Conventional mechanical ventilation

Even if the proportion of neonates undergoing MV has reduced significantly in recent years due to the increased use of noninvasive respiratory support techniques, there are specific clinical situations that require the use of this form of support.

When the clinician has established that a patient requires MV, several decisions need to be made.

Great attention must be paid in choosing the method to provide respiratory support. In fact, criteria include the gestational age of the baby, the underlying lung condition, and the need to minimize VILI and other organ damage (e.g., avoiding hyperoxia in babies at risk of retinopathy of prematurity).

Currently, thanks to progresses in biomedical engineering, there is a wide range of devices available, which are applicable to a large variety of clinical scenarios. These improvements, however, have given birth to a whole host of definitions and modes that may be confusing for the neonatologist.

Given the wide variety of techniques available, guidelines for ventilating babies are not necessarily absolute indications and are likely to vary between NICUs [2].

Basic principles of ventilation modes

The rationale through which the ventilator supports the baby's breathing is characterized by three key points:
1. The way the support of each breath begins (trigger)
2. The way the gas flow during breathing is controlled (limit or control)
3. The way the breathing support finishes (cycle)

1. In the so-called "conventional ventilation", inflations are delivered regardless of the synchronism with the infant's breath. The neonatologist sets frequency and ventilation parameters (pressure and time) in order to obtain the optimal minute ventilation.

   Alternatively, when mechanical inflations are delivered in synchrony with the patient's respiratory effort, we refer to "synchronized mechanical ventilation." In this modality, the ventilation frequency control is subject to the synchronized MV technique in use and to the trigger that the neonatologist has set.

2. The main gas flow delivery mechanism during each breath is alternatively the pressure and/or the volume (tidal volume [V_t]).

3. The end of the respiratory support occurs at predetermined time (time-cycle) or depending on the flow rate decrease (flow-cycle).

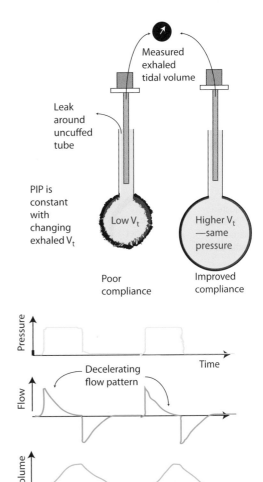

Pressure control ventilation (Fig. 14.2)

Pressure limiting ventilation was the gold standard in neo-natal ventilation for years, since volume control ventilation in extremely premature infants was difficult to use. This type of respiratory support continues to be widely used because of its relative simplicity, the possibility to effectively ventilate the baby despite large leaks from the endotracheal tube (ETT), and for the improvement of intrapulmonary gas exchange due to the decelerating gas flow and the direct control of peak inspiratory pressure (PIP). The limit of this technique is the lack of control on volumes due to rapid changes in lung compliance.

Volume-targeted ventilation (Fig. 14.3)

Volume targeted ventilation (VTV) is a form of MV where the primary target variable is the tidal volume. In order to reach this set volume, fluctuation of pressure is permitted. However, the pressure control acts if delivered pressure exceeds a safety limit, that is, usually set at around 40 cmH$_2$O.

This type of ventilation is usually combined with:
- Intermittent mandatory ventilation (IMV)
- Synchronized intermittent mandatory ventilation (SIMV) (alone or plus pressure support [PS])
- Assist control (AC) or synchronized intermittent positive pressure ventilation (SIPPV)
- Pressure support ventilation (PSV)

During VTV, the continuous inspiratory flow produces the typical ramping of pressure, with peak pressure and volume delivery occurring at the *end* of inspiration. This is a relevant difference in respect to pressure target ventilation, where they occur *early* in inspiration.

Fig. 14.2 Pressure Control Ventilation with Decelerating Flow Pattern. PIP is attained early resulting in better intrapulmonary gas exchange in conditions associated with poor compliance. However, if compliance rapidly changes, tidal volume also changes resulting in hypo- or hypercapnia. Copyright: Satyan Lakshminrusimha.

One of the main concerns regarding VTV is related to loss of delivered volume from leaks. This is particularly evident in very small infants, and with the use of uncuffed ETTs.

VTV is, at least theoretically, the optimal technique to treat heterogeneous lung disease, since it provides slower inflations which lead to a better gas flow uniformity. Its clinical indications include RDS, ventilator-dependent heart disease and BPD, but it is applicable to virtually all lung diseases.

In this mode of ventilation, the volume control is based on the volume released by the ventilator, and not on the

Synchronization of ventilation

Synchronization of the ventilator with the infant's breaths, limiting the use of deep sedation and muscle relaxants, has been shown to be useful in avoiding frequent desaturations; delivery of excessive air pressure in the airways; and in reducing ventilation duration, cerebral hemorrhage, and pneumothorax [5]. However, a deep understanding of the interaction between the patient's effort and the ventilator's inflation is needed in order to avoid a suboptimal ventilation. In fact, the V_t entering the lung is determined by the combination of the patient's inspiratory effort (negative intrapleural pressure) and the positive pressure generated by the ventilator, which together form the transpulmonary pressure.

When used with extremely preterm infants, however, this mode of ventilation has to face the difficulty in synchronizing all breaths, including those producing minimal signals.

The detection sensitivity (the so-called "trigger") must be very high and it must have a rapid response time (less than 50 ms) to follow the short inspiratory time and high respiratory rates typical of preterm infants. In addition, the variability of flow loss due to the use of noncuffed ETT further complicates the synchronization.

The first technique for synchronization used a change in the pressure in the ventilator circuit, which depends on the baby making a sufficiently large inspiration to modify the circuit pressure (~0.5 cmH$_2$O). However, it is inaccurate if the baby is very small or has a low inspiratory effort.

Another option is a capsule (Graseby capsule) stuck on the abdomen to detect abdominal movements. This technique may be unreliable and the effectiveness and accuracy depends on where the capsule is placed on the abdomen.

Presently, in the majority of the devices in use, triggering is made through a hot wire flow sensor placed between the wye piece of the ventilator circuit and the ETT.

Two tungsten wires heated to $400\,^\circ$C detect the gas flow through the cooling effect of the gas. It detects inspiratory gas flow, and when this has reached about 0.2 L/min, around 30 ms after the beginning of inspiratory flow, an inflation is started. The delay time depends on the set trigger sensitivity on a scale ranging from 1 to 10 (1 is the most sensitive). This sensitivity should always be set to 1 so that the inflation occurs as close as possible to the onset of the baby's inspiration. A higher number will mean a longer delay between the onset of inspiration and the start of inflation, resulting in a nonsynchronous inflation.

Some clinicians are concerned that adding a flow sensor increases the dead space and thereby increases the infant's PaCO$_2$. For this reason, for very preterm babies <1 kg, the V_{te} can be slightly increased to 5–6 mL/kg.

Increased dead space is rarely a significant problem because, as uncuffed ETTs are used, there are almost always leaks around the tube. Even in the case of no leaks, the

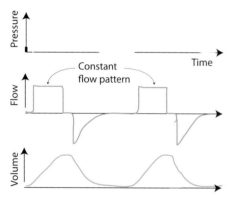

Fig. 14.3 Volume Control Ventilation with a Constant Flow Pattern. Intraalveolar pressure slowly builds up attaining peak pressures toward the end of inspiration. This mode maintains constant volume in spite of changing compliance (as after surfactant therapy or surgery). Copyright: Satyan Lakshminrusimha.

volume actually delivered to the patient, which is probably the main limitation of this technique.

The most widely studied VTV application in newborns is volume guarantee (VG) ventilation.

It has been shown that volume targeting and synchronization reduces mortality and the risk of BPD compared with nonsynchronized and pressure-limited modalities [3].

Although there is strong evidence that the main determinant for VILI development is uncontrolled delivery of volume, only about 50% of large neonatal units use this technique [4].

effect on $PaCO_2$ is small and not of clinical significance compared with the clinical gain from using the sensor.

There may be autotriggering problems when

1. The leakage around the ETT is detected by the sensor but misinterpreted, and so this outflow can wrongly start the cycle.

2. The sensor detects gas flow from condensed water bubbling in the ventilator circuit and this triggers an inflation—even though the baby may not be inspiring at this time, the humidity in the circuit activates the trigger, causing an excessive increase in the ventilation frequency. Some people reduce the sensitivity to prevent this; however, this causes an unacceptable delay between the onset of inspiration and the inflation. This can be avoided by ensuring the ventilator circuit is free of condensed water.

Recently, a new form synchronization has been introduced, called neurally adjusted ventilatory assist (NAVA).

Although it is contraindicated in specific clinical conditions (e.g., esophageal malformations, coagulation disorders, apnea), NAVA has been shown to be a promising approach in preterm and term infants.

Using electrodes on a specially designed nasogastric tube, it detects and analyzes the diaphragmatic EMG and uses this signal to trigger ventilator inflations in proportion and in synchrony with the phasic inspiratory diaphragmatic electrical activity. Backup pressure control is provided when there is no diaphragm signal.

To date, there is no consensus about which modality of synchronization is optimal.

Principal ventilation techniques

Synchronized intermittent mandatory ventilation

The SIMV is a form of patient-triggered ventilation (PTV) characterized by a predetermined number of inflations (= backup rates) which are synchronized with the onset of spontaneous infant breath or delivered automatically if the patient effort is inadequate or absent. In SIMV, spontaneous breaths exceeding the predetermined number are not assisted and supported by the baseline pressure (PEEP).

This means that the smallest infants ventilated through extremely small caliber ETTs are subjected, especially during the weaning phase, to an excessive work of breathing (WOB) with an ineffective minute ventilation. In fact, this occurs when the fixed rate is decreased to favor spontaneous breathing and what was previously considered a "pre-extubation training" is now judged a useless respiratory effort.

The high airway resistance, which includes narrow ETTs, limited strength of the respiratory muscles and a compliant chest wall, results in an ineffective tidal ventilation.

Moreover, since the device's dead space is fixed, in the case of shallow and/or ineffective breaths, a rebreathing of the anatomical dead space gas occurs, affecting the alveolar minute ventilation.

Weaning is probably the best application of SIMV, although some clinicians prefer to use it as an alternative mode to AC.

SIMV can be combined with PS. In that case, the ventilator delivers a set number of mandatory ventilations per minute. Between those mandatory inflations, the infant can take spontaneous breaths and the ventilator will provide PS (e.g., 2–3 cmH_2O) above PEEP values, reducing the WOB.

Assist control (SIPPV)

This technique is another form of PTV. It supports any respiratory effort, either initiated by the patient ("assist") or by the ventilator ("control"), capable of overcoming the trigger threshold set by the clinician.

Compared to SIMV, it reduces WOB and it is the most useful mode in acute phase. For this reason, it is a good ventilator strategy for virtually all patients. However, this technique requires a "dynamic" setting. In fact, during the different phases of RDS lung compliance changes and shallow breathing affects the respiratory rate. Therefore, a careful management of the parameters is needed.

Usually, a backup rate is set to provide a minimum rate in case of apnea. It is usually slightly below the spontaneous rate (30–40 inflations/min).

The V_t should range from 4 to 6 mL/kg, according to the RDS phase (acute/weaning), and pressure parameters should be set with this aim.

The goal is to synchronize the baby's breathing effort with the ventilator as much as possible, thus requiring lower ventilation pressures.

During the weaning phase, the inspiratory peak is gradually lower and the ventilation frequency is not initially changed. In this way, reducing the support provided to each breath, the infant gradually increase the WOB as a compensation for the reduced volume provided by the ventilator.

Especially in very preterm baby, particular attention should be paid to the risk of hypocapnia.

Pressure support ventilation (Fig. 14.4)

PSV is a pressure-controlled mode that partially or fully supports every infant's breath, like AC, but it is flow cycled. This means that in PSV the support is terminated when inspiratory flow decreases its velocity as a consequence of progressive lung filling. This flow cycle ends when a threshold (usually ranging from 5% to 20% of the flow peak)

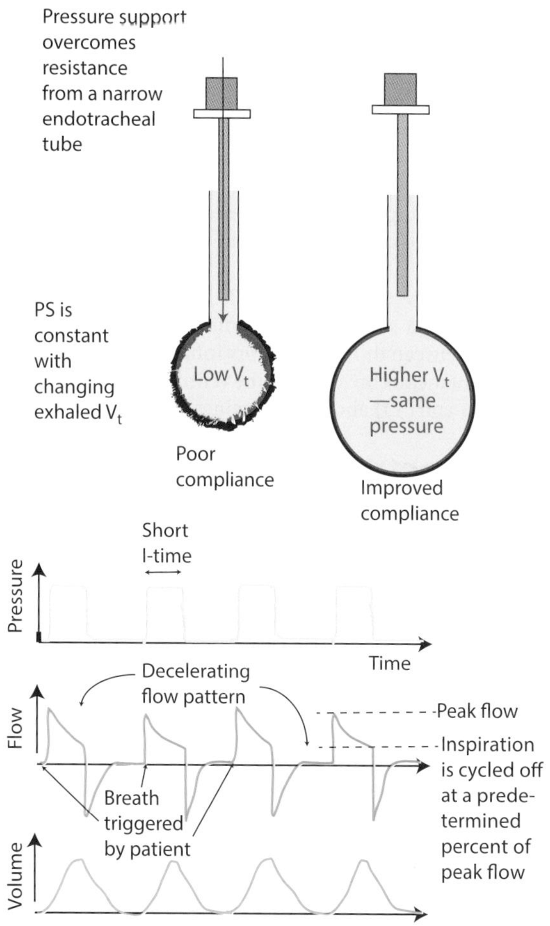

Pressure support
overcomes
resistance
from a narrow
endotracheal
tube

PS is
constant
with
changing
exhaled V_t

Low V_t

Higher V_t
—same
pressure

Poor
compliance

Improved
compliance

Short
I-time

Decelerating
flow pattern

Peak flow

Inspiration
is cycled off
at a prede-
termined
percent of
peak flow

Breath
triggered
by patient

Fig. 14.4 Pressure Support (PS) Ventilation Helps Overcome Airway (Including Endotracheal Tube) Resistance. The breath is triggered by the patient. Inspiration is terminated (cycled off) when the flow reaches a prespecified % of peak flow (usually 5%–20%). Copyright: Satyan Lakshminrusimha.

is reached. This technique eliminates the PS for prolonged inspiration times and theoretically provides greater adherence to the ventilation synchronization. Further advantages may involve the reduction of intrathoracic and intracranial pressure fluctuations.

This technique can be used alone with a backup frequency or, in some ventilators, alternating with the SIMV. This "hybrid" mode tends to better support the spontaneous respiratory effort of the patient.

To date, despite the wide use of SIMV and AC, there is no evidence of superiority of one technique compared to the other with regard to outcomes such as air-leak syndrome, BPD, or shortened ventilation duration. Several pilot studies

highlighted a slight variation in the tidal volume, a lower incidence of tachypnea, a slight fluctuation in the blood pressure and quicker weaning using AC compared to SIMV.

High-frequency ventilation

Despite the availability of the most sophisticated devices to deliver conventional MV, in addition to surfactant replacement therapy and other pharmacological treatments, there are still some neonates who cannot be adequately ventilated. Moreover, atelectotrauma, barotrauma, and volutrauma are still concerns that neonatologists have to face when using conventional MV.

High-frequency ventilation was first described by Lunkenheimer in the early seventies, and during the 1980s, this method of ventilation was introduced in neonatal clinical practice.

High-frequency ventilation has been extensively studied in preterm infants, while in full-term babies this ventilation modality needs to be further investigated, even if it has been shown to be useful to treat severe conditions such as persistent pulmonary hypertension of the newborn and aspiration syndromes.

It includes high-frequency oscillatory ventilation (HFOV), high-frequency jet ventilation (HFJV), and high-frequency percussive ventilation (HFPV) (also known as high-frequency flow interruption [HFFI]).

High-frequency ventilation consists of generating low tidal volume, providing a mean airway pressure (MAP) around which the pressure oscillates at very high rate.

The rate ranges from 5 to 50 Hz, but the most commonly used parameters in clinical practice are 6–15 Hz.

The efficacy of HFV is primarily due to improvement in pulmonary gas exchange, and it is believed to be a result of the reduced pressure and volume swings transmitted to the periphery of the lung.

The main advantage of HFOV is to potentially be lung protective. While atelectotrauma is not significantly lessened, barotrauma and volutrauma can be reduced since HFOV uses lower transpulmonary pressure and smaller tidal volumes than any other modality of assisted ventilation. However, even if lung damage prevention is the primary goal of HFOV, it is applied mostly when pulmonary injury has already occurred.

To be fully effective, HFOV should be delivered to an entirely recruited lung, and this is the reason why the "optimal lung volume strategy" is routine with this technique.

With respect to mortality and neurodevelopmental outcomes, in contrast to what had been demonstrated in initial studies, prophylactic HFOV for preterm infants is now known not to be superior to conventional ventilation, although BPD prevalence was inferior, since air leak with HFOV was most common [6].

There is no consensus on the use of HFOV instead of MV for RDS. However, there are specific clinical conditions which seem to particularly benefit from this technique (e.g., congenital diaphragmatic hernia [CDH], pulmonary interstitial emphysema [PIE], pulmonary hypoplasia, PPHN, meconium aspiration syndrome [MAS], cardiac surgery patients).

HFJV is a variant of HFOV that delivers highly accelerated inspirations (0.020 s) at similar or slightly lower frequencies. In the past, this technique was suspected to cause trachea injury (the so-called "rheotrauma," in which the shear forces of high gas flow rates provoke damage to the airway), but recent randomized controlled trials found no evidence for such concern.

Bhuta and colleagues [7] showed that HFJV used as an alternative to conventional ventilation slightly reduced the risk of BPD but significantly increased the risk of acute brain injury. Moreover, as a rescue therapy, HFJV did not change the risk of BPD or mortality [8]. HFJV is mostly reserved for infants with severe cystic lung disease or evolving BPD.

Recently, some ventilators can combine HFOV with VG. There is still a lack of evidence about its application in clinical practice. Further discussion on high frequency ventilation is provided in chapters - High Frequency Ventilation Basics, High Frequency Oscillatory Ventilation (HFOV): Management Strategy, Management of HFJV.

Importance of the "open lung strategy" (Fig. 14.5)

There is convincing evidence that high tidal volumes are more damaging than pressure by itself, and for this reason neonatologists' focus has shifted to providing a more protective ventilation for the lung. As early as late-1980s, Dreyfuss and colleagues highlighted the role of large tidal volume in occurrence of lung damage regardless of whether that volume was generated by positive or negative pressure [9].

Subsequent experiments emphasized the concept that tidal volume should be distributed evenly throughout the lung to provide a lung-protective ventilation. However, the relevance of achieving and maintaining uniform lung aeration to reduce VILI has been underestimated for years.

In fact, if there are large areas of atelectasis, the tidal volume aerates predominantly already open alveoli and, as a consequence, causes their overdistension with subsequent volu/biotrauma. In the meantime, overdistension provokes the mechanical entrapment of the atelectasic areas, which are going to be even less aerated. Moreover, atelectasis causes exudation in the alveoli of a liquid enriched in proteins that inactivate surfactant and induce the releasing of inflammatory mediators. In addition, between overstretched and atelectasic areas, so-called strain and stress forces are generated and this process enormously increases the pulmonary damage, with a significant increase of transpulmonary pressures and interstitial edema.

Hence, to reduce VILI in ventilated premature infants, we should, at least theoretically, aim to ventilate a recruited or "open lung" with an adequate V_t [10].

The target is to set the lung volume on the deflation limb of the pressure/volume (P/V) curve and above the lower inflection point.

In clinical practice, it means using appropriate PEEP values that prevent recruited alveoli from closing [11]. Thus, PEEP is not just the critical point above which the lung gets open, but also that at which the lung does not get closed.

It was believed for years that high PEEP values were responsible for inadequate venous return and hypercapnia. This "PEEP phobia" probably found its origin in animal experimental studies, which were conducted on normal and then compliant lungs, which substantially differ from premature pulmonary parenchyma.

If applied with adequate PEEP values, the open lung strategy allows homogeneous distribution of tidal volume, and this may be assumed from the results obtained with HFOV recruitment strategies.

It is important, however, to emphasize that there is no one PEEP threshold value which is protective and sufficient to ensure a homogeneous distribution of ventilation. The optimal PEEP should be reached in every patient through alveolar recruitment procedures that nowadays seem to be possible also in conventional MV [12]. The RDS stage, the compliance, as well as the phase of the disease (acute/chronic/weaning) are all criteria which must be considered.

It is indeed clear that a PEEP value of 6 cmH$_2$O in a normal lung can create overdistension, but in a less compliant lung can be insufficient. Since in very premature infants the lung has characteristics which are far from physiology, using PEEP below 5 cmH$_2$O should be the exception to the rule. If PEEP requirement exceeds 8 cmH$_2$O, then other ventilation strategies (e.g., HFOV) or intervention (e.g., surfactant) should be considered. In addition, the neonatologist must keep in mind that RDS is a "dynamic" disease, and for this reason, ventilation parameters must be adapted according to clinical conditions, radiology and, if available, ventilation graphs that may help identifying lung compliance changes in real time.

Clinical tips

As is evident from prior discussion, it is quite difficult to provide guidelines for when and how to initiate MV which is suitable for any clinical situation.

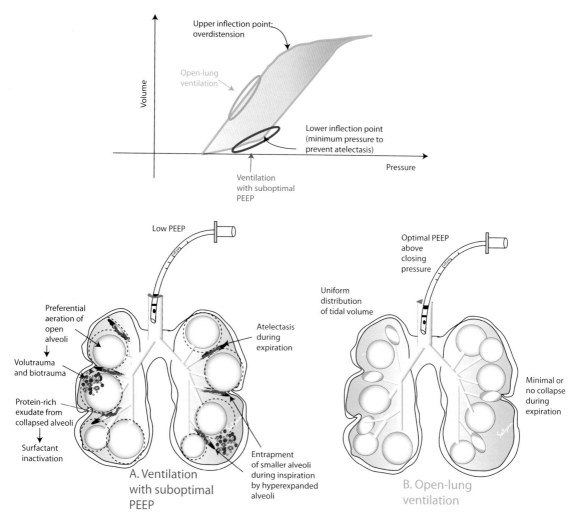

Fig. 14.5 Open-Concept Ventilation. (A) Heterogeneous lung disease with areas of overdistension and atelectasis inducing volutrauma, atelectotrauma, and biotrauma. (B) Open-lung ventilation where PEEP is higher than the lower inflection point. Copyright: Satyan Lakshminrusimha.

Given the wide variety of clinical conditions, types of ventilators, and modes of ventilation, standard recommendations are of limited utility.

First of all, assessment of the baby must be done immediately at NICU entry. In infants with respiratory distress, we suggest starting with:

- clinical evaluation of WOB and respiratory mechanics (e.g., Silvermann score)
- performance of chest X-ray to evaluate lung conditions and make diagnosis
- blood gases for staging the severity of the disease
- echocardiography to detect cardiovascular impairment and/or underlying congenital heart diseases

- considering prenatal history (e.g., prematurity, IUGR, twin pregnancies complicated by twin-to-twin transfusion syndrome, and so on)

Respiratory distress is mainly caused by prematurity and then by surfactant deficiency. The best ventilation management starts in the delivery room, with the optimization of lung volume with recruitment maneuvers (sustained inflations and/or adjustments of CPAP level).

In mechanically ventilated infants, we usually start with AC + VG and we set the following initial parameters:

1. RR 40–60 bpm
2. IT 0.25–0.40 s
3. V_t 5–7 mL/kg

4. PEEP 5 cmH$_2$O
1. RR should be adjusted in order to optimize the comfort of the baby during ventilation and according to CO$_2$ levels.
2. IT is adjusted several times in a day according to lung compliance, searching for the time constant.
3. The exhaled V_t initially set at 5–7 mL/kg should be adjusted in order to reduce WOB, and according to the degree of lung inflation.
   We administer surfactant immediately at NICU entry when gestational age of the patient is below 24 weeks. Above this gestational age, we follow the most recent guidelines on the management of RDS [13] regarding timing of surfactant replacement therapy (when FiO$_2$ requirement is >0.30 in babies less than 26 weeks, when it is >0.40 in neonates above 26 weeks' gestation).
   When using VG ventilation, we usually set the flow at 5–8 L/min. In specific conditions, before deciding to change ETT size, it can be increased up to 10 L/min when compensating leaks is necessary. Higher flow is not used in order to avoid rheotrauma.
   When ventilating patients for prolonged time (e.g., patients affected by BPD), it could be appropriate to increase V_t up to 8–10 mL/kg to overcome the raised functional dead space and trachea enlargement. In this clinical condition, setting IT and backup rates on low values (e.g., 10–15 RR) is useful to avoid overtrapping.
4. PEEP is adjusted according to blood gases values (especially CO$_2$), FiO$_2$ requirement, and lung inflation visible at chest X-ray. PEEP values higher than 8 cmH$_2$O are rarely used.

In the acute phase of RDS, HFOV as early rescue treatment can be considered. High-frequency ventilation is our first choice in CDH, MAS, PIE, or pulmonary hypoplasia with or without lung malformations. All of these clinical conditions are treated with the open lung strategy with incremental and decreasing CDP.

PSV + VG is our preferred modality of ventilation in neonates with respiratory failure:
- in the postabdominal surgery period
- after deep sedation or in severe neurological impairment
- due to heart diseases with ventilator dependence
- with normal lung compliance

PSV + VG ventilation mode is used as a first-line treatment in very premature infants only if they dramatically respond to surfactant replacement therapy.

If the patient is not affected by chronic lung disease, during the weaning phase from VTV, we usually avoid changes in ventilation modality. We maintain AC, and we attempt to reduce RR, V_t (not lower than 4 mL/kg), and PEEP (not lower than 4 cmH$_2$O), trying for extubation when the peak needed to reach the V_t set is around 14–16 cmH$_2$O and FiO$_2$ requirement is less than 0.30.

The use of SIMV + VG is usually limited to the weaning phase of very preterm infants in order to avoid the risk of metabolic acidosis caused by the increase of WOB. However, if the WOB excessively increases using this modality, a PS (e.g., 2–5 cmH$_2$O) over PEEP is often associated and then gradually reduced according to WOB in order to avoid derecruitment.

In the course of PCV as well, clinicians should aim at maintaining a safe and effective V_t, adjusting PEEP and PIP values based on variations of clinical conditions and lung mechanics.

References

[1] Owen LS, Manley BJ, Davis PG, Doyle LW. The evolution of modern respiratory care for preterm infants. Lancet 2017;389:1649–1659.

[2] Keszler M. Mechanical ventilation strategies. Semin Fetal Neonatal Med 2017;22:267–274.

[3] Wheeler KI, Klingenberg C, Morley CJ, Davis PG. Volume-targeted versus pressure-limited ventilation for preterm infants: a systematic review and meta-analysis. Neonatology 2011;100:219–227.

[4] Klingenberg C, Wheeler KI, Owen LS, Kaaresen PI, Davis PG. An international survey of volume-targeted neonatal ventilation. Arch Dis Child Fetal Neonatal Ed 2011;96:F146–F148.

[5] Greenough A, Rossor TE, Sundaresan A, Murthy V, Milner AD. Synchronized mechanical ventilation for respiratory support in newborn infants. Cochrane Database Syst Rev 2016;9:CD000456.

[6] Cools F, Offringa M, Askie LM. Elective high frequency oscillatory ventilation versus conventional ventilation for acute pulmonary dysfunction in preterm infants. Cochrane Database Syst Rev 2015;3:CD000104.

[7] Bhuta T, Henderson-Smart DJ. Elective high frequency jet ventilation versus conventional ventilation for respiratory distress syndrome in preterm infants. Cochrane Database Syst Rev 2000;2:CD000328.

[8] Rojas-Reyes MX, Orrego-Rojas PA. Rescue high-frequency jet ventilation versus conventional ventilation for severe pulmonary dysfunction in preterm infants. Cochrane Database Syst Rev 2015;10:CD000437.

[9] Dreyfuss D, Soler P, Basset G, Saumon G. High inflation pressure pulmonary edema. Respective effects of high airway pressure, high tidal volume, and positive end-expiratory pressure. Am Rev Respir Dis 1988;137:1159–1164.

[10] Lista G, Maturana A, Moya FR. Achieving and maintaining lung volume in the preterm infant: from the first breath to the NICU. Eur J Pediatr 2017;176(10):1287–1293.

[11] Lista FC G. Optimizing lung volume Manual of neonatal respiratory care. Berlin-Heidelberg: Springer; 2017. pp 627–631.

[12] Castoldi F, Daniele I, Fontana P, Cavigioli F, Lupo E, Lista G. Lung recruitment maneuver during volume guarantee ventilation of preterm infants with acute respiratory distress syndrome. Am J Perinatol 2011;28:521–528.

[13] Sweet DG, Carnielli V, Greisen G, Hallman M, et al. European consensus guidelines on the management of respiratory distress syndrome—2016 update. Neonatology 2017;111(2): 107–125.

Chapter | **15A** |

Patient-Triggered Ventilation: Synchronized Intermittent Mandatory Ventilation (SIMV), Assist–Control, Pressure-Support Ventilation (PSV), Neurally Adjusted Ventilatory Assist (NAVA)

Helmut Hummler, MD, MBA

CHAPTER POINTS

- Synchronized modes adapt the ventilator breaths to the infant's breathing pattern and thus improve efficiency of respiratory support
- A proximal flow-sensor is the most commonly used trigger device as it has both high sensitivity and specificity
- Large leaks (>50%) may impair proper function of a flow sensor as a trigger device

- Assist-control (A/C) is the most commonly used mode of synchronized ventilation in the neonate
- Weaning during A/C is done by decreasing the peak pressure of ventilator breaths
- Pressure Support Ventilation (PSV) can be used alone or to support spontaneous breaths if the patient is weaned using Synchronized-Intermittent Mandatory Ventilation (SIMV) with a stepwise decrease in the SIMV rate

Introduction

This chapter reviews synchronized invasive ventilation. Noninvasive ventilation is covered in Chapter 16.

The development of synchronized ventilator modes for neonates was clearly delayed in comparison to developments in adult intensive care, and this was related to the fact that technology to measure very small flows and tidal volumes for premature infants needed to be developed. The almost uniform presence of leaks around the endotracheal tube (Fig. 15A.1), which often vary in size over time and can be very large, had to be considered.

Different types of interaction between spontaneous respiratory breaths and mechanical inflations have been observed in neonates and include the Hering–Breuer reflex, resulting in relaxation of respiratory muscles, augmented breaths (Head' paradoxical reflex), and forced expirations [1]. Although during mechanical ventilation, a close timely interaction of the mechanical inflation with the patients' inspiratory effort

215

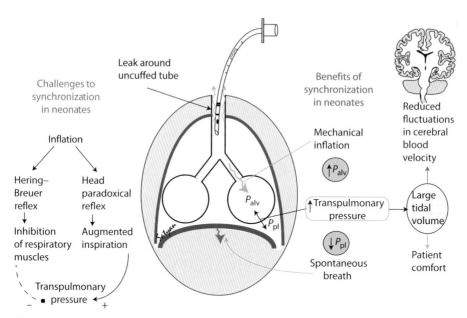

Fig. 15A.1 Challenges and Benefits of Synchronization of Ventilation in Neonates. Transpulmonary pressure is the difference between P_{alv} and P_{pl}; see text for details. P_{alv}, Alveolar pressure; P_{pl}, pleural pressure. Copyright: Satyan Lakshminrusimha.

usually decreases the effort due to the Hering–Breuer reflex and, thus, results in a lower transpulmonary pressure, it may also increase the transpulmonary pressure if a Head' paradoxical reflex occurs (Fig. 15A.1) [2]. It is believed that this reflex plays a critical role in recruitment and maintenance of lung volume in the neonatal age. When being placed on mechanical ventilation, some infants may adapt to the ventilator rhythm [1], and some may respond to mechanical inflation with a few rapid very shallow breaths, whereas others respond with active expiration, which seems to occur predominantly if mechanical inflation occurs at the end of the inspiratory or during the expiratory phase of the infants' spontaneous breath [1]. Active expiration was observed to be associated with the occurrence of pneumothorax in preterm infants with RDS by some authors [1]. Another response may be phase locking in expiration, where mechanical inflation is "locked" in the expiratory phase of spontaneous ventilation [3]. This response seems to be related to the vagal respiratory reflexes [3,4]. Mechanical inflations during the spontaneous expiratory phase prevent exhalation and disturb the infants' breathing pattern and do not contribute to a useful mechanical ventilator support.

larger transpulmonary pressure and thus a larger tidal volume (Fig. 15A.1) [5–7]. This may improve oxygenation in preterm infants with RDS [8]. Synchronization may reduce intrathoracic pressure fluctuations and decrease blood pressure fluctuations [6,7], which have been suggested to be associated with fluctuations of cerebral blood flow velocity and the occurrence of intraventricular hemorrhage [9]. Indeed neuromuscular paralysis has been shown to decrease fluctuations of cerebral blood velocity and may reduce the occurrence of intraventricular hemorrhage and air leaks in ventilated preterm infants [9,10], but it delays weaning and has its inherent side effects, including loss of FRC and negative effects on cardiac output. Thus, routine use of muscular paralysis in ventilated preterm infants with RDS is currently not recommended [10]. Improved efficiency of synchronized ventilation allows the preterm infant to decrease its respiratory effort resulting in improved work of breathing [11,12]. Avoiding to breathe out of phase with the ventilator does seem to decrease agitation and stress as indicated by decreased epinephrine levels found by the authors [13]. In fact, one clinical study suggested that the use of synchronized ventilation may decrease the use of sedation and paralysis, at least in some subgroups [14].

Applied physiology of synchronized mechanical ventilation in the newborn

The physiological effect of spontaneous inspiratory effort being in phase with the mechanical inflation results in a

Effects of the different types of ventilation

Physiological effects of synchronizing mechanical inflations to spontaneous breaths are described in the Section:

Applied physiology of synchronized mechanical ventilation in the newborn.

Modes of synchronized ventilation

A mechanical inflation synchronized to the beginning of inspiration of the spontaneous breath may be applied with a preset pressure or flow profile. Most commonly, a pressure-limited breath with a fixed or variable inspiratory time (time-cycled, pressure-limited inflation) is applied with a preset pressure profile. If the ventilator device measures airflow and terminates the inflation once decreasing flow crosses a certain threshold (i.e., 5%–10% of peak flow), the inspiratory time becomes variable and the (decreasing) flow cycles the inflation off. The two most commonly used modes are synchronized intermittent mandatory ventilation (SIMV) and assist–control (A/C). Pressure-support ventilation (PSV) is being used also in clinical practice, but proportional assist ventilation (PAV) has not gained widespread acceptance in neonatal respiratory support at this time.

Synchronized intermittent positive pressure ventilation; SIMV

During SIMV, a user-defined preset number of mechanical inflations per minute is provided, which are synchronized to the infant's spontaneous breaths. This mode is often used for weaning when there is already a good respiratory effort and a large proportion of work of breathing that is already being done by the infant breathing during the expiratory phase of the ventilator and supported by positive-end expiratory pressure (PEEP) (Fig. 15A.2). The ventilator

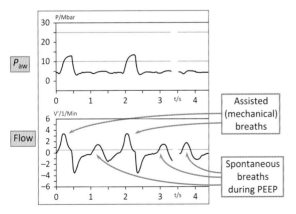

Fig. 15A.2 Synchronized Intermittent Mandatory Ventilation (SIMV) Mode Showing (Larger) SIMV Inflations With Spontaneous Breaths in Between These Breaths During PEEP. P_{aw}, Airway pressure; *PEEP*, positive-end expiratory pressure.

opens a preset window of time during which a spontaneous breath can trigger an inflation given by the ventilator. This window of time is usually a certain percentage of one complete respiratory cycle. If no effort is detected during this window of time, the ventilator provides a nonsynchronized (mandatory) inflation. If the rate of the infants' spontaneous breaths is low, this may result in a situation where no spontaneous breath is detected during this trigger window; by definition, the mechanical inflation is a nonsynchronized backup breath which may actually disrupt the infant's own breathing pattern.

Assist–control

During A/C, mechanical inflations are either *"assisted,"* if the infant has spontaneous efforts, or *"controlled"* (in the absence of patient effort). Every patient breath passing the trigger threshold is supported by the ventilator and the rate of ventilator inflations follows the respiratory rate of the infant (Fig. 15A.3) unless the infants breathes so fast that the next breath is within the default expiratory time, when the ventilator is refractory for another breath (usually 0.20 s). This mode gives the infant more liberty to drive up the ventilator support, if needed, by increasing its own respiratory rate. During A/C, a backup rate is selected to maintain FRC and gas exchange during periods of low respiratory effort of the infant. Some manufacturers use the term "synchronized intermittent positive pressure ventilation" (SIPPV) for this mode.

Pressure-support ventilation

PSV is an assisted mode where spontaneous breaths are either fully or partially supported by an increase in airway pressure. It may be used alone (full support) or in combination with SIMV, where spontaneous breaths between SIMV inflations are supported (partial support). During PSV, a preset peak inspiratory pressure (PIP) is applied, as long as there is a positive inspiratory airflow. Thus, the infant determines the inspiratory time of the inflation supported by the ventilator. Inflation is terminated once one of the following conditions is met first: it may be flow if flow cycling is chosen, or time, if flow cycling is "off" (chosen inspiratory time will be applied).

Proportional assist ventilation

During PAV the ventilator measures airflow and adjusts airway pressure throughout the respiratory cycle every few milliseconds in proportion to the inspired volume to compensate for elastic forces (elastic unloading), and in proportion to the airflow to compensate for resistive forces (resistive unloading) (Fig. 15A.4).

217

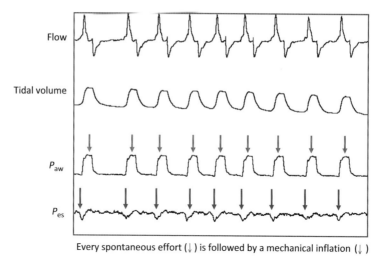

Every spontaneous effort (↓) is followed by a mechanical inflation (↓)

Fig. 15A.3 Assist–Control (A/C) Mode. Every patient effort (*blue arrows* in P_{es} trace) is supported by the ventilator (P_{aw} increase, *red arrows*). P_{aw}, Airway pressure; P_{es}, esophageal pressure.

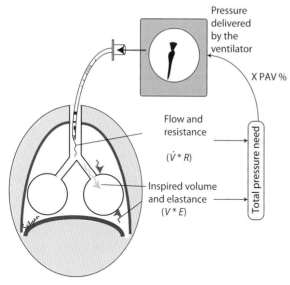

Fig. 15A.4 Proportional Assist Ventilation (PAV). The ventilator measures airflow and volume and adjusts airway pressure throughout the respiratory cycle in proportion to the inspired volume to compensate for elastic forces (elastic unloading), and to the airflow to compensate for resistive forces (resistive unloading). Copyright: Satyan Lakshminrusimha.

Cycling (trigger) techniques for synchronized ventilation

Although many signals have been investigated to trigger ventilator breaths in neonates (esophageal pressure, abdominal wall capsule, thoracic impedance, induction,

airway pressure, and airflow), almost exclusively airflow and sometimes airway pressure are being used clinically. Thoracic impedance was used clinically for some time until the signal was proven to be not very reliable. A phase shift in the impedance signal secondary to chest wall distortion, causing a time lag of the trigger signal, was observed, which could result in long trigger delays or even in trigger during expiration [15]. Unfortunately, those infants needing respiratory support have the highest risk for a low lung compliance and chest wall distortion. The abdominal pressure capsule was commonly used with the Infantstar ventilator, which is not available any more. However, more recently, there is increased interest in using abdominal motion for triggering using noninvasive ventilation [16]. Table 15A.1 lists advantages and disadvantages of different trigger techniques.

Airflow is being used most commonly as the trigger signal as this is the most specific signal available for clinical use at this time. Furthermore, this signal allows monitoring of flow and tidal volume and thus to use volume-targeted ventilator modes (Chapter 15). The additional dead space imposed by the flow sensor has been of some concern, especially for the most immature infants [17]. However, recent data suggests that instrumental dead space secondary to a flow sensor being introduced between the ventilator circuit and the endotracheal tube is not always affecting gas exchange or may affect PCO_2 far less than expected. This may be related to the presence of an endotracheal tube leak and to the fact that air is probably not transported as bulk volume, but rather in parabolic profiles or in a nonlinear fashion allowing to mix during transition from the ventilator circuit to the alveoli [18,19]. From a clinical point of view, the use of a flow sensor should always be favored, and

Table 15A.1 Different trigger techniques for synchronized ventilation (Fig. 15A.5)

Trigger techniques	Advantages	Disadvantages/Problems
Airflow	Very specific signal, low risk of autocycling or trigger failure	Dead space Artifacts due to secretions Air leaks may cause autocycling
Hot wire anemometer	Less problems with secretions	Less sensitive for small flows
Pneumotachograph	Very sensitive, can detect very small flows	Rainout and secretions affect signal
Airway pressure	No dead space	Very immature infants may not be able to trigger Artifacts secondary to secretions in the circuit
Impedance	No dead space	Phase shift causing trigger delay due to chest wall distortion (dependent on positioning of electrodes)
Esophageal pressure	No dead space	Peristalsis of the esophagus causes trigger Cardiac artifacts
Abdominal pressure capsule	Very sensitive No dead space	Autocycling secondary to movement artifacts
Diaphragmatic EMG	No dead space	Requires a specific sensor to detect EMG

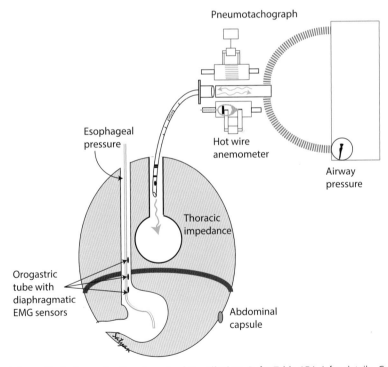

Fig. 15A.5 Different Trigger Techniques for Synchronized Ventilation. Refer Table 15A.1 for details. Copyright: Satyan Lakshminrusimha.

if there are concerns about additional dead space ventilation, the effect of its introduction can always be tested by eliminating/reintroducing the sensor while closely observing the PCO$_2$. Heated circuits help to reduce water rainout and thus decrease the risk for autocycling due to artifacts.

Detection of autocycling and trigger failure

Clinical evaluation of the infants' thorax and abdomen can be very useful to evaluate the origin of a breath; a

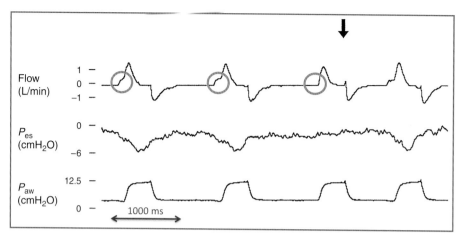

Fig. 15A.6 Autotrigger. Note that the third inflation (*arrow*) does not show the small inspiratory airflow (*red circles*) before the airway pressure increases and the esophageal pressure (P_{es}) curve does not show a deflection indicating that there is no patient effort. P_{aw}, Airway pressure.

spontaneous breath causes abdominal expansion secondary to the contraction of the diaphragm. The latter may cause subcostal (and intercostal and jugular) retractions. However, a spontaneous breath causes only a small expansion of the chest. In supine position, a mechanical inflation (without spontaneous respiratory effort) is directed more toward the cranial and anterior parts of the chest and usually there is no chest wall distortion.

Graphical display of flow and pressure may be very helpful to detect autocycling. Triggered breaths show a small inspiratory airflow before the airway pressure increases with the mechanical inflation causing an acceleration of airflow. The third inflation (*arrow*) in Fig. 15A.6 does not show the small inspiratory airflow before the airway pressure increases to cause inspiratory flow acceleration, and the esophageal pressure (P_{es}) curve does not show a deflection clearly indicating that there is no patient effort. However, a small positive airflow not followed by a mechanical inflation indicates trigger failure (*arrow* in Fig. 15A.7). If autocycling occurs, the trigger threshold has to be increased above leak flow. Some ventilators compensate for leaks automatically.

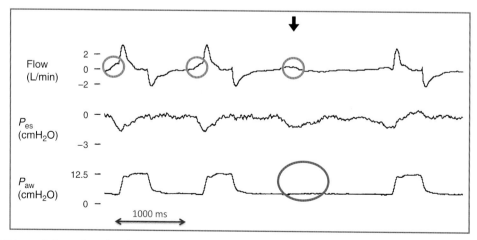

Fig. 15A.7 Trigger Failure. Note that the *arrow points* to a small inspiratory airflow (*red circles*), but there is no mechanical inflation as indicated in the airway pressure (P_{aw}) curve (*blue marker*). The P_{es} curve proves that there is a spontaneous effort. P_{es}, Esophageal pressure.

Indications and contraindications

In infants with spontaneous respiratory effort, synchronized ventilation should be considered the standard mode to take advantage of at least the physiological benefits. However, introduction of a flow sensor causes additional dead space, which may result in CO_2 retention, especially in very small infants. To keep the PCO_2 in the desired reference range, alveolar minute ventilation has to be increased in this situation, which may require an increase in the infants' effort, or in the ventilator rate and/or tidal volume. Risks (increased volutrauma) and benefits (Section, Applied physiology of synchronized mechanical ventilation in the newborn) will have to balance against each other. This decision should be individualized (Section, Detection of autocycling and trigger failure).

More mature preterm or full-term infants with severe lung disease often do not tolerate the presence of an endotracheal tube and mechanical inflations very well and often receive analgesia/sedation or even paralysis in clinical practice. Although there are no studies to confirm the efficacy of this approach, it seems reasonable to try these infants on a synchronized mode before medications are used. Presence of the infants' own respiratory effort helps to maintain FRC, allows to lower ventilator settings, and supports cardiac output.

SIMV

This is very often used as weaning mode, although many clinicians prefer A/C during the acute and weaning phase. During SIMV, the patient has less capability to receive additional support by the ventilator as compared to A/C.

A/C

This mode can be used for many patients during the acute phase or during weaning. In comparison to SIMV, the patient can increase the support given by the ventilator by increasing his/her own breathing rate. Thus, it gives more liberty to the patient to control the degree of ventilator support.

PSV

PSV can be used for full support where every spontaneous inspiration is assisted by additional airway pressure above PEEP, or as a hybrid mode during SIMV where spontaneous breaths between SIMV breaths are usually supported with a lower pressure. This approach is often used as a weaning mode with the PIP chosen only a few cmH_2O above PEEP to support spontaneous breaths to overcome the resistance imposed by the endotracheal tube in place.

Protocol of use

SIMV

The clinician sets the PIP (if pressure targeted), or the desired tidal volume (if volume targeted), the inspiratory time (if time-cycled), and the SIMV rate (similar to IMV). If flow cycling is used (termination of inspiration with the flow decreasing to a certain percentage of the peak flow), the inspiratory time chosen is the maximum inspiratory time. During flow cycling, the beginning and the end of the ventilator inflation is synchronized. For flow cycling, usually 5%–10% of peak flow, to cycle the inflation off, is suggested. Use minimal sensitivity to allow for a short response time. Set trigger threshold just above any artifacts seen in the flow trace and readjust if needed.

A/C

Similar to SIMV, the clinicians set the PIP or the targeted tidal volume. If flow cycling is chosen, the percentage of peak flow to cycle the breath off is chosen (often 5%–10%). Trigger threshold is set similar as during SIMV. The inspiratory time is chosen by the clinician, which is the maximum inspiratory time, if flow cycling is used. A backup for episodes of low respiratory effort is chosen depending on the severity of lung disease and the stability of gas exchange.

PSV

PSV can be used as the primary mode of ventilator support alone. This mode is almost identical to pressure-controlled A/C with flow cycling. However, some ventilators allow hybrid-synchronized modes. SIMV may be used along with PSV, where PSV supports those breaths occurring between SIMV inflations. In this case, the PIP or tidal volume is chosen separately for SIMV and PSV inflations. Inspiratory time and backup rate is chosen similar to A/C.

Bedside application of the technology

If not present already, the trigger device is attached to the baby and the mode is chosen as directed by the manufacturer of the device used.

Adjustment of trigger threshold

External signals like the abdominal pressure capsule or impedance are more prone to artifacts than airflow. If the

intercostal, supraclavicular, and subcostal retractions, and increasing oxygen requirement, despite suctioning of the upper airway and increasing the CPAP pressure to 7 cmH$_2$O. Intermittent nasal IPPV did not result in any clinical improvement, and the FiO$_2$ needed to maintain SpO$_2$ above 85% was gradually increasing over 10 min to 0.45. The infant was then intubated and received surfactant replacement therapy, which resulted in improved oxygenation allowing to decrease the FiO$_2$ to 0.21 and applying a PIP of 18–22 cmH$_2$O and a PEEP of 6 cmH$_2$O initially with a rate of 60 inflations/min during regular pressure-controlled mode; the PIP was weaned to 14 cmH$_2$O and the PEEP to 5 cmH$_2$O over the following night.

The infant's own respiratory rate was 40–50 breaths/min; and in the morning of the 2nd day of life, the FiO$_2$ requirements went up to 0.25–0.30 and the rate had to be increased by 10 inflations/min because of mild CO$_2$ retention. A control chest X-ray showed some mild homogeneous decrease in transparency. The infant was reported by the nurses to need suctioning frequently because of secretions in the endotracheal tube and was also reported to be agitated and "fighting the ventilator" intermittently, breathing out of phase with the ventilator resulting in desaturations, but also seemed to have intermittently poor respiratory effort. The options discussed during rounds were to:

• give morphine for analgesia/sedation intermittently, or
• extubate and place on nasal CPAP or nasal IPPV, or
• place the infant on a synchronized mode.

The final team decision was to leave the infant intubated at this time as the infant had required higher ventilator settings more recently and it was expected that a second dose of surfactant may be needed soon. Sedation was to be avoided and the infant was placed on A/C with a backup rate of 40 breaths/min, as phases of poor respiratory drive were observed before. The infant tolerated this mode very well and was extubated on the 3rd day of life after the PIP was reduced further and FiO$_2$ could be reduced to 0.25.

Comment: Clearly, other clinicians may have used PSV instead of A/C or SIMV. However, SIMV always has the risk of synchronization failure if the patients' effort just does not match nicely with the trigger window. Clearly, A/C or PSV gives the patient more liberty to increase the support provided by the ventilator by just increasing the own respiratory rate, which would not be possible with SIMV. In the absence of appropriate clinical trials to test the different strategies in specific situations, thorough knowledge of the pathophysiology of the disease and the modes available and experience is necessary to select the best mode using a physiology-based approach.

New directions including neurally adjusted ventilatory assist (NAVA)

Microprocessor techniques have allowed to measure small flows and tidal volume and to develop sophisticated assisted modes of ventilator support for small preterm infants such as synchronized modes. The need for invasive ventilation is decreasing with clinicians favoring noninvasive modes of respiratory support. Weaning is traditionally initiated once clinicians feel that the babies are "ready" for weaning. This readiness is rather subjective and actually the absence of standardized criteria and being "ready" to initiate the next step may severely delay weaning. Closed-loop systems may help to standardize weaning in the future and ensure at the same time adequate gas exchange [26].

NAVA

Neurally adjusted ventilatory assist (NAVA) is a more recently developed technique for assisted ventilation for both invasive and noninvasive respiratory support, which uses the electrical activity of the diaphragm (EAdi) (Chapter 30). This signal is obtained within the esophagus using a specifically designed gastric tube, which has electrodes incorporated in its wall. This part of the gastric tube needs to be placed at the proper position in the distal esophagus. The phasic component of the signal is closely related to diaphragmatic activity and allows a shorter response time than airflow, airway pressure, or any other external trigger system. The EAdi signal can be used to monitor the electrical activity of the diaphragm, or trigger a mechanical inflation, and to determine the amount of pressure being delivered throughout the spontaneous respiratory cycle. The degree of assistance is user adjustable, proportional to the signal, and dependent of the selected gain, called "NAVA level" (cmH$_2$O/μV). Thus, the change in airway pressure above PEEP is proportional to the NAVA level.

This system has some similarities to PAV [27]. However, in comparison to PAV, NAVA does not have the problem of overcompensation in case the gain is adjusted too high. An increasing lung volume during inspiration will downregulate diaphragmatic EMG, which will decrease airway pressure, if the system works properly. However, overcompensation during PAV can self-perpetuate the support unless there is a safety limit for inspired tidal volume or pressure.

NAVA is available with the Servo-i ventilator (Maquet Critical Care, Rastatt, Germany) for clinical use in neonates. This ventilator offers many conventional modes and allows synchronized mechanical ventilation using flow or pressure trigger, and can be used for invasive or noninvasive NAVA.

Backup ventilation is available to maintain alveolar ventilation and gas exchange during periods of apnea. The ventilator then continues with NAVA once the EAdi signal returns. Thus, the airflow, PIP, and tidal volume are controlled by the patient and the NAVA level. Airway pressure is decreased to PEEP level once the EAdi signal decreases to a certain percentage of the peak EAdi level.

- **Advantages**: The system provides synchrony throughout the respiratory cycle with the airway pressure in proportion to the spontaneous effort and is not affected by leak. There is no dead space if used for invasive respiratory support and it can be used for noninvasive ventilator support.
- **Disadvantages**: The system is not useful for infants with poor or variable respiratory drive. Thus, usefulness is limited to extremely low birth weight infants or requires frequent backup ventilation. The sensor device is quite expensive.

Clinical studies looking at physiological variables have proven functionality of the NAVA system [28–30]. However, there is limited information available from clinical controlled studies. One randomized crossover study found better synchrony between patient effort and the ventilator and other short-term physiological benefits in comparison to other synchronized modes [31], and there are promising reports on long-term use [32]. Some authors believe that NAVA may be particularly useful for noninvasive ventilation to avoid intubation or for weaning after extubation [33,34].

In summary, NAVA is a feedback control system, which synchronizes mechanical ventilator support to patient effort throughout the spontaneous respiratory cycle, which clearly has many attractive physiological advantages. Clinical studies will have to show whether or not these physiological advantages translate into better clinical outcomes.

References

[1] Greenough A, Morley CJ, Davis JA. Respiratory reflexes in ventilated premature babies. Early Hum Dev 1983;8:65–75.

[2] Hummler H, Gerhardt T, Gonzalez A, Claure N, Everett R, Bancalari E. Increased incidence of sighs (augmented inspiratory efforts) during synchronized intermittent mandatory ventilation (SIMV) in preterm neonates. Pediatr Pulmonol 1997;24:195–203.

[3] Graves C, Glass L, Laporta D, Meloche R, Grassino A. Respiratory phase locking during mechanical ventilation in anesthetized human subjects. Am J Physiol 1986;250:R902–R909.

[4] Petrillo GA, Glass L, Trippenbach T. Phase locking of the respiratory rhythm in cats to a mechanical ventilator. Can J Physiol Pharmacol 1983;61:599–607.

[5] Bernstein G, Heldt GP, Mannino FL. Increased and more consistent tidal volumes during synchronized intermittent mandatory ventilation in newborn infants. Am J Respir Crit Care Med 1994;150:1444–1448.

[6] Amitay M, Etches PC, Finer NN, Maidens JM. Synchronous mechanical ventilation of the neonate with respiratory disease. Crit Care Med 1993;21:118–124.

[7] Hummler H, Gerhardt T, Gonzalez A, Claure N, Everett R, Bancalari E. Influence of different methods of synchronized mechanical ventilation on ventilation, gas exchange, patient effort, and blood pressure fluctuations in premature neonates. Pediatr Pulmonol 1996;22:305–313.

[8] Cleary JP, Bernstein G, Mannino FL, Heldt GP. Improved oxygenation during synchronized intermittent mandatory ventilation in neonates with respiratory distress syndrome: a randomized, crossover study. J Pediatr 1995;126:407–411.

[9] Perlman JM, Goodman S, Kreusser KL, Volpe JJ. Reduction in intraventricular hemorrhage by elimination of fluctuating cerebral blood-flow velocity in preterm infants with respiratory distress syndrome. N Engl J Med 1985;312:1353–1357.

[10] Cools F, Offringa M. Neuromuscular paralysis for newborn infants receiving mechanical ventilation. Cochrane Database Syst Rev 2005;14: CD002773.

[11] Jarreau PH, Moriette G, Mussat P, Mariette C, Mohanna A, Harf A, et al. Patient-triggered ventilation decreases the work of breathing in neonates. Am J Respir Crit Care Med 1996;153:1176–1181.

[12] Kapasi M, Fujino Y, Kirmse M, Catlin EA, Kacmarek RM. Effort and work of breathing in neonates during assisted patient-triggered ventilation. Pediatr Crit Care Med 2001;2:9–16.

[13] Quinn MW, de Boer RC, Ansari N, Baumer JH. Stress response and mode of ventilation in preterm infants. Arch Dis Child Fetal Neonatal Ed 1998;78:F195–F198.

[14] Bernstein G, Mannino FL, Heldt GP, Callahan JD, Bull DH, Sola A, et al. Randomized multicenter trial comparing synchronized and conventional intermittent mandatory ventilation in neonates. J Pediatr 1996;128:453–463.

[15] Hummler HD, Gerhardt T, Gonzalez A, Bolivar J, Claure N, Everett R, et al. Patient-triggered ventilation in neonates: comparison of a flow- and an impedance-triggered system. Am J Respir Crit Care Med 1996;154:1049–1054.

[16] Huang L, Mendler MR, Waitz M, Schmid M, Hassan MA, Hummler HD. Effects of synchronization during noninvasive intermittent mandatory ventilation in preterm infants with respiratory distress syndrome immediately after extubation. Neonatology 2015;108: 108–114.

225

[17] Estay A, Claure N, D'Ugard C, Organero R, Bancalari E. Effects of instrumental dead space reduction during weaning from synchronized ventilation in preterm infants. J Perinatol 2010;30:479–483.

[18] Nassabeh-Montazami S, Abubakar KM, Keszler M. The impact of instrumental dead-space in volume-targeted ventilation of the extremely low birth weight (ELBW) infant. Pediatr Pulmonol 2009;44:128–133.

[19] Keszler M, Montaner MB, Abubakar K. Effective ventilation at conventional rates with tidal volume below instrumental dead space: a bench study. Arch Dis Child Fetal Neonatal Ed 2012;97:F188–F192.

[20] Greenough A, Rossor TE, Sundaresan A, Murthy V, Milner AD. Synchronized mechanical ventilation for respiratory support in newborn infants. Cochrane Database Syst Rev 2016;9:CD000456.

[21] Baumer JH. International randomised controlled trial of patient triggered ventilation in neonatal respiratory distress syndrome. Arch Dis Child Fetal Neonatal Ed 2000;82:F5–F10.

[22] Osorio W, Claure N, D'Ugard C, Athavale K, Bancalari E. Effects of pressure support during an acute reduction of synchronized intermittent mandatory ventilation in preterm infants. J Perinatol 2005;25:412–416.

[23] Patel D-S, Rafferty GF, Lee S, Hannam S, Greenough A. Work of breathing during SIMV with and without pressure support. Arch Dis Child 2009;94:434–436.

[24] Gupta S, Sinha SK, Donn SM. The effect of two levels of pressure support ventilation on tidal volume delivery and minute ventilation in preterm infants. Arch Dis Child Fetal Neonatal Ed 2009;94:F80–F83.

[25] Reyes ZC, Claure N, Tauscher MK, D'Ugard C, Vanbuskirk S, Bancalari E. Randomized, controlled trial comparing synchronized intermittent mandatory ventilation and synchronized intermittent mandatory ventilation plus pressure support in preterm infants. Pediatrics 2006;118:1409–1417.

[26] Claure N, Gerhardt T, Hummler H, Everett R, Bancalari E. Computer-controlled minute ventilation in preterm infants undergoing mechanical ventilation. J Pediatr 1997;131:910–913.

[27] Schulze A, Bancalari E. Proportional assist ventilation in infants. Clin Perinatol 2001;28:561–578.

[28] Gibu CK, Cheng PY, Ward RJ, Castro B, Heldt GP. Feasibility and physiological effects of noninvasive neurally adjusted ventilatory assist in preterm infants. Pediatr Res 2017;82:650–657.

[29] Shetty S, Hunt K, Peacock J, Ali K, Greenough A. Crossover study of assist control ventilation and neurally adjusted ventilatory assist. Eur J Pediatr 2017;176:509–513.

[30] Jung YH, Kim H-S, Lee J, Shin SH, Kim E-K, Choi J-H. Neurally adjusted ventilatory assist in preterm infants with established or evolving bronchopulmonary dysplasia on high-intensity mechanical ventilatory support: a single-center experience. Pediatr Crit Care Med 2016;17:1142–1146.

[31] Lee J, Kim H-S, Jung YH, Shin SH, Choi CW, Kim E-K, et al. Non-invasive neurally adjusted ventilatory assist in preterm infants: a randomised phase II crossover trial. Arch Dis Child Fetal Neonatal Ed 2015;100:F507–F513.

[32] Lee J, Kim H-S, Jung YH, Choi CW, Jun YH. Neurally adjusted ventilatory assist for infants under prolonged ventilation. Pediatr Int 2017;59:540–544.

[33] Firestone KS, Beck J, Stein H. Neurally adjusted ventilatory assist for noninvasive support in neonates. Clin Perinatol 2016;43:707–724.

[34] Stein H, Beck J, Dunn M. Non-invasive ventilation with neurally adjusted ventilatory assist in newborns. Semin Fetal Neonatal Med 2016;21:154–161.

Chapter | 15B |

Neurally Adjusted Ventilatory Assist (NAVA) in Neonates

Howard Stein, MD, Kimberly S. Firestone, MSc, RRT

CHAPTER POINTS

- Neurally adjusted ventilatory assist (NAVA) is a mode of mechanical ventilation. NAVA delivers assistance in proportion to and in synchrony with the patient's respiratory efforts, as reflected by the diaphragmatic electrical signal (Edi).
- NAVA improves patient-ventilator interaction and synchrony even in the presence of significant air leaks and therefore may be the best option for invasive ventilation with uncuffed endotracheal tubes and for non-invasive ventilation in neonates.
- Short term data available for comparison of NAVA to conventional ventilation demonstrates lower peak ventilator pressures required, improved oxygen levels, and lower airway pressures with no adverse events attributable to NAVA.
- NAVA is neurally integrated with lung protective reflexes such as Hering-Breuer reflex which is evident in neonates.
- NAVA is a unique mode that offers personalized ventilation for the neonate permitting them to customize their own ventilatory support based on biophysical and biochemical feedback.

Neurally adjusted ventilatory assist basics

What is neurally adjusted ventilatory assist

Neurally adjusted ventilatory assist (NAVA) is a mode of ventilation that allows the patient to control the initiation, size, and termination of each mechanical breath on a breath-by-breath basis [1,2]. The ventilator incorporates a neural trigger that detects the electrical activity of the diaphragm (Edi) via a specialized nasogastric tube positioned at the level of the crural diaphragm. Once the Edi signal is detected, the ventilator delivers flow to achieve a peak pressure that is proportional to the amount of Edi activity (Fig. 15B.1). Once the Edi signal ceases (at end-inspiration), the breath is terminated.

Normal range for the Edi signal

The Edi peak is a marker of respiratory drive. The concept of "normal" Edi in a ventilated patient can be challenging. If the patient is undersupported, the Edi peak can be very high, and if the patient is oversupported, the Edi peak can be suppressed. Edi min is a marker of tonic activity of the diaphragm to prevent derecruitment during expiration (Fig. 15B.1). Inadequate PEEP will raise the Edi min and excess PEEP will suppress it [3]. To determine goal Edi peak and min values in the ventilated neonate, stable term and preterm neonates off all ventilatory support were evaluated. These studies showed that Edi peak goal should be 5–15 mcV and Edi min should be 2–5 mcV [4,5].

How NANA works

Synchronous for:
Initiation, size, termination of each breath even with ETT/NIV leaks
Responds to respiratory **drive**
Advantages:
Lower PIP, V_t, WOB
Improved blood gases
Improved COMFORT scores
Lower sedation requirements

Edi catheter

NAVA software

Mechanical diaphragm

Phrenic nerve

Hering–Breuer prevents overinflation

Edi min (2–5 μV)

Tonic activity during expiration

Biologic diaphragm

Peak inspiration

Edi max (5–15 μV)

Airway pressure above PEEP (cmH$_2$O)

"NAVA level" (cmH$_2$O/μV)

X

Edi signal (max–min μV)

> Threshold (Edi trigger) ~ 0.5 μV

Gastric tube with diaphragmatic EMG sensors

Fig. 15B.1 The Physiologic Basis and Advantages of NAVA. The electrical activity of the diaphragm (Edi) is detected by sensors embedded in a specialized nasogastric tube. The Edi min value corresponds to the tonic activity of the diaphragm during expiration and the typical values in preterm infants are shown in parenthesis. The Edi peak is generated during inspiration. When the Edi value exceeds a preset trigger value, this initiates a mechanical breath from the ventilator. The ventilator provides flow to generate a peak pressure above PEEP for the mechanical breath as determined by the product of Edi (peak–min) and the NAVA level (see text for details). Copyright: Satyan Lakshminrusimha.

How NAVA works

NAVA improves patient–ventilator interaction

Studies in children showed that patient–ventilator interaction improved from 12%–29% asynchrony during conventional modes to 0%–11% during NAVA [6–14]. Synchrony was not only improved for initiation of the breath but also for size and termination. Asynchrony, as evidenced by false triggering, autotriggering, and missed triggering, was also reduced. This improved synchrony was present even in the presence of large air leaks [15]. This is especially significant in neonates when using uncuffed endotracheal tubes or in noninvasive (NIV) NAVA with large air leaks around the nasal interface.

NAVA allows neonates to control peak pressure and tidal volume

Neonates breathing on NAVA chose lower peak inspiratory pressures (PIP) and tidal volume (V_t) compared with conventional ventilation which were targeted by the bedside clinician [8,16–23]. NAVA is neurally integrated with lung protective reflexes such as Hering–Breuer reflex. As lung inflation progresses, vagally mediated stretch receptors in the lungs sense an adequate level of lung distension and turn off inspiration, so the ventilator breath will be cycled off when neural exhalation begins.

Specific evidence for functional lung reflexes in premature infants comes from NAVA-level titrations (systematic increases from 0.5 to 4 cmH$_2$O/μV) in premature neonates (mean weight at study was 795g, range 500–1441g). Initially, PIP and V_t increased with increasing NAVA levels as the work of breathing was unloaded from the neonate to

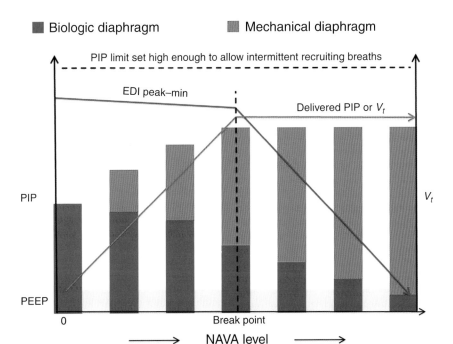

Fig. 15B.2 The Relationship Between NAVA Level and Peak Inspiratory Pressure (PIP) and Tidal Volume (V_t). Increasing NAVA level represents higher workload by the ventilator ("mechanical" diaphragm) and less workload by the patient ("biologic" diaphragm). A NAVA level of 0 provides no mechanical support above PEEP. As NAVA level increases, the workload by the mechanical diaphragm increases until the PIP and V_t plateau. This inflection point is called the 'breakpoint'. NAVA levels higher than the "break point" result in reduction in the contribution of the biologic diaphragm, as shown by Edi *(red line)*, to continue to generate optimal PIP and V_t.

the ventilator. This was followed by a plateau phase where the PIP and V_t did not increase further but the Edi was downregulated (Fig. 15B.2). The NAVA level at which the plateau was evident was termed the "break point" and was considered the optimal NAVA level [24].

Outcomes of neonates on NAVA

Only short-term data (hours to days) are available for NAVA. When changing from conventional ventilation to NAVA, PIP decreased [7,8,10,12,16,18–20,25]. Despite lower PIP and V_t, blood gases improved when on NAVA for more than 4 h [19,20,22]. NAVA improved oxygenation even at lower airway pressures and led to reduced use of sedatives during longer periods of treatment [21] and improved comfort [9]. Neonates on NAVA showed better median weight gain (30 g/day) compared with conventional ventilation (13 g/day), despite the same average caloric intake [26]. No adverse events attributable to NAVA have been noted. Specifically, in one retrospective

review, there was no change in the rate of intraventricular hemorrhage, pneumothorax, or necrotizing enterocolitis [20]. Randomized controlled trials with developmental follow-up are needed to determine the long-term outcomes of neonates ventilated with NAVA.

NAVA and specific neonatal diseases

NAVA has shown to be feasible and effective in neonates with respiratory distress syndrome (RDS) [18–20,27–29], bronchopulmonary dysplasia (BPD) [30], respiratory syncytial virus (RSV) [6,22], congenital diaphragmatic hernia (CDH) [31,32], pulmonary interstitial emphysema (PIE) [33,34], and those undergoing surgery for congenital heart disease (CHD) [8,35–37]. NAVA has also been helpful in the diagnosis of central hypoventilation syndrome [38]. The bedside clinician should use the same method to set up NAVA for all the different neonatal respiratory conditions as described in the next section. Ventilation with NAVA will then allow the neonate to personalize their own ventilatory needs to accommodate their specific respiratory condition on an ongoing breath-to-breath basis.

Set up of NAVA

How to place the Edi catheter

The catheter-positioning screen is utilized to position the Edi catheter electrodes at the level of the crural diaphragm in order to detect the optimal Edi signal. Correct placement of the Edi catheter is vital though it is easily maintained and monitored. Appropriate placement is achieved when the retrocardiac ECG signal with large p and QRS complexes in the upper leads progressing to small or absent complexes in the lower leads (Fig. 15B.3). The blue tracing in the middle 2 leads represents the Edi signal (also seen in the bottom tracing) superimposed over the retrocardiac ECG tracing. This signal can drift to the upper and lower tracings without affecting the signal quality [39].

How to set the NAVA level

The NAVA level is a proportionality factor that converts the quantitative Edi into a delivered inspiratory pressure. It is helpful to imagine the NAVA level as a determinant of how much work of breathing the patient does compared with the ventilator. The patient's respiratory center controls both the biologic diaphragm and the mechanical diaphragm (the ventilator), and the NAVA level determines the proportion of work each diaphragm does. The higher the NAVA level, the more respiratory effort is unloaded from the patient to the ventilator, whereas conversely the lower the NAVA level, the more work of breathing is assumed by

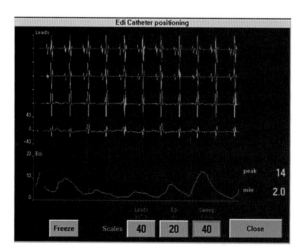

Fig. 15B.3 Edi Catheter Positioning Screen From the Servo-i Ventilator. Note that the p-waves become smaller and disappear from the top tracing to the lower tracing while the QRS complexes get smaller but are still evident in the lower tracings.

the patient. The goal is to unload the work of breathing from the patient to the ventilator without overassisting the patient (and suppressing the respiratory drive) acknowledging that the patient continues to determine the frequency, size, and termination of each breath. Practically, as the NAVA level increases, delivered inspiratory pressure will increase proportionally until a "break point" is reached. At this point the inspiratory pressure will remain steady and the Edi peak (respiratory drive) will decrease with further increases in the NAVA level [24]. It is suggested initiating NAVA with a level of 2 cmH$_2$O/mcV; then observe the patient's Edi peak and work of breathing. If the Edi peak is consistently high (>15–20 mcV) and/or the neonate is having significant work of breathing, increase the NAVA level every few minutes in increments of 0.5 H$_2$O/mcV until the Edi peak decreases to 10–15 mcV and work of breathing improves [39]. When extubating from NAVA to NIV NAVA (typically at a NAVA level of 1 cmH$_2$O/mcV), it is important to increase the NAVA level again to 2 cmH$_2$O/mcV to account for the loss of flow at the nasal interface, and then adjust the NAVA level as described earlier [40].

How to set the Edi trigger

The Edi trigger is comparable to the sensitivity setting in flow- or pressure-triggered ventilation. The Edi trigger is the amount of Edi increase that is needed for the ventilator to initiate the NAVA-supported spontaneous breath. When the Edi trigger is set too low, the ventilator reacts to insignificant small signals and delivers small, ineffective breaths resulting in clinical decompensation. If the Edi trigger is set appropriately (usually at the factory default of 0.5 mcV), the small Edi signals are ignored by the ventilator, interpreted as apnea, and backup ventilation is delivered until the respiratory drive improves and a more robust Edi signal occurs [39].

How to set apnea time

Although located in the alarm section of the ventilator setup, the apnea time is a pertinent ventilator setting. Apnea time is the time the neonate can have a respiratory pause after which the ventilator initiates backup ventilation. In the literature, apnea is defined as no respiratory effort for longer than 15–20 s [41]. However, this may be too long for a ventilated neonate to be without respiratory support and may result in worsening clinical status. Apnea time should be thought of as minimum respiratory rate. For example, an apnea time of 2 s gives a minimum rate of 30 breaths/min. This is unrelated to the backup rate, which is the rate at which the neonate is ventilated during the apneic event, and is preset by the bedside clinician. Providing a minimum rate is a safety feature to ventilate the neonate with recurrent apnea [42].

How to set the peak pressure limit

With conventional ventilation, the peak pressure alarm is typically set slightly higher than the peak pressure to protect the lung from inadvertent high inspiratory pressure and risk of overdistention. However with NAVA ventilation, setting the peak pressure limit at a comparable level to conventional ventilation will restrict the neonate from taking occasional recruiting or sigh breaths and will be at risk for underventilation from progressive atelectasis. Premature neonates show the capacity to regulate their minute ventilation and adjust their ventilator peak pressure demands and respiratory rate on an ongoing basis as long as the peak pressure limit is set high enough to allow them to take occasional recruiting breaths [39]. Therefore, it is recommended to set the peak pressure alarm limit between 30 and 40 cmH$_2$O to allow these occasional recruiting breaths.

Initial setting for invasive and NIV NAVA

The initial setting for invasive and NIV NAVA is listed in Table 15B.1. Extensive clinical experience suggests that a starting NAVA level of 2 cmH$_2$O/mcV is appropriate for most neonates. This includes both those intubated and those who are escalating from CPAP to NIV NAVA. Once the intubated neonate has weaned to a NAVA level of 1 cmH$_2$O/mcV and remains stable, extubation to NIV

NAVA can occur. The NAVA level should be increased again to 2 cmH$_2$O/mcV and adjusted as described in Table 15B.1. The key to successful implementation of NAVA is to reevaluate the neonate frequently and use clinical assessment in addition to the parameters described later to manage the ventilated neonate.

Management of neonates on NAVA

Most neonates will stabilize on NAVA and wean themselves as their disease process improves. There is little variation between disease processes on how to approach the initial setup and management of NAVA. This has been shown in neonates with RDS [18–20,27–29], RSV [6,22], CDH [31,32], PIE [33,34], and those undergoing surgery for CHD [8,35–37]. The exception to this is BPD and apnea, which are discussed in separate sections later.

How to escalate NAVA

After NAVA ventilation has been initiated as described earlier, some neonates will continue to have increased work of breathing and require escalation in their ventilatory support. Table 15B.2 describes how to escalate NAVA in neonates with increased work of breathing using the Edi and blood gases.

Table 15B.1 Recommended initial settings for both NAVA and NIV NAVA in neonates

Parameter	Settings	Management
NAVA level (0–4 cmH$_2$O/mcV)	2.0 cmH$_2$O/mcV	Titrate to neonate's comfort and Edi peak 10–15 mcV: • If there is increased work of breathing and Edi peak >20 mcV, increase the NAVA level in 0.5 cmH$_2$O/mcV increments until the patient is comfortable and the Edi peaks are <15 mcV • If the patient is comfortable and the Edi peaks are <5 mcV, decrease the NAVA level in 0.5 cmH$_2$O/mcV increments until the Edi peak values are >5 mcV
Edi trigger (0–2 mcV)	0.5 mcV	Manufacturer default
Pressure alarm	30–40 cmH$_2$O	Set high enough to allow recruiting breaths Increase if peak pressure limited is consistently reached
Apnea time (2–20 s)	2 s	Set short enough so that the patient gets a rescue (backup) breath before any clinical decompensation noted.
Backup settings	PC 15–25 cmH$_2$O PS = PC PEEP 4–8 cmH$_2$O Rate 40–60 breaths/min IT 0.3–0.4 s	Adjust to maintain clinical stability when the neonate is apneic

IT, Inspiratory time; *PC*, pressure control; *PS*, pressure support (for invasive NAVA only).

Table 15B.2 Escalating NAVA and NIV/NAVA in neonates

Presentation	Issue	Solution
Edi peaks consistently >20 mcV and/or acidosis or hypercapnia	Mostly in backup ventilation	Increase backup rate Increase backup PIP Optimize caffeine
Edi peaks consistently >20 mcV and/or acidosis or hypercapnia	Mostly in NAVA ventilation	Increase NAVA level Decrease apnea time
Edi min >5 mcV	FiO$_2$ high	Increase PEEP by 1 cmH$_2$O

How to wean NAVA

Once the neonate has clinically improved, it is time to wean ventilatory support. As lung compliance increases, their respiratory drive will decrease as manifested by lower Edi and improved blood gases. The neonate autoweans by decreasing their respiratory drive (Edi), thereby spontaneously decreasing the delivered PIP and V_t. Table 15B.3 describes how to wean NAVA using the Edi and blood gases. Neonates with RDS will wean rapidly and ventilator changes can be made 2–3 times a day as tolerated. Most neonates, including those as premature as 23–24 weeks, can be extubated from NAVA to NIV NAVA successfully within the first 3 days. Seventy-four percent of neonates of 23–28 weeks were successfully extubated to NIV NAVA for a median of 8 days after which they were transitioned to CPAP [43].

Troubleshooting on NAVA

Some neonates will have periods of clinical instability and need adjustment of their ventilatory support. Table 15B.4 is a troubleshooting guide that will assist the bedside clinician to adjust the ventilatory support. Of importance is the need always to start with checking catheter position. Because premature neonates can be very small, it does not take much movement for the catheter to become malpositioned and thus results in loss of the Edi signal.

NAVA and BPD

In neonates with BPD, lung development that would have normally occurred in utero takes place postnatally under altered conditions, such as breathing with strain and stretch of immature intrathoracic structures. This results in areas of atelectasis, hyperinflation with multiple course densities, and fibrosis in addition to the development of abnormal pulmonary architecture [44].

When transitioning the neonate with BPD onto NAVA, initial NAVA follows the guidelines described earlier including determining the NAVA level using Edi peak values and the patient's clinical work of breathing [30].

Minimum respiratory rate should be set higher for these infants as the concern for apnea is not an issue in this older and neurologically more mature population. The apnea time can be set as long as 5 s to provide a minimum rate of 12 breaths/min.

The peak pressure alarm limit is one of the most critical settings in neonates with BPD on NAVA. Keep in mind that BPD lungs are stiff and fibrotic and will require much higher peak pressures to deliver appropriate V_t. During

Table 15B.3 Weaning NAVA and NIV NAVA in neonates

Presentation	Issue	Solution
Edi peaks <5 mcV and/or acceptable pCO$_2$ and pH	Mostly in NAVA	Decrease NAVA level by 0.5 cmH$_2$O/mcV until a level of 1 cmH$_2$O/mcV is reached: • If intubated, extubate to NIV NAVA • If on NIV NAVA, change to CPAP/HFNC
Edi peaks <5 mcV and/or acceptable pCO$_2$ and pH	Mostly in backup ventilation	Decrease NAVA level Decrease backup rate Decrease backup PIP Optimize caffeine
Edi min <2 mcV	Low FiO$_2$	Wean PEEP by 1 cmH$_2$O
Edi min >5 mcV	Clinically stable	No change

Table 15B.4 Troubleshooting NAVA and NIV NAVA in neonates

Presentation	Issue	Solution
Baby retracting and/or Edi peak >20 mcV and/or FiO$_2$ rising	Catheter malpositioned	Reposition catheter position
	Peak pressure limit alarming: Needs increased PIP to recruit lung	Increase pressure limit
	Increased WOB: Insufficient unloading to ventilator	Increase NAVA level
	In backup ventilation often: Insufficient back up support	Increase backup pressure
	Failing noninvasive support at maximum support	Intubate and place on invasive NAVA
FiO$_2$ rising and/or desaturations and/or Edi peak <5 mcV	Catheter malpositioned	Reposition and adjust catheter
Undersupported	Spontaneous breathing rate is low or periods of apnea	Apnea time set too long
	Trend Screen-switches to backup often and/or % time in backup high	Increase backup pressure and/or rate
	Failing noninvasive support at maximum support	Needs invasive ventilation
Oversupported	Low Edi peaks Low pCO$_2$	Decrease NAVA level
	High % of time in backup	Decrease backup pressure or rate
	Edi peaks low Spontaneous rate suppressed	
	Edi low or absent Excessive chest rise	

"BPD spells," the neonate with BPD demands high peak pressures and requires high pressure alarms as much as 60–100 cmH$_2$O. Typically starts with pressure limit of 40 cmH$_2$O and increases as needed until the neonate no longer triggers the pressure alarm.

Whether transitioning these patients to home ventilators or planning a weaning program for them, it behooves the care giver to acknowledge that this disease process did not happen overnight and will not resolve rapidly. These neonates need to repair and grow new lung as they are weaned from their ventilator support. Clinical experience suggests that, when weaning neonates with BPD using NAVA, the NAVA level needs to be decreased slowly and deliberately. Weaning occurs slowly with changes as small as 0.1 cmH$_2$O/mcV once or twice per week as tolerated. Careful attention needs to be paid to the neonate's work of breathing, clinical status, and Edi peaks during the weaning process.

NAVA and apnea

Severe and frequent apnea is a major challenge in premature neonates. Some neonates respond to CPAP, but many continue to have apnea severe enough to require NIV or even invasive support. Ideally, CPAP with backup could provide sufficient support when the neonate becomes apneic. However, this is not possible with current CPAP modes. A novel approach is to use NIV NAVA as CPAP [42,43]. The NAVA level is set at zero, and adequate backup support is provided for those periods of apnea. The neonate receives CPAP when there is an Edi signal present. However, when apneic for a predetermined amount of time (apnea time), backup ventilation begins and the neonate is ventilated with predetermined PIP and rate until an Edi signal returns. CPAP then resumes as long as spontaneous breathing is present. This allows sufficient support during episodes of apnea to prevent clinical decompensation.

Contraindications for NAVA

Contraindications for the use of NAVA are complete lack of respiratory drive or inability to place the NAVA nasogastric catheter. Any condition that severely impairs respiratory drive, including hypoxic ischemic encephalopathy or stroke affecting the respiratory center in the brainstem, overwhelming sepsis, and oversedation or paralysis, would result in absence of Edi and the neonate ventilating exclusively in backup. In these cases it is advisable to use conventional ventilation until the respiratory drive begins to return. Once the Edi is present, even intermittently, NAVA can be used. In this way, the ventilator supports any breathing the neonate does synchronously. The other limitation to the use of NAVA is the inability to place the NAVA catheter typically in conditions such as tracheal–esophageal fistula, recent upper airway surgery, esophageal perforation or surgery, abnormal esophagus, or known phrenic nerve lesions. The Edi catheter is not approved for use in the MRI environment, so it would need to be removed from the patient before entering the MRI area.

Conclusion

NAVA is the next step in personalizing ventilation for each neonate on a breath-by-breath basis. This chapter presented NAVA basics and described the essential concepts that make NAVA a unique ventilatory mode. No specific guidelines were offered for each type of neonatal respiratory disease or phase of disease process because the neonate now has the ability to customize their own ventilatory support based on biophysical and biochemical feedback that appears to be superior to what the clinician is able to provide.

Case 1

Two-day-old, 29-week gestation age with diagnosis of RDS. The infant received artificial surfactant (via Insure) and has been placed on NCPAP of 7 cmH$_2$O with FiO$_2$ of 35%. Infant has increasing oxygen requirements and shows clinical signs of increased work of breathing. An Edi catheter was placed to escalate to NIV NAVA. The infant remains tachypneic and the Edi signal does not correlate with the respiratory effort.

Trouble shooting

After examination of the Edi catheter positioning screen seen in Fig. 15B.4, it is noted that the EKG tracings decrease in size to the third tracing but the fourth tracing is large again. This is the typical finding for an Edi catheter that is coiled. Fig. 15B.5 labels the location of each lead and shows how the catheter loops in the stomach and goes back into the esophagus. The catheter will need to be removed and reinserted for correct placement. This will enable proceeding with correct use of NIV NAVA.

Lesson learned

If the neonate continues to have increased work of breathing despite appropriate NAVA settings, it is important to check catheter position prior to changing any ventilator settings. Correct placement of the catheter is essential for appropriate ventilation with NAVA.

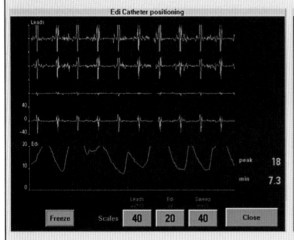

Fig. 15B.4 Edi Catheter Positioning Screen for Patient With RDS and Increased Work of Breathing.

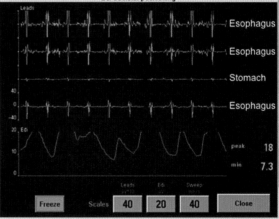

Fig. 15B.5 Labeled Leads Showing How the Edi Catheter Loops From the Esophagus into the Stomach (Third and Smallest Tracing) and Back into the Esophagus Again.

Case 2

Five-month-old with BPD and ventilator dependence with tracheostomy was recently placed on NAVA but had periods where she "would not do well" (consisting of tachypnea, increased work of breathing, and significant desaturations) and required volume ventilation to recover. Ventilator settings were NAVA level 1.5 cmH$_2$O/mcV, PEEP 5 cmH$_2$O, apnea time 4 s, pressure alarm 20 cmH$_2$O; backup settings: PC 25 cmH$_2$O, rate 35 bpm, IT 0.35 s.

Analyzing trends

Fig. 15B.6 shows the peak pressure (PIP) and respiratory rate (RR) trends. Seeing the pressure limit is set at 20 cmH$_2$O, the peak pressure average is 15 cmH$_2$O (5 cmH$_2$O below the pressure limit). The PIP (and V_t) were being limited, so the neonate compensated by increasing the RR to achieve adequate minute ventilation. The pressure limit was increased to 35 cmH$_2$O and, as seen in Fig. 15B.7, the average PIP increased (with increased V_t) and the RR rapidly decreased. Over the next 30 min, as seen on the screen in Fig. 15B.8, the PIP decreased to 10–15 cmH$_2$O with occasional periods of recruiting breaths. The RR remained within the normal range.

Lessons learned

Analyzing the trend screen allows evaluation of the neonate's response over time to interventions. It is important to set the pressure limit high enough to allow neonates to take recruiting breaths as need to maintain adequate lung volumes. This is especially important in neonates with BPD who have stiff, noncomplaint lungs and may need very high pressure limits to meet their respiratory demands.

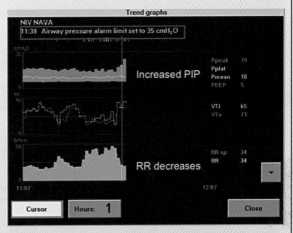

Fig. 15B.7 Increased PIP and Decreased RR Noted Within Minutes After Increasing the Pressure Limit to 35 cmH$_2$O.

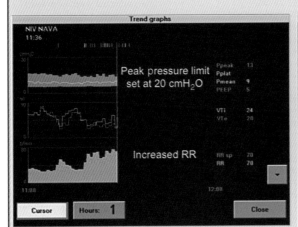

Fig. 15B.6 Trend Screen Showing the Respiratory Rate and the Peak Pressure With the Pressure Limit Set at 20 cmH$_2$O.

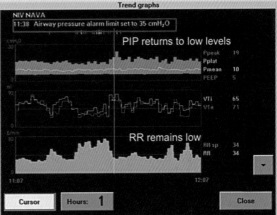

Fig. 15B.8 Mostly Low PIP With Occasional Recruiting Breaths and Continued Normal RR Over the Next 30 min.

Disclosure statement

Dr. Stein and Ms. Firestone are members of the Speakers Bureau for Maquet Getinge Group.

Box 15B.1

Synchronous for:
  Initiation, size, and termination of each breath even with ETT/NIV leaks
  Based on respiratory drive
Advantages:
  Lower PIP, V_t, and WOB
  Improved blood gases
  Improved COMFORT scores
  Lower sedation requirements

References

[1] Sinderby C, Navalesi P, Beck J, Skrobik Y, Comtois N, Friberg S, et al. Neural control of mechanical ventilation in respiratory failure. Nat Med 1999;5(12):1433–1436.

[2] Sinderby C, Spahija J, Beck J. Neurally-adjusted ventilatory assist. In: Vincent J-L, Slutsky AS, Brochard L, editors. Mechanical ventilation. Update in intensive care medicine. 1st ed. Heidelberg: Springer; 2005. p. 125–134.

[3] Emeriaud G, Beck J, Tucci M, Lacroix J, Sinderby C. Diaphragm electrical activity during expiration in mechanically ventilated infants. Pediatr Res 2006;59(5):705–710.

[4] Stein H, Hall R, Davis K, White DB. Electrical activity of the diaphragm (Edi) values and Edi catheter placement in non-ventilated preterm neonates. J Perinatol 2013;33(9):707–711.

[5] Stein HM, Wilmoth J, Burton J. Electrical activity of the diaphragm in a small cohort of term neonates. Resp Care 2012;57(9):1483–1487.

[6] Clement K, Thurman T, Holt S, Heulitt M. Neurally triggered breaths reduce trigger delay and improve ventilator response times in ventilated infants with bronchiolitis. Intensive Care Med 2011;37(11):1826–1832.

[7] Bengtsson JA, Edberg KE. Neurally adjusted ventilatory assist in children: an observational study. Pediatr Crit Care Med 2010;11:253–257.

[8] Zhu L, Shi Z, Ji G, Xu Z, Zheng J, Xu Z, et al. [Application of neurally adjusted ventilatory assist in infants who underwent cardiac surgery for congenital heart disease].

Zhongguo Dang Dai Er Ke Za Zhi 2009;11(6):433–436.

[9] de la Oliva P, Schüffelmann C, Gómez-Zamora A, Villa J, Kacmarek RM. Asynchrony, neural drive, ventilatory variability and COMFORT: NAVA versus pressure support in pediatric patients. A non-randomized cross-over trial. Intensive Care Med 2012;38(5):838–846.

[10] Alander M, Peltoniemi O, Pokka T, Kontiokari T. Comparison of pressure-, flow-, and NAVA-triggering in pediatric and neonatal ventilatory care. Pediatr Pulmonol 2012;47:76–83.

[11] Vignaux L, Grazioli S, Piquilloud L, Bochaton N, Karam O, Jaecklin T, et al. Optimizing patient-ventilator synchrony during invasive ventilator assist in children and infants remains a difficult task. Pediatr Crit Care Med 2013;14(7):e316–e325.

[12] Breatnach C, Conlon NP, Stack M, Healy M, O'Hare BP. A prospective crossover comparison of neurally adjusted ventilatory assist and pressure-support ventilation in a pediatric and neonatal intensive care unit population. Pediatr Crit Care Med 2010;11(1):7–11.

[13] Bordessoule A, Emeriaud G, Morneau S, Jouvet P, Beck J. Neurally adjusted venitlatory assist (NAVA) improves patient-ventilator interaction in infants compared to conventional ventilation. Pediatr Res 2012;72(2):194–202.

[14] Longhini F, Ferrero F, De Luca D, Cosi G, Alemani M, Colombo D, et al. Neurally adjusted ventilatory assist in preterm neonates with acute respiratory failure. Neonatology 2014;107(1):60–67.

[15] Beck J, Reilly M, Grasselli G, Mirabella L, Slutsky AS, Dunn MS, et al. Patient-ventilator interaction during neurally adjusted ventilatory assist in low birth weight infants. Pediatr Res 2009;65(6):663–668.

[16] Duyndam A, Bol B, Kroon A, Tibboel D, Ista E. Neurally adjusted ventilatory assist: assessing the comfort and feasibility of use in neonates and children. Nursing in Critical Care 2013;18(2):86–92.

[17] Piastra M, De Luca D, Costa R, Pizza A, De Sanctis R, Marzano L, et al. Neurally adjusted ventilatory assist vs pressure support ventilation in infants recovering from severe acute respiratory distress syndrome: nested study. J Crit Care 2014;29(2). 312. e1–315.e1.

[18] Lee J, Kim H, Sohn J, Choi C, Kim E, Kim B, et al. Randomized crossover study of neurally adjusted ventilatory assist in preterm infants. J Pediatr 2012;161(5):808–813.

[19] Stein HM, Alosh H, Ethington P, White DB. Prospective crossover comparison between NAVA and pressure control ventilation in premature neonates less than 1500 grams. J Perinatol 2013;33(6):452–456.

[20] Stein HM, Howard D. Neurally adjusted ventilatory assist (NAVA) in neonates less than 1500 grams: a retrospective analysis. J Pediatr 2012;160(5):786–789.

[21] Kallio M, Peltoniemi O, Anttila E, Pokka T, Kontiokari T. Neurally adjusted ventilatory assist (NAVA) in pediatric intensive care—a randomized controlled trial. Pediatr Pulmonol 2015;50(1):55–62.

[22] Liet J, Dejode J, Joram N, Gaillard-LeRouz B, Roze J. Respiratory support by neurally adjusted ventilatory assist (NAVA) in severe RSV-related bronchiolitis: a case series report. BMC Pediatr 2011;11:92.

[23] Gentili A, Masciopinto F, Mondardini M, Ansaloni S, Reggiani M, Baroncini S. Neurally adjusted ventilatory assist in weaning of neonates affected by congenital diaphragmatic hernia. Matern Fetal Neonatal Med 2013;26(6):598–602.

[24] Firestone KS, Fisher S, Reddy S, White DB, Stein H. Effect of changing NAVA levels on peak inspiratory pressures and electrical activity of the diaphragm in premature neonates. J Perinatol 2015;35(8):612–616.

[25] Lee J, Kim H, Jung Y, Shin S, Choi C, Kim E, et al. Non-invasive neurally adjusted ventilatory assist in preterm infants: a randomised phase II crossover trial. Arch Dis Child Fetal Neonatal Ed 2015;100(6):F507–F513.

[26] Rahmani A, Imran A, Boats U, Chedid F, Woodworth S, Kahn J. Can utilizing neurally adjusted ventilatory assist in the ventilation support of critically ill neonates results in shorter hospital stay? J Clin Neonatol 2015;4(1):32–37.

[27] Chen Z, Luo F, Ma X, Lin H, Shi L, Du L. Application of neurally adjusted ventilatory assist in preterm infants with respiratory distress syndrome. Zhongguo Dang Dai Er Ke Za Zhi 2013;15(9):709–712.

[28] Longhini F, Ferrero F, De Luca D, Cosi G, Alemani M, Colombo D, et al. Neurally adjusted ventilatory assist in preterm neonates with acute respiratory failure. Neonatology 2015;107(1):60–67.

[29] Stein HM. NAVA ventilation allows for patient determination of peak pressures facilitating weaning in response to improving lung compliance during respiratory distress syndrome: a case report. Neonatol Today 2010;5(7):1–4.

[30] Jung Y, Kim H, Lee J, Shin S, Kim E, Choi J. Neurally adjusted ventilatory assist in preterm infants with established or evolving bronchopulmonary dysplasia on high-intensity mechanical ventilatory support: a single-center experience. Pediatr Crit Care Med 2016;17(12):1142–1146.

[31] Durrani N, Chedid F, Rahmani A. Neurally adjusted ventilatory assist mode used in congenital diaphragmatic hernia. J Coll Physicians Surg Pak 2011;21(10):637–639.

[32] Oda A, Lehtonen L, Soukka H. Neurally adjusted ventilatory assist can be used to wean infants with congenital diaphragmatic hernias off respiratory support. Acta Paediatr Rev Bras Ter Intensiva 2017;29(4):408–413.

[33] Lee S. Application of selective bronchial intubation versus neurally adjusted ventilatory assist in the management of unilateral pulmonary interstitial emphysema: an illustrative case and the literature review. AJP Rep 2017;7(2):e101–e105.

[34] Lee S, Shek C. Resolution of pulmonary interstitial emphysema in two neonates: why does NAVA work? J Clin Neonatol 2015;4(2):115–118.

[35] Houtekie L, Moerman D, Bourleau A, Reychler G, Dataille T, Derycke E, et al. Feasibility study on neurally adjusted ventilatory assist in noninvasive ventilation after cardiac surgery in infants. Resp Care 2015;60(7):1007–1014.

[36] Zhu L, Xu Z, Gong X, Zheng J, Sun Y, Liu L, et al. Mechanical ventilation after bidirectional superior cavopulmonary anastomosis for single-ventricle physiology: a comparison of pressure support ventilation and neurally adjusted ventilatory assist. Pediatr Cardiol 2016;37(6):1064–1071.

[37] Crulli B, Khebir M, Toledano B, Vobecky S, Poirier N, Emeriaud G. Neurally adjusted ventilatory assist after pediatric cardiac surgery: clinical experience and impact on ventilation pressures. Resp Care 2018;63(2):208–214.

[38] Sinclair R, Teng A, Jonas C, Schindler T. Congenital central hypoventilation syndrome: a pictorial demonstration of absent electrical diaphragmatic activity using non-invasive neurally adjusted ventilatory assist. J Paediatr Child Health 2018;54(2):200–202.

[39] Stein HM, Firestone KS. Nava ventilation in neonates: clinical guidelines and management strategies. Neonatol Today 2012;7(4):1–8.

[40] Loverde B, Firestone KS, Stein H. Comparing changing neurally adjusted ventilatory assist (NAVA) levels in intubated and recently extubated neonates. J Perinatol 2016;36(12):1097–1100.

[41] Stokowski LA. A primer on apnea of prematurity. Adv Neonatal Care 2005;5(3):155–170.

[42] Firestone KS, Beck J, Stein H. Neurally adjusted ventilatory assist for non-invasive support in neonates. Clin Perinatol 2016;43(4):707–724.

[43] Stein H, Beck J, Dunn M. Non-invasive ventilation with neurally adjusted ventilatory assist in newborns. Semin Fetal Neonatal Medicine 2016;21(3):154–161.

[44] Jobe AH, Bancalari E. Bronchopulmonary dysplasia. Am J Respir Crit Care Med 2001;163(7):1723–1729.

Chapter | **16** |

Volume-Targeted and Volume-Controlled Ventilation

Martin Keszler, MD

CHAPTER POINTS

- Excessive volume, not pressure is the key element in ventilator-associated lung injury
- Volume-targeted ventilation reduces lung and brain injury and leads to faster weaning from mechanical ventilation
- Adequate lung volume recruitment is essential to ensure even distribution of tidal volume into an open lung
- One size DOES NOT fit all. Correct tidal volume target depends on patient size, postnatal age and nature of lung disease

Pressure-controlled (PC) ventilation has been the standard approach to mechanical ventilation of newborn infants for more than 40 years because early attempts at volume-controlled ventilation in small preterm neonates were disappointing. The advantages of PC ventilation are the ability to directly control the inflation pressure and time (Fig. 16.1), and to ventilate despite large leaks around the standard uncuffed endotracheal tubes (ETT—Fig. 16.2). The conviction that high inflation pressure is the chief culprit in ventilator-associated lung injury and air leak is the basis of the deeply ingrained "barophobia" that has persisted despite growing evidence that excessive tissue stretch, not pressure, is the culprit (Fig. 16.3). The evidence from preclinical and clinical studies indicates clear benefits of volume-targeted modes of ventilation, but the acceptance of this approach into clinical practice has been uneven, despite strong evidence of benefit.

Rationale for volume-targeted ventilation

A series of animal studies clearly demonstrated that tidal volume (V_t), rather than inflation pressure, is the most important element in ventilator-associated lung injury. Severe acute lung injury occurred in animals ventilated with large V_t, regardless of whether that volume was generated by a high or low inflation pressure [1]. In contrast, animals whose chest wall and diaphragmatic excursion were limited by external binding experienced much less lung damage despite being exposed to the same high inflation pressure [1,2]. Pressure, without correspondingly high V_t, is not by itself injurious to the lungs, although it likely is injurious to immature airways.

The large number of clinical studies documenting both hypercapnia and hypocapnia associated with neonatal brain injury are an equally compelling reason for attempting to control V_t [3–6]. Despite increasing awareness of its adverse consequences, inadvertent hyperventilation remains a common problem with PC ventilation, especially in the first hours after birth when lung compliance changes most rapidly.

A systematic review by Peng et al. [7] and an updated Cochrane meta-analysis [8] that included a combination

Pressure control   Volume control

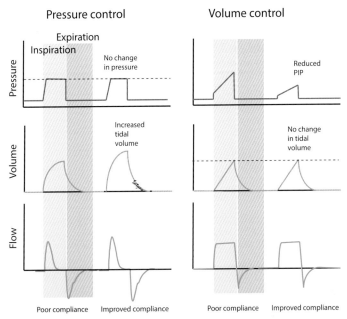

Fig. 16.1 Differences Between Pressure-Controlled and Volume-Controlled Ventilation. The *yellow shade* represents inspiration and *purple shade* represents exhalation. The first waveform in each category reflects low compliance state (such as before surfactant) and the second waveform is representative of improved compliance (such as after surfactant administration). With pressure control, improved compliance results in higher tidal volume increasing the risk of hypocarbia, volutrauma, and tissue injury. With volume control, improved compliance results in lower PIP and the same tidal volume minimizing the risk of tissue injury. Copyright: Satyan Lakshminrusimha.

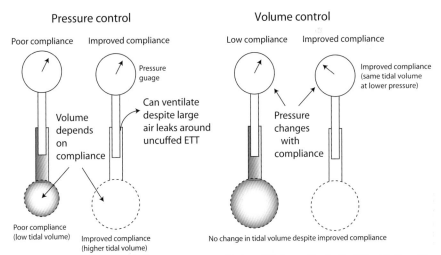

Fig. 16.2 Advantages and Disadvantages of Pressure-Controlled and Volume-Controlled Ventilation. Please refer to text for details.

of several different modalities of volume-controlled (VC) and volume-targeted ventilation (VTV) documented a number of advantages when compared to PC ventilation, including increased survival free of bronchopulmonary dysplasia (BPD), decreased air leak, lower rate of neuroimaging abnormalities, and shorter duration of ventilation (Table 16.1). However, it should be noted that these studies focused on short-term physiologic outcomes, rather than BPD as a primary outcome, and with the exception of one follow-up study based on parental questionnaire, no long-term pulmonary or developmental outcomes have been reported.

Table 16.1 Benefits of VTV/VC ventilation

	Relative risk or mean difference	95% CI	NNTB (95% CI)
Death or BPD at 36-week PMA	0.75	0.53–1.07	NA
BPD at 36-week PMA	0.73	0.59–0.89	8 (5–20)
Grade 3–4 IVH	0.53	0.37–0.77	11 (7–25)
PVL ± severe IVH	0.47	0.27–0.80	11 (7–33)
Pneumothorax	0.52	0.31–0.87	20 (11–100)
Hypocapnia	0.49	0.33–0.72	3 (2–5)
Days of mechanical ventilation	−1.35	−1.83 to −0.86	

BPD, Bronchopulmonary dysplasia; *CI*, confidence interval; *IVH*, intraventricular hemorrhage; *NNTB*, number needed to benefit; *PMA*, postmenstrual age; *PVL*, periventricular leukomalacia; *VC*, volume-controlled ventilation; *VTV*, volume-targeted ventilation. Data from Klingenberg C, Wheeler KI, McCallion N, Morley CJ, Davis PG. Volume-targeted versus pressure-limited ventilation in neonates. Cochrane Database Syst Rev 2017;10:CD003666 [8].

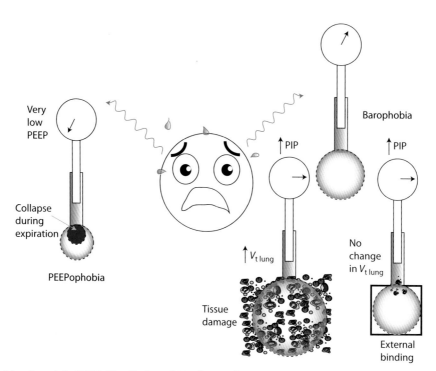

Fig. 16.3 Phobias Associated With Ventilation of Newborn Infants. "PEEPophobia" refers to the use of very low PEEP leading to collapse of the alveoli during expiration. "Barophobia" refers to the use of low PIP to avoid delivering increased pressure to the alveolus. Evidence suggests that increased tidal volume leads to tissue damage and inflammation (volutrauma) and that alveolar damage is not directly due to increased pressure. If external binding is provided to limit lung volume, increased pressure alone without does not increase tissue injury in the absence of high tidal volume. Copyright: Satyan Lakshminrusimha.

Volume-controlled versus volume-targeted ventilation

Many authors refer to all modalities that attempt to control V_t delivered into the lungs as VTV, failing to distinguish between VC ventilation of the "adult" type (VC) and volume-targeted modalities (VTV) that are specifically designed for ventilating extremely low birth weight (ELBW) infants. The term VTV should be limited to PC modalities of ventilation with automatic adjustment of inflation pressure to target a user-set V_t [9]. Thus, VTV is fundamentally different from VC modes of ventilation that are widely used in adult and pediatric applications. In VC ventilation (also known as volume-cycled ventilation), a user-set volume of gas (V_{set}) is introduced into the ventilator end of the patient circuit. Circuit pressure rises passively, in inverse proportion to lung compliance, reaching its peak just before exhalation. In larger patients with cuffed ETT, there is a close correlation between the V_{set} and the V_t that reaches the patients' lungs (V_{del}). In ELBW infants whose lung volume is only a fraction of the volume of the circuit and humidifier, much of the V_{set} is lost to compression of gas in the circuit and leak around uncuffed ETT. Thus, a substantially higher V_{set} must be used, often around 10–12 mL/kg, compared to what would be used with VTV in order to deliver a physiologic V_{del} of 4–5 mL/kg (Fig. 16.4). Because ETT leak fluctuates with head position and the degree of volume loss to compression varies with inflation pressure, the relationship between V_{set} and V_{del} is not constant. Most modern ventilators have provisions to compensate for circuit compliance/gas compression in the circuit, but this ability breaks down with the ubiquitous and highly variable leak around uncuffed ETTs. Some of these limitations can be overcome by using a flow sensor at the airway opening to monitor exhaled V_t, allowing the operator to manually adjust the V_{set} to achieve the desired V_{del}. Because the ETT leak is usually variable, frequent monitoring and adjustment are necessary, making this approach less attractive. An alternate approach is to rely on clinical assessment of chest rise and breath sounds to set the V_{set}, and to make subsequent adjustments based on blood gas measurement. Despite these limitations, VC has been shown to be feasible, at least under research conditions, even in small preterm infants when a flow sensor at the airway opening [10].

How does VTV work?

Several varieties of VTV were developed specifically to address the limitations of VC ventilation when applied to ELBW infants. Volume Guarantee (VG) on the Babylog 8000+ and VN 500 ventilators (Draeger Medical GmbH, Lubeck, Germany) is the most extensively studied VTV modality, and

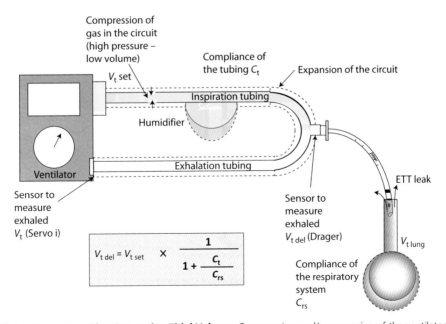

Fig. 16.4 Ventilator Parameters That Determine Tidal Volume. Compression and/or expansion of the ventilator tubing, endotracheal tube (ETT) leak play an important role in determining the delivered tidal volume ($V_{t\,set}$). $V_{t\,del}$ is the delivered tidal volume. Copyright: Satyan Lakshminrusimha.

Table 16.2 Recommended initial V_t settings for VTV

Condition	Initial V_t (mL/kg)	Rationale	References
Term, late preterm, normal lungs	4–4.5	Baseline	Dawson et al. [14]
Preterm RDS, 1250–2500 g	4–4.5	Low alveolar dead space	Dawson et al. [14]
Preterm RDS, 700–1249 g	4.5–5	Dead space of the flow sensor	Nassabeh-Montazami et al. [15]
Preterm RDS, <700 g	5.5–6	Dead space of the flow sensor	Nassabeh-Montazami et al. [15]
Preterm evolving BPD, 3 weeks old	5.5–6.5	Increased anatomical and alveolar dead space	Keszler et al. [16]
Term MAS with classic CXR*	5.5–6	Increased alveolar dead space	Sharma et al. [17]
Term MAS with whiteout CXR	4.5–5	Alveolar dead space less of a problem	Keszler [18]
Term CDH	4–4.5	Normal CO_2 production requires normal alveolar minute ventilation	Sharma et al. [19]
Established severe BPD	7–12	Greatly increased alveolar and anatomical dead space; lower respiratory rate due to long time constants needs larger V_t	Abman et al. [20]

Individual patients may need slightly smaller or larger V_t. The assumption is the V_t that is measured at the airway opening and VTV is used with assist/control or pressure support ventilation, except in the established severe BPD where synchronized intermittent mandatory ventilation is assumed. Typical anatomical dead space is 2 mL/kg. Flow sensor adds between 0.7 and 1.2 mL of dead space (absolute), depending on the type used. This added dead space becomes progressively more impactful as the infant's size decreases. Conditions like bronchopulmonary dysplasia and meconium aspiration syndrome with hyperinflation/heterogeneous inflation increase alveolar dead space and therefore also require large V_t in order to achieve equivalent alveolar minute ventilation. Some infants with meconium aspiration have less heterogeneity and more surfactant inactivation and behave more like infants with respiratory distress syndrome.

BPD, Bronchopulmonary dysplasia; *CDH*, congenital diaphragmatic hernia; *CXR*, chest radiograph; *MAS*, meconium aspiration syndrome; *RDS*, respiratory distress syndrome.
*Classic CXR in MAS shows heterogeneous inflation and air trapping.

malposition, or abdominal distention (see Table 16.4 for specific recommendations).

When to increase V_t?

Respiratory acidosis is an obvious reason for increasing the V_t target. However, ventilator settings should never be based on blood gas measurement alone; acceptable blood gas is not synonymous with adequate support. Persistence of tachypnea and retractions indicate inadequate support and a need for a larger V_t, especially when coupled with relatively low PIP and measured V_t that exceeds the target V_t. When a baby is in distress and "fighting the ventilator," some clinicians mistakenly administer sedatives. This action only masks the symptoms of inadequate respiratory support and prolongs ventilator dependence. The appropriate response is to make necessary ventilator adjustments to allow the infant to relax and work in synchrony with the ventilator. When the set V_t is substantially below the baby's true need, the PIP may drop

down to the level of PEEP. This is because, as long as the patient is able to generate spontaneously a V_t that exceeds the V_t target, the microprocessor will continue to drop the PIP as per the aforementioned algorithm. With time, the baby can no longer sustain the effort and becomes apneic. The ventilator will take over at the set backup rate and the PIP returns to whatever is needed to reach target V_t. With rising PCO_2 and falling pH, the infant will again begin to respond to his/her respiratory drive and attempt to normalize the pH. It is important to recognize that pH, not PCO_2, is the primary driver of respiratory control; the response to metabolic acidosis is hyperventilation and thus PCO_2 values need to be interpreted in the context of pH. ELBW infants with immature renal tubular function and high protein intake tend to have a moderate base deficit in the first few days of life and thus need a relatively lower PCO_2 target to maintain a good pH and avoid excessively high work of breathing and loss of lung volume recruitment when the PIP falls intermittently to or near the level of PEEP.

Table 16.3 Guidelines to initiation of VTV

Recommendation	Rationale
• Start VTV as soon as possible after intubation • Select A/C or PSV as basic mode • If using SIMV + PSV, know that only the SIMV inflations are volume-targeted • Select backup rate about 10/min below spontaneous breathing rate: 30/min for term, 40/min for preterm infants • Select inspiratory time appropriate for the patient's size and diagnosis. Typically, 0.25–0.3 s for <1000 g, <28-week GA infant with RDS; 0.3–0.35 for larger preterm infants with RDS; 0.35–0.5 for infants with evolving BPD; and 0.5–0.6 s for large infants with MAS or established severe BPD • Verify appropriateness of inspiratory time setting by observing flow waveform. Ensure that inspiratory flow is completed before the ventilator cycles off and there is no excessive gap between completion of inspiration and onset of expiration • Select PEEP appropriate to the infant's diagnosis, current condition, and FiO_2 • Optimize lung recruitment to ensure even distribution of V_t • Ensure that flow sensor is calibrated and functioning properly • Select target V_t (refer to Table 16.3) • Set PIP limit 3–5 cmH_2O above expected PIP need • If V_t target not met, ensure ETT is in good position, then increase PIP limit, if needed • Observe chest rise, auscultate breath sounds, assess respiratory rate and retractions, monitor SPO_2, and adjust V_t target as needed • If converting from PC to VTV, match the V_t generated by PC mode if $PaCO_2$ was satisfactory and increase PIP limit by 3–5 cmH_2O	• Compliance and respiratory effort change rapidly with surfactant administration, lung volume recruitment • More stable and smaller V_t, lower work of breathing • The PSV pressure is a set value, not subject to volume-targeting • Backup rate is a safety net in case of apnea. Low rate causes larger fluctuation in SPO_2 and minute ventilation; if too high, there will be more untriggered inflations [21] • Appropriate inspiratory time is based on the time constants of the respiratory system (product of compliance and resistance). ELBW infants with RDS have short time constants; large infants with high airway resistance have long time constants • The suggested values for inspiratory time are averages; individual infants may need longer or shorter times. Flow waveform interpretation indicates if settings are correct for the specific baby • PEEP should always be individualized. Because VTV uses lowest possible PIP, sufficient PEEP is essential to maintain FRC • Controlling delivered V_t is not sufficient to prevent lung injury. Lung volume recruitment ensures its even distribution • Accurate V_t measurement is essential for safe and effective VTV • V_t is now the primary control variable • This allows adjustment of working pressure both up and down • ETT in the main stem bronchus or obstructed on carina would lead to high PIP/volutrauma • Recommended V_t targets are population means; individual patients may need higher or lower V_t • Changing primary control variable does not affect relationship between compliance, PIP, and V_t. Allow PIP to float both up and down as needed. Average PIP will be lower than with pressure-controlled ventilation

A/C, Assist/control; *ETT*, endotracheal tube; *FRC*, functional residual capacity; *PEEP*, positive end-expiratory pressure; *PIP*, peak inflation pressure; *PSV*, pressure support ventilation; *SIMV*, synchronized intermittent mandatory ventilation; *SPO₂*, arterial oxygen saturation by pulse oximetry; *V*$_t$, tidal volume; *VTV*, volume-targeted ventilation.

When to lower V_t?

The set V_t may be too high when a baby who was previously breathing spontaneously becomes apneic some minutes after initiation of VTV. Unless there is another explanation, such as respiratory depression from medications given for intubation, lowering the V_t target is indicated, even before a blood gas is obtained. V_t should also be weaned if the blood gas shows normal (>7.36) or alkalotic pH and the infant does not consistently breathe above the backup rate.

Weaning from VTV

Automatic lowering of PIP in response to improved lung compliance and greater spontaneous respiratory effort makes VTV a self-weaning modality. Weaning occurs in real time, rather than intermittently in response to blood gases and thus results in shorter duration of mechanical ventilation. This effective closed-loop system is counterintuitive to some clinicians who are accustomed to manual adjustments of ventilator settings and they want to decrease the

Table 16.4 Guidelines for subsequent adjustment of VTV

Recommendation	Explanation
• Assess chest rise, breath sounds, respiratory rate and retractions, PIP and SPO_2; adjust V_t target as needed before obtaining initial blood gas	• Recommended V_t targets are population means; individual patients may need higher or lower V_t. Good clinical assessment avoids need for extra blood gases
• Once working PIP range is known, set PIP limit 25%–30% above upper end of the range	• Important safety feature that signals change in compliance or patient effort
• Document range of working PIP, not just PIP limit	• PIP limit does not accurately reflect actual level of support
• If indicated, adjust V_t by 0.3–0.5 mL/kg	• This is about 10% change in most cases
• Consider both pH and $PaCO_2$; do not lower V_t target if pH is not alkalotic and accept higher PCO_2 if pH is OK	• pH, not $PaCO_2$, is the primary control of respiratory drive. Infants compensate for a base deficit by hyperventilating
• Adjust PIP limit as needed to keep it 25%–30% above upper end of the range of PIP	• As compliance and respiratory effort improve, working PIP comes down
• Always assess patient's respiratory rate, comfort, oxygen requirement, and working pressure when considering ventilator change. Increase V_t if necessary to achieve adequate support	• Tachypnea and retractions indicate increased work of breathing. If V_t is set too low, the ventilator lowers the PIP and the infant has to work harder to maintain their minute ventilation
• Adjust PEEP as needed to maintain lung volume	• Ensure adequate distending pressure to keep lungs open
• Always verify appropriateness of support by clinical assessment, especially if large increase in support appears to be needed or blood gas is not consistent with settings	• Machines are fallible. Do not blindly trust any mechanical device. Have a low threshold to recalibrate flow sensor
• Base V_t on birth weight in first week. Remember to adjust for weight gain if the baby remains ventilated	• Short-term changes in weight after birth reflect fluid shifts. Once baby starts to grow, the V_t needs to keep up with current weight

PEEP, Positive end-expiratory pressure; *PIP*, peak inflation pressure; *SPO₂*, arterial oxygen saturation by pulse oximetry; *V_t*, tidal volume.

target V_t in an effort to wean the patient off the ventilator. This is not appropriate because the physiologic V_t required by the patient does not decrease (over time it may actually increase); what goes down is the pressure required to achieve that V_t because of improved compliance of the respiratory system and the infant breathing more effectively. Decreasing V_t target below the patient's physiologic need will increase the work of breathing [22] and may delay successful extubation. It is essential to make sure the V_t target is not excessive and that the infant has a pH low enough to stimulate a good respiratory drive (<7.35). When working pressure is consistently <12 to 15 cmH$_2$O (higher in larger infants), FiO$_2$ is <0.30, and the infant is breathing comfortably without retractions or tachypnea, extubation to non-invasive support is indicated (see Table 16.5 for details).

Caveats, pitfalls, and troubleshooting

An important issue in the use of VTV is ETT leak, which is present to some degree in most intubated ELBW infants and tends to increase with time as the trachea and larynx stretch due to positive pressure ventilation (acquired tracheomegaly) [23] and as the infant grows. While the exhaled V_t is less subject to leak-related underestimation of V_t, when the leak exceeds about 40%, it begins to substantially affect accuracy of V_t measurement, potentially resulting in inadvertent hypocapnia. The reason for this is that some of the gas that entered the lungs escapes around the ETT during the expiratory phase (more when higher PEEP is used) and thus is not measured by the flow sensor as exhaled V_t. The ventilator will detect a below-target V_t and increase working pressure to achieve a larger V_t. Thus, many VTV devices cannot be safely used when the ETT leak approaches this limit. The choice then is to replace the ETT electively to eliminate the leak, or to abandon VTV in favor of PC ventilation, which is not affected by ETT leak. Some of the newest specialty infant ventilators have the ability to calculate an estimated value for the true V_t even in the face of a very large leak, thus avoiding this common problem. Understanding the capabilities of the ventilator being used is therefore crucial to optimal care.

The relationship between lung compliance, PIP, and V_t is the same, whether the PIP is adjusted manually or automatically. Some clinicians are reluctant to "increase PIP" when changing to VTV. It is important to understand that the ventilator must be able to adjust PIP both up and down in order to maintain target V_t. On average, the PIP is same or lower with VTV, compared to PC [24], but when the patient fails to breathe or the lung compliance deteriorates, higher PIP may be needed. Given that volume, not pressure is the key to lung injury, this should not cause alarm. Documentation must include actual working pressure, not just the PIP limit.

Table 16.5 Weaning and extubation

Recommendation	Explanation
• Ensure that pH is <7.35, to provide respiratory drive. Weaning is automatic; do not lower target V_t, unless patient is alkalotic • Withhold/reduce sedation/analgesia if used • Do not reduce V_t below 3.5–4 mL/kg • Consider raising PEEP to maintain adequate distending pressure as PIP comes down • Avoid using SIMV without PSV; do not wean backup rate on A/C or PSV • Observe the graphic display to detect excessive periodic breathing or apnea • Consider extubation if PIP is <12 to 15 cmH$_2$O with satisfactory blood gas, low FiO$_2$, absence of tachypnea/retractions • Readiness for extubation can be assessed using the spontaneous breathing test (SBT) • If not given earlier, caffeine should always be used prior to extubation of preterm infants <32 weeks • Distending pressure with CPAP, NIPPV, or HHHFNC should always be used for at least 24 h postextubation	• Physiologic V_t does not decrease, the PIP needed to achieve it does—self-weaning • Avoid suppressing the respiratory drive • Setting the V_t below what the infant needs imposes excessive WOB • Automatic lowering of PIP may lead to atelectasis if PEEP is relatively low • As PIP comes down, the WOB is gradually shifted from ventilator to infant. The infant controls the ventilator rate • Inconsistent respiratory effort may set up the infant for extubation failure • These pressures are sufficiently low so that most infants are able to take over • The SBT has been shown to accurately predict extubation readiness • Caffeine reduces extubation failure in preterm infants • The use of distending airway pressure after extubation reduces the risk of extubation failure

A/C, Assist/control; *CPAP*, continuous positive airway pressure; *ETT*, endotracheal tube; *FRC*, functional residual capacity; *HHHFNC*, high-humidity, high-flow nasal cannula; *NIPPV*, nasal intermittent positive pressure ventilation; *PEEP*, positive end-expiratory pressure; *PIP*, peak inflation pressure; *PSV*, pressure support ventilation; *SIMV*, synchronized intermittent mandatory ventilation; *SPO$_2$*, arterial oxygen saturation by pulse oximetry; *V$_t$*, tidal volume; *WOB*, work of breathing.

The most common complaint when using VTV is that there are more alarms. VTV is an interactive mode that provides the clinician with valuable feedback. When the V_t target cannot be met with the set PIP limit, the clinician needs to make an assessment of the cause of this change. Excessive alarms can be avoided by setting the PIP limit high enough (~25% above usual working pressure) and setting the alarm delay at maximum; failure to meet V_t for a brief period is not a problem, but if the situation persists, an assessment for any change in ETT position, abdominal distention, and asymmetry of breath sounds must be made. Large leak around ETT that has become too small due to stretching of the immature tissue of the larynx and trachea is a common and correctable source of annoying alarms. The remedy, as suggested earlier, is to reintubate with an appropriate-sized ETT. Subglottic stenosis does not result from the use of appropriately fitting ETT that is inserted easily. There is no evidence from the modern era that a large leak around ETT is beneficial in preventing subglottic stenosis (see Table 16.6 for trouble-shooting suggestions).

Table 16.6 Troubleshooting

Concern	Additional information	Possible explanation	Action
Tachypnea/retractions	PIP is low, occasionally at PEEP, increasing FiO$_2$, pH normal or low, normal V_t	V_t set too low, failure to adjust for weight gain	Reassess V_t target
PIP is too low (near PEEP)	Baby is tachypneic, retracting, normal V_t pH normal or low, rising FiO$_2$	V_t set too low, failure to adjust for weight gain	Reassess V_t target
PIP is too low (near PEEP)	Baby is comfortable, normal RR, low FiO$_2$	Baby is ready to extubate	Extubate

Table 16.6 Troubleshooting (*cont.*)

Concern	Additional information	Possible explanation	Action
PIP is low, not increasing	Baby in distress, falling FiO_2, low or absent V_t	ETT obstruction; some devices drop PIP when complete obstruction is noted	Clear obstruction
PCO_2 is too low	Patient not breathing, pH >7.4	V_t set too high, large ETT leak, flow sensor malfunction	Reassess V_t target, advance ETT if high, Calibrate flow sensor, reintubate with larger ETT if leak is > 40%
PCO_2 is too low	Patient breathing actively, pH >7.4, distorted loops	Agitation, pain, excessive noise, discomfort	Provide better positioning, nesting, sedate if necessary
PCO_2 is too low	pH <7.35, BE −3 or more, patient breathing actively	Infant is compensating for metabolic acidosis	Accept normal physiology, correct acidosis as needed
PCO_2 is too high	pH <7.3, patient tachypneic, fluctuating PIP, occasional low V_t alarm	Inadequate V_t, air trapping, PIP limit too low, increased CO_2 production	Reassess V_t target, evaluate ETT position (CXR), abdominal exam, increase PIP limit
PCO_2 is too high	pH <7.3, patient apneic	Inadequate V_t + sepsis/oversedation	Increase V_t target, evaluate patient's condition
PCO_2 is too high	pH is normal, patient comfortable	Metabolic alkalosis (e.g., diuretics)	Correct underlying cause
PIP is higher than expected	Poor gas exchange, high FiO_2, patient is breathing actively, V_t target is not reached, low V_t alarm sounding	ETT in main stem bronchus, ETT obstructed on carina, atelectasis, pneumothorax, abdominal distention	Evaluate ETT position, rule out pneumothorax, atelectasis, evaluate abdomen, address underlying condition; increase PIP limit in the meantime
Low V_t alarm	Worsening gas exchange, patient breathing actively	Indicates worsening compliance; causes as earlier	As earlier
Low V_t alarm	Patient apneic	Oversedation, sepsis	Reassess need for sedation and dose, evaluate for sepsis, increase PIP limit

BE, Base excess; *ETT*, endotracheal tube; *PEEP*, positive end-expiratory pressure; *PIP*, peak inflation pressure; *RR*, respiratory rate; V_t, tidal volume.

References

[1] Dreyfuss D, Saumon G. Ventilator-induced lung injury: lessons from experimental studies. Am J Respir Crit Care Med 1998;157:294–323.

[2] Hernandez LA, Peevy KJ, Moise AA, Parker JC. Chest wall restriction limits high airway pressure-induced lung injury in young rabbits. J Appl Physiol 1989;66:2364–2368.

[3] Fujimoto S, Togari H, Yamaguchi N, Mizutani F, Suzuki S, Sobajima H. Hypocarbia and cystic periventricular leukomalacia in premature infants. Arch Dis Child Fetal Neonatal Ed 1994;71:F107–F110.

[4] Fabres J, Carlo WA, Phillips V, Howard G, Ambalavanan N. Both extremes of arterial carbon dioxide pressure and the magnitude of fluctuations in arterial carbon dioxide pressure are associated with severe intraventricular hemorrhage in preterm infants. Pediatrics 2007;119:299–305.

[5] Wiswell TE, Graziani LJ, Kornhauser MS, Stanley C, Merton DA, McKee L, et al. Effects of hypocarbia on the development of cystic periventricular

leukomalacia in premature infants treated with high-frequency jet ventilation. Pediatrics 1996;98:918–924.

[6] Kaiser JR, Gauss CH, Pont MM, Williams DK. Hypercapnia during the first 3 days of life is associated with severe intraventricular hemorrhage in very low birth weight infants. J Perinatol 2006;26:279–285.

[7] Peng W, Zhu H, Shi H, Liu E. Volume-targeted ventilation is more suitable than pressure-limited ventilation for preterm infants: a systematic review and meta-analysis. Arch Dis Child Fetal Neonatal Ed 2014;99: F158–F165.

[8] Klingenberg C, Wheeler KI, McCallion N, Morley CJ, Davis PG. Volume-targeted versus pressure-limited ventilation in neonates. Cochrane Database Syst Rev 2017;10: CD003666.

[9] Keszler M. Update on mechanical ventilatory strategies. NeoReviews 2013;14:e237–e251.

[10] Sinha SK, Donn SM, Gavey J, McCarty M. Randomised trial of volume controlled versus time cycled, pressure limited ventilation in preterm infants with respiratory distress syndrome. Arch Dis Child Fetal Neonatal Ed 1997;77:F202–F205.

[11] Keszler M, Abubakar K. Volume guarantee: stability of tidal volume and incidence of hypocarbia. Pediatr Pulmonol 2004;38:240–245.

[12] Keszler M, Sant'Anna G. Mechanical ventilation and bronchopulmonary dysplasia. Clin Perinatol 2015;42: 781–796.

[13] Wheeler KI, Davis PG, Kamlin CO, Morley CJ. Assist control volume guarantee ventilation during surfactant administration. Arch Dis Child Fetal Neonatal Ed 2009;94:F336–F338.

[14] Dawson C, Davies MW. Volume-targeted ventilation and arterial carbon dioxide in neonates. J Paediatr Child Health 2005;41:518–521.

[15] Nassabeh-Montazami S, Abubakar KM, Keszler M. The impact of instrumental dead-space in volume-targeted ventilation of the extremely low birth weight (ELBW) infant. Pediatr Pulmonol 2009;44: 128–133.

[16] Keszler M, Nassabeh-Montazami S, Abubakar K. Evolution of tidal volume requirement during the first 3 weeks of life in infants <800 g ventilated with Volume Guarantee. Arch Dis Child Fetal Neonatal Ed 2009;94:F279–F282.

[17] Sharma S, Clark S, Abubakar K, Keszler M. Tidal volume requirement in mechanically ventilated infants with meconium aspiration syndrome. Am J Perinatol 2015;32:916–919.

[18] Keszler M. Mechanical ventilation strategies. Semin Fetal Neonatal Med 2017;22:267–274.

[19] Sharma S, Abubakar KM, Keszler M. Tidal volume in infants with congenital diaphragmatic hernia supported with conventional mechanical ventilation. Am J Perinatol 2015;32:577–582.

[20] Abman SH, Collaco JM, Shepherd EG, Keszler M, Cuevas-Guaman M, Welty SE, Bronchopulmonary Dysplasia Collaborative. et al. Interdisciplinary care of children with severe bronchopulmonary dysplasia. J Pediatr 2017;181:12–28.

[21] Wheeler KI, Morley CJ, Hooper SB, Davis PG. Lower back-up rates improve ventilator triggering during assist-control ventilation: a randomized crossover trial. J Perinatol 2012;32:111–116.

[22] Patel DS, Sharma A, Prendergast M, Rafferty GF, Greenough A. Work of breathing and different levels of volume-targeted ventilation. Pediatrics 2009;123:e679–e684.

[23] Bhutani VK, Ritchie WG, Shaffer TH. Acquired tracheomegaly in very preterm neonates. Am J Dis Child 1986;140:449–452.

[24] Abubakar KM, Keszler M. Patient-ventilator interactions in new modes of patient-triggered ventilation. Pediatr Pulmonol 2001;32:71–75.

Chapter | 17 |

Noninvasive Ventilation and High-Flow Nasal Cannula

Rangasamy Ramanathan, MBBS, MD, DCH, FAAP, Manoj Biniwale, MBBS, MD, MRCP, MRCPCH, FAAP

CHAPTER POINTS

Non invasive ventilation holds the key to success in neonatal intensive care units. Optimized use of non invasive ventilation leads to better neonatal pulmonary outcomes. This chapter compares and contrasts various strategies of non invasive ventilation in neonatal intensive are units as well as delivery room. Further how to initiate non invasive ventilation strategies and effectively use in different phases of illness are highlighted.

Noninvasive ventilation

Noninvasive ventilation (NIV) refers to administration of positive pressure support using a flow resistor or positive pressure generator without the use of a laryngeal or tracheal interface. Its use in the world of neonatology is widespread with various modes, patient nasal interfaces, and settings used with the goal of keeping infants from getting intubated. Invasive mechanical ventilation especially in premature infants is lifesaving but remains as one of the leading causes for the development of bronchopulmonary dysplasia (BPD) and ventilator-induced lung injury [1]. Most neonatologists now prefer to use NIV either as a primary mode or after a brief period of invasive ventilation in infants with respiratory insufficiency.

History and timeline

First reports of using NIV were published by Donald and Lord in 1953 while carrying out augmented respiratory studies in newborn infants born with atelectasis of lungs [2]. Science has advanced after Gregory et al. applied continuous positive airway pressure (CPAP) successfully in 30 infants

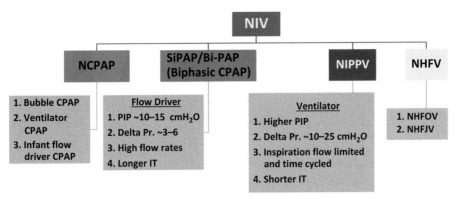

Fig. 17.1 Four Different Modes of Noninvasive Ventilation (NIV) Used in the NICU. *CPAP*, Continuous positive airway pressure; *NCPAP*, nasal continuous positive airway pressure; *NIPPV*, nasal intermittent positive pressure ventilation; *NHFV*, nasal high frequency ventilation; *PIP*, peak inspiratory pressure; *IT*, inspiratory time; *Pr*, pressure; *NHFOV*, nasal high frequency oscillatory ventilation; *NHFJV*, nasal high frequency jet ventilator.

with idiopathic respiratory distress syndrome (RDS) [3]. Negative pressure ventilation was studied simultaneously with some initial benefits [4]. Central nervous system bleeding [5] and gastric perforations [6] marked the era of reluctance for the use of NIV due to the fear of causing more harm than good. For decades, NIV was limited to using CPAP as either bubble CPAP or a flow driver. Concept of using the ventilator to provide NIV support without endotracheal tube gave a new dimension to clinicians working toward decreasing BPD. NIV was revived after revolutionized studies using nasal intermittent positive pressure ventilation (NIPPV) showed decreased frequency of apnea of prematurity and need for intubation or reintubation [7,8]. Multiple studies using NIPPV since then have shown promising results.

Key elements of NIV:

1. modes of NIV (Fig. 17.1)
2. nasal interfaces (Fig. 17.2)
3. settings during different modes

Four most common modes that provide support with NIV in newborn infants are nasal CPAP (NCPAP), SIPAP/Bi-PAP/Duo-PAP, NIPPV, and nasal high-frequency ventilation (NHFV) [9]. There are major differences between these modes.

Indications of NIV

- Apnea of prematurity—prevention or treatment
- Primary respiratory support in newborn intensive care for infants with RDS, transient tachypnea of newborn, meconium aspiration syndrome, pneumonia, congestive heart failure, pulmonary edema, and patent ductus arteriosus
- Primary respiratory support in the delivery room to provide positive pressure ventilation (PPV) and CPAP
- Rescue for patients with difficult intubation
- Postextubation respiratory support
- Postoperative respiratory support

Contraindications of NIV

- Infants with unoperated diaphragmatic hernia
- Nasal obstruction/anomalies
- Tracheoesophageal fistula
- Immediate postoperative period for gastrointestinal surgery

Nasal interfaces

Fig. 17.2 Nasal Interfaces Providing NIV.

NCPAP

NCPAP decreases upper airway resistance, maintains functional residual capacity, decreases chest wall distortion, augments spontaneous breathing efforts, preserves endogenous surfactant, decreases the need for exogenous surfactant administration, and decreases the need and/or duration of invasive ventilation. Prolonged NCPAP has been shown to minimize supplemental oxygen administration and promote lung growth [10,11]. NCPAP is typically generated by using constant or variable flows. Pressures may be provided using a water column (bubble CPAP), a flow generator (infant flow driver), or a conventional ventilator. All these systems generate flow-dependent pressures, including bubble CPAP.

Bubble CPAP

This system uses a constant gas flow rate that is set by the user, and the CPAP generated is equal to the length of expiratory tubing that is immersed under water. Even during bubble CPAP, increasing the flow rate also increases the intraprong pressures at the level of the patient's nasal interface. Typical flow rates used during bubble CPAP are between 6 and 10 L/min. Some studies have suggested that because of small low amplitude (~3–4 cmH$_2$O) oscillations during bubble CPAP, CO$_2$ elimination may be more effective during bubble CPAP. However, randomized, controlled trials have shown no difference in extubation failures between bubble CPAP, infant flow driver CPAP, and ventilator CPAP. In an attempt to increase the amplitude of oscillations, high-amplitude bubble CPAP (HABCPAP) has been developed by creating 135-degree angle at the end of the expiratory tube immersed in the water column [12]. However, no clinical studies have been published using HABCPAP. No backup rate is provided during any of these

types of NCPAP. Studies comparing different means of providing NCPAP have shown extubation failure rates to be similar [13–15].

SiPAP/Bi-PAP/DuoPAP

Infant flow drivers are variable flow devices that generate up to two levels of pressure [a high pressure or peak inspiratory pressure (PIP), and a low pressure or positive end-expiratory pressure (PEEP)] by varying the flow rates. These devices use dedicated flow drivers and generators with a patented fluidic flip mechanism that allows variable flow rates throughout the respiratory cycle. Also known as the Coanda effect, it provides stable baseline pressures and has been shown to decrease expiratory work of breathing [16,17] (Fig. 17.3). Delta pressure (PIP–PEEP) is around 4–6 cmH$_2$O. Because of high resistance, a longer inspiratory time is needed to overcome the resistance. These biphasic CPAP modes essentially mimic NCPAP. Randomized clinical trials comparing Si-PAP/DuoPAP/Bi-PAP with NCPAP as either a primary mode or following a period of invasive ventilation have not shown any difference in clinical outcomes [18] (Table 17.1).

NCPAP in the NICU

A multicenter, randomized trial from the South American Neocosur Network showed that early bubble CPAP and

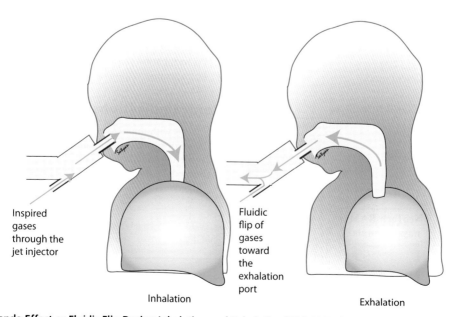

Inspired gases through the jet injector

Fluidic flip of gases toward the exhalation port

Inhalation

Exhalation

Fig. 17.3 Coanda Effect or Fluidic Flip During Inhalation and Exhalation With NCPAP. Copyright: Satyan Lakshminrusimha.

Table 17.1 Results of the randomized control trial comparing Bi-PAP and CPAP

	Bi-PAP (n = 270)	NCPAP (n = 270)	P
BW (g), mean (<28 weeks; n = 334)	870	910	NS
BW (g), mean (>28 weeks; n = 236)	1185	1173	NS
Reintubated within 48 h	21%	20%	0.97
Reintubated within 7 days	34%	31%	0.65
BPD—O_2 at 36 weeks PMA	50%	54%	0.18

Bi-PAP versus NCPAP: RCT (n = 540; GA < 30 and <2 weeks old; 8 NICUs; 2011–14). Bi-PAP: PIP 8; PEEP 4; IT 1.0 s. Rate, 30 breaths/min; NCPAP = CPAP 6. Primary outcome: Failure of extubation within 48 h of randomization; infant flow advance by CareFusion. BPD, Bronchopulmonary dysplasia; BW, birth weight; CPAP, continuous positive airway pressure; NCPAP, nasal continuous positive airway pressure; PEEP, positive end-expiratory pressure; PIP, peak inspiratory pressure; RCT, randomized controlled trial. Source: Based on data from Victor S, Roberts SA, Mitchell S, et al. Biphasic positive airway pressure or continuous positive airway pressure: a randomized trial. Pediatrics 2016;138:e20154095 [18].

selective surfactant administration by the intubation surfactant extubation (INSURE) technique reduced the need for mechanical ventilation and surfactant, but showed no difference in the rates of death or BPD [19]. A major reason for the lack of benefit seen in this trial is secondary to the high rates of NCPAP failures, requiring intubation within 3–7 days of randomization. The most common reasons for NCPAP failures are repeated episodes of apnea, bradycardia or desaturation, hypopnea, need for higher pressures (NCPAP > 8 cmH$_2$O), and/or severe respiratory acidosis. NCPAP when used as a primary mode, or following a period of invasive ventilation, has been shown to result in failure rates of 19.7% to as high as 80%, requiring intubation or reintubation [9] (Fig. 17.4).

Biphasic CPAP in NICU: Si-PAP/Bi-PAP/DuoPAP

The Infant Flow System (Vyaire Medical Inc., Mettawa, IL, USA) is the most widely utilized variable flow device. It uses high-velocity jet flows that can entrain gas on demand during inspiration and thus keep the CPAP level constant. On exhalation, the design of the nasal prongs results in some of the new gas being shunted away through an expiratory outlet (Fig. 17.3) rather than continuing to the nares reducing the expiratory work [17,20–22]. As against regular

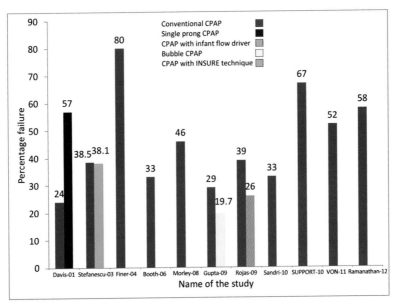

Fig. 17.4 NCPAP Failure Rates From Studies (2001–12). Modified from Ramanathan R. Nasal respiratory support through the nares: its time has come. J Perinatol 2010;30:S67–S72 [9].

NCPAP that provides a continuous distending pressure, biphasic NCPAP (BP-NCPAP) cycles between upper and lower (baseline) level pressures as determined by the following four parameters: (1) lower CPAP level, (2) upper CPAP level, (3) time at upper level, and (4) rate (cycles/min at upper level). Theoretically, functional residual capacity is recruited by the upper CPAP level and maintained with the lower baseline CPAP level, leading to decrease in the work of breathing. There are few studies comparing the use of these two modes of NIV in preterm infants to facilitate sustained extubation following an initial period of intubation and PPV at birth. Earlier study by Migliori et al. showed promising results with BP-NCPAP group infants who had improved gas exchange compared to infants receiving CPAP [23]. Further study by Lista et al. in a larger group of 40 premature infants showed decrease in days of respiratory support, oxygen dependency, and duration of NICU stay in BP-NCPAP group compared to NCPAP group [24]. In the study by O'Brien et al., the incidence of sustained extubation was not statistically different between the BP-NCPAP versus NCPAP group (67% vs. 58%, $P = 0.27$). The incidence of adverse events and short-term neonatal outcomes were similar between the two groups ($P > 0.05$) except for retinopathy of prematurity that was noted to be higher ($P = 0.02$) in the BP-NCPAP group. The study was stopped half way because of slow recruitment and shift toward increasing use of NIPPV [25]. In the largest pragmatic clinical trial comparing NCPAP versus NIPPV by Kirpalani et al., Si-PAP instead of NIPPV was used by many study centers. In the centers that used "NIPPV," PIP was limited to 18 cmH_2O, essentially, making this study a study of NCPAP versus Si-PAP. Results of this study did not show any significance in BPD rates in NCPAP group compared to Si-PAP group [26] (Tables 17.2 and 17.3).

Suggested guidelines for use of CPAP and Si-PAP

Single-level CPAP given by conventional ventilator, bubble CPAP, or through infant flow driver are usually started at 5–6 cmH_2O and adjusted in increments 1 to provide adequate lung expansion to prevent alveolar atelectasis. Maximum pressure of 8–10 cmH_2O can be used based on compliance of the lungs. Si-PAP mode cycles between high and low CPAP levels on a timed basis. Small incremental pressure increases of 2–3 cmH_2O above CPAP is used to generate a sigh breath that, in turn, augments functional residual capacity and decreases work of breathing. The switch to the high CPAP level can usually be set for a duration of 0.1–30 s to produce a sigh. High CPAP is weaned based on CO_2 clearance (Table 17.4).

Table 17.2 Results of the largest randomized control trial comparing CPAP and Si-PAP

	Si-PAP (n = 504)	NCPAP (n = 503)	P
BW (g), mean (SD)	802 (131)	805 (127)	NS
GA (weeks)	26.1 (1.5)	26.2 (1.5)	NS
Reintubated postrandomization	59.5%	61.8%	NS
Prior intubation	46.5%	45.4%	0.70
Caffeine R_x	82.9%	82.9%	NS
Survived with BPD	33.9%	31%	0.32
Death or BPD at 36 weeks PMA	38.4%	36.7%	0.56

Si-PAP versus NCPAP: RCT (n = 1009; <1000 g BW; GA < 30 weeks). NIPPV: most centers used Si-PAP; suggested settings: PIP 9–10; vent: PIP 2–4 above PEEP; max PIP 18; rate 10–40; IT 0.3–1 s; no data on surfactant R_x.
Source: Based on data from Kirpalani H, Millar D, Lemyre B, et al. A trial comparing noninvasive ventilation strategies in preterm infants. N Engl J Med 2013;369:611–620 [26].

Table 17.3 Devices used to provide NIV in Kirpalani study

Ventilator type	NIPPV (%)	NCPAP (%)
Babylog 8000/8000+	21	18
Bird VIP/VIP Gold	9	1
Bubble nCPAP	—	9
Evita 4/XL	7	2
Infant flow/infant flow advance	**10**	**30**
Servo 300/900C/I	5	1
Viasys Si-PAP	**43**	**31**
Others	5	8

Bold indicates those infants who received Si-PAP and not NIPPV.
NIPPV, Nasal intermittent positive pressure ventilation.
Source: Based on data from Kirpalani H, Millar D, Lemyre B, et al. A trial comparing noninvasive ventilation strategies in preterm infants. N Engl J Med 2013;369:611–620 [26].

NIPPV

By providing backup rates along with two levels of pressure, namely, PIP and PEEP, NIPPV has been shown to significantly decrease the intubation or reintubation needs. NIPPV mimics invasive ventilation without an

Table 17.4 Suggested settings for use of Si-PAP

Setting	Start	Increase	Maximum	Decrease	Minimum
Baseline CPAP	5 cmH$_2$O	FiO$_2$ > 30% or signs of respiratory distress	10 cmH$_2$O	FiO$_2$ 21%	4 cmH$_2$O
High CPAP (Si-PAP)	7 cmH$_2$O	CO$_2$ retention or signs of respiratory distress	11 cmH$_2$O	Hyperventilation	6 cmH$_2$O
FiO$_2$	21%	For desaturations	100%	Preductal saturation >90%	21%
Time high	0.5 s	Hypoxia	1 s	Hyperoxia	0.3 s
Cycle rate	10 cycles/min	CO$_2$ retention or apnea	30 cycles/min	Hyperventilation	10 cycles/min
Temperature	34–37°C				
Humidity	100% relative humidity				

FiO$_2$, Fraction of inspired oxygen.

endotracheal tube. Minimizing the duration of invasive ventilation by using NIPPV decreases BPD risk. Both face mask and nasal prongs have been used during NIPPV. Binasal prongs placed in both the nostrils have been shown to be more effective than a single prong [27].

NIPPV in the NICU

NIPPV is the preferred mode to provide NIV in large number of centers across the world. The five variables adjusted during NIPPV include ventilator rate, PIP, inspiratory time, PEEP, and flow rate (Fig. 17.5).

Spontaneous inspiratory effort is augmented when a patient receives a positive pressure breath while receiving NIPPV [28]. The recommended PIP during NIPPV varies from 15 to 25 cmH$_2$O above the PEEP. Use of higher PIP is associated with reduced work of breathing [29] (Table 17.5).

NIPPV: controls/limits

1. **Baseline CPAP level (PEEP)**
2. **A sigh level of CPAP (PIP)**
3. **Duration of high pressure** (inspiratory time = 4–5 × time constant)
4. **Number of sighs (rate)**
5. **Flow rate**

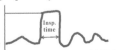

$$20/5 \times 40 \times 0.5 \text{ s}$$

Fig. 17.5 NIPPV Controls. *PEEP*, Positive end-expiratory pressure; *PIP*, peak inspiratory pressure.

Typical rates used during NIPPV range from 20 to 40 breaths/min. However, use of higher rates results in better respiratory unloading as compared to lower rates. Decrease in inspiratory efforts occurs with synchronization (Fig. 17.6A), although tidal volumes are maintained in nonsynchronized NIPPV [30] (Fig. 17.6B).

Due to the high resistance found in the nasal interfaces, the pressure transmitted to the hypopharynx is always lower than set pressures. As the time constant becomes longer due to higher resistance in the circuit, a longer inspiration time (∼0.5 s) is recommended to transmit the pressures set on the ventilator. Many ventilators are now available that have a built-in mode for providing NIPPV. Most of these ventilators automatically adjust flow rates. Leak compensation is also available. In conventional mechanical ventilators without the NIV mode, flow rates of 14–20 L/min are needed to compensate for leaks. For all practical purposes, NIPPV works as a time-cycled, pressure-limited mode of ventilation. Both synchronized and nonsynchronized modes of NIPPV have been studied. At present, there are no devices in the United States that are capable of providing synchronized NIPPV, except for neurally adjusted ventilatory assist (NAVA). However, there are devices available in other parts of the world where flow synchronization as well as Graseby capsule are used to provide synchronized form of NIPPV and are available for clinical use. Multiple randomized, controlled trials comparing NCPAP versus NIPPV have been published to date [8,31–39]. Most of the trials showed a significant reduction in extubation failures with NIPPV [9] (Fig. 17.7), and three of the studies that used NIPPV as a primary mode of respiratory support and selective surfactant administration using INSURE technique also resulted in significantly lower rates ($P < 0.05$) of BPD when compared to NCPAP [33,38,40] (Fig. 17.8).

Table 17.5 Decreased work of breathing with higher PIP in synchronized NIPPV (sNIPPV)

| BW (g) 1367 ± 325 | GA (weeks) 29.5 ± 2.4 | | Age at study (days) 4 ± 4 | |
	NCPAP 5	sNIPPV 10	sNIPPV 12	sNIPPV 14
V_t (mL/kg)	2.9 ± 1.2	2.8 ± 1.32	2.81 ± 1.1	2.9 ± 1.0
RR (per min)	53 ± 23	58 ± 22	53 ± 26	59 ± 23
MV (mL/min/kg)	115 ± 72	119 ± 67	114 ± 70	127 ± 62
Phase angle (degree)	46 ± 58	49 ± 38	47 ± 53	56 ± 54
WOB Insp, per mL (cmH₂O)	2.69 ± 2.24	2.26 ± 1.94	2.29 ± 2.29*	1.91 ± 1.68*
WOB E, per mL (cmH₂O)	1.81 ± 1.67	1.32 ± 1.10	1.50 ± 1.56	1.01 ± 0.95*
RWOB, per mL (cmH₂O)	2.16 ± 2.04	1.71 ± 1.79*	1.79 ± 2.05*	1.56 ± 1.61*
CL (mL/kg/cmH₂O)	1.61 ± 1.68	1.38 ± 2.73	3.37 ± 4.89	2.42 ± 2.86

sNIPPV and work of breathing ($n = 15$). Ventilator-delivered PIP during sNIPPV decreases WOB.
V_t, tidal volume; RR, respiratory rate; Insp, inspiratory; E, expiratory; RWOB, resistive work of breathing; CL, compliance of lung; PIP, peak inspiratory pressure; NCPAP, nasal CPAP; sNIPPV, synchronized NIPPV; MV, minute ventilation; BW, birth weight; GA, gestational age; WOB, work of breathing.
*$P < 0.05$.
Source: Based on data from Aghai ZH, Saslow JG, Nakhla T, et al. Synchronized nasal intermittent positive pressure ventilation (SNIPPV) decreases work of breathing (WOB) in premature infants with respiratory distress syndrome (RDS) compared to nasal continuous positive airway pressure (NCPAP). Pediatr Pulmonol 2006;41:875–881 [29].

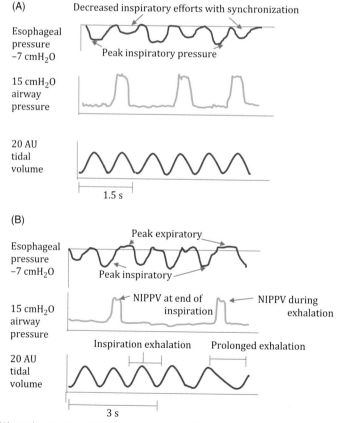

Fig. 17.6 Comparison of (A) synchronized and (B) nonsynchronized NIPPV demonstrating typical esophageal pressures *(red)*, airway pressures *(green)*, and tidal volumes *(blue)* with NIPPV. Modified from Chang HY, Claure N, D'ugard C, et al. Effects of synchronization during nasal ventilation in clinically stable preterm infants. Pediatr Res 2011;69:84–89 [30].

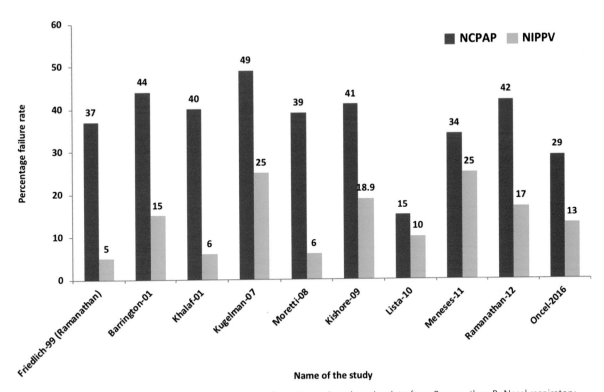

Fig. 17.7 NCPAP Versus NIPPV Studies Comparing Failure Rates. Based on the data from Ramanathan R. Nasal respiratory support through the nares: its time has come. J Perinatol 2010;30:S67–S72.

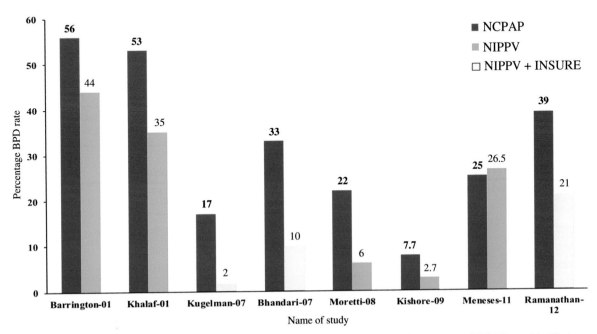

Fig. 17.8 NIPPV With Intubation Surfactant Extubation (INSURE) Technique Showing Decreased BPD Rates. Modified from Ramanathan R. Nasal respiratory support through the nares: its time has come. J Perinatol 2010;30:S67–S72 [9].

In a systematic review and meta-analysis of five studies comparing NCPAP with NIPPV, significant decrease in the need for invasive ventilation (risk ratio: 0.44; 95% confidence interval: 0.33–0.59) [41].

Of all the interventions to improve rates of successful extubation in preterm infants, NIPPV appears to be superior to NCPAP [42] (Table 17.6). An another recent Cochrane review authors that early NIPPV does appear to be superior to NCPAP alone for decreasing respiratory failure and the need for intubation, and endotracheal tube ventilation among preterm infants with RDS [43]. Ventilator-generated NIPPV as well as nonsynchronized NIPPV were the most

significant factors leading to less respiratory failure in the same meta-analysis (Table 17.7).

In summary, NCPAP when used in the delivery room or after a period of invasive mechanical ventilation has not been shown to improve pulmonary outcomes in any of the individual studies. Furthermore, NCPAP use has not been shown to improve pulmonary function at 8 years of age [44] (Table 17.8). This is very likely due to high rates of NCPAP failures, especially in extremely low–birth weight infants, needing prolonged invasive mechanical ventilation. NIPPV has been consistently shown to decrease the need for intubation and may be

Table 17.6 Systematic review and meta-analysis of interventions to improve successful extubation rates in preterm infants

Preventing extubation failures	Risk ratio (95% CI)	NNT (95% CI)
NCPAP versus Head Box	0.59 (0.48–0.72)	6 (3–9)
NCPAP versus HFNC	1.11 (0.84–1.47)	—
Methylxanthines	0.48 (0.32–0.71)	4 (2–7)
DOXAPRAM	0.80 (0.22–2.97)	—
NIPPV versus NCPAP	0.70 (0.60–0.81)	8 (5–13)
NS-NIPPV or Bi-PAP versus NCPAP	064 (0.44–0.95)	8 (4–50)
sNIPPV versus NCPAP	0.25 (0.15–041)	4 (2–5)
NS-NIPPV or sNIPPV versus NCPAP	0.28 (0.18–043)	4 (2–5)

Conclusions and relevance: Preterm infants should be extubated to noninvasive respiratory support. Caffeine should be used routinely. NIPPV is superior to NCPAP.

CI, Confidence interval; HFNC, high flow nasal cannula; NS-NIPPV, non synchronized NIPPV; sNIPPV, synchronized NIPPV.
Source: Based on data from Ferguson KN, Roberts CT, Manley BJ, Davis PG. Interventions to improve rates of successful extubation in preterm infants: a systematic review and meta-analysis. JAMA Pediatr 2017;171:165–174 [42].

Table 17.7 Early NIPPV versus NCPAP in preterm infants with RDS Cochrane review and meta-analysis (10 studies; n = 1061) by device and synchronization

Respiratory failure by device and synchronized versus nonsynchronized	No. of studies	No. of patients	Risk ratio (95% CI)	NNTB
Ventilator-generated NIPPV	6	606	0.63 (0.47–0.86)	13 (7–50)
Bilevel NIPPV	2	160	1.0 (0.44–2.27)	
Mixed devices	2	294	0.59 (0.38–0.93)	
Nonsynchronized NIPPV	5	572	0.60 (0.44–0.83)	
Synchronized NIPPV	4	304	0.65 (0.41–1.02)	
Mixed methods	1	184	0.74 (0.44–1.22)	

RDS, Respiratory distress syndrome; NNTB, number needed to treat for benefit.
Source: Modified from Lemyre B, Laughon M, Bose C, Davis PG. Nasal intermittent positive pressure ventilation (NIPPV) versus nasal continuous positive airway pressure (NCPAP) for preterm neonates after extubation. Cochrane Database Syst Rev 2017;2:CD003212 [43].

Table 17.8 Changes in ventilation mode and lung function at 8 years of age

	1991–92 (n = 225)	1997 (n = 151)	2005 (n = 170)	P
BW (g)	891 ± 176	824 ± 177	867 ± 195	<0.05
GA (weeks)	25.9 ± 1.1	25.6 ± 1.2	25.8 ± 1.2	NS
AS (%)	71	89	85	<0.05
Surfactant R_x (%)	43	84	87*	<0.05*
Postnatal steroids (%)	40	46	23[†]	<0.05[†]
ET ventilation (median days)	21	19	10	
NCPAP (median days)	5	24	31.5[†]	<0.05[†]
BPD—O_2 at 36 weeks (%)	46	43[‡]	56	<0.05[‡]
FEV_t (% of predicted value)	87.9 ± 13.4	94.4 ± 14.9	91.0 ± 14.2[‡]	<0.05[‡]
FEV_1: FVC (% of predicted value)	98.3 ± 10.0	96.8 ± 10.1	93.4 ± 9.2[†]	<0.05[†]

Changes in ventilation modes and O_2 use and lung function at 8 years of age. *BW*, birth weight; *GA*, gestational age; *AS*, antenatal steroids; *Rx*, treatment; *ET*, endotracheal; *BPD*, bronchopulmonary dysplasia; *FEV1*, forced expiratory volume in 1 second; *FVC*, forced vital capacity. Despite substantial increases in the use of less-invasive ventilation (NCPAP only).
*Comparison of 1991-92 and 2005.
[†]Comparison of 2005 to both 1991–92 and 1997.
[‡]Comparison of 2005 to 1997.
Modified from Doyle LW, Carse E, Adams AM, Ranganathan S, Opie G, Cheong JLY Ventilation in preterm infants and lung function at 8 years. N Engl J Med 2017;377:1601–1602.

lung protective. It is likely that using NIPPV in the delivery room may improve pulmonary and nonpulmonary outcomes in preterm infants.

Patient nasal interfaces

Interfaces predominantly consist of either prongs or masks (Fig. 17.2). One of the major issues with NIV is the application of patient nasal interface. Binasal prongs that are currently used are difficult to secure and results in significant nasal injury.

Nasal injuries

The most common side effect of using NIV is nasal injuries. The incidence could be as high as 60% with 5.5% patients getting columellar necrosis leading to long-term nasal septal problems [45,46].

We use specially designed simple nasal interface (Neotech RAM NC) to minimize nasal injuries and have safely used this interface in over 1,000 neonates for over 10,000 days of NIV.

NIV in the delivery room

Lung-protective strategies should be implemented immediately after birth. Establishment of functional residual capacity using NIV is the most important step during the initial stabilization period in preterm infants [47]. Prenatal as well as interventions in the delivery room may impact long-term respiratory outcomes especially in preterm infants (Fig. 17.9). The current Neonatal Resuscitation Program (NRP) guidelines recommend using a T-piece device to deliver consistent CPAP and PPV, rather than using a self-inflating or flow-inflating bag [48]. Bag and mask resuscitation may result in significant mask leaks and airway obstruction especially in premature infants [49–52]. Bag and mask ventilation can cause upper airway obstructions by inadvertently pushing the tongue and soft tissues posteriorly, and the increase in dead space caused by the accumulation of gas in the oropharynx that is not contributing to gas exchange (Fig. 17.10). Capasso et al. compared face mask with nasal cannula during primary neonatal resuscitation in a large randomized controlled trial and concluded that nasal cannula was more effective than bag and mask ventilation in the delivery room [53]. We have successfully used modified nasal cannula in the delivery room [54] (Table 17.9). Although CPAP in the delivery room has improved outcomes of premature infants, the failure rates could be as high as 67% [19, 55–60] (Fig. 17.11). Our retrospective study showed less failure rates in the form of intubation or chest compressions in very low–birth weight infants when cannula was used to provide NIV compared to PPV provided by face mask [61] (Table 17.10). The need for intubation significantly decreased for gestational ages

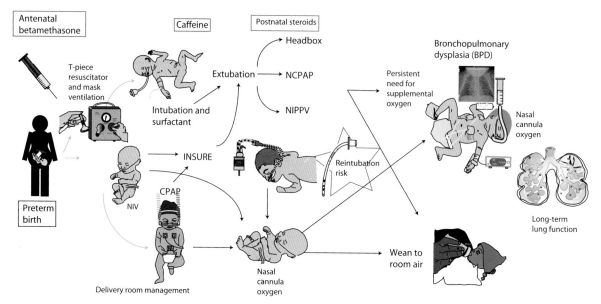

Fig. 17.9 Prenatal and Postnatal Interventions and Impact on Long-Term Respiratory Outcome. Copyright: Satyan Lakshminrusimha.

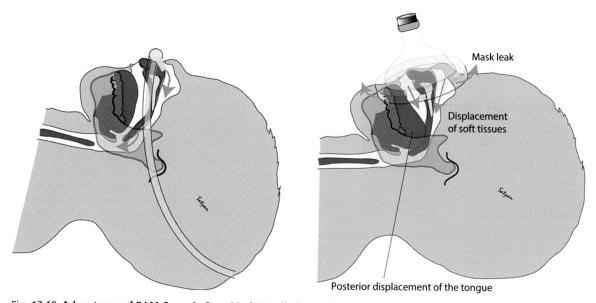

Fig. 17.10 Advantages of RAM Cannula Over Mask Ventilation in the DR. Copyright: Satyan Lakshminrusimha.

between 24 and 30 weeks with use of cannula in the delivery room (Fig. 17.12). Further it was easier for the team to transport infants on cannula to NICU from delivery room. We have also shown that using NIPPV from the delivery room for larger preterm and term infants with respiratory distress results in less need for intubation in the delivery room or at 24 h of age rather than using mask [62]

(Table 17.11). Current NRP guidelines recommend using nasal interface for stabilizing the premature infants in the delivery room who are expected to need NIV in NICU [48].

Based on our experience, we routinely use NIPPV using RAM cannula as a primary mode of respiratory support in all neonates needing positive pressure support during transitional period in the delivery room.

Table 17.9 Our experience with use of RAM cannula in delivery room

	Range
BW (g)	270–4675 (2106 ± 1094)
GA (weeks)	23–41 (32 ± 5)
BW <1000 g, n (%)	20 (19.6)
BW 1000–2000 g, n (%)	29 (28.4)
BW 2001–3000 g, n (%)	28 (27.4)
BW >3000 g, n (%)	25 (24.5)
Chest compressions, n (%)	5 (4.9)
Intubated in DR, n (%)	8 (7.8)
Pneumothorax incidental on CXR, n (%)	5 (4.9)
INSURE R$_x$, n (%)	28 (27.4)

RAM-Nasal Cannula (Bi-Nasal) for primary neonatal resuscitation in the delivery room (n = 102). *BW*, birth weight; *GA*, gestational age; *CXR*, chest xray; *DR*, delivery room; *INSURE*, intubation surfactant extubation
Source: Based on data from Paz P, Ramanathan R, Hernandez R, Biniwale M. Neonatal resuscitation using a nasal cannula: a single-center experience. Am J Perinatol 2014;31: 1031–1036 [54].

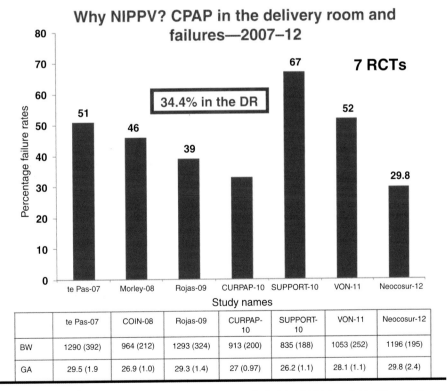

	te Pas-07	COIN-08	Rojas-09	CURPAP-10	SUPPORT-10	VON-11	Neocosur-12
BW	1290 (392)	964 (212)	1293 (324)	913 (200)	835 (188)	1053 (252)	1196 (195)
GA	29.5 (1.9	26.9 (1.0)	29.3 (1.4)	27 (0.97)	26.2 (1.1)	28.1 (1.1)	29.8 (2.4)

Fig. 17.11 CPAP Failure Rates in DR Studies. *RCT*, Randomized controlled trial. *BW*, birth weight; *GA*, gestational age; *DR*, delivery room; *VON*, Vermont Oxford Network

Table 17.15 Outcomes of direct extubation from high-frequency ventilation to noninvasive positive pressure ventilation in very low birth weight infants (n = 82)

	HFV to SIMV (Indirect) (n = 48)	Direct (n = 34)	P
BW (g)	709 ± 254	729 ± 238	0.785
GA (weeks)	26 ± 2	26 ± 2	0.97
Weight at extubation (g)	1299 ± 705	1163 ± 679	0.104
Reintubation within 72 h (%)	10.4	11.8	1.00
Duration of invasive ventilation (days) (mean ± SD)	39.4 ± 17	27.5 ± 14	0.002
Length of stay (days) (mean ± SD)	101 ± 26	105 ± 32	0.749
Direct extubation from HFV to NIPPV may be safe and feasible.			

BW, birth weight; GA, gestational age; HFV, high frequency vnetilator; SIMV, synchronized intermitent mandatory ventilation; NIPPV, non-invasive positive pressure ventilation.
Source: Based on the data from Bhatt P, Ramanathan R, Barton L, Biniwale M. Direct extubation from high frequency ventilation to noninvasive positive pressure ventilation in very low birth weight infants: a retrospective study. Pediatric Academic Societies Annual Meeting, San Francisco, CA, USA, May 2017; Abstract [71].

Invasive HFV to Noninvasive ventilation

Case scenario: SIMV-fails — HFOV/HFJV. When baby is stable, DO NOT go back to SIMV. Extubate to NIPPV

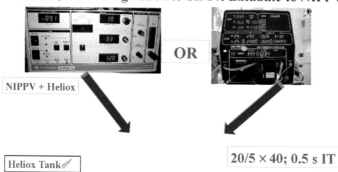

NIPPV + Heliox

OR

Heliox Tank

20/5 × 40; 0.5 s IT

Fig. 17.16 Weaning From High-Frequency Ventilation. *SIMV,* Synchronized intermittent mandatory ventilation *HFOV,* high frequency oscillatory ventilation; *HFJV,* high frequency jet ventilation; *NIPPV,* non-invasive positive pressure ventilation.

that these infants should be intubated before transporting to other facilities. During air transport (or ground transport in mountains), one may need to adjust NIV support due to increases in lung volumes or abdominal gas volumes.

High-flow nasal cannula

HFNC are small, thin, tapered binasal tubes that deliver oxygen or blended oxygen and air mixture at gas flows of more than 2 L/min. HFNC are increasingly popular because of their ease of use. This form of NIV specifically refers to the delivery of blended, heated, and humidified gas. Devices providing HFNC along with recommended flow rates are shown in Table 17.16.

Table 17.16 Devices providing high-flow nasal cannula and recommended flow rates

Device trade name	Flow rate (L/min)	Relative humidity (%)	Gas temperature (°C)
Standard nasal cannula	1–4	Not humidified	Not warmed
Vapotherm precision 2000i high-flow therapy	5–40	95–100	33–43
Fisher and Paykel optiflow high-flow nasal cannula	1–60	100	37

Physiologic principles

A key feature that separates HFNC from standard nasal cannula is the preconditioning of the inspired gas. As it would normally take metabolic energy for the body to warm and humidify the air we breathe, HFNC has the advantage of reducing resting energy expenditure.

The clinically important respiratory benefits of HFNC include decreased work of breathing and reduced supplemental oxygen requirement. There are several proposed mechanisms of action to explain these findings. These include (1) reduction of inspiratory resistance [76], (2) washout of nasopharyngeal dead space [77], and (3) provision of positive airway distending pressure [78,79]. With tightly fitting nasal prongs, high flow rates, and closed mouth, HFNC can generate high nasopharyngeal airway pressures [78,80].

Advantages of using HFNC

Ease of application and minimization of nasal trauma are two big factors that favor use of cannula over CPAP (Fig. 17.21). Nasal trauma is mainly reduced by gas heating and humidification [81–83]. Other factor that aide in use of high-flow cannula include provision of some amount of positive pressure, augmentation of spontaneous tidal volumes, stabilization in patient's work of breathing, and improved gas exchange via dead space washout [84–86]. It also improves patient comfort [87,88].

Disadvantages and safety concerns

Very high pressures can be generated when flow rates higher than 2 L/min are used (Fig. 17.17). Even at 2 L/min, the CPAP generated could be as high as 10 cmH$_2$O [89]. Serious complications due to traumatic air dissection, such as scalp emphysema, pneumoorbitis, and pneumocephalus, have been reported with use of HFNC in the past [90]. As pressures generated are neither measured nor controlled by the user, flow rates more than 2 L/min should not be used in preterm neonates. Unpredictable pressures may be generated by both the most commonly used devices [91] (Fig. 17.18). Pressure-relief valves incorporated into some of the HFNC devices may not be sufficient to avoid excessive pressure [80]. Careful attention should be given to the size of the prongs as recommended by the manufacturers to allow an adequate leak between the prongs and the infant's nares, as well as the use of the lowest effective flow rates. Prolonged use of HFNC with exposure to high pressures results in many adverse outcomes in extremely low–birth

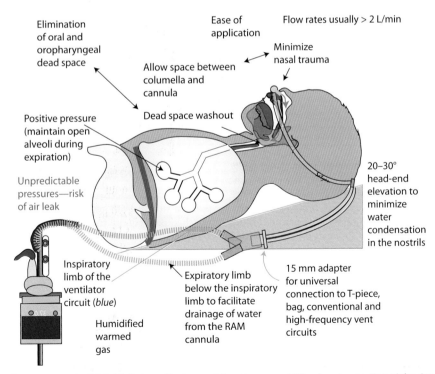

Fig. 17.17 Use of RAM Cannula With High–Low System—Advantages and Disadvantages. Copyright: Satyan Lakshminrusimha.

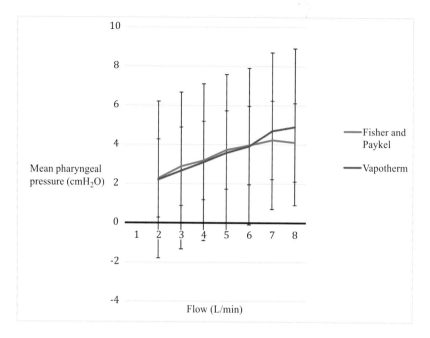

Fig. 17.18 Comparison of two devices delivering high-flow nasal cannula, namely, Fisher and Paykel *(blue)* and Vapotherm *(red)* demonstrating variable CPAP effect shown in *bold* lines (*n* = 9). *Error bar* shows two standard deviations. At 7–8 L/min, pharyngeal pressures are unpredictable and may vary from 1 to 9 cmH$_2$O. Based on the data from Collins CL, Holberton JR, König K. Comparison of the pharyngeal pressure provided by two heated, humidified high-flow nasal cannulae devices in premature infants. J Paediatr Child Health 2013;49:554–556 [91].

weight infants [92]. One must exercise extreme caution when using HFNC, especially in preterm infants. We do not use HFNC in preterm infants.

HFNC versus CPAP

Several studies have been performed for efficacy and safety check while comparing HFNC and CPAP. The study conducted by Lavizzari et al. enrolled 316 patients of more than 29 weeks of gestation age with mild-to-moderate RDS. HFNC showed similar efficacy with regard to failure in 10.8% compared to 9.5% in CPAP group [93]. In a study by Manley et al., infants less than 32 weeks of gestation age were randomized after extubation to CPAP or HFNC. In this study of 303 infants, treatment failure in the HFNC group of 34.2% was comparable to 25.8% in the CPAP group [83]. Whereas in a retrospective study involving more than 2000 infants, Taha et al. found that HFNC was associated with increased respiratory morbidities, delayed oral feeding, and prolonged hospitalization in infants less than 1000 g birth weight [92] (Table 17.17). The HIPSTER trial was an unblended, international, multicenter random-ized noninferiority trial involving infants of 28 weeks and

higher comparing HFC to NCPAP as a primary support for providing NIV. Of proposed enrollment of 750 infants, trial was stopped after enrolling 278 infants because of higher percentage of failure in the HFNC group (25.5% vs. 13.3%) [94] (Table 17.18). Meta-analysis of studies involving HFNC comparing it to CPAP has not shown any difference in BPD rates [95].

HFNC for weaning from NCPAP

There are no prospective, randomized studies of HFNC in preterm infants with regard to weaning from NCPAP. A matched-pair cohort study involving 79 preterm infants ≤28 weeks of gestation age compared while weaning from NCPAP to low-flow cannula versus HFNC and revealed that infants in the HFNC group weaned from NCPAP significantly quicker but had no difference in overall duration of respiratory support [96].

HFNC versus LFNC

Typically, flow rates 2 L/min or less is considered low-flow nasal cannula (LFNC). Majority of centers use LFNC as a

Table 17.17 Study demonstrating morbidity associated with high-flow nasal cannula use in extremely low birth weight infants

	CPAP (941)	HFNC (333)	HFNC ± CPAP (1546)	P
CPAP days (median, IQR)	15 (5–28)		7 (1–19)	
FNC days (median, IQR)		14 (5–25)	13 (6–23)	
Mean BW (g)	**787 ± 145**	776 ± 149	**773 ± 146**	**<0.05**
Mean GA (weeks)	**26.7 ± 2.1**	26.5 ± 1.9	**26.3 ± 1.8**	**<0.05**
Ventilated any time (%)	**799 (84.9)**	284 (85.3)	**1387 (89.7)**	**<0.05**
HFNC ± CPAP (median, IQR)	**15 (5–28)**	14 (5–25)	**26 (14–39)**	**<0.001** Linear regression
BPD or death (%)	**474 (50.4)**	189 (56.8)*	**950 (61.5)**	**<0.05** Logistic regression
BPD (%)	**397 (42.2)**	174 (52.2)*	**912 (59.0)**	**<0.05** Logistic regression
Multiple ventilation courses (%)	**481 (51.1)**	177 (53.1)	**1000 (64.7)**	**<0.05** Logistic regression
More than 3 ventilation courses (%)	**166 (17.6)**	70 (21.0)	**454 (29.4)**	**<0.05** Logistic regression
Ventilator (days) (median, IQR)	18 (5–42)	25 (6–52)*	30 (10–58)†	
Postnatal steroids (%)	**115 (12.2)**	71 (21.3)*	**387 (25.0)**	**<0.05** Logistic regression
Days to room air (median, IQR)	**62 (39–90)**	76 (51–103)*	**72 (51–96)**	**<0.001** Linear regression
Discharge home on oxygen (%)	201 (21.4)	70 (21.0)	432 (27.9)	NS
Severe IVH (grade 3/4) (%)	79 (8.4)	31 (9.3)	170 (11.0)	NS
PDA requiring medical therapy	445 (47.3)	145 (43.5)	797 (51.5)	NS
NEC Bell's stage 2 or higher	74 (7.7)	30 (9.0)	126 (8.1)	NS
ROP requiring laser	81 (8.6)	36 (10.8)	208 (13.4)	NS
Length of hospitalization (days)	**82 (64–104)**	89 (69–111)‡	**95 (75–119)**	**<0.05** Linear regression

Bold values indicate CPAP versus HFNC ± CPAP significant values; *Bw*, birth weight; *GA*, getsaitonal age; *FNC*, flow nasal cannula; *BPD*, bronchopulmonary dysplasia; *D*, days; *IQR*, interquartile range; *IVH*, intraventricular hemorrhage; *PDA*, patent ductus arteriosus; *NEC*, necrotizing enterocolitis; *ROP*, retinopathy of prematurity; *NS*, not significant.
*$P < 0.05$, CPAP versus HFNC.
†$P < .05$, CPAP vs HFNC ± CPAP.
‡$P < 0.001$, CPAP versus HFNC.
Source: Modified from Taha DK, Kornhauser M, Greenspan JS, et al. High flow nasal cannula use is associated with increased morbidity and length of hospitalization in extremely low birth weight infants. J Pediatr 2016;173:50–55 [94].

Table 17.18 Highlights of HIPSTER trial for comparing high-flow nasal cannula to CPAP in premature infants

- Multinational, RCT noninferiority design—Australia and Norway
- HFNC versus NCPAP; no Surf. R_x; BW: 1737 versus 1751 g; GA: 32 versus 32 weeks
- Trial stopped early per DSM Committee because of a significant difference in primary outcome of failure within 72 h of randomization
- Treatment failure: HFNC versus NCPAP: 25.5% versus 13.3%; $P < 0.001$
- Conclusions: When used for primary support for preterm infants with respiratory distress, HFNC resulted in a significantly higher rate of treatment failure than did CPAP

HFNC for primary respiratory support in preterm infants ($n = 564$; GA ≥ 28 weeks) (HIPSTER trial) in VLBW infants; *RCT*, randomized control trial; *Rx*, treatment; *BW*, birth weight; *DSM*, data safety monitoring; *GA*, gestational age; *HFNC*, high flow nasal cannula; *NCPAP*, nasal CPAP.
Source: Based on the data from Roberts CT, Owen LS, Manley BJ, et al. Nasal high-flow therapy for primary respiratory support in preterm infants. N Engl J Med 2016;375:1142–1151 [94].

step-down process from weaning CPAP of 4–5 cmH$_2$O. Main advantage of LFNC is that infants can be fed by mouth rather than gavage tube as against in CPAP or HFNC wherein majority of infants are fed through gavage tube. Also flow rates at 1 L/min or less may not need heated or humidified gas. Furthermore, if needed, LFNC can be easily converted to home oxygen therapy if infant cannot be weaned any further.

Recommendations

HFNC may be effective for support of preterm infants following extubation. As a primary NIV treatment, HFNC did not perform as well as NCPAP. Further studies are needed to assess which clinical conditions are most amenable to HFNC support, the most effective flow rates, and escalation and weaning strategies. Its suitability as first-line treatment needs to be further evaluated [97].

Guidelines for using HFNC

Indications in NICU

- Postextubation ≥28 weeks of gestation age
- Stable infants on CPAP (not "weaning" per se)
- Nasal trauma
- Recommencing respiratory support after
- Weaning off CPAP

Initiation of high and low-flow cannula

Set initial gas flow for HFNC of 6–8 L/min, from either the Optiflow Junior (Fisher and Paykel Healthcare) or Precision Flow (Vapotherm) device (Table 17.19). The size of the nasal cannula is determined according to the manufacturers' instructions to maintain a leak at the nares. The maximum permissible gas flow is 8 L/min, as recommended by the manufacturer. Typically, flow rate at 2 L/min is started when switched to LFNC. Consider using heated, humidified gas when flow rates are ≥1 L/min.

Stable phase for HFNC

In the stable phase for HFNC, following parameters have to be monitored carefully.
- Work of breathing/apnea
- Blood gases
- Oxygen saturations

Table 17.19 High and low-flow nasal cannula initiation settings

Setting	Start	Increase	Maximum	Decrease	Minimum
High flow rate (L/min)	6–8	By 0.5–1 for FiO$_2$ > 30% or signs of respiratory distress	8	By 0.5–1 when FiO$_2$ 21%	2–4
Low flow rate (L/min)	2	—	2	By 0.5 when FiO$_2$ 21%	0.5
FiO$_2$ (%)	21–30	Preductal saturation <88%	50	Preductal saturation >90%	21
Temperature	34–37°C				
Humidity	100% Relative humidity				

FiO$_2$, Fraction of inspired oxygen.

- Nasopharyngeal patency
- Feeding tolerance

If it continues to have increased work of breathing, severe apneic episodes, or FiO_2 more than 40%, then may switch to CPAP or NIPPV.

Stable phase for LFNC

- Keep at 2 L/min while FiO_2 is more than 21%.
- May need to go to CPAP or HFNC if FiO_2 persistently is more than 40%.
- Check the work of breathing before adjusting flow rate.
- Monitor apnea, bradycardia, and desaturations episodes.
- Consider keeping the cannula for premature infants if growth is suboptimal.

Weaning phase for HFNC

We recommend weaning FiO_2 before flow rates and wean flow after FiO_2 is down to 25% for 24 h (Table 17.20).

Weaning phase for LFNC

- Wean FiO_2 before flow rates.
- Weaning no more than 0.5 L/min/day.
- Convert to home oxygen if infant cannot be weaned off from 0.5 L/min and if infant is otherwise ready for discharge.
- Home oxygen settings are usually 1/8 L/min or 1/4 L/min with FiO_2 of 100%.

Precautions when using NIV

1. Do not occlude the nasal passages completely. Allow at least ~30% leak to minimize expiratory resistance and to avoid nasal mucosal or septal injury. One may need to compensate by using slightly high pressures to

Table 17.20 Weaning guidelines for HFNC

Parameter	Wean by	Lowest settings to convert to low-flow or standard nasal cannula
High flow rate (L/min)	0.5–1	2–4
FiO_2 (%)	2%–5%	21–30
Temperature	34–37°C	
Humidity	100% Relative humidity	

Practical issues with NCPAP/SiPAP/NIPPV

1. Nasal septal or columella injury
2. Nosocomial infections postnasal mucosal injury

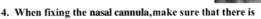

1. STAY AWAY / STAY AWAY ... FROM COLUMELLA
2. Make "NOSE ROUNDS"
3. Use a septal guard, duo derm, T-piece
4. When fixing the nasal cannula, make sure that there is a GAP between the columella and the nasal interface

Fig. 17.19 Precautions Using Nasal Interface While Providing NIV.

Practical issues: Fixing RAM NC: Patient on HFJV and another patient with congenital glaucoma

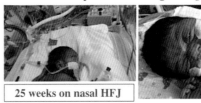

25 weeks on nasal HFJ

Stay away from the columella

Fig. 17.20 Practical Issues While Fixing RAM Cannula.

compensate for the leak. Many devices will be able to provide synchronized NIPPV when the leak is <30%. With sNIPPV for >60% of the time, effort of breathing using pressure–rate product was significantly lower than during HFNC at 6 L/min flow in neonates and young infants [98].

2. Always keep a "gap" between the nasal interface and the columella part of the nose. When fixing the nasal interface, make sure that there is this "gap" between nasal interphase and the columella (Figs. 17.19 and 17.20).

Summary and future of NIV

Based on the randomized, controlled trials, use of NCPAP as a primary mode of support has not decreased the need for intubation or reintubation. Furthermore, both short-term outcomes, such as BPD, and long-term outcomes, such as pulmonary function, at 8 years of age have not improved. A number of studies using true mode of "NIPPV" has clearly shown to decrease the need for intubation or reintubations.

can be achieved by several techniques and a variety of nasal CPAP systems. The delivery devices can be broadly grouped into *continuous-flow* and *variable-flow* systems. With continuous-flow devices this is achieved by using water-seal bubble CPAP (Fisher and Paykel Healthcare, NZ; Babi-Plus [A Plus Medical, CA]; Home-made) systems or via flow opposition, where the patient's expiratory flow opposes a set resistance in the ventilator. In the conventional ventilator-provided CPAP, the pressure fluctuates with infants' expiratory flow and could be higher during crying periods. Ventilator delivered CPAP variable-flow devices that include the Infant Flow Driver (IFD, Infant Flow nasal CPAP system, Care Fusion, Yorba Linda, CA), Benveniste gas jet valve CPAP, Aladdin, and Arabella systems utilize flow opposition with fluidic flow reversal during expiration, where gas is entrained during inspiration to maintain stable pressure and expiratory flow is diverted via a separate fluidic "flip-flop."

Bubble CPAP represents the simplest form of CPAP, requiring only provision of a constant bias flow of blended gas that is heated and humidified, a patient interface and creation of flow opposition and pressure by submerging the tip of the expiratory limb a set distance under the surface of the liquid. Varying the depth of the underwater expiratory tube thus varies the CPAP pressure. Flow escapes beneath the liquid surface via creation of bubbles. Pressure oscillation created by the bubbles is transmitted back to the nares, delivering a variable rather than constant pressure to the airway opening. The generation of bubbling in the water chamber by exhaled gas has been hypothesized to produce chest vibrations that may enhance gas exchange [28]. The applied gas flow rate has been observed to affect the degree of bubbling, and it has been suggested that oscillations from bubbling affect the pressure amplitude and contribute to gas exchange by delivering low-amplitude, high-frequency oscillations to the lungs [14,15,29].

The principle of IFD CPAP is the Bernoulli effect, which directs gas flow toward each naris, and the Coanda effect to cause the inspiratory flow to flip and exit the generator chamber via the expiratory limb. This may assist spontaneous breathing and reduce the work of breathing by decreasing expiratory resistance and maintaining stable airway pressure throughout the respiratory cycle [30]. The Benveniste gas jet valve CPAP is an alternative variable-flow system that consists of two coaxially positioned tubes connected by a ring. It works via the Venturi principle to generate pressure. It is connected to a blended gas source and then to the patient via nasal prongs, generating variable-flow CPAP [31]. Compared with constant pressure flow opposition CPAP, variable-flow opposition CPAP systems may offer important and relevant clinical advantage in the infants with chronic respiratory disease, particularly in the presence of impaired respiratory muscle contractility and susceptibility to fatigue.

Randomized trials comparing continuous positive airway pressure devices

Randomized controlled trials performed at birth

Mazzella et al. [32] compared IFD CPAP with binasal prongs and bubble CPAP through a single nasopharyngeal tube in preterm infants with RDS at less than 12 h of age. They reported a significant beneficial effect on both oxygen requirement and respiratory rate with IFD CPAP, compared to bubble CPAP, and a trend toward a decreased need for mechanical ventilation. Tagare et al. [33] compared the efficacy and safety of bubble CPAP with ventilator-derived CPAP in preterm neonates with RDS. A higher percentage of infants was successfully treated with bubble CPAP (83% vs. 63%, P = 0.03), suggesting superiority of bubble CPAP. Mazmanyan et al. [34] randomized preterm infants to bubble CPAP or IFD CPAP after stabilization at birth in a resource-poor setting. They reported bubble CPAP equivalent to IFD CPAP in the total number of days CPAP was required.

Randomized trials of continuous positive airway pressure after extubation

In a study by Sun et al. [35] among infants greater than 30 weeks' gestation and birth weight greater than 1250 g, the results favored IFD CPAP over ventilator-derived CPAP. In another study, Stefanescu et al. examined extremely low birth weight infants and compared IFD CPAP with ventilator-derived CPAP using INCA prongs and found no difference in the extubation success rate between the two groups [20]. These trials suggest that IFD CPAP is either superior to or has similar efficacy to ventilator-derived CPAP when used after extubation. In a subsequent trial, Gupta et al. [21] randomized preterm infants 24–29 weeks' gestation or 600–1500 g at birth to receive bubble CPAP or IFD CPAP following the first attempt at extubation. Infants were stratified according to duration of initial ventilation (≤14 days or >14 days). Although there was no statistically significant difference in the extubation failure rate (16.9% on bubble CPAP, 27.5% on IFD CPAP) for the entire study group, the median duration of CPAP support was 50% shorter in the infants on bubble CPAP, median 2 days (95% CI, 1–3 days) on bubble CPAP versus 4 days (95% CI, 2–6 days) on IFD CPAP (P = 0.03). In infants ventilated for less than or equal to 14 days, the extubation failure rate was significantly lower with bubble CPAP (14.1%; 9/64) compared to IFD

CPAP (28.6%; 18/63) ($P = 0.046$). This well-designed clinical trial suggests the superiority of postextubation bubble CPAP over IFD CPAP in preterm babies less than 30 weeks, who are initially ventilated for less than 14 days.

There seems to be only a slight difference between continuous- or variable-flow CPAP devices, but there is a trend in favor of bubble CPAP for postextubation support, especially in infants ventilated for ≤2 weeks. The nasal interface is important for optimal delivery of pressure and CPAP delivery while limiting untoward effects, which also requires close monitoring and good nursing care. With increasing use of CPAP devices, it is important that units use the evidence to select an appropriate CPAP device and minimize complications.

Practical aspects of nasal CPAP application and strategies for success

The use of nasal CPAP as the initial mode of respiratory support in critically ill very low birth weight infants is associated with a lower incidence of chronic lung disease [8]. Many institutions have attempted to replicate the practices and results at Columbia University. However, success rates with nasal CPAP are highly variable, which may, in part, be attributable to how well it is utilized. With recent renewed interest in noninvasive respiratory support, particularly bubble nasal CPAP, it is essential to evaluate strategies for success that may depend on the most optimal use of CPAP devices, attention to detail and bedside caregiver experience. Detailed below are strategies that address the issues with the use of bubble nasal CPAP system as practiced at

Columbia University and share the practical aspects for replicating success with bubble nasal CPAP use.

Choose the appropriate size of nasal prongs

It is important to choose the correct size nasal prongs in order to provide effective nasal CPAP and avoid erosion of nasal septum. Smaller size prongs are more likely to move up and rub against septum. Furthermore, they increase airway resistance and allow air to leak around them, making it difficult to maintain a desired optimal pressure. If prongs are too large, they can blanch nares and also cause erosive damage. The correct size prongs should snugly fit the infant's nares without pinching the septum or cause blanching as shown in Fig. 18.2. The nasal prongs should be placed in the nares with the curved side facing down at a 45-degree angle to the infant's face. The prongs may need to be moistened with sterile water or saline, especially in extremely low birth weight infants when first introduced.

Proper fixation of the nasal interface

An appropriate size snug premade cap or stockinet is essential to securely hold the inspiratory and expiratory tubing in place. The rim of the cap should be located above the eyebrows and over the top of the ears. The tubing are then secured on both sides of the cap with Velcro or safety pins and rubber bands, as shown in Fig. 18.2. It is important to have the nasal prongs and tubing properly positioned to reduce pressure on the nose and face. When properly positioned the corrugated tubing should not touch infant's skin, there should be no lateral pressure on the nasal

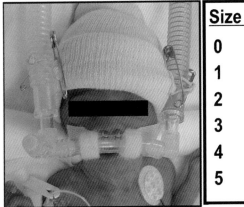

Size	Birth weight
0	<700 g
1	~1000 g
2	~2000 g
3	~3000 g
4	~4000 g
5	Infant

Fig. 18.2 Nasal CPAP interface (Hudson prongs) used at Columbia University showing correct size prongs that snugly fit in infant's nares without pinching the septum or cause blanching and the cannula is held securely in place without touching and compressing the nasal septum with the help of Velcro. Note the tubing secured on both sides of the cap with safety pins and rubber bands. Also included is a table of birth weight and corresponding best size of Hudson prong to be used.

septum and a small space should be present between the tip of the septum and the cannula connecting the prongs. If necessary, self-adhesive Velcro can be used to ensure that the cannula remains away from the nasal septum at all times. The elbows of the nasal prongs should be adjusted so that the corrugated tubing lie along both sides of the face and head.

Optimizing nasal CPAP delivery by using chin straps and pacifiers

A small neck roll can be placed under the infant to prevent neck flexion and airway obstruction. Additionally, chinstraps can be applied as needed to maintain airway pressure, decrease leakage of gases from the mouth, and promote bubbling. A pacifier can provide the same effect as a chin strap so long as the infant can tolerate sucking on it without any signs of distress or discomfort.

Infant care and positioning while on nasal CPAP

Vigilant care is needed to ensure correct positioning of the nasal CPAP prongs to avoid septal irritation and to keep the CPAP cannula off the nasal septum at all times. The nasal cavities, oropharynx, and stomach should be gently suctioned every 3–4 h as needed to improve ventilation and decrease abdominal distension. When performing nasal or oral suctioning, prior to removing the prongs, the infant's eyes should be covered with a dry cloth to prevent contamination from nasal secretions.

The infant's position should be changed at least every 3 h; prone, supine, or lateral positions are all acceptable. However, after changing infant's position one must always ensure that there is no additional pressure on the nasal septum or face from the corrugated tubing.

Frequent systematic check of delivery system and nasal prong position

For nasal CPAP to be effective and successful, it is essential to systematically check the CPAP delivery system including the oxygen blender and flowmeter settings, humidifier water content, inspired gas temperature, and air bubbling out of the solution. The inspiratory oxygen concentration should be titrated to maintain the oxygen saturation between 90% and 95%. The inspired gas should be well humidified and the temperature should be kept around 37°C to prevent irritation of the mucous membranes, avoid mucous plugging, mobilize secretions, and make suctioning less damaging. It is important to ensure that the temperature sensor is always outside the heated isolette. The condensed water in

the circuit should be periodically drained as needed. Flow rates between 5 and 10 L/min should be used to provide adequate flow and prevent rebreathing of carbon dioxide, compensate for leakage from tubing connectors and around CPAP prongs, and generate desired CPAP pressure. The distal end of the expiratory tubing should be inserted to an appropriate length (usually 5–6 cm) below the liquid surface in the "bubbler" to generate the desired CPAP (5–6 cmH$_2$O). Higher CPAP pressures are rarely needed as physiological PEEP of 3 cmH$_2$O is well preserved at those pressures in a nonintubated infant. Higher CPAP pressure may be associated with increased incidence of pneumothorax [8]. The liquid in the bubbler can be sterile water or 0.25% acetic acid. It is recommended that the nasal CPAP circuit be changed once each week.

Avoiding gastric distension

A short length feeding tube is usually placed to permit gastric venting and decompression of the swallowed air. This decreases excessive pressure from the diaphragm and improves lung expansion. The tube should be suctioned periodically as needed whether or not the infant is being fed enterally. The tube position and patency need to be checked periodically.

Nipple feeding and skin-to-skin care during nasal CPAP

Infants on nasal CPAP therapy can be fed by nipple, gavage, or continuous tube feeding if they are clinically stable. No clinically significant aspiration has been demonstrated during the period of the oral feeding while the infant is receiving nasal CPAP [36]. Controlled introduction of oral feedings in infants with BPD during nasal CPAP is safe and may accelerate the acquisition of oral feeding milestones [36]. In infants with good suck–swallow coordination and stable respiratory status, nipple feeding should be encouraged. Early parental involvement in nipple feeding while the infant is still on nasal CPAP also facilitates bonding. Similarly, skin-to-skin care is to be encouraged when patient is on nasal CPAP (Fig. 18.3).

Weaning nasal CPAP

As the infant's respiratory distress improves, the fractional oxygen concentration should be lowered in decrements of 0.02–0.05, keeping the CPAP pressure constant at 5 cmH$_2$O and maintaining oxygen saturation in the optimal range (targeted range at Columbia University is 90%–95%). When the oxygen concentration is 21%, and the infant is without signs of respiratory distress, apnea, or bradycardia, they are eligible for a "trial off" CPAP. This may be achieved by completely discontinuing the CPAP support and closely

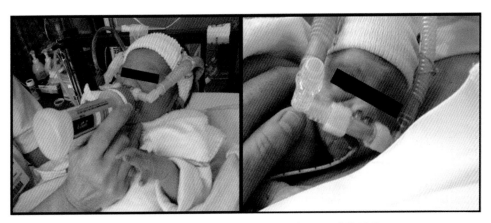

Fig. 18.3 Infants Being Bottle-Fed and Receiving Skin-to-Skin Care During Nasal CPAP Treatment.

monitoring the infant for signs of increasing respiratory distress (tachypnea, retractions, oxygen desaturation, bradycardia, or apnea). If respiratory distress worsens, the infant should be placed back on nasal CPAP. A recent multicenter randomized controlled trial [37] compared three weaning strategies for CPAP (either abrupt discontinuation, weaning CPAP over several days with increasing time off CPAP or cycled on and off CPAP with nasal cannula oxygen at 0.5 L/min during CPAP OFF periods). This study showed that taking "OFF" CPAP with the view to stay "OFF" significantly shortens the weaning time, the duration of CPAP, oxygen duration, incidence of BPD, and length of hospitalization.

Identifying and managing nasal CPAP failure

CPAP failure may occur during the acute phase of RDS or during recovery when nasal CPAP is being weaned. CPAP failure during the acute phase of RDS may occur if nasal CPAP is not sufficient to maintain adequate oxygenation (with an FiO_2 ≥ 0.6) or ventilation (pH <7.2 and PCO_2 ≥ 65 mmHg); or when infant has frequent episodes of apnea requiring repeated stimulation or bag-mask ventilation despite adequate CPAP delivery and oxygenation, the infant may need to be intubated, mechanically ventilated, and perhaps given exogenous surfactant. Prior to initiation of mechanical ventilation, it is important to observe the infant's clinical condition. If the blood gas results are not compatible with the clinical appearance, further investigation is needed before abandoning nasal CPAP therapy. It is important to rule out the improper application of nasal CPAP, poor fit of the CPAP prongs, nasal obstruction due to secretions, airway obstruction caused by a flexed neck, gastric distention, or too frequent handling of the unstable infant. If the CPAP system is felt to be working properly and oxygenation is not adequate, rarely some infants may

benefit from an increase in the end-expiratory pressure. CPAP failure during weaning may occur within minutes of coming off nasal CPAP or as much as 12–24 h later. If the infant is experiencing frequent episodes of apnea and bradycardia or develops respiratory distress while off nasal CPAP, the nasal CPAP should be reinstituted.

Avoiding potential complications with nasal CPAP

Complications of CPAP therapy depend on the interface used. With the nasal prong CPAP described above [1], they may include (1) nasal obstruction from secretions or improper application of nasal prongs; (2) gastric distention from swallowing excessive air, or (3) nasal septum erosion or necrosis. This last complication can be prevented by choosing the appropriate size nasal prongs, ensuring that the cannula is held securely in place without touching and compressing the nasal septum and with vigilant care to keep the cannula off the nasal septum (Fig. 18.2).

Randomized clinical trials of nasal CPAP versus intubation and surfactant

There have been five, large, randomized clinical trials published [8,38–41] comparing early/prophylactic use of nasal CPAP with intubation and surfactant. With the exception of the trial from South America [41], study infants were all <30 weeks' gestation. In two of the trials [38,40], infants were randomized to the treatment arm (CPAP or surfactant) antenatally. In the remaining three trials, the infant's condition was assessed at birth before randomization. Overall, there was only a modest reduction in death or BPD

(29.2% with CPAP vs. 33.5% with intubation and surfactant). Importantly, there was no difference in the incidence of air leak between the treatment arms (5.7% with CPAP and 6.2% with intubation and surfactant). Long-term respiratory outcomes have only been published for SUPPORT [42]. The authors interviewed 918/922 eligible infants at 6-month intervals up until 18–22 months' corrected age. Infants randomized to CPAP versus intubation/surfactant had fewer episodes of wheezing without a cold (28.9% vs. 36.5%; $P < 0.05$), respiratory illnesses diagnosed by a doctor (47.5% vs. 55.2%; $P < 0.05$), and physician or emergency room visits for breathing problems (68.0% vs. 72.9%; $P < 0.05$) at 18–22 months' corrected age.

The question has been raised why the outcomes for nasal CPAP were only marginally better than those following administration of surfactant. There are several possibilities, including (1) inexperience with CPAP at the participating centers, (2) thresholds for discontinuing CPAP were lower than those used routinely at Columbia, (3) the duration of CPAP was very short making it difficult to using BPD as an end point, and (4) some CPAP systems may be more effective than others. Aly et al. have published their experience with nasal CPAP over a 4-year time period, and demonstrated that the incidence of nasal CPAP failure, surfactant use, and BPD all declined significantly over time, suggesting a "learning curve" to the use of nasal CPAP [43]. Much of that "learning curve" is the increase in the comfort level of nurses who are using nasal CPAP for the first time. In addition, the percentage of infants who were intubated and who received surfactant in the two treatment arms of the five randomized clinical trials and the FiO_2 threshold used to define treatment failure were different. With the exception of the NEOCOSUR trial, a high percentage of infants in the "CPAP arm" was intubated (33%–67.1%) and received surfactant (38%–67.1%) in the other clinical trials. As discussed in the subsequent section, those percentages are higher than routinely occur at Columbia. In three of the trials, the FiO_2 used to define treatment failure was <60%; the threshold for intubation at Columbia is an $FiO_2 \geq 60\%$. Finally, the mean duration of CPAP in all five studies was less than 2 weeks, limiting the utility of BPD as an end point and not utilizing the advantage of lung growth stimulation [13] with extended CPAP use.

CPAP in meconium aspiration syndrome

The practice at Columbia regarding the management of MAS is as follows:

1. CPAP is very useful for MAS. Airway diameter is larger during inspiration and smaller during expiration. If airway is plugged with meconium, air may get into lung during inspiration but cannot exhale leading to air trapping. CPAP increases airway diameter. With CPAP, air can get in and out preventing air trapping. CPAP prongs are placed on neonates with MAS as soon as possible in DR. With this strategy, there has not been a single mortality with MAS since 1980 at Columbia, and it is unusual for babies to require intubation and mechanical ventilation.

2. Almost all nasal CPAP pressures are initiated at 5 cmH_2O. Most infants have a physiologic PEEP of +3 cmH_2O without intubation. Very sick neonates with MAS (FiO_2 >0.6) are intubated and receive surfactant. Neonates with mild-to-moderate illness (FiO_2 <0.6) are managed with CPAP alone and pressures of +5 cmH_2O are adequate. High pressures (≥ 8 cmH_2O) are avoided to minimize the risk of air leaks.

3. During initial phases of weaning, only FiO_2 is weaned and CPAP pressure is not weaned.

4. The Columbia protocol allows the infant to be maintained on CPAP +5 cmH_2O as long as the infant is still requiring supplemental oxygen or having respiratory distress.

5. We discontinue CPAP from +5 cmH_2O when infant is on room air and no respiratory distress (no tachypnea, retraction or apnea, bradycardia). If CPAP is discontinued too early, the FRC gradually decreases. If patient becomes distressed again, CPAP is reinstated.

Experience with nasal CPAP at Columbia University

Nasal CPAP has been used for more than 40 years at Columbia University Medical Center and the incidence of chronic lung disease is around 5% [17,44,45]. There is increasing interest at other centers in evaluating this technology and replicating the results. The policy at Columbia is to use nasal CPAP on every spontaneously breathing preterm infant with respiratory distress or supplemental oxygen requirement. CPAP is usually initiated within 10 min of life. At Columbia, CPAP is used more liberally; fewer infants are mechanically ventilated; and less sedation, postnatal steroids and surfactant are used resulting in much lower incidence of chronic lung disease. Our success with nasal CPAP is due to a number of variables, which extend far beyond the cognitive decision to initiate it in an infant with respiratory distress.

We have published two retrospective analyses of preterm infants with RDS admitted to the NICU at Columbia to identify clinical variables predicting CPAP failure [17,45]. Study infants weighed <1250 g in the Ammari study [17] and <1000 g in the Tagliaferro study [45]. We defined success with CPAP when infants were maintained on nasal

CPAP for at least 72 h. The CPAP failure group required intubation within the first 72 h of postnatal age. CPAP failure was defined as worsening oxygenation with an FiO_2 ≥ 0.6 or inadequate ventilation (arterial pH <7.20 and a $PaCO_2$ >65 mmHg or frequent episodes of apnea requiring repeated stimulation or bag/mask ventilation). Infants without any spontaneous ventilation at birth, despite resuscitative efforts, were intubated and ventilated. In the study by Ammari et al., 76% of infants were successfully maintained on nasal CPAP [17]. Success with nasal CPAP was directly related to postmenstrual age. None of the infants in the nasal CPAP success group received surfactant and those infants were significantly less likely to develop chronic lung disease (defined as need for supplemental O_2 at 36-week postconceptional age) than those failing CPAP or ventilated immediately. In the study by Tagliaferro et al., 64% of the infants started on nasal CPAP were successfully maintained for at least 72 h and the incidence of BPD defined, as an oxygen need at 36 weeks' gestation was 4.2% in the CPAP success group, 17.9% in the CPAP failure group, and 15.2% in infants requiring ventilation in the delivery room [45].

Summary

The success with the use of nasal CPAP for respiratory failure in newborn is contingent upon the thorough understanding of the device and astute assessment of the infant during the treatment in order to provide optimal respiratory support that results in minimal volutrauma or barotrauma and reduces the development of chronic lung disease. Not all CPAP devices are created equal, and there is a learning curve for nasal CPAP therapy. The more you do it, the easier it will feel, the better your outcomes will be, and the less complications you will encounter. Existing literature shows conflicting results with nasal CPAP therapy due to variable guidelines for use, different devices and ventilator modes, and variations in training and experience. More recently, there has been a wealth of experimental and clinical data supporting the effectiveness of using early nasal CPAP therapy for respiratory failure in very low birth weight infants to reduce the need for intubation and surfactant replacement therapy. Nasal CPAP also facilitates weaning from mechanical ventilation to reduce lung injury. For preterm infants with immature lungs, prolonged periods of nasal CPAP support, even without oxygen supplementation, enhances lung growth, and can potentially reduce the incidence of BPD. NICUs not using nasal CPAP are encouraged to gain training and experience from an experienced center that uses nasal CPAP appropriately and has proven superior respiratory outcomes. Units implementing "best practices" have demonstrated improved patient outcomes [46,47].

Key strategies for the successful use of nasal CPAP therapy include the following:

1. Choose the right nasal CPAP device.
2. Familiarize caregivers with the device.
3. Learn to use nasal CPAP correctly and troubleshoot.
4. Maintain nasal CPAP with meticulous airway care.
5. Pay attention to details and minimize complications.
6. Gain experience (as there is a learning curve).
7. Initiate nasal CPAP as early as possible (usually in the delivery room) to all infants (no birth weight or gestational age limits) having spontaneous breathing with respiratory distress.
8. Tolerate permissive hypercarbia ($PaCO_2$ 50–65) if oxygenation is adequate.
9. Extended use of nasal CPAP support to enhance the growth of the premature lung.
10. Team work.

Appendix: video of nasal CPAP application at birth in a 480 g preterm infant with RDS

Please visit MedEnact to access the above mentioned video.

References

[1] Wung JT, Driscoll JM, Epstein RA, et al. A new device for CPAP by nasal route. Crit Care Med 1975;3:76–78.

[2] Harrison VC, Heese Hde V, Klein M. The significance of grunting in hyaline membrane disease. Pediatrics 1968;41(3):549–559.

[3] Llewellyn MA, Swyer, PR. Positive Expiratory Pressure During Mechanical Ventilation in the Newborn. Abstract 1970 SPR/APS meeting.

[4] Gregory GA, Kitterman JA, Phibbs RH, Tooley WH, Hamilton WK. Treatment of the idiopathic respiratory distress syndrome with continuous positive airway pressure. N Engl J Med 1971;284:1333–1340.

[5] Avery ME, Tooley WH, Keller JB, Hurd SS, Bryan MH, Cotton RB, et al. Is chronic lung disease in low birth weight infants preventable?

A survey of eight centers. Pediatrics 1987;79(1):26–30.

[6] Van Marter LJ, Allred EN, Pagano M, Sanocka U, Parad R, Moore M, et al. Do clinical markers of barotrauma and oxygen toxicity explain interhospital variation in rates of chronic lung disease? The Neonatology Committee for the Developmental Network. Pediatrics 2000;105(6):1194–1201.

[7] Stevens TP, Harrington EW, Blennow M, Soll RF. Early surfactant administration with brief ventilation vs. selective surfactant and continued mechanical ventilation for preterm infants with or at risk for respiratory distress syndrome. Cochrane Database Syst Rev 2007;4:CD003063.

[8] Morley CJ, Davis PG, Doyle LW, Brion LP, Hascoet J-M, Carlin JB. for the COIN Trial Investigators. Nasal CPAP or intubation at birth for very preterm infants. N Engl J Med 2008;358(7):700–708.

[9] Schmolzer GM, Kumar M, Pichler G, Aziz K, O'Reilly M, Cheung P-Y. Non-invasive versus invasive respiratory support in preterm infants at birth: systematic review and meta-analysis. BMJ 2013;347:f5980.

[10] Rojas-Reyes MX, Morley CJ, Soll R. Prophylactic versus selective use of surfactant in preventing morbidity and mortality in preterm infants. Cochrane Database Syst Rev 2012;3:CD000510.

[11] Stoll BJ, Hansen NI, Bell EF, Walsh MC, Carlo WA, Shankaran S, et al. Trends in care practices, morbidity, and mortality of extremely preterm neonates, 1993–2012. JAMA 2015;314(10):1039–1051.

[12] Elgellab A, Riou Y, Abbazine A, et al. Effects of nasal continuous positive airway pressure (NCPAP) on breathing pattern in spontaneously breathing premature newborn infants. Intensive Care Med 2001;27:1782–1787.

[13] Zhang S, Garbutt V, McBride JT. Strain-induced growth of the immature lung. J Appl Physiol 1996;81:1471–1476.

[14] Lee KS, Dunn MS, Fenwick M, Shennan AT. A comparison of underwater bubble continuous positive airway pressure with ventilator-derived continuous positive airway pressure in premature neonates ready for extubation. Biol Neonate 1998;73:69–75.

[15] Pillow JJ, Travadi JN. Bubble CPAP: is the noise important? An in vitro study. Pediatr Res 2005;57(6):826–830.

[16] Spain CL, Silbajoris R, Young SL. Alterations of surfactant pools in fetal and newborn rat lungs. Ped Res 1987;21:5–8.

[17] Ammari A, Suri MS, Milisavljevic V, et al. Variables associated with the early failure of nasal CPAP in very low birth weight infants. J Pediatr 2005;147:341–347.

[18] Cox JMR, Boehm JJ, Millare EA. Individual nasal masks and intranasal tubes: a non-invasive neonatal technique for the delivery of continuous positive airway pressure (CPAP). Anesthesia 1974;29:597–600.

[19] Kieran EA, Twomey AR, Molloy EJ, Murphy JF, O'Donnell CP. Randomized trial of prongs or mask for nasal continuous positive airway pressure in preterm infants. Pediatrics 2012;130(5):e1170–e1176.

[20] Stefanescu BM, Murphy WP, Hansell BJ, et al. A randomized, controlled trial comparing two different continuous positive airway pressure systems for the successful extubation of extremely low birth weight infants. Pediatrics 2003;112:1031–1038.

[21] Gupta S, Sinha SK, Tin W, et al. A randomized controlled trial of post-extubation bubble continuous positive airway pressure versus Infant Flow Driver continuous positive airway pressure in preterm infants with respiratory distress syndrome. J Pediatr 2009;154(5):645–650.

[22] Ahluwalia JS, White DK, Morley CJ. Infant Flow Driver or single prong nasal continuous positive airway pressure: short-term physiological effects. Acta Paediatr 1998;87(3):325–327.

[23] Kavvadia V, Greenough A, Dimitriou G. Effect on lung function of continuous positive airway pressure administered either by infant flow driver or a single nasal prong. Eur J Pediatr 2000;159(4):289–292.

[24] Bushell T, McHugh C, Meyer MP. A comparison of two nasal continuous positive airway pressure interfaces—a randomized crossover study. J Neonatal Perinatal Med 2013;6(1):53–59.

[25] Kamper J, Ringsted C. Early treatment of idiopathic respiratory distress syndrome using binasal continuous positive airway pressure. Acta Paediatr Scand 1990;79:581–586.

[26] Courtney SE, Pyon KH, Saslow JG, Arnold GK, Pandit PB, Habib RH. Lung recruitment and breathing pattern during variable versus continuous flow nasal continuous positive airway pressure in premature infants: an evaluation of three devices. Pediatrics 2001;107:304–308.

[27] Pandit PB, Courtney SE, Pyon KH, Saslow JG, Habib RH. Work of breathing during constant- and variable-flow nasal continuous positive airway pressure in preterm neonates. Pediatrics 2001;108:682–685.

[28] Martin S, Duke T, Davis P. Efficacy and safety of bubble CPAP in neonatal care in low and middle income countries: a systematic review. Arch Dis Child Fetal Neonatal Ed 2014;99:F495–F504.

[29] Poli JA, Richardson CP, DiBlasi RM. Volume oscillations delivered to a lung model using 4 different bubble CPAP systems. Respir Care 2015;60:371–381.

[30] Moa G, Nilsson K, Zetterstrom H, Jonsson LO. A new device for administration of nasal continuous positive airway pressure in the newborn: an experimental study. Crit Care Med 1988;16:1238–1242.

[31] Benveniste D, Pedersen JE. A valve substitute with no moving parts, for artificial ventilation in newborn and small infants. Br J Anaesth 1968;40:464–470.

[32] Mazzella M, Bellini C, Calevo MG, et al. A randomised control study comparing the Infant Flow Driver with nasal continuous positive airway pressure in preterm infants. Arch Dis Child Fetal Neonatal Ed 2001;85:F86–F90.

[33] Tagare A, Kadam S, Vaidya U, et al. Bubble CPAP versus ventilator CPAP in preterm neonates with early onset respiratory distress—a randomized controlled trial. J Trop Pediatr 2013;59:113–119.

[34] Mazmanyan P, Mellor K, Dore CJ, et al. A randomised controlled trial of flow driver and bubble continuous positive airway pressure in preterm infants in a resource-limited setting. Arch Dis Child Fetal Neonatal Ed 2016;101:F16–F20.

[35] Sun SC, Tien HC, Banabas S. Randomized controlled trial of two methods of nasal CPAP (NCPAP): flow driver vs conventional CPAP [abstract 1898]. Pediatr Res 1999;45:322A.

[36] Hanin M, Nuthakki S, Malkar MB, Jadcherla SR. Safety and efficacy of oral feeding in infants with BPD on nasal CPAP. Dysphagia 2015;30(2):121–127.

[37] Todd DA, Wright A, Broom M, Chauhan M, Meskell S, Cameron C, et al. Methods of weaning preterm babies <30 weeks gestation off NCPAP: a multicentre randomised controlled trial. Arch Dis Child Fetal Neonatal Ed 2012;97:F236–F240.

[38] Finer NN, Carlo WA, Walsh MC, Rich W, Gantz MG, SUPPORT Study Group of the Eunice Kennedy Shriver NICHD Neonatal Research Network. et al. Early CPAP versus surfactant

in extremely preterm infants. N Engl J Med 2010;362(21): 1970–1979.

[39] Sandri F, Plavka R, Ancora G, Simeoni U, Stranak Z, Martinelli S, et al. Prophylactic or early selective surfactant combined with nCPAP in very preterm infants. Pediatrics 2010;125(6):e1402–e1409.

[40] Dunn MS, Kaempf J, de Klerk A, de Klerk R, Reilly M, Vermontal Oxford Network DRM Study Group. et al. Randomized trial comparing 3 approaches to the initial respiratory management of preterm neonates. Pediatrics 2011;128(5):e1069–e1076.

[41] Tapia JL, Urzua S, Bancalari A, Meritano J, Torres G, Fabres J, et al. Randomized trial of early bubble continuous positive airway pressure for very low birth weight infants. J Pediatr 2012;161(1):75–80.

[42] Stevens TP, Finer NN, Carlo WA, Szilagyi PG, Phelps DL, Walsh MC, et al. Respiratory outcomes of the surfactant positive pressure and oximetry randomized trial (SUPPORT). J Pediatr 2014;165(2):240–249.

[43] Aly H, Milner JD, Patel K, El-Mohandes AA. Does the experience with the use of nasal continuous positive airway pressure improve over time in extremely low birth weight infants? Pediatrics 2004;114(3):697–702.

[44] Sahni R, Ammari A, Suri MS, et al. Is the new definition of bronchopulmonary dysplasia more useful? J Perinatol 2005;25:41–46.

[45] Tagliaferro T, Bateman DA, Ruzal-Shapiro C, Polin RA. Early radiologic evidence of severe respiratory distress syndrome as a predictor of nasal continuous positive airway pressure failure in extremely low birth weight newborns. J Perinatol 2015;35(2):99–103.

[46] Birenbaum HJ, Dentry A, Cirelli J, et al. Reduction in the incidence of chronic lung disease in very low birth weight infants: results of a quality improvement process in a tertiary level neonatal intensive care unit. Pediatrics 2009;123:44–50.

[47] Levesque BM, Kalish LA, LaPierre J, et al. Impact of implementing 5 potentially better respiratory practices on neonatal outcome and cost. Pediatrics 2011;128:e218–e226.

Chapter | **18B** |

Continuous Positive Airway Pressure in the Treatment of Meconium Aspiration Syndrome

Rakesh Sahni, MD, Jen-Tien Wung, MD, FCCM

CHAPTER POINTS

- A good understanding of the underlying complicated pathophysiology and pulmonary mechanics is needed to manage infants with meconium aspiration syndrome (MAS) successfully.
- Use of early nasal CPAP in infants with MAS can reduce the need for subsequent mechanical ventilation.
- Majority of infants with MAS do not need innovative ventilatory support that includes use of HFOV, inhaled nitric oxide or surfactant.

Introduction

Meconium aspiration syndrome (MAS) is a complex syndrome that ranges in severity from mild respiratory distress to severe respiratory failure, persistent pulmonary hypertension of the newborn (PPHN), and sometimes death.

Accordingly, the respiratory support should be tailored depending on the severity of respiratory distress from continuous positive airway pressure (CPAP) to conventional mechanical ventilation (MV), high-frequency oscillatory ventilation (HFOV), and extracorporeal membrane oxygenation (ECMO). Approximately 30%–50% of infants diagnosed with MAS have severe disease, defined as the need for MV [1–3]. Bhutani et al. reported that only 20% of infants with MAS requiring positive pressure assistance needed "innovative ventilatory support" (defined as the use of high-frequency ventilation, inhaled nitric oxide, or surfactant) and no infants died or required ECMO [4]. It seems that when used optimally, conventional therapies (CPAP and MV) are adequate to improve oxygenation in the majority of infants with this disease. However, MV though life-saving can result in ventilation-induced lung injury, and is associated with prolonged duration of hospitalization and subsequent increased burden on the health care system [5,6]. Neonatal MAS challenges the caretakers to make the correct diagnosis, understand the syndrome's complicated pathophysiology and alterations in pulmonary mechanics, and then tailor the appropriate treatment strategy, including the use of early nasal CPAP, and other therapies.

Diagnosing meconium aspiration syndrome

Approximately 8%–19% of all term deliveries occur through meconium-stained amniotic fluid and MAS develops in 5%–33% of these infants [3]. The respiratory signs of MAS are similar to other neonatal respiratory diseases

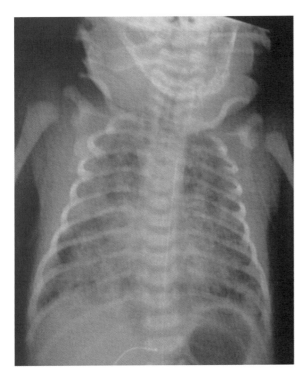

Fig. 18B.1 Classic radiographic picture in meconium aspiration syndrome showing diffuse patchy infiltrates with areas of atelectasis mixed with areas of hyperinflation throughout the lung fields.

and include tachypnea, retractions, grunting, nasal flaring, and cyanosis. If the meconium has been present in utero for greater than 3 h, the infant may have meconium staining of the skin, nails, and umbilical cord. The anterior–posterior diameter of the chest may be increased if there is significant air trapping. The classic radiographic picture of MAS includes diffuse patchy infiltrates with areas of atelectasis mixed with areas of hyperinflation throughout the lung fields (Fig. 18B.1). Other findings on X-ray include possible air leaks and cardiomegaly, if significant perinatal asphyxia has resulted in cardiomyopathy.

Despite the classic clinical and radiological appearance of MAS, it may be difficult in certain cases to distinguish MAS from other neonatal respiratory diseases such as transient tachypnea of newborn, aspiration of amniotic fluid, respiratory distress syndrome, pneumonia, sepsis with pulmonary edema, PPHN, and congenital heart disease [7]. It is important diagnostically and physiologically to determine if PPHN is secondary to MAS or may be present by itself (primary PPHN) with concurrent meconium-stained amniotic fluid but no true aspiration [8]. Importantly, the

treatment of the infant's respiratory disease will depend on the presence and severity of pulmonary hypertension.

Pathophysiology of meconium aspiration syndrome

Pulmonary pathophysiology of MAS is complex as it involves multiple mechanisms. Meconium has deleterious effects on the airways, injures the pulmonary parenchyma and alveoli, inhibits surfactant function, and may cause hypoxic pulmonary vasoconstriction resulting in PPHN [9]. The most common disturbance of lung function in MAS is hypoxemia and decreased lung compliance. Poor oxygenation is attributable to a combination of ventilation–perfusion mismatching, intrapulmonary shunting related to regional atelectasis, and extrapulmonary shunting due to PPHN. Infants may manifest any one or more of these effects and the respiratory distress may change depending on the severity of the underlying pathophysiology.

One common mechanism of MAS is due to obstruction of airways with meconium in the lung. When the obstruction is partial, a "ball-valve" mechanism may lead to air trapping and air leaks (Fig. 18B.2) [10]. If meconium plug is in the airway, during inspiration the dilated airway allows the gas to enter the lung, but during expiration when the airway constricts around the obstruction, air is trapped inside the lung. This may result in overexpansion of the lung, ventilation–perfusion mismatch, decreased compliance, and possibly air leak. Complete obstruction of the airway by meconium may result in atelectasis and resultant hypoxemia and hypercapnia.

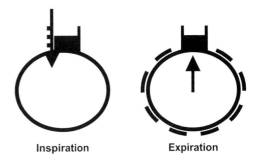

Inspiration   Expiration

Fig. 18B.2 The airway is bigger during inspiration (left) compared with expiration (right). In the presence of meconium plug, the bigger airway allows for air to enter the lung during inspiration. However, during expiration with a smaller airway, exhalation of air is difficult resulting in air trapping and hyperinflation.

Chapter | 19 |

Nasal Intermittent Positive Pressure Ventilation

Vikramaditya Dumpa, MD, Vineet Bhandari, MD, DM

CHAPTER POINTS

- NIPPV is an intermediate mode of noninvasive respiratory support between endotracheal tube ventilation and CPAP
- NIPPV is different from BiPAP, and when synchronized, is referred to as SNIPPV
- Early use of NIPPV has been proven to be superior to CPAP in decreasing the need for intubation and endotracheal tube ventilation
- Indications and guidelines for the ventilator settings for primary and secondary modes of NIPPV are different
- A decompression orogastric tube should be present in all babies on NIPPV

Introduction

Noninvasive ventilation strategies are becoming increasingly popular in the care of preterm infants across the globe

due to the potential for less barotrauma, volutrauma, and oxygen toxicity—all being the factors that contribute to the development of bronchopulmonary dysplasia (BPD). Early initiation of continuous positive airway pressure (CPAP) has become a standard in the care of the spontaneously breathing preterm infant. However, CPAP failure occurs in up to 50% of extremely low birth weight infants, most often due to apnea of prematurity and progressive respiratory acidosis [1–4]. Nasal intermittent positive-pressure ventilation (NIPPV) is a form of noninvasive ventilatory assistance using a nasal interface to deliver intermittent peak inspiratory pressures (PIP) above positive end-expiratory pressure (PEEP). NIPPV is an intermediate approach between invasive ventilation with an endotracheal tube and noninvasive CPAP.

History

NIPPV has been used as a form of noninvasive respiratory support in newborn infants since the 1970s [5]. Its use was described to be an effective mode of ventilation in intractable apnea of prematurity [6]. However, the technique went into disfavor in the 1980s after reports of increased gastrointestinal perforations in infants ventilated with facemask or nasal prongs [7]. It was in the early 2000s that there was a renewed interest in this technique after randomized controlled trials (RCT) proved it to be effective without an increased incidence of gastrointestinal perforations [8–10].

Mechanism(s) of action (Fig. 19.1)

NIPPV theoretically works by recruitment of collapsed alveoli establishing functional residual capacity (FRC) and improved gas exchange [11,12]. Other reported physiological effects include improved stability of the chest wall,

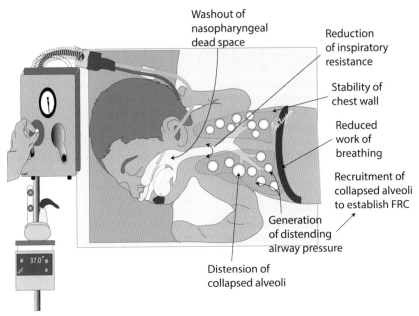

Washout of
nasopharyngeal
dead space

Reduction
of inspiratory
resistance

Stability of
chest wall

Reduced
work of
breathing

Recruitment of
collapsed alveoli
to establish FRC

Generation
of distending
airway pressure

Distension of
collapsed alveoli

Fig. 19.1 Benefits of Nasal Intermittent Positive Ventilation (NIPPV) With Nasal Prongs. Nasal ventilation is easy to use and results in washout of nasopharyngeal dead space and distends collapsed alveoli establishing functional residual capacity (FRC). It reduces work of breathing and inspiratory resistance. Modified from a graphic abstract MHNP journal. Copyright: Satyan Lakshminrusimha.

improved pulmonary mechanics and thoracoabdominal motion synchrony, decreased flow resistance [13], increased tidal and minute volumes [14], decreased work of breathing, and reduced chest wall distortion [15–17], and addition of increased intermittent distending pressure above PEEP, with increased flow delivery in the upper airway [8]. Use of NIPPV has also been shown to decrease pulmonary inflammation in newborn piglets managed with NIPPV compared with invasive ventilation [18]. A majority of the studies noted above were conducted with NIPPV being delivered in the synchronized mode, that is, SNIPPV, using the Infant Star ventilator in the StarSync mode (Infrasonics Inc., San Diego, CA). This ventilator (no longer available in the United States) used the Graseby capsule, which was placed on the abdominal region over the surface of the liver in the neonate to detect the respiratory efforts by changes in the abdominal excursion.

Types of NIPPV—primary mode versus secondary mode

Primary mode of NIPPV refers to its use soon after birth with or without a short period (≤2 h) of intubation for surfactant delivery, followed by extubation. The secondary mode refers to its use after a longer period (>2 h to days to weeks) of intubation [12].

NIPPV versus BiPAP

BiPAP or bilevel CPAP or biphasic CPAP is not to be confused with NIPPV. In BiPAP, flow drivers are used to deliver alternating high- and low-level CPAP pressures. The high-level pressure is usually in the range of 9–11 cmH_2O with the difference in the two pressure levels being <5 cmH_2O, and the inflation times are prolonged. On the other hand, the aim in NIPPV is to mimic invasive ventilation with peak inspiratory pressures and positive-end expiratory pressures similar to those used in invasive ventilation with an endotracheal tube and the inflation times are usually short. A subgroup analysis of a large multicenter randomized trial comparing infants who received treatment with NIPPV versus bilevel CPAP did not show a significant difference in the composite outcome of death/BPD or BPD alone, but morbidity was higher in the bilevel CPAP group [19]. It is recommended that these two modalities should not be considered equivalent until further evidence is available from large RCTs.

NIPPV versus SNIPPV

Synchronized NIPPV (SNIPPV) refers to the use of NIPPV with synchronization to the patient's inspiratory efforts. Clinical trials have demonstrated the effectiveness of SNIPPV over NIPPV and NCPAP in reducing need for intubation in respiratory distress syndrome (RDS), improving the success of extubation, and treating apnea of prematurity, with a reassuring absence of relevant side effects [8–10,15,20]. As mentioned earlier, synchronization was achieved using the Infant Star ventilator using the StarSync mode with a Graseby capsule placed on the anterior abdominal wall. However, this ventilator was phased out of production and this technique of synchronization has become obsolete in the United States. Some European manufacturers are introducing ventilators with incorporated flow-synchronization mechanisms showing encouraging results with synchronization in published studies [21]. A retrospective study comparing clinical outcomes in infants managed with SNIPPV versus NIPPV showed that use of NIPPV was not associated with increased BPD/death or other common neonatal morbidities after adjusting for significant confounding variables [22].

Clinical use of NIPPV

Respiratory distress syndrome (RDS)

In the management of spontaneously breathing preterm infants with clinical/radiological evidence of RDS, we recommend the early use of NIPPV at settings as described (Section: Practical guidelines for the use of NIPPV). However, it is important to consider the use of early surfactant in extremely preterm infants (≤ 26 weeks of gestational age) and in infants with severe RDS requiring fraction of inspired oxygen (FiO_2) > 0.4, as surfactant deficiency is a major contributing factor to the failure of NIPPV.

Early surfactant therapy by minimally invasive surfactant therapy (MIST) or intubation, surfactant, extubation (INSURE) approach is recommended, whenever feasible in this population. The MIST approach seems to be a safe and an effective alternative to INSURE in RCTs conducted to date [23]. In a RCT comparing early NIPPV versus NCPAP in preterm infants, early NIPPV decreased the use of invasive mechanical ventilation and the need for surfactant treatment (given as MIST) within 72 h of life [24].

Two recent Cochrane reviews with meta-analysis of multiple RCTs comparing NIPPV to NCPAP concluded that early NIPPV is superior to NCPAP alone in decreasing respiratory failure and the need for intubation and endotracheal tube ventilation [25,26].

Prevention of postextubation failure

Use of NIPPV after invasive mechanical ventilation and extubation decreases the risk of meeting respiratory failure criteria and the need for reintubation, compared to NCPAP [25,26]. Early surfactant replacement as needed, early caffeine therapy, and maintaining an optimal hematocrit are vital for preventing postextubation failure. Please refer to Section, Practical guidelines for the use of NIPPV, for further details on management of infants on secondary mode of NIPPV.

Apnea of prematurity

Immature pulmonary reflexes to hypoxia and hypercapnia are involved in the pathophysiology of apnea of prematurity [27]. Apnea is one of the main causes of noninvasive ventilation failure [28]. NIPPV is known to augment the beneficial effects of CPAP in preterm infants with frequent or severe apnea [25,26]. Increasing the frequency on the NIPPV settings is helpful in preterm infants presenting with apneic episodes. However, if the episodes of apnea are frequent (≥ 2 episodes/h) or require manual bag-mask ventilation, it is recommended to intubate and place on invasive mechanical ventilation (see criteria for reintubation in Section: Practical guidelines on use of NIPPV).

BPD

Invasive endotracheal tube ventilation is a critical contributing factor to the pathogenesis of BPD. Invasive ventilation induces mechanical stretch injury and generates an inflammatory response characterized by an increase in the proinflammatory cytokines, such as interleukin-6 (IL-6), IL-8, tumor necrosis factor-alpha (TNF-α), and decrease in antiinflammatory cytokines, for example, IL-10. This inflammatory response in the setting of hyperoxia leads to a multiple hit pathway predisposing to BPD [29]. In particular, during the first 3 postnatal days in the life of a preterm infant there is a high proinflammatory environment as measured by increased levels of cytokines IL-6, IL-8, and granulocyte-colony-stimulating factor (G-CSF) in the tracheal secretions in neonates ≤ 30 weeks of gestational age [30]. Any additional inflammation secondary to invasive mechanical ventilation with subsequent barotrauma and/or volutrauma during this critical period may contribute to further lung damage and development of BPD. Thus, emphasis should be placed on aggressive weaning and early extubation to a noninvasive mode of ventilation within the first postnatal week, preferably within the first 72 h, as early extubation is associated with decreased BPD/death [31,32].

An attempt toward extubation should always be considered as soon as the infant is weaned to appropriate settings [12]. In an interesting retrospective study, it was noted that infants who were extubated early but had to be reintubated later have a lower incidence of BPD/death compared to infants who remained intubated and were extubated later [32].

Multiple small RCTs comparing the use of NIPPV to NCPAP have shown a decreased incidence of BPD with NIPPV [33–36]. However, the meta-analysis from the recent Cochrane reviews did not demonstrate a significant reduction in chronic lung disease with the use of NIPPV compared to CPAP [25,26]. The RCT conducted by Kirpalani et al. also showed no significant differences in survival or BPD between the two groups [37]. However, in a recent RCT, comparing early NIPPV versus NCPAP, the NIPPV group had significantly decreased moderate-to-severe BPD [24].

NIPPV failures

In a large retrospective study analyzing the characteristics of infants who failed NIPPV, it was noted that female gender, increased gestational age, and weight at the time of extubation were protective against NIPPV failure. The most common reasons attributed to NIPPV failure are work of breathing, increasing FiO_2 requirement (in the first 6 h after extubation), and apnea (after 24 h of extubation) [28].

Additional modes of synchronization to provide noninvasive support: NIV-NAVA

Synchronization utilizing neurally adjusted ventilatory assist (NAVA) in noninvasive ventilation is a relatively newer concept in neonatal ventilation. In NAVA, the electrical activity of the diaphragm is measured and is used to trigger and control the ventilator. The ventilator delivers mechanical breaths that are synchronized with the patient's inspiratory effort and also provides pressure support proportional to the patient's inspiratory effort. This eliminates the asynchrony between the infant's respiratory efforts and the ventilator-delivered breaths, theoretically leading to improvement in the work of breathing [38]. Published studies using NIV-NAVA are showing promising results in small trials [39,40]. However, large, multicenter RCTs are required to determine the short- and long-term effects of NIV-NAVA before it can be recommended as the primary mode of noninvasive ventilation.

Flow synchronization

Another mode of synchronization reported in a European unit utilizes a flow sensor to detect spontaneous inspiratory flow with the help of a pressure transducer pneumotachograph and specially designed ventilator software (Giulia flow trigger). Studies comparing flow SNIPPV to NIPPV and NCPAP using this device showed a reduced need for intubation, decreased extubation failure, and improvement in apnea of prematurity in the SNIPPV group [21,41,42]. Additional studies and more adequately powered trials are needed to confirm these data.

Practical guidelines for the use of NIPPV

Indications

1. A method of noninvasive ventilatory assistance in the spontaneously breathing infant with impending or existing ventilatory failure because of increased work of breathing.
2. A form of weaning from invasive conventional mechanical ventilation in the spontaneously breathing patient with increased work of breathing [12].

Contraindications

1. Upper airway abnormalities
   a. Choanal atresia
   b. Cleft palate
   c. Tracheoesophageal fistula
2. Severe cardiovascular instability

Potential hazards/complications

1. Obstruction of prongs because of mucus plugging
2. Feeding intolerance
3. Abdominal distension
4. Gastrointestinal perforation
5. Ventilator-induced lung injury including air-leak syndromes
6. Hypoventilation
7. Infection
8. Nose bleed/nasal irritation
9. Skin irritation and pressure necrosis

Equipment and supplies

1. Ventilator
2. Nasal prongs (or mask)
3. Tape
4. Hydrocolloid dressing, for example, DuoDerm
5. Orogastric tube (8 or 9 Fr)
6. Suction catheter

Table 19.1 Recommended initial and maximum support in primary and secondary modes with extubation criteria prior to secondary mode of nasal intermittent positive-pressure ventilation (NIPPV)

	Primary mode—initial settings	Primary mode—maximum support	Extubation criteria prior to secondary mode	Secondary mode—initial settings	Secondary mode—maximum support
PIP (cmH$_2$O)	4 cm above that required for manual ventilation		≤16	2–4 cm above that required on conventional ventilator	
PEEP (cmH$_2$O)	4–6	6–8	≤5	≤5	6–8
MAP (cmH$_2$O)		<1000 g–≤14 ≥1000 g–≤16			<1000 g–≤14 ≥1000 g–≤16
Frequency (per min)	30	45	15–25	15–25	40
T_i (sec)	0.45	0.55	0.45	0.45	0.55
Flow (L/min)	8–10	12	8–10	8–10	12

PIP, peak inspiratory pressure; *PEEP*, positive end-expiratory pressure; *MAP*, mean airway pressure; *Ti*, inspiratory time.

Procedure

1. Estimate appropriate size prongs for the infant.
2. Place DuoDerm strips in front of the nostrils, after making holes in the strips that will fit the nasal prongs snugly. Additionally, place a Duoderm strip over the upper lip, if the prongs are going to be resting there.
3. Position the prongs in the infant's nose. The short binasal prongs should fit fully inside the nostrils.
4. Place the headcap over the infant's head and secure the nasal interface with Velcro straps, if appropriate.
5. Insert an orogastric tube; connect the other end of the tube to a 10 mL syringe, remove plunger, and place it higher than the infant and open to the atmosphere.
6. Connect the nasal interface setup to the ventilator.
7. See Table 19.1 for initial and maximal NIPPV settings.
8. After initial placement of NIPPV, it is necessary to auscultate to check for air entry and oxygenation (SpO$_2$). Increase PIP in steps of 2 cmH$_2$O till you get good air entry, appropriate chest rise, and SpO$_2$ is being maintained in the desired range. The rate may need to be increased, as needed.
9. It is imperative to start caffeine therapy as soon as possible; at least 1 h prior to extubation.
10. Maintain a hematocrit ≥35%

Monitoring on NIPPV

1. Monitor: SpO$_2$, heart rate (HR), and respiratory rate (RR). Target SpO$_2$ within the desired range as per the individual unit's protocol.

2. Obtain a blood gas in 15–30 min.
3. Adjust ventilator settings to maintain blood gases (Table 19.2).
4. Suction mouth and pharynx as necessary.

NIPPV—maintenance

1. Attempt to minimize air leak from the mouth
   a. Use a pacifier
   b. Use a chin strap
2. Attempt to keep PIP/MAP within 4/2 cmH$_2$O of the targeted value
3. Orogastric (large bore) decompression tube
   a. Connect to an empty 10 mL syringe, with the plunger removed, open to the atmosphere
   b. Keep at a higher level than the infant to decrease abdominal distension
   c. Can be used for feeding via gravity drip method
4. If requiring continuous feeds, a 6 Fr orogastric tube can be placed (passed along the large-bore decompression tube and can be taped to it) and connected to a syringe pump

NIPPV: consideration for reintubation despite maximal support settings

1. Blood gas: pH < 7.25 and PaCO$_2$ ≥60 mmHg
2. Severe apnea: Any episode requiring bag and mask resuscitation

Table 19.2 Suggested changes in nasal intermittent positive-pressure ventilation (NIPPV) settings based on blood gases/apnea

	Hypoxemia	Hypercarbia	Hypercarbia + Hypoxemia	Apnea
T_i^* (s)	↑ (max 0.55)	↓ (min 0.4)	↑ (max of 0.55)	0.4–0.5
Rate* (/min)	↑ (max 40)	↑ (max 40)	↑ (max 40)	↑ (max of 40)
PIP* (cmH_2O)	↑	↑	↑	Usually 15–20
PEEP* (cmH_2O)	↑ (max 8)	–/↓	↑ (max 8)	Usually 4–6

↑, Increase; ↓, decrease; *MAP*, mean airway pressure; *max*, maximum; *min*, minimum; *PEEP*, positive end expiratory pressure; *PIP*, peak inspiratory pressure; T_i, inspiratory time.
*Variables determining MAP. Adjust these parameters to increase MAP to a maximum of 14 cmH_2O in <1000 g and 16 cmH_2O in ≥1000 g weight infants.

3. Frequent (>2–3 episodes/h) of apnea/bradycardia (cessation of respiration for >20 s associated with a HR <100/min) not responding to caffeine
4. Frequent desaturation (SpO_2 ≤85%): ≥3 episodes/h, not responding to increased ventilator settings
   Adjust FiO_2 to maintain O_2 saturations in the desired range. If FiO_2 ≥0.6:
   - **Step 1**: Increase PIP by 2, minimize pressure leaks by closing the mouth.

- **Step 2**: If unable to wean FiO_2, increase T_i by 0.05.
- **Step 3**: If unable to wean FiO_2, increase PEEP by 1.
- **Step 4**: if unable to wean FiO_2, repeat steps 1–3 *in the same sequence*, until maximum MAP is reached.
   In clinical practice, we do not have a maximum value for the PIP. PIP is adjusted to achieve adequate chest expansion, equal and good breath sounds. PEEP is adjusted based on FiO_2 requirement. We do not routinely obtain chest X-rays in patients on NIPPV (Fig. 19.2).

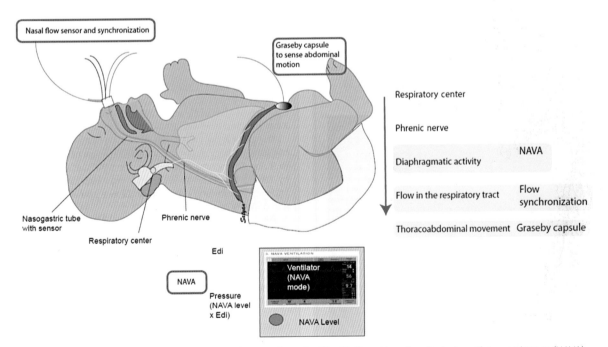

Fig. 19.2 Mechanisms of Synchronization During Noninvasive Ventilation. Neurally adjusted ventilatory assistance (NAVA) detects diaphragmatic electrical activity (Edi). Flow detectors sense spontaneous inspiratory flow. Graseby capsule detects abdominal movement during inspiration (see text for details). Copyright: Satyan Lakshminrusimha.

Online supplementary material

Please visit MeDEnact to access the video on NIPPV

References

[1] Finer NN, Carlo WA, Walsh MC, et al. Early CPAP versus surfactant in extremely preterm infants. N Engl J Med 2010;362(21):1970–1979.

[2] Morley CJ, Davis PG, Doyle LW, Brion LP, Hascoet JM, Carlin JB. Nasal CPAP or intubation at birth for very preterm infants. N Engl J Med 2008;358(7):700–708.

[3] Stefanescu BM, Murphy WP, Hansell BJ, Fuloria M, Morgan TM, Aschner JL. A randomized, controlled trial comparing two different continuous positive airway pressure systems for the successful extubation of extremely low birth weight infants. Pediatrics 2003;112(5):1031–1038.

[4] Waitz M, Mense L, Kirpalani H, Lemyre B. Nasal intermittent positive pressure ventilation for preterm neonates: synchronized or not? Clin Perinatol 2016;43(4):799–816.

[5] Helmrath TA, Hodson WA, Oliver TK Jr. Positive pressure ventilation in the newborn infant: the use of a face mask. J Pediatr 1970;76(2):202–207.

[6] Moretti C, Marzetti G, Agostino R, et al. Prolonged intermittent positive pressure ventilation by nasal prongs in intractable apnea of prematurity. Acta Paediatrica Scandinavica 1981;70(2):211–216.

[7] Garland JS, Nelson DB, Rice T, Neu J. Increased risk of gastrointestinal perforations in neonates mechanically ventilated with either face mask or nasal prongs. Pediatrics 1985;76(3):406–410.

[8] Friedlich P, Lecart C, Posen R, Ramicone E, Chan L, Ramanathan R. A randomized trial of nasopharyngeal-synchronized intermittent mandatory ventilation versus nasopharyngeal continuous positive airway pressure in very low birth weight infants after extubation. J Perinatol 1999;19(6 Pt 1):413–418.

[9] Barrington KJ, Bull D, Finer NN. Randomized trial of nasal synchronized intermittent mandatory ventilation compared with continuous positive airway pressure after extubation of very low birth weight

infants. Pediatrics 2001;107(4):638–641.

[10] Khalaf MN, Brodsky N, Hurley J, Bhandari V. A prospective randomized, controlled trial comparing synchronized nasal intermittent positive pressure ventilation versus nasal continuous positive airway pressure as modes of extubation. Pediatrics 2001;108(1):13–17.

[11] Jackson JK, Vellucci J, Johnson P, Kilbride HW. Evidence-based approach to change in clinical practice: introduction of expanded nasal continuous positive airway pressure use in an intensive care nursery. Pediatrics 2003;111(4 Pt 2):e542–547.

[12] Bhandari V. Nasal intermittent positive pressure ventilation in the newborn: review of literature and evidence-based guidelines. J Perinatol 2010;30(8):505–512.

[13] Kiciman NM, Andreasson B, Bernstein G, et al. Thoracoabdominal motion in newborns during ventilation delivered by endotracheal tube or nasal prongs. Pediatr Pulmonol 1998;25(3):175–181.

[14] Moretti C, Gizzi C, Papoff P, et al. Comparing the effects of nasal synchronized intermittent positive pressure ventilation (nSIPPV) and nasal continuous positive airway pressure (nCPAP) after extubation in very low birth weight infants. Early Hum Dev 1999;56(2–3):167–177.

[15] Chang HY, Claure N, D'Ugard C, Torres J, Nwajei P, Bancalari E. Effects of synchronization during nasal ventilation in clinically stable preterm infants. Pediatr Res 2011;69(1):84–89.

[16] Ali N, Claure N, Alegria X, D'Ugard C, Organero R, Bancalari E. Effects of non-invasive pressure support ventilation (NI-PSV) on ventilation and respiratory effort in very low birth weight infants. Pediatr Pulmonol 2007;42(8):704–710.

[17] Aghai ZH, Saslow JG, Nakhla T, et al. Synchronized nasal intermittent positive pressure ventilation (SNIPPV) decreases work of breathing (WOB)

in premature infants with respiratory distress syndrome (RDS) compared to nasal continuous positive airway pressure (NCPAP). Pediatr Pulmonol 2006;41(9):875–881.

[18] Lampland AL, Meyers PA, Worwa CT, Swanson EC, Mammel MC. Gas exchange and lung inflammation using nasal intermittent positive-pressure ventilation versus synchronized intermittent mandatory ventilation in piglets with saline lavage-induced lung injury: an observational study. Crit Care Med 2008;36(1):183–187.

[19] Millar D, Lemyre B, Kirpalani H, Chiu A, Yoder BA, Roberts RS. A comparison of bilevel and ventilator-delivered non-invasive respiratory support. Arch Dis Child Fetal Neonatal Ed 2016;101(1):F21–25.

[20] Huang L, Mendler MR, Waitz M, Schmid M, Hassan MA, Hummler HD. Effects of synchronization during noninvasive intermittent mandatory ventilation in preterm infants with respiratory distress syndrome immediately after extubation. Neonatology 2015;108(2):108–114.

[21] Gizzi C, Montecchia F, Panetta V, et al. Is synchronised NIPPV more effective than NIPPV and NCPAP in treating apnoea of prematurity (AOP)? A randomised cross-over trial. Arch Dis Child Fetal Neonatal Ed 2015;100(1):F17–23.

[22] Dumpa V, Katz K, Northrup V, Bhandari V. SNIPPV vs NIPPV: does synchronization matter? J Perinatol 2012;32(6):438–442.

[23] Kribs A. Minimally invasive surfactant therapy and noninvasive respiratory support. Clin Perinatol 2016;43(4):755–771.

[24] Oncel MY, Arayici S, Uras N, et al. Nasal continuous positive airway pressure versus nasal intermittent positive-pressure ventilation within the minimally invasive surfactant therapy approach in preterm infants: a randomised controlled trial. Arch Dis Child Fetal Neonatal Ed 2016;101(4):F323–328.

[25] Lemyre B, Davis PG, De Paoli AG, Kirpalani H. Nasal intermittent positive pressure ventilation (NIPPV) versus nasal continuous positive airway pressure (NCPAP) for preterm neonates after extubation. Cochrane Database Syst Rev 2017;2:Cd003212.

[26] Lemyre B, Laughon M, Bose C, Davis PG. Early nasal intermittent positive pressure ventilation (NIPPV) versus early nasal continuous positive airway pressure (NCPAP) for preterm infants. Cochrane Database Syst Rev 2016;12:Cd005384.

[27] Zhao J, Gonzalez F, Mu D. Apnea of prematurity: from cause to treatment. Eur J Pediatr 2011;170(9):1097–1105.

[28] Mehta P, Berger J, Bucholz E, Bhandari V. Factors affecting nasal intermittent positive pressure ventilation failure and impact on bronchopulmonary dysplasia in neonates. J Perinatol 2014;34(10):754–760.

[29] Balany J, Bhandari V. Understanding the impact of infection, inflammation, and their persistence in the pathogenesis of bronchopulmonary dysplasia. Front Med 2015;2:90.

[30] Chang BA, Huang Q, Quan J, et al. Early inflammation in the absence of overt infection in preterm neonates exposed to intensive care. Cytokine 2011;56(3): 621–626.

[31] Dumpa V, Northrup V, Bhandari V. Type and timing of ventilation in the first postnatal week is associated with bronchopulmonary dysplasia/death. Am J Perinatol 2011;28(4):321–330.

[32] Berger J, Mehta P, Bucholz E, Dziura J, Bhandari V. Impact of early extubation and reintubation on the incidence of bronchopulmonary dysplasia in neonates. Am J Perinatol 2014;31(12):1063–1072.

[33] Jasani B, Nanavati R, Kabra N, Rajdeo S, Bhandari V. Comparison of non-synchronized nasal intermittent positive pressure ventilation versus nasal continuous positive airway pressure as post-extubation respiratory support in preterm infants with respiratory distress syndrome: a randomized controlled trial. J Matern Fetal Neonatal Med 2016;29(10):1546–1551.

[34] Bhandari V, Gavino RG, Nedrelow JH, et al. A randomized controlled trial of synchronized nasal intermittent positive pressure ventilation in RDS. J Perinatol 2007;27(11):697–703.

[35] Kugelman A, Feferkorn I, Riskin A, Chistyakov I, Kaufman B, Bader D. Nasal intermittent mandatory ventilation versus nasal continuous positive airway pressure for respiratory distress syndrome: a randomized, controlled, prospective study. J Perinatol 2007;150(5):521–526. 526.e521.

[36] Ramanathan R, Sekar KC, Rasmussen M, Bhatia J, Soll RF. Nasal intermittent positive pressure ventilation after surfactant treatment for respiratory distress syndrome in preterm infants <30 weeks' gestation: a randomized, controlled trial. J Perinatol 2012;32(5):336–343.

[37] Kirpalani H, Millar D, Lemyre B, Yoder BA, Chiu A, Roberts RS. A trial comparing noninvasive ventilation strategies in preterm infants. N Engl J Med 2013;369(7):611–620.

[38] Firestone KS, Beck J, Stein H. Neurally adjusted ventilatory assist for noninvasive support in neonates. Clin Perinatol 2016;43(4):707–724.

[39] Colaizy TT, Kummet GJ, Kummet CM, Klein JM. Noninvasive neurally adjusted ventilatory assist in premature infants postextubation. Am J Perinatol 2017;34(6):593–598.

[40] Gibu C, Cheng P, Ward RJ, Castro B, Heldt GP. Feasibility and physiological effects of non-invasive neurally adjusted ventilatory assist (NIV-NAVA) in preterm infants. Pediatr Res 2017;82(4):650–657.

[41] Gizzi C, Papoff P, Giordano I, et al. Flow-synchronized nasal intermittent positive pressure ventilation for infants <32 weeks' gestation with respiratory distress syndrome. Crit Care Res Pract 2012;2012: 301818.

[42] Moretti C, Giannini L, Fassi C, Gizzi C, Papoff P, Colarizi P. Nasal flow-synchronized intermittent positive pressure ventilation to facilitate weaning in very low-birthweight infants: unmasked randomized controlled trial. Pediatr Int 2008;50(1):85–91.

Chapter | 20A |

High Frequency Ventilation

Payam Vali, MD, Donald M. Null, MD

CHAPTER POINTS

- Avoiding excessive tidal volumes and ensuring adequate lung volume recruitment are imperative to mitigate ventilator-induced lung injury and reduce the risk of bronchopulmonary dysplasia.
- High frequency ventilation provides low tidal volumes and is a very effective mode of ventilation for neonates with severe lung disease.
- Understanding the mechanics of high frequency ventilation leads to improved ventilation strategies for newborns with lung pathology.

Introduction

Respiratory support remains an indispensable therapy in the care of most patients admitted to the neonatal intensive care unit (NICU). Ventilator support, positive pressure, and/or supplemental oxygen are required to manage the most vulnerable extremely premature infants with respiratory distress syndrome (RDS), as well as term newborns suffering from hypoxic respiratory failure (HRF). Remarkable advancements in ventilation support have been made since the first reported cases, in the early 1950s, of a respiratory device used to provide positive pressure breaths to

newborns in respiratory distress [1]. Despite extraordinary technological advancements in ventilator devices and neonatal respiratory care, bronchopulmonary dysplasia (BPD) remains the most prevalent chronic morbidity in premature newborns, 50 years following its first description [2,3].

One of the most important conceptual breakthroughs in managing patients with respiratory failure is that mechanical ventilation may exacerbate lung injury [4], and ongoing research continues to expand our understanding of ventilator-induced lung injury (VILI) [5,6]. Experimental studies have clearly demonstrated that the lungs (particularly diseased lungs) are very susceptible to overdistension (volutrauma) [4,7]. Furthermore, repeated opening and closing of terminal lung units (atelectotrauma) [8,9], and release of inflammatory markers (biotrauma) [10], also contribute to VILI. In an attempt to improve the management of patients with severe respiratory disease who died of intractable hypoxia complicated by multisystem organ failure, high frequency ventilation gained substantial interest in the management of adult RDS [11], as well as newborn RDS [12,13].

High-frequency ventilation (HFV) represents a generic term that encompasses any mode of assisted ventilation operating at a frequency at least 4 times the natural breathing rate [14]. HFV can be categorized into three general types: (1) high-frequency positive-pressure ventilation (HFPPV) produced by modified conventional ventilation operating at rapid rates, (2) high-frequency jet ventilation (HFJV) produced by ventilators that deliver a high-velocity jet of gas by means of a flow-interrupter, and (3) high-frequency oscillatory ventilation (HFOV), produced by moving air back and forth at the airway opening, while generating minimal bulk gas flow. The chapter focuses on HFOV, which is defined by any device that uses reciprocating pumps of a piston, diaphragm, or generates sinusoidal waveforms and vibrates air in and out of the lungs at frequencies ranging from 180 to 3000 breaths/min

(3–50 Hz) [15,16]. Characteristically, gas is both driven into the lung and actively withdrawn by the pump stroke. HFJV will also be briefly discussed.

Brief history on HFOV

Conventional pulmonary physiology dictates that the partial pressure of arterial carbon dioxide ($PaCO_2$) is inversely related to alveolar ventilation (V_a), and that the gas available for gas exchange, the alveolar volume, is derived from the tidal volume (V_t) minus the anatomic dead space (V_d); $V_a = V_t - V_d$. However, the notion that V_t needs to be greater than the V_d to allow adequate ventilation was challenged over a century ago by Henderson et al. who speculated by observing panting dogs that "there may easily be gaseous exchange sufficient to support life, even when V_t is considerably less than dead space" [17]. To support their claim, in a simple experiment, they demonstrated that when blowing tobacco smoke down a transparent elongated tube, a long thin spike formed and that "the quicker the puff, the thinner and sharper the spike." When the puff stopped "the spike breaks instantly, everywhere, and the tube is seen to be filled from side to side with a mixture of smoke and air," [17] so as flow stopped, diffusion occurred.

Not until several decades later, did the concept of high frequency oscillation spark the interest of scientist anew [18–20]. During experiments measuring the effects of muscle relaxants on lung impedance using loudspeakers, a group of researchers were astounded that CO_2 appeared at the mouthpiece during a breath-hold in increasing amounts with each beat of the loudspeaker. In the same year, Lunkenheimer et al. demonstrated that the oscillator dramatically lowered $PaCO_2$ [19,20]. In the following years, a group of dedicated researchers devised a piston pump and started a systematic study on the effects of oscillations on beagle dogs; the results were presented at the Federation of American Societies for Experimental Biology in 1979 [18,21]. Henceforth, to this day, a surge of experimental and clinical studies exploring the mechanism and effects of high-frequency oscillations has emerged in the scientific literature.

Physiology of HFOV

Mechanisms of HFOV

The physiology responsible for gas transport during HFOV remains theoretical and is believed to involve several contributing mechanisms [22–24], which are briefly reviewed:

1. Bulk convection: Even with small tidal volumes, gas flow may reach proximal alveoli and participate in direct alveolar ventilation.
2. Pendelluft: At high frequencies, gas distribution is strongly influenced by time-constant inequalities, and there is redistribution from full, fast-filling units to slower-filling units (hence augmenting gas exchange) [25].
3. Asymmetric inspiratory and expiratory velocity profiles: Inspiratory gas tends to stream along the center of the airway toward the alveoli, while expiratory gas streams along the outer wall [26].
4. Taylor dispersion: When convective flow is superimposed on a diffusive process, there is an increased dispersion of tracer molecules (diffusion of the high-velocity central gases to the margins of the airway—primarily in smaller airways) [27].
5. Cardiogenic mixing: Beating action of the heart promotes gas mixing in the pericardial regions of the lungs [28].
6. Molecular diffusion: As in normal ventilation, there is a movement of molecules from higher concentration to lower concentration.

The key concept underlying the aforementioned mechanisms is that increased energy of the gas molecules at high frequencies and high flows leads to augmented mixing of gas in the airways [29]. In more practical terms, the success in using HFOV depends on understanding the strategies aimed at oxygenating and, especially, ventilating the patients.

Oxygenation in HFOV

Similar to conventional ventilators, high-frequency oscillator devices function to improve oxygenation and ventilation, and while the factors affecting oxygenation and ventilation are interrelated, they are distinct. The two factors that determine oxygenation are mean airway pressure and fraction of inspired oxygen (FiO_2). The cause for hypoxemia in neonatal lung disease is primarily due to atelectasis, and therefore increasing mean airway pressure decreases the degree of atelectasis and improves ventilation-perfusion matching. In HFOV, the way the pressure and flow waveform move down the airway is very different from the characteristic pressure and flow patterns in conventional ventilation. During conventional ventilation, bulk flow essentially generates the pressure at the airway opening, which is transmitted to the endotracheal tube and ultimately the alveoli; whereas in HFOV the pressure at the airway opening is considerably higher but significantly attenuates at the alveolar level [30]. Additionally, the way the pressure is transmitted or attenuated is not even across the lung. Some airways will get a higher-pressure transmission than other ones, which is dependent on their physical location in the respiratory

system and their disease state [31]. Therefore, alveolar pressure in HFOV usually ranges between 0.1 and 5 cmH$_2$O. Owing that there is no means in monitoring respiratory function on HFOV to determine pressure–volume curves as is the case in conventional ventilation, a crude way to assess adequate inflation volume is with the help of chest radiographs to look for lung expansion and diaphragm position.

Other factors that influence blood oxygen content include pulmonary vascular resistance, extrapulmonary shunts, cardiac output, hemoglobin concentration, and FiO$_2$. Mean airway pressure needs to be carefully adjusted to avoid hyperinflation, which restricts venous return, compromises cardiac output and consequently impairs oxygenation [32,33]. When lung volume is excessive, airway pressures exert compressive forces against the capillaries within respiratory units and may also increase pulmonary vascular resistance and impede pulmonary blood flow [34,35]. Conversely, a low mean airway pressure leads to hypoventilation, increases atelectatic areas in the lungs, and results in worsening ventilation/perfusion mismatch and decreased oxygenation.

Ventilation in HFOV

In conventional ventilation, there is a proportional relationship between CO$_2$ elimination (alveolar ventilation) and tidal volume ($V_a = f \times V_t$). In HFOV, tidal volume has a greater effect on CO$_2$ removal than frequency and appears to be a linear function of $(f)^a \times (V_t)^b$, where "a" is approximately 0.7–1 and "b" is between 1.5 and 2.2, depending on the circuit or species [23,36]. Therefore, during conventional ventilation, if we assume a frequency of 40 breaths/min and a V_t of 8 mL/breath, the volume of exhaled CO$_2$ (VCO$_2$) per minute is proportional to the minute ventilation of 320 mL/min. Increasing either the f or V_t on the conventional ventilator by 25%, for example, proportionally increases minute ventilation to 400 mL/min and increase VCO$_2$ by 25%. In comparison, in HFOV, if f is 600 breaths/min (10 Hz) and V_t is 2 mL/breath, minute ventilation = 2400 mL/min (600 × 2^2). Increasing f by 25% increases minute ventilation to 3000 mL/min (750 × 2^2), while an increase in V_t by 25% leads to a greater increase in minute ventilation to 3750 mL/min (600 × 2.25^2). Altering frequency on an oscillator, changes effective V_t as described later and further complicates this relationship.

During HFOV, V_t is determined by the stroke volume the ventilator applies to the system (Fig. 20A.1). The distance that the piston/diaphragm moves creates the amplitude. This movement results in a gas volume displacement and a visual chest wiggle. It may also be described as the peak-to-through swing around the mean airway pressure. The area under the curve of the volume-time curve represents the stroke volume, which increases by increasing amplitude (tidal pressure range) or decreasing frequency (longer cycle time).

Amplitude

Amplitude has the greatest effect on V_t and is, therefore, the primary control to enhance CO$_2$ removal. Amplitude controls the "force" with which the piston moves and is measured in units of pressure (cmH$_2$O). When setting the amplitude, the mean airway pressure needs to be considered first, as CO$_2$ elimination is not efficient without adequate lung recruitment [37]. There is no set rule on how to choose the initial amplitude. The best way to assess adequacy of the amplitude is by visualizing the chest wiggle. A rough estimate for setting the initial amplitude is twice the HFOV mean airway pressure. Any further changes in amplitude will, thereafter, depend on the PaCO$_2$. An early gas should be obtained and, subsequently, transcutaneous CO$_2$ readings have been shown to be reliable in trending CO$_2$ in infants on HFOV [38].

Frequency

Frequency can provide secondary control of CO$_2$ removal. The frequency controls the time allowed for the piston to move. The lower the frequency is set, the greater the volume displacement is achieved, and conversely, the higher the frequency, the lower the displaced volume. Therefore, lower frequencies result in greater stroke volume and, hence, greater CO$_2$ removal. Unlike conventional or jet ventilation, no inspiratory or expiratory time is set for HFOV. Instead, a percentage of time spent in inspiration and expiration (I:E ratio) is set (e.g., I:E ratio of 1:1 or 1:2, 50 or 33%, respectively). The I:E ratio is rarely adjusted in HFOV and is usually set at 1:2.

The most important aspect of lung mechanics in determining optimal frequency is the time constant, which equals the product of dynamic compliance and airway resistance. In general, patients with short time constants (low lung compliance or low airway resistance) can be ventilated effectively at higher frequencies than those with longer time constants (high lung compliance or high airway resistance) [39]. Different compliances within the lung affect the effect frequency has on V_t because the compliance of the respiratory system affects the transmission of the pressure down the airway (Fig. 20A.2) [40,41]. Pressure amplitude transmission decreases with increasing compliance and increasing frequency. In the compliant lung, there is marked dampening of the pressure waveform in HFOV. Lung disease affects the diffusion of gas in the alveolus and, thus, affects the optimum range of frequency for efficient gas exchange. In the noncompliant lung (e.g., RDS), the dampening of pressure down the airways is decreased and, consequently, the frequency can have a much larger effect on V_t. With less dampening of pressure down the pulmonary system, there is a potential for barotrauma in the poorly recruited lung at low frequency [42].

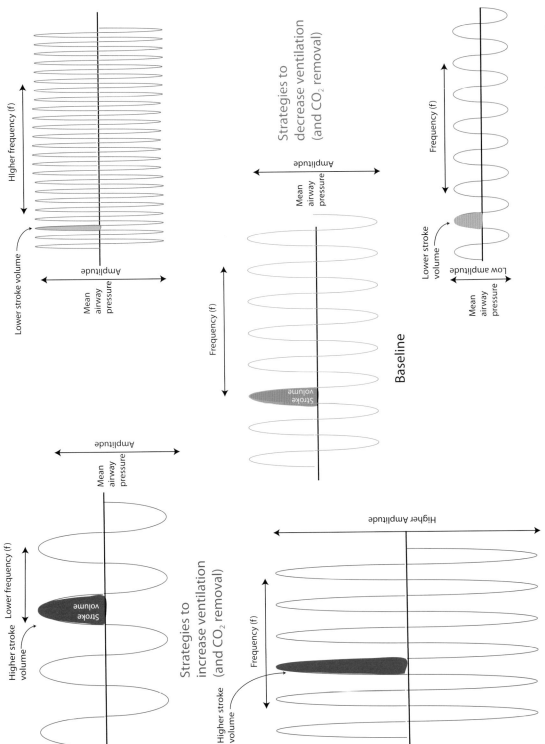

Fig. 20A.1 Volume-Time Curve in High-Frequency Oscillatory Ventilation (HFOV). Tidal volume (V_t) is determined by the stroke volume, which represents the area under the curve of the volume-time curve. Increasing the amplitude increases the tidal pressure ranges, while decreasing the frequency (f) leads to a longer cycle time; both changes increase the stroke volume and, therefore, V_t. Conversely, increasing f or lowering the amplitude will decrease V_t and thus decrease CO_2 removal.

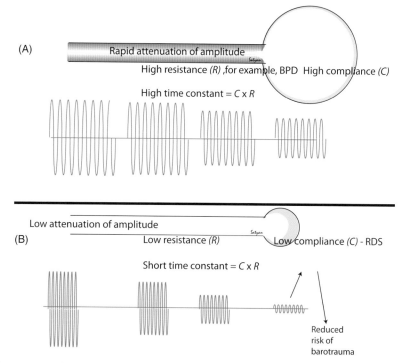

Fig. 20A.2 Time Constants and Amplitude Attenuation in HFOV. (A) Lung pathology with high airway resistance and low airway compliance, such as BPD, has a high time constant with a rapid attenuation of amplitude. Optimal ventilation mode: Lower frequency = Prevents attenuation of amplitude. A low frequency would optimize ventilation to prevent attenuation of the amplitude. (B) Lung pathology with low airway resistance and low airway compliance, such as RDS, has a short time constant with a rapid attenuation of amplitude. Optimal ventilation: High frequency = Rapid attenuation of amplitude. Higher frequencies optimize ventilation in neonates with low airway resistance and low airway compliance. Copyright: Satyan Lakshminrusimha.

During HFOV, several factors can influence tidal volume (Fig. 20A.3). Changes that lead to increased V_t and facilitate CO_2 elimination include increasing the amplitude, decreasing the frequency, decreasing resistance, and optimizing mean airway pressure. The disease state and the compliance of the lung also impact the efficiency of HFOV. Independent of the intrinsic airway disease of the patient, the resistance created by the endotracheal tube is also very significant. Assuming laminar flow, the resistance in the endotracheal tube (ETT) is derived from the equation $R = 8\eta L/\pi r^4$ (where R is resistance, η represents viscosity of the gas, and L represents the length of the tube). Knowingly, exchanging the ETT from a 2.5-mm internal diameter tube to a 3.5-mm tube decreases resistance by a factor of approximately 4.

Clinical application of HFOV

The evidence behind HFOV

HFOV has been studied in animal models for almost 4 decades and the majority of animal data supports the superiority of HFOV over conventional ventilation. Of particular interest, HFOV used in primate models have demonstrated improved gas exchange and lung mechanics, uniform inflation, reduced air leak, and decreased concentration of inflammatory mediators in the lung, as compared with conventional mechanical ventilation [43,44]. Unfortunately, the National Institutes of Health-sponsored trial of HFOV in neonatal RDS (HIFI trial) came at a time when optimal HFOV application was not completely understood [37,45]. The final HIFI protocol tested the low-volume/low-pressure strategy of HFOV and found no pulmonary benefit. In this trial, HFOV actually appeared to increase the incidence of intraventricular hemorrhage.

Around the time of the HIFI trial, emerging evidence supported favorable outcomes in clinical and animal models when applying a high-pressure open-lung strategy with HFOV [44,46], which led to ongoing experiments and trials, despite the poor outcomes of the HIFI trial. Owing to the ongoing interest in HFOV by the San Antonio group in North America who continued to champion this mode of ventilation and the advent of the SensorMedics oscillator, HFOV use has now become widespread in NICUs around the world [18].

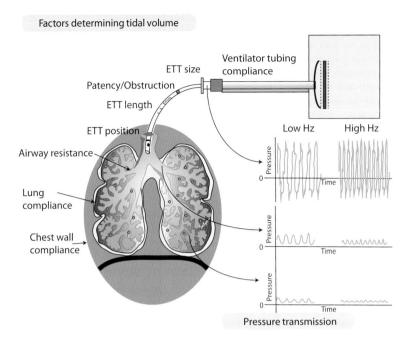

Fig. 20A.3 Factors Influencing Tidal Volume and Pressure Transmission in HFOV. *ETT*, Endotracheal tube. Copyright: Satyan Lakshminrusimha.

In the two more recent, largest, randomized clinical trials, significant benefit from HFOV was only seen in the study that restricted entry to very low birth weight infants who met set FiO_2 and mean airway pressure requirements after surfactant administration [12]. In that population, HFOV increased survival without chronic lung disease and infants managed with HFOV were extubated successfully 1 week earlier than those receiving lung-protective ventilation at conventional frequencies. The other study found no substantial benefit and no adverse effects of HFOV compared with conventional ventilation when all premature newborns within a given range of gestational age were randomized irrespective of the degree of parenchymal disease [13]. Despite the enormous number of publications on HFOV, substantial variability remains about when and how to use HFOV. At one end of the spectrum, HFOV is used as the primary mode of ventilation; whereas at the other extreme HFOV is reserved as a rescue technique, only after conventional ventilation has failed. HFOV should be reserved for a subset of infants with moderate to severe disease, and in the words of Dr. Alison Froese "in mild disease it is not needed. In end-stage disease, it will be useless" [37].

High-frequency jet ventilation

The concept of high-frequency jet ventilation (HFJV) was first introduced in 1967 by Sanders when he demonstrated

the ability to maintain adequate oxygenation and ventilation during bronchoscopy using periodic jets of compressed gas [47]. Subsequently, extensive experimental and clinical studies using the delivery of gases through a small-bore cannula under high pressure confirmed adequacy of CO_2 elimination and improved oxygenation [48–51]. The Bunnell Life Pulse jet ventilator (Bunnell Inc., Salt Lake City, Utah) was designed specifically for infants and remains the most widely used jet ventilator in NICUs. HFJV is primarily used in patients with air-leak syndromes or in cases of nonhomogeneous lung disease.

Mechanism of HFJV and ventilator adjustments

HFJV introduces small volumes typically less than 1 ml/kg (range 0.35 to 1 ml/kg) [52] of gas into the patient's airway at a frequency of 150–600 breaths/min, typically 360–420 breaths/min in the neonatal population. Short pulses of pressurized gas are directly delivered into the upper airway through a narrow-bore cannula or jet injector. The jet gas entering the restricted side port of the adapter accelerates and creates transitional flow (jet streams) into the airway. The jet gas penetrates through the center of the airways and thus limits the pressure exerted on the outside wall of the airway. The high velocity of the jet gas entrains or drags gas from the surrounding airway distally by the Venturi Principle [53]. Exhalation occurs passively as a result of lung recoil along the outer walls of the airway and CO_2 is ultimately expelled

through the expiratory port—an open ventilator-patient circuit is therefore essential.

HFJV can only be used in tandem with a conventional ventilator, whereby ventilation (amplitude) is provided by the jet ventilator and oxygenation (mean airway pressure) is provided by the conventional ventilator. The conventional ventilator can provide recruitment (sigh) breaths to open the lungs, maintains a positive end-expiratory pressure (PEEP), and is the main source of gas through the circuit. A triple-lumen ETT adapter interfaces the two ventilators and consists of (1) a pressure monitoring line that measures pressures at the ETT and feeds back that information to the ventilator, (2) a jet injection port where the jet gas enters, and (3) a standard lumen for connection to a CMV. This adapter avoids the need for reintubation prior to HFJV initiation.

When transitioning from CMV to HFJV, the ETT hub needs to be exchanged for the triple-lumen ETT adapter, and the patient can be reconnected to the previous CMV settings. Then the jet injector and pressure monitoring lines are connected to their respective ports on the adapter. The rate on the jet ventilator is usually set at 420 breaths/min, but can be decreased to as low as 240 breaths/min. Compared to HFOV, HFJV has a set time cycle (default at 0.02 s) and thus a variable I:E ratio, depending on the set frequency. In addition, as the time cycle is fixed, V_t stays constant with changes in frequency and can only be adjusted by a change in delta P (e.g., increase in PIP). The PIP is initially set at the same level as the CMV (and can be increased to a maximum of 50 cmH$_2$O). Once the HFJV settings are set, the PIP and rate on the CMV can be taken off.

The conventional ventilator is necessary to provide PEEP and is usually set 2–3 cmH$_2$O higher when used with the jet. The jet ventilator also allows larger volume breaths (sigh breaths) to be delivered using the conventional ventilator. Sigh breaths may be beneficial in patients suffering from cardiac dysfunction who need to be ventilated with lower Paw and PEEP compared to the higher level of PEEP used during HFOV. Sigh breaths can also help recruit atelectatic lung areas, especially in nonhomogenous lung disease, but should not exceed 5–10 breaths/min. Using excessive conventional breaths rather than a higher Paw is less lung protective. Once the patient is stable, an attempt should be made to decrease the sigh breaths to avoid volutrauma.

Clinical cases

Case of severe pneumomediastinum and pneumoperitoneum

A 36-week gestation late-preterm male born vaginally to a 30-year-old primigravida mother with gestational diabetes. Mother presented in preterm labor and there was no history of chorioamnionitis or prolonged rupture of membranes. The newborn was noted to have increased work of breathing and had persistent hypoxia. He was intubated shortly following birth and received two doses of surfactant in the first 24 h of age. He was placed on CMV on a V_t of 4.5 cc/kg, PEEP of 7 cmH$_2$O, a rate of 20 breaths/min and T_i of 0.35 s. On the second day, he was noted to have worsening respiratory distress requiring an increase in FiO$_2$ and the X-ray

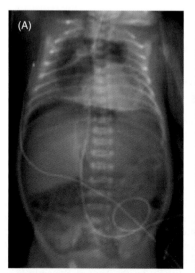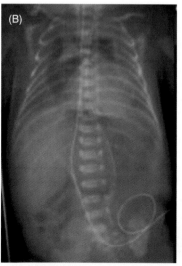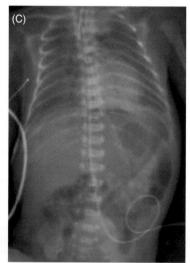

Fig. 20A.4 A 36-week gestation male with RDS at 2 days of age with large pneumomediastinum and pneumoperitoneum on CMV (A). Improvement shown 10 h (B) and 48 h (C) following initiation of HFOV.

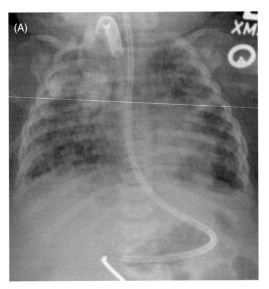 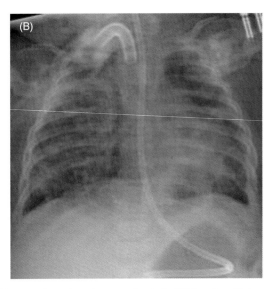

Fig. 20A.5 Former extreme premature infant corrected to term with severe bronchopulmonary dysplasia (BPD) and ventilator acquired pneumonia (A). Improvement in aeration and oxygenation following switch to HFOV (B).

revealed development of a large pneumomediastinum and pneumoperitoneum (Fig. 20A.4A)

The patient was transitioned to HFOV on the following settings: Paw, 20 cmH$_2$O; f, 10 Hz; and amplitude of 20A. The patient's hemoglobin saturations improved quickly and within the first hour FiO$_2$ was weaned from 0.75 to 0.4, and the Paw was decreased to 18 cmH$_2$O. By 10 h, the FiO$_2$ had decreased to 0.26 (Fig. 20A.4B) and the Paw had been gradually weaned to 14 cmH$_2$O. By 48 h, the Paw was down to 12 cmH$_2$O and FiO$_2$ remained <0.25 (Fig. 20A.4C). The following day the patient was extubated from HFOV (Paw, 10 cmH$_2$O; f, 12 Hz; amplitude 18) to a noninvasive positive pressure ventilation.

Case of severe BPD

Former 24-week gestation extreme premature male at corrected gestational age of 40 weeks with severe BPD complicated by ventilator acquired pneumonia. Patient's hemoglobin oxygen saturation deteriorated on CMV settings of V_t 6 cc/kg, PEEP of 8 cmH$_2$O, and rate of 20 (Fig. 20A.5A). The patient was switched to HFOV: Paw, 13 cmH$_2$O; amplitude 30; and f, 9 Hz; and within 1 h FiO$_2$ decreased from 0.93 to 0.72. After 48 h, the patient's FiO$_2$ was 0.4 on a Paw of 15 cmH$_2$O (amplitude of 33 and f of 8). Following the treatment of his pneumonia he was transitioned back to CMV (Fig. 20A.5B).

References

[1] Donald I, Lord J. Augmented respiration studies in atelectasis neonatorum. Lancet 1953;261:9–17.

[2] Northway WH, Rosan RC, Porter DY. Pulmonary disease following respirator therapy of hyaline-membrane disease. Bronchopulmonary dysplasia. N Engl J Med 1967;276:357–368.

[3] Owen LS, Manley BJ, Davis PG, Doyle LW. The evolution of modern respiratory care for preterm infants. Lancet 2017;389:1649–1659.

[4] Webb HH, Tierney DF. Experimental pulmonary edema due to intermittent positive pressure ventilation with high inflation pressures. Protection by positive end-expiratory pressure. Am Rev Respir Dis 1974;110:556–565.

[5] Parker JC, Hernandez LA, Peevy KJ. Mechanisms of ventilator-induced lung injury. Crit Care Med 1993;21:131–143.

[6] Slutsky AS, Ranieri VM. Ventilator-induced lung injury. N Engl J Med 2013;369:2126–2136.

[7] Dreyfuss D, Soler P, Basset G, Saumon G. High inflation pressure pulmonary edema. Respective effects of high airway pressure, high tidal volume, and positive end-expiratory pressure. Am Rev Respir Dis 1988;137:1159–1164.

[8] Sandhar BK, Niblett DJ, Argiras EP, Dunnill MS, Sykes MK. Effects of positive end-expiratory pressure on hyaline membrane formation in a rabbit model of the neonatal respiratory distress syndrome. Intensive Care Med 1988;14:538–546.

[9] Muscedere JG, Mullen JB, Gan K, Slutsky AS. Tidal ventilation at low airway pressures can augment lung injury. Am J Respir Crit Care Med 1994;149:1327–1334.

[10] Tremblay LN, Slutsky AS. Ventilator-induced injury: from barotrauma to biotrauma. Proc Assoc Am Physician 1998;110:482–488.

[11] Oba Y, Salzman GA. Ventilation with lower tidal volumes as compared with traditional tidal volumes for acute lung injury. N Engl J Med 2000;343:813. 813–814.

[12] Courtney SE, Durand DJ, Asselin JM, Hudak ML, Aschner JL, Shoemaker CT. Group NVS. High-frequency oscillatory ventilation versus conventional mechanical ventilation for very-low-birth-weight infants. N Engl J Med 2002;347:643–652.

[13] Johnson AH, Peacock JL, Greenough A, Marlow N, Limb ES, Marston L, Group UKOS. et al. High-frequency oscillatory ventilation for the prevention of chronic lung disease of prematurity. N Engl J Med 2002;347:633–642.

[14] Slutsky AS, Brown R, Lehr J, Rossing T, Drazen JM. High-frequency ventilation: a promising new approach to mechanical ventilation. Med Instrum 1981;15:229–233.

[15] Froese AB, Bryan AC. High frequency ventilation. Am Rev Respir Dis 1987;135:1363–1374.

[16] Butler WJ, Bohn DJ, Bryan AC, Froese AB. Ventilation by high-frequency oscillation in humans. Anesth Analg 1980;59:577–584.

[17] Henderson Y, Chillingworth F, Whitney J. The respiratory dead space. Am J Physiol 1915;38:1–19.

[18] Bryan AC. The oscillations of HFO. Am J Respir Crit Care Med 2001;163:816–817.

[19] Lunkenheimer PP, Rafflenbeul W, Keller H, Frank I, Dickhut HH, Fuhrmann C. Application of transtracheal pressure oscillations as a modification of "diffusing respiration". Br J Anaesth 1972;44:627.

[20] Lunkenheimer PP, Frank I, Ising H, Keller H, Dickhut HH. Intrapulmonary gas exchange during simulated apnea due to transtracheal periodic intrathoracic pressure changes. Anaesthesist 1973;22:232–238.

[21] Bohn D. The history of high-frequency ventilation. Respir Care Clin N Am 2001;7:535–548.

[22] Drazen JM, Kamm RD, Slutsky AS. High-frequency ventilation. Physiol Rev 1984;64:505–543.

[23] Kolton M. A review of high-frequency oscillation. Can Anaesth Soc J 1984;31:416–429.

[24] Chang HK, Harf A. High-frequency ventilation: a review. Respir Physiol 1984;57:135–152.

[25] Lehr JL, Butler JP, Westerman PA, Zatz SL, Drazen JM. Photographic measurement of pleural surface motion during lung oscillation. J Appl Physiol (1985) 1985;59:623–633.

[26] Haselton FR, Scherer PW. Bronchial bifurcations and respiratory mass transport. Science 1980;208:69–71.

[27] Fredberg JJ. Augmented diffusion in the airways can support pulmonary gas exchange. J Appl Physiol Respir Environ Exerc Physiol 1980;49:232–238.

[28] Slutsky AS. Gas mixing by cardiogenic oscillations: a theoretical quantitative analysis. J Appl Physiol Respir Environ Exerc Physiol 1981;51:1287–1293.

[29] Slutsky AS, Drazen JM. Ventilation with small tidal volumes. N Engl J Med 2002;347:630–631.

[30] Gerstmann DR, Fouke JM, Winter DC, Taylor AF, deLemos RA. Proximal, tracheal, and alveolar pressures during high-frequency oscillatory ventilation in a normal rabbit model. Pediatr Res 1990;28:367–373.

[31] Pillow JJ. High-frequency oscillatory ventilation: mechanisms of gas exchange and lung mechanics. Crit Care Med 2005;33:S135–S141.

[32] Reller MD, Donovan EF, Kotagal UR. Influence of airway pressure waveform on cardiac output during positive pressure ventilation of healthy newborn dogs. Pediatr Res 1985;19:337–341.

[33] Tana M, Polglase GR, Cota F, Tirone C, Aurilia C, Lio A, et al. Determination of lung volume and hemodynamic changes during high-frequency ventilation recruitment in preterm neonates with respiratory distress syndrome. Crit Care Med 2015;43:1685–1691.

[34] Whittenberger JL, McGregor M, Berglund E, Borst HG. Influence of state of inflation of the lung on pulmonary vascular resistance. J Appl Physiol 1960;15:878–882.

[35] Polglase GR, Morley CJ, Crossley KJ, Dargaville P, Harding R, Morgan DL, et al. Positive end-expiratory pressure differentially alters pulmonary hemodynamics and oxygenation in ventilated, very premature lambs. J Appl Physiol (1985) 2005;99:1453–1461.

[36] Slutsky AS, Drazen FM, Ingram RH, Kamm RD, Shapiro AH, Fredberg JJ, et al. Effective pulmonary ventilation with small-volume oscillations at high frequency. Science 1980;209:609–671.

[37] Froese AB, Kinsella JP. High-frequency oscillatory ventilation: lessons from the neonatal/pediatric experience. Crit Care Med 2005;33:S115–S121.

[38] Berkenbosch JW, Tobias JD. Transcutaneous carbon dioxide monitoring during high-frequency oscillatory ventilation in infants and children. Crit Care Med 2002;30:1024–1027.

[39] Keszler M, Durand DJ. Neonatal high-frequency ventilation. Past, present, and future. Clin Perinatol 2001;28:579–607.

[40] Pillow JJ, Wilkinson MH, Neil HL, Ramsden CA. In vitro performance characteristics of high-frequency oscillatory ventilators. Am J Respir Crit Care Med 2001;164:1019–1024.

[41] Pillow JJ, Sly PD, Hantos Z. Monitoring of lung volume recruitment and derecruitment using oscillatory mechanics during high-frequency oscillatory ventilation in the preterm lamb. Pediatr Crit Care Med 2004;5:172–180.

[42] Venegas JG, Fredberg JJ. Understanding the pressure cost of ventilation: why does high-frequency ventilation work? Crit Care Med 1994;22:S49–S57.

[43] Yoder BA, Siler-Khodr T, Winter VT, Coalson JJ. High-frequency oscillatory ventilation: effects on lung function, mechanics, and airway cytokines in the immature baboon model for neonatal chronic lung disease. Am J Respir Crit Care Med 2000;162:1867–1876.

[44] Meredith KS, deLemos RA, Coalson JJ, King RJ, Gerstmann DR, Kumar R, et al. Role of lung injury in the pathogenesis of hyaline membrane disease in premature baboons. J Appl Physiol (1985) 1989;66:2150–2158.

[45] Rigatto H, Davi M, Frantz ID, Boynton B, Mannino F, Heldt G, et al. High-frequency oscillatory ventilation compared with conventional mechanical ventilation in the treatment of respiratory failure in preterm infants. The HIFI Study Group. N Engl J Med 1989;320:88–93.

[46] Froese AB, Butler PO, Fletcher WA, Byford LJ. High-frequency oscillatory ventilation in premature infants with respiratory failure: a preliminary report. Anesth Analg 1987;66:814–824.

[47] Sanders R. Two ventilating attachments for bronchoscopes. Del State Med J 1967;39:170–175.

[48] Weisberger SA, Carlo WA, Fouke JM, Chatburn RL, Tillander T, Martin RJ. Measurement of tidal volume during high-frequency jet ventilation. Pediatr Res 1986;20:45–48.

[49] Carlo WA, Chatburn RL, Martin RJ. Randomized trial of high-frequency jet ventilation versus conventional ventilation in respiratory distress syndrome. J Pediatr 1987;110:275–282.

[50] Keszler M, Donn SM, Bucciarelli RL, Alverson DC, Hart M, Lunyong V, et al. Multicenter controlled trial comparing high-frequency jet ventilation and conventional mechanical ventilation in newborn infants with pulmonary interstitial emphysema. J Pediatr 1991;119:85–93.

[51] Keszler M, Modanlou HD, Brudno DS, Clark FI, Cohen RS, Ryan RM, et al. Multicenter controlled clinical trial of high-frequency jet ventilation in preterm infants with uncomplicated respiratory distress syndrome. Pediatrics 1997;100:593–599.

[52] Musk GC, Polglase GR, Bunnell JB, McLean CJ, Nitsos I, Song Y, Pillow JJ. High positive end-expiratory pressure during high-frequency jet ventilation improves oxygenation and ventilation in preterm lambs. Pediatr Res 2011;69:319–324.

[53] Standiford TJ, Morganroth ML. High-frequency ventilation. Chest 1989;96:1380–1389.

Chapter |20B|

High-Frequency Oscillatory Ventilation Management Strategy

Dushyant Batra, MRCPCH, Craig Smith, MRCPCH, Bernard Schoonakker, MRCPCH, P.K. Rajiv, DCH, MD

CHAPTER POINTS

- HFOV is often used as a rescue mode of ventilation when conventional ventilation is failing or requiring very high pressures
- Optimizing lung volume with adequate MAP important for the success of HFOV
- In non-homogeneous lung disease, a low volume strategy should be used
- Volume targeting, if available, can help avoid CO_2 fluctuations

Introduction

High-frequency oscillatory ventilation (HFOV) is a type of high-frequency ventilation produced by applying sinusoidal oscillations at a frequency typically ranging from 8 to 15 Hz, with volumes of gas near or below the physiological dead space at the airway opening [1]. The gas exchange is thought to be reliant on different processes including bulk convection, asymmetric inspiratory and expiratory velocity profiles, pendelluft, Taylor dispersion and turbulence, molecular dispersion, and collateral ventilation [2].

Different HFOV ventilators use different mechanisms (piston, membrane, venturi, or reverse jet) to achieve HFOV, for example, SensorMedics, Draeger, SLE, Accutronics, Hummingbird, and so on [3]. The manner in which an oscillatory waveform is generated is less important than the waveform it produces. A true oscillator is a device that generates an equal positive and negative pressure; in other words, it has an active expiratory phase. In contrast, flow interrupters such as the Infant Star have only a small negative pressure deflection. These differences should be accounted for when choosing a strategy for HFOV, as their effectiveness may vary in different patient groups or disease states.

Patient groups and indications

While some centers may use HFOV as the primary mode of neonatal ventilation, there is insufficient evidence to support the routine use of this mode in all preterm infants needing invasive respiratory support [4]. HFOV is more commonly used as a rescue mode when conventional ventilation fails or uncomfortably high pressures are needed. Rescue use should occur early enough to avoid serious complications of conventional ventilation. Indications for HFOV include the following conditions:
- Moderate–severe homogeneous lung disease
  - Respiratory distress syndrome
  - Pulmonary hypoplasia
- Nonhomogeneous lung disease
  - Meconium aspiration
  - Congenital lobar emphysema
  - Severe bronchopulmonary dysplasia (BPD)
  - Atelectasis

- Congenital diaphragmatic hernia
- Persistent pulmonary hypertension of newborn (PPHN)
- Air leaks
  - Pulmonary interstitial emphysema (PIE)
  - Pneumothorax

In homogeneous lung disease, optimizing lung volumes is strategically important to minimize ventilator-induced lung injury (VILI) and improve gas exchange. In nonuniform lung disease, for example, congenital lobar emphysema, compliance varies throughout the lungs, creating areas of variable expansion, affecting gas exchange, and increasing the risk of air leak. In this situation it may be useful to adopt a "low-volume" lung strategy (Fig. 20B.1). Close monitoring of the effect and safety of HFOV is essential.

When using HFOV, underinflation and overinflation are problematic and are associated with VILI and ventilation–perfusion mismatch (Fig. 20B.2).

Initiation of HFOV

For initiation of HFOV, refer to Fig. 20B.1.

Patient preparation

- Consider arterial access for invasive BP monitoring and arterial blood gas (ABG) analysis.
- Blood pressure and perfusion should be optimized prior to HFOV; any volume replacement contemplated should be completed and inotropes commenced, if necessary.
- Use analgesia and sedation as appropriate.
- Muscle relaxants are not routinely indicated unless previously in use or clinically indicated.

Initial settings

The HFOV parameters that need setting include mean airway pressure (MAP), amplitude (or power), frequency and inspiration to expiration (I:E) ratio. The initial settings will depend on the clinical condition of the patient and the management strategy being used. These settings are described later and in Fig. 20B.1.

Rescue therapy with optimal lung volume strategy

- **MAP**: Start at 2 cm above the MAP on conventional ventilation when using *I*:E ratio of 1:2 to maintain a comparable tracheal pressure [6].
- **Amplitude**: Start at a number twice the MAP (generally 20–25) and then slowly increase in increments of

3–5 cmH_2O until the chest wall is seen to gently bounce (wiggle). Some ventilators use the term Power to describe the pressure amplitude generated and thus volume of gas displaced during the oscillation. The initial power should be set at 2 and this should be modified on the basis of the chest bounce and CO_2 levels on ABG (range 1–10). It is useful to note the starting diffusion coefficient of carbon dioxide (DCO_2) when available, and follow the trend as you stabilize the baby on HFOV.

- **Frequency**: Start at 10–12 Hz in most infants, but lower (6–8) if treating MAS or BPD.
- **I:E ratio**: Start the ratio at 1:2.
- Stay with the patient and slowly increase MAP in 1–2 cmH_2O increments every 5–10 min (escalating recruitment maneuver), observing oxygenation (saturations and arterial PaO_2) and blood pressure. These should improve as the lungs are better recruited [7]. It is unusual to need MAP above 20 cmH_2O.
- Once the FiO_2 has stabilized to an acceptable level, for example, <0.4 (ideally <0.3), lower the MAP by decrements of 1 cmH_2O while maintaining oxygen saturations and FiO_2 within target limits until the oxygenation just begins to deteriorate (closing pressure), then go back up 1–2 cmH_2O [8].
- Watch blood pressure and perfusion carefully. Hemodynamic impairment may occur if MAP is excessive. Recognize that once the lung is recruited, it becomes more compliant and thus needs less MAP than was needed for the initial recruitment (Fig. 20B.2).
- Arrange for a chest X-ray (CXR) after the recruitment maneuver, to assess lung volumes, aiming for 8–9 posterior ribs at the dome of the diaphragm.
- Once stability is achieved, consider the addition of volume targeting when available. Adequate tidal volumes (VThf) are typically between 1 and 3 mL/kg. Close observation of ventilator-measured parameters (VThf, DCO_2), clinical examination, and blood gases will guide the tidal volume setting (VThf).

Rescue therapy with "low" lung volume strategy (e.g., air leak, nonhomogeneous lung disease)

- **MAP**: Start at the MAP on conventional ventilation. High MAP can worsen the air leaks and can be counterproductive. Permissive hypercapnia and optimal oxygenation with minimum possible MAP are key to the success of HFOV in these situations. FiO_2 may need to be higher to maintain the target O_2 saturations. If available, high-frequency jet ventilation may be preferable for this indication.

Assess
- Has conventional ventilation been optimized?
- Review CXR and clinical parameters to assess nature of lung disease.
- Assess hemodynamic status including blood pressure and lactate.
- Ensure adequate monitoring: *consider arterial access.*
- Identify the appropriate lung volume strategy: **optimal lung volume strategy** or a **low volume strategy** (appropriate for certain clinical situations like PIE or air leaks, see text)

Set MAP
- **Optimal lung volume strategy**: Start with a MAP 2 cmH_2O above the MAP used on conventional ventilation.
- **Low volume lung strategy**: Start at the same MAP value as on conventional ventilation.

Set frequency, amplitude, and I:E ratio
- Set **frequency** to 10 Hz.
- Set amplitude (**ΔPhf**): Start at twice the set MAP value (or 20–25 cmH_2O). Adjust in increments of 3–5 until the chest wall is seen to gently bounce. If chest movement is excessive, reduce amplitude promptly to avoid the risk of hypocapnia.
- Set I:E ratio to 1:2.
- Alarm settings (e.g., minute ventilation) may need adjusting.

Optimize

Optimal lung volume strategy:
- Stay with the patient and slowly increase MAP in 1–2 cmH_2O increments while closely monitoring O_2 saturations, BP and PaO_2. These should slowly improve. Reduce MAP if they deteriorate. It is rare to need MAP above 20 cmH_2O.
- Once the observations and FiO_2 have stabilized to an acceptable level (typically <40%), consider lowering MAP by 1–2 cmH_2O while continuing to observe the patient; to achieve the optimal volume and avoid over distension.
- Continue close monitoring including ABG.
- Consider addition of volume targeting based on VThf, DCO_2, and $PaCO_2$. Usually a VThf of 1.5–3 mL/kg is adequate.
- CXR after recruitment (sooner if clinically indicated) to assess lung volumes; aim for 8–9 posterior ribs above the diaphragm.

Low volume strategy:
- Stay at lower MAP, accept higher FiO_2 and $PaCO_2$. Consider volume targeting, start at 1.5–2 mL/kg.
- Close monitoring with a CXR in 1–2 h, aiming for 6–8 posterior ribs above the diaphragm.

Fig. 20B.1 Initiation of High-Frequency Oscillatory Ventilation (HFOV) [5]. *ABG,* Arterial blood gas; *CXR,* chest X-ray; *DCO₂,* diffusion coefficient of carbon dioxide; *MAP,* mean airway pressure; *PIE,* pulmonary interstitial emphysema.

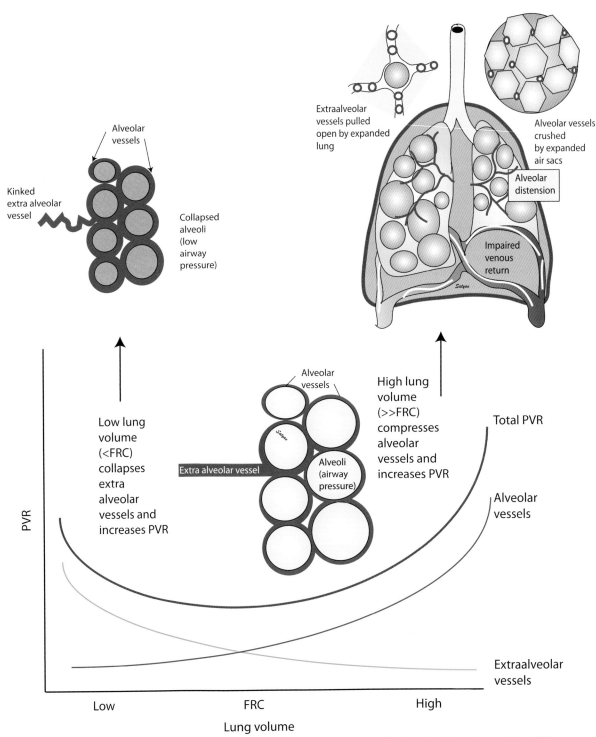

Fig. 20B.2 Pulmonary vascular resistance (PVR) is lowest at functional residual capacity (FRC). At low lung volumes below FRC, extra-alveolar vessels get kinked and offer high resistance increasing PVR. When lung volumes are extremely high, venous return is impaired reducing right ventricular preload and alveolar vessels are compressed leading to high PVR. Copyright: Satyan Lakshminrusimha.

- **Amplitude**: Start at a number twice the MAP (generally 20–25) and then slowly increase in increments of 3–5 until the chest wall is seen to gently bounce/wiggle. Some ventilators use the term Power to describe the volume of gas during the oscillation. The initial power should be set at 2 (range 1–10) and this should be modified on the basis of the chest bounce, DCO_2 trend, CO_2 levels on ABG.
- **Frequency**: Start at 10–12 Hz.
- **I:E**: Start at a ratio of 1:2.
- If there is no improvement in oxygenation, carefully consider small increments in MAP (1 cmH_2O) observing oxygenation (saturations and arterial PaO_2) and blood pressure. These should improve as the lungs are recruited [7].
- Once the FiO_2 has stabilized consider lowering the MAP by 1 cmH_2O continuing to observe the patient, before weaning the FiO_2.
- Watch blood pressure and perfusion carefully.
- Arrange for a CXR after the recruitment maneuver, to assess lung volumes, aiming for 6–8 posterior ribs at the dome of the diaphragm.
- Once stability is gained, consider the addition of volume targeting. Adequate tidal volumes are typically between 1.5 and 2 mL/kg, but some infants require substantially larger VThf. Emerging evidence indicates that factors that cause larger VT requirement with conventional ventilation also apply to HFOV [9,10]. Thus, the tiniest infants, sicker infants, and older infants with BPD may need as much as 3 mL/kg. Close observation of ventilator-measured parameters (e.g., VThf, DCO_2), clinical examination, and blood gases will guide adjustments of volume targets.

Adjusting settings during HFOV

Refer to Fig. 20B.3 for guidance on adjusting settings in response to blood gas results.

Oxygenation

- Oxygenation is controlled by adjusting the MAP and FiO_2, and the lungs must be optimally inflated.
- MAP may be increased or decreased in 1–2 cmH_2O increments.
- Generally, it is rare to use MAP levels >20 cmH_2O.
- Increasing the MAP will initially improve lung inflation (recruitment), but if the lungs become overdistended, then oxygenation will worsen and paradoxically MAP will need to be reduced (Fig. 20B.2) [11]. Overinflation can be assessed clinically and by X-ray. Bedside indicators like a drop in blood pressure and poor perfusion may be seen beyond the trough of the J curve (Fig. 20B.2) [11].

Ventilation

- Lungs must be optimally inflated.
- Changes in $PaCO_2$ may be affected by changing
  - amplitude of oscillation (ΔPhf);
  - VThf (in volume targeted mode); and
  - frequency (f).
- Chest wall bounce should be assessed clinically and the amplitude adjusted to achieve a gentle "wiggle" of the chest. If chest movement is excessive reduce the amplitude promptly to avoid the risk of hypocapnia.
- Frequency is usually set at 10 Hz. It is not common to change this though some ELBW infants with RDS may require higher frequencies (11–15 Hz) and some term infants may require a lower frequency (6–8 Hz). Some oscillators are less powerful at higher frequencies, for example,12–15 Hz. Refer to the instruction manual of the ventilator in your unit and discuss with experienced senior staff. In conventional ventilation, reducing the frequency of breaths reduces CO_2 clearance, assuming the tidal volume stays the same. In HFOV, decreasing the frequency will increase the tidal volume (VThf) and therefore increase CO_2 clearance at the same amplitude. However, if volume targeting is being used, decreasing the frequency will decrease the CO_2 clearance, because the VThf is fixed and thus unaffected by frequency.
- DCO_2 is a measure of alveolar ventilation during HFOV. It is derived from the calculation $DCO_2 = VThf^2 \times f$ and expressed as mL^2/s. Regular monitoring of this parameter can guide CO_2 clearance. Trends are more important than the absolute numbers though most neonates will have adequate CO_2 clearance between 40 and 100 mL^2/s.

I:E ratio

The normal starting ratio is 1:2, that is, 33% inspiration to 67% expiration. At 10 Hz it is equivalent to a T_i of 0.03 s. Increasing the ratio to 1:1 may be used to improve oxygenation or to increase the power of some oscillators at high MAP and/ or amplitude. This may, however, lead to air trapping and eventually poorer CO_2 clearance and impedance of venous return. If oxygenation is satisfactory but CO_2 clearance is poor, a ratio of 1:3 may be tried. However, this can only be successfully achieved with a lower frequency range (5–10 Hz).

Volume targeting

Once stability is achieved and the lungs are recruited, then the volume targeting function may offer optimal control over CO_2 clearance. Start with a VThf value typically 1.5–2 mL/kg or use the value associated with recent stability and good gas exchange. The amplitude will then vary to deliver this volume and a maximal value for ΔPhf should

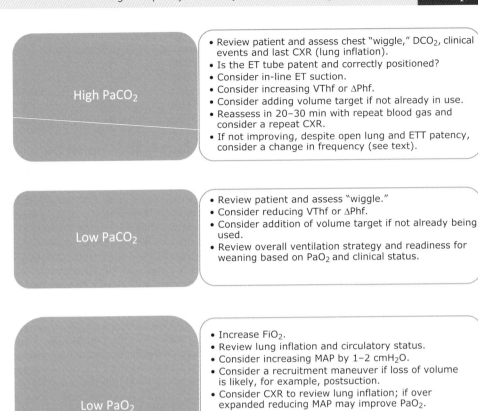

High PaCO$_2$
- Review patient and assess chest "wiggle," DCO$_2$, clinical events and last CXR (lung inflation).
- Is the ET tube patent and correctly positioned?
- Consider in-line ET suction.
- Consider increasing VThf or ΔPhf.
- Consider adding volume target if not already in use.
- Reassess in 20–30 min with repeat blood gas and consider a repeat CXR.
- If not improving, despite open lung and ETT patency, consider a change in frequency (see text).

Low PaCO$_2$
- Review patient and assess "wiggle."
- Consider reducing VThf or ΔPhf.
- Consider addition of volume target if not already being used.
- Review overall ventilation strategy and readiness for weaning based on PaO$_2$ and clinical status.

Low PaO$_2$
- Increase FiO$_2$.
- Review lung inflation and circulatory status.
- Consider increasing MAP by 1–2 cmH$_2$O.
- Consider a recruitment maneuver if loss of volume is likely, for example, postsuction.
- Consider CXR to review lung inflation; if over expanded reducing MAP may improve PaO$_2$.
- Consider factors associated with pulmonary hypertension (BP and perfusion) as well as need for adjuncts such as surfactant and nitric oxide.
- Consider the possibility that the MAP is excessive, leading to impairment of pulmonary blood flow.

Fig. 20B.3 **HFOV: Adjusting the Ventilator Settings in Response to the Blood Gas Findings.**

be set for the range of values required. Monitoring the trend in the DCO$_2$ will help identify the optimum VThf.

During HFOV, the I:E ratio remains constant regardless of VThf. At higher frequencies the time available to deliver VThf reduces. This explains the reduction in VThf and CO$_2$ elimination with an increase in frequency, opposite to the effect of increasing the respiratory rate in conventional ventilation [12]. However, in the volume targeted mode, the ventilator maintains a constant VThf up to its performance limit, therefore increasing frequency leads to an increase in minute ventilation and better CO$_2$ clearance, as long as the VThf can be maintained.

Radiology

Radiological assessment of lung inflation is very important for safe and effective use of HFOV. Consider requesting an initial CXR after a recruitment maneuver to assess lung inflation and lung fields. It may be necessary to perform CXR 6–12 hourly, especially if oxygenation, gas exchange or blood pressure is unstable. Normal inflation on HFOV should show the diaphragm to be at 8–9 posterior ribs with no intercostal bulging of pleura.

Overinflation is demonstrated on a CXR by [13]
- Flattening of diaphragm below the 9th rib
- Intercostal pleural bulging of lungs
- Air is visible as a crescent under the cardiac shadow

The assessment of inflation should be considered in the context of the clinical condition and other ventilatory and bedside parameters. For example, in babies with pulmonary hypoplasia or congenital diaphragmatic hernia, hyperinflation should not solely rely on diaphragm position but also on the appearance of the hypoplastic lungs, intercostal bulges, and heart size.

Underinflation is indicated by a high diaphragm. Lung volumes are difficult to assess in the presence of pulmonary hypoplasia, diaphragmatic hernia, or abdominal distension, for example, postgastroschisis repair. When managing patients with air leak or congenital diaphragmatic hernia, consider maintaining normal PaO_2 levels with the minimum possible MAP and accept higher FiO_2 levels.

Monitoring

All babies on HFOV need close continuous monitoring. The electronic record or paper observation chart should include the values and trends of the following:
- O_2 saturations (consider pre- and postductal for PPHN)
- ECG and heart rate
- Blood pressure (consider arterial access for invasive BP and PaO_2 monitoring)
- Blood gases and oxygenation index (OI = FiO_2 × MAP/ PaO_2(in kPa) × 7.5)
- Ventilator measurements, such as VThf, DCO_2, amplitude, MAP, and frequency
- Clinical observations of the baby such as chest wiggle and pain score
- Consider using transcutaneous CO_2 monitoring when DCO_2 is not available to avoid the risk of hypocapnia

Disconnection and suction

- Maintenance of optimal lung volumes is critical, and disconnections should be discouraged.
- Ensure the ventilator circuit is kept free from water condensation as this can impair oscillation. Position the tubing to ensure that the water does not drain down the tubing to the baby.
- Babies on HFOV should have inline/verso adapter suctioning.
- Repositioning of the baby should be performed by two nurses to avoid disconnection from the ventilator.
- Whenever the MAP falls, for example, following disconnection and/or suctioning, it may be necessary to increase the MAP for a short period to reestablish lung volume.

Surfactant therapy during HFOV

Surfactant may be administered in the routine manner to babies receiving HFOV, including bolus administration followed by a short period of ventilation using a T-piece. Surfactant may improve compliance rapidly, and the ventilator requirements should be altered accordingly.

Potential complications of HFOV

- Hypotension due to reduced venous return [14,15]
- Hyperinflation (focal or generalized)

- Inadvertent overventilation (even small increases in VThf can drop PCO_2 substantially, due to the f × $VThf^2$ relationship)
- Air leak [16]
- Lack of improvement or further deterioration (see Figure 20B.3)
- Necrotizing tracheobronchitis [17] (very rare)

Assessing failure on HFOV

HFOV will at least temporarily improve the respiratory status in the majority of neonates. The common iatrogenic reasons for apparent HFOV failure include failure to achieve optimal lung volumes, inappropriate ventilation settings, small ETT diameter, long ETT and ETT leak, as well as secretions or water in the ETT or tubing.

HFOV is considered failed if after 2 h the OI and $PaCO_2$ are rising or oxygen saturations are worsening in spite of good recruitment and "wiggle." Severe respiratory disease, coexistent high inotropic requirements, and presence of nonhomogeneous lung disease are also known as risk factors for HFOV failure. A common cause of apparent failure of HFOV is excessive MAP that results in hemodynamic impairment and increased pulmonary vascular resistance (Fig. 20B.2). In some infants who are not oxygenating, lowering, not increasing MAP is the correct move. CXR is not always helpful, so a trial of lower MAP is usually indicated if oxygenation is a problem. Some patients deteriorate immediately on transfer to HFOV and need to be stabilized back on a conventional mode of ventilation.

Weaning from HFOV and extubation

Weaning of HFOV

Once the patient is stable with improving oxygenation (typically FiO_2 <0.4) and improved systemic status, an active weaning process can start. Each change should be closely monitored with clinical parameters, including oxygen saturations, heart rate, and blood pressure. Arterial blood gases should be performed 20–60 min after each change depending on the magnitude of change.
- MAP: Reduce in 1 cmH_2O steps every 4–6 h as tolerated
- Amplitude: If volume targeting is being used, the amplitude will "autowean" as the lung mechanics improve. In the absence of volume targeting, amplitude can be weaned in steps of 1–2 cmH_2O every 4 h guided by $PaCO_2$ and DCO_2. If instead of amplitude, power is used to determine the volume of gas-driving oscillations, these can be weaned by 0.2–0.3 every 4 h. The target $PaCO_2$ will depend on the clinical situation: it will be higher when managing patients with established chronic lung disease.

Sudden deterioration with loss of chest wobble/bounce	• Check ventilator connections and tubing. • Check ETT position and patency; consider suction. • Is there a pneumothorax or other clinical change (BOLDPEEP)? • ***BOLDPEEP—B**ad lung disease, **O**bstructed ETT, **L**ong ETT, **D**islodged ETT, **P**neumothorax, **E**quipment malfunction or **E**quipment-**P**atient. asynchrony.* • Consider manual ventilation through ETT to assess tube position, patency, and chest rise.
Set ΔPhf or VThf is not achieved or MV is low	• Consider ET tube obstruction and need for suction. • Consider CXR to assess lung inflation and disease. • Consider a recruitment maneuver. • If on high MAP (>14 cmH₂O), consider changing *I:E* ratio to 1:1. • Some babies may benefit from a change in frequency.
MV is high	• Are the alarm limits appropriate? • Review patient, assess chest wobble and VThf. • Check ABG and if appropriate wean ΔPhf or VThf. • Consider volume-targeted HFOV.
Lack of improvement	• Stay at bedside, review clinical and ventilator parameters. • Consider increasing MAP by 1–2 cmH₂O. • Consider BOLDPEEP (see above). • Consider using muscle relaxation; treat hypotension if present. • Some babies do not improve with HFOV and may benefit from switching to conventional ventilation.
Hypotension	• Consider overdistension: Can MAP be weaned? • Is baby hypovolemic? • Consider cause of hypotension and need for inotropes.

Fig. 20B.4 HFOV Troubleshooting and Alarm Management [5].

Extubation

Centers vary in their practice with regards to extubation from HFOV. Babies can be successfully extubated from HFOV or switched to conventional ventilation before extubation. Typical settings suggesting readiness for extubation are:

• MAP < 9–10 cmH₂O
• FiO₂ < 0.3–0.4

Troubleshooting and alarms

Fig. 20B.4 provides a framework for troubleshooting and responding to alarms. At the outset the clinical team should be aware that successful use of HFOV is highly dependent upon the following:

• Optimal lung volumes
• Minimal or no ETT leak
• Patent ventilator tubing and ETT lumen

- Experience of clinicians with the ventilator in HFOV mode
- Skilled nursing staff

Supporting parents and careers

- Explain how HFOV is different to other forms of ventilation in a language that the parents understand.

- Cuddles or kangaroo care are possible in stable babies receiving HFOV but may be constrained by the type of ventilator and ventilator circuit.
- Ensure the parents are encouraged to talk to their baby and use containment holding to provide comfort.

References

[1] Bohn DJ, et al. Ventilation by high-frequency oscillation. J Appl Physiol 1980;48:710–716.

[2] Pillow J. High-frequency oscillatory ventilation: mechanisms of gas exchange and lung mechanics. Crit Care Med 2005;33:S135–S141.

[3] Keszler M, Pillow JJ, Courtney S. High frequency oscillatory ventilation in the neonate. In: Rimensberger PC, editor. Pediatric and neonatal mechanical ventilation: from basics to clinical practice. Heidelberg, Berlin: Springer; 2015: 1161–1172.

[4] Cools F, Offringa M, Askie LM. Elective high frequency oscillatory ventilation versus conventional ventilation for acute pulmonary dysfunction in preterm infants. In: Cools F, editor. Cochrane database of systematic reviews. Chichester, UK: John Wiley & Sons, Ltd; 2015. doi: 10.1002/14651858.CD000104.pub4.

[5] Swamy K, Batra D, Schoonakker B, Smith C, Hillyard D. High frequency oscillatory ventilation in neonates. 2017;1–18. Available from: https://www.nuh.nhs.uk/download.cfm?doc=docm93jijm4n927.pdf&ver=5027.

[6] Pillow JJ. High-frequency oscillatory ventilation: theory and practical applications. Perth: Drägerwerk AG & Co; 2016.

[7] Murthy BV, Petros AJ. High-frequency oscillatory ventilation combined with intermittent mandatory ventilation in critically ill neonates and infants. Acta Anaesthesiol Scand 1996;40:679–683.

[8] De Jaegere A, van Veenendaal MB, Michiels A, van Kaam AH. Lung recruitment using oxygenation during open lung high-frequency ventilation in preterm infants. Am J Respir Crit Care Med 2006;174:639–645.

[9] Akita, D. et al. Optimal high-frequency tidal-volume in very low birth weight infants. In: Paediatric Academic Society conference; 2014.

[10] Korzan, S. et al. Tidal volume during high frequency oscillatory ventilation with the VN-500 ventilator. In: Paediatric Academic Society conference; 2014.

[11] Keszler M, Abubakar KM. Physiologic principles. In: Goldsmith J, Karotkin E, Keszler M, Suresh G, editors. Assisted ventilation of the neonate: an evidence-based approach to newborn respiratory care. 6th ed. Philadelphia: Elsevier; 2017. p. 8–30.

[12] Pillow JJ. Tidal volume, recruitment and compliance in HFOV: Same principles, different frequency. Eur Respir J 2012;40:291–293.

[13] Johnson AH, et al. High-frequency oscillatory ventilation for the prevention of chronic lung disease of prematurity. N Engl J Med 2002;347:633–642.

[14] Traverse JH, Korvenranta H, Merrill Adams E, Goldthwait DA, Carlo WA. Impairment of hemodynamics with increasing mean airway pressure during high-frequency oscillatory ventilation. Pediatr Res 1988;23:628–631.

[15] Traverse JH, Korvenranta H, Adams EM, Goldthwait DA, Carlo WA. Cardiovascular effects of high-frequency oscillatory and jet ventilation. Chest 1989;96:1400–1404.

[16] Children F, Hospital M, Springs C, Valley U, Medical R. Randomized study of high-frequency oscillatory ventilation in infants with severe respiratory distress syndrome. HiFO Study Group. J Pediatr 1993;122:609–619.

[17] Ong WW, Ok TFF, G PCN, Heung KLC. High frequency ventilation in neonates. HK J Paediatr 2003;8:113–120.

Chapter |20C|

High-Frequency Jet Ventilation: Guide to Patient Management

J. Bert Bunnell, ScD FAIMBE

CHAPTER POINTS

- Conventional mechanical ventilation (CMV) aims to breathe for patients who cannot breathe on their own. High-frequency ventilation (HFV) takes a different approach: it is designed to facilitate gas exchange. While we use the same terminology to describe the settings used on both types of machines (e.g., rate, tidal volume, peak inspiratory pressure, pressure amplitude, and so on), high-frequency jets and oscillators operate at rates and deliver "tidal" volumes (i.e., the volume between inspiration and expiration) that can be orders of magnitude higher and smaller, respectively, than those used during CMV.

- The way in which jets and oscillators deliver tidal volumes reduces physiologic dead space to the point that it can be less than anatomic dead space [1,2]. Oscillators push gas in and pull gas back out of the lungs, usually in a 1:2 duty cycle. Jets deliver the gas in short, high-velocity spurts, allowing more time for passive exhalation. When used properly, both modalities offer the opportunity to prevent lung injury in preterm babies [3,4].

- As inflammation is typically triggered by mechanical ventilation of any sort, as well as tracheal intubation, jets are more effective in treating lung injury, as demonstrated in the success of HFJV for the treatment of pulmonary interstitial emphysema (PIE) [5]. Injured areas of the lungs have increased airway resistance as well as poor perfusion. Thus, CMV using higher rates and shortened inspiratory times improves ventilation/perfusion ratios in patients with PIE. HFJV provides

an extension of that approach by operating at much higher rate and shorter inspiratory time with I:E ratios as small as 1:12, which provides even better ventilation/perfusion ratios as well as adequate time for passive exhalation.

- CMV can provide some things that HFV cannot, such as tidal volumes of size and duration sufficient to open up collapsed alveoli. CMV can also control mean airway pressure (MAP) by regulating positive end-expiratory pressure (PEEP) and provide gas for spontaneous breathing.

- The following charts and flowcharts are designed to aid HFJV operators in developing treatment strategies for infants and children with various pathophysiologies. The goal of these teaching aids is to provide lung protective ventilation by facilitating gas exchange in the most gentle ways possible, including enabling infants to breathe spontaneously. (Needless sedation should be avoided.)

- While certain HFJV and CMV settings are recommended, operators are urged to use the principles of these recommendations to determine how to best apply HFJV. Certain settings and conditions that would dictate, for example, when to wean an infant from HFJV to a less invasive form of respiratory support, are left vague on purpose. Clinicians should evaluate each patient individually based upon their abilities to breathe spontaneously without periodic apnea spells to make such setting decisions.

- The first chart is designed to serve as a general guide to applying HFJV in circumstances and conditions commonly found in newborn and pediatric intensive care units. The other flowcharts assist in optimizing PEEP and MAP.

Circumstances— complications	Goals	Actions (vent settings)
General HFJV startup	Get lungs open. Keep them open.	HFJV rate: Set by baby size and condition: • At least 420 bpm for infants <1 kg. • <420 for bigger babies, gas trapping, severe PIE, and babies >2 weeks old. HFJV PIP: Adjust as needed to control PCO_2. HFJV I-time: 0.02 s CMV rate: Start with 5 bpm until baby is stable and discontinue to find optimal PEEP (see later). CMV PIP: Set to achieve moderate chest rise. CMV I-time: Sufficient to recruit alveoli. CMV PEEP: Adjust to maintain pre-HFJV MAP.
Provide adequate ventilation	PCO_2 <55 mmHg	Transcutaneous CO_2 monitoring is helpful. Adjust HFJV PIP until ineffective in reducing $PaCO_2$, and then alleviate by increasing I-time in 0.004 increments to enable V_T delivery. Compare HFJV-displayed PEEP with set CMV PEEP to assess gas trapping (inadvertent PEEP); if monitored PEEP > set PEEP, alleviate by reducing HFJV rate in 60 bpm increments.
Optimize PEEP	Keep lungs open without impeding pulmonary perfusion while minimizing CMV rate and V_T to decrease lung injury.	Once baby is stable, discontinue 5 bpm CMV; use CPAP only, or as close as possible by minimizing CMV rate, PIP, and I-time. Raise PEEP incrementally to avoid raising FiO_2. Reinstitute 5 bpm CMV temporarily if necessary, until PEEP has been adjusted to the point where CMV breaths are no longer needed.
General maintenance	Keep lungs open. Maintain good blood gases with FiO_2 <0.30 if possible.	Use CMV for alveolar recruitment only (e.g., after suctioning). Use PEEP to maintain adequate MAP and avoid atelectasis. Use lower PEEP and low CMV rate if high PEEP impedes cardiac output.
RDS	Maintain adequate lung volume; gently provide adequate ventilation (PCO_2 <55 mmHg).	HFJV rates >420 may be used for preterm babies. Use HFJV PIP as primary control of ventilation (PCO_2). CMV should be used for alveolar recruitment only. Find and use optimal PEEP (see later).
RDS, surfactant deficiency	Facilitate surfactant delivery.	Surfactant may be administered via catheter downstream of LifePort adapter during HFJV to improve distribution. Alternatively, put jet in standby and deliver per hospital CMV policy.
CDH, pulmonary hypoplasia	Maintain adequate lung volume; provide adequate ventilation (PCO_2 <55 mmHg) in gentlest way possible.	HFJV rate: At least 420 bpm; increase in 60 bpm increments if PIP >40 cmH_2O. HFJV PIP: Set as needed to control PCO_2. HFJV I-time: 0.02 s; increase as needed when raising PIP no longer seems capable to reducing $PaCO_2$. CMV: CPAP only, or as close to CPAP as you can get by minimizing CMV rate, PIP, and I-time. PEEP: Raise as necessary to counteract abdominal pressure and maintain appropriate lung volume postsurgery.

Circumstances— complications	Goals	Actions (vent settings)
PIE, other air leaks, and early BPD	Facilitate healing and normal lung growth. Minimize CMV rate and V_T by optimizing lung volume, PEEP.	Use HFJV rates <420 bpm to lengthen exhalation time. Use CPAP only or adjust CMV as close to CPAP as you can get by minimizing CMV rate, PIP, and I-time. Adjust PEEP upward to enable lower FiO_2 (<0.30 if possible).
MAS, PPHN, bronchiolitis	Facilitate mucociliary clearance, reduce gas trapping.	Use optimal PEEP (see above) and low HFJV rate (240–300). Raise HFJV PIP and/or I-time to enable $PaCO_2$ = 35–40 torr. Low CMV rate may be helpful. Delivering inhaled NO via HFJV may be effective.
Pulmonary hyperinflation	Avoid and remedy gas trapping.	Reduce HFJV rate incrementally by 60 bpm toward 240 bpm if X-ray reveals hyperinflation. HFJV rate reduction may require increases in PEEP and HFJV PIP to maintain adequate blood gases. Continue to optimize rather than minimize PEEP to avoid airway collapse and worse gas trapping.
Severe BPD, pulmonary hyperinflation	Reduce hyperinflation and hypercapnia.	Reduce HFJV rate to 240 bpm. Increase PEEP and HFJV PIP as necessary to enable adequate oxygenation and ventilation, respectively. If HFJV PIP >40, increase HFJV I-time in 0.004 increments to maximum = 0.034 s.
Cardiac patients in respiratory distress	Improve hemodynamics, cardiac index.	Moderately hyperventilate at low MAP using HFJV PIP and rate appropriate for patient size (at least 420 bpm for preterms, lower rates for larger patients). Use low-rate CMV and lower PEEP, as needed for control of lung volume.
Surgery patients (CDH, cardiac)	Facilitate surgical repair.	HFJV may be used before, during (improves field of view), and after surgery, which enables chest closure due to low MAP capability.
Wean (applicable to all disorders)	Minimize mechanical ventilation time. Maintain gentlest ventilation on HFJV all the way to extubation. Extubate ASAP.	Minimize CMV rate, PIP, and I-time unless temporary alveolar recruitment is necessary. Reduce HFJV PIP as PCO_2 allows. Reduce FiO_2 and MAP as PO_2 allows. Reduce FiO_2 before MAP until FiO_2 <0.40 to 0.30. Reduce MAP before FiO_2 when PEEP is impeding cardiac output. Reduce PEEP cautiously to avoid atelectasis. Encourage spontaneous breathing via reduction of HFJV rate and PIP; do not oversedate. Once baby is sufficiently spontaneously breathing and MAP can be maintained via CPAP, extubate directly to nasal CPAP near last recorded MAP.

BPD, Bronchopulmonary dysplasia; *bpm*, breaths per minute; *CMV*, conventional mechanical ventilation; *CPAP*, continuous positive airway pressure; *HFJV*, high-frequency jet ventilation; *I-time*, inspiratory time; *MAP*, mean airway pressure; *PEEP*, peak end-expiratory pressure; *PIE*, pulmonary interstitial emphysema; *PIP*, peak inspiratory pressure; *RDS*, respiratory distress syndrome; V_T, tidal volume. Copyright: Bert Bunnell.

*Finding optimal PEEP during HFJV ***

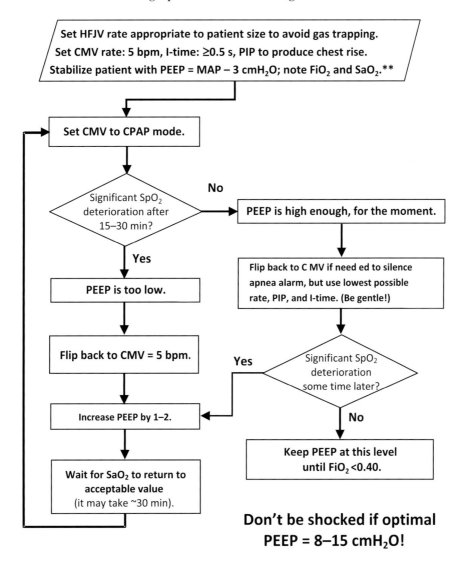

Set HFJV rate appropriate to patient size to avoid gas trapping.
Set CMV rate: 5 bpm, I-time: ≥0.5 s, PIP to produce chest rise.
Stabilize patient with PEEP = MAP – 3 cmH$_2$O; note FiO$_2$ and SaO$_2$.**

Set CMV to CPAP mode.

Significant SpO$_2$ deterioration after 15–30 min?

No

PEEP is high enough, for the moment.

Yes

PEEP is too low.

Flip back to C MV if need ed to silence apnea alarm, but use lowest possible rate, PIP, and I-time. (Be gentle!)

Flip back to CMV = 5 bpm.

Yes

Significant SpO$_2$ deterioration some time later?

Increase PEEP by 1–2.

No

Wait for SaO$_2$ to return to acceptable value (it may take ~30 min).

Keep PEEP at this level until FiO$_2$ <0.40.

Don't be shocked if optimal PEEP = 8–15 cmH$_2$O!

*Optimal PEEP may be lower in patients with active air leaks.

**Assumes patient is being transitioned from CMV or HFOV.

Optimizing MAP during HFJV

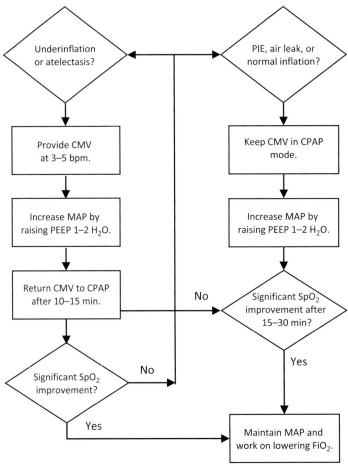

MAP may be too low if FiO_2 >0.5 or SpO_2 <85%.

Underinflation or atelectasis?

PIE, air leak, or normal inflation?

Provide CMV at 3–5 bpm.

Keep CMV in CPAP mode.

Increase MAP by raising PEEP 1–2 H_2O.

Increase MAP by raising PEEP 1–2 H_2O.

Return CMV to CPAP after 10–15 min.

Significant SpO_2 improvement after 15–30 min?

No

Significant SpO_2 improvement?

No

Yes

Yes

Maintain MAP and work on lowering FiO_2.

Copyright: Bert Bunnell.

References

[1] Henderson Y, Chillingworth FP, Whitney JL. The respiratory dead space. Am J Physiol 1915;38:1–19.

[2] Musk GC, Polglase GR, Bunnell JB, McLean CJ, Nitsos I, Song Y, et al. High positive end-expiratory pressure during high-frequency jet ventilation improves oxygenation and ventilation in preterm lambs. Pediatr Res 2011;69:319–324.

[3] Keszler M, et al. Multicenter controlled clinical trial of high-frequency jet ventilation in preterm infants with uncomplicated respiratory distress syndrome. Pediatrics 1997;100:593–599.

[4] Courtney SE, Durand DJ, Asselin JM, Hudak ML, Aschner JL, Shoemaker CT. Early high-frequency oscillatory ventilation versus conventional ventilation in

very-low-birth-weight-infants. N Engl J Med 2002;347:643–653.

[5] Keszler M, Donn SM, Bucciarelli RL, et al. Multicenter controlled trial comparing high-frequency jet ventilation and conventional mechanical ventilation in newborn infants with pulmonary interstitial emphysema. J Pediatr 1991;119:85–93.

Chapter | 21 |

Pulmonary Vasodilators in the Treatment of Persistent Pulmonary Hypertension of the Newborn

Ru-Jeng Teng, MD, G. Ganesh Konduri, MD

CHAPTER POINTS

- PPHN remains a challenging clinical problem, associated with significant morbidity and mortality for the affected infants
- The introduction of inhaled nitric oxide and other pulmonary vasodilators have greatly improved the outcomes in PPHN
- This chapter summarizes our current knowledge of pulmonary vasodilator therapy, the challenges that remain and future directions for research

Introduction

Persistent pulmonary hypertension of the newborn (PPHN) is a syndrome caused by failure of the pulmonary vascular resistance (PVR) to decrease at birth. Elevated PVR can be secondary to pulmonary vasoconstriction, structural thickening of pulmonary arterial wall, or dysmorphic angiogenesis in the lung. Prompt recognition and management of underlying lung disease is an integral part of the overall approach to PPHN [1]. The overall prevalence of PPHN remains constant at 2 per 1000 live births [2,3]. However, the lung diseases contributing to PPHN have changed over the last 20 years with the decreasing incidence of meconium aspiration syndrome [4]. Congenital diaphragmatic hernia is now the leading cause of severe PPHN among infants needing ECMO cannulation for neonatal respiratory failure (Fig. 21.1). This is followed by meconium aspiration syndrome, primary PPHN, and surfactant deficiency due to pneumonia or respiratory distress syndrome. Genetic causes of respiratory failure are increasingly being recognized among infants with severe PPHN. These include surfactant protein B and ABCA3 deficiency and alveolar capillary dysplasia. Additionally, PPHN can complicate the course of infants being treated with hypothermia for hypoxic ischemic encephalopathy [5]. The appropriate treatment depends on the underlying lung disease contributing to PPHN. Echocardiography is an essential tool to rule out congenital heart disease as a cause of cyanosis and to document pulmonary hypertension.

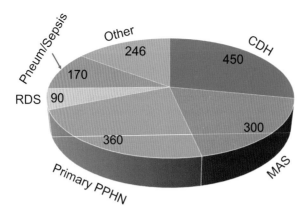

ELSO registry for neonatal respiratory diseases for 2010 and 2011; *n* = 1616

Fig. 21.1 Incidence of Lung Diseases Associated With Hypoxic Respiratory Failure in Term and Late Preterm Infants Who Required ECMO Cannulation During the Years 2010 and 2011. Data are from the ELSO Registry for neonatal respiratory indications for ECMO, shown for this 2-year period. Congenital diaphragmatic hernia *(CDH)* was the most common indication, followed by primary PPHN *(PPHN)*, meconium aspiration syndrome *(MAS)*, respiratory distress syndrome *(RDS)*, and pneumonia/sepsis. Other includes hypoxic ischemic injury, genetic causes, and other causes of lung hypoplasia.

Regulation of vascular tone in pulmonary circulation

Vascular tone is determined by the continuous balance between vasoconstrictor and vasodilator influences that operate on these vessels. The pulmonary vessels are capable of autonomous regulation of tone, although various neural, endocrine, and paracrine factors influence the regulation of tone. Fetal pulmonary circulation is in relatively low oxygen tension (20–39 torr), which facilitates pulmonary vasoconstriction. This tilt in balance toward vasoconstriction is reversed during postnatal transition, favoring rapid onset of pulmonary vasodilation. During fetal life, increased levels of endothelin-1 (ET-1) and thromboxane A$_2$ (TxA$_2$) contribute to increased tone. Endothelin, a potent peptide released by vascular endothelial cells [6], exists in at least three isoforms: ET-1, ET-2, and ET-3, which interact with at least four known endothelin receptors: ETA, ETB$_1$, ETB$_2$ and ETC [7]. ET-1 is the most extensively studied vasoconstrictor in PPHN; elevated levels have been demonstrated in PPHN infants [8]. The ETA receptor is primarily located on vascular smooth muscle cells and mediates vasoconstriction. ET-1 also induces vasoconstrictor effects by the generation of endothelium-derived TxA$_2$ [9]. The ETB receptor is primarily located on endothelial cells and its activation leads to release of NO and prostacyclin when activated, to cause vasodilatation [6]. However, ETB receptor on vascular smooth muscle cells mediates vasoconstriction and stimulates cell proliferation. In healthy vasculature, ET

can mediate vasorelaxation due to its site-specific effect on endothelial ETB receptor, but causes vasoconstriction in diseased vasculature due to different expression patterns of the ET receptors [7]. Increased expression of ETA and ETB receptors on the vascular smooth muscle cells may be a contributing factor for PPHN. TxA$_2$, the vasoconstrictor eicosanoid, is a product of PGH$_2$ metabolism by thromboxane synthase. Since prostacyclin synthase and thromboxane synthase compete for PGH$_2$, decreased expression or activity of one can lead to higher levels of vasodilator PGI$_2$ or constrictor, TxA$_2$. Studies in fetal lamb model of PPHN demonstrated that reciprocal decrease in PGI$_2$ synthase expression and activity is associated with increased expression and activity of thromboxane synthase and higher levels of TxB$_2$, the stable metabolite of TxA$_2$ [10]. These studies demonstrate that the vascular tone balance is shifted toward vasoconstriction in PPHN.

Vasodilation in the perinatal pulmonary circulation is largely mediated by cGMP- and cAMP-dependent signaling mechanisms (Fig. 21.2). These two complementary systems are activated by the release of endothelium derived nitric oxide for cGMP and prostacyclin for cAMP. Nitric oxide is the catalytic by-product of the oxidation of L-arginine on the terminal amino group by the enzyme, nitric oxide synthase, which generates L-citrulline. The levels of lung endothelial NOS protein increase in late gestation to ensure that pulmonary circulation is primed for the release of NO immediately after onset of respiration [11]. Both lung distension and increase in oxygen tension at birth activate eNOS either directly or indirectly by release of paracrine factors, such as vascular endothelial growth factor (VEGF)

and ATP. NO diffuses to adjacent vascular smooth muscle cell to activate soluble guanylate cyclase, which initiates synthesis of cGMP from GTP (Fig. 21.2). Cyclic GMP activates protein kinase G to decrease the contractility of vascular smooth muscle cell, which leads to vasodilation. The levels of cGMP in the cell are tightly regulated by the activity of type V phosphodiesterase in the vascular smooth muscle which breaks down cGMP to limit the duration of vasodilation (Fig. 21.2). Studies in neonates with PPHN and the fetal lamb model of PPHN demonstrated downregulation of NO-cGMP signaling at multiple levels due to increased oxidative stress. The expression of eNOS and plasma levels of NO metabolites are decreased in neonates with PPHN [12,13]. Studies in the fetal lamb model of PPHN demonstrated that both the expression of endothelial NOS and its function are decreased with depletion of NOS cofactor, tetrahydrobiopterin (BH_4) and the interaction of eNOS with its chaperone, Hsp90 [14,15]. Additionally, oxidation of heme component of soluble guanylate cyclase leads to decreased sensitivity to NO in PPHN [16]. Increased activity of PDE-5 also leads to accelerated degradation of cGMP in the VSM and promotes vasoconstriction [17].

Prostacyclin initiates vasodilation through the activation of adenylate cyclase, which converts ATP to cAMP, and activation of protein kinase A (Fig. 21.2). The effects of PKA activation are similar to PKG activation and leads to decreased VSM contractility and vasodilation. The levels of cAMP are also tightly regulated by rapid breakdown of cAMP by type III phosphodiesterase (Fig. 21.2). Previous studies in the endothelial cells from fetal lamb model of PPHN demonstrated decreases in the expression of cyclo-oxygenase and PGI_2 synthase and the levels of PGI_2 [10], suggesting a coordinated downregulation of both cGMP- and cAMP-dependent signaling in PPHN.

The development of pulmonary vasodilators for PPHN parallels our understanding of vascular biology of perinatal circulation as summarized earlier. The available agents targeting the cGMP signaling include inhaled NO, sGC activators, cinaciguat [16] and riociguat and PDE-5 inhibitors, sildenafil and tadalafil. Both inhaled nitric oxide (iNO) and sildenafil have been investigated in neonates with PPHN through randomized controlled trials (RCTs) and are currently being used. The sGC activators have been tested in adults with pulmonary hypertension, but no case reports or

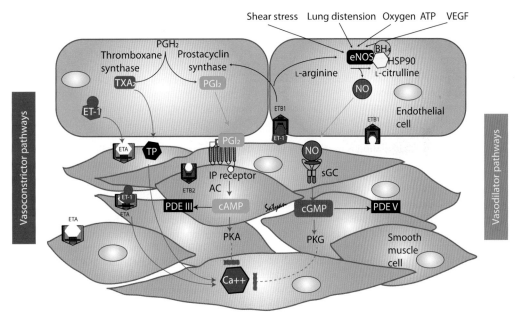

Fig. 21.2 Mechanism of Endothelium-Dependent Pulmonary Vasodilation and Vasoconstriction During Birth-Related Transition. Birth-related stimuli, including oxygen and lung distension, activate endothelial nitric oxide synthase (eNOS) and cyclooxygenase directly or indirectly through release of paracrine factors, VEGF and ATP. Release of NO and prostacyclin (PGI_2) leads to activation of guanylate cyclase and adenylate cyclase, respectively in vascular smooth muscle cell. These enzymes in turn generate cGMP and cAMP, respectively. The cyclic nucleotides then activate their corresponding protein kinases, which lead to decreased Ca++ and smooth muscle cell relaxation. The phosphodiesterases-V and III breakdown cGMP and cAMP, respectively, to limit the duration of vasodilation. Two important vasoconstrictor pathways are conversion of PGH_2 to thromboxane A_2 (TxA₂) by thromboxane synthase and synthesis and release of endothelin-1 (ET-1). Both TxA_2 and ET-1 are potent vasoconstrictors released in response to hypoxia, elevated pressure, or inflammation. Copyright: Satyan Lakshminrusimha.

clinical trials have been published about their use in neonates. Among cAMP-targeted therapies, intravenous, inhaled, and subcutaneous PGI$_2$ or its analogs have been studied in pulmonary hypertension as discussed in detail later. Additionally, limited data suggest that milrinone, a phosphodiesterase-3 (PDE-3) inhibitor, improves oxygenation in PPHN and is currently being used in neonates who fail to respond to iNO therapy. ETA inhibitor, bosentan has been tested in case reports and a pilot randomized trial in neonates with PPHN; current experience with this agent is very limited and is not recommended as a primary vasodilator in PPHN.

General management of PPHN

Optimum response to pulmonary vasodilator therapy requires adequate expansion of the lung, proper acid–base balance, sufficient preload for the left heart, and optimum cardiac performance (Fig. 21.3). Appropriate use of the adjunct therapies is as important as the selection of right vasodilator for the infant (Fig. 21.3). These therapies should be targeted to the underlying lung disease associated with PPHN. For parenchymal lung disease secondary to RDS, pneumonia or perinatal aspiration syndrome, early surfactant therapy can rapidly improve oxygenation and decrease the level of ventilator support needed for lung recruitment. Additionally, use of higher PEEP on conventional mechanical ventilation (CMV) or high frequency oscillation (HFO) in the presence of parenchymal lung disease may enhance the response to iNO therapy. These two approaches are discussed further in following sections. The traditional practice of targeting a high PO$_2$ (>100 torr) and low PCO$_2$ (<40 torr) to achieve pulmonary vasodilation has not been shown to improve outcomes and is potentially harmful to the developing lung and cerebral perfusion. While achieving a normal PaO$_2$ of 60–90 torr is important for restoring postnatal adaptation, there is no evidence that a PaO$_2$

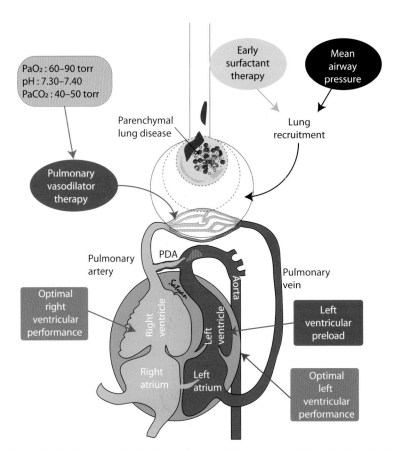

Fig. 21.3 A Schematic for the Initial Approach to Management of Hypoxic Respiratory Failure. An integrated approach, including lung recruitment, pulmonary vasodilation, and optimizing cardiac function with attention to preload, inotropic state, and afterload is needed for relieving hypoxemia. Copyright: Satyan Lakshminrusimha.

>100 causes a greater reduction in PVR [18]. Similarly, it is important to maintain normal acid–base balance (pH 7.30–7.40 and PCO_2 40–50 torr) to optimize the responses to pulmonary vasodilator therapy; however, hypocarbia and alkalosis should be avoided [19].

Use of surfactant therapy for PPHN

A number of previous studies have demonstrated that surfactant improves oxygenation and decreases the need for ECMO in term and late preterm infants with hypoxic respiratory failure and PPHN [20]. Findlay and coworkers demonstrated in a pilot RCT in 40 term infants with meconium aspiration syndrome that surfactant improves oxygenation and decreases the need for ECMO [21]. Neonates treated with surfactant in this study also had decreased length of stay on the ventilator, oxygen therapy, and hospital stay. A subsequent multicenter trial by Lotze et al. randomly assigned 328 term infants (gestational age >36 weeks) with respiratory failure to either surfactant therapy or placebo [22]. The infants treated with surfactant had decreased need for ECMO. The best responses were observed for infants with meconium aspiration syndrome or sepsis/pneumonia and no response was seen for infants with a diagnosis of primary PPHN. Best responses were also seen when surfactant was given early in respiratory failure, at an oxygenation index (OI) of 15–23. Surfactant was less effective when given at an OI of 23–30 and ineffective when given at an OI >30, suggesting the need for early treatment with surfactant for these infants. These two studies were done before the wide availability of iNO therapy, which was not used in the study patients. The RCT of early iNO study done by Konduri et al. reported that infants treated with surfactant at an OI of 15–25 had a twofold reduction in the risk of mortality/need for ECMO, compared to infants that did not receive surfactant [23]. No improvement in outcome was observed with surfactant therapy for primary PPHN in this study also. However, infants with any parenchymal lung disease showed a highly significant ($P < 0.001$), threefold reduction in the risk of mortality/need for ECMO. Additionally, surfactant-treated infants were also significantly more likely to be discharged home at 30 and 60 days, compared to untreated infants. Surfactant-treated babies in this study also had a decreased length of stay on the ventilator. These data suggest that surfactant therapy given early in respiratory failure for parenchymal lung disease improves the outcomes for the affected infants. Based on the strength of these data, we recommend that any late preterm or term neonate requiring intubation and mechanical ventilation for respiratory failure secondary to parenchymal lung disease should be given surfactant, early in the course of illness. A consistent need for FiO_2 >40%

on positive pressure support should trigger an evaluation of underlying lung disease and lung expansion to assess the need for surfactant therapy.

High frequency ventilation

Although high frequency ventilation (HFV) has been extensively studied in the management of RDS in preterm infants, few studies were done in term and late preterm infants with respiratory failure and PPHN. Clark et al. conducted a rescue study of HFV versus CMV in a group of 79 neonates with respiratory failure who met ECMO criteria [24]. They randomized 40 infants to CMV and 39 to HFV. The treatment failure criteria were met more often by the infants randomized to CMV, although the difference between the two groups was not significant. The study included a crossover design for infants who met treatment failure criteria; 16/24 infants who failed CMV and crossed over to HFV improved their oxygenation, compared to 4/17 who failed HFV and crossed over to CMV; the difference between the two groups was significant. An RCT of prophylactic use of HFO early in respiratory failure did not show a difference in mortality risk or incidence of air leak, compared to CMV group [25]. Kinsella et al. randomly assigned neonates with respiratory failure and PPHN to conventional ventilation with iNO or HFV alone [26]. Infants who failed to respond to either therapy crossed over to HFV + iNO. They reported greater oxygenation response to iNO with HFV for infants with meconium aspiration syndrome or RDS. Infants with primary PPHN responded to iNO equally whether it was given with CMV or HFV. These data suggest that a lung recruitment strategy with the application of HFV, with its higher mean airway pressure, led to better responses to iNO, when PPHN is secondary to parenchymal lung disease. These studies with surfactant and HFV demonstrate broadly the importance of lung recruitment for optimizing the outcomes for infants with PPHN. Based on these data, HFO should be considered for infants with parenchymal lung disease who fail to improve their oxygenation despite a trial of surfactant replacement and iNO or other pulmonary vasodilator therapy. HFO merits consideration when the OI is >15 despite these measures, since it provides a safe way to use higher distending pressure, to distribute the vasodilator more uniformly and reduce V/Q mismatch in the lung.

Inhaled nitric oxide therapy

The introduction of iNO therapy had a dramatic impact on the outcome of babies with PPHN [27]. Hageman et al. reported 30% mortality risk for infants with PPHN in a

study published in 1984 [28]. The mortality risk decreased to <10% in the most recent RCT of iNO therapy, when this therapy was given early in respiratory failure [29]. Development of this approach for PPHN is a remarkable example of the bench-to-bedside translational biology research done by several investigators. Shortly after the discovery of NO as the endothelium-derived relaxing factor was reported in 1987, inhalation of NO as a therapy for pulmonary hypertension was tested in animal models. Inhaled NO was shown to cause selective pulmonary vasodilation at doses <100 parts per million (ppm) in a sheep model of pulmonary hypertension [30]. Inhaled NO gas reaches alveolar space quickly and diffuses to the vascular smooth muscle of the adjacent pulmonary artery from the abluminal side (Fig. 21.4). In the smooth muscle cell, NO causes relaxation by increasing the intracellular cGMP levels. As NO continues to diffuse into the lumen of pulmonary artery, it is rapidly bound and inactivated by Hb, limiting its effect to the pulmonary circulation. Inhaled NO is also preferentially distributed to the ventilated segments of the lung,

resulting in increased perfusion of the ventilated segments, thereby optimizing the VQ match (Fig. 21.4). The effect of iNO on pulmonary circulation is also not limited by the presence of extra-pulmonary right–left shunts, which often lead to hypotension with intravenous vasodilators. These properties make iNO the ideal pulmonary vasodilator in neonatal respiratory failure. Recent studies demonstrated that NO levels in the nasal cavity of premature infants can reach 50–100 parts per billion [31,32]. Significant exhaled NO concentrations are measured in these infants, suggesting that inhalation of NO occurs physiologically during tidal respiration [32] in neonates. Pilot studies in neonates with PPHN reported a rapid and sustained improvement in oxygenation with iNO [33,34]. The improvement in oxygenation is usually evident within a few minutes of starting iNO, which facilitates the rapid stabilization of a severely hypoxic and compromised neonate. Several large randomized clinical trials demonstrated that iNO therapy decreases the need for ECMO/risk of mortality in full term and late preterm (≥34 weeks gestation) infants with severe

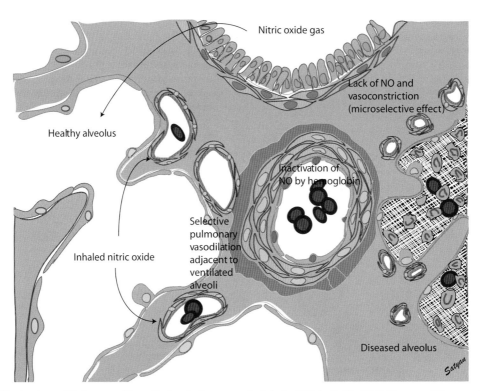

Fig. 21.4 Mechanism of Pulmonary Vasodilation in Response to Inhaled Nitric Oxide (NO) Therapy. NO gas enters alveolar space and diffuses freely across the alveolar epithelium to come in contact with the adjacent pulmonary arteries. Here, NO initiates vasodilation by increasing cGMP levels in the smooth muscle cells. As NO continues to diffuse into the blood, it binds and gets inactivated by Hb, restricting the vasodilator effect to pulmonary circulation. Additionally, NO enters only ventilated segments of the lung and dilates blood vessels only in the ventilated segments, improving VQ match. These properties make it the ideal pulmonary vasodilator. Copyright: Satyan Lakshminrusimha.

hypoxic respiratory failure and pulmonary hypertension [32,35–38]. Inhaled NO improves oxygenation in ≥70% of the infants with PPHN, with the best responses observed in idiopathic PPHN [36,37]. Based on the results of these trials, iNO therapy has been approved for clinical use in term/late preterm newborn infants (≥34 weeks gestation) with hypoxic respiratory failure since 2000 by FDA [1]. Randomized clinical trials suggested that the ideal starting dose for iNO is 20 ppm with the effective doses between 5 and 20 ppm [29]. Doses >20 ppm did not increase the efficacy and were associated with more adverse effects in these infants [37,39].

The timing of initiation of iNO therapy is an important consideration in the management of PPHN. The RCT of early iNO for hypoxic respiratory failure has randomized neonates with moderate respiratory failure (OI 15–25) to iNO therapy at this OI or to a placebo group that received standard iNO therapy at OI >25. The group randomized to early iNO had decreased progression of respiratory failure to OI >30 or OI >40. On a subgroup analysis of the study results [23], neonates who received iNO at an OI of 15–20 had a 2.5-fold reduction in the need for ECMO/mortality risk, which was significant, compared to treatment at OI of 20–25 ($P = 0.015$). Early iNO also decreased the composite outcome of progression to OI >30 and/or need for ECMO/ mortality risk [23]. Treatment of neonates with iNO at an OI of 15–20 also decreased the time to discharge from the hospital, with an overall decrease in the cost of hospital care for infants treated at OI of 15–20 compared to those

treated at an OI of 20–25 [40]. Additionally, a review of the previous clinical trials of iNO therapy shows that decrease in ECMO/mortality risk parallels the OI at the time of initiation of iNO therapy (Fig. 21.5). The ECMO rates observed for iNO-treated infants in these trials correlate well with the OI at the time of initiation of iNO and range from 40% to 11% (Fig. 21.5). The optimum time for initiation of iNO is before the infant develops severe respiratory failure secondary to progression of lung disease and/or lung injury. Taking these data together, we recommend the initiation of iNO therapy when respiratory failure progresses and OI reaches 15–20 on at least two blood gases. The randomized controlled studies of iNO also demonstrated both short- and long-term safety of this therapy in infants with PPHN. Inhaled NO therapy can be associated with three potential adverse events: methemoglobinemia generated by oxidation of Hb by NO, exposure to NO_2 generated by reaction of NO and O_2, and inhibition of platelet aggregation by NO. Previous iNO trials reported low methemoglobin levels and no significant exposure to NO_2 when doses ≤20 ppm are used. Davidson et al. reported that at doses of 80 ppm, the average methemoglobin levels peak at >5% with up to one-third of babies having levels >7% [39]. Significant levels of NO_2 were also measured at the 80 ppm dose. Generally, methemoglobin levels <5% are well-tolerated by neonates and levels ≥5% should trigger a weaning of iNO dose and frequent checks of repeat metHb levels until these levels return to safer range. Abrupt discontinuation of iNO dose should be avoided. Levels ≥10% lead to tissue

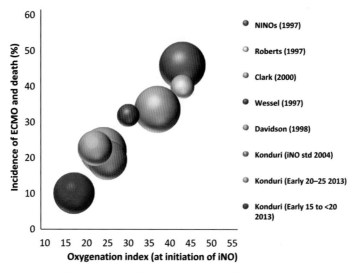

Fig. 21.5 **Relationship of Severity of Respiratory Failure, Indicated by Oxygenation Index (OI) at the Time of Initiation of iNO Therapy and the Requirement for ECMO and/or Mortality Risk.** The outcome of ECMO/mortality incidence is shown for the iNO arm of the published randomized trials of iNO therapy in term and late preterm infants with respiratory failure. The rate of ECMO/mortality risk for the treated infants correlates directly with the OI at the time of initiation of iNO therapy.

hypoxia from inability to adequately saturate the Hb and lead to lowering of pulse oximeter-measured O_2 saturation despite having a normal or near normal PaO_2. This disparity between PaO_2 and pulse oximetry measured-O_2 saturation should lead to suspicion of altered Hb affinity for O_2 and metHb is a leading cause of decreased O_2 affinity of Hb. In view of the risk of metHb in the babies on iNO therapy, the level of metHb should be checked 12–24 h after starting this therapy and periodically while the infant remains on this therapy. In our practice, if the first two checks show low metHb values, we will monitor them once a week for the duration of iNO therapy. NO_2 levels should be ≤1 ppm while receiving iNO therapy. Although a spike in NO_2 levels in the circuit can be transiently observed, these levels should quickly return to ≤1 ppm. Persistence of higher levels should lead to rapid weaning of iNO and checking of the equipment and tanks of NO gas for potential leak with mixing of ambient air with NO. Although altered platelet function is a potential complication, Christou et al. found no difference in platelet activation by ADP in babies receiving 40 ppm of iNO and placebo group [35]. Inhaled NO therapy is contraindicated in neonates with congenital heart disease with ductal-dependent systemic blood flow and in total anomalous pulmonary venous return. In congenital heart defects where the systemic blood flow is only maintained by right ventricular blood flow coming across the PDA (hypoplastic left heart syndrome, interrupted aortic arch, and severe coarctation), pulmonary vasodilation can rapidly decompensate the infant. In total anomalous pulmonary venous return with obstruction of pulmonary veins, pulmonary vasodilation can worsen the pulmonary edema and rapidly worsen the respiratory failure. It is important to use echocardiography to rule out these defects in a setting where iNO therapy is being used for hypoxic respiratory failure.

Once an infant's oxygenation is stabilized, FiO_2 and ventilator settings can be weaned before weaning the iNO dose. Weaning of iNO can commence once FiO_2 is decreased to 60% or less. A concern about weaning of the iNO dose after obtaining oxygenation response is a decrease in PaO_2. The NINOS study used the approach of weaning the dose in 20–10–5–4–3–2–1–0 ppm algorithm. A secondary analysis of arterial blood gas data from the NINOS study by Sokol et al. reported that weaning from 20 to 10 ppm and to 5 ppm led to only modest decreases in PaO_2 [41]. They also reported that weaning below 5 ppm in 1 ppm decrements led to small decreases in PaO_2, while weaning from 5 to 0 ppm was associated with significant drop in PaO_2. Based on this analysis, iNO should be weaned by 1 ppm decrements at doses below 5 ppm until the dose is finally weaned from 1 to 0.5 ppm and then off [41]. Increasing the FiO_2 by 20% at the time of discontinuation can also moderate the decrease in PaO_2. Generally, the endogenous eNOS activity is restored after 30 min to 1 h.

Exposure to iNO even for a brief period can sensitize the pulmonary circulation to rebound vasoconstriction during discontinuation of iNO therapy, even in the absence of oxygenation response. A significant drop in PaO_2 during withdrawal of iNO can be avoided by weaning the dose gradually in steps from 20 ppm to the lowest dose possible (0.5–1 ppm) for a period of time before its discontinuation [41]. Even in babies that show no response to iNO, sudden discontinuation can precipitate pulmonary vasoconstriction and rapid deterioration [1]. When iNO therapy is used in non-ECMO centers, it should be continued during transport of the infant to ECMO center [1]. Non-ECMO centers should establish treatment failure criteria for iNO in collaboration with the nearest ECMO center so that transfer of an ill infant is not delayed while waiting for a response to iNO [1].

Based on the efficacy and safety of iNO from controlled clinical trials, we recommend using this therapy early, before prolonged exposure to high FiO_2 or maximal ventilator support (Fig. 21.6). Exposure to 100% O_2 even for a brief period can induce vascular dysfunction, increase oxidative stress, and impair subsequent response to iNO [18]. Inhaled NO facilitates rapid weaning of FiO_2 and decreases oxidative stress from O_2 in an animal model of PPHN [42]. The recommended starting dose for iNO is 20 ppm. The dose can be weaned once the infant's oxygenation is stabilized. Monitoring the metHb levels and NO_2 levels to avoid side effects is important during iNO therapy. Discontinuation of iNO therapy should be done carefully while monitoring the oxygenation of the infant.

Use of iNO therapy in premature infants for hypoxic respiratory failure and prevention of BPD

Since iNO improves oxygenation in neonates with parenchymal lung disease and VQ mismatch, a number of studies have been done to investigate its use in premature infants in RDS. These studies have shown that up to 60% of extremely preterm infants with RDS show improved oxygenation with iNO therapy [43]. However, iNO therapy did not improve either survival rate or survival free of BPD [43]. Several multicenter RCTs investigated the use of iNO administered in early prophylaxis approach [44,45] or for prevention of BPD in infants at higher risk for this complication [46,47]. Ballard et al. conducted a multicenter RCT in premature infants still requiring mechanical ventilation at 1–3 weeks of postnatal age, which indicates an increased risk of BPD [48]. They observed a 7% improvement in survival free of BPD for infants who received iNO compared to placebo. On subgroup analysis, most of the improvement occurred in infants who were given iNO therapy starting at 1–2 weeks of postnatal age [46]. A subsequent multicenter

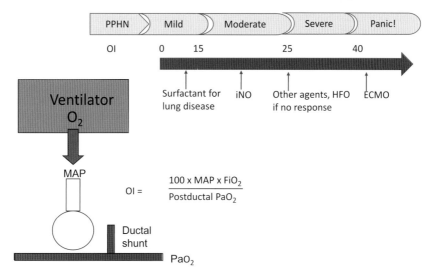

Fig. 21.6 Suggested Timing of Interventions for the Management of Respiratory Failure in Relation to the OI. Early administration of surfactant, before the infant reaches moderate degree of respiratory failure facilitates optimum lung recruitment. Early inhaled NO therapy in moderate degree of respiratory failure (OI 15–25) will alleviate pulmonary hypertension early and shorten the exposure to hyperoxia and barotrauma. If the respiratory failure progresses despite the use of these therapies, additional lung recruitment measures, such as high frequency ventilation and alternate vasodilators should be considered.

study has attempted to verify the potential benefit of iNO therapy suggested in this subgroup analysis, with a larger sample size [49]. The trial has randomized premature infants requiring mechanical ventilation at 1–2 weeks of postnatal age to iNO or placebo. This recent study did not observe a difference in rates of survival, free of BPD in the two study groups [49]. Based on these large RCTs, iNO therapy cannot be recommended for prevention of BPD in premature infants with respiratory distress. However, some premature infants present with severe hypoxemia secondary to PPHN physiology, despite adequate lung recruitment with surfactant therapy [50–53]. These infants typically have pulmonary hypoplasia secondary to premature prolonged rupture of membranes, oligohydramnios, and/or intrauterine growth restriction [50–53]. Limited observational studies suggest that the use of iNO therapy in these high-risk infants can be of benefit in relieving hypoxemia and in lowering mortality risk [50].

Use of vasodilators in BPD pulmonary hypertension

Pulmonary hypertension has also been recognized as a late complication of bronchopulmonary dysplasia. The risk of this complication is higher in infants with IUGR, prenatal infection, postnatal sepsis or necrotizing enterocolitis, and prolonged patency of ductus arteriosus [54]. The prevalence of pulmonary hypertension in BPD has been estimated to be from 14% to 18% [55–57] in prospective or

retrospective screening studies where PH was identified by echocardiography done at 32–36 weeks of postmenstrual age. PH increases the risk of morbidity and mortality in BPD infants. The current vasodilator management of PH in BPD is largely based on experience extrapolated from term PPHN infants. There are currently no RCTs that tested the efficacy of vasodilator therapy in BPD-PH. The agents currently used target NO-cGMP system or PGI_2-cAMP system and ET-receptor antagonists [54]. Since BPD-PH is a chronic condition in contrast to PPHN in term infants, therapies that can be used in ambulatory setting are generally preferred for management of these infants. The commonly used agents include enteric sildenafil and bosentan and subcutaneous treprostinil, a PGI_2 analog [54]. Among these available agents, the largest clinical experience is with the use of sildenafil. There are no RCTs that tested the efficacy of sildenafil in improving outcomes for BPD infants with PH. There are four observational cohort studies that described the outcomes for BPD-PH after sildenafil therapy [58–61]. These studies had small cohorts ranging from 21 to 25 patients per series. Sildenafil was started at 3–6 months postnatal age in these reports and the duration of therapy ranged from 2 to 8 months. Some of the infants were on other vasodilator medications, including iNO, bosentan, or milrinone, which makes it hard to assess the response to sildenafil. Response was evaluated by echocardiography parameters for pulmonary hypertension, including TR jet velocity when present, septal flattening, and RV hypertrophy. The studies were consistent in reporting improved

hemodynamic parameters in two-thirds of infants after initiation of sildenafil therapy. However, whether the improvement occurred from the natural evolution of PH or as a result of sildenafil therapy remains undetermined until a prospective RCT is done. The evidence for the use of bosentan and treprostinil is even more limited with a few case reports and small case series describing the dose and route of administration of these agents. PH remains a long-term complication of BPD and is accelerated by hypoxia and hypercarbia spells that these infants undergo. PH appears to be a marker for and contributor to worse outcomes in BPD and its overall management requires identification of other BPD complications related to airway disease, GE reflux, and parenchymal lung disease. Addressing these comorbidities can often improve the trajectory of PH in BPD and should be attempted first before vasodilator therapy is considered. Additionally, presence of significant contributors to PH, such as systemic to pulmonary collaterals and pulmonary vein stenosis should be carefully evaluated. Since vasodilator agents can have significant side effects, initiation of these therapies should be done only in a setting where multidisciplinary care and follow-up for infants with BPD and PH are available. Recently, guidelines for the identification and care of infants with PH secondary to BPD have been published by investigators from pediatric pulmonary hypertension network [62].

Phosphodiesterase-5 inhibitors

The PDE-5 inhibitors, sildenafil and tadalafil, have been investigated widely in adult pulmonary hypertension. Sildenafil has been investigated to a more limited extent in neonatal respiratory failure [63,64] and PPHN [65]. Enteric sildenafil was successfully used in an infant with PPHN with improved oxygenation by the Chief Editor (RP) in 2002 (*BMJ* 2002;325:181). Subsequent randomized trials have demonstrated its efficacy in improving oxygenation and decreasing mortality. A pilot RCT of enteric sildenafil done in Colombia in a setting where ECMO was not available showed that it improves oxygenation in neonates with severe PPHN compared to placebo-treated infants [65]. The trial was halted early after five out of six infants in the placebo group died compared to one out of seven infants in the sildenafil group [65]. Improvement in oxygenation occurred in the sildenafil-treated infants 6–12 h after the first dose. An RCT of sildenafil given by enteric route was also done in 51 neonates with PPHN with 20 infants assigned to placebo group and 31 to oral sildenafil in a dose of 3 mg/kg/dose in Mexico [66]. This study reported that sildenafil decreased the mortality risk significantly from 40% in the placebo group to 6% in the sildenafil-treated neonates. Improvement in oxygenation

was observed 7 h after the first oral dose of sildenafil. Systemic hypotension was not observed in these studies with oral/enteric sildenafil. These RCTs show that sildenafil, used as the primary therapy for PPHN, is effective and safe in a resource constrained setting where iNO therapy is not available. A clinical trial of open label IV sildenafil therapy was done in 36 neonates with PPHN; 29 of the infants were already receiving iNO therapy [67]. Sildenafil administration was associated with a significant decrease in OI, starting 4 h after beginning the infusion. In seven neonates who received sildenafil infusion without iNO, oxygenation improved with a decrease in OI from a mean of 24.6–14.7. Overall, one neonate needed ECMO therapy in this trial. The results of this study suggest that IV sildenafil can be an alternative or useful adjunct to iNO, when oral/enteric therapy cannot be given due to the critical nature of the infant's illness or side effects from oral sildenafil. Since hypotension occurred more frequently with IV sildenafil, we recommend oral/enteric therapy first and attempt IV infusion when administration by enteric route is not practical. Initial bolus dose of IV sildenafil also should be given over 3 h to decrease the risk of hypotension, as shown in Table 21.1. Tadalafil is a long acting PDE-5 inhibitor that can be given once a day. An RCT was reported recently comparing oral sildenafil 1 mg/kg 3 times/day and oral tadalafil 1 mg/kg once a day; both agents showed similar efficacy [47]. The dose was chosen based on a recent study [68]. Once-a-day administration offers better compliance and ease of administration in practice, when these agents are used in an ambulatory setting for chronic pulmonary hypertension. The wide availability and low cost of PDE-5 inhibitors make them ideal alternatives to iNO therapy and their synergistic effects on NO-cGMP pathway make them useful adjuncts for infants not responding to iNO therapy (Fig. 21.6). A suggested algorithm for the application of the available therapies in neonates with hypoxic respiratory failure and PPHN is shown in Fig. 21.6.

Prostaglandins in PPHN

Prostacyclin (PGI_2) and its analogs relax pulmonary artery by increasing intracellular cAMP in the smooth muscle cells [82]. These agents were used as the primary treatment modality in adults with pulmonary arterial hypertension for over 3 decades. Most of the experience with prostaglandins in adult patients comes from IV administration of epoprostenol through a central venous catheter by continuous infusion. However, their use in neonates with PPHN was more limited since parenteral administration of these agents can lead to systemic hypotension in the presence of right to left shunts across PFO or PDA. Additionally, in the presence of parenchymal lung disease, a global increase in

Table 21.1 Vasodilators in PPHN management

Drugs	Administration route/dose	Mechanism of action	Use in PPHN
General treatment			
Oxygen	To achieve **PaO$_2$ 60–90 mmHg or SpO$_2$ 90%–97%**	Generates ATP in circulation, enhances NO formation from endothelium	The first line of treatment
Tolazoline [69,70]	IV: 0.5–2 mg/kg hr after 1 mg/kg loading over 10 minutes; Neb: 1–2.5 mg/kg	Nonspecific endothelium-independent vasodilation and α-adrenergic inhibitor	Currently not recommended due to high risk of systemic hypotension
Adenosine [71]	IV: 25–50 µg/kg/min	Stimulates A2 adenosine receptor to induce NO release from endothelium	• Extremely short half-life • Needs to be given continuously through a venous line
Calcium channel blockers			
MgSO$_4$ [72]	IV: 200 mg/kg bolus over 30 min then 20–150 mg/kg/h	Nonspecific smooth muscle relaxant	• Slow onset of response • Muscle relaxation [73] and sedative effect
Diltiazem [74]	IV: 1–2 mg/kg q 12–6 h	Block calcium channel	Not recommended in neonates due to adverse cardiac effects
Nitric oxide and nitric oxide donor			
Nitric oxide	Inhalation: 5–20 ppm	Produced in the vascular endothelium; causes vasodilation through increase in intracellular cGMP in the smooth muscle cells	• The standard treatment for PPHN • Selective pulmonary vasodilator • Needs to monitor methemoglobin and NO$_2$ during use [75]
Nitroglycerine [76]	IV: 2–10 µg/kg/min	NO donor	Not recommended; high risk of hypotension
Nitroprusside [77]	IV: 0.2–6.0 µg/kg/min	NO donor	Monitoring thiocyanate level is recommended
Prostaglandins			
PGI$_2$ [78]	IV: 2–5 ng/kg/min; increments of 2–5 ng/kg/min q 15 min; aerosol inhalation of 50 ng/kg/min continuous [57,69,79,86]: iloprost 0.5–2 µg/kg/dose q 2–4 h as inhalation	Produced from arachidonic acid; causes vasodilatation by increasing intracellular cAMP in lung smooth muscle	• Vasodilatation through alternative and complementary pathway • May enhance NO action • A nonspecific pulmonary vasodilator • May have systemic effects
PGE$_1$ [80]	IV: 0.01–0.1 µg/kg/min	Similar to PGI$_2$	Similar to PGI$_2$
PGE$_1$	Aerosol inhalation: 100–300 ng/kg/min	Similar to PGI$_2$	Similar to PGI$_2$
Treprostinil [96]	IV or SC: Start 1-2ng/kg/min; increase 1-2ng/kg/min Q12 h based on tolerance until target dose 20ng/kg/min	Similar to PGI$_2$	Similar to PPHN
Phosphodiesterase inhibitors			
Sildenafil	IV: loading 0.14 mg/kg/h for 3 h followed by 0.07 mg/kg/h; PO/NG: 0.5–2 mg/kg/dose q 6 h	Inhibitor of phosphodiesterase enzyme type V (responsible for cGMP degradation)	• It may potentiate nitric oxide • Safe and easy to administer • May worsen oxygenation due to vasodilation of unventilated areas

(Continued)

Table 21.1 Vasodilators in PPHN management (*cont.*)

Drugs	Administration route/dose	Mechanism of action	Use in PPHN
Tadalafil [68]	PO/NG: 1 mg/kg/day once daily	Similar to sildenafil	Similar to sildenafil
Milrinone	**Term**: IV: loading: 50 µg/kg over 60 min; maintenance: 0.25–0.75 µg/kg/min or continuous infusion only at 0.25-0.75 µg/kg/min [100] **GA <30 weeks**: IV: loading: 50 µg/kg over 3 h; maintenance: 0.2 µg/kg/min	Inhibitor of the phosphodiesterase enzyme type III (responsible for degradation of cAMP)	• May potentiate the action of prostaglandins • Improves right cardiac output by reducing afterload
Dipyridamole [46,81]	IV: 0.3–0.6 mg/kg	Nonspecific PDE inhibition	Use together with iNO to prevent rebound vasoconstriction
Endothelin receptor inhibitor			
Bosentan	Oral: 1–2 mg/kg twice daily	Nonspecific antagonist A and B endothelin receptors	Seldom used in newborns due to the potential for damage to liver function

pulmonary blood flow can worsen the VQ match and oxygenation. Aerosolized PG given into the lungs can overcome these limitations; however, their penetration to alveolar and vascular compartments is uneven due to the deposition of droplets in ET tube or upper airway, resulting in variable responses. For these reasons, they are not currently used as the primary agents in PPHN, but can be important alternate agents when PPHN infants fail to respond to the combination of mechanical ventilation, surfactant, and iNO. In our experience, prostaglandins have been more effective in neonates with PPHN secondary to CDH or alveolar capillary dysplasia. There are three different prostacyclin analogs that are currently available and their use and route of administration in neonates is discussed in following sections, with the manufacturer given names in the parentheses.

Epoprostenol (Flolan, Veletri)

Epoprostenol can be given either through IV or aerosol route. It is one of the most commonly prescribed vasodilators for pulmonary hypertension. The effects of epoprostenol last only a few minutes; consequently, it requires continuous IV infusion or continuous aerosol administration. In one retrospective study in neonatal PPHN, it was initiated at 1–2 ng/kg/min and subsequently titrated up by 0.5–2 ng/kg/min, intravenously [78,83]. Eronen et al. reported starting it at a higher dose of 20 ng/kg/min IV, which was later increased stepwise to a mean dose of 60 ng/kg/min (30–120 ng/kg/min) [84]. Systemic hypotension was noted in some patients, which required volume expansion and inotropic support. There are currently no RCTs to determine its efficacy, optimum dose, or frequency of side effects in neonates

with PPHN. Aerosol administration of epoprostenol has been shown to improve oxygenation in pilot studies and in case reports [85–87]. Bindl et al. reported that a dose of 20–30 ng/kg/min of continuous aerosolized PGI_2 administration has improved oxygenation in one term infant with PPHN but was less effective in another infant [88]. Kelly et al. reported that continuous epoprostenol aerosol administration has improved oxygenation in four infants with PPHN unresponsive to iNO [86]. They administered the drug by continuous nebulization at a dose of 50 ng/kg/min, diluted into a volume of 8 mL/h. One concern with inhaled epoprostenol treatment is that the diluent buffer has an alkaline pH of 10. Kelly et al. reported no adverse effects in their pilot study; however, no data on the potential impact of high pH on the neonatal lungs are available.

Iloprost (Ventavis)

Iloprost is a synthetic PGI_2 analog with a half-life of 20–30 min and can be given by inhaled route up to 6–9 times a day through a nebulizer or can be also given intravenously. A retrospective study compared inhaled iloprost with oral sildenafil in term infants with PPHN in a setting where iNO, ECMO, and HFV were not available. This study observed better responses in the Iloprost treatment group [89]. The dose for inhaled Iloprost was 1–2.5 µg/kg every 2–4 h through the endotracheal tube via a nebulizer [88]. In another retrospective study, 15 premature infants who were treated with surfactant and ventilator support continued to have OI above 25 with suspected PPHN. Inhaled Iloprost was given at a dose of 0.5–1.0 µg/kg/day. The mean maximal OI decreased from 38 to 8 by the end of the treatment.

No cessation of treatment was needed for side effects in this report [90]. There were a few other case reports using Iloprost nebulization at doses 2 μg/kg in extremely premature infants with PPHN [91] or a total dose of 20 μg/kg/day in term infants [92]. For intravenous administration, a starting dose of 0.5–3.0 ng/kg/min with maintenance doses of 1–10 ng/kg/min of Iloprost was reported in severe PPHN [93]. The dosage was then titrated up by the clinical response and was adjusted by 0.5–1 ng/kg/min increments in this study [93]. We prefer to use agents, such as Iloprost by aerosol route, to take advantage of the preferential pulmonary vascular effects and avoidance of hypotension (Fig. 21.7). Inhaled PG also overcomes the presence of right to left extra-pulmonary shunts, which interfere with the delivery of IV agents to pulmonary circulation (Fig. 21.7).

Treprostinil (Tyvaso, Remodulin and Orenitram)

Treprostinil, a stable prostacyclin analog, was initially approved by the FDA for subcutaneous use and subsequently approved for intravenous and inhaled use. Compared to epoprostenol, treprostinil is [54] stable at room temperature, [94] has longer half-life, [42] fewer side effects, and [46] a smaller pump size as an option for continuous infusion. Subcutaneous treprostinil offers the advantage of not requiring a central venous catheter [95]. In our limited experience and published case series, SC administration of treprostinil is well tolerated by neonates with very few of the local complications previously reported in older children and adults. This route makes ambulatory administration feasible with appropriate training of the parents [96]. Our longest experience with SC treprostinil administration in an ambulatory setting is 9 months in a premature infant with BPD who had persistent elevation of PVR, despite oral sildenafil therapy.

Prostaglandin E$_1$ (Alprostadil)

Prostaglandin E$_1$ (PGE$_1$) has been used in infants with ductus arteriosus–dependent congenital heart disease at doses of 0.01–0.1 μg/kg/min as IV continuous infusion [97]. Once ductal patency is established, the infusion can be titrated down to the lowest effective dose (generally at 0.01 μg/kg/min). PGE$_1$ also can cause pulmonary vasodilation and has been used for this indication in PPHN. PGE$_1$ can improve right ventricular function in CDH patients by providing patent ductus arteriosus as an outlet to decompress the stressed right ventricle and to assist the systemic blood flow in the presence of LV dysfunction. PGE$_1$ can be also aerosolized

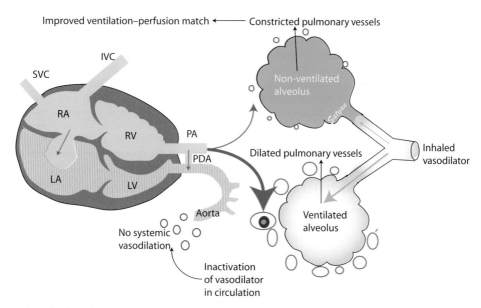

Fig. 21.7 Benefits of Inhaled Vasodilators in Neonates with PPHN Secondary to Parenchymal Lung Disease. Inhaled vasodilators, iNO, and prostacyclin are preferentially distributed to ventilated segments of the lung, where they dilate the adjacent pulmonary vessels. They do not reach the atelectatic segments of the lung where pulmonary vessels remain constricted. This property improves the matching of ventilation with perfusion. In case of inhaled NO, inactivation of NO by Hb limits the vasodilation to pulmonary circulation, leading to highly selective effect on the lung. Inhaled vasodilators also are not affected by presence of right to left extra-pulmonary shunts at PFO and PDA, which reduce the delivery of IV agents to pulmonary circulation. Copyright: Satyan Lakshminrusimha.

and administered into the lung, similar to epoprostenol. Sood et al. reported that a safe and effective dose of inhaled PGE_1 is 150–300 ng/kg/min in their phase I/II open label clinical trial [98]. However, a planned RCT of PGE_1 for PPHN was terminated early due to low enrollment.

Phosphodiesterase-3 inhibitors

Milrinone (Primacor)

Milrinone is the only available PDE-3 inhibitor which has been used in PPHN treatment. Milrinone increases the bioavailability of cAMP and may indirectly also increase cGMP levels through some inhibitory effect on PDE-5 [99]. McNamara et al. reported an open label trial of milrinone in 11 term neonates with PPHN. Milrinone was given in a loading dose of 50 µg/kg over 30–60 min, followed by a maintenance infusion at 0.33–0.99 µg/kg/min for 24–72 h [100]. They observed improvement in PaO_2 and sustained reductions in FiO_2, OI, mean airway pressure, and iNO dose. They also demonstrated decreases in PA pressure and right to left shunts and improvement in LV and RV output by echocardiography. Although hypotension was observed, they noted an improvement in base deficit and reduction in blood lactate levels. Bassler et al. reported their experience with milrinone in four neonates with severe PPHN unresponsive to iNO, with mean OI of 40 ± 12. They observed an improvement in oxygenation, with a reduction in OI to 28 ± 16 followed by extubation and survival of all four infants. However, two infants developed severe IVH and one other infant had a small IVH. Since this is not an RCT, it is unclear whether the IVH was secondary to severe underlying illness or to milrinone administration [79]. We currently use milrinone in neonates with CDH, where its combination of pulmonary vasodilator and inotropic effects are beneficial in some infants with PPHN and poor LV function. However, RCTs are needed to define its indications, efficacy, and potential side effects. We advise against using both sildenafil and milrinone simultaneously in the same infant due to the potential for severe hypotension associated with blocking both PDE isoforms in the vascular smooth muscle.

Endothelin receptor antagonist

There are three oral medications (bosentan, ambrisentan, and macitentan) in the endothelin receptor antagonist (ERA) class. These medications block the endothelin receptors, thereby reducing the vasoconstrictor effects of endothelin. Bosentan is the first ERA available to treat PPHN, and it blocks both type A and type B receptors. Ambrisentan is another oral ERA that preferentially blocks the ETA receptor, and is a pill which is taken once daily. Macitentan is the most recently approved once daily pill that blocks both the type A and the type B ET receptors. Bosentan is the only one studied in neonates with PPHN. It is a competitive antagonist of ET-1 at both ETA and ETB receptors with slightly higher affinity for ETA than ETB [101]. Nakwan et al. have previously reported the benefits of bosentan in neonates with PPHN [102]. An RCT in PPHN infants less than 7 days of age, in a setting where iNO and ECMO were not available, showed an 88% response rate with improved oxygenation in the treatment group, compared to 20% response rate in the placebo group [103]. The dose used in that study was 1–2 mg/kg twice daily, via nasogastric tube. No detectable side effect was observed in this report, but liver injury has been reported in adult patients with pulmonary arterial hypertension. A recent randomized trial of Bosentan in a group of neonates already on iNO therapy for respiratory failure [104] was stopped early due to slow recruitment. Bosentan was found to be safe, but no significant improvement in oxygenation, time to wean from iNO, or ventilator support was noted in the Bosentan-treated group compared to placebo. Although systemic blood pressure and hepatic transaminases were not different between the groups, more infants treated with Bosentan had anemia and peripheral edema. The study also found low serum levels of the drug for the first 5 days after beginning nasogastric administration, possibly due to poor absorption from the gut in these ill neonates. Based on this limited evidence and the availability of agents that are more widely studied, bosentan is not recommended as first or second line therapy and should be reserved for occasions where iNO, PDE inhibitors, and prostacyclin analogs failed to provide improvement or are unavailable in PPHN.

Other vasodilators tested in PPHN

Magnesium sulfate

Magnesium sulfate was previously used to treat PPHN in settings where inhaled NO and PDE-5 inhibitors were not available [72,94,105]. The reported doses of $MgSO_4$ were 20–100 mg/kg/h, following a loading dose of 200 mg/kg over 30 min. Magnesium is believed to inhibit NMDA receptors in the central nervous system [106] to offer protection to the brain and to induce muscle relaxation by blocking the neuromuscular junction [73]. Magnesium antagonizes calcium in the smooth muscle cells, which leads to muscle relaxation. However, only observational studies are available in newborn infants. Magnesium sulfate should be only rarely used in PPHN since it can be

associated with systemic hypotension. Owing to the lack of adequate RCTs and the availability of more effective pulmonary vasodilators, we currently do not recommend the use of $MgSO_4$ in this setting.

Adenosine

Adenosine is a purine nucleoside and vasodilator of systemic and pulmonary vasculature in both fetal and neonatal vessels [107,108]. Adenosine causes vasodilatation by activation of endothelial A2a adenosine receptors and subsequent release of NO [78]. From a randomized, placebo-controlled trial of 18 infants, Konduri et al. showed an improvement in oxygenation in 45% of term infants with PPHN [109]. The dosage used was 25–50 µg/kg/min given as continuous infusion. This study did not report any systemic side effects, presumably due to the rapid metabolism of adenosine at these doses by pulmonary vascular endothelial cells, as previously shown in the lamb model of neonatal pulmonary hypertension [108]. However, the improvement in oxygenation was not sustained and it did not decrease the need for ECMO or mortality in neonatal PPHN [109]. In a single-center prospective observation study, nine infants on mechanical ventilation and receiving iNO at 20 ppm were given continuous intravenous infusion of adenosine at 50 µg/kg/min; six of these infants responded favorably with improved oxygenation [110]. Owing to its extremely short half-life, adenosine should be given through continuous infusion, preferably in the upper part of the body, since SVC flow is less likely to be shunted across the PFO.

Steroids

A randomized controlled study showed benefit to the use of glucocorticoids in managing PPHN caused by meconium aspiration [111]. Improved oxygenation was also shown with antenatal betamethasone or postnatal hydrocortisone in a sheep model of PPHN [112–114]. The possible mechanisms include increase in eNOS expression and function in the endothelial cells or normalization of PDE-5 activity in pulmonary artery smooth muscle cells [114]. Although steroids are commonly used in neonatal intensive care unit to manage systemic hypotension, its efficacy in relaxing pulmonary arteries in PPHN remains to be determined. There are currently no RCTs of this therapy in PPHN. Based on the studies in premature infants, there is a concern of possible neurodevelopmental effects when they are administered early in life.

Conclusions

PPHN occurs in 2/1000 live births and the affected infants are often the sickest in the neonatal intensive care units. The introduction of iNO therapy led to dramatic improvements in the outcomes for the neonates with PPHN [115]. However, about 20%–30% of these infants do not improve their oxygenation sufficiently with iNO, creating a need for alternate agents to manage refractory PPHN. The incidence of PPHN remains high and the survival rate for affected infants remains low in the resource-constrained areas of the world where surfactant, HFV, and iNO therapy are not readily available. The use of alternate agents like oral sildenafil or inhaled prostaglandins may offer benefit in these areas (Table 21.1). However, many of these alternate vasodilators lack high quality RCTs to establish their efficacy. Some newer agents showed promising effects in animal studies, but no human experience is available [16]. In future, conducting these trials specifically in the settings where iNO is not available, may provide important evidence to define their indications, appropriate dose, and weaning strategies. Adaptive trial designs with crossover component need to be developed as alternatives to 1:1 randomization traditionally used in RCTs to allow the benefit of potentially useful therapies in the affected infants with PPHN in these settings. Finally, future studies need to explore the genetic factors that contribute to the development of PPHN and variability in the response to different vasodilators.

References

[1] American Academy of Pediatrics Committee on Fetus and Newborn. Use of inhaled nitric oxide. Pediatrics 2000;106:344–345.

[2] Steurer MA, Jelliffe-Pawlowski LL, Baer RJ, Partridge JC, Rogers EE, Keller RL. Persistent pulmonary hypertension of the newborn in late preterm and term infants in California. Pediatrics 2017;139:e20161165.

[3] Walsh-Sukys MC, Tyson JE, Wright LL, et al. Persistent pulmonary hypertension of the newborn in the era before nitric oxide: practice variation and outcomes. Pediatrics 2000;105:14–20.

[4] Paden ML, Conrad SA, Rycus PT, Thiagarajan RR. ELSO Registry. Extracorporeal life support organization registry report 2012. ASAIO J 2013;59(3):202–210.

[5] Shankaran S, Pappas A, Laptook AR, McDonald SA, Ehrenkranz RA, Tyson JE, et al. Outcomes of safety and effectiveness in a multicenter randomized, controlled trial of whole-body hypothermia for neonatal hypoxic-ischemic encephalopathy. Pediatrics 2008;122:e791–e798.

[6] DeNucci G, Thomas R, D'Orleans-Juste P, et al. Pressor effects of

circulating endothelin are limited by its removal in the pulmonary circulation and by the release of prostacyclin and endothelium-derived relaxing factor. Proc Natl Acad Sci USA 1988;85:9797–9800.

[7] Böhm F, Pernow J. The importance of endothelin-1 for vascular dysfunction in cardiovascular disease. Cardiovasc Res 2007;76:8–18.

[8] Rosenberg AA, Kennaugh J, Koppenhafer SL, Loomis M, Chatfield BA, Abman SH. Elevated immunoreactive endothelin-1 levels in newborn infants with persistent pulmonary hypertension. J Pediatr 1993;123:109–114.

[9] Taddei S, Vanhoutte PM. Endothelium-dependent contractions to endothelin in the rat aorta are mediated by thromboxane A2. J Cardiovasc Pharmacol 1993;22(S8):S328–S331.

[10] Mahajan CN, Afolayan AJ, Eis A, Teng RJ, Konduri GG. Altered prostanoid metabolism contributes to impaired angiogenesis in persistent pulmonary hypertension in a fetal lamb model. Pediatr Res 2015;77:455–462.

[11] North AJ, Star RA, Brannon TS, et al. Nitric oxide synthase type I and type III gene expression are developmentally regulated in rat lung. Am J Physiol Lung Cell Mol Physiol 1994;266:L635–L641.

[12] Dollberg S, Warner BW, Myatt L. Urinary nitrite and nitrate concentrations in patients with idiopathic persistent pulmonary hypertension of the newborn and effect of extracorporeal membrane oxygenation. Pediatr Res 1995;37:31–34.

[13] Villanueva ME, Zaher FM, Svinarich DM, Konduri GG. Decreased gene expression of endothelial nitric oxide synthase in newborns with persistent pulmonary hypertension. Pediatr Res 1998;44:338–343.

[14] Konduri GG, Ou J, Shi Y, Pritchard KA. Decreased association of Hsp90 impairs endothelial nitric oxide synthase in fetal lambs with persistent pulmonary hypertension. Am J Physiol Heart Circ Physiol 2003;285:H204–H211.

[15] Teng RJ, Du J, Xu H, Bakhutashvili I, Eis A, Shi Y, et al. Sepiapterin improves angiogenesis of pulmonary artery endothelial cells with in utero pulmonary hypertension by recoupling endothelial nitric oxide synthase. Am J Physiol Lung Cell Mol Physiol 2011;301:L334–L345.

[16] Chester M, Seedorf G, Tourneux P, et al. Cinaciguat, a soluble guanylate cyclase activator, augments cGMP after oxidative stress and causes pulmonary vasodilation in neonatal pulmonary hypertension. Am J Physiol Lung Cell Mol Physiol 2011;301:L755–L764.

[17] Farrow KN, Wedgwood S, Lee KJ, et al. Mitochondrial oxidant stress increases PDE5 activity in persistent pulmonary hypertension of the newborn. Respir Physiol Neurobiol 2010;174:272–281.

[18] Lakshminrusimha S, Swartz DD, Gugino SF, Ma CX, Wynn KA, Ryan RM, et al. Oxygen concentration and pulmonary hemodynamics in newborn lambs with pulmonary hypertension. Pediatr Res 2009;66:539–544.

[19] Wung JT, James LS, Kilchevsky E, James E. Management of infants with severe respiratory failure and persistence of the fetal circulation, without hyperventilation. Pediatrics 1985;76:488–494.

[20] Gadzinowski J, Kowalska K, Vidyasagar D. Treatment of MAS with PPHN using combined therapy: SLL, bolus surfactant and iNO. J Perinatol 2008;28(Suppl. 3):S56–S66.

[21] Findlay RD, Taeusch HW, Walther FJ. Surfactant replacement therapy for meconium aspiration syndrome. Pediatrics 1996;97:48–52.

[22] Lotze A, Mitchell BR, Bulas DI, Zola EM, Shalwitz RA, Gunkel JH. Multicenter study of surfactant (beractant) use in the treatment of term infants with severe respiratory failure. Survanta in Term Infants Study Group. J Pediatr 1998;132:40–47.

[23] Konduri GG, Sokol GM, Van Meurs KP, Singer J, Ambalavanan N, Lee T, et al. Impact of early surfactant and inhaled nitric oxide therapies on outcomes in term/late preterm neonates with moderate hypoxic respiratory failure. J Perinatol 2013;33:944–949.

[24] Clark RH, Yoder BA, Sell MS. Prospective, randomized comparison of high-frequency oscillation and conventional ventilation in candidates for extracorporeal membrane oxygenation. J Pediatr 1994;124:447–454.

[25] Rojas MA, Lozano JM, Rojas MX, et al. Randomized, multicentre trial of conventional ventilation versus high-frequency oscillatory ventilation for the early management of respiratory failure in term or near-term infants in Colombia. J Perinatol 2005;25:720–724.

[26] Kinsella JP, Truog WE, Walsh WF, et al. Randomized, multicenter trial of inhaled nitric oxide and high frequency oscillatory ventilation in severe persistent pulmonary hypertension of the newborn. J Pediatr 1997;131:55–62.

[27] Finer NN, Barrington KJ. Nitric oxide for respiratory failure in infants born at or near term. Cochrane Database Syst Rev 2000;2:CD000399.

[28] Hageman JR, Adams MA, Gardner TH. Persistent pulmonary hypertension of the newborn: trends in incidence, diagnosis, and management. Am J Dis Child 1984;138:592–595.

[29] Konduri GG, Solimano A, Sokol GM, et al. A randomized trial of early versus standard inhaled nitric oxide therapy in term and near-term newborn infants with hypoxic respiratory failure. Pediatrics 2004;113:559–564.

[30] Frostell C, Fratacci MD, Wain JC, et al. Inhaled nitric oxide: a selective pulmonary vasodilator reversing hypoxic pulmonary vasoconstriction. Circulation 1991;83:2038–2047.

[31] Leipala JA, Williams O, Sreekumar S, et al. Exhaled nitric oxide levels in infants with chronic lung disease. Eur J Pediatr 2004;163:555–558.

[32] Williams O, Rafferty GF, Hannam S, et al. Nasal and lower airway levels of nitric oxide in prematurely born infants. Early Hum Dev 2003;72:67–73.

[33] Kinsella JP, Neish SR, Shaffer E, et al. Low-dose inhalation nitric oxide in persistent pulmonary hypertension of the newborn. Lancet 1992;340:819–820.

[34] Roberts JD, Fineman JR, Morin FC, et al. Inhaled nitric oxide and persistent pulmonary hypertension of the newborn. N Engl J Med 1997;336:605–610.

[35] Christou H, Van Marter LJ, Wessel DL, et al. Inhaled nitric oxide reduces the need for extracorporeal membrane oxygenation in infants with persistent pulmonary hypertension of the newborn. Crit Care Med 2000;28:3722–3727.

[36] Clark RH, Kueser TJ, Walker MW, et al. Low-dose nitric oxide therapy for persistent pulmonary hypertension of the newborn. N Engl J Med 2000;342:469–474.

[37] The Neonatal Inhaled Nitric Oxide Study Group. Inhaled nitric oxide in

full-term and nearly full-term infants with hypoxic respiratory failure. N Engl J Med 1997;336:597–604.

[38] Roberts JD, Polaner DM, Lang P, et al. Inhaled nitric oxide in persistent pulmonary hypertension of the newborn. Lancet 1992;340:818–819.

[39] Davidson D, Barefield ES, Kattwinkel J, et al. Inhaled nitric oxide for the early treatment of persistent pulmonary hypertension of the term newborn: a randomized, double-masked, placebo-controlled, dose-response, multicenter study. The I-NO/PPHN Study Group. Pediatrics 1998;101:325–334.

[40] Konduri GG, Menzin J, Frean M, Lee T, Potenziano J, Singer J. Inhaled nitric oxide in term/late preterm neonates with hypoxic respiratory failure: estimating the financial impact of earlier use. J Med Econ 2015;18: 612–618.

[41] Sokol GM, Fineberg NS, Wright LL, Ehrenkranz RA. Changes in arterial oxygen tension when weaning neonates from inhaled nitric oxide. Pediatr Pulmonol 2001;32:14–19.

[42] Afolayan AJ, Eis A, Alexander M, Michalkiewicz T, Teng RJ, Lakshminrusimha S, et al. Decreased endothelial nitric oxide synthase expression and function contribute to impaired mitochondrial biogenesis and oxidative stress in fetal lambs with persistent pulmonary hypertension. Am J Physiol Lung Cell Mol Physiol 2016;310:L40–L49.

[43] Van Meurs KP, Wright LL, Ehrenkranz RA, Lemons JA, Ball MB, Poole WK, et al. Inhaled nitric oxide for premature infants with severe respiratory failure. N Engl J Med 2005;353(1):13–22.

[44] Kinsella JP, Cutter GR, Walsh WF, et al. Early inhaled nitric oxide therapy in premature newborns with respiratory failure. N Engl J Med 2006;355: 354–364.

[45] Mercier JC, Hummler H, Durrmeyer X, et al. Inhaled nitric oxide for prevention of bronchopulmonary dysplasia in premature babies (EUNO): a randomised controlled trial. Lancet 2010;376:346–354.

[46] Al-Alaiyan S, Al-Omran A, Dyer D. The use of phoshodiestersae inhibitor (dipyridamole) to wean from inhaled nitric oxide. Intensive Care Med 1996;22:1093–1095.

[47] Alipour MR, Lookzadeh MH, Namayandeh SM, Pezeshkpour Z, Sarebanhassanabadi M. Comparison

of tadalafil and sildenafil in controlling neonatal persistent pulmonary hypertension. Iran J Pediatr 2017;27:e6385.

[48] Ballard RA, Truog WE, Cnaan A, et al. Inhaled nitric oxide in preterm infants undergoing mechanical ventilation. N Engl J Med 2006;355:343–353.

[49] Hasan SU, Potenziano J, Konduri GG, Perez JA, Van Meurs KP, Walker MW, et al. Effect of inhaled nitric oxide on survival without bronchopulmonary dysplasia in preterm infants: a randomized clinical trial. JAMA Pediatr 2017;171(11):1081–1089.

[50] Baczynski M, Ginty S, Weisz DE, McNamara PJ, Kelly E, Shah P, et al. Short-term and long-term outcomes of preterm neonates with acute severe pulmonary hypertension following rescue treatment with inhaled nitric oxide. Arch Dis Child Fetal Neonatal Ed 2017;102(6):F508–F514.

[51] Dani C, Corsini I, Cangemi J, Vangi V, Pratesi S. Nitric oxide for the treatment of preterm infants with severe RDS and pulmonary hypertension. Pediatr Pulmonol 2017;52(11):1461–1468.

[52] Jorge AS, Javier CM, Diaz-Quijano FA. Inhaled nitric oxide in preterm neonates with refractory hypoxemia associated to oligohydramnios. Curr Drug Discov Technol 2018;15: 156–160.

[53] Kinsella JP, Steinhorn RH, Krishnan US, Feinstein JA, Adatia I, Austin ED, et al. Recommendations for the use of inhaled nitric oxide therapy in premature newborns with severe pulmonary hypertension. J Pediatr 2016;170:312–314.

[54] Abman SH, Hansmann G, Archer SL, Ivy DD, Adatia I, Chung WK, et al. Pediatric pulmonary hypertension. Circulation 2015;132:2037–2099.

[55] Backes CH, Reagan PB, Smith CV, Jadcherla SR, Slaughter JL. Sildenafil treatment of infants with bronchopulmonary dysplasia-associated pulmonary hypertension. Hosp Pediatr 2016;6(1):27–33.

[56] Bhat R, Salas AA, Foster C, Carlo WA, Ambalavanan N. Prospective analysis of pulmonary hypertension in extremely low birth weight infants. Pediatrics 2012;129(3):e682–e689.

[57] Mourani PM, Sontag MK, Younoszai A, Miller JI, Kinsella JP, Baker CD, et al. Early pulmonary vascular disease in preterm infants at risk for bronchopulmonary dysplasia. Am J Respir Crit Care Med 2015;191:87–95.

[58] Mourani PM, Sontag MK, Ivy DD, Abman SH. Effects of long-term sildenafil treatment for pulmonary hypertension in infants with chronic lung disease. J Pediatr 2009;154(3). 379.e2-384.e2.

[59] Nyp M, Sandritter T, Poppinga N, Simon C, Truog WE. Sildenafil citrate, bronchopulmonary dysplasia and disordered pulmonary gas exchange: any benefits? J Perinatol 2012;32(1):64–69.

[60] Tan K, Krishnamurthy MB, O'Heney JL, Paul E, Sehgal A. Sildenafil therapy in bronchopulmonary dysplasia-associated pulmonary hypertension: a retrospective study of efficacy and safety. Eur J Pediatr 2015;174(8):1109–1115.

[61] Trottier-Boucher MN, Lapointe A, Malo J, Fournier A, Raboisson MJ, Martin B, et al. Sildenafil for the treatment of pulmonary arterial hypertension in infants with bronchopulmonary dysplasia. Pediatr Cardiol 2015;36(6):1255–1260.

[62] Krishnan U, Feinstein JA, Adatia I, et al. Evaluation and management of pulmonary hypertension in children with bronchopulmonary dysplasia. J Pediatr 2017;188. 24.e1-34.e1.

[63] Daga SR, Verma B, Valvi C. Sildenafil for pulmonary hypertension in non-ventilated preterm babies. Internet J Pediatr Neonatol 2007;8(1):1–4.

[64] Francis SH, Blount MA, Corbin JD. Mammalian cyclic nucleotide phosphodiesterases: molecular mechanisms and physiological functions. Physiol Rev 2011;91: 651–690.

[65] Baquero H, Soliz A, Neira F, Venegas ME, Sola A. Oral sildenafil in infants with persistent pulmonary hypertension of the newborn: a pilot randomized blinded study. Pediatrics 2006;117:1077–1083.

[66] Vargas-Origel A, Gomez-Rodriguez G, Aldana-Valenzuela C, Vela-Huerta MM, Alarcon-Santos SB, Amador-Licona N. The use of sildenafil in persistent pulmonary hypertension of the newborn. Am J Perinatol 2009;27:225–230.

[67] Steinhorn RH, Kinsella JP, Pierce C, Butrous G, Dilleen M, Oakes M, et al. Intravenous sildenafil in the treatment of neonates with persistent pulmonary hypertension. Pediatrics 2009;155:841–847.

[68] Shiva A, Shiran M, Rafati M, et al. Oral tadalafil in children with pulmonary arterial hypertension. Drug Res 2016;66:7–10.

[69] Stevens DC, Schreiner RL, Bull MJ, et al. An analysis of tolazoline therapy in the critically-ill neonate. J Pediatr 1980;15:964–970.

[70] Welch JC, Bridosn JM, Gibbs JL. Endotracheal tolazoline for severe persistent pulmonary hypertension of the newborn. Br Heart J 1995;73: 99–100.

[71] Kappa P, Jahnukainen T, Grinlund J, Rautanen M, Halkola L, Välimäki I. Adenosine triphosphate treatment for meconium aspiration-induced pulmonary hypertension in pigs. Acta Physiol Scand 1997;160: 283–289.

[72] Wu TJ, Teng RJ, Yau KIT. Persistent pulmonary hypertension of the newborn treated with magnesium sulfate in premature neonates. Pediatrics 1995;96:472–474.

[73] Snyder SW, Cardwell MS. Neuromuscular blockade with magnesium sulfate and nifedipine. Am J Obs Gynecol 1989;161:35–36.

[74] Islam S, Masiakos P, Schnitzer JJ, Doody DP, Ryan DP. Diltiazem reduces pulmonary arterial pressures in recurrent pulmonary hypertension associated with pulmonary hypoplasia. J Pediatr Surg 1999;34:712–714.

[75] Gardner PR. Nitric oxide dioxygenase function and mechanism of flavohemoglobin, hemoglobin, myoglobin and their associated reductases. J Inorg Biochem 2005;99:247–266.

[76] Tamura M, Kawano T. Effects of intravenous nitroglycerin on hemodynamic in neonates with refractory congestive heart failure or PFC. Acta Paediatr Jpn 1990;32: 291–298.

[77] Benitz WE, Malachowski N, Cohen RS, Stevenson DK, Ariagno RL, Sunshine P. Use of sodium nitroprusside in neonates: efficacy and safety. J Pediatr 1985;106:102–110.

[78] Kaapa P, Koivisto M, Ylikorkala O, Kouvalainen K. Prostacyclin in the treatment of neonatal pulmonary hypertension. J Pediatr 1985;107: 951–953.

[79] Bassler D, Choong K, McNamara P, Kirpalani H. Neonatal persistent pulmonary hypertension treated with milrinone: four case reports. Biol Neonate 2006;89:1–5.

[80] Thanopoulos BD, Andreou A, Frimas C. Prostaglandin E2 administration in infants with ductus-dependent cyanotic congenital heart disease. Eur J Pediatr 1987;146:279–282.

[81] Ivy DD, Kinsella JP, Ziegler JW, Abman SH. Dipyridamole attenuates rebound pulmonary hypertension after inhaled nitric oxide withdrawal in postoperative congenital heart disease. J Thorac Cardiovasc Surg 1998;115:875–882.

[82] Soifer SJ, Clyman RI, Heymann MA. Effects of prostaglandin D2 on pulmonary arterial pressure and oxygenation in newborn infants with persistent pulmonary hypertension. J Pediatr 1988;112:774–777.

[83] McIntyre CM, Hanna BD, Rintoul N, Ramsey EZ. Safety of epoprostenol and treprostinil in children less than 12 months of age. Pulm Circ 2013;3:862–869.

[84] Eronen M, Pohjavuori M, Andersson S, Pesonen E, Raivio KO. Prostacyclin treatment for persistent pulmonary hypertension of the newborn. Pediatr Cardiol 1997;18:3–7.

[85] Brown AT, Gillespie JV, Miquel-Verges F, et al. Inhaled epoprostenol therapy for pulmonary hypertension: improves oxygenation index more consistently in neonates than in older children. Pulm Circ 2012;2:61–66.

[86] Kelly LK, Porta NF, Goodman DM, Carroll CL, Steinhorn RH. Inhaled prostacyclin for term infants with persistent pulmonary hypertension refractory to inhaled nitric oxide. J Pediatr 2002;141:830–832.

[87] Soditt V, Aring C, Groneck P. Improvement of oxygenation induced by aerosolised prostacyclin in a preterm infant with persistent pulmonary hypertension of the newborn. Intensive Care Med 1997;23:1275–1278.

[88] Bindl L, Fahnenstich H, Peukert U. Aerosolised prostacyclin for pulmonary hypertension in neonates. Arch Dis Child Fetal Neonatal Ed 1994;71:F214–F216.

[89] Kahveci H, Yilmaz O, Avsar UZ, et al. Oral sildenafil and inhaled iloprost in the treatment of pulmonary hypertension of the newborn. Pediatr Pulmonol 2014;49:1205–1213.

[90] Yilmaz O, Kahveci H, Zeybek C, Ciftel M, Kilic O. Inhaled iloprost in preterm infants with severe respiratory distress syndrome and pulmonary hypertension. Am J Perinatol 2014;31:321–326.

[91] Eifinger F, Sreeram N, Mehler K, Huenseler C, Kribs A, Roth B. Aerosolized iloprost in the treatment of pulmonary hypertension in extremely preterm infants: a pilot study. Klin Padiatr 2008;220:66–69.

[92] Ehlen M, Wiebe B. Iloprost in persistent pulmonary hypertension of the newborn. Cardiol Young 2003;13:361–363.

[93] Janjindamai W, Thatrimontrichai A, Maneenil G, Chanvitan P, Dissaneevate S. Effectiveness and safety of intravenous iloprost for severe persistent pulmonary hypertension of the newborn. Indian Pediatr 2013;50:934–938.

[94] Abu-Osba YK, Galal O, Manasra K, Rejjal A. Treatment of severe persistent pulmonary hypertension of the newborn with magnesium sulfate. Arch Dis Child 1992;67: 31–35.

[95] Levy M, Celermajer DS, Bourges-Petit E, Del Cerro MJ, Bajolle F, Bonnet D. Add-on therapy with subcutaneous treprostinil for refractory pediatric pulmonary hypertension. J Pediatr 2011;158:584–588.

[96] Ferdman DJ, Rosenzweig EB, Zuckerman WA, Krishnan U. Subcutaneous treprostinil for pulmonary hypertension in chronic lung disease of infancy. Pediatrics 2014;134:e274–e278.

[97] Heymann MA. Pharmacologic use of prostaglandin E1 in infants with congenital heart disease. Am Heart J 1981;101:837.

[98] Sood BG, Delaney-Black V, Aranda JV, Shankaran S. Aerosolized PGE1: a selective pulmonary vasodilator in neonatal hypoxemic respiratory failure results of a Phase I/II open label clinical trial. Pediatr Res 2004;56:579–585.

[99] Travadi JN, Patole SK. Phosphodiesterase inhibitors for persistent pulmonary hypertension of the newborn: a review. Pediatr Pulmonol 2003;36:529–535.

[100] McNamara PJ, Shivananda SP, Sahni M, Freeman D, Taddio A. Pharmacology of milrinone in neonates with persistent pulmonary hypertension of the newborn and suboptimal response to inhaled nitric oxide. Pediatr Crit Care Med 2013;14:74–84.

[101] Funke C, Farr M, Werner B, et al. Antiviral effect of Bosentan and Valsartan during coxsackievirus B3 infection of human endothelial cells. J Gen Virol 2010;91:1959–1970.

[102] Nakwan N, Choksuchat D, Saksawad R, Thammachote P, Nakwan N. Successful treatment of persistent pulmonary hypertension of the newborn with bosentan. Acta Paediatr 2009;98:1683–1685.

[103] Mohamed WA, Ismail M. A randomized, double-blind, placebo-controlled, prospective study of bosentan for the treatment of persistent pulmonary hypertension of the newborn. J Perinatol 2012;32:608–613.

[104] Steinhorn RH, Fineman J, Kusic-Pajic A, Cornelisse P, Gehin M, Nowbakht P, et al. Bosentan as adjunctive therapy for persistent pulmonary hypertension of the newborn: results of the randomized multicenter placebo-controlled exploratory trial. J Pediatr 2016;177:90–96.

[105] Chandran S, Haque ME, Wickramasinghe HR, Wint Z. Use of magnesium sulphate in severe persistent pulmonary hypertension of the newborn. J Trop Pediatr 2004;50:219–223.

[106] Ruppersberg JP, Kitzing EV, Schoepfer R. The mechanism of magnesium block of NMDA receptors. Semin Neurosci 1994;6:87–96.

[107] Konduri GG, Theodorou AA, Mukhopadhyay A, Deshmukh DR. Adenosine triphosphate and adenosine increase the pulmonary blood flow to postnatal levels in fetal lambs. Pediatr Res 1992;31:451–457.

[108] Konduri GG, Woodard LL, Mukhopadhyay A, Deshmukh DR. Adenosine is a pulmonary vasodilator in newborn lambs. Am Rev Respir Dis 1992;146:670–676.

[109] Konduri GG, Garcia DC, Kazzi NJ, Shankaran S. Adenosine infusion improves oxygenation in term infants with respiratory failure. Pediatrics 1996;97:295–300.

[110] Ng C, Franklin O, Vaidya M, Pierce C, Petros A. Adenosine infusion for the management of persistent pulmonary hypertension of the newborn. Pediatr Crit Care Med 2004;5:10.

[111] Tripathi S, Saili A. The effect of steroids on the clinical course and outcome of neonates with meconium aspiration syndrome. J Trop Pediatr 2007;53:8–12.

[112] Chandrasekar I, Eis A, Konduri GG. Betamethasone attenuates oxidant stress in endothelial cells from fetal lambs with persistent pulmonary hypertension. Pediatr Res 2008;63:67–72.

[113] Konduri GG, Bakhutashvili I, Eis A, Afolayan A. Antenatal betamethasone improves postnatal transition in late preterm lambs with persistent pulmonary hypertension of the newborn. Pediatr Res 2013;73:621–629.

[114] Perez M, Wedgwood S, Lakshminrusimha S, Farrow KN, Steinhorn RH. Hydrocortisone normalizes phosphodiesterase-5 activity in pulmonary artery smooth muscle cells from lambs with persistent pulmonary hypertension of the newborn. Pulm Circ 2014;4:71–81.

[115] Konduri GG, Kim UO. Advances in the diagnosis and management of persistent pulmonary hypertension of the newborn. Pediatr Clin North Am 2009;56:579–600.

Further Reading

[116] Christou H, Magnani B, Morse DS, et al. Inhaled nitric oxide does not affect adenosine 5'-diphosphate-dependent platelet activation in infants with persistent pulmonary hypertension of the newborn. Pediatrics 1998;102:1390–1393.

[117] Davidson D, Barefield ES, Kattwinkel J. Safety of withdrawing inhaled nitric oxide therapy in persistent pulmonary hypertension of the newborn. Pediatrics 1999;104:231–236.

[118] Elliott RB, Starling MB, Neutze JM. Medical manipulation of the ductus arteriosus. Lancet 1975;1:140–142.

[119] Keller R. Pulmonary hypertension and pulmonary vasodilators. Clin Perinatol 2016;43:187–202.

[120] Kinsella JP, Toricelli F, Ziegler JW, Ivy DD, Abman SH. Dipyridamole augmentation of response to nitric oxide. Lancet 1995;346:647–648.

[121] Lakshminrusimha S, Keszler M. Persistent pulmonary hypertension of the newborn. NeoReviews 2015;16:e680–e692.

[122] Lakshminrusimha S, Konduri GG, Steinhorn RH. Considerations in the management of hypoxemic respiratory failure and persistent pulmonary hypertension in term and late preterm neonates. J Perinatol 2016;36(Suppl. 2):S12–S19.

[123] Nuntnarumit P, Korones SB, Yang W, Bada HS. Efficacy and safety of tolazoline for treatment of severe hypoxemia in extremely preterm infants. Pediatrics 2002;109:852–856.

[124] Perez M, Lakshminrusimha S, Wedgwood S, Czech L, Gugino SF, Russell JA, et al. Hydrocortisone normalizes oxygenation and cGMP regulation in lambs with persistent pulmonary hypertension of the newborn. Am J Physiol Lung Cell Mol Physiol 2012;302:L595–L603.

[125] Santak B, Schreiber M, Kuen P, Lang D, Radermacher P. Prostacyclin aerosol in an infant with pulmonary hypertension. Eur J Pediatr 1995;154:233–235.

[126] Wessel DL, Adatia I, Van Marter LJ, et al. Improved oxygenation in a randomized trial of inhaled nitric oxide for persistent pulmonary hypertension of the newborn. Pediatrics 1997;100:E7.

Chapter | 22 |

Extracorporeal Membrane Oxygenation for Refractory Respiratory Failure

Laurance Lequier, MD, FRCPC, Karunakar Vadlamudi, MD

CHAPTER POINTS

- Extracorporeal membrane oxygenation (ECMO) is an invaluable tool and means of providing short-term cardiopulmonary support.
- ECMO is appropriate, only if underlying pathology is reversible.
- ECMO can be categorized according to the circuit used Veno-Venous and Veno- Arterial
- Oxygenation index and alveolar–arterial oxygen gradient are well standardized indicators for initiating ECMO, after the failure of optimal non-ECMO support.
- Strict Monitoring of antithrombotic therapy is essential and can be challenging.
- Complications and outcomes of ECMO support varies by gestational age, type of support, indications, and underlying diagnosis.

Introduction

Extracorporeal membrane oxygenation (ECMO) has been used to support 30,000 neonates with severe refractory respiratory failure over the past 40 years. According to the Extracorporeal Life Support Organization (ELSO) database registry, neonates with respiratory failure have the highest survival across all patient indications of ECMO [1]. It is considered as the standard of care for the newborn with respiratory failure or shock and has failed to respond to less invasive therapies [2]. Neonatal respiratory diseases that result in respiratory failure and require ECMO therapy after failed ventilation and vasodilator therapies include congenital diaphragmatic hernia (CDH), meconium aspiration syndrome (MAS), persistent pulmonary hypertension of the newborn

(PPHN), neonatal pneumonia, sepsis with respiratory compromise, hyaline membrane disease accompanied by PPHN, and other congenital lung disorders. The use of ECMO to treat these disease states is usually limited to the neonate within the first 10–14 days of life, who is greater than 34 weeks gestation and/or greater than 2 kg birth weight, without a major bleeding complication, including a significant intraventricular or intracranial hemorrhage (ICH) [3].

Indications

ECMO therapy should be considered in term and late preterm infants with hypoxic respiratory failure and have failed to improve with other medical interventions. Understanding of optimal medical management in newborns with respiratory failure has changed tremendously over the years. Inhaled nitric oxide (iNO), surfactant, and high-frequency ventilation (HFV) are now used routinely, while hyperventilation, hyperoxia, and several other therapies have become obsolete. The most commonly used quantifier of disease severity for neonatal hypoxic respiratory failure remains the oxygenation index (OI). Calculation of OI is as follows:

$$OI = \frac{MAP \times FiO_2}{PaO_2} \times 100$$

where MAP = mean airway pressure in cm H_2O and PaO_2 is measured in mmHg.

Indications for ECMO enrollment

Severe hypoxemic respiratory failure: The initial trials used an OI greater than 40 as enrollment criteria for ECMO. Many centers still use an OI range of 40–45 as the primary indication for ECMO support. Grist et al. reviewed neonatal patients to determine whether cannulation timing correlated to increased mortality. Elevated CO_2 gradient [$P(v–a)CO_2$], anion gap corrected for BUN and albumin level (AG_c), and viability index ($AG_c + P(v–a)CO_2$) correlated with a higher mortality in patients on ECMO [4]. The authors concluded that starting ECMO too late may cause reperfusion injury that reduces survival. Thus, it is recommended that any neonate with respiratory failure and an OI of greater than 25 be cared for in an ECMO center, where timely initiation can occur if the patient's condition warrants ECMO. Therapeutic options including surfactant and iNO have decreased the need for ECMO in neonates with respiratory failure [5]. While patients should be given the opportunity to respond to less invasive therapies, delaying ECMO cannulation is

unacceptable. Regional ECMO centers should work with the non-ECMO centers in their area to establish a standard protocol regarding transfer criteria in order to prevent untimely delays.

Contraindications

Certain patients with complicating pathologies should not be considered for ECMO. This includes patients with lethal chromosomal disorders (such as trisomy 13 or trisomy 18), severe preexisting brain damage, or significant ICH (grade III or IV). Neonates with irreversible, extrapulmonary organ injury are ineligible for ECMO unless they are being considered for transplantation. Even with technical progress, ECMO remains a high-risk and resource-intense intervention; it should only be utilized in those patients with a high likelihood of a meaningful survival.

Weight less than 2 kg

For the past 4 decades, weight less than 2 kg has been a relative contraindication to ECMO. In 2004, Rozmierek et al. hypothesized that ECMO was effective and safe in babies less than 2 kg and sought to examine outcome. Neonatal patients (less than 30 days old) in the ELSO registry ($n = 14,305$) were divided into those less than 2 kg ($n = 663$) and those greater than 2 kg ($n = 13,642$). Overall, survival rate reached 76% but was lower in infants less than 2 kg. Regression analysis determined that the lowest weight at which a survival rate of 40% could be achieved was 1.6 kg. A 40% survival compares to that seen in patients with congenital heart disease receiving ECMO [6].

Gestational age less than 34 weeks

Some centers feel comfortable providing ECMO to infants less than 34 weeks if they are otherwise deemed good candidates, but this degree of prematurity remains a relative contraindication. A review of 21,218 neonatal ECMO cases in the ELSO registry from 1986 to 2006 evaluated the gestational age and outcome. Infants were divided into three groups: late preterm (34 0/7 to 36 6/7), early term (37 0/7 to 38 6/7), and full term (39 0/7 to 42 6/7). Neonates with CDH and other major congenital disorders including cardiac defects, chromosomal, and genetic abnormalities, were excluded. Late preterm infants experienced the highest mortality on ECMO (late preterm 26.2%, early term 18%, full term 11.2%, $P < 0.001$) and had longer ECMO runs; they also had higher rates of ICH (late preterm 12.3%, early term

7.6%, full term 3.6%, $P < 0.0001$) and other neurological complications on ECMO. Furthermore, they experienced increased mechanical, metabolic, and infectious complications on ECMO [7].

Intracranial hemorrhage

Grade III or IV ICH can be detected by head ultrasound (HUS) and this degree of hemorrhage is associated to poor long-term prognosis [8]. Thus, ECMO should not be offered in this population. Patients with pre-ECMO grade I or II ICH have been successfully managed on ECMO without extension of hemorrhage. Even in this less severe situation, diligent monitoring of hemodynamics, clotting factors, platelets, bleeding times, anticoagulation, and imaging is required. In cases where there is strong evidence of hypoxic injury on MRI, abnormal EEG findings, significant metabolic acidosis, and low Apgar scores, strong consideration for withholding ECMO should occur.

ECMO cannulation: venovenous or venoarterial? (Fig. 22.1)

Once it has been decided that a baby needs ECMO support, the next decision is whether it should be venovenous (VV) or venoarterial (VA) support. In neonates, VV ECMO is almost always via a dual lumen cannula (VVDL). Dual lumen cannulas provide VV ECMO support via a single jugular venous access site. Blood is removed from the patient via one lumen and then returned to the patient via a smaller lumen. Although VV ECMO does not provide direct cardiac support, the delivery of well-oxygenated blood to the right atrium invariably improves cardiac output even in unstable neonates requiring high-dose inotropic support [9].

Many experienced ECMO centers now prefer to support all neonates with VV ECMO where possible. Each center will need to determine their comfort with initiating VV ECMO in such patients. However, VV ECMO patients can be converted

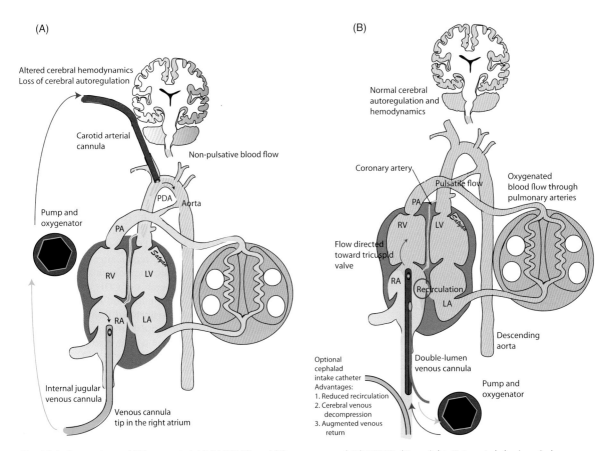

Fig. 22.1 Comparison of (A) venoarterial (VA) ECMO and (B) venovenous (VV) ECMO. (Copyright: Satyan Lakshminrusimha; modified from Workbook in Practical Neonatology.)

to VA ECMO support, if VV support proves inadequate. Occasions where VA support is required include infants less than 2.5 kg where the right internal jugular vein is unlikely to accommodate the smallest VVDL cannula (presently the 13 F OriGen cannula). Low cardiac output state as the result of sepsis or a cardiac anomaly usually requires VA support. Traditionally, neonates with CDH have received VA ECMO support, partly because they are often unstable at the time of cannulation, but also because the neck veins in CDH tend to be smaller than equivalent weight of neonates and are displaced from their normal anatomical position, particularly in right-sided CDH [10]. However, VV ECMO can and should be considered in selected cases [11].

Congenital diaphragmatic hernia

The use of ECMO in CDH was first reported in 1977 by German et al. [12]. In the late 1980s, the role of pulmonary hypertension in CDH was recognized and clinicians transitioned to a delayed surgical strategy, waiting until the infant was hemodynamically stable and/or pulmonary hypertension had stabilized. ECMO is commonly reserved for patients who are failing optimal medical management. When incorporated with a strategy of relatively gentle pressure-limited ventilation and permissive hypercapnia, early use of ECMO may help minimize ventilator-associated lung injury (VALI). Unfortunately, entry criteria that accurately predict high mortality prior to the initiation of ECMO in infants with CDH have not been published. Multiple parameters have been used to predict those who may benefit from ECMO [13]. However, none of these criteria have been validated in multicenter studies. ECMO use in CDH varies according to the location of providers; for example, ECMO is utilized more frequently in the United States compared to the United Kingdom [14]. ECMO survival for CDH infants was 46% in the United States and 53% in the United Kingdom. Currently, ECMO is predominantly used to provide a period of preoperative stabilization [15].

Efficacy of ECMO for CDH

Reversibility of the underlying pulmonary derangement in CDH is a key criterion when considering ECMO therapy. However, this criterion presents a challenging dilemma as the degree of respiratory failure in CDH depends on the severity of the existing pulmonary hypertension, pulmonary hypoplasia, and the degree of VALI. The intrinsic problems related to CDH have led to poor outcomes compared to other neonatal indications for ECMO. The overall survival of infants with CDH reported to the ELSO is approximately 50%, the lowest among all etiologies of neonatal respiratory failure requiring ECMO [1].

Considering the above observations, the evaluation of pulmonary development may improve patient selection, optimizing morbidity and mortality associated with ECMO in infants with CDH. Pulmonary hypoplasia, an important factor that affects outcome of CDH, represents a challenging condition to accurately assess prenatally. Surrogate indicators of lung development include the observed-to-expected lung:head ratio, measured with repeated fetal ultrasound during pregnancy and total fetal lung volume assessed by maternal magnetic resonance imaging in the second and third trimesters of pregnancy. Postnatally, the use of alveolar arterial oxygen gradient, pre-ductal hemoglobin saturations, post-ductal arterial PaO_2, OI, and hypercarbia have been utilized by some centers to create algorithms for identification of children with the best chance of survival and who would benefit most from ECMO therapy [16,17].

A recent CDH Study Group report identified predictors of survival in infants with CDH who received ECMO. In ECMO-treated patients, survivors were born at a greater estimated gestational age, had greater birth weights, were less likely to be diagnosed with CDH prenatally, and were on ECMO for a shorter length of time [18]. Others have also tried to identify factors that predict progression to ECMO and survival in CDH infants. One group found that lung area to head circumference ratio (LHR < 1.0) and gestational age at delivery predicted the use of ECMO and survival [19]. While a recent report identified pre-ECMO $PaCO_2$ as a predictor of survival, another group described difficulty identifying pre-ECMO predictors of survival [20,21].

CDH surgery on ECMO

The optimal timing of repair of CDH on ECMO remains unclear due to inadequate study and variability among centers. Operations performed on ECMO are high risk because of the potential for bleeding complications. A recent update from the CDH Study Group found that surgical repair of CDH while on ECMO was associated with decreased survival relative to repair after ECMO therapy [22]. This was found to be significant even after controlling for factors associated with severity of CDH, but meaningful comparisons without confounding are impossible. Quite clearly, patients who can be liberated from ECMO have a far better prognosis, while those who cannot and have not undergone an early repair are relegated to a late repair or remain unrepaired and do not survive.

ECMO circuit and components

A standard ECMO circuit consists of a mechanical blood pump, gas exchange device, and a heat exchanger, all connected together with circuit tubing between the venous

access cannula and either the venous (VV) or arterial (VA) infusion cannula (Fig. 22.1) [23]. Individual centers customize their ECMO circuits to suit their patient population and program needs. A pump is an essential component of the ECMO circuit. Semiocclusive roller pumps have been the standard for decades but have mainly been replaced by novel centrifugal pumps. ECMO circuits have a gas exchange device called a membrane oxygenator to add O_2 and remove CO_2 from blood. ECMO circuits usually have a variety of monitors including an integrated blood pump flow monitor that measures total circuit blood flow, as well as separate ultrasonic flow detectors that can be placed on venous drainage and arterial infusion limbs of the circuit (Fig. 22.2).

A survey of neonatal ECMO centers revealed a shift from roller head to centrifugal pumps in the past decade [24]. Prior to this time, roller pumps were used in almost all neonatal ECMO programs. Centrifugal pumping systems have the benefit of smaller circuit size, less blood-prosthetic surface area, and inherent protection against cavitation and over-pressurization of the circuit. They do not require gravity drainage and can be placed closer to the patient. In contrast, roller pumps are less expensive and simpler in design, but have the potential complication of tubing rupture. Hemolysis occurs commonly with centrifugal pumps, especially with small cannula, due to the shearing force on blood components created by the vortex in the pump head.

Newer generation centrifugal pumps have been designed to have less stagnation in the pump head with decreased hemolysis. Despite design improvements there remain recent reports of patients supported on centrifugal pumps exhibiting hemolysis during ECMO [25].

Patients supported with centrifugal pumps should have routine screening of plasma free hemoglobin (pfHb). If the pfHb level exceeds 50 mg/dL, the cause should be investigated [26]. Barrett et al. compared outcomes of neonates supported with centrifugal or roller pumps [27]. The centrifugal pump group had higher rates of hemolysis, hyperbilirubinemia, hypertension, and acute renal failure than the roller pump group. They separated the centrifugal group into older versus newer generation pumps and found the same morbidities, but at a lower rate with the newer pumps [28].

For neonatal ECMO, the circuit is primed with packed red blood cells (PRBCs) and fresh frozen plasma (FFP) to a hematocrit of 35%–45% [26]. The blood prime is heparinized, and then calcium added to correct the hypocalcemia caused by citrate anticoagulation. Acidosis is corrected by adding sodium bicarbonate as a buffer. The blood prime is warmed to 37 °C, unless the infant is undergoing hypothermia therapy. In that case, the blood should be warmed to a temperature of 34 °C. Once ECMO is initiated, pump flow should be increased over a period of several minutes in order to determine the maximal

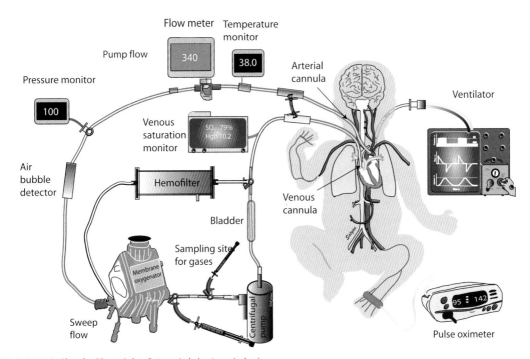

Fig. 22.2 ECMO Circuit. (Copyright: Satyan Lakshminrusimha.)

flow that can be achieved. When initiating VV ECMO, it is important to increase pump flow slowly, as prime blood may have elevated potassium levels that can cause myocardial dysfunction and even asystole. On VV ECMO, support is adequate if arterial saturation is in an acceptable range on low ventilator settings and any hypotension or acidosis resolves. Pump flow can range from 80–150 mL/kg/min. Once cannula position is optimized, suboptimal ECMO support can be addressed with a second cephalad cannula in the jugular vein to augment venous drainage. An 8 or 10 F arterial cannula is used for this technique. The use of a cephalad jugular drain in the setting of VV ECMO has several theoretical advantages including augmented venous return, reduced recirculation, and cerebral venous decompression (Fig. 22.1).

The medical gas flow from the blender to the oxygenator (sweep gas flow) is initiated in a 1:1 ratio of blood flow to gas flow. If pump flow is 300 mL/min then sweep flow is 0.3 L/min (Fig. 22.2). Sweep flow is adjusted to target an arterial PCO_2 of 40–50 mmHg unless there is significant pre-cannulation hypercarbia. When initiating ECMO support, it is critical to correct hypercapnia slowly. Hypocapnia in the newborn is associated with cerebral vasoconstriction and an increased incidence of periventricular leukomalacia, intraventricular hemorrhage, cerebral palsy, and poor neurodevelopmental outcome.

Neurologic system

Neonatal ECMO patients have high risk of brain injury with resulting adverse neurodevelopmental outcome (Fig. 22.3). Potential injury can be attributed to the underlying disease process leading to ECMO as well as to accompanying hypoxia, hypotension, and hypocarbia [29]. Cannulation produces further alterations in cerebral blood flow related to ligation of the right jugular vein and the right carotid artery that can result in cerebral ischemia, reperfusion injury, and loss of cerebral autoregulation. Neonatal ECMO survivors have a significant incidence of neuroimaging abnormalities and neurodevelopmental disability. Thus, regular assessment of the neurologic exam, daily HUS, and consideration of other diagnostic modalities are advisable. Prompt recognition of potentially treatable conditions is important to optimize outcome.

Neuromonitoring on ECMO

Current techniques for neuromonitoring of the neonatal ECMO patient include neurologic exam, HUS, EEG, amplitude-integrated EEG (aEEG), and near-infrared spectroscopy (NIRS). Close and frequent monitoring of the

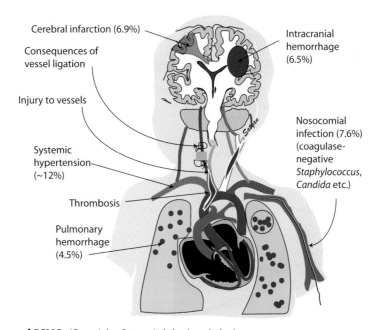

Fig. 22.3 Complications of ECMO. (Copyright: Satyan Lakshminrusimha.)

Cerebral infarction (6.9%)
Consequences of vessel ligation
Injury to vessels
Systemic hypertension (~12%)
Thrombosis
Pulmonary hemorrhage (4.5%)
Intracranial hemorrhage (6.5%)
Nosocomial infection (7.6%) (coagulase-negative *Staphylococcus*, *Candida* etc.)

neurologic exam is warranted on ECMO. ICH, the most significant complication in neonates on ECMO, occurs in 7.5% of patients, and the incidence of cerebral infarction is also noteworthy at 6.9% [1]. In an analysis of the ELSO registry, gestational age was the strongest predictor of ICH in neonates on ECMO, but pre-ECMO factors included acidosis, primary diagnosis of sepsis, coagulopathy, and treatment with epinephrine [30]. The strongest predictor of disability in ECMO survivors is the extent and severity of abnormality on post-ECMO neuroimaging [31]. HUS studies should be performed prior to the initiation of ECMO, with serial daily HUS commencing 12–24 h after cannulation. Khan et al. have reported that over 90% of ICHs occur in the first 5 days of ECMO therapy [32]. Some ECMO centers perform HUS less frequently after day 5 or perform daily HUS only in high-risk infants or infants with abnormal HUS pre-ECMO or immediately following cannulation [33].

Earlier detection of neurologic injury permits therapeutic intervention and potentially can improve outcomes. Conventional EEG is not routinely used in the neonatal ECMO population unless seizure activity is suspected. The ELSO registry reports clinical seizures in 8.8% of neonates [1]. The aEEG is being used with increasing frequency in the NICU; abnormal aEEG predicted death or moderate to severe intracranial injury [34]. Interestingly, infants with adverse outcome had abnormal tracings before or within the first 24 h on ECMO. NIRS has emerged as an effective, noninvasive technique for neuromonitoring in a variety of intensive care settings. NIRS monitoring on ECMO may help to identify poor cerebral oxygen delivery and infants at highest risk of adverse developmental outcome.

Therapeutic hypothermia has been shown, in large randomized controlled trials and meta-analyses, to result in a statistically significant and clinically important reduction in the combined outcome of mortality or major neurodevelopmental disability for term newborns greater than 36 weeks gestation, with moderate to severe encephalopathy. Cooling on ECMO is easily performed using a temperature probe in the blood path proximal to the arterial cannula, adjusting the ECMO heater/cooling device to reach and maintain a core patient temperature of 33–34°C [35]. The Neonatal ECMO Study of Temperature (NEST) determined that mild hypothermia to 34°C did not improve the outcome at 2 years of age in newborns requiring ECMO when compared to normothermia [36].

Sedation and analgesia

Infants with severe respiratory failure are frequently heavily sedated, given analgesics, and paralyzed prior to ECMO. However, after cannulation, paralysis is not required and should be discontinued. Similarly, excessive sedation limits the ability to interpret the neurologic status and may inappropriately add to concerns regarding neurologic injury. Prolonged high cumulative doses of opioids and benzodiazepines have been associated with tolerance, physical dependency, and subsequent withdrawal. Commonly used drugs for analgesia and sedation include morphine and midazolam. The pharmacokinetics of midazolam, lorazepam, and fentanyl are altered on ECMO due to sequestration of the drug by ECMO circuit components [37]. Morphine may be a good choice for patients on ECMO as drug levels are unaffected.

Respiratory support

While on ECMO, the lungs are allowed to rest and recover from the underlying lung disease and from barotrauma caused by pre-ECMO management. Rest settings on VV ECMO are usually higher than those used on VA. Typical VA settings are PIP (cm H20) 15–20, PEEP 5, rate 15–20, and FiO_2 0.21 and typical VV settings are PIP 15–25, PEEP 5–10, rate 20–30, and FiO_2 0.30–0.50 [38]. Some advocate for higher PEEP to prevent alveolar collapse without compromising venous return. An older multicenter study found that high PEEP of 12–14 cm H_2O versus low PEEP of 3–5 cm H_2O facilitated lung recovery and resulted in shorter ECMO runs [39]. Continued use of surfactant while on ECMO in the setting of neonatal respiratory failure has demonstrated benefit. One small single-center study administered surfactant or placebo at 2, 8, 20, and 32 h, and found significantly decreased duration of ECMO, improved pulmonary mechanics, and reduced complications when compared with a placebo group [40].

Patient arterial blood gases, along with circuit pre- and post-oxygenator blood gases, are obtained every 6–12 h. Daily chest radiographs are obtained to confirm ECMO catheter and tube position; assess lung volume changes following significant atelectasis or collapse; and to diagnose air leak syndromes. Air leaks can be managed with lower ventilator settings including low CPAP settings, decreasing until no further air leaks are present, with gentle re-expanding of lung over longer period of time. A large or tension pneumothorax, particularly if obstructing venous return, requires placement of a thoracostomy tube. Radiograph findings combined with frequent or continuous tidal volume measurements and blood gases provide the ECMO practitioner with the data needed to formulate a weaning plan.

Routine pulmonary clearance is essential while on ECMO. Endotracheal suctioning is recommended every 4–6 h. Changes in secretions should be noted, including watching for blood-tinged secretions. Pulmonary

hemorrhage was reported in 4.5% of neonatal patients undergoing ECMO [1]. Studies in the pediatric population on ECMO have illustrated the usefulness of bronchoscopy in patients with persistent atelectasis including removal of secretions and identifying infectious etiology [41]. Overall, the procedure was well tolerated with only minimal complications of bleeding, similar to other studies. Treatment of pulmonary hemorrhage varies with the severity of the event and includes limitation of suctioning, increasing PEEP, decreasing anticoagulation parameters, increasing platelet count target, and instillation of dilute epinephrine. Prone positioning should be considered in patients on prolonged ECMO support, with benefits including reducing the risk of development of pressure ulcers as well as improving aeration to posterior portions of the lungs and in alveolar ventilation–perfusion matching.

Cardiovascular supports

Neonates with respiratory failure being considered for ECMO often require inotropic or vasopressor support. Patients with decreased cardiac function may still be considered for VV ECMO. Studies have found that use of inotropes substantially decrease both in patients with VV ECMO and VA ECMO [42,43]. One institution evaluated cardiac function in 15 infants on VV ECMO and found borderline or normal cardiac indices prior to ECMO, with normalization of function on ECMO [44]. The authors concluded that VV ECMO did not worsen cardiac function, potentially due to avoidance of an increase in LV afterload as seen with VA ECMO, as well as increased oxygen content provided to coronary arteries with VV ECMO.

Hypertension occurs commonly on ECMO; 12% of neonatal ECMO patients, reported to the ELSO registry database, had systolic hypertension requiring vasodilators [1]. One institution noted systemic hypertension in 93% of their neonatal ECMO population, with an associated increase in ICH and plasma renin activity [45]. Prior to a protocol that medically managed systemic hypertension on ECMO, 50% of neonates at the institution had clinically significant intracranial bleeds, compared with 9% after initiation of the protocol. The authors found captopril to be the most effective in lowering blood pressure.

Echocardiography may be a useful tool throughout the ECMO course. Prior to cannulation, echocardiography may unmask underlying cardiac pathology, including total anomalous pulmonary venous return. It has been utilized during or after cannulation to evaluate cannula position [46].

Fluids, electrolytes, and nutrition

Initial daily fluid intake on ECMO is usually limited to 60–100 mL/kg/day as the typical neonatal ECMO patient is edematous due to substantial fluid overload prior to cannulation. Transient renal dysfunction with oliguria is common but usually spontaneously resolves over the first 48–72 h. A natural diuresis phase occurs as cardiac output improves, capillary leak resolves, and fluid mobilization takes place.

Renal function and fluid balance in newborns with severe cardiorespiratory failure managed with VV ECMO was compared to neonates managed without ECMO [47]. VV ECMO was associated with positive fluid balance, lower urine output, and higher BUN and creatinine values in the first 96 h of bypass without any differences in blood pressure or diuretic use. Diuretics are commonly used following ECMO initiation. If urine output does not improve, continuous renal replacement therapy (CRRT) may be utilized to accomplish solute clearance and fluid removal.

Historically, neonates on ECMO were not fed enterally due to concerns regarding intestinal perfusion prior to ECMO, intestinal ischemia, and the risk of necrotizing enterocolitis. Gut barrier function and intestinal distension due to obstruction are other concerns. A single-center study over a 5-year period demonstrated that neonates on ECMO tolerated enteral feedings well without any serious adverse effects; a notable finding is that 80% of newborns fed enterally were receiving inotropic support [48]. Over the duration of the study the use of enteral feedings increased from 71% to 94% and the time to initiation of feeds dropped from 67 to 37 h. Serum electrolytes are monitored at least daily and glucose every 12 h. Calcium and magnesium requirements may also be higher than usual. Metabolic alkalosis may become evident due to exposure to large amounts of blood products containing the anticoagulant citrate-phosphate-dextran.

Infection

Infections acquired during ECMO are not uncommon and can significantly increase ECMO duration and decrease survival. A review of ELSO data from 1998 to 2008 found that the overall infection rate for neonates was 7.6% with the incidence increasing with longer runs and in VA ECMO patients [49]. Coagulase negative *Staphylococci* were the most common organisms, followed by *Candida*. The commonly identified organisms had associations with invasive

support including central lines, endotracheal tubes, and urinary catheters. Thus, continuing strategies to prevent catheter-associated and ventilator-associated infections should decrease the nosocomial infection rate of these neonates. Although reducing nosocomial infections on ECMO is important, there is no benefit to the administration of prophylactic antibiotics [50].

Anticoagulation

Anticoagulation of the neonate on ECMO is challenging due to immaturity of the coagulation system and the propensity for ICH in the neonate. Historically, unfractionated heparin (UNFH) has been the anticoagulant of choice for the vast majority of ECMO indications. UNFH undergoes hepatic metabolism, renal excretion, and has a plasma half-life of 30–60 min [51]. A bolus dose of UNFH ranging from 50 to 100 units/kg is given after the exposure of the vessels and before insertion of the cannulas for ECMO. Subsequently, UNFH is administered as a continuous intravenous infusion. The activated clotting time (ACT) provides a measure of clotting of whole blood, and has long been the standard measure of anticoagulant activity of UNFH for ECMO. Advantages of ACT are that it can be done at the bedside, requires a drop of blood, and results are available within a few minutes. The UNFH infusion is typically started once ACT reaches 300 s or less. Some ECMO centers have a minimum and maximum UNFH infusion rate that typically ranges from a minimum of 10 units/kg/h, to a maximum of 60 units/kg/h. The standard, initial ACT range is 160–200 s, with the UNFH infusion dose and goal ACT range adjusted based on factors including patient bleeding and circuit clotting. The anti-factor Xa assay has become an important supplementary means of titrating UNFH for ECMO [52]. The anti-Xa assay is not a measure of UNFH concentration, but rather a measure of UNFH effect, based on the ability of UNFH to catalyze antithrombin inhibition of factor-Xa. In contrast to the ACT, the anti-Xa assay is specific to the anticoagulant effect of UNFH and is not influenced by coagulopathy, thrombocytopenia, or dilution. Administration of anticoagulants place patients at risk of bleeding and therefore it can be a challenge to provide enough anticoagulant effect while minimizing bleeding and thrombotic complications.

Hematologic issues

Whenever possible, factor depletion, thrombocytopenia, and hypofibrinogenemia should be corrected. It is also important to verify that the infant received vitamin K at birth. Daily monitoring of coagulation factors, platelet count, and hematocrit are done every 8–12 h and deficiencies corrected. ECMO goals include maintaining a platelet count greater than 80,000, hematocrit greater than 35%–40%, fibrinogen greater than 150 mg/dL, and normal PT and INR.

Weaning ECMO

Weaning from VV and VA ECMO support is indicated with improvement of chest radiograph, tidal volumes, patient venous saturation, and patient arterial blood gases. ECMO pump flow is decreased by 5–10 mL/kg/h every 2–4 h as long as arterial saturation is >90%, until approximately 50 mL/kg/min flows are reached. Sweep FiO_2 can also be weaned and the mechanical ventilator rate may be increased. Further weaning from VV ECMO is made to a minimum of approximately 30 mL/kg/min, the sweep flow can be weaned until off, ventilator FiO_2 should be increased. On VA ECMO pump flow can be weaned until a flow rate of 20 mL/kg/min is reached, where the patient is considered to be "idling" on ECMO. For both VV and VA weaning, if blood gases are adequate, decannulation should be scheduled. In patients who have had a long ECMO run, or have serious complications, such as ICH, it may be necessary to use HFV, surfactant replacement, inotropes or steroids, or iNO to wean off.

Neonatal ECMO survival

Almost 30,000 neonates have been treated with ECMO for neonatal respiratory failure with an overall survival to discharge or transfer of 74% as reported to the ELSO registry [1]. The survival outcome of neonates supported on ECLS for acute hypoxemic respiratory failure varies with the primary diagnosis, and can be as high as 95% in neonates with MAS and as low as 50% in those with CDH. In a retrospective study of neonates with PPHN supported on ECMO between 2000 and 2010, Lazar and coworkers identified that prematurity, acidosis, and profound hypoxemia were independently associated with increased mortality [53]. Similarly, a UK study of 718 neonates over a 13-year period identified that lower birth weight, lower gestational age, older age at ECMO, and higher OI were associated with increased risk of death in non-CDH neonates; whereas, in neonates with CDH, lower birth weight and younger age at ECMO were significant risk factors for death [54].

Long-term neurodevelopmental outcomes

The excellent survival outcomes from neonatal ECMO have produced a growing population of childhood survivors; however, the long-term medical and neurodevelopmental outcomes remain of some concern, particularly in certain diagnostic groups, such as CDH [55,56]. In the latest ELSO registry report, cerebral infarction and hemorrhage, diagnosed by ultrasound or computed tomography scan, was seen in 6.9 and 6.5% of neonates with corresponding survival rates of 53 and 43%, respectively [1]. Although these short-term complications are not an accurate representation of long-term problems, they identify a cohort of patients with higher risk. Neurodevelopmental consequences are commonly described in ECMO follow-up studies [57]. The mental development scores of neonatal ECMO survivors when tested at the preschool age are generally favorable, with several reporting normal development both with respect to overall cognition and language development [58]. Studies of children tested at 5 years of age, report intelligence in the normal range with one reporting language development above average population norms [59]. Neonatal ECMO survivors without severe neurologic impairment usually have a neuropsychological profile characterized by average intelligence, with significantly lower scores on attention, concentration, and memory tasks [60].

CDH

Infants with CDH who received ECMO support appear to have a higher risk and greater severity of neurological morbidity compared to those who did not receive ECMO and those who received ECMO for other non-CDH diagnoses. McGahren et al. reported survival of 75%, with 67% of the survivors exhibiting neurologic compromise [61]. A recent study from the Netherlands considered the motor and cognitive status at 5 years of patients who had received ECMO. The CDH cohort demonstrated the lowest survival and lowest rate of functionally normal children compared to patient children with meconium aspiration [62]. The lower overall survival and higher rates of morbidities affirm that neonates with CDH requiring ECMO therapy are a very challenging category of patients.

Recommendations for long-term follow-up

Routine standardized follow-up programs are offered by very few ECMO programs. Longitudinal studies from the Netherlands have demonstrated unequivocally the value and benefit of early identification and intervention to the children and the families [63]. Children with neurologic complications are usually recognized to be at risk for adverse outcome at an early stage and are referred appropriately for post-discharge care. However, for neonatal ECMO survivors without evident acute neurologic events, it is important to receive adequate long-term aftercare. Neonatal ECMO survivors without overt neurologic complications usually have favorable outcomes in the first years of life, but they are at risk for academic, behavioral, and motor function problems at later age for which they need to be monitored [64]. Long-term follow-up should focus on early recognition and providing timely interventions. Arranging for consistent, multidisciplinary follow-up of patients who have received ECMO support is important to engage families, community health, and educational psychology services. The availability of a structured, longitudinal follow-up for all neonates receiving complex invasive therapies, such as ECMO, from hospital discharge to adolescence, will allow for interventions tailored to the needs of the child and family. A neonate with an identified risk factor or who has developed a neurological complication on ECMO should receive a more targeted follow-up after discharge so that all issues are identified appropriately and managed promptly.

Summary

Therapies, such as iNO, surfactant, gentle ventilation strategies, and HFOV have led to a decrease in the utilization of ECMO for certain neonatal disease states. This trend has resulted in fewer, more complicated patients receiving ECMO treatment, resulting in longer, more complicated courses. Decades of clinical experience and innovation have resulted in the provision of ECMO as a standard of care for neonates with severe refractory respiratory failure in qualified centers. Novel equipment and protocols have allowed the deployment of ECMO safely and efficiently with very good survival and overall outcome for the majority of patients.

References

[1] Extracorporeal Life Support Organization. ECLS registry report international summary. Ann Harbor, MI; January 2016.

[2] Firmin RK, Peek GL, Sosnowski AW. Role of extracorporeal membrane oxygenation. Lancet 1996;348(9030):824.

[3] Suttner DM. Indications and contraindications for ECLS in neonates with respiratory failure. In: Brogan T, Lequier L, Lorusso R, MacLaren G, Peek G, editors. Extracorporeal life support: the ELSO redbook. 5th ed. Ann Arbor, MI: ELSO; 2017. p. 151–158.

[4] Grist G, Whittaker C, Merrigan K, Fenton J, Pallotto E, Lofland G. Defining the late implementation of extracorporeal membrane oxygenation (ECMO) by identifying increased risk using specific physiologic cut-points in neonatal and pediatric respiratory patients. J Extra Corpor Technol 2008;41(4):213–219.

[5] Hintz SR, Suttner DM, et al. Decreased use of neonatal extracorporeal membrane oxygenation (ECMO): how new treatment modalities have affected ECMO utilization. Pediatrics 2000;106(6):1339–1343.

[6] Rozmiarek AJ, Qureshi FG, Cassidy L, et al. How low can you go? Effectiveness and safety of extracorporeal membrane oxygenation in low-birth-weight neonates. J Pediatr Surg 2004;39(6):845–847.

[7] Reoma JL, Rojas A, Kim AC, et al. Development of an artificial placenta I: pumpless arterio-venous extracorporeal life support in a neonatal sheep model. J Pediatr Surg 2009;44(1):53–59.

[8] Ancel PY, Livinec F, Larroque B, et al. Cerebral palsy among very preterm children in relation to gestational age and neonatal ultrasound abnormalities: the EPIPAGE cohort study. Pediatrics 2006;117(3):828–835.

[9] Roberts N, Westrope C, Pooboni SK, et al. Venovenous extracorporeal membrane oxygenation for respiratory failure in inotrope dependent neonates. ASAIO J 2003;49(5):558–571.

[10] Frenckner B, Palmar K, Linden V. Neonates with congenital diaphragmatic hernia have smaller neck veins than other neonates–an alternative route for cannulation. J Pediatr Surg 2002;37(6):906–908.

[11] Davis CF, Walker G. ECLS cannulation for neonates with respiratory failure. In: Brogan T, Lequier L, Lorusso R, MacLaren G, Peek G, editors. Extracorporeal life support: the ELSO redbook. 5th ed. Ann Arbor, MI: ELSO; 2017. p. 159–167.

[12] German JC, Gazzaniga AB, Amlie R, Huxtable RF, Bartlett RH. Management of pulmonary insufficiency in diaphragmatic hernia using extracorporeal circulation with a membrane oxygenator (ECMO). J Pediatr Surg 1977;12(6):905–912.

[13] Somaschini M, Locatelli G, Salvoni L, Bellan C, Colombo A. Impact of new treatments for respiratory failure on outcome of infants with congenital diaphragmatic hernia. Eur J Pediatr 1999;158(10):780–784.

[14] Brown KL, Sriram S, Ridout D, et al. Extracorporeal membrane oxygenation and term neonatal respiratory failure deaths in the United Kingdom compared with the United States: 1999 to 2005. Pediatr Crit Care Med 2010;11(1):60–65.

[15] Harting MT, Davis CF, Lally KP. Congenital diaphragmatic hernia on ECMO. In: Brogan T, Lequier L, Lorusso R, MacLaren G, Peek G, editors. Extracorporeal life support: the ELSO redbook. 5th ed. Ann Arbor, MI: ELSO; 2017. p. 133–150.

[16] Boloker J, Bateman DA, Wung JT, Stolar CJ. Congenital diaphragmatic hernia in 120 infants treated consecutively with permissive hypercapnea/spontaneous respiration/elective repair. J Pediatr Surg 2002;37(3):357–366.

[17] Sebald M, Friedlich P, Burns C, et al. Risk of need for extracorporeal membrane oxygenation support in neonates with congenital diaphragmatic hernia treated with inhaled nitric oxide. J Perinatol 2004;24(3):143–146.

[18] Seetharamaiah R, Younger JG, Bartlett RH, Hirschl RB. Factors associated with survival in infants with congenital diaphragmatic hernia requiring extracorporeal membrane oxygenation: a report from the Congenital Diaphragmatic Hernia Study Group. J Pediatr Surg 2009;44(7):1315–1321.

[19] Odibo AO, Najaf T, Vachharajani A, Warner B, Mathur A, Warner BW. Predictors of the need for extracorporeal membrane oxygenation and survival in congenital diaphragmatic hernia: a center's 10-year experience. Prenat Diagn 2010;30(6):518–521.

[20] Tiruvoipati R, Vinogradova Y, Faulkner G, Sosnowski AW, Firmin RK, Peek GJ. Predictors of outcome in patients with congenital diaphragmatic hernia requiring extracorporeal membrane oxygenation. J Pediatr Surg 2007;42(8):1345–1350.

[21] Hoffman SB, Massaro AN, Gingalewski C, Short BL. Predictors of survival in congenital diaphragmatic hernia patients requiring extracorporeal membrane oxygenation: CNMC 15-year experience. J Perinatol 2010;30(8):546–552.

[22] Bryner BS, West BT, Hirschl RB, et al. Congenital diaphragmatic hernia requiring extracorporeal membrane oxygenation: does timing of repair matter? J Pediatr Surg 2009;44(6):1165–1171. discussion 1171–1162.

[23] Lequier L, Hoerton SB, McMullan DM, Bartlett RH. Extracorporeal membrane oxygenation circuitry. Pediatr Crit Care Med 2013;14:S7–S12.

[24] Lawson S, Ellis C, Butler K, McRobb C, Mejak B. Neonatal extracorporeal membrane oxygenation devices, techniques and team roles: 2011 survey results of the United States' Extracorporeal Life Support Organization centers. J Extra Corpor Technol 2011;43(4):236–244.

[25] Neal JR, Quintana E, Pike RB, Hoyer JD, Joyce LD, Schears G. Using daily plasmafree hemoglobin levels for diagnosis of critical pump thrombus in patients undergoing ECMO or VAD support. J Extra Corpor Technol 2015;47(2):103–108.

[26] Bhombal S, Sheehan AM, Van Meurs KP. Medical management of the neonate with respiratory failure on ECLS. In: Brogan T, Lequier L, Lorusso R, MacLaren G, Peek G, editors. Extracorporeal life support: the ELSO redbook. 5th ed. Ann Arbor, MI: ELSO; 2017. p. 183–199.

[27] Barrett CS, Jaggers JJ, Cook EF, et al. Outcomes of neonates undergoing extracorporeal membrane oxygenation

support using centrifugal versus roller blood pumps. Ann Thorac Surg 2012;94(5):1635–1641.

[28] Clark JB, Guan Y, McCoach R, Kunselman AR, Myers JL, Undar A. An investigational study of minimum rotational pump speed to avoid retrograde flow in three centrifugal blood pumps in a pediatric extracorporeal life support model. Perfusion 2011;26(3):185–190.

[29] Short BL. The effect of extracorporeal life support on the brain: a focus on ECMO. Semin Perinatol 2005;29(1):45–50.

[30] Hardart GE, Fackler JC. Predictors of intracranial hemorrhage during neonatal extracorporeal membrane oxygenation. J Pediatr 1999;134(2):156–159.

[31] Glass P, Bulas DI, Wagner AE, et al. Severity of brain injury following neonatal extracorporeal membrane oxygenation and outcome at age 5 years. Dev Med Child Neurol 1997;39(7):441–448.

[32] Khan AM, Shabarek FM, Zwischenberger JB, et al. Utility of daily head ultrasonography for infants on extracorporeal membrane oxygenation. J Pediatr Surg 1998;33(8):1229–1232.

[33] Heard ML, Clark RH, Pettignano R, Dykes FD. Daily cranial ultrasounds during ECMO: a quality review/cost analysis project. J Pediatr Surg 1997;32(8):1260–1261.

[34] Pappas A, Shankaran S, Stockmann PT, Bara R. Changes in amplitude-integrated electroencephalography in neonates treated with extracorporeal membrane oxygenation: a pilot study. J Pediatr 2006;148(1):125–127.

[35] Massaro A, Rais-Bahrami K, Chang T, Glass P, Short BL, Baumgart S. Therapeutic hypothermia for neonatal encephalopathy and extracorporeal membrane oxygenation. J Pediatr 2010;157(3):499–501.

[36] Field D. Neonatal ECMO study of temperature (NEST): a randomized controlled trial. Pediatrics 2013;132(5):e1247–e1256.

[37] Harthan AA, Buckley KW, Heger ML, Fortuna RS, Mays K. Medication adsorption into contemporary extracorporeal membrane oxygenator circuits. J Pediatr Pharmacol Ther 2014;19(4):288–295.

[38] Rais-Bahrami K, Van Meurs KP. Venoarterial versus venovenous ECMO for neonatal respiratory failure. Semin Perinatol 2014;38(2):71–77.

[39] Keszler M, Ryckman FC, McDonald JV, et al. A prospective, multicenter, randomized study of high versus low positive end-expiratory pressure during extracorporeal membrane oxygenation. J Pediatr 1992;120(1):107–113.

[40] Lotze A, Knight GR, Martin GR, et al. Improved pulmonary outcome after exogenous surfactant therapy for respiratory failure in term infants requiring extracorporeal membrane oxygenation. J Pediatr 1993;122(2):261–268.

[41] Kamat PP, Popler J, Davis J, et al. Use of flexible bronchoscopy in pediatric patients receiving extracorporeal membrane oxygenation (ECMO) support. Pediatr Pulmonol 2011;46(11):1108–1113.

[42] Roberts N, Westrope C, Pooboni SK, et al. Venovenous extracorporeal membrane oxygenation for respiratory failure in inotrope dependent neonates. ASAIO J 2003;49(5):568–571.

[43] Knight GR, Dudell GG, Evans ML, Grimm PS. A comparison of venovenous and venoarterial extracorporeal membrane oxygenation in the treatment of neonatal respiratory failure. Crit Care Med 1996;24(10):1678–1683.

[44] Strieper MJ, Sharma S, Dooley KJ, Cornish JD, Clark RH. Effects of venovenous extracorporeal membrane oxygenation on cardiac performance as determined by echocardiographic measurements. J Pediatr 1993;122(6):950–955.

[45] Sell LL, Cullen ML, Lerner GR, Whittlesey GC, Shanley CJ, Klein MD. Hypertension during extracorporeal membrane oxygenation: cause, effect, and management. Surgery 1987;102(4):724–730.

[46] Stewart DL, Sobczyk WL, Bond SJ, Cook LN. Use of two-dimensional and contrast echocardiography for venous cannula placement in venovenous extracorporeal life support. ASAIO J 1996;42(3):142–145.

[47] Roy BJ, Cornish JD, Clark RH. Venovenous extracorporeal membrane oxygenation affects renal function. Pediatrics 1995;95(4):573–578.

[48] Hanekamp MN, Spoel M, Sharman-Koendjbiharie I, et al. Routine enteral nutrition in neonates on extracorporeal membrane oxygenation. Pediatr Crit Care Med 2005;6(3):275–279.

[49] Bizzarro MJ, Conrad SA, Kaufman DA, Rycus P. Extracorporeal Life Support Organization Task Force on Infections, Extracorporeal Membrane Oxygenation. Infections acquired during extracorporeal membrane oxygenation in neonates, children, and adults. Pediatr Crit Care Med 2011;12(3):277–281.

[50] O'Horo JC, Cawcutt KA, De Moraes AG, Sampathkumar P, Schears GJ. The evidence base for prophylactic antibiotics in patients receiving extracorporeal membrane oxygenation. ASAIO J 2016;62(1):6–10.

[51] Sinauridze EI, Panteleev MA, Ataullakhanov FI. Anticoagulant therapy: basic principles, classic approaches and recent developments. Blood Coagul Fibrinolysis 2012;23(6):482–493.

[52] Bridges BC, Ranucci M, Lequier L. Anticoagulation and disorders of hemostasis. In: Brogan T, Lequier L, Lorusso R, MacLaren G, Peek G, editors. Extracorporeal life support: the ELSO redbook. 5th ed. Ann Arbor, MI: ELSO; 2017. p. 93–104.

[53] Lazar DA, Cass DL, Olutoye OO, et al. The use of ECMO for persistent pulmonary hypertension of the newborn: a decade of experience. J Surg Res 2012;177(2):263–267.

[54] Karimova A, Brown K, Ridout D, et al. Neonatal extracorporeal membrane oxygenation: practice patterns and predictors of outcome in the UK. Arch Dis Child Fetal Neonatal Ed 2009;94:F129–F132.

[55] McNally H, Bennett CC, Elbourne D, Field DJ. United Kingdom collaborative randomized trial of neonatal extracorporeal membrane oxygenation: follow-up to age 7 years. Pediatrics 2006;117(5):e845–e854.

[56] Ijsselstijn H, Madderom MJ, Hoskote A. Outcomes, complications, and follow-up of neonates with respiratory failure. In: Brogan T, Lequier L, Lorusso R, MacLaren G, Peek G, editors. Extracorporeal life support: the ELSO redbook. 5th ed. Ann Arbor, MI: ELSO; 2017. p. 217–230.

[57] Polito A, Barrett CS, Peter RT, Netto R, Cogo PE, Thiagarajan RR. Acute neurologic injury in neonates supported with extracorporeal membrane oxygenation: an analysis of ELSO registry data. Intensive Care Med 2012;38:S57.

[58] Khambekar K, Nichani S, Luyt DK, et al. Developmental outcome in

newborn infants treated for acute respiratory failure with ECMO: present experience. Arch Dis Child Fetal Neonatal Ed 2006;91(1): F21–F25.

[59] Hanekamp MN, Mazer P, van der Cammenvan Zijp MH, et al. Follow-up of newborns treated with extracorporeal membrane oxygenation: a nationwide evaluation at 5 years of age. Crit Care 2006;10(5):R127.

[60] Madderom MJ, Schiller RM, Gischler SJ, et al. Growing up after critical illness: verbal, visual-spatial and working memory problems in neonatal ECMO survivors. Crit Care Med 2016;44:1182–1190.

[61] McGahren ED, Mallik K, Rodgers BM. Neurological outcome is diminished in survivors of congenital diaphragmatic hernia requiring extracorporeal membrane oxygenation. J Pediatr Surg 1997;32(8):1216–1220.

[62] Nijhuis-van der Sanden MW, van der Cammen-van Zijp MH, Janssen AJ, et al. Motor performance in five-year-old extracorporeal membrane oxygenation survivors: a population-based study. Crit Care 2009;13(2):R47.

[63] Madderom MJ, Reuser JJCM, Utens EMWJ, et al. Neurodevelopmental, educational and behavioral outcome at 8 years after neonatal ECMO: a nationwide multicenter study. Intensive Care Med 2013;39(9): 1584–1593.

[64] van der Cammen-van Zijp MH, Janssen AJ, Raets MM, et al. Motor performance after neonatal extracorporeal membrane oxygenation: a longitudinal evaluation. Pediatrics 2014;134(2):e427–e435.

Section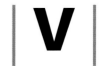

Clinical Management

Chapter | **23** |

Principles of Mechanical Ventilation and Strategies of Ventilatory Support in Neonatal Lung Disease

Manimaran Ramani, MD, Namasivayam Ambalavanan, MD

CHAPTER POINTS

- General strategies to reduce lung injury include avoiding invasive mechanical ventilation using non-invasive techniques, and if intubation is inevitable to limit the duration of invasive ventilation as much as possible.
- During conventional mechanical ventilation, oxygenation is influenced by mean airway pressure (PEEP being the primary factor along with PIP and inspiratory time) and inspired oxygen concentration.
- Removal of CO_2 during conventional ventilation is proportional to alveolar minute ventilation ([tidal volume-dead space] x rate). However, inadequate expiratory time at high rates may lead to gas trapping and CO_2 retention.
- Among infants on supplemental oxygen, targeting oxygen saturations in the low-90s in preterm infants and mid-90s in term infants appears to be a prudent approach.

- $PaCO_2$ targets vary based on the phase and nature of respiratory pathology. A target in the 40s to low 50s is appropriate for neonates with acute respiratory disease such as RDS but higher targets (permissive hypercapnia) to minimize lung injury are beneficial in conditions such as severe BPD and CDH.

Introduction

Development of new ventilator technologies, improved understanding of neonatal lung mechanics, and the increasing use of antenatal steroids and of postnatal surfactant have significantly reduced the mortality of premature infants over the past 4 decades. However, with the increasing survival of very preterm infants, respiratory sequelae such as bronchopulmonary dysplasia (BPD) continue to lead to significant morbidity and late mortality. Similarly, with improvements in obstetric care and reductions in the incidence of meconium aspiration syndrome (MAS), the use of high-frequency ventilation, and the introduction of inhaled nitric oxide and extracorporeal membrane oxygenation (ECMO), the morbidity and mortality of term and near-term infants due to respiratory failure have been markedly reduced. However, the mortality and longer-term morbidity due to some conditions such as congenital diaphragmatic hernia (CDH), lung hypoplasia associated with severe oligohydramnios, and developmental disorders of the lung continue to remain high. Despite several advances in ventilator technology,

it is still not clear in many clinical scenarios which mode of ventilation is the optimal approach and has the best chance of reducing ventilator-associated lung injury that may potentially contribute to long-term respiratory morbidity. In neonates, the risk of acute and chronic lung injury increases with longer duration of assisted ventilation. The smallest and more extremely premature infants are at highest risk of developing long-term complications of prolonged assisted ventilation. It is likely that an individualized ventilatory approach based on the underlying lung pathophysiology may significantly improve the long-term pulmonary outcome.

Positive pressure ventilation involves movement of a gas mixture (usually air enriched with oxygen) into the lungs using an external source of pressure to create a pressure gradient, with exhalation being usually passive (except in high-frequency oscillatory ventilation). Ventilation can be achieved by either invasive (conventional and high frequency) or noninvasive modes of ventilation. This chapter will discuss the principles of conventional assisted ventilation (invasive and noninvasive) and provide the potential ventilator strategies in neonates with respiratory distress syndrome (RDS) and respiratory disorders other than RDS.

The basic principles of ventilator strategies can be summarized as follows:

1. Avoid initiation of mechanical ventilation as much as possible—use noninvasive strategies first, and intubation only when absolutely necessary.
2. Use the ventilation settings that would damage the lungs the least (lowest pressures required for adequate functional residual capacity [FRC] and tidal volume), and lead to adequate but not excessive gas exchange.
3. Minimize the duration of mechanical ventilation and attempt extubation as early as possible.
4. Careful monitoring of physiologic status and gas exchange is essential, with initiation and adjustment of settings based on disease pathophysiology and responses to changes in therapy.
5. Excellent nursing and respiratory care.

Basics of conventional positive pressure ventilation

Regardless of the mode (volume cycled, pressure cycled, or dual ventilation) and method of support (continuous mandatory ventilation, assist/control ventilation, intermittent mandatory ventilation, synchronous intermittent mandatory ventilation, pressure support ventilation, and noninvasive ventilation), the basic concepts of conventional positive pressure ventilation remain the same. The basic parameters of conventional positive pressure ventilation are peak inspiratory pressure (PIP), positive end-expiratory pressure (PEEP), ventilator rate, inspiratory–expiratory ratio (*I:E*), inspiratory fractional oxygen concentration (FiO_2), and the flow rate. Below are the brief discussions about each components and their impact on ventilation and oxygenation, and an illustration of their relationships on oxygenation is shown in Fig. 23.1.

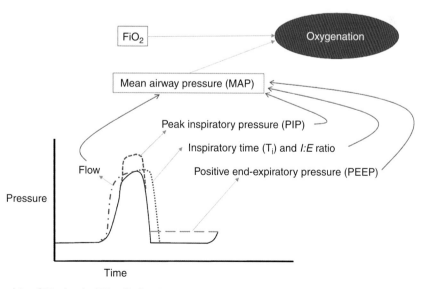

Fig. 23.1 Relationship of Mechanical Ventilation Parameters to Oxygenation.

Peak inspiratory pressure

PIP is the highest proximal airway pressure delivered during inhalation. PIP directly affects the delta pressure (difference between PIP and PEEP) and thereby it determines the tidal volume delivered to the neonate. As carbon dioxide elimination is directly proportional to the amount of tidal volume delivered, increasing the PIP will increase the carbon dioxide elimination. Changes in PIP also affect the oxygenation by altering the mean airway pressure (MAP). Suboptimal levels of PIP lead to inadequate tidal volume and result in hypercapnia and hypoxemia. On the other hand, higher levels of PIP will cause overdistension of the alveoli, volutrauma, air leak, hypocapnia, lower lung and cardiac perfusion, and acute and chronic lung injury. In addition, delivering higher levels of PIP when the airway resistance is high and time constant is prolonged also results in significant volutrauma and gas trapping. Most neonates may not need a tidal volume more than 4–6 mL/kg for ventilation and oxygenation. The amount of PIP required to deliver the optimal tidal volume depends on the compliance of the lungs. The degree of chest wall expansion during inspiration can fairly correlate with the compliance of the lungs [1]. A useful clinical indicator of adequate PIP is gentle rise in the chest wall with every ventilator-delivered breath that is similar to the chest expansion seen in a comfortable spontaneously breathing neonate. It is advisable to use the lowest effective PIP that maintains adequate gas exchange but minimizes volutrauma and reduces the risk of air leak. Physiological impact of changes in PIP is included in Table 23.1.

Positive end-expiratory pressure

PEEP is pressure in the airway above ambient pressure at the end of passive expiration. PEEP is the distending pressure which helps lungs maintain their FRC by keeping alveoli inflated. By reducing surface tension, surfactant prevents the alveoli from collapsing during each

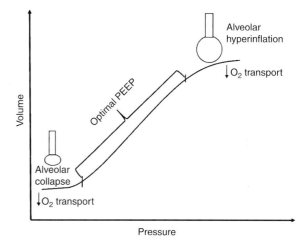

Fig. 23.2 Relationship of PEEP to Alveolar Inflation and Oxygen Transport.

exhalation and maintains FRC. During conditions of surfactant deficiency (e.g., RDS), adequate PEEP is required to overcome the increase in surface tension and maintain FRC. Providing PEEP during ventilation reduces the workload of respiratory muscle by keeping the alveoli at the optimal distension after exhalation and reducing airway resistance. Although increasing PEEP increases FRC, a very high PEEP results in poor lung compliance and reduces tidal volume and leads to accumulation of carbon dioxide. On the other hand, suboptimal PEEP causes alveolar collapse and requires higher PIP during each inspiration to open atelectatic alveoli. Both alveolar atelectasis and overdistension cause alveolar capillary constriction, thereby leading to pulmonary shunting and causing decreased oxygen transport (Fig. 23.2). For many premature infants with RDS, PEEP levels between 4 and 5 cmH_2O are well tolerated and adequate to improve oxygenation. Physiological impact of changes in PEEP is included in Table 23.2.

Table 23.1 Effects of changes in PIP

Changes in PIP	Physiological impact
Optimal PIP	Adequate tidal volume $PaCO_2$ in target range Minimal lung injury
Higher PIP	Increases tidal volume Decreases $PaCO_2$ Volutrauma Air leaks
Lower PIP	Decreases tidal volume Increases $PaCO_2$

Table 23.2 Effects of changes in PEEP

Changes in PEEP	Physiological impact
Optimal PEEP	Maintains FRC Increases oxygenation Prevents atelectasis
Low PEEP	Atelectasis Pulmonary shunting
High PEEP	Over distension Air leak Pulmonary shunting

Table 23.3 Effects of changes in Ventilator Rate

Changes in ventilator rate	Physiological impact
Optimal rate	Adequate minute ventilation $PaCO_2$ in target range
Low rate	Decrease minute ventilation CO_2 retention
Higher rate	Inadvertent PEEP Gas trapping CO_2 retention

Ventilator rate

The ventilator rate is the number of breaths delivered by the ventilator per minute. The minute ventilation is the product of tidal volume and rate, whereas alveolar minute ventilation is the product of (tidal volume minus dead space) and rate. Lower ventilator rates decrease minute ventilation. Higher ventilator rates (with inspiratory time kept constant) reduces the duration of exhalation which in turn results in gas trapping and carbon dioxide accumulation. The threshold at which the tidal volume decreases with increase in rate depends on the time constant of the respiratory system. A single time constant is defined as the amount of time taken for the alveolar pressure or volume to reach 63% of peak alveolar pressure or volume [2]. Lung compliance and resistance determine the time constant as follows:

$$\text{Time constant} = \text{Compliance} \times \text{Resistance}$$

Infants with immature lungs have surfactant deficiency, resulting in poor lung compliance and thereby have shorter time constants. Infants with RDS, wherein pulmonary time constant is short, can tolerate higher ventilator rates without compromising the minute ventilation. Rates higher than 60/min are usually well tolerated in infants with RDS [3,4]. However, even in disease states with short time constants, very rapid rate may lead to inadvertent PEEP and gas trapping resulting from inadequate time for exhalation. Careful attention should be paid to the changes in the chest wall movement while increasing the ventilator rate to prevent gas trapping and carbon dioxide retention. The absence of brief pause in the chest wall movement at the end-expiration may indicate inadequate expiratory time. Physiological impact of changes in rate is included in Table 23.3.

Inspiratory–expiratory ratio

The time constant of the respiratory system determines the inspiratory time T_i and expiratory time T_e. Time constant for exhalation is longer than the inhalation. Usually once the ventilator rate and the T_i are set, T_e and the $I{:}E$

are automatically determined. The usual $I{:}E$ ratio is 1:3. Increasing the ventilator rate without decreasing the T_i will compromise the exhalation time and leads to gas trapping. T_i of 0.3–0.5 s is sufficient for most of the neonates. Extreme T_i (less than 0.2 s or greater than 0.7 s) can lead to poor tidal volume and gas trapping. Reversed $I{:}E$ ratios (with inspiration longer than expiration) may improve oxygenation, but at the expense of impaired venous return, gas trapping and air leaks are no longer recommended.

Inspiratory fractional oxygen concentration

As may be anticipated, changes in the inspiratory fractional oxygen concentration (FiO_2) have a direct proportional effect on alveolar oxygen content. In the absence of right to left shunting, increases in FiO_2 would also increase systemic oxygenation. It is important to remember that as both changes in FiO_2 and MAP increase oxygenation (Fig. 23.1), the clinician must evaluate their relative contribution to oxygenation and adjust the correct parameter. In general, if the MAP is inadequate (lung volumes below FRC), a higher FiO_2 is required. One may attempt to identify optimal lung expansion, which is the FRC when the FiO_2 is the lowest required. In preterm infants during the acute phase of RDS, FiO_2 is usually adjusted to keep target oxygen saturation between 91% and 95%. In infants with established BPD, if there is evidence of pulmonary hypertension, the target saturation is often increased slightly to 92%–97%. In preterm infants, it is important to avoid very high oxygen saturations (>95%) in order to reduce the risk of retinopathy of prematurity (ROP), and hence frequent changes in FiO_2 are often required. In term infants, FiO_2 higher than that required to maintain PaO_2 70–100 mmHg should be avoided. It is necessary to use pulse oximetry (less commonly, transcutaneous oxygen oximetry, or near-infrared oximetry) to adjust oxygen delivery, rather than infrequent arterial blood gases. Both increased pressures, volumes (barotrauma and volutrauma), and a high FiO_2 are capable of inducing lung injury, and their exact contributions to chronic lung disease in an infant may vary depending upon multiple variables. However, it is generally believed that at $FiO_2 < 0.6$ or 0.7, the risk of oxygen toxicity is less than that of volutrauma. During episodes of oxygen desaturation procedures such as repositioning, suctioning, and so on, the FiO_2 may need to be transiently increased. Recent advances in ventilator care to include closed loop systems that automatically adjust FiO_2 based on SpO_2 may potentially minimize periods of oxygen desaturation and hyperoxemia.

Flow rate

In most modern ventilators, changes in the flow rate minimally affect gas exchange, as long as sufficient flow is used to generate the ventilator pressures and rate.

Effect of dead space

Dead space reduces the tidal volume that reaches the alveoli. While physiological dead space may be countered by efforts to improve lung inflation and reduce unventilated areas, anatomical dead space can be reduced by shortening endotracheal tubes and removing other contributors to dead space. For example, some ventilators use a pneumotachograph with a dead space of 0.8 mL, which is perceived as a small volume. However, for a 0.5 kg infant with a tidal volume of 4 mL/kg (anatomic dead space of 1.5 mL/kg), the usual tidal volume of 2 mL ($0.5 \times 4 = 2$ mL, with

anatomic dead space of 0.75 mL) needs to be increased by a substantial amount (to 2.8 mL, or by 40%) to overcome this additional dead space, which may increase volutrauma.

Ventilator management of common respiratory conditions in the neonate

Ventilator management of common respiratory conditions in the neonate is listed below, and is summarized in Table 23.4.

Table 23.4 Mechanical ventilation strategies used in common neonatal respiratory diseases (management must be individualized as many infants require strategies outside common ranges)

Disorder	Goals	Rate (/min)	FiO$_2$	PIP (cmH$_2$O)	PEEP (cmH$_2$O)	T_i (s)
Preterm infants						
Respiratory distress syndrome (RDS)—early	pH 7.25–7.30, PaO$_2$ 50–70 mmHg (SpO$_2$ 91%–95%), and PaCO$_2$ 45–55 mmHg	50–70	0.4–0.7 (minimum needed)	10–20 (minimum needed)	4–5	0.25–0.4
RDS—pre-extubation	pH 7.20–7.30, SpO$_2$ 91%–95%, and PaCO$_2$ <60 in first week, <70 in week 2	≤20	<0.4	<15	<6	0.25–0.4
Apnea of prematurity (AoP)	pH 7.25–7.4, SpO$_2$ 91%–95%, and PaCO$_2$ 50–70 mmHg	10–20	0.21–0.3; as low as needed	10–15 (minimum needed)	3–5	0.3–0.5
Bronchopulmonary dysplasia (BPD)—early	pH 7.20–7.25, SpO$_2$ 91%–95%, and PaCO$_2$ 50–60 mmHg	20–40	0.3–0.8 (minimum needed)	15–25 (minimum needed)	4–6	0.35–0.5
BPD—severe	pH 7.20–7.25, SpO$_2$ 91%–95%, and PaCO$_2$ 50–65 mmHg	20–30	0.3–0.8 (minimum needed)	May be as high as 30–40; use minimum needed	5–8	0.4–0.7
Term infants						
Normal lungs (e.g., mechanical ventilation during surgery)	pH 7.3–7.40, PaO$_2$ 70–100 mmHg (SpO$_2$ 93%–98%), and PaCO$_2$ 40–55 mmHg (35–45 mmHg in infants with hypoxic-ischemic encephalopathy)	30–50	0.21– minimum needed	10–15	3–5	0.35–0.45
Persistent pulmonary hypertension of newborn (PPHN)	pH 7.35–7.45, PaO$_2$ 60–100 mmHg, SpO$_2$ 93%–98%, and PaCO$_2$ 35–45 mmHg	50–70	0.3–0.8	15–25	3–5	0.3–0.4
Meconium aspiration syndrome (MAS)	pH 7.35–7.45, PaO$_2$ 60–120 mmHg, SpO$_2$ 93%–98%, and PaCO$_2$ 40–60 mmHg	30–50	0.3–0.8	15–25	2–4	0.4–0.5
Congenital diaphragmatic hernia (CDH)	pH >7.25, preductal SpO$_2$ 85%–95%, and PaCO$_2$ 50–70 mmHg	40–80	0.5–0.9	15–25	3–4	0.25–0.35

Ventilator management of respiratory distress syndrome

RDS due to surfactant deficiency and inactivation is relatively common in preterm infants. The surfactant deficiency leads to microatelectasis of alveoli, a reduction in lung compliance, and lower lung volume. The reduced lung compliance is associated with very short time constants (0.05–0.1 s) during the acute phase of RDS. Attempts to expand atelectatic areas of the lung using higher peak pressures may result in volutrauma to both airways and distal lung parenchyma.

Respiratory support of preterm infants with RDS usually consists of escalation from either supplemental oxygen without pressure (oxyhood, oxygen environment, etc.) or CPAP to mechanical ventilation.

The indications for mechanical ventilation consist of clinical criteria and blood gas criteria.

Clinical criteria

- Respiratory distress with tachypnea (respiratory rate in excess of 60–70/min) or severe retractions (intercostal, subcostal, and suprasternal).
- Inadequate oxygenation (SpO_2 <91% with oxygen hood or CPAP with FiO_2 >0.4 to 0.7).
- Apnea unresponsive to medical management (CPAP, and methylxanthines such as aminophylline or caffeine).

Blood gas criteria

- Severe hypercapnia with $PaCO_2$ >55 to 60 mmHg and arterial pH <7.2.
- Severe hypoxemia with PaO_2 <40 mmHg at FiO_2 >0.4 to 0.7.

The clinical course of RDS in individual infants is variable. Some infants, especially those who are depressed at birth, are intubated and receive surfactant soon after birth. Other infants who are placed on CPAP in the delivery room may be unable to maintain oxygenation on CPAP and are intubated rapidly, while other infants require gradually escalating CPAP/FiO_2 or develop severe apnea and are intubated at a later time point. Decisions to intubate are frequently made on clinical criteria soon after birth, and upon blood gas criteria after initial stabilization. The initial mechanical ventilator settings and strategy have to be individualized, based upon the severity of lung disease, magnitude of spontaneous ventilation, and other variables (e.g., clinical course until then, presence of air leaks). The presence of retractions per se is generally not sufficient as an indicator of the need for mechanical ventilation.

Recent clinical trials indicate that a conservative approach to intubation and mechanical ventilation is better. Prophylactic nasal CPAP when compared to mechanical ventilation in very preterm infants reduces the need for mechanical ventilation and surfactant, and also reduces the incidence of BPD and death or BPD [5]. Recent large trials in which antenatal steroid use is common and there is routine postdelivery stabilization on CPAP demonstrate less risk of BPD or death when using early stabilization on CPAP with selective surfactant administration to infants requiring intubation [6]. Hence, most clinicians use prophylactic nasal CPAP in extremely preterm infants, and early initiation of CPAP in larger preterm infants, with resort to intubation, surfactant administration, and mechanical ventilation only in infants who cannot be supported on CPAP. As mentioned in the criteria earlier, inadequate oxygenation (clinically or on blood gas criteria) or apnea is generally considered failure of CPAP. The FiO_2 threshold for "CPAP failure" is variable, depending upon clinician preference and clinical characteristics (gestational age, postnatal age, severity of RDS), but in general, a lower threshold (FiO_2 >0.3 to 0.4) is used for smaller sicker preterm infants (<28-week GA, <1 kg) soon after birth (<24 h of age) and a higher threshold (FiO_2 >0.6 to 0.7) for larger preterm infants (>32-week GA, >1.5 to 2 kg) and at later time points (beyond 48–72 h of postnatal age).

Initial settings for conventional pressure-limited, time-cycled ventilation for neonates with RDS are a respiratory rate of 50–70 breaths/min, with PIP enough to achieve chest inspiratory excursions similar to a normal spontaneous breath (usually 10–20 cmH_2O) and moderate PEEP (4–5 cmH_2O). The inspiratory time usually ranges from 0.25 to 0.4 s, and the FiO_2 from 0.4 to 0.7 (depending upon FiO_2 on CPAP at time of transition). These settings are not dependent upon factors such as the birth weight or gestational age or postnatal age of the infant, but upon lung pathophysiology, gas exchange, and lung mechanics. The blood gas targets for the initial phase of RDS are usually a pH 7.25–7.30, PaO_2 50–70 mmHg (SpO_2 91%–95%), and $PaCO_2$ 45–55 mmHg.

Following administration of surfactant, pulmonary mechanics may change rapidly, and it may be necessary to make ventilator settings adjustments frequently, based upon chest excursions, change in oxygen saturation, transcutaneous O_2/CO_2 measurements, end-tidal CO_2 ($ETCO_2$), and blood gas measurements. Initial ventilator settings usually consist of rapid rates and shorter inspiratory times due to the short time constants. The combination of rapid rates and short inspiratory times, as opposed to shorter rates and longer inspiratory times, has been shown to reduce air leaks in human infants, and to reduce lung injury in animal models. The required tidal volume for infants with RDS is often in the range of 4–6 mL/kg. It is often preferable to lower $PaCO_2$ by increasing minute ventilation, through increases in ventilator rate rather than by increasing PIP (unless PIP is low to begin with), in order to reduce volutrauma. Similarly, if an infant has a low $PaCO_2$, it is advisable to first reduce PIP to lowest required pressure for adequate chest movement (and tidal volume), and then reduce rate.

The initial PIP required (between 10 and 20 cmH$_2$O) is usually determined at the time of initiating mechanical ventilation by observing the pressures required to produce adequate chest movement. If excessive chest movement is observed, PIP should be reduced quickly for lung damage can happen rapidly. If inadequate chest movement is noted, PIP should be increased rapidly for hypoxemia is also detrimental. If PIP increases do not increase chest movement or tidal volume, evaluation of potential etiologies is needed (e.g., tube occlusion by mucus plugging, tube dislodgement, pneumothorax) before increasing PIP to much higher levels. If tidal volume can be measured, the PIP can be adjusted subsequently to use the lowest PIP required that produces adequate tidal volume (usually 4–6 mL/kg) to provide sufficient gas exchange.

Unless an infant has very severe RDS, the duration of mechanical ventilation is usually brief (1–3 days). Once the infant has been stabilized with appropriate ranges of pH, PaO$_2$, and PaCO$_2$, weaning from mechanical ventilation should be aggressively performed. Many clinicians find it beneficial to restrict fluid intake (maintaining serum sodium in 140–150 mEq/L range, and with 10%–15% weight loss in the first few days after birth, which usually can be attained by a total fluid intake of 70 mL/kg/day in a well-humidified environment such as an incubator) [7], and provide methylxanthines (caffeine or aminophylline) for infants with RDS in the initial postnatal days to assist with extubation [8,9]. Weaning of the ventilator can be performed relatively rapidly (every few hours), if close monitoring such as with transcutaneous CO$_2$ monitoring or frequent blood gases is provided. During weaning, once the PIP has been brought down to relatively low levels (e.g., 10–12 cmH$_2$O), the FiO$_2$ can be decreased. Maintenance of an adequate lung volume (FRC) by use of sufficient MAP will ensure ventilation/perfusion (V/Q) matching, enabling reductions in FiO$_2$. If reductions in MAP are not possible, it is likely that V/Q matching is not adequate and the cause may need investigation—it is possible that additional doses of surfactant are required, or there are complications such as atelectasis. After the first few days, when the risk of intraventricular hemorrhage (IVH) is lower, many clinicians choose to tolerate a higher PaCO$_2$ (permissive hypercapnia), as long as pH is more than 7.2, and the PaCO$_2$ is not too high (generally <60 mmHg in the first week, and <70 in the second week). It is important to reduce extremes of PaCO$_2$ (hypocapnia or hypercapnia), as both extremes are associated with neurologic injury [10,11], and hypocapnia associated with excessive ventilation may be associated with volutrauma and sensorineural deafness.

Infants can generally be extubated from mechanical ventilation to CPAP, once they are on sufficiently low settings (rate of less than 20/min, PIP <15 cmH$_2$O, PEEP <6 cmH$_2$O, and FiO$_2$ usually <0.40), and have good spontaneous respiratory effort. Infants who accidentally extubate at settings higher than (but close to) these settings can also be placed on CPAP to evaluate their ability to stay off the ventilator. In the acute phase of RDS, PEEP levels of 5–6 cmH$_2$O may be needed to maintain lung inflation and prevent end-expiratory atelectasis. As RDS resolves, the PEEP can be reduced slowly to 4-5 cm H$_2$O before extubation to CPAP. Reduction of PEEP below 3 is not recommended while intubated, in order to prevent reduction of FRC. During the process of weaning, once the PIP has been reduced, and the rate is being reduced slowly, the magnitude of spontaneous respiratory effort needs to be observed. Infants with good spontaneous effort can be weaned faster, while those with inadequate effort may need to be evaluated further (excessive PEEP will suppress spontaneous ventilator efforts; lack or inadequate dosage of methylxanthines; CNS injury; overventilation with low PaCO$_2$ that suppresses spontaneous breathing). Techniques such as patient-triggered ventilation (PTV), pressure support (PS), and synchronized IMV (SIMV) may facilitate weaning. Extubation is generally done to NCPAP, although extubation to NCPAP in combination with non-invasive positive pressure ventilation (NIPPV), which may be synchronized (SNIPPV), may reduce extubation failure (need for reintubation soon after extubation) as well [12]. Larger preterm infants with less respiratory distress can sometimes be extubated directly to oxygen hood or nasal cannula.

There are various alternative techniques of ventilation, in addition to conventional pressure-limited, time-cycled ventilation, including various methods of volume-targeted ventilation (e.g., volume guarantee), high-frequency ventilation (e.g., jet ventilation, oscillatory ventilation), but these methods probably offer no advantage and have some limitations for the average infant with RDS. For example, measurement of tidal volume is rather imprecise and inaccurate at very low volumes (<5 mL), and hence the infants who may benefit the most (ELBW infants at highest risk of BPD) may not benefit as much as hoped for by the clinician. High-frequency ventilation is usually attempted as a rescue therapy in case of hypoxemic respiratory failure despite maximal conventional ventilation, or in cases of air leak syndrome (pulmonary interstitial emphysema—PIE or pneumothorax).

Management of refractory apnea of prematurity

Preterm infants are at high risk of apnea of prematurity (AoP), and are usually managed with methylxanthines (caffeine or aminophylline) or CPAP, or a combination of CPAP with methylxanthines. However, some infants (especially extremely preterm infants or those with CNS injury) have severe apneic episodes that may require resuscitative efforts despite CPAP and methylxanthine therapy, and may

require a trial of NIPPV, and subsequently may require intubation and mechanical ventilation if noninvasive ventilation is not sufficient. As such infants being ventilated primarily for apnea have relatively less lung disease, they may be ventilated using lower pressures (10–15 cmH$_2$O; sufficient for normal chest excursions) and low rates (10–20/min) and low FiO$_2$ to keep SpO$_2$ 91%–95%.

Management of established bronchopulmonary dysplasia

While BPD is generally defined at the age of 28 postnatal days or 36 weeks' postmenstrual age, clinicians are generally aware that an infant is not improving rapidly and is at high risk of BPD by 1 or 2 weeks after birth. Most infants who have RDS improve rapidly and are extubated before the end of the first postnatal week with appropriate care. Infants who do not show such rapid improvement and still require high IMV settings are at high risk of developing BPD. The main objective of ventilator management in BPD is to maintain adequate gas exchange while minimizing ventilator-associated lung injury. The exact ventilator settings will depend upon the lung mechanics and the status of gas exchange. Infants with BPD may have varying injury and remodeling to lung parenchyma, vasculature, and airways. Infants with relatively homogeneous lung disease may require settings similar to that for RDS, with relatively faster rates and lower pressures, while those with patchy atelectasis and areas of hyperinflation may do better with a strategy of lower rates and higher pressures (and resulting higher tidal volumes), with longer inspiratory times (T_i 0.35–0.5 s; due to longer time constants) as compared to infants with RDS. Some infants with severe chronic BPD may benefit from volume-targeted ventilation, and with tolerance of a higher PaCO$_2$, as long as pH is maintained >7.2. Infants with BPD often have better V/Q matching with higher levels of PEEP (5–8 cmH$_2$O) as compared to infants with RDS. Infants with severe BPD sometimes require very high peak pressures (e.g., 30–40 cmH$_2$O) and high tidal volumes (e.g., 10 mL/kg) despite relatively lower rates (e.g., 20/min) to maintain oxygenation due to severe V/Q mismatch, but clinicians should try to reduce these settings whenever possible.

It is important to emphasize to the entire clinical team the need to wean ventilator support whenever possible, despite frequent swings in clinical status. The default technique is usually to increase ventilator settings rapidly during episodes of deterioration, but wean settings very slowly in between such episodes, which leads to a progressive increase in ventilator settings over time that aggravates ventilator-induced lung injury. Infants with severe BPD can often be extubated to CPAP/noninvasive PPV at reasonably high MAPs (7–10 cmH$_2$O), rates (10–20/min), and high FiO$_2$ (>0.4). A key determinant for whether extubation

will be successful or not in such infants is the magnitude of spontaneous respiratory effort (which often generates pressures and tidal volumes exceeding those provided by the ventilator).

Infants with BPD are at high risk for pulmonary hypertension, and it is recommended that preterm infants be screened regularly (probably starting at about a month of age, and then monthly, if still on substantial respiratory support) by echocardiography for the development of this complication. Infants diagnosed with pulmonary hypertension in the setting of BPD may need additional specialized investigation (e.g., CT angiography, cardiac catheterization) and therapy (e.g., inhaled nitric oxide, sildenafil, higher oxygen saturation targets). In a few patients with severe BPD, who remain mechanically ventilated for months, tracheostomy may benefit in maintenance of an airway, assisting pulmonary toilet, and reducing dead space. Some infants may also benefit from neutrally adjusted ventilatory assist (NAVA) in which ventilator assistance is provided in proportion to and in synchrony with the patient's respiratory efforts as indicated by electrodes that pick up the electrical activity of the diaphragm.

Alternative modes of ventilation such as high-frequency ventilation are generally not superior to conventional ventilation in severe chronic BPD, due to higher airway resistance that reduces the efficacy of gas exchange during high-frequency ventilation.

Term infants requiring mechanical ventilation

1. Term infants with normal lungs (e.g., infants requiring mechanical ventilation due to need for general anesthesia or due to neurologic issues)
   Term infants who have normal lungs but need mechanical ventilation either briefly (e.g., during surgical procedures) or for a prolonged duration (e.g., for neuromuscular conditions) need to be ventilated using low pressures (10–15 cmH$_2$O; just sufficient for normal chest excursions) and moderate rates (30–50/min) and low FiO$_2$ (if lungs are normal, and there is no major systemic illness, the required FiO$_2$ is usually <0.25). It is important to monitor for apnea and desaturation after extubation, even after brief ventilation.
   Infant with hypoxic-ischemic encephalopathy (HIE) may occasionally have lung pathology, but more often have impaired control of breathing. They may be apneic due to severe brain injury, or tachypneic due to metabolic acidosis. Infants with HIE are often treated with therapeutic hypothermia, and in such cases, it is important to remember that hypothermia shifts the oxyhemoglobin dissociation curve to the left (increases oxygen saturation for a given PaO$_2$). To

avoid disruptions in cerebral blood flow, it is necessary to maintain $PaCO_2$ in the 35–45 mmHg range as much as possible. To avoid additional brain injury due to either hypoxia or hyperoxemia, it is also necessary to maintain oxygenation in the normal range (PaO_2 70–100 mmHg). The ventilator settings required in such infants is usually that required for infants with normal lungs (low pressures, moderate rates, and low FiO_2, as indicated in the previous paragraph), unless the infant develops fluid overload, ARDS, pulmonary hemorrhage, or other morbidity associated with HIE.

2. Term infants with abnormal lungs or pulmonary circulation (e.g., infants with persistent pulmonary hypertension of the newborn (PPHN), MAS, CDH, or other disorders)

Term infants with PPHN usually have severe hypoxemia out of proportion to clinically or radiographically lung disease, due to extrapulmonary shunting (usually at ductal level, and sometimes at the atrial level). As hypoxemia and acidosis are known to increase pulmonary vascular resistance and increase right to left shunting, the strategy is to avoid hypoxemia and acidosis. The usual goal is to maintain PaO_2 60–100 mmHg, and a pH in the 7.35–7.45 range. Initially, infants may be provided oxygen by hood or CPAP to prevent hypoxemia, but if hypoxemia is persistent (e.g., SpO_2 <90%, PaO_2 <50 mmHg) or respiratory acidosis is present (e.g., pH <7.2 with $PaCO_2$ >55 mmHg), infants may need to be intubated and mechanically ventilated. Mechanical ventilation with faster rates (50–70/min) and relatively short inspiratory times (T_i 0.3–0.4 s) may help reduce $PaCO_2$, preventing respiratory acidosis. In infants with persistent hypoxemia or hypercapnia, it is better to start inhaled nitric oxide (induces pulmonary vasodilation, improves V/Q matching) early (e.g., at Oxygenation Index of 15–20), rather than increase ventilator pressures and rates very high before initiating nitric oxide. This is because use of very high ventilator pressures or rates in the setting of PPHN may lead to excessive MAP and further reduce pulmonary circulation.

Infants with MAS may have areas of atelectasis, gas trapping, and areas of chemical pneumonitis. Many of the infants with MAS also have pulmonary hypertension, and the general goals of therapy are the same. However, if gas trapping is noted, the expiratory time should be increased (>0.5 s, perhaps as much as 0.7–1 s), and PEEP decreased (to 2–4 cmH_2O). If oxygenation is borderline but adequate (e.g., SpO_2 88–92, PaO_2 45–60 mmHg) and there is no pulmonary hypertension, it may be preferable to conservatively manage such infants without further increases in ventilator settings (in order to reduce the risk of air leaks). Adjunct therapies such as iNO and surfactant therapy should be considered early, rather than later. Infants with MAS and pulmonary hypertension should have higher oxygen saturations (e.g., SpO_2 93%–98%) and PaO_2 (e.g., PaO_2 70–120 mmHg) targeted, in order to reduce hypoxemic episodes that may exacerbate pulmonary hypertension. In general, most clinicians prefer to increase FiO_2 before increasing ventilator pressures (as long as tidal volume and chest excursions are adequate), in the setting of MAS, in order to reduce the risk of air leaks. Infants with CDH require specialized management in collaboration with pediatric surgeons. Most centers now use a strategy of "gentle ventilation" with initial cardiopulmonary stabilization followed by delayed surgical repair (sometimes while on ECMO). The general goals of therapy are often to maintain sufficient preductal oxygenation (preductal SpO_2 >90% preferably, or at least 85%) while tolerating higher $PaCO_2$ (up to 60–65 mmHg) as long as pH is adequate (>7.25). The initial settings are usually rapid rates (40–80/min), adequate PIP for tidal volume delivery/chest movement (usually 15–25 cmH_2O), short inspiratory times (T_i 0.25–0.35 s), with FiO_2 as needed to maintain adequate oxygenation (often >0.70).

Conclusion

The principles of ventilation for neonates vary with lung pathology, size of the infant, and associated morbidities (such as cardiac dysfunction and pulmonary hypertension). Close monitoring using noninvasive (SpO_2, $ETCO_2$, transcutaneous monitoring) and invasive techniques (blood gases) with frequent adjustment of ventilator settings will reduce morbidity and mortality. Lung protective strategies include optimizing ventilator support with gentle ventilator techniques to limit barotrauma, volutrauma, and atelectotrauma. Reducing the duration of invasive mechanical ventilation, especially in extremely preterm infants, is likely to decrease the extent of lung injury and BPD.

References

[1] Aufricht C, Huemer C, Frenzel C, Simbruner G. Respiratory compliance assessed from chest expansion and inflation pressure in ventilated neonates. Am J Perinatol 1993;10(2):139–142.

[2] Carlo WA, Martin RJ. Principles of neonatal assisted ventilation. Pediatr Clin North Am 1986;33(1):221–237.

[3] Mireles-Cabodevila E, Chatburn RL. Mid-frequency ventilation: unconventional use of conventional mechanical ventilation as a lung-protection strategy. Respir Care 2008;53(12):1669–1677.

[4] Bhat R, Kelleher J, Ambalavanan N, Chatburn RL, Mireles-Cabodevila E, Carlo WA. Feasibility of mid-frequency ventilation among infants with respiratory distress syndrome. Respir Care 2017;62(4):481–488.

[5] Subramaniam P, Ho JJ, Davis PG. Prophylactic nasal continuous positive airway pressure for preventing morbidity and mortality in very preterm infants. Cochrane Database Syst Rev 2016;6:CD001243.

[6] Rojas-Reyes MX, Morley CJ, Soll R. Prophylactic versus selective use of surfactant in preventing morbidity and mortality in preterm infants. Cochrane Database Syst Rev 2012;3:CD000510.

[7] Bell EF, Acarregui MJ. Restricted versus liberal water intake for preventing morbidity and mortality in preterm infants. Cochrane Database Syst Rev 2014;12:CD000503.

[8] Henderson-Smart DJ, Davis PG. Prophylactic methylxanthines for endotracheal extubation in preterm infants. Cochrane Database Syst Rev 2010;12:CD000139.

[9] Borszewska-Kornacka MK, Hozejowski R, Rutkowska M, Lauterbach R. Shifting the boundaries for early caffeine initiation in neonatal practice: results of a prospective, multicenter study on very preterm infants with respiratory distress syndrome. PLoS One 2017;12(12):e0189152.

[10] Ambalavanan N, Carlo WA, Wrage LA, Das A, Laughon M, Cotten CM, et al. PaCO2 in surfactant, positive pressure, and oxygenation randomised trial (SUPPORT). Arch Dis Child Fetal Neonatal Ed 2015;100(2):F145–F149.

[11] Fabres J, Carlo WA, Phillips V, Howard G, Ambalavanan N. Both extremes of arterial carbon dioxide pressure and the magnitude of fluctuations in arterial carbon dioxide pressure are associated with severe intraventricular hemorrhage in preterm infants. Pediatrics 2007;119(2):299–305.

[12] Lemyre B, Davis PG, De Paoli AG, Kirpalani H. Nasal intermittent positive pressure ventilation (NIPPV) versus nasal continuous positive airway pressure (NCPAP) for preterm neonates after extubation. Cochrane Database Syst Rev 2017;2:CD003212.

Chapter | **24** |

Respiratory Distress Syndrome and Surfactant Therapy

Manoj Biniwale, MBBS, MD, MRCP, MRCPCH, FAAP, Rangasamy Ramanathan, MBBS, MD, DCH, FAAP

CHAPTER POINTS

- Respiratory distress syndrome is the most common pulmonary problem in premature infants secondary to inadequate surfactant synthesis. Diagnosis is based on classic clinical picture with radiographic evidence supporting uniform opacification of lungs. Mangement strategies include prenatal corticosteroids, non invasive ventilation in the delivery room, early selective surfactant therapy and minimizing exposure to mechanical ventilation. Complications can be prevented by early caffeine therapy, permissive hypercapnia, postnatal steroids in selected patients and optmizing nutrition.

Introduction

Respiratory distress syndrome (RDS), also known as hyaline membrane disease (HMD) due to surfactant deficiency, is the principal cause of respiratory distress in preterm infants who require immediate intervention during fetal to neonatal transition at birth. Surfactant is produced by type II pneumocytes, lining the alveoli. Type II pneumocytes cover approximately 10% of alveolar surface area and play an important role in surfactant metabolism and secretion. Surfactant is composed of phosphatidylcholine (PC), surfactant associated proteins, plasmalogens, phosphatidylglycerol, and other acidic phospholipids [1] (Fig. 24.1). Most important component of surfactant is dipalmitoyl PC or DPPC. Four surfactant-associated proteins, namely, SP-A, SP-B, SP-C, and SP-D, have been identified to date [2]. SP-A and SP-A belong to a group of proteins, called lectins, and work like endogenous antibiotics. SP-A and SP-D are hydrophilic proteins and help to maintain "sterility" of the lung due to their role in host defense. SP-B and SP-B are extremely lipophilic and help to maintain "stability" of the lungs by lowering the surface tension in the lung and help to maintain functional residual capacity. Homozygous SP-B deficiency results in severe respiratory failure and needs lung transplantation for survival. DPPC requires SP-B, SP-C, and antioxidant phospholipid plasmalogen to spread and adsorb onto the entire surface area of the lung to lower the surface tension [3].

Surfactant metabolism

1. **Synthesis**: Synthesized in the microsomes and transported as lamellar bodies. Surfactant proteins are made in the endoplasmic reticulum and glycosylated in the Golgi bodies before storage. Lamellar bodies containing SP-A, SP-B, and SP-C are the intracellular storage form of surfactant [4] (Fig. 24.2).
2. **Transport**: Transporter proteins, such as ATP-binding cassette protein-A3 (ABCA3), are responsible for lamellar body formation and secretion. Patients with ABCA3 splicing mutation have smaller and denser lamellar bodies and develop severe RDS. By a process of exocytosis, lamellar bodies are secreted into the alveolar subphase and in the presence of SP-A form tubular myelin. Tubular myelin unravels to form

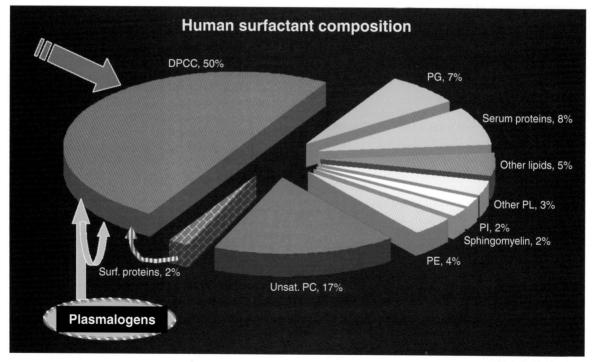

Fig. 24.1 Surfactant Composition. *DPPC*, dipalmitoylphosphatidylcholine; *PC*, phospphatidyl choline; *PE*, phosphatidyl ethanolamine; *PG*, phosphatidyl glycerol; *PI*, phosphatidyl inositol; *PL*, phospholipid; *surf*, surfactant; *unsat*, unsaturated. Modified from Hamm H, Fabel H, Bartsch W. The surfactant system of the adult lung: physiology and clinical perspectives. Clin Invest 1992;70:637–657 [1].

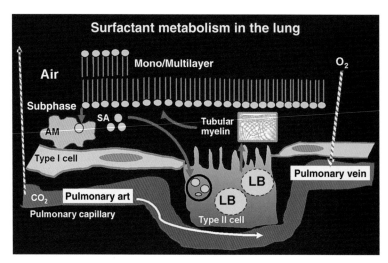

Fig. 24.2 Surfactant Metabolism. *AM*, alveolar macrophage; art; artery; *LB*, lamellar bodies; *SA*, small aggregate surfactant. Modified from Ramanathan R. Surfactants in the management of respiratory distress syndrome in extremely premature infants. J Pediatr Pharmacol Ther 2006;11:132–144 [4].

mono- or multilayers at the air–liquid interface, thus lowering surface tension.

3. **Recycling**: Residual surfactant is effectively recycled by endocytosis into type II pneumocytes, repackaged, and secreted again. Recycling decreases the need for de novo synthesis. Nearly 95% of the secreted surfactant is recycled. Exogenously administered surfactant is also recycled.

4. **Clearance**: Alveolar macrophages catabolize surfactant remnants, and some of the surfactant is lost in the exhaled gas.

5. Highest amount of surfactant is present at birth in term babies with 100 mg/kg, whereas estimated pool size in preterm neonates with RDS is about 3–5 mg/kg.

6. A number of conditions or hormones influence the surfactant metabolism. Factors that accelerate lung maturation are chronic maternal hypertension, intrauterine growth restriction, pregnancy-induced hypertension, chorioamnionitis, corticosteroids, thyroid hormones, beta-agonists, and methylxanthines. Similarly, a number of factors also delay lung maturation or surfactant production. These include uncontrolled or poorly controlled maternal diabetes, Rh isoimmunization, second-born twin, male sex, cesarean delivery, insulin, and androgens.

Surfactant functions

1. Reduction of surface tension
2. Increase in lung compliance
3. Decreased work of breathing
4. Prevention of alveolar collapse at end-expiration
5. Enhanced fluid clearance
6. Decreased opening pressure
7. Decreased precapillary tone
8. Host defense

Surfactant lowers the surface tension at the air–liquid interface dynamically. Surface tension is high when the alveolar diameter becomes smaller at the end of expiration. Infants with surfactant deficiency develop end-expiratory atelectasis. Relationship between collapsing pressure and surface tension is well described by **LaPlace equation: Pressure = 2 × Surface tension/radius**.

Pathophysiology of RDS

Inadequate surfactant synthesis in the premature infants leads to decreased lung compliance and lower end-expiratory volumes. Resulting atelectasis causes ventilation perfusion mismatch. This consequently leads to hypoxia and hypoventilation. Lung injury initiated by positive pressure ventilation and/or supplemental oxygen causes inflammation, mediated through cytokine release. Pulmonary edema is the end result of inflammation, with decreased pulmonary fluid clearance, and low urine output (Fig. 24.3). Surfactant inactivation also contributes toward development of RDS. Inactivation can occur secondary to the presence of blood or meconium in alveoli as well as mechanical ventilation (MV) causing mechanical stress and oxidation injury. Because of the developmental regulation of surfactant production and release, premature delivery is the most common cause of surfactant deficiency. In addition, mutations in the genes encoding surfactant proteins SP-B and

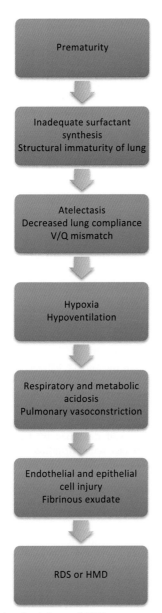

Fig. 24.3 Pathophysiology of RDS.

SP-C [5,6] and ABCA3 [7–10] may also cause surfactant deficiency with dysfunction, and respiratory failure especially in infants born late preterm or at term (Table 24.1).

Epidemiology of RDS

More than half of the infants born before 28 weeks of gestation develop RDS compared to about a third in infants born between 28 and 34 weeks of gestation (Fig. 24.4). RDS is the primary cause of death as well as disability in preterm infants. Extremely premature infants pose the highest risk for development of RDS occurring in more than 95% for infants born less than 26 weeks of gestation [11]. The incidence lowers with advancing gestational age manifesting in about 5%–10% of infants ≥34 weeks of gestation [12]. Additionally, up to 1% of the early term infants at 37 and 38 weeks of gestation also develop RDS (Fig. 24.4). Caucasian race and male sex pose additional risks at 34–39 weeks of gestation. Gestation age less than 39 weeks, operative delivery maternal diabetes, and maternal chorioamnionitis are also other risk factors in this cohort [13].

Prenatal diagnosis of RDS

RDS can be diagnosed prenatally using various tests done on amniotic fluid such as lecithin sphingomyelin ratio, phosphatidyl glycerol levels, and lamellar body counts [14] (Table 24.2). Although fetal lung maturity testing may help identify fetuses at risk of RDS, mature fetal pulmonary test results may not reliably predict other adverse outcomes and should not justify a delivery without other indications [15].

Clinical features

Symptoms can occur in most of the affected infants within minutes of birth in the delivery room as lung function is inadequate necessitating positive pressure support. Some infants in whom the surfactant inactivation occurs may not manifest at birth but slowly deteriorate over first few hours of life.

Presenting features

- Tachypnea
- Nasal flaring
- Grunting
- Intercostal and subcostal retractions
- Severe cases—apnea and cyanosis
- Physical examination—bilaterally decreased breath sounds on auscultation

Clinical course

Natural course of RDS includes deterioration for first 48–72 h followed by improvement due to synthesis of endogenous surfactant. With advent of exogenous surfactant, recovery could be faster with return of lung function within hours of its administration.

Table 24.1 Characteristics of European- and African-descent single ABCA3 mutations for neonatal RDS

Characteristic	European descent		P	African descent		P
	RDS (*n* = 112)	Non-RDS (*n* = 161)		RDS (*n* = 44)	Non-RDS (*n* = 196)	
Gender			0.51			<0.001
Female	47 (0.42)	74 (0.46)		10 (0.23)	101 (0.52)	
Male	65 (0.58)	87 (0.54)		34 (0.77)	95 (0.48)	
Gestational age, mean ± SD (weeks)	37.0 ± 1.7	38.2 ± 1.6	<0.001	37.6 ± 2.7	38.9 ± 1.7	0.003
Birth weight, mean ± SD (kg)	3.1 ± 0.6	3.1 ± 0.7	0.37	2.9 ± 1.0	3.1 ± 0.4	0.08
Route of delivery			0.54			<0.001
Vaginal	55 (0.49)	73 (0.45)		15 (0.34)	133 (0.68)	
Cesarean	57 (0.51)	88 (0.55)		29 (0.66)	63 (0.32)	

Source: Modified from Wambach JA, Wegner DJ, Depass K, Heins H, Druley TE, Mitra RD, et al. Single ABCA3 mutations increase risk for neonatal respiratory distress syndrome. Pediatrics 2012;130:e1575–e1582 [10].

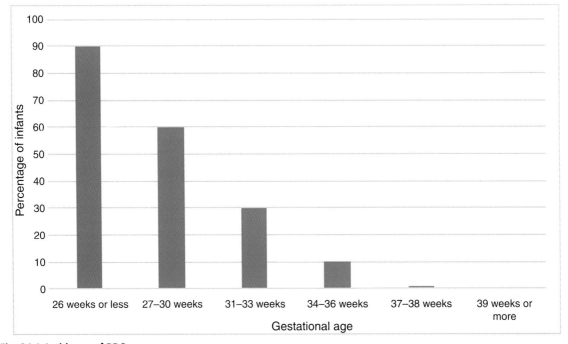

Fig. 24.4 Incidence of RDS.

Laboratory findings and diagnosis

Diagnosis is clinical with classic presentation of deterio-rating lung function after birth supported by radiological findings of homogenous reticulogranular or ground glass pattern in lung parenchyma with air bronchogram and low lung volume (Figs. 24.5 and 24.6). Blood gas findings include hypoxemia and hypercarbia. Lung ultrasound is also increasingly being used to make the diagnosis of RDS.

Table 24.2 Prenatal tests for fetal lung maturity

Amniotic fluid test	Predictive value of RDS (%)
L/S ratio >2.0	<0.5
L/S ratio <1.0	100
Phosphatidylglycerol (PG) present	<0.5
L/S ratio >2.0, no PG	>80
L/S ratio >2.0, PG+	0
L/S ratio >2.0 and diabetes or Rh isoimmunization	13
Lamellar body counts >50,000	0

L/S, Lecithin/Sphingomyelin

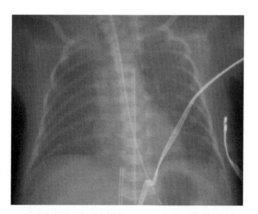

Fig. 24.5 Chest Radiograph Demonstrating Mild RDS.

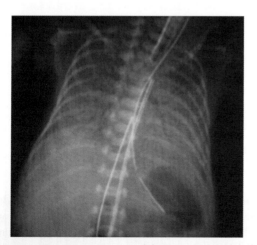

Fig. 24.6 Chest Radiograph Demonstrating Moderate-to-Severe RDS.

Differential diagnosis

Several conditions mimic RDS clinically but can be differentiated by radiologic as well as laboratory tests. Transient tachypnea of newborn usually occurs in more mature infants. It presents with milder symptoms and recovers early without needing much mechanical ventilator support. Pneumothorax is a complication of RDS secondary to rupture of alveoli and can be diagnosed radiologically with the presence of extrapulmonary air leak. Bacterial pneumonia with or without sepsis may have similar presentation and is generally difficult to distinguish, as both clinical and radiologic findings could be similar in both these conditions. Identification of bacteria in tracheal aspirate or blood culture may help point the correct diagnosis. Other rare pulmonary diseases such as congenital surfactant protein deficiency, pulmonary hypoplasia, and other anomalies sometimes mimic RDS presentation (Table 24.3).

Management of RDS

The aim of managing RDS is to enhance survival and minimize long-term adverse outcomes such as bronchopulmonary dysplasia (BPD). Many treatment strategies

Table 24.3 Differential diagnosis of RDS

Condition	How to differentiate
Transient tachypnea of newborn	Mature infants Milder symptoms Quicker recovery
Pneumothorax	Unequal breath sounds Glow on transillumination Air leak on x-ray
Bacterial pneumonia	Patchy infiltrates on chest x-ray; isolation of bacteria from tracheal aspirate Other systems affected Abnormal blood counts, elevated CRP
Pulmonary hypoplasia	History of anhydramnios or oligohydramnios Needs very high pressures Little improvement after surfactant Presence of PPHN
Lung anomalies	Prenatal diagnosis Radiological findings

CRP, C-reactive protein; *PPHN*, persistent pulmonary hypertension of newborn

Table 24.4 Management of RDS	
Timing	Strategies
Prenatal management	Vaginal progesterone in women with short cervix to prevent preterm delivery Antenatal corticosteroids (AS) Tocolysis to gain time to give AS
Delivery room management	Thermoneutral environment Use of blended gas CPAP/NIPPV Sustained inflation
Early treatment in NICU	Rescue surfactant therapy INSURE/minimally invasive technique
Treatment after stabilization	Noninvasive ventilation Caffeine administration Volume guarantee mode to decrease volutrauma Permissive hypercapnia Permissive hypoxemia Postnatal steroids in select cases
Supportive treatment	Maintain temperature 36.5–37.5°C Restricted fluid intake during the first 2 weeks Early optimized nutrition Exclusive breast milk-based nutrition Antibiotics only when necessary Maintain blood pressure and control PDA

INSURE, intubation surfactant extubation; *PDA*, patent ductus arteriosus

have evolved over last 4 decades. Several clinical trials are still continuing evaluating new therapies both for prevention and treatment. Summary of management is shown in Table 24.4.

Prenatal management

Management of RDS begins before birth if preterm delivery cannot be prevented. For impending preterm deliveries, interventions that prolong gestation even by few days may prepare the fetus for a better outcome. Diagnostic measures such as cervical length measurement and fetal fibronectin testing may help identifying imminent delivery and could be managed more aggressively [16]. Use of tocolytic medications may help delay in delivery allowing transfer to a center more equipped with the skilled personnel to take care of premature infants or allow time for the prenatal corticosteroid to have full effect [17].

Antenatal corticosteroid therapy

In 1969, Liggins found that preterm lambs had air in their lungs after pregnant sheep received dexamethasone [18]. The first randomized controlled trial was done by Liggins in 1972 in humans using betamethasone in 282 pregnant women with threatened or planned delivery prior to 37 weeks of gestation. The study showed sixfold decrease in RDS for infants born less than 32 weeks and overall mortality decreased by fivefold [19]. Since then, several studies have shown the benefits of using antenatal steroids in threatened preterm delivery. A recent Cochrane review compared the results from 30 studies which showed that the administration of corticosteroids decreased risk of perinatal death, neonatal death, RDS, and intraventricular hemorrhage in preterm infants [20].

Mechanisms of action

- Maturational changes in fetal lung architecture
- Increased synthesis of surfactant
- Increased release of surfactant

Recommendations

- All pregnant women between 23 and 34 weeks who are at risk of preterm delivery within the next 7 days to prevent or decrease the severity of neonatal RDS [21].
- A single course for pregnant women between 34 0/7 and 36 6/7 weeks of gestation at risk of preterm birth within 7 days, and who have not received a previous course of antenatal corticosteroids [22].
- A single repeat course of steroids may be considered if preterm birth does not occur within a week after the initial course and subsequent assessment demonstrates that there is a high risk of preterm birth in the next 7 days as recommended by WHO [23].

The optimal treatment to delivery interval is more than 24 hours and less than 7 days after the initiation of steroid treatment. Whether steroids should be repeated in 1 or 2 weeks after the first course for women with threatened preterm labor is debatable. Repeat courses have not shown any reduction in neonatal death, but have shown to reduce RDS and other short-term health problems at the cost of reduction in birth weight and paucity of long-term beneficial effects [24]. Repeat courses given after 32 weeks of gestation are unlikely to improve outcome, and have not shown any benefit by 5 years of age with regard to reduction in death or disability [25].

Delivery room management

Infants with RDS have difficulty maintaining oxygenation as well as ventilation after birth. Updated Neonatal

Resuscitation Program Guidelines were published in 2016, highlighting recent evidence-based approaches to assess and support infants during the immediate postnatal period [26]. Resuscitation training courses typically focus on infants with apnea secondary to prolonged hypoxia with the emphasis on achieving positive pressure ventilation by observing adequate chest rise, and identifying a baby to be well while monitoring oxygen saturations. Preterm infants with RDS may require more time to transition, and therefore one must limit exposing them to a minimum number of interventions that may cause harm [27].

Blended air and oxygen

Air is better than oxygen for resuscitation of term infants for reduced mortality, and 100% oxygen is harmful to the preterm infants, due to increased oxidative stress [28]. To achieve normal transitional oxygen saturations measured by pulse oximetry, extremely low birth weight infants usually require oxygen between 30% and 40% [29,30]. One should start with lower supplemental oxygen and increase as needed rather than starting with high and decreasing to reduce oxidative stress, although starting with 21% may not be possible for the most immature infants who may need at least around 30% oxygen. A recent meta-analysis did not show any difference in the risk of death or common preterm morbidities when comparing lower (30% or less) with higher (60% or more) FiO_2 in resuscitation of less than 29 weeks of gestation infants [31]. In our center, we typically start with room air (FiO_2 of 21%) during resuscitation and increase oxygen as needed. Our priority is to establish ventilation and increase heart rate to >100/min during resuscitation.

CPAP and NIV

To provide effective CPAP from birth, the T-piece device is a better choice than a self-inflating bag [32]. CPAP during stabilization can be delivered either by face mask or by a short nasal interface [33]. Our study showed use of modified nasal cannula provided adequate noninvasive support to decrease intubation rates in very low birth weight premature infants with RDS [34]. For spontaneously breathing preterm infants, provision of CPAP alone could be optimal, and use of positive pressure breaths may risk injury to the immature lung [35].

Sustained inflation

Sustained inflation has shown promising results in initial studies with improvement in heart rate and oxygen saturations, decreased need for intubation, and decreased duration MV [36–38]. Currently, use of sustained inflation during neonatal resuscitation has been limited to research studies. The Sustained Aeration of Infant's Lungs trial

involving 600 infants between gestational age of 23 and 26 weeks is currently underway [39].

Surfactant therapy: type, timing, technique for surfactant treatment

Exogenous surfactant therapy acutely improves pulmonary gas exchange until enough endogenous surfactant is produced in preterm infants. The use of exogenous surfactant to prevent and treat RDS has been the standard of care for more than 3 decades [40]. Several commercially available surfactants, both synthetic- and animal-derived, have been shown to be clinically effective for the treatment of RDS [41,42].

Types of surfactant

Synthetic surfactants

First-generation synthetic surfactants. First two studies published in the 1960s did not show any benefit when nebulized DPPC was administered to treat RDS [43,44]. This is because DPPC as a crystalline gel and rigid form at physiologic temperatures had difficulty adsorbing at the air–liquid interface. In 1987, a 10-center trial of a synthetic surfactant, pumactant (artificial lung expanding compound [ALEC]) composed of DPPC, and PG in very preterm infants showed significant reduction in mortality and respiratory support [45]. The development of alternate additives replacing roles of SP-B and SP-C, namely, tyloxapol and hexadecanol, led to production of first FDA-approved protein-free surfactant, colfosceril palmitate (Exosurf, Burroughs Wellcome, London, UK) for the treatment of RDS in the United States. Over next few years, several randomized clinical trials using Exosurf for the prevention and treatment of RDS showed significant reduction in neonatal and infant mortality as well as air leaks [46]. However, a meta-analysis in 2001 showed that treatment with these first-generation synthetic surfactants, such as colfosceril palmitate or pumactant, was associated with increased mortality and a greater risk of pneumothorax when compared to newer animal-derived surfactants [47]. The inferiority of first-generation synthetic surfactants was thought be related to lack of SP-B and SP-C.

Second-generation synthetic surfactants. Due to possibilities of infectious and antigenic complications from animal-derived surfactants, suboptimal response to first-generation synthetic surfactants, and high cost of their production, second-generation synthetic surfactants containing compounds similar to the structure and functions of SP-B or SP-C were developed. The main advantages of such

preparations were the consistency in the amounts of these compounds and the possibility of decreasing risks related to transmission of infections. The two synthetic surfactants that had undergone clinical trials were lusupultide (Venticute, Takeda Pharmaceuticals, Zurich, Switzerland) and lucinactant (Surfaxin; Discovery Laboratories, Warrington, PA). Lusupultide contains recombinant SP-C. It was not studied in neonates and was mainly used in clinical trials in adults with acute lung injury in which short-term benefits were not accompanied by improvements in survival [48]. Lucinactant contains two phospholipids, a fatty acid, and sinapultide (KL4), a 21-amino acid hydrophobic synthetic peptide, which has similar activity to SP-B. The US Food and Drug Administration approved use of lucinactant in 2012 [49]. Lucinactant was available as a gel formulation in single-use vials of 8.5 mL. When ready to administer, it required warming for 15 min in a dry block heater at 44°C. Free flowing suspension was formed after vigorous shaking and then allowed to cool to body temperature. The approved dose was 5.8 mL/kg to be administered intratracheally as frequently as every 6 h for up to 4 doses in the first 48 h of life [50].

Studies with synthetic- versus animal-derived surfactants

Lucinactant was compared to colfosceril palmitate and beractant in a trial enrolling 1294 infants who were ≤32 weeks of gestation [51]. Prophylactic surfactant was administered within the first 30 min of life. Significantly decreased rates of RDS at 24 h after birth were noted along with a significant reduction in RDS-related mortality in the lucinactant group. Lucinactant also reduced BPD rates at 36 weeks when compared to colfosceril palmitate. There was a significant reduction of RDS-related deaths in the lucinactant group when compared to beractant, and overall mortality was also marginally higher with beractant. However, no differences in other morbidities related to prematurity were seen between the lucinactant and beractant groups. The Surfaxin Therapy Against RDS (STAR) study compared lucinactant with poractant alpha in infants with gestational ages ranging from 24 to 28 weeks and birth weights 600–1250 g as a noninferiority trial. The study was stopped midway due to slow recruitment [52]. In these two published randomized trials, lucinactant has been shown to be safe and effective to reduce mortality associated with RDS [51,52]. These data suggest that this second-generation synthetic surfactant was comparable with animal-derived preparations in outcomes, and in fact, superior to first-generation synthetic surfactant. Difficulties with the use of lucinactant were its high viscosity at room temperature, the need for warming before its use, and the requirement of administering large volume. Lucinactant was withdrawn from the market in 2015. Currently, neither the first- nor the second-generation synthetic surfactants are available for intratracheal administration to treat RDS in the United States or elsewhere.

Animal-derived surfactants

Preclinical studies

In 1972, Enhorning and Robertson showed that preterm rabbits treated with natural surfactant containing both phospholipids and proteins improved the signs of RDS [53]. In 1973, they showed that pharyngeal deposition of natural surfactant was effective [54]. Adams et al. also demonstrated beneficial effects when natural bovine surfactant was instilled into the trachea of lambs in 1978 [55].

Clinical studies with animal-derived surfactants

The first successful exogenous surfactant administered in newborn infants with RDS was in 1980 in 10 preterm infants, with a surfactant prepared from minced bovine lungs (surfactant TA) [56]. After this report, several randomized, controlled, clinical trials have been performed involving bovine or porcine surfactants in preterm infants. Different animal-derived surfactants are available worldwide. Three major animal-derived surfactants studied have unique features, for example, lavage versus solvent extraction for calf lung surfactant extract (Infasurf, Forest Labs, New York, NY) and specific additives in the lipid extract of bovine mince, beractant (Survanta, Abbott Laboratories, Columbus, OH). Poractant alpha (Curosurf, Chiesi Farmaceutici, Parma, Italy), a porcine surfactant developed by Bengt Robertson and Tore Curstedt, was used in a pilot clinical trial in 1987 [57]. Poractant alpha undergoes an additional step, called liquid gel chromatography, resulting in pure form of polar lipids with a phospholipid concentration of 76 mg/mL. Furthermore, poractant alpha contains the highest concentration of DPPC, SP-B, and plasmalogen compared to beractant and calfactant [58] (Table 24.5). Poractant alpha is also the lowest viscosity surfactant making it ideal for less invasive surfactant treatment (LIST) techniques, with less reflux of the drug and better tolerance.

Bovine surfactants

Trials comparing beractant and calfactant have not demonstrated any significant differences in clinical outcomes or dosing-related complications. However, among infants treated for RDS, a subgroup of those who received calfactant had clinical improvement with longer interval between doses, a lower inspired oxygen concentration, and a lower mean airway pressure in the first 72 h of life compared to infants treated with beractant [59–61] (Table 24.6).

383

Table 24.5 Composition of commonly used surfactants worldwide

Surfactant	Preparation	Phospholipids (mg/mL)	DPPC (mg/mL)	Total proteins (mg/mL)	SP-B (mg/mL)	PLMGN (mol% total PL)
Poractant alpha (Curosurf)	Minced porcine lung extract—purified via liquid gel chromatography	76	30	1	0.45	3.8 ± 0.1
Beractant (Survanta)	Minced bovine lung extract/DPPC, palmitic acid, tripalmitin	25	11–15.5	<1	Not specified	1.5 ± 0.24
Calfactant (Infasurf)	Bovine lung lavage/DPPC, cholesterol	35	16	0.7	0.26	Not specified
CLSE BLES	Bovine lung lavage	27	Not Specified	0.176–0.5	Not Specified	Not specified

Composition of natural, modified surfactants.

DPPC, Dipalmytoylphosphatidylcholine; *PLMGN*, plasmalogen.

Source: Modified from Sardesai S, Biniwale M, Wertheimer F, Garingo A, Ramanathan R. Evolution of surfactant therapy for respiratory distress syndrome: past, present, and future. Pediatr Res 2017; 81:240–248 [58].

Table 24.6 Comparison of bovine versus bovine surfactant preparation: beractant versus calfactant

Trials (3)	N	Arm	GA	BW	Results
Bloom et al. [59]	374	Prophylaxis	≤29 weeks	<1250 g	Primary—no difference in need for second dose Secondary—CA: longer dosing interval after second dose
	608	Rescue	N/A	≤2000 g	Primary—no difference in need for third dose Secondary—CA: lower average FiO_2 requirement and MAP 0–72 h
Attar et al. [60]	40	Rescue	<37 weeks	N/A	Primary—no difference in lung compliance
Bloom and Clark [61]	749/2000	Prophylaxis	23–29 weeks	N/A	Primary—no difference in BPD at 36 weeks Early trial closure*
	1361/2080	Rescue	N/A	401–2000 g	Primary—no difference in BPD at 36 weeks Early trial closure*

Clinical outcomes in three comparative studies (rescue = 648). *Beractant (Survanta) versus Calfactant (Infasurf)*.

BW, birth weight; *GA*, gestational age.

*Early trial closure prevents us from either accepting or rejecting our null hypothesis.

Porcine surfactant

The first multicenter trial of poractant alpha showed reduced neonatal mortality as well as incidence of pulmonary interstitial emphysema (PIE) and pneumothorax after comparison with control group in preterm infants with severe RDS [62]. A second trial by Speer demonstrated efficacy of multiple doses of poractant alpha. There was a rapid improvement in oxygenation as reflected by a threefold increase in arterial to alveolar oxygen tension ratio within 5 min after surfactant instillation noted with additional doses. In addition, ventilatory requirement was reduced in the multiple-dose group [63]. Subsequent studies of poractant alpha showed that early treatment was favored than later administration [64–66].

Bovine versus porcine surfactant

Six randomized clinical trials comparing poractant alpha and beractant have been published to date [67–72] (Table 24.7).

All these studies showed faster weaning of oxygen and mean airway pressure, less need for 2 or more doses, less days on MV, lower mortality in ≤32 weeks of gestation infants, less air leaks and patent ductus arteriosus (PDA), and higher rates of survival without BPD with use of poractant alpha when compared to beractant treated infants. In a systematic review and meta-analysis of five randomized controlled trials, 529 infants were compared while receiving poractant alpha or beractant for rescue treatment. The incidence of oxygen dependence at a postmenstrual age of 36 weeks was similar in both groups. Infants treated with poractant alpha at 100 mg/

kg (low dose) or 200 mg/kg (high dose) showed statistically significant reductions in death, the need for redosing, oxygen requirements, duration of oxygen treatment, and duration of MV. The test of heterogeneity yielded positive results for the duration of oxygenation and ventilation. Deaths remained significantly low with poractant alpha compared to beractant. The need for redosing with high-dose poractant alpha was significantly less but not when low-dose of poractant alpha was used [73]. Many studies have shown that use of a higher dose is associated with better clinical outcomes with different surfactant preparations [74–77] (Table 24.8). Use of

Table 24.7 Clinical outcomes between bovine versus porcine surfactant: beractant versus poractant alpha

Trials (6)	Surfactant	N	Type	Patients	Results
Speer et al. [67]	PA versus BE	73	Tx	700–1500 g	PA: Lower FiO$_2$ PIP and MAP at 12–24 h
Baroutis et al. [68]	PA versus BE versus BO	80	Tx	<2000 g	PA: Fewer days on O$_2$ and PPV; decreased LOS
Ramanathan et al. [69]	PA versus BE	293	Tx	750–1750 g	PA: Lower FiO$_2$, fewer doses, decreased mortality <32 weeks
Malloy et al. [70]	PA versus BE	58	Tx	<37 weeks	PA: Lower FiO$_2$ up to 48 h, fewer doses, lower volume
Fujii et al. [71]	PA versus BE	52	Tx	<30 weeks	PA: Faster weaning, less air leaks, PDA, and MV at 72 h
Dizdar et al. [72]	PA versus BE	126	Tx	<37 weeks	PA: Faster weaning, fewer doses, rapid extubation, and higher survival free of BPD

Clinical outcomes in six comparative studies (rescue = 682). Poractant alpha (PA) (*Curosurf*) *versus* Beractant (BE) (*Survanta*).

BO, Bovactant (Alveofact); BPD, bronchopulmonary dysplasia; LOS, length of stay; MAP, mean airway pressure; MV, mechanical ventilation; PDA, patent ductus arteriosus; PIP, peak inspiratory pressure; PPV, positive pressure ventilation; Tx, rescue surfactant therapy.

Table 24.8 Better clinical outcomes with higher dose of surfactant preparations

Studies (5)	Low versus high dose	Surfactant studied	Results with high dose
Konishi et al. [74]	60 versus 120 mg/kg	Surfactant TA	Lower BPD ($P = 0.01$), IVH ($P = 0.047$) and longer duration of action ($P < 0.05$)
Dunn et al. [75] (single versus multiple doses—up to 4 doses), 30–36 weeks of GA	Single versus multiple doses	BLES 100 mg/kg	Multiple dose group: Faster weaning of oxygen, improved a/A ratio (70%—2 doses; 41%—3 doses; 11%—4 doses)
Speer et al. [63] (single vs. multiple doses)	Single versus multiple doses	Poractant alpha	Multiple dose group: Less PTX (18% vs. 9%; $P < 0.001$) and mortality 21% versus 13%; $P < 0.05$)
Halliday et al. [76] (mean dose in the low-dose group: 242 mg/kg)	Up to 300 versus 600 mg/kg	Poractant alpha	Less points on O$_2$ >40%; 48.4% versus 42.6%, $P < 0.01$
Gortner et al. [77]	50 versus 100 mg/kg	Alveofact	Improved oxygenation and less PIE

Higher dose is associated with better outcomes. Based on the evidence, European Consensus Guidelines (2016) recommends initial dose of 200 mg/kg of poractant alpha for early, rescue Rx of RDS. Also endorsed by European Association of Perinatal Medicine. "Dose-related response exists."

BPD, bronchopulmonary dysplasia; IVH, intraventricular hemorrhage; PTX, pneumothorax.

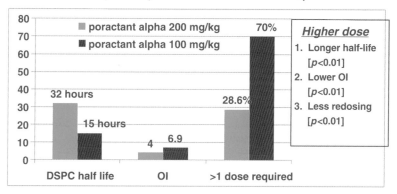

Fig. 24.7 Higher Dose of Poractant Alpha and Outcomes. *DSPC*, disaturated phosphatidylcholine; *OI*, oxygenation index. Modified from Cogo PE, Facco M, Simonato M, Verlato G, Rondina C, Baritussio A, et al. Dosing of porcine surfactant: effect on kinetics and gas exchange in respiratory distress syndrome. Pediatrics 2009;124:e950–e957 [78].

a higher dose of poractant alpha also results in longer half-life, lower oxygenation index and less need for redosing [78] (Fig. 24.7).

Another meta-analysis concluded that results of randomized, controlled trials of different preparations of animal-derived surfactants where poractant alpha reduced the need for repeat dosing, associated with fewer complications of administration, led to better short-term oxygenation and reduced the risk of mortality compared to beractant [79]. In the most recent (2015) Cochrane reviews, significant differences in outcomes were noted when trials of beractant were compared with poractant alpha including a significant increase in the risk of mortality prior to discharge, death, or oxygen requirement at 36 weeks of postmenstrual age, PDA requiring treatment, and patients receiving more than 1 dose of surfactant in infants treated with beractant compared with poractant alpha [80]. The difference in these outcomes was observed only in the studies using a higher initial dose of poractant alpha. Although these studies suggest that the differences observed between poractant alpha and beractant are related to the higher phospholipid dosage of the former, one cannot exclude that other factors such as animal source (porcine vs. bovine) or chemical composition may also have contributed to those findings (Table 24.9).

In a large retrospective study, Ramanathan et al. compared 14,173 infants treated with poractant alpha, calfactant, or beractant, and reported significantly higher mortality rates in infants treated with calfactant or beractant compared to poractant alpha-treated infants [81]. Overall mortality was lower in infants treated with poractant alpha (3.61%) compared to beractant (4.58%, $P = 0.053$) or calfactant (5.95%, $P = 0.043$). In infants with birth weights 500–749 g, a

Table 24.9 Bovine versus porcine surfactants: clinical outcomes—Cochrane reviews 2015

	RR (95% CI)	NNTH
Death before hospital discharge (9 studies, 901 infants)	1.44 (1.04–2.00)	20
Death before hospital discharge (with higher initial dose of PA)	1.62 (1.11–2.38)	16
Death or O_2 at 36 weeks' PMA (3 studies, 448 infants)	1.30 (1.04–1.64)	9
Death or O_2 at 36 weeks' PMA (with higher initial dose ≥100 mg/kg of PA)	1.39 (1.08–1.79)	7
>1 Dose of surfactant (6 studies, 786 infants)	1.57 (1.29–1.92)	7
PDA needing Rx (3 studies, 137 infants)	1.86 (1.28–2.70)	4

Beractant versus poractant alpha: Cochrane review 2015.

NNTH, Number needed to harm, with use of beractant; *PA*, poractant alpha; *PMA*, post menstrual age; *PDA*; patent ductus arteriosus; *RR*, relative risk.

Source: Modified from Singh N, Halliday HL, Stevens TP, Suresh G, Soll R, Rojas-Reyes MX. Comparison of animal-derived surfactants for the prevention and treatment of respiratory distress syndrome in preterm infants. Cochrane Database Syst Rev 2015;12:CD010249 [80].

significantly decreased mortality rate was observed for those treated with poractant alpha (11.72%) when compared with those treated with calfactant (20.67%, $P < 0.001$), or beractant (17.39%, $P < 0.011$). Another retrospective study evaluating comparative effectiveness between these three surfactants in 51,282 infants showed no differences in mortality [82]. However, more than 50% of the infants in this study were more than 31 weeks of gestation. In addition, all known confounders were not accounted for.

Third-generation synthetic surfactant

In animal studies, third-generation synthetic surfactant containing DPPC, 1-palmitoyl-2-oleoyl-PG (POPG), and SP-B and SP-C analogs has been shown to be superior, when compared to calfactant [83]. In a study with preterm lambs, a synthetic surfactant containing both SP-B and SP-C analogues (CHF 5633) resisted inactivation better than poractant alpha [84]. Phase I human clinical trial on synthetic surfactant CHF 5633 in RDS involved 40 preterm infants between gestational age of 27 and less than 34 weeks of gestation. The first 20 infants received CHF 5633 at the dose of 100 mg/kg and next 20 infants received the medication at 200 mg/kg. Both doses were well tolerated showing promising clinical efficacy [85]. A phase II multicenter double-blinded randomized controlled clinical trial comparing CHF 5633 with poractant alpha for RDS treatment is currently ongoing in the United States (ClinicalTrials.gov NCT02452476) [86].

Indications of surfactant administration

In 2014, American Academy of Pediatrics (AAP) and updated 2016 European Consensus Guidelines (ECG) recommended to initially provide nCPAP to all patients with RDS, and intubate and administer surfactant to those with persistent severe respiratory distress or who are apneic [87–89] (Table 24.10).

Subsequent surfactant administration may decrease mortality and morbidity in infants less than 30 weeks of gestation with RDS. Multiple doses using INSURE technique has

Table 24.10 Indications of surfactant treatment

Gestation age	FiO$_2$ requirement with CPAP/PPV
≤26 weeks	>30%
>26 weeks	>40%
Subsequent dose in all infants	Persistent requirement for oxygen >30%

also been successfully used and has not shown to worsen outcome [90]. Predicting who is likely to fail INSURE using clinical criteria and blood gases may help define a population that would be reasonable to maintain on MV [91].

European Consensus Guidelines for RDS management (2016 update) [89]

Babies with RDS should be given a natural surfactant:
1. Early rescue surfactant Rx if there is evidence of RDS or for ELBW infants whose mothers had not received AS or those intubated for stabilization.
2. ≤26 weeks with FiO$_2$ >0.30 and >26 weeks with FiO$_2$ >0.40 should be considered for early rescue surfactant.
3. Poractant alpha 200 mg/kg is better than 100 mg/kg of PA or beractant.
4. Consider INSURE and early extubation to NCPAP/NIPPV.
5. Less invasive surfactant administration (LISA) or minimally invasive surfactant (MIST) may be used as alternatives to INSURE for spontaneously breathing infants.
6. Caffeine should be considered for all babies <1250 g BW, who are on NCPAP/NIPPV.

Type of surfactant: Based on evidence, use of porcine surfactant, poractant alpha, at an initial dose of 200 mg/kg results in better outcomes and cost-effective, especially, in resource limited countries, mainly due to decreased need for redosing, less number of days on oxygen and MV, and less need for PDA treatment. All of these benefits contribute to reduce the cost of caring premature infant.

Timing of surfactant administration: prophylaxis versus rescue

Earlier studies in the 1990s when less than half of mothers received corticosteroids for lung maturity prior to delivery showed that prophylactic surfactant given within first 15 min of life in a fluid-filled lung had better distribution of surfactant and was associated with better outcomes than rescue therapy. With greater use of antenatal steroids and routine use of CPAP during the transitional period in the delivery room, prophylactic surfactant Rx is associated with more risk of death or BPD (risk ratio [RR]: 1.13, 95% CI: 1.02–1.25) [92]. In this population with a high usage of antenatal steroids and routine use of noninvasive ventilation (NIV) in the delivery room, **prophylactic surfactant therapy is no longer recommended.**

Timing of surfactant administration: early versus delayed rescue/selective surfactant Rx

In 1999, Verder in a clinical trial comparing early versus late selective surfactant administration in preterm infants on nasal CPAP randomized to receive intratracheal surfactant treatment when reaching lower versus higher oxygen requirement (FiO_2 0.37–0.55 vs. 0.56–0.77 for more than 30 min) showed that early rescue treatment was associated with significantly less need for intubation and/or death before 7 days of life or before discharge from the hospital [93] (Fig. 24.8A). Ten years later, in 2009, a similar clinical trial published from South America demonstrated significantly less need for intubation as well as less air leaks with early rescue treatment [94] (Fig. 24.8B). Decrease in the duration of MV is an important outcome especially when medical resources are limited and may result in less BPD in both developed and low resource areas.

Exact timing for administering surfactant remains unclear, especially in the infants receiving noninvasive ventilation. Less need for supplemental oxygen may not reflect the severity of RDS due to use of high pressures during NIPPV. We have observed faster weaning of oxygen when babies are on NIPPV compared to patients on NCPAP, likely due to use of higher mean airway pressure and better recruitment of alveoli (personal observation). Studies evaluating the timing based on oxygen requirement while on NIPPV are currently being evaluated. Future research should focus on optimizing timing for individual patients with not only oxygen requirement but also taking into the consideration of pressures required to keep alveoli open, adequacy of ventilation as well as oxygenation, and radiologic findings.

Timing of surfactant administration: beyond the first week of age

Late surfactant administration after the first week of life was recently evaluated in two randomized controlled trials [95,96]. Study by Ballard et al. in infants receiving inhaled nitric oxide (iNO) did not show any difference in BPD at 36 or at 40 weeks of corrected gestational age with the use of calfactant [95]; however, reduced respiratory morbidity prior to 1 year of age was noted in the study by Hascoe et al. in which these authors used 200 mg/kg of poractant alpha at 14 days of age, raising the possibility for long-term benefits of late surfactant therapy [96]. It appears that higher dose of poractant alpha both during the acute phase of RDS and evolving phase of BPD is beneficial in reducing chronic respiratory morbidity (CRM).

Early versus late selective surfactant Rx

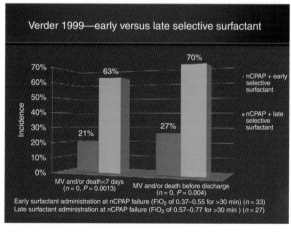

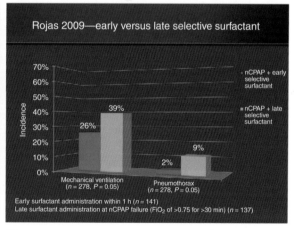

(A)   (B)

Fig. 24.8 (A–B) Comparison of early versus late surfactant therapy. Part A: Modified from Verder H, Albertsen P, Ebbesen F, Greisen G, Robertson B, Bertelsen A, et al. Nasal continuous positive airway pressure and early surfactant therapy for respiratory distress syndrome in newborns of less than 30 weeks' gestation. Pediatrics 1999;103:E24 [93]; part B: Modified from Rojas MA, Lozano JM, Rojas MX, Laughon M, Bose CL, Rondon MA, et al. Very early surfactant without mandatory ventilation in premature infants treated with early continuous positive airway pressure: a randomized, controlled trial. Pediatrics 2009;123:137–142 [94].

Techniques of surfactant administration: INSURE versus modified INSURE

Traditionally, surfactant was given to all preterm infants who were on MV due to respiratory failure from RDS. Currently, most preterm infants are placed on NIV support. The infants are intubated only to administer surfactant. At present, intubation, surfactant, and extubation (INSURE) technique first described more than 24 years ago by Verder has been very popular [97]. INSURE procedure involves intubation and surfactant administration using an endotracheal tube followed by extubation after a brief period of MV. The procedure minimizes the amount of invasive ventilation. But often, premedication with opioids is used during this procedure. Failure or reluctance to extubate following surfactant administration is not unusual. Leone et al. showed that INSURE technique led to more sustained oxygenation compared to rescue surfactant administration during invasive MV. In addition, premature infants treated with INSURE developed less respiratory comorbidities, including pneumothorax, BPD, and BPD or death [98]. A recent meta-analysis included nine clinical trials (1551 infants) and compared INSURE with CPAP alone. There were no statistically significant differences between early INSURE and CPAP alone for all outcomes such as combined outcome of BPD and/or death, BPD, death, air leaks, severe IVH, neurodevelopmental delay, or death and/or neurodevelopmental impairment [99]. Conclusion is that, "currently, no evidence suggests that either early INSURE or CPAP alone is superior to the other." There is concern that even a brief period of ventilation can induce lung injury in the vulnerable preterm lung. Furthermore, surfactant distribution may be suboptimal when surfactant is administered via positive pressure ventilation.

In premature infants with RDS, strategies to avoid intubation leading to invasive positive pressure and MV are now being sought. Intubation procedure may damage the larynx or trachea and requires the use of sedatives as well as pain medications risking undesirable side effects. Also, positive pressure and MV given even for a short period of time can damage the preterm lung and its avoidance altogether may potentially decrease the incidence of BPD.

Surfactant administration via laryngeal mask airway (LMA) has been described in several newer but small studies demonstrating safety and feasibility in larger preterm infants [100]. In a randomized trial of LMA compared to INSURE technique, Pinheiro showed decreased need for MV in the LMA group in preterm infants >29 weeks and birth weight >1000 g with moderate RDS. This technique is a potentially very good option in low-income countries with limited resources to administer surfactant [101] (Table 24.11).

Modified INSURE technique

Modified insure technique (*mINSURE*) typically involves surfactant administration using a small tube, like a feeding tube, angiocatheter, or a specially made small diameter catheter, while the baby is breathing spontaneously on NCPAP or NIPPV without premedication/sedation. This technique, also known as LISA, is currently being studied in many centers around the world. Several alternate names are used by various researchers to describe *mINSURE* technique [102] (Table 24.12). For example, MIST, avoidance of mechanical ventilation (AMV), surfactant without intubation (SWI), nonintubated surfactant application

Table 24.11 Comparison of surfactant administered via laryngeal mask airway to INSURE technique

	LMA (*n* = 30)	INSURE (*n* = 30)	*P*
BW, g	2118 (1150–3984)	1945 (1015–3700)	NS
GA, ≥33 weeks	63%	40%	NS
Antenatal steroids	50%	53%	NS
Mean age at randomization (h)	17.3 (3–43)	15.8 (3–42)	NS
Mean FiO$_2$ at Rx	0.37 (0.30–0.50)	0.38 (0.30–0.50)	0.003
Failure rate	30%	77%*	<0.0001

Surfactant via laryngeal mask airway versus INSURE via ETT (29–36 weeks of GA; BW >1000 g; FiO$_2$ 0.30–0.60; *n* = 60).

BW, birth weight; *GA*, gestational age; *INSURE*, intubation surfactant extubation; *LMA*, laryngeal mask airway; *Rx*, treatment.
*Atropine + morphine; LMA–atropine only; high failure rate in INUSRE is likely due to sedation; early failure = need for mechanical ventilation or use of naloxone (3% vs. 67%).
Source: Modified from Pinheiro JM, Santana-Rivas Q, Pezzano C. Randomized trial of laryngeal mask airway versus endotracheal intubation for surfactant delivery. J Perinatol 2016;36:196–201 [101].

Table 24.12 Techniques studied for minimally or less invasive surfactant therapy in spontaneously breathing preterm infants without using an endotracheal tube

Method	Tube/Catheter	Dose and mode of surfactant delivery	Premedication/Sedation
Cologne method [103]	4 or 5 Fr feeding tube	100 mg/kg, given over 1–3 min	Atropine, sedation and analgesia (optional)
SWI [104]	4 Fr Feeding tube	100 mg/kg given over 1–5 min	Atropine (optional)
Hobart method [105]	16 G Angiocath	100–200 mg/kg, given over 15–30 s	Sucrose
AMV/NINSAPP method [114]	Catheter using Magill forceps	100 mg/kg, given over 1–3 min	Atropine, sedation and analgesia (optional)
LISA [112]	1.3 mm diameter feeding tube using Magill forceps	200 mg/kg, given over 2–5 min	None
Take Care [111]	5 Fr feeding tube	100 mg/kg, given over 30–60 s	None
SONSURE [106]	4 Fr feeding tube	100 mg/kg, given over 1–3 min	Atropine
Karolinska method [107]	5 Fr × 30 cm catheter	Given over 30 s	Atropine, fentanyl
ECALMIST study [108]	17 G vascular catheter, 133 mm long	5 mL/kg, 0.25–0.5 mL bolus over 20–30 s	None
SAINT trial [107]	300 mm long catheter	Not specified	Narcotic analgesia
MiSurf trial [109]	Feeding tube	4 mL/kg	Not specified
Modified MIST procedure [110]	5 Fr orogastric tube	4 mL/kg, over 30–45 s	No sedation

Source: Modified from Sardesai S, Biniwale M, Wertheimer F, Garingo A, Ramanathan R. Evolution of surfactant therapy for respiratory distress syndrome: past, present, and future. Pediatr Res 2017; 81:240–248 [58].

(NINSAPP), Take Care method, Sonda Nasogastrica SURfactante Extubacion (SONSURE), Early CPAP and Large volume MIST (ECALMIST), and Minimally Invasive SURF administration (MISURF) are some of the terms used to describe this technique.

In Take Care technique for preterm infants on CPAP, Kanmaz compared surfactant administration using a 5F sterile flexible nasogastric tube during spontaneous breathing along with NCPAP (Take Care) with the INSURE procedure where brief oral intubation performed for surfactant administration. Duration of CPAP and MV were significantly shorter in the Take Care group compared to INSURE group. With decrease in the need for and duration of MV, there was a reduction of BPD rates in the Take Care group [111]. Klebermass–Schrehof assessed the results of LISA technique in a cohort of 224 between 23 and 27 weeks of gestation infants at a single-center. While comparing to historical controls, they found significantly higher survival rates (75.8% vs. 64.1%), less IVH (28.1% vs. 45.9%), less severe IVH (13.1% vs. 23.9%), and cystic periventricular leukomalacia (1.2% vs. 5.6%) in the infants treated with LISA method [112]. In another similar study by Krajewski, surfactant replacement therapy without intubation while receiving CPAP in preterm infants done with a thin endotracheal catheter was associated with significantly lower need for intubation and MV compared to the INSURE method (19.2% vs. 65%). In addition, better pulmonary outcomes were also noted with this new method of surfactant replacement. BPD in the studied group was significantly lower (15.4%) compared to the INSURE group (40%) [113]. In a recent multicenter trial from German neonatal network, NINSAPP technique in 211 preterm infants 23–26 weeks of gestation resulted in significantly higher combined survival without severe adverse events compared to surfactant via endotracheal tube in infants on MV [114]. In another study, MIST technique using an umbilical catheter inserted 2 cm below the vocal cords has been shown to result in a rapid and homogenous increase in end-expiratory lung volume and improved oxygenation [115].

Systematic review and meta-analysis of six randomized controlled trials using minimally invasive (mINSURE) or less invasive surfactant technique (LIST) to administer poractant alpha in premature infants with RDS resulted in decreased risks of BPD (RR = 0.71 [0.52–0.99]; NNT = 21), death or BPD (RR = 0.74 [0.58–0.94]; NNT = 15), and early CPAP failure or invasive ventilation requirements (RR = 0.67 [0.53–0.84]; NNT = 8 and RR = 0.69 [0.53–0.88]; NNT = 6). Compared to INSURE, LIST decreased the risks of BPD or death (RR = 0.63

[0.44–0.92]; NNT = 11) and of early CPAP failure (RR = 0.71 [0.53–0.96]; NNT = 11) [111,114,116–120].

In another meta-analysis, the use of LISA technique reduced the composite outcome of death or BPD at 36 weeks (RR = 0.75 [95% CI: 0.59–0.94], P = 0.01), BPD at 36 weeks among survivors (RR = 0.72 [0.53–0.97], P = 0.03), need for MV within 72 h of birth (RR = 0.71 [0.53–0.96], P = 0.02), or need for MV anytime during the neonatal intensive care unit stay (RR = 0.66 [0.47–0.93], P = 0.02). There were no differences noted for the outcome of death and other neonatal morbidities. Procedure failure rate on the first attempt and the need for additional doses of surfactant were not different between the intervention groups [121] (Table 24.13).

A large multinational multicenter randomized masked controlled trial in preterm infants 25–28 weeks of gestation comparing surfactant delivery using semirigid surfactant instillation catheter (Horbart method) to sham treatment is currently underway [122].

Collaborative Paired Trial Investigating MIST (OPTIMIST)

1. Multinational RCT
2. 25–28 weeks of gestational age on NCPAP/NIPPV
3. <6 h of age, on FIO$_2$ $\geq$0.30

4. MIST: Curosurf 200 mg/kg initial dose
5. Criteria for intubation: FIO$_2$ $\geq$0.45
6. Sample size: 606 (recruitment ongoing)

Further studies are needed to identify the safest instillation techniques, use of sedation or analgesia, choosing optimal surfactant dose, and selection of preterm infants who would benefit most.

Technique: We recommend *mINSURE* technique using atropine to prevent bradycardia during feeding tube or catheter placement, and also use sucrose for pain management during *mINSURE*.

Noninvasive surfactant treatment (NIST)

Aerosolized surfactant

Current focus is on identifying even more "gentler" methods to deliver surfactant such as via aerosolization, nebulization, or atomization. Potential advantages of administering aerosolized surfactant include ease of administration, avoidance of hypoxemia, more homogenous distribution, less likelihood of airway complications as well as MV, and less volume. Even though the animal studies have demonstrated promising results, there have been only as few

Table 24.13 Characteristics of studies comparing less invasive ventilation and INSURE technique

Studies (6); N = 895	Population/ Surfactant Rx	Criteria for surfactant Rx	LISA group	INSURE protocol	Premedication
Gopel et al. [116]	GA: 26–28 weeks; Germany—12 NICUs Curosurf/bovine 100 [80% Curosurf Rx]	NCPAP + FiO$_2$ $\geq$0.3 for LISA; variable FiO$_2$ for INSURE	N = 108; 2.5–5 Fr catheter; Magill forceps	N = 112; yes	±
Kanmaz et al. [111]	<32 weeks; Turkey— Curosurf 100	NCPAP + FiO$_2$ $\geq$0.4	N = 100; 5 Fr feeding tube	N = 100; yes	None
Mirnia et al. [117]	27–32 weeks; Iran—3 NICUs; Curosurf 200	NCPAP + FiO$_2$ $\geq$0.3	N = 66; 5 Fr feeding tube	N = 70; yes	Atropine
Bao et al. [118]	28–32 weeks; China—Curosurf 200	NCPAP + FiO$_2$ $\geq$0.3 or $\geq$0.35	N = 47; 16 g catheter	N = 43; yes	—
Mohammadizadeh et al. [119]	<34 weeks; Iran—2 NICUs; Curosurf 200	NCPAP + FiO$_2$ $\geq$0.3 and Silverman $\geq$5	N = 19; 4 Fr feeding tube; Magill forceps	N = 19; yes	Atropine
Kribs et al. [114]	23–27 weeks; Germany—13 NICUs; Curosurf 100	NCPAP + FiO$_2$ $\geq$0.3 and Silverman $\geq$5	N = 107; 4 Fr catheter; Magill forceps	N = 104; yes	±

LISA versus INSURE using Curosurf/NCPAP: meta-analysis.
LISA: Less need for PPV, reduction in death or BPD and BPD.

Source: Modified from Aldana-Aguirre JC, Pinto M, Featherstone RM, Kumar M. Less invasive surfactant administration versus intubation for surfactant delivery in preterm infants with respiratory distress syndrome: a systematic review and meta-analysis. Arch Dis Child Fetal Neonatal Ed 2017;102:F17–F23 [121].

clinical studies demonstrating efficacy using this route. Finer et al. published an open-label pilot study of aerosolized lucinactant in preterm neonates on CPAP to prevent RDS in 17 infants. They concluded that aerosolized surfactant could be safely given via CPAP as an alternative to surfactant administration via endotracheal tube [123]. Two doses of beractant administered as an aerosol using 100 mg phospholipid/kg or 200 mg phospholipid/kg is also currently being evaluated (NCT02294630) [124].

Combination therapies with surfactant

CRM can be caused by a combination of persistent inflammation, triggered by infection, MV, as well as oxygen. Resultant release of proinflammatory cytokines may lead to aberrant repair of the developing lung in preterm infants. Anti-inflammatory therapy in combination with surfactant may help decrease BPD, thus reducing CRM.

Surfactant as vehicle

Lung inflammation plays a crucial role in the pathogenesis of BPD and inhaled glucocorticoid treatment is one potential therapy to prevent BPD. In a pilot study by Yeh, early intratracheal instillation of budesonide using surfactant as a vehicle in 116 very low birth weight infants with severe radiographic evidence of RDS requiring MV resulted in significantly less death or BPD compared with infants in the control group who had received surfactant without budesonide [125]. Recently, same investigators completed a randomized multicenter study of using surfactant with budesonide in 265 very low birth weight infants. Death or BPD rate of 42% in the intervention group was significantly less compared to control group (66%) while number needed to treat to prevent death or BPD in intervention group was 4.1 (95% CI: 2.8–7.8, $P \leq 0.001$) [126] (Table 24.14). More studies are needed using this technique since both these studies had high BPD rates in the control population. In the future, intratracheal instillation of budesonide using surfactant as a vehicle may play a role due to anti-inflammatory effects leading to decrease I BPD rates in extremely low-birth-weight infants.

Surfactant with nitric oxide

In a trial, 85 extremely low birth weight infants ventilated at 7–14 days were randomly assigned to receive up to 5 doses of pulmonary surfactant protein B (SP-B) containing surfactant (calfactant) plus prolonged iNO compared with iNO alone. Clinical status and recovery of SP-B from tracheal aspirates were transiently improved. However, these effects waned after 1 day and favorable pulmonary effects were not maintained [127].

Recombinant club cell protein (rhCC-10)

Club cell protein-10 (CC-10) is one of the most abundant protein produced endogenously by airway epithelial cells and plays a significant role in the regulation of inflammatory responses, protection of structural integrity of pulmonary tissue while preserving pulmonary function during various insults by inhibiting NF-kB pathway in the airways. Preterm infants with RDS/BPD are deficient in CC-10. A phase II trial evaluating intratracheal use of rhCC-10 in surfactant treated preterm infants has been completed and results are pending (NCT 01941745) [128].

Pneumonia: Surfactant inactivation has also been associated with pneumonia [129,130]. In a small randomized trial, the subgroup of infants with sepsis showed improvement in oxygenation and decreased need for ECMO. Newborn infants with pneumonia or sepsis receiving surfactant also demonstrated improvement in gas exchange compared with infants who did not receive surfactant [129].

Table 24.14 Effect of intratracheal budesonide to prevent death or BPD				
	Surfactant + budesonide Rx (*n* = 131)	**Surfactant only** (*n* = 134)	**Risk ratio (95% CI)**	*P*
Death or BPD	42%	66%	0.58 (0.44–0.77)	<0.001 (NNT = 4.1 [2.8–7.8])

Early intratracheal budesonide [Pulmicort] (0.25 mg/kg) + surfactant (100 mg/kg) to prevent BPD in VLBW infants: RCT (*n* = 265).
Source: Modified from Yeh TF, Chen CM, Wu SY, Husan Z, Li TC, Hsieh WS, et al. Intratracheal administration of budesonide/surfactant to prevent bronchopulmonary dysplasia. Am J Respir Crit Care Med 2016;193:86–95 [126].

Pulmonary hemorrhage: Surfactant for treating pulmonary hemorrhage has been found to be beneficial in observational studies as the presence of blood in alveoli may inhibit surfactant function [131]. In another study, the surfactant therapy was found to be beneficial for severe pulmonary hemorrhage to improve lung function and shorten the duration of high oxygen requirement [132] (Table 24.15).

Hypoplastic lungs: Congenital diaphragmatic hernia-affected hypoplastic lung may have surfactant deficiency [133]. Surfactant treatment in a large series of infants with congenital diaphragmatic hernia failed to show any improvements in outcomes. On the contrary, the need for ECMO, the incidence of chronic lung disease, and mortality rates were increased when surfactant was administered [134,135].

Surfactant treatment for acute RDS (ARDS)

When to use?
1. Yes: MAS, pneumonia, sepsis-induced ARDS, SP-B deficiency, aspiration pneumonias, ECMO points with ARDS, pulmonary hemorrhage.
2. No: Congenital diaphragmatic hernia.
3. How to use? Bolus instillation.
4. What to use? Poractant alpha due to smaller volume, higher amount of DPPC, SP-B and plasmalogen, and lower viscosity.
5. Dose: 50–100 mg/kg/dose q 6–12 h.

Oxygen supplementation beyond stabilization during RDS management

There is ongoing debate to determine optimal saturation targets for preterm infants, avoiding negative effects of oxygen toxicity such as retinopathy of prematurity (ROP) balancing with negative effects of hypoxia leading to increased mortality or adverse neurodevelopmental outcome. The NeOProM collaboration analyzed the results of five large randomized clinical trials with similar study design from different parts of the world to give greater power to detect small yet important differences in outcomes such as mortality [136]. All these trials were designed comparing saturation targeting in a lower range (85%–89%) to a higher range (91%–95%) with blinded oximeters. The SUPPORT trial from the United States showed the low saturation group had decreased ROP, but a 3.7% increase in mortality [137]. When combined these data along with the UK and Australian BOOST-II trials confirmed the excess mortality in lower saturation group. Hence enrolment was stopped in the UK and Australia/New Zealand study [138]. Canadian Oxygen Trial neither reported any significant differences in death or significant neurodisability, nor any significant difference in ROP rates [139]. NeOProM meta-analysis (Neonatal Oxygenation Prospective Meta-analysis) confirmed that the lower oxygen saturation target range (85%–89%) was associated with a significant increased mortality, but there

Table 24.15 Study with surfactant for pulmonary hemorrhage showing improved oxygenation

	With surfactant Rx (n = 4)		Without surfactant Rx (n = 8)	
	AaDO$_2$	OI	AaDO$_2$	OI
GA (weeks)	27 (1.4)		27 (1.45)	NS
Birth weight (g)	903 (252)		859 (253)	NS
0–I h	563 (122)	37.8 (9.3)	525 (71)	28 (21)
1–2 h	465 (131)	29 (17)	489 (115)	27 (15)
2–4 h	335 (144)*	17 (7)	471 (136)	21 (15)
Time to reach FiO$_2$ <40% (h)	13 (11–16)†		41 (8–108)†	

Rx protocol: Intratracheal spraying of epinephrine (1:10,000) 0.5 mL diluted with 1 mL of air; HFOV, correction of DIC; surfactant Rx within 0.5–1.5 h of Hge.

Surfactant for pulmonary hemorrhage (VLBW; 2006–11; n = 12): improved oxygenation.
*Compared to 0–1 h data; P < 0.05.
†Two group comparison; P = 0.05.
Source: Modified from Yen TA, Wang CC, Hsieh WS, Chou HC, Chen CY, Isao PN. Short-term outcome of pulmonary hemorrhage in very-low-birth-weight preterm infants. Pediatr Neonatol 2013;54:330–334 [132].

Table 24.16 Death or disability risk at 18–24 months from NeOProM meta-analysis

SpO$_2$ (low vs. high)	85–89	91–95	RR (95% CI)	P value
BOOST (Australian trial) [138]	45%	40%	1.11 (0.97–1.27)	0.12
BOOST (UK trial) [138]	52%	47%	1.10 (0.98–1.26)	0.11
BOOST (New Zealand trial) [138]	39%	45%	0.88 (0.69–1.13)	0.31
COT (US and Canada trial) [139]	52%	50%	1.01 (0.91–1.13)	0.80
SUPPORT (US trial) [137]	59%	60%	0.99 (0.90–1.09)	0.89
Overall	51%	49%	1.04 (0.98–1.09)	0.20

RR, Relative risk.
Source: Modified from Askie LM, Darlow BA, Finer N, Schmidt B, Stenson B, Tarnow-Mordi W, et al. Neonatal oxygenation prospective meta-analysis (NeOProM) collaboration. Association between oxygen saturation targeting and death or disability in extremely preterm infants in the neonatal oxygenation prospective meta-analysis collaboration. JAMA 2018;319:2190–2201.

Table 24.17 Significant secondary outcomes from NeOProM meta-analysis

SpO$_2$ (low vs. high)	85–89	91–95	RR (95% CI)	P value
Death at corrected 18–24 months	19.9%	17.1%	1.17 (1.04–1.31)	0.01
ROP requiring treatment	10.9%	14.9%	0.74 (0.63–0.86)	<0.001
Severe NEC	9.2%	6.9%	1.33 (1.10–1.61)	0.003
Surgically treated PDA	11.4%	9.7%	1.18 (1.00–1.39)	0.046
Supplemental oxygen at PMA of 36 weeks	24.9%	30.2%	0.81 (0.74–0.90	<0.001

NEC, Necrotizing enterocolitis; *PMA'*, postmenstual age; *ROP*, retinopathy of prematurity; *RR*, relative risk.
Source: Modified from Askie LM, Darlow BA, Finer N, Schmidt B, Stenson B, Tarnow-Mordi W, et al. neonatal oxygenation prospective meta-analysis (NeOProM) collaboration. Association between oxygen saturation targeting and death or disability in extremely preterm infants in the neonatal oxygenation prospective meta-analysis collaboration. JAMA 2018;319:2190–2201.

was not any difference between both groups with regard to death or disability at 18–24 months. Prospectively planned meta-analysis of individual participant data from the five large randomized clinical trials enrolling infants born before 28 weeks of gestation (4965 infants) confirmed that there was no significant difference between a lower oxygen saturation (85%–89%) target range compared with a higher oxygen saturation (91%–95%) target range on the primary composite outcome of death or major disability at a corrected age of 18–24 months. The lower SpO$_2$ target range was associated with higher risk of death and necrotizing enterocolitis (NEC), but a lower risk of retinopathy of ROP treatment [140] (Tables 24.16 and 24.17).

Follow-up meta-analysis at 18–24 months from BOOST II, COT, and SUPPORT trials did not show any difference in mortality [141].

The ability to maintain saturations within the predefined target could pose a problem especially when saturations are constantly fluctuating. Many infants spend much time outside the target range, with frequent prolonged hypoxic and hyperoxic episodes [142]. Automated controlled oxygen delivery show promise in maintaining babies within the desired target range for more time compared to manual control [143]. We recently reported our results from a large retrospective study with using graded SpO$_2$ targeting. We used 85%–89% during phase I of ROP and 90%–94% during phase II ROP [144] (Table 24.18).

Table 24.18 Incidence of retinopathy of prematurity with graded oxygen saturations

Clinical outcomes	Group 1, 1995–2001 static SpO$_2$	Group 2, 2003–10 graded SpO$_2$	OR*	95% CI*	P*
Primary outcomes	n = 267	n = 220			
Severe ROP (stage III or higher)	48.3%	21.3%	0.18	(0.11–0.30)	<0.001
Laser treatment†	34.9%	19.7%	0.31	(0.18–0.52)	<0.001

Graded SpO$_2$ targeting and ROP.
*Adjusted values by logistic regression.
†One infant was treated with Bevacizumab (Avastin).
Data from Cayabyab R, Arora V, Wertheimer F, Durand M, Ramanathan R. Graded oxygen saturation targets and retinopathy of prematurity in extremely preterm infants. Pediatr Res 2016;80:401–406 [144].

Oxygen

With

Love

Keep my SpO$_2$:

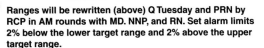

Ranges will be rewritten (above) Q Tuesday and PRN by RCP in AM rounds with MD. NNP, and RN. Set alarm limits 2% below the lower target range and 2% above the upper target range.

BW and/or GA at birth	Target SpO$_2$ from birth (phase I)	Target SpO$_2$ at PMA of: (phase II)
1. Less than 1250 g OR 2. Less than 29 0/7 weeks OR 3. Less than 1250 g and between 29 0/7 and 32 6/7 weeks	85%–89%	**33 0/7 to 35 6/7 weeks:** 90%–94% **36 0/7 weeks and above:** 94%–98%
More than 1250 g and between 29 0/7 and 32 6/7 weeks	90%–94%	
33 0/7 weeks and greater	94%–98%	

Fig. 24.9 Guidelines for Targeting Graded Oxygen Saturations in Newborn Intensive Care Unit.
Courtesy: Dr Ramanathan.

Our guidelines with graded SpO$_2$ targeting is shown in Fig. 24.9.

Caffeine therapy

Caffeine therapy has been the standard practice in many centers in the management of premature infants. The Caffeine for Apnea of Prematurity (CAP) trial showed that caffeine was associated with earlier extubation leading to reduction in BPD, and follow-up at 18 months showed a reduction in neurodisability [145]. Earlier rather than later caffeine administration has been supported by many studies to improve outcomes such as BPD [146–148]. The standard dose of caffeine citrate is 20 mg/kg loading followed by 5–10 mg/kg daily maintenance.

Permissive hypercapnia

Tolerating higher partial pressure of carbon dioxide (pCO_2) in mechanically ventilated, extremely low birth weight infants might reduce ventilator-induced lung injury and BPD. Post hoc analysis of data from the SUPPORT trial showed an association between higher $PaCO_2$ and risk of death, intraventricular hemorrhage, BPD and adverse neurodevelopmental outcome, highlighting the need for further evaluation of ideal $PaCO_2$ targets (SUPPORT trial). The PHELBI trial randomized ventilated preterm babies <29 weeks of gestation and <1000 g birth weight to two target $PaCO_2$ levels for the first 14 days of ventilation, the higher arm reaching about 10 kPa and the lower group about 8 kPa [149]. Targeting a higher pCO_2 did not decrease the rate of BPD or death in ventilated preterm infants. The rates of mortality, intraventricular hemorrhage, and retinopathy did not differ between groups.

Postnatal steroids

Strategies to reduce lung inflammation during the acute stage of RDS may potentially limit the time on MV. Postnatal dexamethasone decreased BPD, but its use declined dramatically with its association leading to increased risk of cerebral palsy [150]. On the contrary, BPD is also associated with adverse neurological outcome and the higher the risk of BPD, the more potential benefit there would come from a course of dexamethasone [151]. Low-dose dexamethasone (<0.2 mg/kg/day) is currently recommended for babies who remain intubated especially after 1–2 weeks [152]. Inhaled budesonide could be a viable alternative to systemic steroids and recent large RCT confirmed use of prophylactic inhaled budesonide reduced both persistent ductus arteriosus (PDA) and BPD [153].

Inhaled nitric oxide

Clinical trials have not shown any benefit when iNO was administered either as rescue or routine therapy in preterm infants with RDS for reducing mortality or the risk of BPD. Nitric oxide should not be used to treat preterm infants with RDS except in rare cases of pulmonary hypertension or hypoplasia [154].

Supportive management

In addition to managing ventilation, the infants with RDS also need to receive essential care in regard to metabolic, nutritional, and cardiovascular aspects. These measures help decrease morbidities by reduction in caloric spending as well as oxygen needs. Additionally, optimization of nutrition remains the key to the success while caring infants to provide not only enough energy for metabolic needs but also to enhance growth.

Temperature control

Maintaining body temperature 36.5 and 37.5 °C during delivery room stabilization as well as NICU admission is extremely important for infants with RDS. At the time of preterm birth, the labor and delivery units are advised to have environmental temperature to be above 25 °C. Initial stabilization of infants less than 32 weeks should be performed using a polyethylene bag under a radiant warmer [26]. Warming and humidification of gases required for stabilization have also shown to improve temperature [155]. Following admission to NICU, the premature infants should be managed in servo-controlled incubators set at 36.5 °C with high relative humidity to reduce insensible water losses [156]. For the very premature infants who have gelatinous skin, the humidity of 60%–80% is required initially and reduced over next 2 weeks as skin integrity improves. Infants should be maintained in a thermoneutral environment while maintaining the core temperature between 36.5 and 37.5 °C throughout the stay in NICU.

Fluid management

Maintaining fluid balance can be challenging as smallest infants may loose a very high amount of fluid through immature skin. Fluids need to be adjusted to maintain in a slightly negative balance. Excessive fluid intake can contribute toward increase the risk of PDA, NEC, and BPD [157]. Routine use of diuretics (particularly furosemide) in preterm infants with RDS should be avoided due to lack of benefit [158]. Often diuretic use leads to electrolyte abnormalities, especially hyponatremia and hypokalemia, due to urinary loss of sodium and potassium as well as hypochloremia which may enhance bicarbonate and carbon dioxide necessitating use of higher ventilator settings.

Nutrition

Parenteral nutrition should be started immediately after admission to NICU. Early initiation of amino acids leads to positive nitrogen balance [159], decreases time to regain

birth weight leading to enhanced weight gain at discharge [160]. Minimal enteral nutrition with breast milk should be initiated as soon as possible. Breast milk is the preferred option for initiation of feeding; however, if unavailable, then donor breast milk has been proven to be better than formula feeding as it has been shown to reduce the risk of NEC [161].

Use of antibiotics

Traditionally, it had been considered good practice to screen infants who present with early respiratory distress for infection as well as due to the fact that maternal infections may lead to premature birth; however, routine prolonged antibiotic use without any evidence of infection may be harmful and hence discouraged [162–164]. Antibiotic should be discontinued with negative blood culture results within 36–48 h along with reassuring serial blood counts and C-reactive protein measurements. It is not unreasonable to avoid routine antibiotics in preterm infants with RDS in low-risk situations such as planned delivery by elective cesarean section for maternal indications.

Cardiovascular management

In premature infants, blood pressure is lower in the first few hours of life and increases gradually over the first 24 h of life [165]. Blood pressure varies with gestational age as well as chronological age [166] (Table 24.19). Hypotension in infants with RDS may be contributed by hypovolemia, large left-to-right ductus shunts, or myocardial dysfunction. Hypovolemia can be minimized by delaying cord clamping. Dopamine has been shown to be more effective than dobutamine in increasing blood pressure and also can improve cerebral blood flow in hypotensive infants [167]. Epinephrine and hydrocortisone are generally required in

refractory hypotension when dopamine and dobutamine have failed to optimize blood pressure and systemic perfusion.

PDA in very preterm infants with RDS can cause low blood pressure, poor systemic tissue perfusion, pulmonary edema, and difficulty weaning from MV. Permissive tolerance of PDA not showing hemodynamic instabilty is an acceptable strategy as long as the infant is thriving, tolerating feeds, and requiring minimal respiratory support [168]. Cyclooxygenase inhibitors such as indomethacin or ibuprofen are usually successful in closing the duct. Surgical ligation of PDA is associated with worse long-term neurodevelopmental outcome. Surgery should only be considered after medical therapy has failed [169]. More recently, paracetamol has been shown to promote ductal closure, although more trials with long-term follow-up are needed before it can be routinely recommended [170].

Complications of RDS

With the advancement of therapies including antenatal steroids and surfactant administration, complications of RDS (Table 24.20) have largely been decreased. Complications may be related to natural progression of disease or due to therapeutic interventions such as placement of arterial catheters, supplemental oxygen, positive pressure ventilation, and the use of endotracheal tubes.

Endotracheal tube complications

Adverse events related to intubation could be as high as 40% in NICU [171]. Displacement or misplacement of the endotracheal tubes may occur on occasions. Endotracheal tube placement into right main stem bronchus is the most common complication, resulting in hyperinflation of the ventilated lung, whereas atelectasis occurs in the contralateral lung. The hyperinflation may further contribute to air leak. Other complications associated with intubation

Table 24.19 Gestational and postnatal age-dependent nomogram for mean blood pressure values in neonates during the first 3 days of life

Gestational age	At birth	12 h of age	24 h of age	36 h of age	48 h of age	60 h of age	72 h of age
23–26	23	24	25	26	28	29	30
27–32	29	30	32	33	34	35	36
33–36	35	36	37	38	40	41	43
37–43	43	44	45	46	47	49	50

Source: Adapted from Nuntnarumit P, Yang W, Bada-Ellzey HS. Blood pressure measurements in the newborn. Clin Perinatol 1999;26:981–996 [166].

Table 24.20 Complications of RDS

Complication	Diagnosis	Management
Endotracheal tube-related complications		
Atelectasis and hyperinflation	X-ray to confirm tube position	Adjust tube
Subglottic stenosis	Laryngoscopy	Best to avoid by limiting duration of intubation
Pulmonary air leak		See Air leaks syndrome chapter (Chapter 13b)
Pneumothorax	X-ray confirmation	Supportive management, needle aspiration or chest tube placement
Pneumomediastinum	X-ray confirmation	Supportive management
Pulmonary interstitial emphysema	X-ray confirmation	High-frequency ventilation preferred over conventional ventilation Low mean airway pressures
Bronchopleural fistula	X-ray confirmation and bubbling of intercostal drain	Supportive management (Section, Ventilatory Management of Complications of RDS)
Bronchopulmonary dysplasia	Oxygen requirement at 36 weeks of corrected gestation	See Bonchopulmonary dysplasia chapter (Chapter 27)

include subglottic stenosis and atelectasis after extubation [172]. Esophageal and pharyngeal perforations rarely occur, especially with inexperienced personnel or extremely fragile infants.

Pulmonary air leak

Pulmonary air leaks are common acute complications of RDS with a reported incidence of around 6.3% in low birth weight infants [173]. Air leaks are due to the rupture of overdistended alveoli, and may occur spontaneously or from positive pressure received with MV. The air may dissect toward the hilum, resulting in a pneumomediastinum, or into the pleural space, resulting in a pneumothorax. Less commonly, air may dissect into the pericardial space, subcutaneous tissue, or peritoneal space, which can lead to pneumopericardium, subcutaneous emphysema, and pneumoperitoneum, respectively. In the preterm infant, the perivascular connective tissue is more abundant and compliant, allowing air trapping in the perivascular space, which may result in PIE.

Pneumothorax can occur spontaneously, secondary to assisted ventilation with higher pressures especially with early gestational age infants or change in compliance after administration of surfactant in patients with RDS. Infants with developing PIE pose additional risk. Spontaneous pneumothorax may occur within first few breaths and may present with tachypnea, grunting, and retractions, and is very difficult to distinguish from RDS. Pneumothorax on patients already receiving ventilatory support is more pronounced with acute deterioration in vitals, namely, hypoxia, hypercapnia along with sudden increase in heart rate and decrease in blood pressure. Pneumothorax should be suspected in patients after receiving surfactant if there is sudden deterioration instead of improvement in oxygenation.

A bronchopleural fistula is a communication between the bronchial tree and pleural space. Clinically, it may be formed as a persistent air leak or a failure to reinflate the lung despite chest tube drainage for 24 h. The main problems with a large fistula in a ventilated patient are unable to deliver set tidal volume, inability to apply set PEEP, persistent lung atelectasis, and delayed weaning from MV.

Ventilator management of RDS

Noninvasive respiratory support

NIV is considered the preferred method of providing support to preterm infants with RDS, and includes CPAP, nasal intermittent positive pressure ventilation (NIPPV), and humidified oxygen delivered by high-flow nasal cannulae (HF). Traditionally, noninvasive methods were used as a step-down from ventilation through an endotracheal

tube, and initially CPAP was the only method used. Further studies showed that initiation of CPAP from delivery room rather than routine intubation for stabilization or prophylactic surfactant administration is better for minimizing lung injury [92].

NIPPV is also used as primary respiratory support in many centers, with conventional ventilators used to deliver peak inspiratory pressures, with or without synchronization, but through nasal prongs [174]. NIPPV has shown to reduce extubation failure, but has not consistently been beneficial in reducing BPD. Studies where NIPPV was most successful used synchronization of inspiratory pressure delivered through a signal from an abdominal Graseby capsule. These ventilators are not widely available, and delivering effective synchronization using flow sensors is challenging due to large leaks during CPAP, and it is unclear whether nonsynchronized NIPPV is effective [175].

The use of heated humidified HF as an alternative to CPAP has increased in popularity. A recent meta-analysis of 15 studies comparing HF with other modes of noninvasive respiratory support showed similar rates of efficacy to other forms of noninvasive respiratory support in preterm infants for preventing treatment failure, death, and CLD. Following extubation, HF was associated with less nasal trauma, and might be associated with reduced pneumothorax compared with nasal CPAP [176]. A potential mechanism may be carbon dioxide washout from the nasopharyngeal space; however, with higher flow rates there infant might receive additional CPAP. Flow rates of 4–8 L/min have been typically used, with weaning of flow rate determined clinically by FiO_2 levels remaining low and work of breathing. HF was used as primary mode of respiratory support in the delivery room in a small study showing feasibility [177], but in a large multicenter clinical trial HF used as primary support for preterm infants with respiratory distress, it resulted in a significantly higher rate of treatment failure than did CPAP (25.5% vs. 13.3%) [178]. Further evidence

is also required for evaluating the safety and efficacy of HF in extremely preterm and mildly preterm subgroups, and for comparing different HF devices.

Suggested high-flow cannula, CPAP, and NIPPV settings are shown below (Tables 24.21 and 24.22).

Mechanical ventilation strategies

About half of extremely preterm babies with RDS will not tolerate NIV and need to be intubated [179]. The goal of MV is to provide reasonable blood gas values without risking lung injury, or hypocarbia. The principle of MV is to provide stable airway, recruit lung by inflation and optimize lung volume. Hyperinflation increases the risk of air leaks including pneumothorax and PIE. Lower pressure, on the other hand, leads to atelectasis during expiration. Pressure-limited flow-cycled ventilation and volume-targeted ventilation are the most common modes used. Pressure-limited ventilation does not have any control over volume generated and potentially leads to excess of volume administration especially when the compliance changes after surfactant administration. Excessively high-tidal volumes may injure the lung due to volutrauma and also may lead to hypocarbia which can potentially lead to brain injury such as periventricular leukomalacia or intraventricular hemorrhage [180,181]. In contrast, low-tidal volumes cause uneven distribution, increase work of breathing, agitation of the infant leading to hypoventilation and hypercarbia. Volume-targeted mode may enable clinicians to ventilate with controlled tidal volumes and weaning of pressure as lung compliance improves. When compared to pressure-cycled ventilation, the volume targeted ventilation may reduce BPD or death and intraventricular hemorrhage, and decrease duration of MV [182,183]. Conventional ventilation settings are shown in Table 24.23.

Table 24.21 Continuous positive airway pressure and high-flow nasal cannula settings for RDS

Setting	Start	Increase	Maximum	Decrease	Minimum
CPAP PEEP	5 cmH$_2$O	FiO_2 >30% or signs of respiratory distress	7 cmH$_2$O	FiO_2 21%	4 cmH$_2$O
High flow	4–6 L/min	FiO_2 > 30% or signs of respiratory distress	8 L/min	FiO_2 <21%	
FiO_2	21%	Preductal saturation <85%	40%	Preductal saturation >90%	21%
Temperature			34–37°C		
Humidity			100% Relative humidity		

CPAP, Continuous positive airway pressure; FiO_2, fraction of inspired oxygen; PaO$_2$, partial pressure of arterial oxygen; PEEP, positive end expiratory pressure.

Table 24.22 Nonsynchronized noninvasive positive pressure settings for RDS

Setting	Start	Increase	Maximum	Decrease	Minimum
PEEP (cmH$_2$O)	5	FiO$_2$ > 30% or signs of respiratory distress	7	FiO$_2$ 21%	4
PIP (cmH$_2$O)	20	PCO$_2$ >55 mmHg	30–35	PCO$_2$ <45 mmHg	10
Rate (breaths/min)	40	PCO$_2$ >55 mmHg	50	PCO$_2$ <45 mmHg only after PIP = 10 cmH$_2$O	0 (CPAP)
iTime (s)	0.5	If needed to increase the number of supported breaths	1	Once stable, before weaning rate	0.5
FiO$_2$	21%	Preductal saturation <85%	50% (temporarily) Generally should be <40%	Preductal saturation >90%	21%
Temperature			34–37°C		
Humidity			100% Relative humidity		

FiO$_2$, Fraction of inspired oxygen; *PaO$_2$*, partial pressure of arterial oxygen; *PCO$_2$*, partial pressure of carbon dioxide; *PEEP*, positive end-expiratory pressure; *PIP*, peak inspiratory pressure; *iTime*, inspiratory time.

Table 24.23 Invasive positive pressure settings for RDS

Setting	Start	Increase	Maximum	Decrease	Minimum
PEEP (cmH$_2$O)	5	FiO$_2$ >30% or signs of respiratory distress	7	FiO$_2$ 21%	4
PIP (cmH$_2$O)	16	PCO$_2$ >55 mmHg	24–26	PCO$_2$ <45 mmHg	10
Rate (breaths/min)	30	PCO$_2$ >55 mmHg	40–45	PCO$_2$ <45 mmHg only after PIP = 10 cmH$_2$O	10–15
iTime (s)	0.3	If needed to increase the number of supported breaths	0.4	Once stable, before weaning rate	0.3
FiO$_2$	21%	Preductal saturation <85%	50% (temporarily) Generally should be <40%	Preductal saturation >90%	21%
Temperature			34–37°C		
Humidity			100% Relative humidity		

FiO$_2$, Fraction of inspired oxygen; *PaO$_2$*, partial pressure of arterial oxygen; *PCO$_2$*, partial pressure of carbon dioxide; ; *PEEP*, positive end-expiratory pressure; *PIP*, peak inspiratory pressure.

When high pressures are needed to achieve adequate lung inflation, high-frequency oscillatory ventilation (HFOV) is a preferred alternative to MV. HFOV allows gas exchange at very low-tidal volumes delivered at very fast rates while lungs held open at optimal inflation by a continuous distending pressure. A recently updated meta-analysis of RCTs comparing HFOV with conventional ventilation showed use of elective HFOV compared with CV resulted in a small reduction in the risk of BPD, but the evidence was weakened by the inconsistency of this effect

Table 24.24 High-frequency oscillator settings for RDS

Setting	Start	Increase	Maximum	Decrease	Minimum
MAP (P) (cmH$_2$O)	10–12 or ≥2 MAP on conventional ventilator	Hypoxemia (preductal saturation <85% and/or low lung volume (<8 ribs expanded)	As needed to achieve 10 ribs expansion	Overexpansion (>10 ribs expanded) or FiO$_2$ <30%	9
Amplitude (rP) (cmH$_2$O)	25 (adjust to obtain chest wiggle)	PCO$_2$ >55 mmHg	40–45	PCO$_2$ <45 mmHg	12
Frequency (Hz)	12–15	PCO$_2$ <45 mmHg (after adjusting amplitude)	15	PCO$_2$ >55 mmHg (after adjusting amplitude)	6–8
% Inspiratory time	33	Changes are generally not necessary			
Bias flow (L/min)	15	If unable to maintain desired MAP	20		15

FiO$_2$, Fraction of inspired oxygen; *MAP (P)*, mean airway pressure; *PCO$_2$*, partial pressure of carbon dioxide; *PIP*, peak inspiratory pressure.

across trials. In addition, the benefit could be counteracted by an increased risk of acute air leak. Adverse effects on short-term neurological outcomes had been observed in some studies, but these effects did not achieve overall significance. Most trials reporting long-term outcome had not identified any difference [184].

We found HFOV to be better in more severe cases of RDS in which risk of complication rates are high. Settings for HFOV can be found below (Table 24.24).

Infants refractory to HFOV or the ones more prone to get complications such as air leaks or PIE can be effectively managed with high-frequency jet ventilator (HFJV). Jet ventilators pose several theoretical advantages, including higher expiratory time, additional psi breaths and lower frequencies than HFOV. Following table shows settings for HFJV for managing infants with RDS (Table 24.25).

During ventilation hypocarbia as well as hypercarbia should be avoided because of their association with an increased risk of BPD, periventricular leukomalacia, and intraventricular hemorrhage, and continuous CO$_2$ assessment can be helpful especially during first few days of ventilation. Weaning of ventilation should be started immediately upon effective gas exchange and improvement of compliance. The volume-targeted mode is better as automatic weaning done by ventilator by a decrease in peak inspiratory pressure with improvement in compliance. Infants with RDS improve quickly following surfactant administration and can be extubated to no invasive mode. Extubating to a relatively higher level of CPAP pressure may improve the chance of successfully remaining off the ventilator [185].

Ventilatory management of complications of RDS

Management of pneumothorax is based on the cause and severity of illness. Most of the times pneumothorax is self-resolving and needs to be managed only by adjusting ventilatory support and careful monitoring. In infants receiving noninvasive or conventional ventilatory support, we tend to keep PIP as low as possible to keep tidal volumes around 3.5 mL/kg, decrease inspiratory time (0.3 s), and increase ventilator rate while maintaining on the same modality of respiratory support. Generally, pH is maintained at 7.25–7.3 and permissive hypercapnia with PCO$_2$ between 50 and 60 preferred to minimize further damage to the lungs. Tension pneumothorax requires needle aspiration followed by chest tube placement for reaccumulation of air. Persistent pneumothorax or sudden respiratory deterioration leading to hypoxia or hypercapnia is best managed by high-frequency ventilation. Absence of high PIP, very short absolute inspiratory time and small tidal volumes generated by HFV are key elements aiding the resolution.

Indications for HFOV:
- High PIP (>24 in preterm infants and >26 in term infants)
- MAP >11 to 12 on conventional ventilator
- FiO$_2$ >50% and rising with conventional ventilator with adequate lung expansion
- Persistent or recurrent air leaks
- Worsening PIE

Table 24.25 High-frequency jet ventilator settings for RDS

Setting	Start	Increase	Maximum	Decrease	Minimum
PEEP (cmH_2O)	7–12 or conventional ventilator MAP or <1–2 HFOV MAP	Hypoxemia (preductal saturation <85%), even if hyperexpanded or to maintain MAP when weaning PIP	As needed to achieve lung expansion and saturation goal	If cardiac output is impaired (i.e., small cardiac silhouette, decreased cardiac output) or if oxygenation is stable with FiO_2 <30%	6
Jet PIP (cmH_2O)	20 or <1–2 conventional PIP	PCO_2 >55 mmHg	40-45	PCO_2 <45 mmHg	16
Jet rate (breaths/min)	360	To decrease PCO_2 levels	420	Measured PEEP >2 cmH_2O over set PEEP or PCO_2 >55 mmHg (after adjusting PIP) or airtrapping/PIE changes	240
Jet iTime (s)	0.02	Changes are generally not necessary. May increase to 0.024 if PIP = 40 cmH_2O and PCO_2 >55 mmHg			
Backup PIP (cmH_2O)	Adequate for chest rise	To prevent atelectasis	1 <Jet PIP	Minimize to prevent lung injury	
Backup rate (breaths/min)	0–2	To prevent atelectasis No backup rate for infants with air leak	5	Once optimal PEEP is reached	0
Backup iTime (s)	0.4	Changes are generally not necessary			

HFOV, High-frequency oscillatory ventilator; *MAP*, mean airway pressure; *PaO₂*, partial pressure of arterial oxygen; *PCO₂*, partial pressure of carbon dioxide; *PEEP*, positive end-expiratory pressure; *PIP*, peak inspiratory pressure; *iTime*, inspiratory time.

Suggested starting HFOV settings are MAP same as or slightly lower than conventional ventilator around 8–9 cmH_2O, respiratory rate of 12–15 Hz with amplitude enough to give wiggle. Settings are gradually increased for lack of improvement. Infants are usually kept on HFOV till complete resolution of pneumothorax and quite often extubated directly to noninvasive support [186].

Infants with PIE are managed conservatively. The majority of these infants are extremely premature and already receiving high-ventilatory support. Most often these infants require switching ventilation to HFOV or HFJV. Lower peak pressures provided by high-frequency ventilators aide in decreasing air leak while healing distal airways [187]. Smaller infants may require higher amplitudes for gas exchange as distal airways collapse with lower pressures exacerbating gas trapping. MAP same as conventional ventilator is preferred but not always possible due to immature lungs. We tend to manage these infants by frequently adjusting amplitude to manage PCO_2 while keeping frequency same (12–15 Hz). Occasionally, frequency may need to be changed to 8–10 Hz instead of increasing MAP if oxygenation is not optimized.

We frequently use high-frequency jet ventilation for managing these infants who do not respond to HFOV.

This mode enhances ventilation at lower peak and mean airway pressures while keeping inspiratory time constant with more rapid resolution of PIE. Typically, MAP on HFJV is kept same as of previous modality and PIP is lowered as possible to give just enough delta P (PIP–PEEP) for PCO_2 clearance. Typical starting rates used are 360/min and may have to adjusted depending on PCO_2 and lung inflation while keeping inspiratory time at 0.02 s. One may have to decrease frequency further to 240/min for minimizing air trapping. Target pH is between 7.25 and 7.3, but rarely we tolerate down to 7.20 if infant's condition is critical. Permissive hypercapnia is preferred with PCO_2 values maintained between 55 and 65. Transiently one may have to tolerate increased FiO_2 requirements (0.5–0.75) in order to heal severe PIE while keeping PIP and PEEP low. Sigh breaths are not recommended for managing infants with air leaks. Localized PIE are managed by positioning the infant with affected side down to minimize lung aeration to that side. Severe cases may require selective bronchial intubation.

Management strategies for bronchopleural fistula include mainly conservative measures such as one or more large bore chest. In mechanically ventilated patients, the goal is to maintain adequate ventilation and

oxygenation while minimizing the fistula flow to allow the lung to heal. This may include strategies combining to reduce PIP, tidal volumes, respiratory rate, PEEP, and inspiratory times, and accepting permissive hypercapnia and lower oxygen saturations. Most air leaks will resolve spontaneously over a few days if the patient can be weaned onto spontaneous respiration without high levels of respiratory support. Small tears or punctures usually heal quickly, while larger structural damage to the lung or a major bronchus will not heal with conservative management, particularly if high pressures are required for adequate gas exchange. The use of HFV and differential lung ventilation through double-lumen tubes may be needed. For proximal leaks, fiberoptic bronchoscopy and direct application of sealants have been attempted with some success. Refractory cases may need to be repaired surgically by thoracoplasty, lung resection/stapling, pleural abrasion/decortication, or other techniques.

Summary and recommendations

- RDS is one of the most common diagnoses in premature infants in NICU.
- Diagnosis of RDS is mostly based on oxygen requirements.
- Use of antenatal steroids is essential in threatened preterm delivery.
- Delivery room CPAP and noninvasive ventilation need to be aggressively.
- Exogenous surfactant therapy has become one of the most common procedures performed for the treatment of RDS in preterm infants globally.
- Composition, timing, and techniques of administering surfactant have been evolving over time.
- INSURE method is currently preferable for surfactant administration.
- Prophylactic surfactant therapy may only have a limited role where antenatal corticosteroid administration rates are low.
- At present, animal-derived surfactants are the standard of care for RDS.
- One must limit MV for decreasing morbidities.
- Adjuvant therapies such as caffeine, volume-targeted mode of ventilation in intubated infants, permissive hypercapnia, and conservative use of oxygen remain key elements.
- Comprehensive treatment of infants with RDS includes optimal nutrition based on exclusive breast milk-based diet, thermoregulation and cardiovascular stability.
- Future research of surfactant therapy should focus on using surfactant as a vehicle to deliver anti-inflammatory molecules, and less invasive or noninvasive modes of surfactant administration.

Cases

Case 1

A 38-year-old G3P1 mom admitted to labor and delivery with chronic hypertension and intrauterine growth restricted fetus with absent end-diastolic blood flows at 25 weeks of gestation. Mom was admitted for blood pressure management and rule out preeclampsia. Mom had previous preterm delivery for preeclampsia at 26 weeks of gestational age. Mom reported that previous child was "healthy" and did not have any complications. Mom received 1 dose of betamethasone and magnesium sulfate started for neuroprotection.

Decision to proceed with c-section was secondary to mother's uncontrolled hypertension and HELLP syndrome. Infant was born by classical c-section. Obstetricians removed amniotic bag from uterus and delivered infant with the sac. Patient weighing 400 g was brought to radiant warmer at 25 s of life, placed in polyurethane bag with cord and placenta attached. Infant with weak cry, and so NIPPV initiated with Ram cannula (PIP of 25 and PEEP of 5). Heart rate at 1 min was less than 100. Pulse oximeter probe applied to right radial area, and orogastric tube was placed. The team was unable to acquire good reading from pulse oximeter probe until 2 of life. Unable to maintain adequate saturations despite holding mouth closed, so transitioned to NIPPV with mask and T-piece connector, to which she responded well. She was then transitioned back to NIPPV via Ram cannula requiring FiO_2 of 40% during transport over to NICU, but was quickly weaned back to 21% before moving her to the isolette.

Initially, infant was placed on NIPPV in NICU. Initial ABG on admission was pH 7.20/CO_2 62/BE-8. She developed desaturations increasing FiO_2 requirement to 70%. Intubated with 2.5 ETT and placed on SIMV with pressure support 20/5 rate 40. Infant was administered first dose of surfactant as infant was requiring higher FiO_2 on conventional ventilator. Chest X-ray was suggestive RDS (Fig. 24.10). Initially, baby responded to surfactant with chest X-ray showing better expansion and FiO_2 was weaned (Fig. 24.11).

Over next 2 days baby had CO_2 retention with ABG showing pH 7.14/CO_2 70/BE-8 and at this point infant's settings on conventional ventilator were pressures 24/6 rate 40 and FiO_2 60%. Respiratory support was changed to high-frequency oscillator as infant's mean airway pressure on conventional ventilator was too high (MAP = 11). Infant received additional 2 doses of surfactant over next 48 h secondary to worsening lung disease and increased settings on oscillator (MAP increased from 13 to 15, Amp increased from 20 to 24). Echocardiogram at this point showed large PDA with predominantly left to right shunting. Infant received two courses of indomethacin for PDA.

Infant continued to require high settings on oscillator MAP 15, Amp 24, Hz 12 and received additional dose of

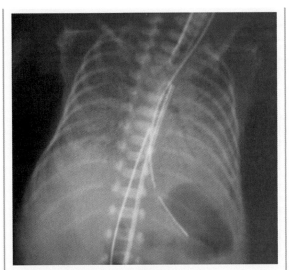

Fig. 24.10 **Intubated Preterm Infant Showing Moderate-to-Severe RDS.**

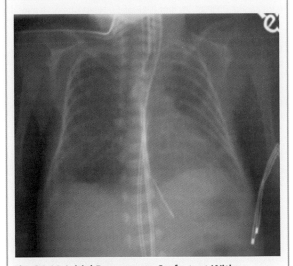

Fig. 24.11 **Initial Response to Surfactant With Improvement of Lung Aeration.**

surfactant as X-ray continued to suggest RDS (Fig. 24.12). Infant responded to this dose with improvement in CO_2 ABG 7.30/52/−2. Infant was weaned gradually to settings on MAP 10, Amp 16, and then was placed on conventional ventilator with settings of 24/6 rate 40. Patient was extubated after several days of stabilization and weaning on conventional ventilator pressures 18/6 rate 20 to NIPPV using Ram cannula at settings of 25/5 rate of 40 in FiO_2 of 30%. Ram cannula pressures were gradually weaned over next month while focusing on nutrition and growth. Feeding

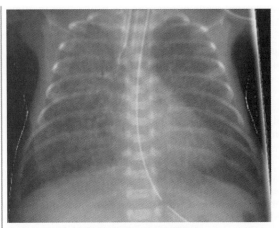

Fig. 24.12 **Worsening RDS on Oscillator.**

was established over next 2 weeks. Once the pressures were 10/5, rate was weaned by 2 every 12 h till rate of 10 was achieved.

Infant was transitioned to CPAP of 6 by 33 weeks of corrected gestation and was weaned to 2 L/min nasal cannula within days of switching to CPAP.

Infant was gradually weaned off nasal cannula over next 2 weeks. Baby had periods of desaturations especially with feeding over next 2 weeks. X-ray revealed residual lung disease (Fig. 24.13). With adequate nutrition and growth, infant improved with no episodes of desaturations by corrected 36 weeks of gestation. Baby passed oxygen challenge test and was discharged home not needing any supplemental oxygen.

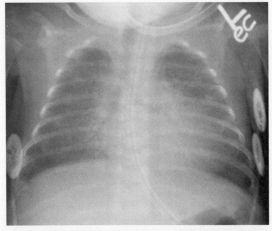

Fig. 24.13 **X-Ray at 2 months of Age Still Shows Residual Lung Disease.**

Case 2

A preterm 24 1/7-week-female child was born to a 16-year-old G2P2 mother. Mother had vaginal bleeding concerning for preterm labor versus vasa previa and was transferred to delivery hospital from outside hospital. She received betamethasone × 2 doses prior to transfer along with magnesium for neuroprotection and ampicillin. On admission to labor and delivery, mother began having contractions every 10–15 min and advanced overnight to every 2–5 min contractions.

Infant was born by spontaneous vaginal delivery. The patient weighing 600 g was brought to the warmer emergently without delayed cord clamping. Nuchal cord was noted upon delivery. The patient was placed in a bag and on a chemical mattress. She was dried and stimulated and bulb suctioned. Ram cannula was placed emergently after baby arrived at warmer, settings of 26/6, FiO_2 increased to 50% and then subsequently decreased with improving oxygen saturation. Heart rate initially less than 100 at 1 min, subsequently improved to more than 100 with NIPPV.

Patient transferred to NICU on NIPPV. Chest X-ray was suggestive of mild RDS (Fig. 24.14). Initial blood gas pH 7.26/50/-5. Infant received surfactant using INSURE technique. Over the first week of life infant's respiratory status improved. Echocardiogram showed moderate-to-large PDA requiring indomethacin treatment.

Second week of life infant was noted to have increased work of breathing requiring intubation (Fig. 24.15) and received two additional doses of surfactant. Infant was placed conventional ventilator SIMV with pressure support on settings of 24/6 rate of 30 FiO_2 between 21% and 30% and I-time 0.3 s. Over next 24 h infant deteriorated with chest radiograph, showing changes suggestive of

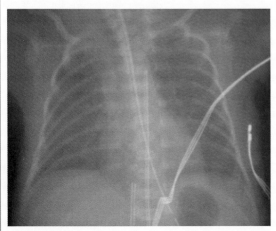

Fig. 24.14 Premature Infant Showing Signs of RDS on First Day of Life.

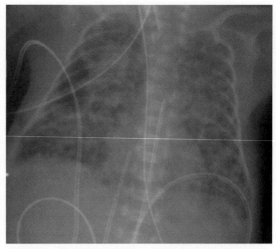

Fig. 24.15 Worsening RDS in Second Week of Life in Premature Infant.

reticulogranular pattern and ABG 7.16/68/−7. Endotracheal tube cultures revealed klebsiella pneumoniae requiring IV cefotaxime.

Infant was switched to high-frequency oscillator due to retained CO_2 (ABG 7.22/66/−6.5) despite high settings on conventional ventilator (pressures 25/6 rate 40, MAP 11, FiO_2 50%). Setting at start of HFOV were MAP 13, Amp 24, Hz 15. Over next week lungs started appearing cystic. High mean airway pressures on high-frequency oscillator (MAP 16, Amp 30, Hz 10) in the infant with high FiO_2 50%–70% warranted switching to high-frequency jet ventilator (Jet PEEP 14, PIP 36, rate 360). Echocardiogram was done at this point revealed large PDA. Despite medical treatment PDA did not close. Surgical ligation of PDA was done secondary to worsening pulmonary and hemodynamic status.

Infant received a 9-day course of dexamethasone (starting dose 0.1 mg/kg/day two divided doses tapering every 3 days) for imminent BPD (Fig. 24.16). Baby responded partially (ABG 7.32/56/+4) and was weaned to conventional ventilator. But infant was placed back on jet ventilator due to respiratory deterioration (ABG 7.26/64/+3). Feeding was established while continuing respiratory support with jet ventilator. With resolution of infection, no PDA and tolerance of feeding infant's condition improved. With another course of dexamethasone infant was gradually weaned off jet ventilator and extubated to NIPPV.

Over next month NIPPV was weaned off to nasal cannula. Infant was also started on diuretics and inhaled steroids with bronchodilators. Infant slowly improved respiratory desaturations and stabilized to go home on low-flow oxygen (Fig. 24.17). Echocardiogram did not show any pulmonary hypertension.

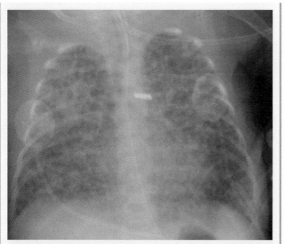

Fig. 24.16 **Cystic Changes in Premature Infant Evolving BPD.**

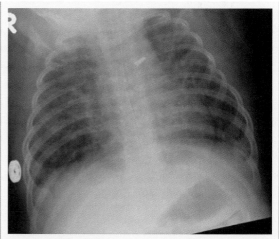

Fig. 24.17 **Mild BPD in Premature Infant Corrected to Term at Discharge.**

References

[1] Hamm H, Fabel H, Bartsch W. The surfactant system of the adult lung: physiology and clinical perspectives. Clin Invest 1992;70: 637–657.

[2] Jobe AH, Ikegami M. Biology of surfactant. Clin Perinatol 2001;28: 655–669.

[3] Whitsett JA, Weaver TE. Hydrophobic surfactant proteins in lung function and disease. N Engl J Med 2002;347:2141–2148.

[4] Ramanathan R. Surfactants in the management of respiratory distress syndrome in extremely premature infants. J Pediatr Pharmacol Ther 2006;11:132–144.

[5] Nogee LM, Garnier G, Dietz HC, Singer L, Murphy AM, deMello DE, et al. A mutation in the surfactant protein B gene responsible for fatal neonatal respiratory disease in multiple kindreds. J Clin Invest 1994;93:1860–1863.

[6] Nogee LM, Dunbar AE 3rd, Wert SE, Askin F, Hamvas A, Whitsett JA. A mutation in the surfactant protein C gene associated with familial interstitial lung disease. N Engl J Med 2001;344:573–579.

[7] Shulenin S, Nogee LM, Annilo T, Wert SE, whitsett JA, Dean M. ABCA3 gene mutations in newborns with fatal surfactant deficiency. N Engl J Med 2004;350:1296–1303.

[8] Somaschini M, Nogee LM, Sassi I, Danhaive O, Presi S, Boldrini R, et al. Unexplained neonatal respiratory distress due to congenital surfactant deficiency. J Pediatr 2007;150:649–653.

[9] Wert SE, Whitsett JA, Nogee LM. Genetic disorders of surfactant dysfunction. Pediatr Dev Pathol 2009;12:253–274.

[10] Wambach JA, Wegner DJ, Depass K, Heins H, Druley TE, Mitra RD, et al. Single ABCA3 mutations increase risk for neonatal respiratory distress syndrome. Pediatrics 2012;130:e1575–e1582.

[11] Stoll BJ, Hansen NI, Bell EF, Shankaran S, Laptook AR, Walsh MC, et al. Neonatal outcomes of extremely preterm infants from the NICHD Neonatal Research Network. Pediatrics 2010;126:443–456.

[12] Hibbard JU, Wilkins I, Sun L, Gregory K, Haberman S, Consortium on Safe Labor. et al. Respiratory morbidity in late preterm births. JAMA 2010;304:419–425.

[13] Anadkat JS, Kuzniewicz MW, Chaudhari BP, Cole FS, Hamvas A. Increased risk for respiratory distress among white, male, late preterm and term infants. J Perinatol 2012;32: 780–785.

[14] Grenache DG, Gronowski AM. Fetal lung maturity. Clin Biochem 2006;39:1–10.

[15] The American College of Obstetricians and Gynecologists Committee on Obstetric Practice and the Society for Maternal–Fetal Medicine. Committee opinion no. 561: nonmedically indicated early-term deliveries. Obstet Gynecol 2013;121:911–915.

[16] Van Baaren GJ, Vis JY, Wilms FF, Oudijk MA, Kwee A, Porath MM, et al. Predictive value of cervical length measurement and fibronectin testing in threatened preterm labor. Obstet Gynecol 2014;123:1185–1192.

[17] Haas DM, Caldwell DM, Kirkpatrick P, McIntosh JJ, Welton NJ. Tocolytic therapy for preterm delivery: systematic review and network meta-analysis. BMJ 2012;345:e6226.

[18] Liggins GC. Premature delivery of foetal lambs infused with glucocorticoids. J Endocrinol 1969;45:515–523.

[19] Liggins GC, Howie RN. A controlled trial of antepartum glucocorticoid treatment for prevention of the respiratory distress syndrome in premature infants. Pediatrics 1972;50:515–525.

[20] Roberts D, Brown J, Medley N, Dalziel SR. Antenatal corticosteroids for accelerating fetal lung maturation for women at risk of preterm birth. Cochrane Database Syst Rev 2017;3:CD004454.

[21] El-Sayed YY, Borders AEB, Gyamfi-Bannerman C. Committee on Obstetric Practice. Committee opinion no. 713: antenatal corticosteroid therapy for fetal maturation. Obstet Gynecol 2017;130:e102–e109.

[22] Gyamfi-Bannerman C, Thom EA, Blackwell SC, Tita AT, Reddy UM, Saade GR, et al. Antenatal betamethasone for women at risk for late preterm delivery. N Engl J Med 2016;374:1311–1320.

[23] World Health Organization. WHO recommendations on interventions to improve preterm birth outcomes. Geneva: WHO; 2015.

[24] Crowther CA, McKinlay CJD, Middleton P, Harding JE. Repeat doses of prenatal corticosteroids for women at risk of preterm birth for improving neonatal health outcomes. Cochrane Database Syst Rev 2015;7:CD003935.

[25] Asztalos EV, Murphy KE, Willan AR, Matthews SG, Ohlsson A, Saigal S, et al. Multiple courses of antenatal corticosteroids for preterm birth study: outcomes in children at 5 years of age (MACS-5). JAMA Pediatr 2013;167:1102–1110.

[26] Wyckoff MH, Aziz K, Escobedo MB, Kapadia VS, Kattwinkel J, Perlman JM, et al. Part 13: neonatal resuscitation: 2015 American Heart Association Guidelines Update for Cardiopulmonary Resuscitation and Emergency Cardiovascular Care. Circulation 2015;132:S543–S560.

[27] Saugstad OD. Delivery room management of term and preterm newly born infants. Neonatology 2015;107:365–371.

[28] Saugstad OD, Aune D, Aguar M, Kapadia V, Finer N, Vento M. Systematic review and meta-analysis of optimal initial fraction of oxygen levels in the delivery room at ≤32 weeks. Acta Paediatr 2014;103: 744–751.

[29] Vento M, Cubells E, Escobar JJ, Escrig R, Aguar M, Brugada M, et al. Oxygen saturation after birth in preterm infants treated with continuous positive airway pressure and air: assessment of gender differences and comparison with a published nomogram. Arch Dis Child Fetal Neonatal Ed 2013;98:F228–F232.

[30] Kapadia VS, Chalak LF, Sparks JE, Allen JR, Savani RC, Wyckoff MH. Resuscitation of preterm neonates with limited versus high oxygen strategy. Pediatrics 2013;132:e1488–e1496.

[31] Oei JL, Vento M, Rabi Y, Wright I, Finer N, Rich W, et al. Higher or lower oxygen for delivery room resuscitation of preterm infants below 28 completed weeks gestation: a meta-analysis. Arch Dis Child Fetal Neonatal Ed 2017;102:F24–F30.

[32] Szyld E, Aguilar A, Musante GA, Vain N, Prudent L, Fabres J, et al. Delivery Room Ventilation Devices Trial Group: comparison of devices for newborn ventilation in the delivery room. J Pediatr 2014;165:234–239.

[33] McCarthy LK, Twomey AR, Molloy EJ, Murphy JF, O'Donnell CP. A randomized trial of nasal prong or face mask for respiratory support for preterm newborns. Pediatrics 2013;132:e389–e395.

[34] Biniwale M, Wertheimer F. Decrease in delivery room intubation rates after use of nasal intermittent positive pressure ventilation in the delivery room for resuscitation of very low birth weight infants. Resuscitation 2017;116:33–38.

[35] Jobe AH, Ikegami M. Mechanisms initiating lung injury in the preterm. Early Hum Dev 1998;53:81–94.

[36] Ngan AY, Cheung PY, Hudson-Mason A, O'Reilly M, van Os S, Kumar M, et al. Using exhaled CO_2 to guide initial respiratory support at birth: a randomised controlled trial. Arch Dis Child Fetal Neonatal Ed 2017;102:F525–F531.

[37] Jiravisitkul P, Rattanasiri S, Nuntnarumit P. Randomised controlled trial of sustained lung inflation for resuscitation of preterm infants in the delivery room. Resuscitation 2017;111:68–73.

[38] El-Chimi MS, Awad HA, El-Gammasy TM, El-Farghali OG, Sallam MT, Shinkar DM. Sustained versus intermittent lung inflation for resuscitation of preterm infants: a randomized controlled trial. J Matern Fetal Neonatal Med 2017;30:1273–1278.

[39] Foglia EE, Owen LS, Thio M, Ratcliffe SJ, Lista G, Te Pas A, et al. Sustained aeration of infant lungs (SAIL) trial: study protocol for a randomized controlled trial. Trials 2015;16:95.

[40] Jobe AH. Pharmacology review: why surfactant works for respiratory distress syndrome. NeoReviews 2006;7:e95–e106.

[41] Soll R. Synthetic surfactant for respiratory distress syndrome in preterm infants. Cochrane Database Syst Rev 1998;3:CD001149.

[42] Seger N, Soll R. Animal derived surfactant extract for treatment of respiratory distress syndrome. Cochrane Database Syst Rev 2009;2:CD007836.

[43] Robillard E, Alarie Y, Dagenais-Perusse P, Baril E, Guilbeault A. Microaerosol administration of synthetic beta-gamma-dipalmitoyl-l-alpha-lecithin in the respiratory distress syndome: a preliminary report. Can Med Assoc J 1964;90:55–57.

[44] Chu J, Clements JA, Cotton EK, Klaus MH, Sweet AY, Tooley WH, et al. Neonatal pulmonary ischemia. I. Clinical and physiological studies. Pediatrics 1967;40:S709–S782.

[45] Ten Centre Study group. Ten centre trial of artificial surfactant (artificial lung expanding compound) in very premature babies. Br Med J 1987;294:991–996.

[46] Soll RF. Prophylactic synthetic surfactant for preventing morbidity and mortality in preterm infants. Cochrane Database Syst Rev 2000;2:CD001079.

[47] Soll RF, Blanco F. Natural surfactant extract versus synthetic surfactant for neonatal respiratory distress syndrome. Cochrane Database of Syst Rev 2001;2:CD000144.

[48] Spragg RG, Lewis JF, Walmrath HD, et al. Effect of recombinant surfactant protein C-based surfactant on the acute respiratory distress syndrome. N Engl J Med 2004;351:884–892.

[49] Discovery Labs. Surfaxin (lucinactant) intratracheal suspension. www.accessdata.fda.gov. (complete prescribing information.) Ref:3097860.

[50] Revak SD, Merritt TA, Cochrane CG, Heldt GP, Alberts MS, Anderson DW, et al. Efficacy of synthetic peptide-containing surfactant in the treatment of respiratory distress syndrome in preterm infant rhesus monkeys. Pediatr Res 1996;39:715–724.

[51] Moya FR, Gadzinowski J, Bancalari E, Salinas V, Kopelman B, Bancalari A, et al. International Surfaxin Collaborative Study Group. A multicenter, randomized, masked, comparison trial of lucinactant, colfosceril palmitate, and beractant for the prevention of respiratory

distress syndrome among very preterm infants. Pediatrics 2005;115:1018–1029.

[52] Sinha SK, Lacaze-Masmonteil T, Valls i Soler A, wiswell TE, Gdzinowski J, Hajdu J, et al. Surfaxin Therapy Against Respiratory Distress Syndrome Collaborative Group. A multicenter, randomized, controlled trial of lucinactant versus poractant alfa among very premature infants at high risk for respiratory distress syndrome. Pediatrics 2005;115: 1030–1038.

[53] Enhörning G, Robertson B. Lung expansion in the premature rabbit fetus after tracheal deposition of surfactant. Pediatrics 1972;50:58–66.

[54] Enhörning G, Grossmann G, Robertson B. Pharyngeal deposition of surfactant in the premature rabbit fetus. Biol Neonate 1973;22:126–132.

[55] Adams FH, Towers B, Osher AB, Ikegami M, Fujiwara T, Nozaki M. Effects of tracheal instillation of natural surfactant in premature lambs. I. Clinical and autopsy findings. Pediatr Res 1978;12:841–848.

[56] Fujiwara T, Maeta H, Chida S, Morita T, Watabe Y, Abe T. Artificial surfactant therapy in hyaline-membrane disease. Lancet 1980;1:55–59.

[57] Noack G, Berggren P, Curstedt T, Grossmann G, Herin P, Mortensson W, et al. Severe neonatal respiratory distress syndrome treated with the isolated phospholipid fraction of natural surfactant. Acta Paediatr Scand 1987;76:697–705.

[58] Sardesai S, Biniwale M, Wertheimer F, Garingo A, Ramanathan R. Evolution of surfactant therapy for respiratory distress syndrome: past, present, and future. Pediatr Res 2017;81:240–248.

[59] Bloom BT, Kattwinkel J, Hall RT, et al. Comparison of Infasurf (calf lung surfactant extract) to Survanta (beractant) in the treatment and prevention of respiratory distress syndrome. Pediatrics 1997;100: 31–38.

[60] Attar MA, Becker MA, Dechert RE, Donn SM. Immediate changes in lung compliance following natural surfactant administration in premature infants with respiratory distress syndrome: a controlled trial. J Perinatol 2004;24:626–630.

[61] Bloom BT, Clark RH. Infasurf Survanta Clinical Trial Group. Comparison of Infasurf (calfactant) and Survanta (beractant) in the prevention and treatment of respiratory distress

syndrome. Pediatrics 2005;116:392–399.

[62] Collaborative European Multicenter Study Group. Surfactant replacement therapy for severe neonatal respiratory distress syndrome: an international randomised clinical trial. Pediatrics 1988;82:683–691.

[63] Speer CP, Robertson B, Curstedt T, et al. Randomized European multicenter trial of surfactant replacement therapy for severe neonatal respiratory distress syndrome: single versus multiple doses of Curosurf. Pediatrics 1992;89:13–20.

[64] Egberts J, de Winter JP, Sedin G, et al. Comparison of prophylaxis and rescue treatment with Curosurf in neonates less than 30 weeks' gestation: a randomized trial. Pediatrics 1993;92:768–774.

[65] Walti H, Paris-Llado J, Bréart G, Couchard M. Porcine surfactant replacement therapy in newborns of 25-31 weeks' gestation: a randomized, multicentre trial of prophylaxis versus rescue with multiple low doses. The French Collaborative Multicentre Study Group. Acta Paediatr 1995;84:913–921.

[66] Bevilacqua G, Parmigiani S, Robertson B. Prophylaxis of respiratory distress syndrome by treatment with modified porcine surfactant at birth: a multicentre prospective randomized trial. J Perinat Med 1996;24:609–620.

[67] Speer CP, Gefeller O, Groneck P, et al. Randomised clinical trial of two treatment regimens of natural surfactant preparations in neonatal respiratory distress syndrome. Arch Dis Child Fetal Neonatal Ed 1995;72:F8–F13.

[68] Baroutis G, Kaleyias J, Liarou T, Papathoma E, Hatzistamatiou Z, Costalos C. Comparison of three treatment regimens of natural surfactant preparations in neonatal respiratory distress syndrome. Eur J Pediatr 2003;162:476–480.

[69] Ramanathan R, Rasmussen MR, Gerstmann DR, Finer N, Sekar K. North American Study Group. A randomized, multicenter masked comparison trial of poractant alfa (Curosurf) versus beractant (Survanta) in the treatment of respiratory distress syndrome in preterm infants. Am J Perinatol 2004;21:109–119.

[70] Malloy CA, Nicoski P, Muraskas JK. A randomized trial comparing beractant and poractant treatment in neonatal

respiratory distress syndrome. Acta Paediatr 2005;94:779–784.

[71] Fujii AM, Patel SM, Allen R, Doros G, Guo CY, Testa S. Poractant alfa and beractant treatment of very premature infants with respiratory distress syndrome. J Perinatol 2010;30:665–670.

[72] Dizdar EA, Sari FN, Aydemir C, et al. A randomized, controlled trial of poractant alfa versus beractant in the treatment of preterm infants with respiratory distress syndrome. Am J Perinatol 2012;29:95–100.

[73] Singh N, Hawley KL, Viswanathan K. Efficacy of porcine versus bovine surfactants for preterm newborns with respiratory distress syndrome: systematic review and meta-analysis. Pediatrics 2011;128:e1588–e1595.

[74] Konishi M, Fujiwara T, Naito T, Takeuchi Y, Ogawa Y, Inukai K, et al. Surfactant replacement therapy in neonatal respiratory distress syndrome. A multi-centre, randomized clinical trial: comparison of high-versus low-dose of surfactant TA. Eur J Pediatr 1988;147:20–25.

[75] Dunn MS, Shennan AT, Possmayer F. Single- versus multiple-dose surfactant replacement therapy in neonates of 30 to 36 weeks' gestation with respiratory distress syndrome. Pediatrics 1990;86:564–571.

[76] Halliday HL, Tarnow-Mordi WO, Corcoran JD, Patterson CC. Multicentre randomised trial comparing high and low dose surfactant regimens for the treatment of respiratory distress syndrome (the Curosurf 4 trial). Arch Dis Child 1993;69:276–280.

[77] Gortner L, Pohlandt F, Bartmann P, Bernsau U, Porz F, Hellwege HH, et al. High-dose versus low-dose bovine surfactant treatment in very premature infants. Acta Paediatr 1994;83: 135–141.

[78] Cogo PE, Facco M, Simonato M, Verlato G, Rondina C, Baritussio A, et al. Dosing of porcine surfactant: effect on kinetics and gas exchange in respiratory distress syndrome. Pediatrics 2009;124:e950–e957.

[79] Fox GF, Sothinathan U. The choice of surfactant for treatment of respiratory distress syndrome in preterm infants: a review of the evidence. Infant 2005;1:8–12.

[80] Singh N, Halliday HL, Stevens TP, Suresh G, Soll R, Rojas-Reyes MX. Comparison of animal-derived surfactants for the prevention and

treatment of respiratory distress syndrome in preterm infants. Cochrane Database Syst Rev 2015;12:CD010249.

[81] Ramanathan R, Bhatia JJ, Sekar K, Ernst FR. Mortality in preterm infants with respiratory distress syndrome treated with poractant alfa, calfactant or beractant: a retrospective study. J Perinatol 2013;33:119–125.

[82] Trembath A, Hornik CP, Clark R, Smith PB, Daniels J, Laughon M. Best Pharmaceuticals for Children Act—Pediatric Trials Network. Comparative effectiveness of surfactant preparations in premature infants. J Pediatr 2013;163. 955.e1–960.e1.

[83] Walther FJ, Hernández-Juviel JM, Gordon LM, Waring AJ. Synthetic surfactant containing SP-B and SP-C mimics is superior to single-peptide formulations in rabbits with chemical acute lung injury. PeerJ 2014;2:e393.

[84] Seehase M, Collins JJ, Kuypers E, Jellema RK, Ophelders DRMG, Ospina OL, et al. New surfactant with SP-B and C analogs gives survival benefit after inactivation in preterm lambs. PLoS One 2012;7:e47631.

[85] Sweet DG, Turner MA, Straňák Z, Plavka R, Clarke P, Stenson BJ, et al. A first-in-human clinical study of a new SP-B and SP-C enriched synthetic surfactant (CHF5633) in preterm babies with respiratory distress syndrome. Arch Dis Child Fetal Neonatal Ed 2017;102:F497–F503.

[86] A Double Blind, randomized, controlled Study to Compare CHF 5633 (Synthetic Surfactant) and Poractant Alfa in RDS. ClinicalTrials. gov NCT02452476.

[87] Committee on Fetus and Newborn, American Academy of Pediatrics. Respiratory support in preterm infants at birth. Pediatrics 2014;133:171–174.

[88] Sweet DG, Carnielli V, Greisen G, Hallman M, Ozek E, Plavka R, et al. European Consensus Guidelines on the Management of Respiratory Distress Syndrome—2016 Update. Neonatology 2017;111:107–125.

[89] Polin RA, Carlo WA. Committee on Fetus and Newborn, American Academy of Pediatrics. Surfactant replacement therapy for preterm and term neonates with respiratory distress. Pediatrics 2014;133:156–163.

[90] Dani C, Corsini I, Poggi C. Risk factors for intubation-surfactant-extubation (INSURE) failure and multiple INSURE strategy in preterm infants. Early Hum Dev 2012;88:S3–S4.

[91] Brix N, Sellmer A, Jensen MS, Pedersen LV, Henriksen TB. Predictors for an unsuccessful INtubation-SURfactant-Extubation procedure: a cohort study. BMC Pediatr 2014;14:155.

[92] Rojas-Reyes MX, Morley CJ, Soll RF. Prophylactic versus selective use of surfactant in preventing morbidity and mortality in preterm infants. Cochrane Database Syst Rev 2012;3:CD000510.

[93] Verder H, Albertsen P, Ebbesen F, Greisen G, Robertson B, Bertelsen A, et al. Nasal continuous positive airway pressure and early surfactant therapy for respiratory distress syndrome in newborns of less than 30 weeks' gestation. Pediatrics 1999;103:E24.

[94] Rojas MA, Lozano JM, Rojas MX, Laughon M, Bose CL, Rondon MA, et al. Colombian Neonatal Research Network. Very early surfactant without mandatory ventilation in premature infants treated with early continuous positive airway pressure: a randomized, controlled trial. Pediatrics 2009;123:137–142.

[95] Ballard RA, Keller RL, Black DM, Ballard PL, Merrill JD, Eichenwald EC, et al. TOLSURF Study Group. Randomized trial of late surfactant treatment in ventilated preterm infants receiving inhaled nitric oxide. J Pediatr 2016;168. 23. e4–29.e4.

[96] Hascoët JM, Picaud JC, Ligi I, Blanc T, Moreau F, Pinturier MF, et al. Late surfactant administration in very preterm neonates with prolonged respiratory distress and pulmonary outcome at 1 year of age: a randomized clinical trial. JAMA Pediatr 2016;170:365–372.

[97] Verder H, Agertoft L, Albertsen P, Christensen NC, Curstedt T, Ebbesen F, et al. [Surfactant treatment of newborn infants with respiratory distress syndrome primarily treated with nasal continuous positive airway pressure. A pilot study]. Ugeskr Laeger 1992;154:2136–2139.

[98] Leone F, Trevisanuto D, Cavallin F, Parotto M, Zanardo V. Efficacy of INSURE during nasal CPAP in preterm infants with respiratory distress syndrome. Minerva Pediatr 2013;65:187–192.

[99] Isayama T, Chai-Adisaksopha C, McDonald SD. Noninvasive ventilation with vs without early surfactant to prevent chronic lung disease in preterm

infants: a systematic review and meta-analysis. JAMA Pediatr 2015;169:731–739.

[100] Attridge JT, Stewart C, Stukenborg GJ, Kattwinkel J. Administration of rescue surfactant by laryngeal mask airway: lessons from a pilot trial. Am J Perinatol 2013;30:201–206.

[101] Pinheiro JM, Santana-Rivas Q, Pezzano C. Randomized trial of laryngeal mask airway versus endotracheal intubation for surfactant delivery. J Perinatol 2016;36:196–201.

[102] More K, Sakhuja P, Shah PS. Minimally invasive surfactant administration in preterm infants: a meta-narrative review. JAMA Pediatr 2014;168:901–908.

[103] Kribs A, Pillekamp F, Hünseler C, Vierzig A, Roth B. Early administration of surfactant in spontaneous breathing with nCPAP: feasibility and outcome in extremely premature infants (postmenstrual age </ = 27 weeks). Paediatr Anaesth 2007;17:364–369.

[104] Vik SD, Vik T, Lydersen S, Støen R. Case-control study demonstrates that surfactant without intubation delayed mechanical ventilation in preterm infants. Acta Paediatr 2017;106:554–560.

[105] Dargaville PA, Aiyappan A, De Paoli AG, et al. Minimally-invasive surfactant therapy in preterm infants on continuous positive airway pressure. Arch Dis Child Fetal Neonatal Ed 2013;98:F122-F126.

[106] Aguar M, Cernada M, Brugada M, Gimeno A, Gutierrez A, Vento M. Minimally invasive surfactant therapy with a gastric tube is as effective as the intubation, surfactant, and extubation technique in preterm babies. Acta Paediatr 2014;103: e229–e233.

[107] Aguar M, Vento M, Dargaville PA. Minimally invasive surfactant therapy: an update. NeoReviews 2014;15:e275–e285.

[108] Seshia M, Ethawi YA, Hussain A, Minski J, Miller J, Alvaro R. Large volume surfactant administration in preterm infants using minimally invasive technique (ECALMIST; Early CPAP and Large Volume Minimal Invasive Surfactant Therapy). Abstract 2012.

[109] El Helou S. MISurf Versus InSurE. A Comparison of Minimally Invasive Surfactant Application Techniques in Preterm Infants

(MIsurf). ClinicalTrials.gov Identifier: NCT01615016.

[110] Tomar RS, Ghuliani R, Yadav D. Effect of surfactant therapy using orogastric tube for tracheal catheterization in preterm newborns with respiratory distress. Indian J Pediatr 2017;84:257–261.

[111] Kanmaz HG, Erdeve O, Canpolat FE, Mutlu B, Dilmen U. Surfactant administration via thin catheter during spontaneous breathing: randomized controlled trial. Pediatrics 2013;131:e502–e509.

[112] Klebermass-Schrehof K, Wald M, Schwindt J, Grill A, Prusa AR, Haiden N, et al. Less invasive surfactant administration in extremely preterm infants: impact on mortality and morbidity. Neonatology 2013;103:252–258.

[113] Krajewski P, Chudzik A, Strzałko-Głoskowska B, Gorska M, Kmiecik M, Wieckowska K, et al. Surfactant administration without intubation in preterm infants with respiratory distress syndrome–our experiences. J Matern Fetal Neonatal Med 2015;28:1161–1164.

[114] Kribs A, Roll C, Göpel W, Wieg C, Groneck P, Laux R, et al. NINSAPP Trial Investigators. Nonintubated surfactant application vs conventional therapy in extremely preterm infants: a randomized clinical trial. JAMA Pediatr 2015;169:723–730.

[115] van der Burg PS, de Jongh FH, Miedema M, Frerichs I, van Kaam AH. Effect of minimally invasive surfactant therapy on lung volume and ventilation in preterm infants. J Pediatr 2016;170:67–72.

[116] Göpel W, Kribs A, Ziegler A, Laux R, Hoehn T, Wieg C, et al. Avoidance of mechanical ventilation by surfactant treatment of spontaneously breathing preterm infants (AMV): an open-label, randomised, controlled trial. Lancet 2011;378:1627–1634.

[117] Mirnia K, Heidarzadeh M, Hoseini MB, Sadeghnia AR, Balila M, Ghojazadeh M. Comparison outcome of surfactant administration via tracheal catheterization during spontaneous breathing with INSURE. Med J Islam World Acad Sci 2013;21:143–148.

[118] Bao Y, Zhang G, Wu M, Ma L, Zhu J. A pilot study of less invasive surfactant administration in very preterm infants in a Chinese tertiary center. BMC Pediatr 2015;15:21.

[119] Mohammadizadeh M, Ardestani AG, Sadeghnia AR. Early administration of surfactant via a thin intratracheal catheter in preterm infants with respiratory distress syndrome: feasibility and outcome. J Res Pharm Pract 2015;4:31–36.

[120] Rigo V, Lefebvre C, Broux I. Surfactant instillation in spontaneously breathing preterm infants: a systematic review and meta-analysis. Eur J Pediatr 2016;175:1933–1942.

[121] Aldana-Aguirre JC, Pinto M, Featherstone RM, Kumar M. Less invasive surfactant administration versus intubation for surfactant delivery in preterm infants with respiratory distress syndrome: a systematic review and meta-analysis. Arch Dis Child Fetal Neonatal Ed 2017;102:F17–F23.

[122] Dargaville PA, Kamlin CO, De Paoli AG, Carlin JB, Orsini F, Soll RF, et al. The OPTIMIST-A trial: evaluation of minimally-invasive surfactant therapy in preterm infants 25–28 weeks gestation. BMC Pediatr 2014;14:213.

[123] Finer NN, Merritt TA, Bernstein G, Job L, Mazela J, Segal R. An open label, pilot study of Aerosurf® combined with nCPAP to prevent RDS in preterm neonates. J Aerosol Med Pulm Drug Deliv 2010;23:303–309.

[124] Aerosolized Surfactant in Neonatal RDS (AS-02). Clinicaltrials.gov NCT02294630.

[125] Yeh TF, Lin HC, Chang CH, Wu TS, Su BH, Li TC, et al. Early intratracheal instillation of budesonide using surfactant as a vehicle to prevent chronic lung disease in preterm infants: a pilot study. Pediatrics 2008;121:e1310–e1318.

[126] Yeh TF, Chen CM, Wu SY, Husan Z, Li TC, Hsieh WS, et al. Intratracheal administration of budesonide/surfactant to prevent bronchopulmonary dysplasia. Am J Respir Crit Care Med 2016;193:86–95.

[127] Keller RL, Merrill JD, Black DM, et al. Late administration of surfactant replacement therapy increases surfactant protein-B content: a randomized pilot study. Pediatr Res 2012;72:613.

[128] Efficacy of recombinant Human Clara Cell 10 Protein (rhCC10) administered to premature neonates with respiratory distress syndrome. Clinicaltrials.gov NCT 01941745.

[129] Tan K, Lai NM, Sharma A. Surfactant for bacterial pneumonia in late preterm and term infants. Cochrane Database Syst Rev 2012;2:CD008155.

[130] Vento GM, Tana M, Tirone C, et al. Effectiveness of treatment with surfactant in premature infants with respiratory failure and pulmonary infection. Acta Biomed 2012;83:33–36.

[131] Aziz A, Ohlsson A. Surfactant for pulmonary haemorrhage in neonates. Cochrane Database Syst Rev 2012;7:CD005254.

[132] Yen TA, Wang CC, Hsieh WS, Chou HC, Chen CY, Tsao PN. Short-term outcome of pulmonary hemorrhage in very-low-birth-weight preterm infants. Pediatr Neonatol 2013;54:330–334.

[133] Cogo PE, Zimmermann LJ, Meneghini L, Mainini N, Bordignon L, Suma V, et al. Pulmonary surfactant disaturated-phosphatidylcholine (DSPC) turnover and pool size in newborn infants with congenital diaphragmatic hernia (CDH). Pediatr Res 2003;54:653–658.

[134] Van Meurs K. Congenital Diaphragmatic Hernia Study Group. Is surfactant therapy beneficial in the treatment of the term newborn infant with congenital diaphragmatic hernia? J Pediatr 2004;145:312–316.

[135] Lally KP, Lally PA, Langham MR, Hirschi R, Moya FR, Tibboel D, et al. Congenital Diaphragmatic Hernia Study Group. Surfactant does not improve survival rate in preterm infants with congenital diaphragmatic hernia. J Pediatr Surg 2004;39:829–833.

[136] Askie LM, Brocklehurst P, Darlow BA, Finer N, Schmidt B, Tarnow-Mordi W. NeOProM Collaborative Group. NeOProM: Neonatal Oxygenation Prospective Meta-analysis Collaboration study protocol. BMC Pediatr 2011;11:6.

[137] Carlo WA, Finer NN, Walsh MC, Rich W, Gantz MG, Laptook AR, et al. SUPPORT Study Group of the Eunice Kennedy Shriver NICHD Neonatal Research Network. Target ranges of oxygen saturation in extremely preterm infants. N Engl J Med 2010;362:1959–1969.

[138] Stenson BJ, Tarnow-Mordi WO, Darlow BA, Simes J, Juszczak E, Askie L, et al. BOOST II United

Kingdom Collaborative Group; BOOST II Australia Collaborative Group; BOOST II New Zealand Collaborative Group. Oxygen saturation and outcomes in preterm infants. N Engl J Med 2013;368:2094–2104.

[139] Schmidt B, Whyte RK, Asztalos EV, Moddemann D, Poets C, Rabi Y, et al. Canadian Oxygen Trial (COT) Group. Effects of targeting higher vs lower arterial oxygen saturations on death or disability in extremely preterm infants: a randomized clinical trial. JAMA 2013;309: 2111–2120.

[140] Askie LM, Darlow BA, Finer N, Schmidt B, Stenson B, Tarnow-Mordi W, et al. Neonatal Oxygenation Prospective Meta-analysis (NeOProM) Collaboration. Association between oxygen saturation targeting and death or disability in extremely preterm infants in the neonatal oxygenation prospective meta-analysis collaboration. JAMA 2018;319: 2190–2201.

[141] Manja V, Lakshminrusimha S, Cook DJ. Oxygen saturation target range for extremely preterm infants: a systematic review and meta-analysis. JAMA Pediatr 2015;169:332–340.

[142] Lim K, Wheeler KI, Gale TJ, Jackson HD, Kihlstrand JF, Sand C, et al. Oxygen saturation targeting in preterm infants receiving continuous positive airway pressure. J Pediatr 2014;164:730–736.

[143] Van Kaam AH, Hummler HD, Wilinska M, Swietlinski J, Lal MK, te Pas AB, et al. Automated versus manual oxygen control with different saturation targets and modes of respiratory support in preterm infants. J Pediatr 2015;167:545–550.

[144] Cayabyab R, Arora V, Wertheimer F, Durand M, Ramanathan R. Graded oxygen saturation targets and retinopathy of prematurity in extremely preterm infants. Pediatr Res 2016;80:401–406.

[145] Schmidt B, Roberts RS, Davis P, Doyle LW, Barrington KJ, Ohlsson A, et al. Caffeine for Apnea of Prematurity Trial Group: long-term effects of caffeine therapy for apnea of prematurity. N Engl J Med 2007;357:1893–1902.

[146] Dobson NR, Patel RM, Smith PB, Kuehn DR, Clark J, Vyas-Read S, et al. Trends in caffeine use and association between clinical

outcomes and timing of therapy in very low birth weight infants. J Pediatr 2014;164:992–998.

[147] Taha D, Kirkby S, Nawab U, Dysart KC, Genen L, Greenspan JS, et al. Early caffeine therapy for prevention of bronchopulmonary dysplasia in preterm infants. J Matern Fetal Neonatal Med 2014;27:1698–1702.

[148] Lodha A, Seshia M, McMillan DD, Barrington K, Yang J, Lee SK, Canadian Neonatal Network. et al. Association of early caffeine administration and neonatal outcomes in very preterm neonates. JAMA Pediatr 2015;169:33–38.

[149] Thome UH, Genzel-Boroviczeny O, Bohnhorst B, Schmid M, Fuchs H, Rohde O, PHELBI Study Group. et al. Permissive hypercapnia in extremely low birthweight infants (PHELBI): a randomised controlled multicentre trial. Lancet Respir Med 2015;3: 534–543.

[150] Doyle LW, Ehrenkranz RA, Halliday HL. Late (>7 days) postnatal corticosteroids for chronic lung disease in preterm infants. Cochrane Database Syst Rev 2014;5:CD001145.

[151] Doyle LW, Halliday HL, Ehrenkranz RA, Davis PG, Sinclair JC. An update on the impact of postnatal systemic corticosteroids on mortality and cerebral palsy in preterm infants: effect modification by risk of bronchopulmonary dysplasia. J Pediatr 2014;165:1258–1260.

[152] Jefferies AL. Postnatal corticosteroids to treat or prevent chronic lung disease in preterm infants. Paediatr Child Health 2012;17:573–574.

[153] Bassler D, Plavka R, Shinwell ES, Hallman M, Jarreau PH, Carnielli V, NEUROSIS Trial Group. et al. Early inhaled budesonide for the prevention of bronchopulmonary dysplasia. N Engl J Med 2015;3(73):1497–1506.

[154] Kumar P. Committee on Fetus and Newborn, American Academy of Pediatrics. Use of inhaled nitric oxide in preterm infants. Pediatrics 2014;133:164.

[155] Meyer MP, Hou D, Ishrar NN, Dito I, te Pas AB. Initial respiratory support with cold, dry gas versus heated humidified gas and admission temperature of preterm infants. J Pediatr 2015;166:245–250.

[156] Sinclair JC. Servo-control for maintaining abdominal skin temperature at 36°C in low birth

weight infants. Cochrane Database Syst Rev 2002;1:D001074.

[157] Bell EF, Acarregui MJ. Restricted versus liberal water intake for preventing morbidity and mortality in preterm infants. Cochrane Database Syst Rev 2014;12:CD000503.

[158] Stewart A, Brion LP, Soll R. Diuretics for respiratory distress syndrome in preterm infants. Cochrane Database Syst Rev 2011;12:CD001454.

[159] Trivedi A, Sinn JKH. Early versus late administration of amino acids in preterm infants receiving parenteral nutrition. Cochrane Database Syst Rev 2013;7:CD008771.

[160] Moyses HE, Johnson MJ, Leaf AA, Cornelius VR. Early parenteral nutrition and growth outcomes in preterm infants: a systematic review and meta-analysis. Am J Clin Nutr 2013;97:816–826.

[161] Quigley M, McGuire W. Formula versus donor breast milk for feeding preterm or low birth weight infants. Cochrane Database Syst Rev 2014;4:CD002971.

[162] Polin RA, Watterberg K, Benitz W, Eichenwald E. The conundrum of early-onset sepsis. Pediatrics 2014;133:1122–1123.

[163] Soll RF, Edwards WH. Antibiotic use in neonatal intensive care. Pediatrics 2015;135:928–929.

[164] Cotton CM. Antibiotic stewardship: reassessment of guidelines for management of neonatal sepsis. Clin Perinatol 2015;42:195–206.

[165] Batton B, Li L, Newman NS, Das A, Watterberg KL, Yoder BA, et al. Eunice Kennedy Shriver National Institute of Child Health and Human Development Neonatal Research Network. Evolving blood pressure dynamics for extremely preterm infants. J Perinatol 2014;34:301–305.

[166] Nuntnarumit P, Yang W, Bada-Ellzey HS. Blood pressure measurements in the newborn. Clin Perinatol 1999;26:981–996.

[167] Subhedar NV, Shaw NJ. Dopamine versus dobutamine for hypotensive preterm infants. Cochrane Database Syst Rev 2003;3:CD001242.

[168] Heuchan AM, Clyman RI. Managing the patent ductus arteriosus: current treatment options. Arch Dis Child Fetal Neonatal Ed 2014;99: F431–F436.

[169] Weisz DE, More K, McNamara PJ, Shah PS. PDA ligation and health

411

outcomes: a meta-analysis. Pediatrics 2014;133:e1024–e1046.

[170] Ohlsson A, Shah PS. Paracetamol (acetaminophen) for patent ductus arteriosus in preterm or low-birth-weight infants. Cochrane Database Syst Rev 2015;3:CD010061.

[171] Hatch LD, Grubb PH, Lea AS, Walsh WF, Markham MH, Whitney GM, et al. Endotracheal intubation in neonates: a prospective study of adverse safety events in 162 infants. J Pediatr 2016;168. 62.e6–66.e6.

[172] Ratner I, Whitfield J. Acquired subglottic stenosis in the very-low-birth-weight infant. Am J Dis Child 1983;137:40–43.

[173] Horbar JD, Badger GJ, Carpenter JH, Fanaroff AA, Kilpatrick S, LaCorte M, et al. Trends in mortality and morbidity for very low birth weight infants, 1991–1999. Pediatrics 2002;110:143–151.

[174] Dumpa V, Katz K, Northrup V, Bhandari V. SNIPPV versus NIPPV: does synchronization matter? J Perinatol 2012;32:438–442.

[175] Bancalari E, Claure N. The evidence for non-invasive ventilation in the preterm infant. Arch Dis Child Fetal Neonatal Ed 2013;98:F98–F102.

[176] Wilkinson D, Andersen C, O'Donnell CP, de Paoli AG, Manley BJ. High flow nasal cannula for respiratory support in preterm infants. Cochrane Database Syst Rev 2016;2:CD006405.

[177] Reynolds P, Leontiadi S, Lawson T, Otunla T, Ejiwumi O, Holland N. Stabilisation of premature infants in the delivery room with nasal high flow. Arch Dis Child Fetal Neonatal Ed 2016;101:F284–F287.

[178] Roberts CT, Owen LS, Manley BJ, Frøisland DH, Donath SM, Dalziel KM, HIPSTER Trial Investigators. et al. Nasal high-flow therapy for primary respiratory support in preterm infants. N Engl J Med 2016;375:1142–1151.

[179] Finer NN, Carlo WA, Walsh MC, Rich W, Gantz MG, Laptook AR, SUPPORT Study Group of the Eunice Kennedy Shriver NICHD Neonatal Research Network. et al. Early CPAP versus surfactant in extremely preterm infants. N Engl J Med 2010;362:1970–1979.

[180] Ambalavanan N, Carlo WA, Wrage LA, Das A, Laughon M, Cotten CM, SUPPORT Study Group of the NICHD Neonatal Research Network. et al. PaCO$_2$ in surfactant, positive pressure, and oxygenation randomised trial (SUPPORT). Arch Dis Child Fetal Neonatal Ed 2015;100:F145–F149.

[181] Erickson SJ, Grauaug A, Gurrin L, Swaminathan M. Hypocarbia in the ventilated preterm infant and its effect on intraventricular haemorrhage and bronchopulmonary dysplasia. J Paediatr Child Health 2002;38:560–562.

[182] Peng W, Zhu H, Shi H, Liu E. Volume-targeted ventilation is more suitable than pressure-limited ventilation for preterm infants: a systematic review and meta-analysis. Arch Dis Child Fetal Neonatal Ed 2014;99:F158–F165.

[183] Wheeler K, Klingenberg C, McCallion N, Morley CJ, Davis PG. Volume-targeted versus pressure-limited ventilation in the neonate. Cochrane Database Syst Rev 2010;11:CD003666.

[184] Cools F, Offringa M, Askie LM. Elective high frequency oscillatory ventilation versus conventional ventilation for acute pulmonary dysfunction in preterm infants. Cochrane Database Syst Rev 2015;3:CD000104.

[185] Buzzella B, Claure N, D'Ugard C, Bancalari E. A randomized controlled trial of two nasal continuous positive airway pressure levels after extubation in preterm infants. J Pediatr 2014;164:46–51.

[186] Ellsbury DL, Klein JM, Segar JL. Optimization of high-frequency oscillatory ventilation for the treatment of experimental pneumothorax. Crit Care Med 2002;30:1131–1135.

[187] Keszler M, Donn SM, Bucciarelli RL, Alverson DC, Hart M, Lunyong V, et al. Multicenter controlled trial comparing high-frequency jet ventilation and conventional mechanical ventilation in newborn infants with pulmonary interstitial emphysema. J Pediatr 1991;119:85–93.

Chapter | 25A |

Meconium Aspiration Syndrome— Part 1: Epidemiology, Pathophysiology, Signs and Symptoms, and Diagnosis

Rama Bhat, MD, Dharmapuri Vidyasagar, MD

CHAPTER CONTENTS HD

CHAPTER POINTS

- MAS is a major cause of respiratory failure and morbidity in term newborn.
- Recent advances in perinatal and neonatal management have steadily decreased the incidence & complications and increased the survival.
- MAS is a multifactorial disease and includes pulmonary and vascular components.
- Pathophysiology of MAS includes airway obstruction, inflammatory response, surfactant inactivation, and development of pulmonary hypertension.
- Improved obstetrical and postnatal care has decreased the mortality for MAS from 40% to <5% in developed countries.

Introduction

Meconium is the first stool of an infant; and it is a tarry/greenish, odorless viscid material containing 70%–80% water and the gastrointestinal secretions, such as bile acids, bile pigments, mucopolysaccharides, fatty acids, and pancreatic enzymes, such as phospholipase A2, various drug metabolites, vernix, lanugo, and swallowed fetal cells. Fetuses from 10%–20% pass first stool in utero and the rest within 48 h of birth.

Aristotle, a philosopher-biologist (380–323 BC) coined the term "meconium," as it resembled crude extract of Opium and the babies born through meconium-stained amniotic fluid (MSAF) were found depressed or sleepy. Obstetric textbooks from the beginning of last century described the passage of meconium in utero as an impending sign of fetal death [1].When aspirated meconium can cause mild to severe respiratory symptoms requiring both respiratory and cardiovascular support in an intensive care nursery. Meconium aspiration syndrome (MAS), once a common cause of respiratory failure with high mortality and morbidity in term and near-term neonates, has been steadily declining in the western world (<5%), but in the developing countries it is still the leading cause of respiratory failure in the newborn period with high (32%) mortality [2,3].

This chapter will focus on the epidemiology, recent advances in pathophysiology of MSAF and MAS, clinical manifestations, and diagnosis.

Significance of MSAF

MSAF is a "fetal environmental hazard" [4]. MSAF occurs in 3%–20% of all pregnancies and 1.5%–5% of these infants born through MSAF develop MAS (7,500–25,000 cases/year in the United States alone). Another 3.4%–5.2% develop other respiratory problems such as transient tachypnea (TTN), delayed adaptation after birth, pulmonary hypertension, sepsis/pneumonia, and pneumothorax. Newborns with MAS from 30% to 50% require ventilator support and treatment for pulmonary hypertension. Meconium in the amniotic fluid indicates the need for close observation of mother and fetus in the intrapartum period for any signs of fetal compromise. It also increases the risk for cesarean birth, the need for additional personnel skilled in neonatal resuscitation at delivery and admission to NICU. Decision to deliver an infant, however, should be based on fetal well-being rather than presence of meconium.

Epidemiology of MSAF

MSAF is seen in 3%–20% of term deliveries. In postterm ($\geq$42 weeks) deliveries, incidence can be as high as 48% [5]. Higher incidence of MSAF has been reported among African-American, southeast Asian, Black African, Pacific Islanders and indigenous populations of Australia [6,7]. This has been attributed to advanced gut maturation, but exact mechanisms are not known. Balchin et al. in a prospective population-based study reported that black and southeast Asian babies have higher risk of being born through MSAF (OR: 8.4, 95% CI: 2.4–28.8) [8]. Other risk factors include postmaturity, maternal smoking, in-utero hypoxia from preeclampsia, drug abuse, intrapartum medications, prolonged rupture of membranes, and chorioamnionitis. Table 25A.1 shows the reported risk factors of MSAF.

In preterm pregnancies (<34 weeks gestation) the incidence of MSAF is around 4%–5% [9]. The low incidence in preterm infants has been attributed to decreased bowel motility and lower amount of meconium in the bowel.

Table 25A.2 shows the incidence of MSAF in various countries around the world.

Pathophysiology of MSAF

Fetal defecation is very common up to 16–20 weeks but it is uncommon between 20 and 32 weeks gestation. One possible explanation for this is the innervation of anal sphincter, which is complete by 20 weeks. Passage of the meconium in utero can be due to maturational/physiological reasons

Table 25A.1 Risk factors for meconium-stained amniotic fluid (MSAF)

	Risk factors	Incidence of MSAF
Maturational	Increasing gestational age	<34 weeks, 5% 38–40 weeks, 10%–20% 41 weeks, 38.7% 42 weeks, 48%
Racial/Ethnic	Racial differences— higher incidence among African-American, Black Africans, South Asians, Pacific Islanders	Black African—22.6% South Asian— 16.8% White—15.7%
Physiological	Breech presentation	
Stress mediated	Smoking during pregnancy	
	Drug abuse	
	IUGR	
	Preeclampsia,	
	Chorioamnionitis	
	Intrapartum oxytocin or misoprostol	
	Prolonged rupture of membranes	

IUGR, Intrauterine growth restriction.

Table 25A.2 Reported global incidence of MSAF*

	Countries	Incidence (%)
Western	United States	10–15
	France	7.93
	United Kingdom	16.3
Southeast Asia	Japan	13
	China	13–16.4
	Korea	4.99
South Asia	India	9.8–14.3
	Nepal	13.4–14.6
	Pakistan	7.7
	Iran	11.6
Africa	Nigeria	20.4
	Ethiopia	15.4

*Data obtained from the published reports during the last 20 years.

or from stress-mediated mechanisms (Fig. 25A.1). Higher motilin levels and increased cholinergic innervation with advancing gestation can explain the higher incidence of MSAF in term and postterm (>294 days) infants [10]. Incidence of MSAF among southeast Asians, African-Americans, and Pacific Islanders compared to Caucasians has been attributed to advanced gut maturation [6,7].

Other factors associated with in utero meconium passage are drug abuse, intrauterine infection, use of vaginal Misoprostol for labor induction, and gestational cholestasis [11–13]. In the later instance, MSAF was attributed to increased fetal colonic stimulation by higher bile acid accumulation in maternal serum. Campos et al. recently reported that infusion of cholic acid into fetal lambs increased colonic motility [14]. In a recent study, Ahanya et al. reported that fetal stress increases corticotropin releasing factor (CRF) and CRF-R1 receptors, which lead to increased colonic contractility [15]. Cortisol and CRF levels in fetuses with MSAF were higher and administration of glucocorticoid and thyroxin to the fetus showed increased colonic contractility and passage of meconium [16]. The low incidence of MSAF in preterm infants may be secondary to low motilin, decreased peristalsis, and small amount of meconium in the gut.

MSAF can be thin or translucent (grade-1), moderately thick (grade-2, opalescent), and thick (grade-3, pea soup) depending on the amount of meconium passed, volume of the amniotic fluid, and its clearance from the amniotic cavity. MAS is more common in infants born through thick viscid MSAF [17].

Meconium aspiration

Definitions of MAS

1. Meconium aspiration is defined as respiratory distress in an infant born through MSAF whose symptoms cannot otherwise be explained [18].
2. Meconium aspiration defined by clinical criteria: (1) respiratory distress (tachypnea, retractions, or grunting) in a neonate born through MSAF; (2) need for supplemental oxygen to maintain oxygen saturation (SaO$_2$) 92% or more; (3) oxygen requirement starting during the first 2 h of life and lasting for at least 12 h; and (4) absence of congenital malformations of the airway, lung, or heart [19].
3. MAS is defined as respiratory distress presenting from immediately after birth to 12 h of age. Hypoxia, tachypnea, gasping respiration, and often underlying asphyxia. Chest X-ray shows overexpansion of lungs widespread coarse fluffy infiltrates [20].

The above three definitions have been used in various clinical reports of MAS.

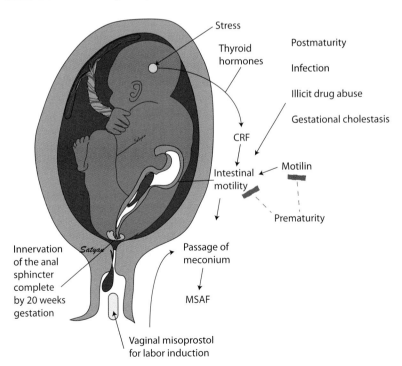

Fig. 25A.1 Risk Factors for Meconium Aspiration Syndrome (MAS): Stress, Thyroid and Glucocorticoid Hormones, and Motilin-Enhanced Intestinal Motility. Prematurity is associated with poor intestinal motility. *CRF*, Corticotrophin releasing factor; *MSAF*, meconium-stained amniotic fluid. Copyright: Satyan Lakshminrusimha.

Incidence

In developed countries, the incidence of MAS ranges from 1.5% to 5% of all babies born through MSAF. During the last 2 decades the incidence of MAS has been steadily decreasing while in the developing countries the reported MAS incidence has ranged from 5% to 21% [21].

Yoder et al. in a single-center prospective study reported that the changing obstetric practices at their institution during the 1990–1998 resulted in decreased incidence of MAS from 5.8% to 1.5% [2]. This reduction in MAS was attributed to more frequent recognition of nonreassuring fetal heart rate (FHR) pattern and significant (33%) reduction in births >41 weeks.

Other recent population reports from the United Kingdom, France, and Australia showed a significant downward trend in MAS incidence [8,22]. Vivian-Taylor et al. reported a 11.3% per year reduction in MAS from a large population-based cohort study from Australia and attributed this decline in MAS to reduction in (1) births ≥40 weeks, (2) birth weight <3rd percentile, (3) maternal smoking, and (4) delivery at small hospitals [23].

Risk factors for MAS include African-American race, infants born through thick MSAF, nonreassuring FHR tracing (category II and III FHR), low 1 and 5 min Apgar score (Table 25A.3).

Pathophysiology of MAS

Despite the recent advances in meconium-induced lung injury, the following question remains as puzzle: namely, why large number of infants who had meconium in trachea and radiological findings suggestive of MAS, remain asymptomatic. Until 1990, the traditional belief was that

Table 25A.3 Risk factors for MAS*

Risk factors	Odds ratio (CI)	P-value
Fetal distress—nonreassuring fetal heart rate patterns (category II and III)	6.9 (1.8–26.9)	0.006
Consistency of MSAF—thick versus thin MSAF	9.85 (4.39–22.08)	
Prolonged labor	5.2 (2.5–10.7)	
Depressed at birth—Apgar <7 at 1 and 5 min		

MSAF, Meconium-stained amniotic fluid.
*Odds ratio obtained from the published reports.

meconium aspiration occurs immediately after birth and aspirated meconium causes obstructive respiratory distress initially which is then followed by chemical pneumonitis. Several studies, both clinical and experimental, carried out during the last 2 decades have shed new light into the pathogenesis of meconium aspiration. The Fig. 25A.2 summarizes the current understanding of meconium-induced lung injury in newborns.

Currently, MAS is considered as a multifactorial disease with many players either acting alone or in combination.

1. **Airway obstruction**
2. **Noninflammatory**
   a. Apoptosis—direct damage to airway and alveolar epithelial cells
   b. Surfactant inactivation and/or decreased synthesis
   c. Epithelial sodium channel (ENaC) inactivation—decreased reabsorption of lung fluid
3. **Inflammatory response**
   a. Production of proinflammatory agents (cytokines, chemokines), phospholipase A2
   b. Activation of compliment (C5a) and Toll-like receptors
   c. Increased production of, prostaglandins and leukotrienes
   d. Increased production of reactive oxygen species (ROS) and reactive nitrogen species (RNS)
   e. Injury to endothelium and epithelium and leakage of protein and fluid to alveoli
4. **Pulmonary hypertension:** In utero hypoxia, muscularization of acinar vessels, meconium aspiration and subsequent postnatal hypoxia hypercarbia, acidosis, and increased thromboxane levels after birth resulting in continuation of fetal circulation

Airway obstruction

Until 1990, respiratory distress seen in term infants born through MSAF was attributed to airway obstruction and chemical pneumonitis from aspirated meconium. Thureen et al. reported autopsy findings in eight infants with fatal meconium aspiration in spite of appropriate perinatal airway management. They showed no airway obstruction but excessive muscularization of pulmonary arteries and intralobular arterioles. The findings let them conclude that MAS occurred in utero [25]. Satoh et al. reported autopsy findings from stillborn infants and infants born through MSAF who died within few days after birth which showed occluded bronchiolar and alveolar spaces in five infants and in three infants small amount of meconium in alveolar spaces [26]. Experimental studies on newborn puppies and young adult rabbits [27,28] have reported pathological and pulmonary functional changes after instilling 20%–50% meconium to trachea. The studies on dogs showed rapid clearance of tantalum-labeled meconium from trachea and main bron-

chi to the peripheral airways and alveoli within 1 h. Instillation of 25% meconium into airway showed early (15 min after instillation) increase in both inspiratory and expiratory respiratory resistance suggestive of large airway obstruction; however, the expiratory resistance was higher than inspiratory resistance indicative of partial obstruction. This was associated with an increase in functional residual capacity (hyperexpanded lung fields), decrease in dynamic compliance, and unchanged static compliance consistent with partial obstruction. By 2 h, airway resistance decreased suggesting distal migration of meconium. Examination of lungs showed widespread areas of atelectasis and emphysematous areas indicating distal small airway obstruction. Atelectasis leads to right-to-left shunting of blood without oxygenation at the alveolar level while air trapping from a ball valve obstruction causes hypoxia, hypercarbia, and acidosis leading to pulmonary hypertension and right-to-left shunting via foramen ovale and ductus arteriosus. Ball valve airway obstruction can also result in pneumothorax and pneumomediastinum in 10%–30% of infants with MAS requiring mechanical ventilation. These observations led to airway intervention strategies, such as intrapartum oropharyngeal suction and laryngoscopic suction of trachea after birth [29,30]. However, recent large multicenter randomized controlled trials of intrapartum oropharyngeal and postnatal airway suctioning conducted during the last 2 decades have failed to prevent MAS and/or alter the course of the disease [31,32]. These findings suggest that meconium-induced lung injury is not due to simple obstruction alone but other factors, such as inflammation, alterations surfactant function, and yet unknown factors may play a role.

Noninflammatory

- **Meconium-induced apoptosis:** Experimental studies from our laboratory on 2-week-old rabbits after intratracheal instillation of 10% meconium solution showed massive epithelial cell death, which peaked at 24 h compared to saline-instilled rabbits. Most of the dead epithelial cells were either apoptotic or necrotic. Apoptosis was evident soon after instillation of meconium. Further morphological studies of lungs showed detachment of airway epithelium into airway lumen indicating direct toxic effect of meconium on airway and alveolar epithelia [33]. Exact mechanisms for meconium-induced apoptosis is not fully understood but cytokines and free radicals released by macrophages, neutrophils, phospholipase A2, and angiotensin II may also play a role in meconium-induced apoptosis [34,35].
- **Meconium-induced surfactant inactivation:** The exact mechanism by which meconium induces surfactant inactivation is not fully understood. Possible mechanisms include (1) meconium-induced concentration-dependent structural alterations in surfactant phospholipids resulting in higher ratio of small round aggregates to large aggregates which has low surface reducing activity [36], (2) meconium contains phospholipase A2a potent initiator of inflammation and an inhibitor of surfactant activity [37], (3) by direct toxicity on type II cells and decrease surfactant production [38]. Change in surfactant function can lead to widespread atelectasis and pulmonary edema. Exogenous high-dose surfactant administration has been shown to decrease the severity of illness and reduced the need for extracorporeal membrane oxygenation (ECMO) [39].
- **Pulmonary edema:** Meconium-induced lung injury and hypoxia can lead to alveolar tight junction damage and leakage of fluid, and inhibition of lung fluid reabsorption [40]. ENac and surfactant dysfunction can also contribute to pulmonary edema. Pulmonary venous hypertension secondary to cardiac dysfunction due to asphyxia can increased pulmonary capillary hydrostatic pressure and cause pulmonary edema (Fig. 25A.2).

Inflammatory response

- **Animal studies:** Meconium contains several proinflammatory cytokines and has strong chemotactic activity (Fig. 25A.3). Recent studies on piglets following instillation of meconium showed massive influx of neutrophils and macrophages within few hours in the lungs and these cells trigger the production of proinflammatory substances, such as TNF α, IL-1β, IL-6, leukotrienes, and thromboxanes, leading to pulmonary and vascular injury. Meconium also contains phospholipase A2 (PLA2), which is a potent inflammatory agent and elevated plasma levels of PLA2, has been reported following intratracheal instillation of meconium [34]. Other studies have reported meconium-induced activation of complement cascade subsequent increase in C5b-9b, cytokines, chemokines, arachidonic metabolites and reactive oxygen species. These inflammatory mediators not only produce meconium pneumonitis but also systemic inflammatory reaction [41].
- **Human studies:** In utero fetal exposure to meconium has been shown to induce inflammation in the chorionic plate of the placenta, ulceration in umbilical cord, vascular injury with medial muscle necrosis, and vasoconstriction [42,43].

Pulmonary hypertension

Pulmonary hypertension is a serious life threatening condition occurring in 30% of newborns with severe MAS. Pulmonary hypertension is more common among infants born to mothers with chronic hypertension, or chronic placental

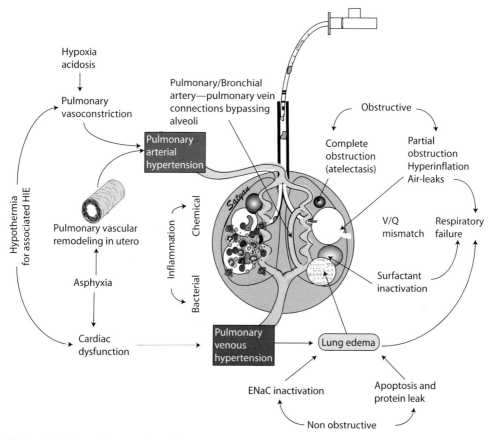

Fig. 25A.2 Pathophysiology of Lung Injury After Aspiration of Meconium in Utero or After Birth. *ENaC*, Epithelial sodium channel. Copyright: Satyan Lakshminrusimha. Modified from the original publication of Vidyasagar D, Harris V, Pildes RS. Assisted ventilation in infants with meconium aspiration syndrome. Pediatrics 1975;56:208–213 [24].

abruption and in utero meconium aspiration. Clinical and autopsy studies on human neonates have reported development of pulmonary hypertension following in utero meconium aspiration or postnatal intratracheal meconium instillation. Chronic hypoxia results in extension of medial musculature to small acinar arterioles (normally not muscular), which is the major contributor for pulmonary hypertension. Other factors inducing pulmonary hypertension are elevated ET-1 levels, thromboxane levels, and direct injury to endothelial cells by inflammatory mediators [44–46].

Pulmonary hypertension cannot be predicted by radiological findings alone. Many MAS infants present with clear overexpanded lung fields on chest X-ray show severe pulmonary hypertension on echocardiogram examination. Thus, it is imperative that all infants requiring mechanical ventilation for poor oxygenation should be screened for pulmonary hypertension early (first 3 days of life).

In summary, the available evidence clearly indicates that MAS is a multifactorial disease and not a simple airway

obstruction or chemical pneumonitis. van Ireland and de Beaufort have renamed the MAS as "meconium-associated pulmonary inflammation (MAPI)" [47].

Clinical features

The classic MAS newborn is a postterm or term infant born through thick MSAF, had fetal decelerations (Type 2 FHR) during labor, depressed at birth (Apgar < 7 at 1 and 5 min), had meconium below vocal cords, and presents soon after birth or within few hours after birth with tachypnea (respiratory rate > 60/min), retractions, grunting, and cyanosis requiring oxygen or ventilator support to maintain oxygen saturation >90%.

Based on clinical severity, oxygen requirement and the need for assisted ventilation MAS has been classified in to three types: mild, moderate, and severe MAS.

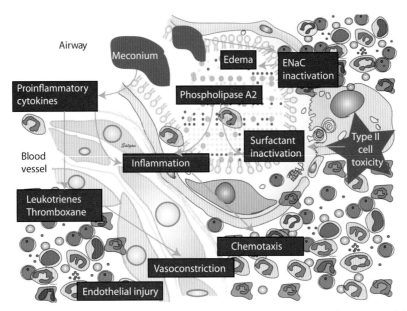

Fig. 25A.3 Cellular Mechanisms Associated With Pulmonary Pathology in MAS. Copyright: Satyan Lakshminrusimha.

- Mild MAS: Oxygen requirement <40% for <48 h
- Moderate MAS: Oxygen requirement >40% for 48 h
- Severe MAS: Infants requiring mechanical ventilation and other therapy for associated pulmonary hyperventilation.

Clinical features include increased anteroposterior diameter of the chest (barrel-shaped chest); decreased air entry and shift of apical impulse (in the presence of pneumothorax), rales, and rhonchi; subcostal and intercostal retractions. Infants from 25%–30% requiring mechanical ventilation may develop pneumothorax.

Other clinical signs include signs of postmaturity—dry peeling skin; long nails; meconium staining (greenish-yellow) of skin, nails, and umbilical cord.

Significant number of infants develop respiratory distress secondary to delayed absorption of lung fluid, and the diagnosis can be made by chest X-ray showing fluid in transverse fissure and perihilar congestion.

Infants born depressed (Apgar score at 1 and 5 min <7) are more likely to have early symptoms of tachypnea and retractions than infants born with normal Apgar scores (> 7 at 1 and 5 min).

Differential diagnosis

- TTN
- Aspiration of amniotic fluid/blood
- Pneumonia/Sepsis
- Diaphragmatic hernia
- Cyanotic heart disease
- Primary persistent pulmonary hypertension

Many of the above conditions can be differentiated by dual saturation monitoring, chest X-ray, echocardiogram, arterial blood gas analysis, complete blood count (CBC), C-reactive protein (CRP), and blood culture. Indications for these tests and the expected findings in MAS are described below.

Initial diagnostic tests

Chest X-ray

Chest roentgenogram is diagnostic and the usual findings include the following (Fig. 25A.4):
- Patchy infiltrates with areas of hyperinflation
- Hyperinflated lung fields—evidence of ball valve obstruction
- Atelectasis on one or both lung fields
- Pneumothorax or pneumomediastinum
- Pleural effusion
- Perihilar congestion with prominent transverse fissure on right lung
- Oligemic lung fields (more common with severe pulmonary hypertension)
- Cardiomegaly—more common in infants born with low 1 and 5 min Apgar scores.

It is important to note that the severity respiratory distress may not correlate with radiological findings.

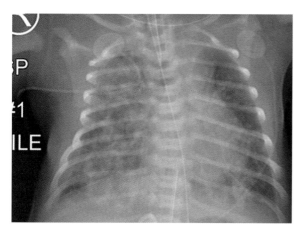

Fig. 25A.4 Typical X-ray in MAS Showing Hyperinflated Lung Fields With Fluffy Infiltrates. Courtesy: Dr. V. Karody.

Lung ultrasonography

The use of ultrasonography to diagnose pulmonary lesions is on the rise. One recent large study involving 117 infants with MAS reported that ultrasonography of the chest can be as reliable as chest X-ray to diagnose MAS (100% sensitivity and 100% specificity) [48].

Ultrasonography findings in MAS cases included:
- Pulmonary consolidation with air bronchogram (100%)
- Atelectasis (16.2%)
- Pleural effusion (13.7%)
- Alveolar interstitial syndrome

Use of ultrasound as a diagnostic tool in NICU has an advantage over repeated X-ray imaging by avoiding radiation. It has been used to diagnose pulmonary hemorrhage in preterm infants. Further studies are needed on sick neonates to validate the aforementioned findings.

Pre- and postductal oxygen saturation

All newborns with MAS requiring mechanical ventilation should have dual continuous oxygen saturation monitoring. The saturation probes should be placed on right hand (preductal) and the second probe in the lower extremity (postductal). A saturation difference of > 10% is highly suggestive of pulmonary hypertension.

Arterial blood gas

Newborns with MAS need a blood gas to rule out other causes of respiratory distress, such as TTN and congenital heart disease (CHD). In MAS, blood gas analysis will show low pO_2 and higher pCO_2, especially the one with asphyxia.

Complete blood count

In newborns with early onset sepsis and infants with pneumonia will show leukocytosis or neutropenia with immature neutrophils and thrombocytopenia. Thrombocytopenia is more common in infants with birth asphyxia

C-reactive protein and procalcitonin

Both peptides, CRP and procalcitonin, are acute phase reactants and produced by liver and the latter also by monocytes in reaction to infection. CRP level increases slowly starting at 6 h; whereas procalcitonin rises within few hours. Normal levels of CRP is less than 0.5 mg/dL and procalcitonin level <0.5 ng/mL. The two tests aforementioned can help the physician at bedside to diagnose neonatal sepsis/pneumonia and differentiate from MAS and CHD.

Blood culture

Newborns admitted with MAS need a blood culture to rule out infection. Many with MAS also have chorioamnionitis in addition during intrapartum period. MSAF, especially thick viscous amniotic fluid, is a good media for bacterial overgrowth.

Hyperoxia test

This test is done to rule out cyanotic heart disease and of value in hospitals without echocardiogram facilities. The test is done by administering 100% oxygen for 15 min and observing pre- and postductal oxygen saturation. In infants with cyanotic CHD and with severe MAS and pulmonary hypertension, oxygen saturation will not increase. Further differentiation can be made by echocardiogram and by arterial blood gas analysis. The latter will show higher pCO_2 in cases with severe MAS but pCO_2 will be normal in CHD cases.

Echocardiography

Indications for echocardiography in infants with MAS include: (1) to rule out congenital cyanotic and acyanotic conditions, (2) cardiac contractility (RV and LV function), tricuspid regurgitation, right to left shunt through ductus arteriosus and foramen ovale. Neonates with MAS requiring >60% oxygen should get an echocardiogram early in the first 2 days to diagnose pulmonary hypertension. Presence of tricuspid jet, right ventricular dilatation, right to left shunt through PDA and/or foramen ovale is very diagnostic for pulmonary hypertension. Follow-up echocardiograms may be necessary to evaluate the response to therapy. Up to 30% of mechanically ventilated MAS infants may develop PPHN.

References

[1] Schultz M. The significance of the passage of meconium during labor. Am J Obstet Gynecol 1925;10:83.

[2] Yoder BA, Kirsch EA, Barth WH, et al. Changing obstetric practice associated with decreasing incidence of meconium aspiration syndrome. Obstet Gynecol 2002;126:712–715.

[3] Anwar Z, Butt TK, Anjum F, et al. Mortality in meconium aspiration syndrome in hospitalized babies. J Coll Physicians Surg Pak 2011;21:695–699.

[4] Ramin KD, Leveno KJ, Kelly MA, et al. Amniotic fluid meconium: a fetal environmental hazard. Obstet Gynecol 1996;87:181–184.

[5] Satomi M, Hiraizumi Y, Suzuki S. Perinatal outcomes associated with meconium stained amniotic fluid in Japanese singleton pregnancies. Open J Obstet Gynecol 2011;1:42–46.

[6] Sedaghatian MR, Othman L, Hossain MM, Vidyasagar D. Risk of meconium stained amniotic fluid in different ethnic groups. J Perinatol 2000;4:257–261.

[7] Dargaville PA, Copnell B. Australian and New Zealand Neonatal Network. The epidemiology of meconium aspiration syndrome: incidence, risk factors, therapies, and outcome. Pediatrics 2006;17:1712–1721.

[8] Balchin I, Whitaker JC, Lamont RF, et al. Maternal and fetal characteristics associated with meconium stained amniotic fluid. Obstet Gynecol 2011;117:828–835.

[9] Tybulewicz AT, Clegg SK, Fonfé GJ, et al. Preterm meconium staining of the amniotic fluid: associated findings and risk of adverse clinical outcomes. Arch Dis Child Fetal Neonatal Ed 2004;89:F328–F330.

[10] Lakshmanan J, Ross MG. Mechanisms of inutero meconium passage. J Perinatol 2008;28:S8–13.

[11] Chasnoff IJ, Burns KA, Burns WJ. Cocaine use in pregnancy; perinatal morbidity and mortality. Neurotoxicol Teratol 1987;9:291–293.

[12] Hofmeyr GJ, Gulmezoglu AM. Vaginal misoprostol for cervical ripening and induction of labor. Cochrane Database Syst Rev 2003; 1: Art no: CD 000941.

[13] Glantz A, Marschall HU, Mattsson LA. Intrahepatic cholestatsis of pregnancy: relationship between bile acid levels, and fetal complication rates. Hepatology 2004;40:467–474.

[14] Campos GA, Guerra FA, Israel EJ. Effects of cholic acid infusion in fetal lambs. Acta Obstet Gynecol Scand 1986;65:23–26.

[15] Ahanya SN, Lakshmanan J, Morgan B, et al. Meconium passage in utero: mechanisms, consequences and management. Obstet Gyneccol Surv 2005;60:45–56.

[16] Ahanya SN, LakshmananJ, Babu J, et al. In utero betamethasone administration induces meconium passage in fetal rabbits. J Soc Gynecol Investig 2004;11:102.

[17] Wiswell TE, Gannon CM, Jacob J, et al. Delivery room management of apparently vigorous meconium stained neonate. Results of multicenter, international collaborative trial. Pediatrics 2000;105:1–7.

[18] Cleary GM, Wiswell TE. Meconium stained amniotic fluid and meconium aspiration: an update. Pediatr Clin North Am 1998;45:511–529.

[19] Vain NE, Szyld EG, Prudent LM, et al. Oropharyngeal and nasopharyngeal suctioning of meconium stained neonates before delivery of their shoulders: multicenter, randomized controlled trial. Lancet 2004;364:597–602.

[20] Abeywardana S. The report of the Australian and New Zealand Neonatal Network 2004. Sydney: ANZNN; 2006.

[21] Khazardoost S, Hantoushzadeh S, Khooshideh M, et al. Risk factors for meconium aspiration in meconium stained amniotic fluid. J Obstet Gynaecol 2007;27:577–579.

[22] Fischer C, Rybakowski C, Ferdinus C, et al. A population based study of meconium aspiration syndrome in neonates born between 37–43 weeks gestation. Int J Pediatr 2012;2012:321545.

[23] Vivian-Taylor J, Sheng J, Hadfield RM, et al. Trends in obstetric practices and meconium aspiration syndrome in a population based study. BJOG 2011;118:1601–1607.

[24] Vidyasagar D, Harris V, Pildes RS. Assisted ventilation in infants with meconium aspiration syndrome. Pediatrics 1975;56:208–213.

[25] Thureen PJ, Hall DM, Hoffenberg A, et al. Fatal meconium aspiration in spite of appropriate perinatal airway management: pulmonary and placental evidence of prenatal disease. Am J Obstet Gynecol 1997;176:967–975.

[26] Satoh F, Kakimoto Y, Miyashita K, et al. Implication of meconium aspirated lung in stillborns and neonatal deaths. Austin J Forensic Sci Crim 2015;2:1034.

[27] Gooding CA, Gregory GA, Taber P, et al. An experimental model for the study of meconium aspiration in the newborn. Radiology 1971;100:137.

[28] Tran N, Lowe C, Sivieri EM, et al. Sequential effects of acute meconium obstruction on pulmonary function. Pediat Res 1980;14:34–38.

[29] Gregory GA, Gooding CA, Phibbs RH, et al. Meconium aspiration in infants—a prospective study. J Pediatr 1974;85:848–852.

[30] Carson BS, Losey RW, Bowes WA, et al. Combined obstetric and pediatric approach to prevent meconium aspiration syndrome. Am J Obstet Gynecol 1976;126:712–715.

[31] Wiswell TE, Gannon CM, Jacob J, et al. Delivery room management of apparently vigorous meconium stained neonate: results of the multicenter international collaborative trial. Pediatrics 2000;105:1–7.

[32] Vain NE, Szyld EG, Prudent IM, et al. Oropharyngeal and nasopharyngeal suctioning of meconium stained neonates before the delivery of their shoulders: multicenter randomized controlled trial. Lancet 2004;364:597–602.

[33] Zagariya A, Bhat R, Uhal B, et al. Cell death and lung cell histology in meconium aspirated newborn rabbit lung. Eur J Pediatr 2000;159:819–826.

[34] Holopainen R, Aho H, Laine J, et al. Human meconium has high phospholipase A2 activity and induces cellular injury and apoptosis in piglet lungs. Pediatr Res 1999;46:626–632.

[35] Vidyasaagar D, Zagariya A. Studies of meconium induced lung injury: inflammatory cytokine expression and apoptosis. J Perinatol 2008;S3:S102–S107.

[36] Ochs M, Schuttler M, Stichtenoth G, et al. Morphological alterations of exogenous surfactant inhibited

by meconium can be prevented by dextran. Respir Res 2006;7:86.

[37] Schrama AJ, de Beaufort AJ, Sukul YR, et al. Phospholipase A2 is present in meconium and inhibits the activity of surfactant: an in vitro study. Acta Paediatr 2001;90:412–416.

[38] Janssen DJ, Carnielli VP, Cogo P, et al. Surfactant phosphatidylcholine metabolism in neonates with meconium aspiration syndrome. J Pediatr 2006;149:634–639.

[39] Findlay RD, Taeusch HW, Walther FJ. Surfactant replacement therapy for meconium aspiration syndrome. Pediatrics 1996;97:48–52.

[40] Chua BA, Chan L, Kindler PM, et al. The association between meconium and the production and reabsorption of lung liquid and lactate loss by in vitro lungs from fetal guinea pigs. Am J Obstet Gynecol 2000;183:235–244.

[41] Lindenskov PH, Castellheim A, Aamodt G, et al. Complement activation reflects severity of meconium aspiration syndrome in newborn pigs. Pediatr Res 2004;56:810–817.

[42] Burgess AM, Hutchins GM. Inflammation of the lungs, umbilical cord, and placenta associated with meconium passage in utero. Review of 123 cases. Pediatr Res 1996;192:1121–1128.

[43] Altshuler G, Arizawa M, Molnar-Nadasdy G. Meconium induced umbilical cord vascular necrosis and ulceration: a potential link between placenta and poor pregnancy outcome. Obstet Gynecol 1992;79:760–766.

[44] Murphy JD, VawterGF, Reid LM. Pulmonary vascular disease in fetal meconium aspiration. J Pediatr 1984;104:758–762.

[45] Shekerdemian LS, Ravn HB, Penny DJ. Intravenous sildenafil lowers pulmonary vascular resistance in a model of neonatal pulmonary hypertension. AM J Respir Critical Care Med 2002;165:1098–1102.

[46] Zagariya A, Doherty J, Bhat R, et al. Elevated immunoreactive endothelin-1 in rabbit lungs after meconium aspiration. Pediatr Crit Care 2002;3:297–302.

[47] van Ireland Y, de Beaufort AJ. Why does meconium cause meconium aspiration syndrome? Current concepts of meconium aspiration syndrome pathophysiology. Early Hum Dev 2009;85:617–626.

[48] Liu J, Cao HY, Fu W. Lung ultrasonography to diagnose meconium aspiration syndrome of newborn. J Int Med Res 2016;44:1534–1542.

Chapter | **25B** |

Meconium Aspiration Syndrome—Part 2: Clinical Management

Mark F. Weems, MD, FAAP, Ramasubbareddy Dhanireddy, MD, FAAP

CHAPTER POINTS

- Provide respiratory support to minimize ventilation-perfusion mismatch and optimize lung volume. Avoid hypoxemia and acidosis.
- Surfactant replacement is appropriate for meconium aspiration patients who require mechanical ventilation or high FiO_2.
- In case of sudden clinical deterioration, consider the high risk of pneumothorax.
- Inotropes, pulmonary vasodilators, and extracorporeal membrane oxygenation (ECMO) may be used to support infants with hypoxic respiratory failure.

Delivery room management

1. **Neonatal resuscitation team.** Meconium-stained amniotic fluid is a high-risk condition, and a neonatal resuscitation team should be present at the time of birth. The initial resuscitation should not differ from the standard steps (temperature control, clear the airway, dry, stimulate), as described in Chapter 4.
2. **Delayed cord clamping.** There is a growing body of evidence to support delayed cord clamping for both term and preterm infants. A delay of 30–60 s is recommended prior to clamping the cord for vigorous infants provided the initial steps of resuscitation can begin during this time [1]. In the preterm lamb animal model, it has been shown that establishing ventilation prior to cord clamping improves cardiovascular function, increases pulmonary blood flow, and smoothens the transition to extrauterine life compared to the traditional practice of cutting the cord before beginning resuscitation [2]. While delayed cord clamping is feasible in infants at risk for resuscitation, there is currently no evidence to suggest that delayed cord clamping improves outcomes for infants who actually require resuscitation at birth [3,4]. It may be, however, that infants who require resuscitation at birth would have the most to gain from delayed cord clamping by facilitating placental transfusion and gas exchange, while the resuscitation team establishes adequate aeration of the lungs. Additional research is needed to determine if delayed cord clamping improves outcomes in infants requiring intubation for meconium aspiration.

In order to balance the benefits of delayed cord clamping for vigorous infants with the current standard practice of immediate cord cutting if resuscitation is needed, it is important for the delivery team to maintain open communication throughout the delivery process. A member of the neonatal team must be able to observe the infant, begin the initial steps of resuscitation, and call for immediate cord cutting if there is concern that additional resuscitation steps are necessary. Fig. 25B.1 illustrates appropriate delivery room management for infants at risk for meconium aspiration.

3. **Routine intubation and suction** are not recommended. For nearly 30 years, it was a standard practice to perform intrapartum suctioning for any infant born with meconium-stained amniotic fluid. This was followed by endotracheal suctioning for infants felt to be high risk for meconium aspiration syndrome (MAS)

Delivery room management of meconium-stained fluid

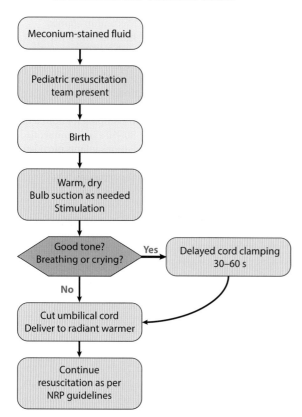

Fig. 25B.1 Delivery Room Management of Infants at Risk for Meconium Aspiration. *NRP*, Neonatal Resuscitation Program.

[5]. Lack of evidence for benefit and concern about potential harm has led to a gradual abandonment of these interventions. For the vigorous infant, clearing of secretions with a bulb syringe may be all that is needed. For the depressed infant with poor respiratory effort, the initial steps of resuscitation remain the same as for any other infant. The routine practice of intubation and tracheal suctioning is no longer recommended. Endotracheal intubation should be performed if bag-mask ventilation is not sufficient to stabilize the infant, and suctioning of the airway may be necessary if the endotracheal tube (ETT) is obstructed [3].

4. **Bulb suction.** In the case that an infant born with meconium-stained fluid has an obstructed airway or is not breathing, it is appropriate to use suction tools to remove the obstruction. The infant's head should be placed in the "sniffing" position, and a bulb syringe can be used to gently remove secretions from the mouth and then the nose.

5. **Suction catheter.** If the bulb syringe is not sufficient, a suction catheter attached to a suction source set between 80 and 100 mmHg (109–136 cmH$_2$O) may be used to clear the airway [6]. Care should be taken to avoid blind deep suctioning with a catheter; this is more likely to result in gastric aspiration than airway clearance. Evidence suggests that gastric aspiration in the delivery room may be harmful and is unlikely to provide any benefit; therefore, this practice should be avoided [7].

6. **Intubation.** If an ETT is placed and becomes obstructed with meconium, a suction catheter may be inserted into the ETT. If meconium cannot be easily removed with a suction catheter set at 80–100 mmHg suction, the ETT should be attached directly to the suction tubing using a meconium aspirator (Fig. 25B.2). With the suction activated, the ETT should be withdrawn over 3–5 s and replaced with a clean ETT. This procedure may be repeated only until there is adequate ventilation; complete removal of meconium should not be expected [6].

Respiratory support—recruitment phase

1. The initial goal of respiratory support is to optimize oxygen delivery and lung volume. This will decrease ventilation–perfusion (V/Q) mismatch, improve gas exchange, and help speed the drop in pulmonary vascular resistance that is expected as the neonate transitions from fetal circulation to neonatal circulation. Fig. 25B.3 and Table 25B.1 illustrate the recommended pathway of respiratory support for infants with meconium aspiration.

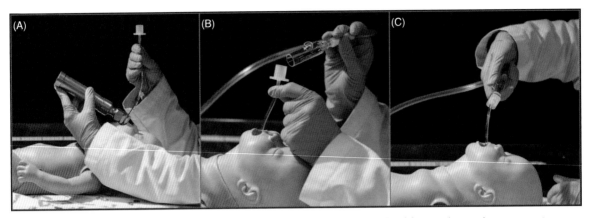

Fig. 25B.2 Use of Meconium Aspirator. (A) Intubate with standard endotracheal tube. (B) Meconium aspirator connects suction tubing to endotracheal tube. (C) Operator obstructs side hole to activate suction and pulls back slowly over 3–5 s until endotracheal tube has been removed. Courtesy: Mark Weems, MD.

2. Oxygen
   a. **Oxygen delivery.** Meconium aspiration is the most common cause of persistent pulmonary hypertension in the newborn; both the presence of meconium and the associated hypoxemia contribute to increased pulmonary vascular resistance [8–10]. Supplemental oxygen is well recognized to be a potent pulmonary vasodilator and should be delivered through a blender with nasal cannula flow of at least 2 L/min to maintain preductal PaO_2 50–70 mmHg and preductal saturation between 90% and 97%. Titrating oxygen delivery within these parameters balances the treatment of pulmonary hypertension with the risks of oxygen toxicity.
   b. **Oxygen hood or tent** to administer oxygen should be avoided, however, because administration of high concentrations of oxygen with a low distending pressure leads to absorption atelectasis [11]. The mechanism is similar to that used by the outdated treatment for pneumothorax. Described as nitrogen washout, highly concentrated oxygen replaces nitrogen within the poorly ventilated alveoli where it gets absorbed quickly. Because of airway obstruction or lack of distending pressure, there is inadequate pressure to prevent alveolar collapse. The progressive atelectasis increases V/Q mismatch, creates an intrapulmonary shunt, and worsens hypoxemia.
   c. **Oxygen toxicity.** Even in the presence of adequate distending pressure, excessive oxygen delivery causes more harm than benefit. In healthy term infants, the oxidative challenge of extrauterine life exceeds the newborn antioxidant capabilities resulting in elevated markers of oxidative stress that decrease over the first year after birth [12]. Data from premature infants and animal models show that administration of 90%–100% oxygen increases oxidative stress, downregulates antioxidant enzyme activity, and increases pulmonary vascular resistance compared to 30% oxygen or less [13–15]. Additional data from a meconium aspiration/antenatal ductal ligation model of PPHN in lambs confirm that pulmonary vascular resistance decreases with increasing oxygen saturation and PaO_2. However, pulmonary vascular resistance begins to increase as oxygen saturation approaches 100%, and there is no additional reduction in pulmonary vascular resistance beyond PaO_2 of 45 mmHg [16].

   There are no human data to determine the optimum oxygen delivery and goal saturation in the case of meconium aspiration. Histologic evaluation of lung tissue in infants with severe meconium aspiration has revealed that there are intrapulmonary bronchopulmonary anastomoses (Fig. 25B.4) formed that are common in other severe respiratory diseases such as alveolar capillary dysplasia, bronchopulmonary dysplasia, and congenital diaphragmatic hernia. These anastomoses contribute to intrapulmonary shunting and intractable hypoxemia that may not be corrected with increased oxygen administration [17].

   If inspired oxygen needs exceed 40%–60%, additional support should be considered to decrease the risk of excessive oxygen exposure.

3. **Noninvasive ventilation**
   a. **Noninvasive respiratory support**, including high-flow nasal cannula, nasal continuous positive

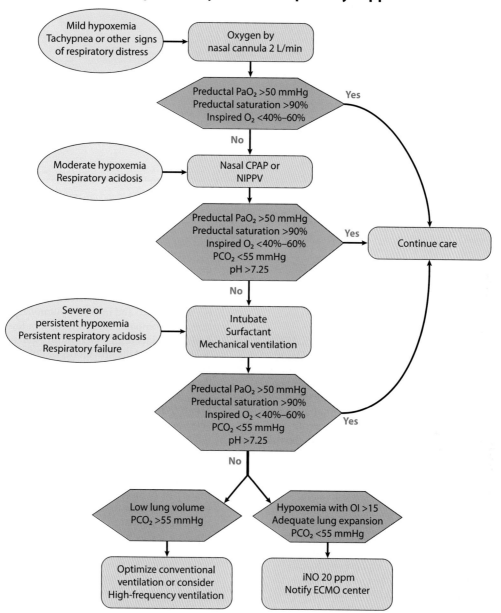

Fig. 25B.3 Respiratory Management of Infants With Respiratory Distress Due to Meconium Aspiration Syndrome. *CPAP,* Continuous positive airway pressure; *ECMO,* extracorporeal membrane oxygenation; *iNO,* inhaled nitric oxide; *NIPPV,* noninvasive positive pressure ventilation; *OI,* oxygen index; *PaO$_2$,* partial pressure of arterial oxygen; *PCO$_2$,* partial pressure of carbon dioxide.

Table 25B.1 Oxygen delivery and titration for meconium aspiration syndrome

Stage	Action	Goal
Initial	Nasal cannula 2 L/min Inspired O_2 40%	Preductal saturation 90%–97% and preductal PaO_2 50–70 mmHg
Saturation <90%	Increase FiO_2 as needed	
Inspired O_2 >60%	Change respiratory support mode	
Saturation >97%	Decrease FiO_2 as tolerated	
Inspired O_2 <30%	Wean respiratory support	

FiO_2, Fraction of inspired oxygen; *PaO_2,* partial pressure of arterial oxygen.

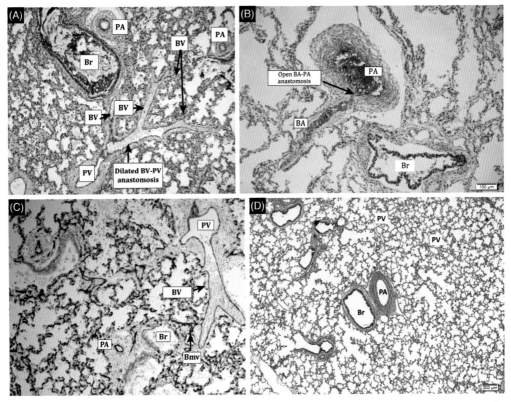

Fig. 25B.4 (A) Periodic acid–Schiff stain shows an enlarged anastomotic connection between the pulmonary vein and dilated bronchial veins (bronchial vein, *arrows*). Bronchial veins are markedly dilated, which may be due to increased blood flow in the bronchial (systemic) circulation. (B) H&E staining illustrates open vascular anastomosis between PA and BA. (C) CD31 immunostaining with the bronchial microvasculature (bronchial microvessels). (D) Histology of lung from young infant who died from nonrespiratory causes. *BA*, Bronchial artery; *Bmv*, bronchial microvessel; *Br*, bronchiole; *BV*, bronchiole vein; *H&E*, hematoxylin and eosin; *PA*, pulmonary artery; *PV*, pulmonary veins. From Ali N, Abman SH, Galambos C. Histologic evidence of intrapulmonary bronchopulmonary anastomotic pathways in neonates with meconium aspiration syndrome. J Pediatr 2015;167(6):1445–7 [17].

airway pressure (CPAP), and noninvasive positive pressure ventilation (NIPPV), is increasingly being used to support term and preterm infants in respiratory distress. These modes are preferred over oxygen delivery without distending pressure, and may be used to prevent intubation in infants with moderate respiratory distress.

There may be hesitation to use such noninvasive modes in the case of meconium aspiration for fear that a continuous distending pressure may increase the risk of pneumothorax. This fear is not unfounded given that increased risk of pneumothorax has been associated with both high-pressure CPAP in preterm infants and meconium aspiration in term infants [18,19]. Furthermore, meconium aspiration often presents with hyperexpansion of the lungs; the ball valve mechanism of partial meconium obstruction may

lead to air trapping beyond the obstruction until alveoli begin to rupture. Evidence, however, does not support this fear.

b. **CPAP** of 5–6 cmH$_2$O should be considered for infants requiring inspired O$_2$ greater than 40%–60% or those with respiratory acidosis (Table 25B.2). CPAP at moderate levels (5–6 cmH$_2$O) does not increase the risk of pneumothorax in term infants with meconium aspiration [20,21]. CPAP in this range may prevent atelectasis in those alveoli with impaired surfactant function and may contribute to distension of partially obstructed airways (Fig. 25B.5), thereby preventing air trapping and improving gas exchange [22].

c. **High-flow nasal cannula** may have a similar effect to CPAP due to the distending pressure associated with high flow rates. However, the relationship between flow and pressure is highly variable. In

Table 25B.2 Continuous positive airway pressure and high-flow nasal cannula settings for meconium aspiration syndrome

Setting	Start	Increase	Maximum	Decrease	Minimum
CPAP PEEP	5 cmH$_2$O	Inspired O$_2$ >40% or signs of respiratory distress	7 cmH$_2$O	Inspired O$_2$ <30%	4 cmH$_2$O
High flow	4–6 L/min	Inspired O$_2$ >40% or signs of respiratory distress	8 L/min	Inspired O$_2$ <30%	
Inspired O$_2$	30%	PaO$_2$ <50 mmHg or preductal saturation <90%	100% (temporarily) Generally should be <40%	PaO$_2$ >70 mmHg or preductal saturation >97%	21%
Temperature			34–37°C		
Humidity			100% Relative humidity		

CPAP, Continuous positive airway pressure; *PaO$_2$*, partial pressure of arterial oxygen.

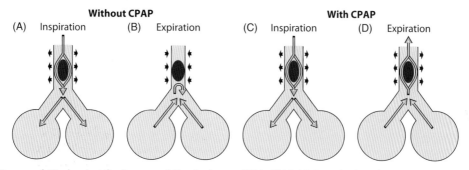

Fig. 25B.5 Proposed Mechanism for Improved Gas Exchange With CPAP. (A) Negative intrathoracic pressure during inspiration allows air to flow around meconium particles in the airway. (B) During expiration, increased intrathoracic pressure compresses the airway around meconium particles and causes air to be trapped beyond the obstruction. (C) With CPAP, inspiratory flow remains as in panel A. (D) When CPAP is applied to the expiratory phase, airway compression is reduced allowing expiratory flow to pass around the meconium particles.

the case of meconium aspiration, the pressure delivered by high-flow nasal cannula may vary as lung compliance evolves over the first several days. Studies are needed to better define the role of high-flow nasal cannula for patients with meconium aspiration; recommendations from a recent consensus report as they might be applied to MAS are presented in Table 25B.2 [23].

d. **NIPPV.** For those infants unable to maintain adequate oxygenation and ventilation with CPAP, the addition of a respiratory rate and peak inspiratory pressure (PIP) may increase the effectiveness of noninvasive support. NIPPV is superior to CPAP in preventing intubation in preterm infants [24]. However, there are no data to guide its use in term infants with meconium aspiration. A significant concern exists regarding the safety of NIPPV with meconium aspiration because lungs affected by meconium aspiration have a prolonged time constant compared to lungs of a healthy, term infant. This puts infants with meconium aspiration at risk for inadvertent positive end-expiratory pressure (PEEP) and hyperexpansion if the expiratory time is insufficient. In the case of synchronized NIPPV, the inspiratory and expiratory times can be adjusted to prevent inadvertent PEEP. However, NIPPV is frequently nonsynchronized, increasing the chance that a breath is delivered during exhalation.

In the case of invasive ventilation, a breath delivered during exhalation causes "breath stacking" and inadvertent PEEP, but this is less of a concern for NIPPV. Ventilator breaths delivered during inspiration successfully increase tidal volume, while breaths delivered during exhalation or apnea have little effect on lung volume [25]. This phenomenon allows a spontaneously breathing infant to regulate the inspiratory and expiratory time. A longer set inspiratory time serves to increase the number of supported breaths without affecting expiratory time or leading to breath stacking. Inspirations synchronized with ventilator breaths are supported with the set PIP, while asynchronous inspirations are supported only with PEEP. The excess pressure delivered by the ventilator is distributed to the path of least resistance, generally out of the mouth. Table 25B.3 describes recommended settings for nonsynchronized NIPPV.

e. **Do not delay intubation.** While CPAP and NIPPV may be useful to prevent intubation in neonates, optimal lung expansion and ventilation are imperative for infants with meconium aspiration to prevent clinical decompensation that may result in a need for extracorporeal membrane oxygenation (ECMO) or death. Three common scenarios may occur that suggest noninvasive support is inadequate. First, there may be persistent respiratory acidosis with pH <7.25 and/or PCO_2 >55 mmHg. In this case, the respiratory support should be quickly increased to the maximum recommended settings for that mode and changed to another mode if there is not rapid improvement. Second,

Table 25B.3 Nonsynchronized noninvasive positive pressure settings for meconium aspiration syndrome

Setting	Start	Increase	Maximum	Decrease	Minimum
PEEP (cmH$_2$O)	5	Inspired O$_2$ >40% or signs of respiratory distress	7	Inspired O$_2$ <30%	4
PIP (cmH$_2$O)	20	PCO$_2$ >55 mmHg	25	PCO$_2$ <45 mmHg	10
Rate (bpm)	40	PCO$_2$ >55 mmHg	50	PCO$_2$ <45 mmHg only after PIP = 10 cmH$_2$O	0 (CPAP)
iTime (s)	0.5	If needed to increase the number of supported breaths	1	Once stable, before weaning rate	0.5
Inspired O$_2$	30%	PaO$_2$ <50 mmHg or preductal saturation <90%	100% (temporarily) Generally should be <40%	PaO$_2$ >70 mmHg or preductal saturation >97%	21%
Temperature			34–37°C		
Humidity			100% Relative humidity		

PaO$_2$, Partial pressure of arterial oxygen; *PCO$_2$*, partial pressure of carbon dioxide.

the patient may appear to be "fighting the vent." This may occur whether the respiratory support driver is a continuous flow or a variable flow device. This situation is a sign the patient is suffering from "air hunger" because the respiratory support mode does not match the patient's needs. Rather than sedating the patient to mask the signs of respiratory distress, it is preferable to intubate and use mechanical ventilation with or without sedation to support the patient's respiratory needs. Finally, the patient may appear stable but require high inspired O_2, often in excess of 60%. This too is a sign that noninvasive respiratory support is insufficient, and the patient should be supported with mechanical ventilation until the respiratory status improves.

4. **Surfactant**
   a. **Surfactant** should be given to any infant with MAS who is intubated or requiring FiO_2 greater than 40%. Meconium is known to impair surfactant function by altering surfactant structure and by inducing inflammation leading to increased surface tension within the alveoli [26]. Surfactant replacement has been shown to reduce the need for ECMO in term infants with respiratory failure associated with surfactant inactivation, and the American Academy of Pediatrics recommends clinicians consider rescue surfactant in the case of hypoxic respiratory failure due to conditions known to cause surfactant inactivation such as meconium aspiration [26,27].
   b. **Dose and frequency** of surfactant administration are dependent on the formulation available in each institution (Table 25B.4).

5. **Mechanical ventilation**
   a. **Ventilation strategies.** MAS is an uneven lung disease characterized by a high respiratory time constant, decreased compliance, and increased resistance. Several ventilation strategies have been used with very little evidence to guide practice. Choosing the best strategy for an individual

patient is complicated by several variables that increase V/Q mismatch, including atelectasis, localized hyperinflation, intrapulmonary shunting, inflammation, and pulmonary hypertension. The optimal ventilation strategy takes these variables into account and may change as the patient shifts from early phases of meconium-induced airway obstruction and surfactant inactivation to later phases of acute respiratory distress syndrome distinguished by the presence of inflammatory pulmonary edema [28].

   b. **PEEP.** To minimize atelectasis that occurs due to surfactant inactivation, administration of appropriate PEEP is necessary. Four to 7 cmH_2O is the optimal range with higher and lower PEEP associated with decreased oxygenation [29].
   c. **Tidal volume.** Either pressure-controlled ventilation or volume-targeted ventilation may be used, but tidal volume and minute ventilation requirements are higher in infants with meconium aspiration due to increased dead space. While tidal volume 4–6 mL/kg is appropriate for most neonates, a tidal volume of 5–7 mL/kg is recommended for infants with meconium aspiration [30].
   d. **Gas trapping.** In order to minimize hyperinflation caused by gas trapping, care should be taken to ensure adequate expiratory time. A respiratory rate between 40 and 60 breaths/min is appropriate for most term neonates with respiratory failure. At this rate, an inspiratory time of 0.3 s will ensure an expiratory time of at least 0.7 s. If there is significant gas trapping, ventilation may improve by lengthening the expiratory time. This can be accomplished by reducing the respiratory rate or shortening the inspiratory time to as little as 0.25 s [31].
   e. **Gentle ventilation.** Among newborns with pulmonary hypertension, often associated with meconium aspiration, the historic strategy was to use hyperventilation to improve oxygenation.

Table 25B.4 Intratracheal surfactant dosing

Trade names	Generic names	Sources	Initial dose (mL/kg)	Repeat dose
Curosurf	Poractant alfa	Porcine-derived minced lung extract	2.5	1.25 mL/kg q12 h, up to 3 doses
Infasurf	Calfactant	Calf lung extract	3	3 mL/kg q12 h, up to 3 doses
Surfaxin	Lucinactant	Synthetic	5.8	5.8 mL/kg q6 h, up to 4 doses
Survanta	Beractant	Modified bovine lung extract	4	4 mL/kg q6 h, up to 4 doses

The hypothesis states that because acidosis increases pulmonary vascular resistance, alkalosis must cause pulmonary vascular relaxation and decrease pulmonary hypertension. In the 1980s, hyperventilation was used frequently without any evidence of improved survival [8]. While it is recognized that hyperventilation may transiently improve oxygenation, the strategy offers no long-term benefit and is believed to cause excessive lung injury [32,33]. Gentle ventilation, currently the standard of care, minimizes barotrauma while maintaining sufficient oxygen delivery [34]. Optimal blood gas parameters and ventilator limits have not been defined for MAS. A gentle ventilation strategy generally limits the PIP to 25 cmH_2O or less. Therapy should be adjusted to target the following blood gas parameters: PCO_2 45–55 mmHg, PaO_2 50–70 mmHg, and pH greater than 7.25.

f. **High-frequency ventilation (HFV)** may be used as a rescue therapy when conventional ventilation fails to achieve or maintain goal blood gas parameters within acceptable pressure limits [35]. It has been proposed that small tidal volumes associated with HFV may protect the newborn from lung injury induced by conventional ventilation. However, it is not clear that routine use of HFV is better than conventional ventilation for newborns with respiratory failure [36]. The success of both conventional and HFV strategies is highly dependent on the ability to reverse atelectasis, maintain optimal lung volume, and minimize intrapulmonary shunting. Compared to conventional ventilation, HFV offers improved CO_2 removal due to increased minute ventilation [37]. This may be of benefit in meconium aspiration as it may allow for adequate CO_2 removal even in the common scenario of mixed atelectasis and hyperexpansion.

- **High-frequency oscillatory ventilation (HFOV)** (Table 25B.5)
  - **Mean airway pressure (MAP)** is used to control oxygenation. When changing from conventional ventilation to HFOV, it is generally recommended to choose a MAP 2 cmH_2O above the previously measured MAP on the conventional ventilator. Following a gentle ventilation strategy, this typically yields a starting HFOV MAP of 13–14 cmH_2O. Be careful to avoid a drop in MAP when switching from conventional ventilation to

Table 25B.5 High-frequency oscillator settings for meconium aspiration syndrome

Setting	Start	Increase	Maximum	Decrease	Minimum
MAP (P_{aw}) (cmH_2O)	13–14 or 2 >MAP on conventional ventilator	Hypoxemia (preductal saturation <90% or PaO_2 <50 mmHg) and/or low lung volume (<8 ribs expanded)	ECMO available*: 25 ECMO not feasible*: as needed to achieve 10 ribs expansion	Overexpansion (>10 ribs expanded) or inspired O_2 <30%	12
Amplitude (ΔP) (cmH_2O)	25 (Adjust to obtain chest wiggle)	PCO_2 >55 mmHg	ECMO available*: 45 ECMO not feasible*: 60	PCO_2 <45 mmHg	13
Frequency (Hz)	10–12	PCO_2 <45 mmHg (after adjusting amplitude)	15	PCO_2 >55 mmHg (after adjusting amplitude)	ECMO available*: 8 ECMO not feasible*: 5
% Inspiratory time	33	Changes are generally not necessary			
Bias flow (L/min)	15	If unable to maintain desired MAP	20		15

ECMO, Extracorporeal membrane oxygenation; MAP (P_{aw}), mean airway pressure; PaO_2, partial pressure of arterial oxygen; PCO_2, partial pressure of carbon dioxide.
*ECMO available centers include those with access to a regional ECMO center; these centers should initiate the ECMO process early to minimize ventilator-associated lung injury. For centers in which transfer for ECMO is not feasible, physicians may increase ventilator support as needed to maintain survival; every effort should be made to wean to lower ventilator settings as quickly as possible.

HFOV as this will worsen atelectasis. Adjust as needed to minimize atelectasis and optimize lung expansion to 8–10 ribs.

- **Amplitude** is used to control CO_2 removal. Start at 25 cmH$_2$O and adjust to obtain good chest wiggle.
- **Frequency** should be optimized for the patient's size and disease. For infants with meconium aspiration should generally be 10–12 Hz. A lower frequency may improve CO_2 removal, partly by increasing expiratory time. A higher frequency will be more appropriate for smaller patients.
- **High-frequency jet ventilation (HFJV)** (Table 25B.6)
  - **PEEP** is the primary variable to control oxygenation and MAP in HFJV. Start at 7–12 cmH$_2$O and adjust to maintain 8–10 ribs expansion. Optimal PEEP has been reached when oxygen saturation remains stable as the backup rate is turned to zero. It is acceptable to allow greater than 10 ribs expansion when using HFJV as long as

there is no hemodynamic impairment from excessive airway pressure.
- **HFJV PIP** should start at 20 cmH$_2$O and may be adjusted to achieve chest wiggle. Further adjustments are needed to maintain PCO_2 45–55 mmHg. The maximum PIP available is 50 cmH$_2$O, but when PIP is greater than 40 cmH$_2$O it may be helpful to slowly increase the HFJV inspiratory time.
- **HFJV rate** is determined by the disease process and the patient size. For infants with meconium aspiration, HFJV rate should start at 360 breaths/min (6 Hz). Gas trapping may be recognized by measuring PEEP more than 1-2 cmH$_2$O above set PEEP. In this case, the rate should be decreased to increase expiratory time, generally in steps of 60 breaths/min (1 Hz).
- **Backup breaths** are used with HFJV to prevent atelectasis. Start with a backup rate of 5 breaths/min. PIP should be set high enough to obtain visible chest rise but should be less than HFJV PIP. If PEEP is adequate, the backup rate may be turned off with no loss of lung

Table 25B.6 High-frequency jet settings for meconium aspiration syndrome

Setting	Start	Increase	Maximum	Decrease	Minimum
PEEP (cmH$_2$O)	7–12 or conventional ventilator MAP or 1–2 <HFOV MAP	Hypoxemia (preductal saturation <90% or PaO$_2$ <50 mmHg), even if hyperexpanded or to maintain MAP when weaning PIP		If cardiac output is impaired (i.e., small cardiac silhouette, decreased cardiac output) or if oxygenation is stable with Inspired O$_2$ <30%	4
Jet PIP (cmH$_2$O)	20 or 1–2 < conventional PIP	PCO$_2$ >55 mmHg	40	PCO$_2$ <45 mmHg	16
Jet rate (bpm)	360	Weight <2 kg	420	Measured PEEP >1-2 cmH$_2$O over set PEEP or PCO$_2$ >55 mmHg (after adjusting PIP) or nearing extubation with PIP <20	240
Jet iTime (s)	0.02	Changes are generally not necessary. May increase to 0.024 if PIP = 40 cmH$_2$O and PCO$_2$ >55 mmHg			
Backup PIP (cmH$_2$O)	Adequate for chest rise	To prevent atelectasis	1 <Jet PIP	Minimize to prevent lung injury	
Backup rate (bpm)	3–5	To prevent atelectasis	10	Once optimal PEEP is reached	0
Backup iTime (s)	0.4	Changes are generally not necessary			

HFOV, High-frequency oscillatory ventilator; *MAP*, mean airway pressure; *PaO$_2$*, partial pressure of arterial oxygen; *PCO$_2$*, partial pressure of carbon dioxide; *PEEP*, positive end-expiratory pressure; *PIP*, peak inspiratory pressure.

expansion. If oxygen saturation drops when the backup rate is turned off, a re-recruitment maneuver is necessary. Increase the PEEP by 1 cmH$_2$O and set the backup rate to 5–10. After 30–60 min, turn the backup rate to zero and observe for a drop in saturation. This maneuver may need to be repeated several times to achieve optimal PEEP. If recurring atelectasis is impossible to prevent with optimal PEEP, a backup rate of 3–5 may be used until atelectasis resolves.

- **Choice of high-frequency mode.** The choice HFOV or HFJV is best determined by the clinician's comfort and experience. There are no clear data to show that one mode is superior to the other for newborns with meconium aspiration. However, several studies suggest there may be clinical differences between these modes. In both animal models and preterm infants with hypoxic respiratory failure, HFJV is associated with improved oxygenation at lower MAPs compared to HFOV [38,39]. Without compelling evidence to support one HFV mode over the other for meconium aspiration, the preferred mode is the one that can most successfully be managed by the bedside clinicians.

Respiratory support—stable phase

1. Once adequate lung expansion and gas exchange have been achieved with FiO$_2$ less than 0.6, patience is required on the part of the physician while the patient recovers from the meconium-induced pulmonary insult. Respiratory support during this phase is focused on maintaining gentle ventilation parameters, optimizing lung expansion, and limiting oxygen toxicity. Adjustments may be needed to maintain goals shown in Table 25B.7, but changes should be made slowly to prevent loss of lung recruitment.

Respiratory support—weaning phase

1. After several days, inflammation from the meconium insult resolves and PVR begins to drop. During this phase, the clinical condition improves allowing for the slow and consistent wean of respiratory support. FiO$_2$ should generally be less than 0.4; an increase in oxygen needs signifies that attempts to wean were too aggressive, and the clinician should move back to the stable or recruitment phase of management. Adjustments should be made in a stepwise fashion to maintain lung recruitment and to prevent the return of pulmonary hypertension. General weaning recommendations are presented in Fig. 25B.6; adjustments may be needed based on individual patient needs.

2. **Mechanical ventilation.** There is little value to weaning from one invasive ventilation mode to another, unless it is done to improve patient comfort or to better match the mode of support to the patient's needs. For example, one does not need to change from HFOV to conventional ventilation simply because certain settings have been reached during the weaning phase.

Table 25B.7 Goal parameters during stable phase of meconium aspiration syndrome

Parameter	Goal	Respiratory mode	Adjustment
Chest X-ray	8–10 Ribs expansion	Noninvasive or conventional mechanical ventilation or HFJV	PEEP
		HFOV	MAP ($P_{\overline{aw}}$)
Preductal oxygen saturation	90%–97%	Noninvasive or conventional mechanical ventilation or HFJV	PEEP or FiO$_2$
		HFOV	MAP ($P_{\overline{aw}}$) or FiO$_2$
PaO$_2$	50–70 mmHg	Noninvasive or conventional mechanical ventilation or HFJV	PEEP or FiO$_2$
		HFOV	MAP ($P_{\overline{aw}}$) or FiO$_2$
PCO$_2$	45–55 mmHg	Noninvasive positive pressure ventilation or HFJV	PIP
		Conventional mechanical ventilation	PIP or rate
		HFOV	Amplitude (ΔP)

FiO$_2$, Fraction of inspired oxygen; *HFJV*, high-frequency jet ventilator; *HFOV*, high-frequency oscillatory ventilator; *MAP*, mean airway pressure; *PaO$_2$*, partial pressure of arterial oxygen; *PCO$_2$*, partial pressure of carbon dioxide; *PEEP*, positive end-expiratory pressure; *PIP*, peak inspiratory pressure.

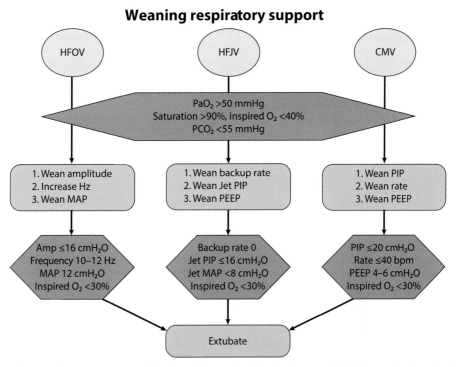

Fig. 25B.6 Weaning Respiratory Support With Meconium Aspiration Syndrome. *CMV,* Conventional mechanical ventilator; *FiO$_2$,* fraction of inspired oxygen; *HFJV,* high-frequency jet ventilator; *HFOV,* high-frequency oscillatory ventilator; *MAP,* mean airway pressure; *PaO$_2$,* partial pressure of arterial oxygen; *PCO$_2$,* partial pressure of carbon dioxide; *PEEP,* positive end-expiratory pressure; *PIP,* peak inspiratory pressure.

Instead, the clinician should focus on continuing to wean until extubation can be achieved.

3. **Noninvasive respiratory support** may be used to facilitate earlier extubation. NIPPV, CPAP, and nasal cannula are frequently used as postextubation support. In addition to adjustments to maintain goals presented in Table 25B.7, it is recommended that weaning proceed only after inspired O$_2$ is less than 30% (Fig. 25B.7) [23]. In the case of nonsynchronized NIPPV, benefit is seen when at least 60% of breaths are supported [40]. This requires that the rate remains high, generally 40–50 bpm. As such, it is preferable to wean the PIP first to a minimum of 10 cmH$_2$O before weaning the rate.

Cardiovascular support

1. **Hypotension**, defined as blood pressure lower than the fifth percentile for age, is common in meconium aspiration. These infants may suffer from decreased right ventricular preload due to systemic inflammatory vasodilation, decreased left ventricular preload due to

pulmonary hypertension, and decreased myocardial contractility due to hypoxic injury. Because there are few normative data available for neonates in the first few days of life, clinicians frequently follow the mean blood pressure, which is expected to increase over the first 3 days after birth. This method, however, does not predict which patients will benefit from intervention to modify the blood pressure [41]. Other clinical observations such as urine output, serum lactate level, capillary refill, acidosis, and functional echocardiography should be considered, although each of these alone is of limited value [42]. If intervention is felt to be indicated, normal blood pressures should be targeted to optimize cardiac function and oxygen delivery. Targeting supraphysiologic blood pressure in an effort to reduce right-to-left shunting is not recommended [32].

2. **Volume resuscitation.** The first step in the treatment of hypotension is to ensure adequate circulatory volume. If volume expansion is needed, an isotonic crystalloid solution may be given slowly in doses of 10 mL/kg [3]. If normal blood pressure is not maintained after volume administration, additional therapy is indicated [32].

Postextubation respiratory support

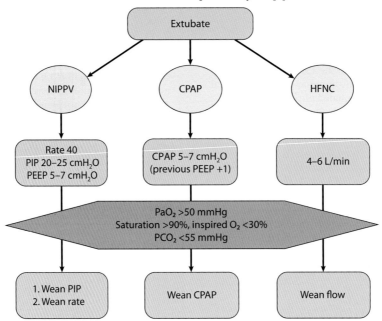

Fig. 25B.7 Weaning Postextubation Respiratory Support With Meconium Aspiration Syndrome. *CPAP*, Continuous positive airway pressure; *FiO₂*, fraction of inspired oxygen; *HFNC*, high-flow nasal cannula; *NIPPV*, noninvasive positive pressure ventilation; *PaO₂*, partial pressure of arterial oxygen; *PCO₂*, partial pressure of carbon dioxide; *PEEP*, positive end-expiratory pressure.

3. **Inotropes and vasopressors** are discussed in detail in Chapter 31 Management of Shock. The most common medications are discussed briefly as follows.
   a. **Dopamine** is the most frequently used medication for increasing blood pressure in the neonatal intensive care unit. Acting on multiple receptors, dopamine has a dose-dependent effect resulting in increased blood pressure by increasing cardiac contractility and raising systemic vascular resistance. Dopamine may also increase pulmonary vascular resistance when used to treat hypotension in infants with pulmonary hypotension; however, dopamine has a greater effect on systemic vascular resistance than on pulmonary vascular resistance [42].
   b. **Epinephrine** increases blood pressure by increasing cardiac contractility and raising systemic vascular resistance. Caution is advised because epinephrine may lead to a rise in lactate levels that may cloud one's assessment of adequate perfusion [43].
   c. **Dobutamine** is preferred in the case of myocardial systolic dysfunction, which may occur with

meconium aspiration due to hypoxia. However, it should be avoided if there is vasodilation or impaired cardiac filling because it may further decrease systemic resistance and limit cardiac relaxation [43].
   d. **Vasopressin** acts as a potent vasoconstrictor in the case of catecholamine-resistant hypotension. Small studies suggest that low-dose vasopressin leads to increase blood pressure and urine output and leads to decrease in both lactate level and inotrope infusion rates. However, its use beyond 24 h is associated with hyponatremia, which may be severe [44–46].
   e. **Hydrocortisone** remains the preferred treatment for catecholamine-resistant hypotension [43]. When used as rescue therapy in neonates receiving dopamine infusions of at least 15 mcg/kg/min, low-dose hydrocortisone is associated with increases in blood pressure, stroke volume, and systemic resistance and decreases in heart rate and dopamine requirement [47].

Bicarbonate infusion

1. **No benefit.** Similar to the hypothesis that contributed to hyperventilation becoming standard therapy for pulmonary hypertension in the 1980s, there was an assumption that alkali infusion may also be beneficial. Prior to the approval of inhaled nitric oxide (iNO), alkali infusion was frequently used, generally in the form of a continuous infusion of sodium bicarbonate [8]. To date, there has been no randomized clinical trial to demonstrate the safety or efficacy of sodium bicarbonate for neonates with meconium aspiration or other syndromes commonly associated with acidosis.
2. **Possible harm.** While there is no proven benefit of bicarbonate infusion, multiple studies have illustrated risks of harm associated with bicarbonate infusion, including increased mortality with rapid infusion [48], increased risk of death and intraventricular hemorrhage in preterm infants [49], and increased risk of ECMO in infants with pulmonary hypertension [8]. Until there is compelling evidence to support the use of sodium bicarbonate in neonates with meconium aspiration, it should be avoided. Therapeutic efforts should instead focus on improving oxygen delivery, reducing V/Q mismatch, and minimizing intrapulmonary shunting.

Antibiotics

1. **Antibiotic stewardship.** In the current era of antibiotic stewardship, there is a struggle between providing life-saving antibiotic therapy when indicated and preventing the inappropriate use of antibiotics. Some NICUs start antibiotics for nearly every admission, even without suspicion for infection [50]. This practice likely contributes to antibiotic resistance, and prolonged treatment may alter the infant's developing microbiome, increasing the risk of death and necrotizing enterocolitis [51]. The decision to give antibiotics to infants with meconium aspiration is complicated by several prenatal and postnatal factors.
2. **Inflammation or infection.** Meconium aspiration is associated with inflammation that may mimic signs of infection. It is often preceded by intra-amniotic and fetal inflammation, and may induce inflammation in the neonate when aspirated [52–54]. Perinatal passage of meconium may also be a marker of intra-amniotic infection and may enhance bacterial growth [55,56]. Furthermore, it is difficult to distinguish respiratory distress due to pneumonia or sepsis from respiratory distress due to meconium aspiration.

3. **Routine antibiotics** should be avoided. Recent data show that antibiotics offer no benefit to infants born through meconium-stained fluid or with MAS [56–59]. It may be reasonable to start antibiotics in infants with meconium aspiration who require significant respiratory support, but antibiotics should not be continued beyond 36–48 h without compelling evidence of infection such as a positive blood culture. Antibiotics should not be given to infants born through meconium-stained fluid without respiratory distress unless there are other maternal risk factors for which testing and empiric treatment for early onset sepsis are indicated.

Chest physiotherapy

1. **Chest physiotherapy**, including postural drainage, percussion, vibration, suction, and lavage, may reduce atelectasis and secretions in neonates [60,61]. However, in cases of meconium aspiration, these potential benefits must be balanced by frequent decompensation that occurs with even minimal stimulation.
2. **Saline lavage.** Due to the thick nature of meconium, it can be difficult to remove with a standard suction catheter. To assist with removal of secretions, normal saline is often instilled into the ETT prior to suctioning. However, this is not recommended because meconium is not easily dislodged by small aliquots of saline and it is associated with transient hypoxemia [62].
3. **Surfactant lavage.** There is some reported benefit from the use of diluted surfactant lavage. Additional research is needed to determine the best method and effect of this therapy [63].

Pulmonary vasodilators

Pulmonary vasodilators are discussed in detail in Chapter 21. The most common medications are discussed briefly as follows.

1. **iNO** has been shown to reduce the need for ECMO in term and near-term infants with hypoxic respiratory failure, including those with pulmonary hypertension due to meconium aspiration [64]. The recommended starting dose is 20 ppm and has been shown to be safe with no increase in neurodevelopmental, behavioral, or medical problems at 18–24-month follow-up [65]. In the case of meconium aspiration, it is important to recognize that iNO is delivered via respiratory gases so it is only effective in those areas of the lung receiving adequate ventilation. iNO will have

no effect on alveoli which are not available for gas exchange due to atelectasis or on alveoli which are preventing pulmonary flow due to overexpansion. iNO may, however, decrease V/Q mismatch by increasing pulmonary flow in those areas with optimal ventilation. Therefore, one should focus on optimizing ventilation before adding iNO.

This is not to suggest that iNO should be delayed when indicated because iNO therapy is more effective when started early, before the progression to more severe respiratory failure. While studies have not demonstrated a difference in mortality or need for ECMO, fewer patients progress to more severe disease when iNO is started for moderate disease (oxygenation index [OI] 15–25) compared to when started for severe disease (OI >35) [64].

2. **Echocardiogram.** If treatment with iNO is started, it is recommended to ensure that an echocardiogram is available to rule out congenital heart disease.

3. **ECMO center.** If resources are available to allow transport to an ECMO center, open communication with the nearest ECMO center is necessary so expedient transfer without discontinuation of iNO can be arranged if the patient worsens [66].

4. **Discontinuation.** If the patient does not respond to iNO, it should be discontinued. Even without adequate response, iNO should be weaned off over several hours to prevent rebound pulmonary hypertension that may occur from abrupt discontinuation.

5. **Other pulmonary vasodilators**
   a. **Other specific and nonspecific pulmonary vasodilators** have been used for neonates with pulmonary hypertension, although there is little supportive evidence of benefit for infants with MAS.
   b. **Sildenafil.** There is growing interest in using sildenafil and other phosphodiesterase 5 (PDE-5) inhibitors to treat pulmonary hypertension in neonates. Several small studies found that sildenafil was associated with improved survival in neonates with pulmonary hypertension without access to advanced therapies such as iNO or HFV [67]. The benefits of adding sildenafil for meconium aspiration patients already being treated with iNO and optimal ventilation are not clear. There is a plausible hypothesis that sildenafil may enhance the effect of iNO by blocking breakdown of cyclic GMP. Animal studies suggest that brief hyperoxia increases PDE-5 activity, which is responsible for cyclic GMP breakdown and could limit the effectiveness of iNO [68]. Sildenafil may help facilitate weaning of iNO if the infant remains on iNO beyond 5 days, and it may improve oxygenation in infants with pulmonary hypertension who are unresponsive to iNO. It

seems to be well tolerated in the short term without associated hypotension that may be seen in other disease states [69–71]. However, there are no large randomized control trials to describe short-term or long-term effects of sildenafil in patients with meconium aspiration. As such, its use should be considered investigational and used with caution.

c. **Prostacyclin.** The prostacyclin—cyclic AMP—PDE-3 pathway runs in parallel to NO—cyclic GMP—PDE-5 and contributes to pulmonary vasodilation. Prostacyclin and its analogs have been used in both inhaled and enteral forms with short-term benefit, but no long-term data are available [72].

d. **Milrinone** inhibits PDE-3 leading to increased prostacyclin-induced pulmonary vasodilation by increased cyclic AMP levels. Effects in the neonate are variable because PDE-3 expression is low at birth and naturally increases over time. In the case of meconium aspiration, milrinone may become more effective after treatment with iNO because iNO increases PDE-3 activity in an animal model [43,73]. There are no data to determine the safety or efficacy of milrinone for patients with meconium aspiration. Milrinone may be beneficial if pulmonary hypertension is accompanied by ventricular dysfunction secondary to asphyxia or sepsis.

e. **Tolazoline** has been used historically prior to the approval of iNO. However, tolazoline is no longer recommended for the treatment of pulmonary hypertension due to meconium aspiration because there is a risk of extreme systemic hypotension.

f. **Magnesium sulfate** has been used to treat pulmonary hypertension without any randomized control trials to show benefit; it also carries a high risk of systemic hypotension [74].

g. **Nitroprusside** may be tolerated in infants with pulmonary hypertension; however, it is not recommended because response is variable and it is not associated with improved survival [75].

Extracorporeal membrane oxygenation

1. **ECMO** offers a survival advantage to neonates with severe hypoxic respiratory failure caused by reversible pulmonary disease [76]. Among neonates placed on ECMO for respiratory failure, MAS is the most common indication, representing 31% of cases. It is also associated with the best ECMO outcomes with 94% survival [77]. More recently, ECMO use

for meconium aspiration has decreased due to improvements in pre-ECMO respiratory management and other available therapies [72,78].

2. **Therapeutic goal.** The goal of ECMO is to support the respiratory and/or cardiovascular needs of the infant while the lungs recover from the meconium-induced injury and simultaneously minimizing further lung injury due to aggressive mechanical ventilation.

3. **Indications** for ECMO vary from institution to institution, but general recommendations include severe hypoxic respiratory failure defined by an OI (Fig. 25B.8) greater than 40 for 4 h, moderate respiratory failure defined by an OI greater than 20 for 24 h with maximal medical therapy, or severe or progressive respiratory failure unresponsive to interventions [79]. Maximal medical therapy is open to interpretation and variable depending on local resources.

4. **Do not delay ECMO.** One should keep in mind the goals of gentle ventilation and use of ECMO as part of a lung protection strategy rather than as a rescue therapy of last resort. ECMO is recognized to be a high-risk therapy, but follow-up data show long-term morbidity is related to the underlying illness rather than to the use of ECMO [80]. Therefore, neonates with MAS who do not improve with optimal ventilation and iNO should be offered ECMO before a prolonged course of hypoxia and instability contributes to long-term morbidities.

$$OI = \frac{100 \times FiO_2 \times MAP}{PaO_2}$$

Fig. 25B.8 *FiO$_2$*, Fraction of inspired oxygen; *MAP*, mean airway pressure (mmHg); *OI*, oxygenation Index; *PaO$_2$*, partial pressure of postductal arterial oxygen (mmHg).

Air leak syndromes

1. **Increased risk.** MAS increases the risk of air leak syndromes, both pulmonary interstitial emphysema and pneumothorax, because compliance and resistance are variable through the affected lungs due to heterogeneous distribution of meconium and surfactant deactivation. Mechanical ventilation with excessive pressure or gas trapping increases these risks. In the case of meconium aspiration, it is imperative to consider PIE or pneumothorax as a cause for clinical worsening and respond quickly.

2. **Pneumothorax.** Transillumination may help with a presumptive diagnosis. However, the presence of extrapulmonary air on chest radiograph will confirm the diagnosis. Needle thoracentesis is indicated in the case of confirmed or suspected pneumothorax with hemodynamic compromise or respiratory failure. However, the placement of a thoracostomy tube attached to suction will allow continued removal of extrapulmonary air until there is resolution of the air leak (Fig. 25B.9).

3. **Respiratory adjustments.** Both PIE and pneumothorax warrant adjustments to respiratory management, as described in Chapter 13B. If one lung is affected by airleak, rotation of the infant so the affected side is down improves ventilation in the unaffected side. The weight of surrounding structures partially compresses the airways in the affected lungs and allows for resolution of the air leak over time. Adjustments to the ventilator should be made to minimize tidal volume, maximize exhalation time, and prevent inadvertent PEEP. The high-frequency jet ventilator is effective in supporting gas

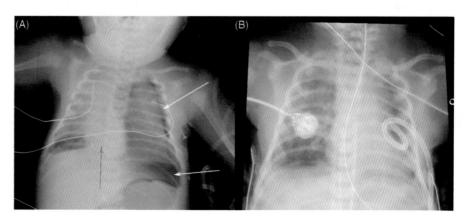

Fig. 25B.9 (A) Chest radiograph demonstrating the present of pneumothorax *(white arrows)* with mediastinal shift to the right *(red arrow)*. (B) Placement of a thoracostomy tube with resolution of the left-sided pneumothorax.

exchange in the presence of an air leak syndrome; a rate of 60–120 breaths/min lower than typical for the patient's size will increase exhalation time and may hasten resolution of the air leak. It is also recommended to minimize backup PIP, rate, and inspiratory time [81]. If conventional ventilation is used in the case of an air leak, it is appropriate to choose a higher rate with the minimal PIP that will allow sufficient gas exchange. As the rate increases, however, the risk of breath stacking increases. This can be limited by shortening the inspiratory time [31].

Cases

Case 1

A 23-year-old gravida 1 mother with a normal prenatal course presents for induction of labor at 41 weeks of gestation. Upon artificial rupture of membranes, the mother passes meconium-stained amniotic fluid, and the fetus is found to have persistent category 3 fetal heart tracing. The newborn resuscitation team is called to the operating room for the delivery of a 3.9 kg infant male via urgent cesarean section.

The infant is flaccid at birth without respiratory effort. The umbilical cord is cut immediately and the infant is brought to the radiant warmer. The infant is dried and stimulated, and the airway is cleared with bulb suction. Despite the initial steps of resuscitation, however, the infant remains apneic. The initial assessment reveals a heart rate of 70 beats/min. Mask ventilation is initiated with the following parameters: PIP 18 cmH$_2$O, PEEP 5 cmH$_2$O, rate 40 bpm, and FiO$_2$ 0.3. Adequate chest rise is noted, but the pulse oximeter now reads pulse 53 and oxygen saturation 48%. The FiO$_2$ is turned up to 1.0 without clinical improvement, and the decision is made to intubate.

The ETT passes easily between the vocal cords and is used with a meconium aspirator to remove additional meconium from the airway (Fig. 25B.2). A second ETT is placed between the vocal cords and attached to the resuscitation circuit for ventilation with PIP 20 cmH$_2$O, PEEP 5 cmH$_2$O, rate 40 breaths/min, and FiO$_2$ 1.0. The heart rate increases to 160 and the saturation begins to increase. FiO$_2$ is titrated, so the saturation remains 92%–97%, and the infant is transported to the NICU on PIP 20 cmH$_2$O, PEEP 5 cmH$_2$O, rate 50 breaths/min, inspiratory time 0.3 s, and FiO$_2$ 0.65.

Upon arrival in the NICU, a chest radiograph reveals coarse interstitial opacities consistent with meconium aspiration (Fig. 25B.10) and the results of an arterial blood gas (ABG) are pH 7.03, PCO$_2$ 71 mmHg, PaO$_2$ 38 mmHg, bicarbonate 18, and base deficit 11. The FiO$_2$ has been turned

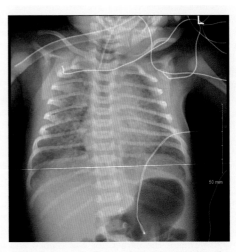

Fig. 25B.10 Chest Radiograph Demonstrating the Endotracheal Tube in Good Position and Coarse Central Interstitial Opacities Compatible With the Clinical History of Meconium Aspiration.

up to 0.75, and the measured tidal volume is 4 mL/kg. After surfactant is given (poractant alfa 2.5 mL/kg via ETT), the tidal volume increases to 5 mL/kg and FiO$_2$ is weaned to 0.5. Increasing the PIP to 25 cmH$_2$O increases the tidal volume to 6 mL/kg, and a follow-up ABG is pH 7.28, PCO$_2$ 48 mmHg, PaO$_2$ 52 mmHg, bicarbonate 22 mEq/L, and base deficit 4 mEq/L.

Over the next 4 h, FiO$_2$ is slowly titrated up to 1.0, and a follow-up ABG is pH 6.95, PCO$_2$ 88 mmHg, PaO$_2$ 36 mmHg, bicarbonate 19 mEq/L, and base deficit 12 mEq/L. A repeat chest radiograph confirms there is no air leak, and the ventilator is changed to HFOV with MAP 14 cmH$_2$O, amplitude 25 cmH$_2$O, and frequency 10 Hz. FiO$_2$ is weaned down to 0.7, and the blood gas improves. An echocardiogram now shows right heart dilation and suggests near-systemic pulmonary pressure. Over the next 2 h, the blood pressure drops to 42/25 (mean 31) mmHg and FiO$_2$ is turned up to 1.0 for persistent hypoxemia.

Dopamine is started at 5 mcg/kg/min continuous IV drip and slowly titrated up to maintain a goal mean blood pressure between 40 and 50 mmHg. As the dopamine infusion approaches 15 mcg/kg/min, hydrocortisone is added at a starting dose of 10 mg/m^2 IV every 8 h.

Despite maintaining mean blood pressure between 40 and 50 mmHg and increasing the HFOV MAP as high as 25 cmH$_2$O, the FiO$_2$ remains 1.0. Oxygen saturation at the right wrist has generally been 90%–94%, but now drops as low as 75%. The oxygen saturation at the left foot drops to 59%. iNO is added to the respiratory circuit at 20 ppm with immediate improvement of saturation (preductal 89%, postductal 86%). ABG now results pH 6.84, PCO$_2$ 71, PaO$_2$ 50, bicarbonate 12, and base deficit 20. In response, the

HFOV amplitude is titrated up to 45 cmH$_2$O. Although the PCO$_2$ improves slightly, oxygenation continues to worsen. Sildenafil 0.8 mg/kg/day continuous IV drip is started, and the ECMO team is called.

The infant is placed on veno-venous ECMO without complications. ABG after cannulation is pH 7.45, PCO$_2$ 36 mmHg, PaO$_2$ 254 mmHg, bicarbonate 24 mEq/L, and base deficit 0. Blood pressure increases to 85/60 (mean 68) mmHg, and dopamine is slowly weaned off. The HFOV is changed to a conventional ventilator with PIP 20 cmH$_2$O, PEEP 7 cmH$_2$O, rate 30, iTime 0.4 s, and FiO$_2$ 0.4 for the duration of the ECMO course. iNO was weaned off and sildenafil was discontinued. Finally, hydrocortisone was discontinued.

Throughout the ECMO course, flow was titrated to maintain oxygenation targets PaO$_2$ 50–70 mmHg. After 5 days, the infant was tolerating ECMO flow of 60 mL/kg/min (230 mL/min). The oxygenator was capped and the patient was decannulated.

After decannulation, he had a transient increase in FiO$_2$ to 0.55 that was weaned to 0.35 the following day. Over the next several days, the PIP is weaned to 18 cmH$_2$O, the rate is weaned to 30, the PEEP is weaned to 6, and FiO$_2$ is weaned to 0.28. The infant is extubated to HFNC 4 L/min and weaned to room air over the next 4 days because FiO$_2$ remained <0.3. The infant is discharged home on room air once he is able to meet his nutritional goals.

Case 2

A 28-year-old gravida 2, para 1 mother with a normal prenatal course presents in labor at 40 weeks of gestation. After spontaneous rupture of membranes, the mother passes meconium-stained amniotic fluid. The newborn resuscitation team is called to the delivery room for the birth of a 4.2 kg infant female via spontaneous vaginal delivery.

The infant is active at birth and cutting the umbilical cord is delayed while the infant is dried and stimulated. After 60 s, the umbilical cord is cut and the infant is brought to the radiant warmer for evaluation. The infant remains vigorous, and the airway is cleared with bulb suction. The heart rate remains greater than 100 bpm, and the oxygen saturation is rising appropriately without respiratory support.

At 7 min after birth, the infant becomes tachypneic and begins to have subcostal retractions. The heart rate remains greater than 100 bpm, but the oxygen saturation at the right wrist drops to 75%. This infant is placed on supplemental oxygen 2 L/min via nasal cannula and oxygen delivery is titrated up to 80% to maintain oxygen saturation at least 90%. The infant is transported to the NICU where a chest radiograph reveals a large left-sided pneumothorax (Fig. 25B.9A).

Preductal oxygen saturation has dropped to 75%, although the infant is now on 100% oxygen via nasal cannula at 2 L/min. A left-sided chest tube is placed and the extrapleural air is removed. Oxygen saturation increases to 87%, but the nurse is unable to wean the oxygen below 100%. The patient is intubated, umbilical catheters are placed, and surfactant (poractant alfa 2.5 mL/kg via ETT) is given. The ventilator is set on SIMV Volume Guarantee with rate 40 bpm, inspiratory time 0.3 s, tidal volume 6 mL/kg, pressure limit 25 cmH$_2$O, and PEEP 5 cmH$_2$O.

The chest radiograph (Fig. 25B.9B) shows resolution of the pneumothorax, and the ABG shows pH 7.03, PCO$_2$ 48 mmHg, PaO$_2$ 30, bicarbonate 12, and base deficit 16. The OI is 28, and an echocardiogram reveals normal cardiac anatomy with suprasystemic pulmonary pressure. iNO is started at 20 ppm, and a follow-up ABG is pH 7.12, PCO$_2$ 50 mmHg, PaO$_2$ 48 mmHg, bicarbonate 16 meq/L, and base deficit 12 mEq/L.

Over the next 24 h, the infant remains stable on conventional ventilation and iNO, but the nurse is unable to wean FiO$_2$ below 0.7 due to frequent desaturation events that resolve with sedation. Sildenafil is started at a dose of 0.5 mg/kg via NG tube every 6 h. After 24 h of sildenafil, the infant is having fewer desaturation events and FiO$_2$ has been weaned to 0.6. She tolerates weaning iNO off over 6 h followed by a further reduction in oxygen administration.

There is no evidence of continued air leak, and the chest tube is removed. With continued clinical improvement, the infant is tolerating FiO$_2$ 0.3, tidal volume 5 mL/kg which requires a PIP of 17 cmH$_2$O, and rate 30 bpm. She is extubated to nasal CPAP 6 cmH$_2$O and weaned to room air over the next 3 days.

Once on room air, a follow-up echocardiogram shows resolution of pulmonary hypertension and sildenafil is discontinued. The infant is discharged home, and an echocardiogram 3 weeks after discharge shows there is no recurrence of pulmonary hypertension.

References

[1] Committee on Obstetric Practice. Committee Opinion No. 684: delayed umbilical cord Clamping after birth. Obstet Gynecol 2017;129(1):e5–e10.

[2] Bhatt S, Alison BJ, Wallace EM, et al. Delaying cord clamping until ventilation onset improves cardiovascular function at birth in preterm lambs. J Physiol 2013;591(8):2113–2126.

[3] Wyckoff MH, Aziz K, Escobedo MB, et al. Part 13: neonatal resuscitation: 2015 American Heart Association guidelines update for cardiopulmonary resuscitation and emergency cardiovascular care. Circulation 2015;132(18 Suppl. 2):S543–S560.

[4] Katheria AC, Brown MK, Faksh A, et al. Delayed cord clamping in newborns born at term at risk for resuscitation: a feasibility randomized clinical trial. J Pediatr 2017;187:313–317.

[5] Emergency Cardiac Care Committee and Subcommittees, American Heart Association. Guidelines for cardiopulmonary resuscitation and emergency cardiac care. Part VII. Neonatal resuscitation. JAMA 1992;268(16):2276–2281.

[6] Weiner GM, Zaichkin J, Kattwinkel J. American Academy of Pediatrics, American Heart Association. Textbook of neonatal resuscitation. 7th ed. Elk Grove Village, IL: American Academy of Pediatrics; 2016.

[7] Kiremitci S, Tuzun F, Yesilirmak DC, Kumral A, Duman N, Ozkan H. Is gastric aspiration needed for newborn management in delivery room? Resuscitation 2011;82(1):40–44.

[8] Walsh-Sukys MC, Tyson JE, Wright LL, et al. Persistent pulmonary hypertension of the newborn in the era before nitric oxide: practice variation and outcomes. Pediatrics 2000;105(1 Pt. 1):14–20.

[9] Ban R, Ogihara T, Mori Y, Oue S, Ogawa S, Tamai H. Meconium aspiration delays normal decline of pulmonary vascular resistance shortly after birth through lung parenchymal injury. Neonatology 2011;99(4):272–279.

[10] Lakshminrusimha S, Swartz DD, Gugino SF, et al. Oxygen concentration and pulmonary hemodynamics in newborn lambs

with pulmonary hypertension. Pediatr Res 2009;66(5):539–544.

[11] Derosa S, Borges JB, Segelsjo M, et al. Reabsorption atelectasis in a porcine model of ARDS: regional and temporal effects of airway closure, oxygen, and distending pressure. J Appl Physiol (1985) 2013;115(10):1464–1473.

[12] Friel JK, Friesen RW, Harding SV, Roberts LJ. Evidence of oxidative stress in full-term healthy infants. Pediatr Res 2004;56(6):878–882.

[13] Vento M, Moro M, Escrig R, et al. Preterm resuscitation with low oxygen causes less oxidative stress, inflammation, and chronic lung disease. Pediatrics 2009;124(3):e439–e449.

[14] Kumar VH, Patel A, Swartz DD, et al. Exposure to supplemental oxygen and its effects on oxidative stress and antioxidant enzyme activity in term newborn lambs. Pediatr Res 2010;67(1):66–71.

[15] Patel A, Lakshminrusimha S, Ryan RM, et al. Exposure to supplemental oxygen downregulates antioxidant enzymes and increases pulmonary arterial contractility in premature lambs. Neonatology 2009;96(3):182–192.

[16] Lakshminrusimha S, Konduri GG, Steinhorn RH. Considerations in the management of hypoxemic respiratory failure and persistent pulmonary hypertension in term and late preterm neonates. J Perinatol 2016;36(Suppl. 2):S12–S19.

[17] Ali N, Abman SH, Galambos C. Histologic evidence of intrapulmonary bronchopulmonary anastomotic pathways in neonates with meconium aspiration syndrome. J Pediatr 2015;167(6):1445–1447.

[18] Morley CJ, Davis PG, Doyle LW, et al. Nasal CPAP or intubation at birth for very preterm infants. N Engl J Med 2008;358(7):700–708.

[19] Duong HH, Mirea L, Shah PS, Yang J, Lee SK, Sankaran K. Pneumothorax in neonates: trends, predictors and outcomes. J Neonatal Perinatal Med 2014;7(1):29–38.

[20] Panton L, Trotman H. Outcome of neonates with meconium aspiration syndrome at the University Hospital of the West Indies, Jamaica: a resource-limited setting. Am J Perinatol 2017;34(12):1250–1254.

[21] Malik RK, Gupta RK. A two year experience in continuous positive airway pressure ventilation using nasal prongs and pulse oximetry. Med J Armed Forces India 2003;59(1):36–39.

[22] Murki S, Mehta A, Oleti T, Gannavaram D, Bhagwat P. Continuous positive airway pressure in meconium aspiration syndrome: an observational study. J Clin Neonatol 2015;4(2):96.

[23] Yoder BA, Manley B, Collins C, et al. Consensus approach to nasal high-flow therapy in neonates. J Perinatol 2017;37(7):809–813.

[24] Lemyre B, Laughon M, Bose C, Davis PG. Early nasal intermittent positive pressure ventilation (NIPPV) versus early nasal continuous positive airway pressure (NCPAP) for preterm infants. Cochrane Database Syst Rev 2016;12:CD005384.

[25] Owen LS, Morley CJ, Dawson JA, Davis PG. Effects of non-synchronised nasal intermittent positive pressure ventilation on spontaneous breathing in preterm infants. Arch Dis Child Fetal Neonatal Ed 2011;96(6):F422–F428.

[26] Polin RA, Carlo WA. Committee on Fetus and Newborn, American Academy of Pediatrics. Surfactant replacement therapy for preterm and term neonates with respiratory distress. Pediatrics 2014;133(1):156–163.

[27] Lotze A, Mitchell BR, Bulas DI, Zola EM, Shalwitz RA, Gunkel JH. Multicenter study of surfactant (beractant) use in the treatment of term infants with severe respiratory failure. Survanta in Term Infants Study Group. J Pediatr 1998;132(1):40–47.

[28] De Luca D, van Kaam AH, Tingay DG, et al. The Montreux definition of neonatal ARDS: biological and clinical background behind the description of a new entity. Lancet Respir Med 2017;5(8):657–666.

[29] Fox WW, Berman LS, Downes JJ Jr, Peckham GJ. The therapeutic application of end-expiratory pressure in the meconium aspiration syndrome. Pediatrics 1975;56(2):214–217.

[30] Sharma S, Clark S, Abubakar K, Keszler M. Tidal volume requirement in mechanically ventilated infants

with meconium aspiration syndrome. Am J Perinatol 2015;32(10):916–919.

[31] Goldsmith JP, Karotkin EH. Assisted ventilation of the neonate. 5th ed. Philadelphia, PA: Elsevier; 2011.

[32] Abman SH, Hansmann G, Archer SL, et al. Pediatric pulmonary hypertension: guidelines from the American Heart Association and American Thoracic Society. Circulation 2015;132(21):2037–2099.

[33] Sosulski R, Fox WW. Transition phase during hyperventilation therapy for persistent pulmonary hypertension of the neonate. Crit Care Med 1985;13(9):715–719.

[34] Wung JT, James LS, Kilchevsky E, James E. Management of infants with severe respiratory failure and persistence of the fetal circulation, without hyperventilation. Pediatrics 1985;76(4):488–494.

[35] Clark RH, Yoder BA, Sell MS. Prospective, randomized comparison of high-frequency oscillation and conventional ventilation in candidates for extracorporeal membrane oxygenation. J Pediatr 1994;124(3):447–454.

[36] Rojas MA, Lozano JM, Rojas MX, et al. Randomized, multicenter trial of conventional ventilation versus high-frequency oscillatory ventilation for the early management of respiratory failure in term or near-term infants in Colombia. J Perinatol 2005;25(11):720–724.

[37] Bancalari E, Polin RA. The newborn lung. 1st ed. Philadelphia, PA: Saunders/Elsevier; 2008.

[38] Friedlich P, Subramanian N, Sebald M, Noori S, Seri I. Use of high-frequency jet ventilation in neonates with hypoxemia refractory to high-frequency oscillatory ventilation. J Matern Fetal Neonatal Med 2003;13(6):398–402.

[39] Boros SJ, Mammel MC, Coleman JM, Horcher P, Gordon MJ, Bing DR. Comparison of high-frequency oscillatory ventilation and high-frequency jet ventilation in cats with normal lungs. Pediatr Pulmonol 1989;7(1):35–41.

[40] Kamerkar A, Hotz J, Morzov R, Newth CJL, Ross PA, Khemani RG. Comparison of effort of breathing for infants on nasal modes of respiratory support. J Pediatr 2017;185:26–32.e3.

[41] Sahni M, Jain S. Hypotension in neonates. NeoReviews 2016;17(10):e579-e589.

[42] Seri I. Systemic and pulmonary effects of vasopressors and inotropes

in the neonate. Biol Neonate 2006;89(4):340–342.

[43] Noori S, Seri I. Neonatal blood pressure support: the use of inotropes, lusitropes, and other vasopressor agents. Clin Perinatol 2012;39(1):221–238.

[44] Meyer S, Gortner L, McGuire W, Baghai A, Gottschling S. Vasopressin in catecholamine-refractory shock in children. Anaesthesia 2008;63(3):228–234.

[45] Ikegami H, Funato M, Tamai H, Wada H, Nabetani M, Nishihara M. Low-dose vasopressin infusion therapy for refractory hypotension in ELBW infants. Pediatr Int 2010;52(3):368–373.

[46] Acker SN, Kinsella JP, Abman SH, Gien J. Vasopressin improves hemodynamic status in infants with congenital diaphragmatic hernia. J Pediatr 2014;165(1):53–58.e1.

[47] Noori S, Friedlich P, Wong P, Ebrahimi M, Siassi B, Seri I. Hemodynamic changes after low-dosage hydrocortisone administration in vasopressor-treated preterm and term neonates. Pediatrics 2006;118(4):1456–1466.

[48] Usher R. Comparison of rapid versus gradual correction of acidosis in RDS of prematurity. Pediatr Res 1967;3:221.

[49] Berg CS, Barnette AR, Myers BJ, Shimony MK, Barton AW, Inder TE. Sodium bicarbonate administration and outcome in preterm infants. J Pediatr 2010;157(4):684–687.

[50] Hauge C, Stalsby Lundborg C, Mandaliya J, Marrone G, Sharma M. Up to 89% of neonates received antibiotics in cross-sectional Indian study including those with no infections and unclear diagnoses. Acta Paediatr 2017;106(10):1674–1683.

[51] Cotten CM, Taylor S, Stoll B, et al. Prolonged duration of initial empirical antibiotic treatment is associated with increased rates of necrotizing enterocolitis and death for extremely low birth weight infants. Pediatrics 2009;123(1):58–66.

[52] Lee J, Romero R, Lee KA, et al. Meconium aspiration syndrome: a role for fetal systemic inflammation. Am J Obstet Gynecol 2016;214(3). 366.e1–369.e1.

[53] Salvesen B, Stenvik J, Rossetti C, Saugstad OD, Espevik T, Mollnes TE. Meconium-induced release of cytokines is mediated by the TRL4/MD-2 complex in a CD14-

dependent manner. Mol Immunol 2010;47(6):1226–1234.

[54] Hofer N, Jank K, Strenger V, Pansy J, Resch B. Inflammatory indices in meconium aspiration syndrome. Pediatr Pulmonol 2016;51(6):601–606.

[55] Romero R, Hanaoka S, Mazor M, et al. Meconium-stained amniotic fluid: a risk factor for microbial invasion of the amniotic cavity. Am J Obstet Gynecol 1991;164(3):859–862.

[56] Goel A, Nangia S, Saili A, Garg A, Sharma S, Randhawa VS. Role of prophylactic antibiotics in neonates born through meconium-stained amniotic fluid (MSAF)—a randomized controlled trial. Eur J Pediatr 2015;174(2):237–243.

[57] Basu S, Kumar A, Bhatia BD. Role of antibiotics in meconium aspiration syndrome. Ann Trop Paediatr 2007;27(2):107–113.

[58] Natarajan CK, Sankar MJ, Jain K, Agarwal R, Paul VK. Surfactant therapy and antibiotics in neonates with meconium aspiration syndrome: a systematic review and meta-analysis. J Perinatol 2016;36(Suppl. 1): S49–S54.

[59] Kelly LE, Shivananda S, Murthy P, Srinivasjois R, Shah PS. Antibiotics for neonates born through meconium-stained amniotic fluid. Cochrane Database Syst Rev 2017;6:CD006183.

[60] Finer NN, Moriartey RR, Boyd J, Phillips HJ, Stewart AR, Ulan O. Postextubation atelectasis: a retrospective review and a prospective controlled study. J Pediatr 1979;94(1):110–113.

[61] Etches PC, Scott B. Chest physiotherapy in the newborn: effect on secretions removed. Pediatrics 1978;62(5):713–715.

[62] O'Leary J, Mitchell ML, Cooke M, Schibler A. Efficacy and safety of normal saline instillation and paediatric endotracheal suction: an integrative review. Aust Crit Care 2018;31(1):3–9.

[63] Hahn S, Choi HJ, Soll R, Dargaville PA. Lung lavage for meconium aspiration syndrome in newborn infants. Cochrane Database Syst Rev 2013;(4):CD003486.

[64] Barrington KJ, Finer N, Pennaforte T, Altit G. Nitric oxide for respiratory failure in infants born at or near term. Cochrane Database Syst Rev 2017;1:CD000399.

[65] The Neonatal Inhaled Nitric Oxide Study Group. Inhaled nitric oxide

in term and near-term infants: neurodevelopmental follow-up of the neonatal inhaled nitric oxide study group (NINOS). J Pediatr 2000;136(5):611–617.

[66] American Academy of Pediatrics. Committee on fetus and newborn. Use of inhaled nitric oxide. Pediatrics 2000;106(2 Pt. 1):344–345.

[67] Shah PS, Ohlsson A. Sildenafil for pulmonary hypertension in neonates. Cochrane Database Syst Rev 2011;(8):CD005494.

[68] Farrow KN, Lee KJ, Perez M, et al. Brief hyperoxia increases mitochondrial oxidation and increases phosphodiesterase 5 activity in fetal pulmonary artery smooth muscle cells. Antioxid Redox Signal 2012;17(3):460–470.

[69] Limjoco J, Paquette L, Ramanathan R, Seri I, Friedlich P. Changes in mean arterial blood pressure during sildenafil use in neonates with meconium aspiration syndrome or sepsis. Am J Ther 2015;22(2):125–131.

[70] Steinhorn RH, Kinsella JP, Pierce C, et al. Intravenous sildenafil in the treatment of neonates with persistent pulmonary hypertension. J Pediatr 2009;155(6). 841.e1–847.e1.

[71] Stocker C, Penny DJ, Brizard CP, Cochrane AD, Soto R, Shekerdemian LS. Intravenous sildenafil and inhaled nitric oxide: a randomised trial in infants after cardiac surgery. Intensive Care Med 2003;29(11):1996–2003.

[72] Fuloria M, Aschner JL. Persistent pulmonary hypertension of the newborn. Semin Fetal Neonatal Med 2017;22(4):220–226.

[73] Chen B, Lakshminrusimha S, Czech L, et al. Regulation of phosphodiesterase 3 in the pulmonary arteries during the perinatal period in sheep. Pediatr Res 2009;66(6):682–687.

[74] Asad A, Bhat R. Pharmacotherapy for meconium aspiration. J Perinatol 2008;28(Suppl. 3):S72–S78.

[75] Benitz WE, Malachowski N, Cohen RS, Stevenson DK, Ariagno RL, Sunshine P. Use of sodium nitroprusside in neonates: efficacy and safety. J Pediatr 1985;106(1):102–110.

[76] UK Collaborative ECMO Trial Group. UK collaborative randomised trial of neonatal extracorporeal membrane oxygenation. Lancet 1996;348(9020):75–82.

[77] Extracorporeal Life Support Organization. ECLS Registry Report International Summary. https://www.elso.org/Registry/Statistics/InternationalSummary.aspx. Updated July, 2016. Accessed July 18, 2016.

[78] Barbaro RP, Paden ML, Guner YS, et al. Pediatric Extracorporeal Life Support Organization Registry International Report 2016. ASAIO J 2017;63(4):456–463.

[79] ELSO. Guidelines for neonatal respiratory failure; 2013. Available from: https://www.elso.org/Portals/0/IGD/Archive/FileManager/8588d1a580cusersshyerdocumentselsoguidelinesforneonatalrespiratoryfailure13.pdf.

[80] McNally H, Bennett CC, Elbourne D, Field DJ. UK Collaborative ECMO Trial Group. United Kingdom collaborative randomized trial of neonatal extracorporeal membrane oxygenation: follow-up to age 7 years. Pediatrics 2006;117(5):e845–e854.

[81] General guidelines for life pulse HFV; 2017. Available from: http://www.bunl.com/uploads/4/8/7/9/48792141/hfjvguidelines.pdf.

Chapter | **26**

Persistent Pulmonary Hypertension of the Newborn (PPHN)

Satyan Lakshminrusimha, MD, P.K. Rajiv, MBBS, DCH, MD (Fellowship in Australia)

CHAPTER POINTS

- Labile hypoxemia and/or differential cyanosis are classic clinical features of PPHN.
- Severity of PPHN is assessed by echocardiography and hypoxemia by oxygenation index (OI) and oxygen saturation index (OSI).
- Management includes optimizing lung recruitment and ventilation, pulmonary vasodilator therapy and hemodynamic stabilization.
- Gentle ventilation targeting $PaCO_2$ between 50 to 60 mmHg and PaO_2 between 50 and 80 mmHg while avoiding acidosis (pH > 7.25) appears to be rational approach.

- Inhaled nitric oxide is a selective pulmonary vasodilator but does not lead to sustained improvement in a third of patients.

Introduction

Neonatal respiratory failure affects 2% of all live births and is responsible for more than one-third of all neonatal deaths. Persistent pulmonary hypertension of the newborn (PPHN) is a frequent complication of respiratory disease in neonates. PPHN can develop in approximately 10% of infants with hypoxemic respiratory failure (HRF) and can lead to severe respiratory distress and hypoxemia associated with considerable mortality (close to 7.6%) and morbidity [1,2]. Recent estimates suggest an incidence for PPHN of 1.9/1000 live births [1]. Newborns with PPHN are at risk for severe asphyxia and its complications, including death, chronic lung disease, neurodevelopmental sequelae, and other problems.

Definition

PPHN is a cardiopulmonary disorder characterized by labile systemic arterial hypoxemia secondary to elevated pulmonary vascular resistance (PVR) in relation to systemic vascular resistance (SVR) with resultant right-to-left shunting through persistent fetal channels such as the ductus arteriosus and foramen ovale, bypassing the lungs. Inadequate pulmonary blood flow leads to refractory hypoxemia, respiratory distress, and finally acidosis.

Pathophysiology

The pathophysiology of PPHN can be discussed under three subheadings—changes in pulmonary vasculature, lung, and heart (Fig. 26.1).

Pulmonary vasculature

During fetal life, pulmonary blood flow (Q_p) is low (5%–10% of combined ventricular cardiac output [CO] from both ventricles in lambs and 13%–21% in humans). This is due to high PVR and the presence of shunts (foramen ovale, ductus arteriosus) which permit blood to bypass the pulmonary vascular bed (Fig. 26.1). At birth, PVR decreases significantly, Q_p increases to 100% of right ventricular output, and, by 24 h after birth, pulmonary artery pressure (PAP) typically decreases to about 50% of systemic arterial pressure. In infants with PPHN, pulmonary vascular transition is not successful resulting in persistently elevated PVR. In cases of severe PPHN, pulmonary vasculature demonstrates increased muscularization of pulmonary arteries and peripheral extension of vascular smooth muscle cell layer.

Lungs

PPHN is classified as secondary when there is associated lung diseases (Fig. 26.2) such as meconium aspiration syndrome (MAS), pneumonia or sepsis, respiratory distress syndrome (RDS), transient tachypnea of newborn (TTN), and congenital diaphragmatic hernia (CDH). In these conditions, the lung parenchymal pathology leads to PPHN. If there is no underlying lung disease and PPHN is predominantly due to vascular changes, it is called primary, idiopathic, or black-lung PPHN (absence of lung disease and less vascularity make the lungs look black on chest X-ray).

Cardiac changes

Extrapulmonary right-to-left shunting of blood secondary to high PVR is the hallmark of PPHN. Right-to-left or bidirectional shunt is commonly seen at the level of patent foramen ovale (PFO, from right atrium to left atrium) or across the patent ductus arteriosus (PDA, from pulmonary artery to aorta). Elevated pulmonary arterial pressure can also result in pulmonary insufficiency, right ventricular hypertrophy (and dysfunction), tricuspid regurgitation (TR), bowing of the interventricular septum to the left, and

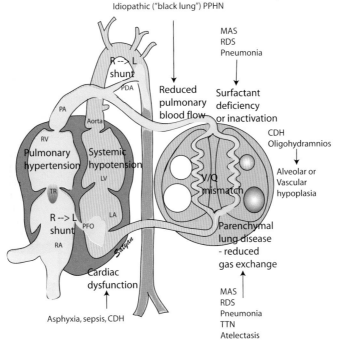

Fig. 26.1 **Etiology of PPHN and Hemodynamic Changes in PPHN/HRF.** *CDH*, Congenital diaphragmatic hernia; *LA*, left atrium; *LV*, left ventricle; *MAS*, meconium aspiration syndrome; *PA*, pulmonary artery; *PDA*, patent ductus arteriosus; *PFO*, patent foramen ovale; *RA*, right atrium; *RV*, right ventricle; *RDS*, respiratory distress syndrome; *TR*, tricuspid regurgitation; *TTN*, transient tachypnea of the newborn. Modified from Polin R, Fox W. Fetal and neonatal physiology. 5th ed. Philadelphia, PA, USA: Elsevier; 2016. Copyright: Satyan Lakshminrusimha.

445

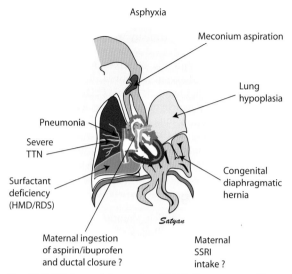

Asphyxia

Meconium aspiration

Lung hypoplasia

Pneumonia

Severe TTN

Congenital diaphragmatic hernia

Surfactant deficiency (HMD/RDS)

Satyan

Maternal ingestion of aspirin/ibuprofen and ductal closure ?

Maternal SSRI intake ?

Fig. 26.2 Etiology of Secondary PPHN. Common conditions associated with secondary PPHN are shown in this figure. Some controversy exists regarding maternal intake of nonsteroidal anti-inflammatory medications (NSAIDs) and selective serotonin reuptake inhibitors (SSRI) and PPHN. Copyright: Satyan Lakshminrusimha.

left ventricular dysfunction. The absence of structural heart disease and the presence of some of the above findings on echocardiogram confirm the diagnosis of PPHN.

Hemodynamic changes (Fig. 26.1)

1. Elevated PVR results in shunting of poorly oxygenated blood across the PDA and PFO. If right-to-left shunt occurs predominantly at the ductal level, differential cyanosis (the lower extremities are more cyanotic with lower pulse oximeter readings than the head and upper extremities) is present. It is important to evaluate patients with suspected PPHN by dual pulse oximetry. The preductal pulse oximetry should always be placed on the right upper extremity as the left subclavian artery may be postductal in some infants. If the shunt across the PFO is the primary cause of hypoxemia, both upper and lower extremities will have similar low oxygen saturations by pulse oximetry (SpO_2).
2. Relatively low systemic blood pressure and SVR are commonly observed in PPHN, especially in the presence of sepsis. Low SVR enhanced right-to-left shunting in the presence of high PVR (Fig. 26.3).

SVR > PVR

PVR > SVR

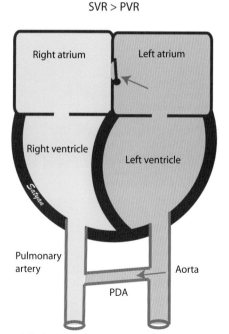

Right atrium

Left atrium

Right ventricle

Left ventricle

Satyan

Pulmonary artery

Aorta

PDA

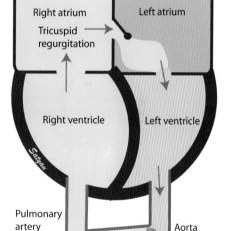

Right atrium

Tricuspid regurgitation

Left atrium

Right ventricle

Left ventricle

Satyan

Pulmonary artery

Aorta

PDA

Fig. 26.3 Labile Oxygenation in PPHN. The relationship between systemic vascular resistance (SVR) and pulmonary vascular resistance (PVR) determines oxygenation in PPHN. During postnatal life, normally, SVR is higher than PVR. However, in PPHN, PVR is higher or equal to SVR resulting in right-to-left or bidirectional shunt at PDA and PFO. Correcting systemic hypotension with fluids and inotropes will reduce right-to-left shunt and improve oxygenation. However, maintaining systemic blood pressure at supraphysiological levels adds to ventricular strain and is not recommended. Copyright: Satyan Lakshminrusimha.

Maintaining normal systemic blood pressure is important during management of PPHN. However, elevating systemic blood pressure to supraphysiologic values using vasoconstrictor medications to limit shunting in the presence of elevated PVR is likely to be counterproductive for the following reasons.

a. Most vasoconstrictor medications such as dopamine are not selective to systemic vasculature and cause significant pulmonary vasoconstriction further elevating PVR.

b. Very high SVR can result in left ventricular strain and dysfunction.

c. PDA and PFO act as pop-off valves in the presence of high PVR. Attempts to limit shunt and increase Q_p in the presence of a constricted pulmonary vascular circuit are likely to lead to pulmonary endothelial dysfunction and exacerbation of PPHN. Increasing Q_p in PPHN should preferably be achieved by dilating the pulmonary vascular bed.

Mechanism of PPHN

Based on etiology, PPHN can be assigned to one of four types (Fig. 26.4):

1. *Poor adaptation secondary to lung disease*: The presence of parenchymal diseases such as RDS, meconium (or blood or amniotic fluid) aspiration syndrome (MAS), or pneumonia. *(Maladaptation)*

2. *Remodeled pulmonary vasculature* with normal parenchyma, also known as idiopathic PPHN or black-lung PPHN. *(Maldevelopment)*

3. *Hypoplasia*: Hypoplastic vasculature as seen in pulmonary hypoplasia (CDH, oligohydramnios secondary to kidney disease or chronic leakage of amniotic fluid). *(Underdevelopment)*

4. *Obstruction*: Polycythemia and hyperviscosity leading to intravascular sludging and elevated PVR.

Etiology of PPHN

1. MAS is common in term newborns and is often associated with birth asphyxia and leads to hypoxic respiratory failure with high morbidity and mortality [3]. It is often associated with birth asphyxia. Meconium-stained amniotic fluid (MSAF) is observed in 3%–14% of pregnancies. Neonates (5%–10%) born through MSAF are at risk of developing MAS. Chemical pneumonitis and surfactant inactivation triggered by meconium are associated with ventilation–perfusion (V/Q) mismatch.

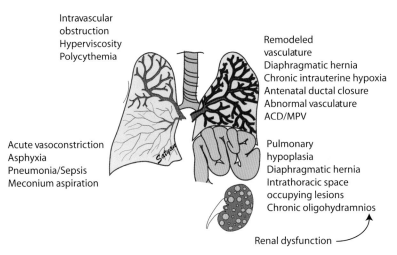

Intravascular obstruction
Hyperviscosity
Polycythemia

Remodeled vasculature
Diaphragmatic hernia
Chronic intrauterine hypoxia
Antenatal ductal closure
Abnormal vasculature
ACD/MPV

Acute vasoconstriction
Asphyxia
Pneumonia/Sepsis
Meconium aspiration

Pulmonary hypoplasia
Diaphragmatic hernia
Intrathoracic space occupying lesions
Chronic oligohydramnios

Renal dysfunction

Fig. 26.4 Mechanisms of PPHN. Elevated pulmonary vascular resistance (PVR) is typically secondary to four mechanisms. Parenchymal lung disease, such as hyaline membrane disease (HMD), resulting in acute alveolar hypoxia leads to pulmonary vasoconstriction. Intravascular obstruction secondary to hyperviscosity often due to polycythemia can lead to PPHN. Remodeled vasculature (*maladaptation* of pulmonary circulation) due to congenital diaphragmatic hernia, intrauterine closure of ductus arteriosus, and chronic intrauterine hypoxia leads to PPHN. Pulmonary hypoplasia secondary intrathoracic space occupying lesions such as congenital pulmonary malformations, diaphragmatic hernia, and oligohydramnios due to renal disease or chronic leakage leads to PPHN. Finally, infants born with malformations of alveolar and vascular development such as alveolar capillary dysplasia (ACD) with malalignment of pulmonary veins (MPV) have intractable and often lethal PPHN. Copyright: Satyan Lakshminrusimha.

2. *Pneumonia and infection* are associated with decreased SVR and elevated PVR. Sepsis leads to hypotension exacerbating right-to-left shunting and cyanosis. Septic infants suffer from myocardial dysfunction leading to elevated left atrial pressures and pulmonary venous hypertension [4]. Recent epidemiological studies suggest that infection is an important cause of PPHN accounting for 30% of cases [2].

3. *Pulmonary hypertension in premature infants* [5]. Pulmonary hypertension (PH) in preterm infants is associated with RDS or bronchopulmonary dysplasia (BPD) and has a bimodal postnatal age distribution. Early PH in preterm infants is associated with RDS and responds poorly to conventional vasodilator therapy. Late PH is associated with BPD and considerably increases mortality associated with BPD.

4. *Idiopathic PPHN (also known as "black-lung PPHN")*: In the absence of parenchymal lung disease, PPHN can result from remodeling of pulmonary arteries. Given the dark lung fields secondary to pulmonary oligemia, this condition is labeled as "black-lung" PPHN. Some cases can be secondary to intrauterine stress, premature closure of the ductus arteriosus, maternal ingestion of SSRI, or NSAID medications. The association between maternal ingestion of these medications and PPHN is controversial.

5. *CDH* causes intractable and chronic PPHN and is associated with approximately 30% mortality. A combination of lung hypoplasia, remodeling of pulmonary arteries, and cardiac dysfunction contribute to high morbidity and mortality in this condition. Further details of this condition are described in Chapter 28.

6. *Alveolar capillary dysplasia or* misalignment of the pulmonary veins (ACD/MPV) results in severe hypoxic respiratory failure and is often fatal. More recently, mild forms that survive beyond the neonatal period have been described. Impaired gas exchange secondary to poorly formed alveolocapillary interphase leads to hypoxia. The diagnosis is often confirmed with a lung biopsy.

Clinical features

1. **Index of suspicion**: A neonate with *labile hypoxemia* (SpO_2 fluctuating without any significant changes in ventilation settings and with minimal stimulation) out of proportion to lung disease should be suspected to have PPHN. These infants readily drop their SpO_2 with routine handling such as suctioning, diaper change, stimulation by parents, and so on. Other factors consistent with the diagnosis of PPHN include the following:

a. Oxygen requirement disproportional to lung disease and pressure settings on the ventilator.
b. History of a disease such as asphyxia, MAS, or CDH commonly associated with PPHN.
c. Differential cyanosis—SpO_2 in the right arm is higher than values obtained from the legs.
d. Onset of symptoms within the first few hours of life (late onset is common in preterm infants and infants with CDH).
e. Cardiac examination demonstrates right ventricular heave, a loud second heart sound, and a harsh systolic murmur heard best at the left lower sternal border secondary to TR.

2. **Diagnosis**: PPHN is suspected in infants with labile hypoxemia with or without differential cyanosis. Occasionally, they are asymptomatic and detected during pulse oximetry for congenital heart disease screening. A chest X-ray, CBC with differential and a blood gas analysis, are the first steps in finding an etiology for PPHN. An echocardiogram confirms the diagnosis and rules out structural heart disease.

3. **Differential cyanosis**: Right-to-left shunt can occur at the level of PFO or PDA. Infants with PPHN whose right-to-left shunt is predominantly at the PDA present with SpO_2 5%–10% higher in the right upper limb compared with the lower limbs. However, if the shunt is predominantly at the PFO level, differential cyanosis may not be perceived. Infants with coarctation or interrupted aortic arch can present with low saturations in the lower limbs.

4. **Hyperoxia–hyperventilation test**
a. **Hyperoxia test:** The patient is placed in 100% oxygen for 15 min. An arterial blood gas is obtained to differentiate pulmonary parenchymal or respiratory depression (where PaO_2 typically increases >150 mmHg) from cyanotic heart disease or PPHN (PaO_2 does not exceed 150 mmHg). False positive conclusion (PaO_2 does not exceed 150 mmHg) may result from severe parenchymal disease, especially if oxygen is delivered through a hood without any positive pressure. False negative conclusion (where PaO_2 typically increases >150 mmHg) may be derived in some cases of PPHN and total anomalous pulmonary venous return (TAPVR) due to oxygen-induced decrease in PVR and alteration of shunts.
b. **Hyperoxia–hyperventilation** (hyperoxia and hypocapnia to induce alkalosis and pulmonary vasodilation to improve PaO_2) may be helpful in some cases of PPHN. Infants with reactive pulmonary vasculature and PPHN may improve oxygenation in response to hypocapnia. Infants with severe PPHN with remodeled pulmonary vasculature and cyanotic CHD patients do not respond to hyperoxia and hyperventilation. It is

important to remember that hyperventilation-induced hypocapnia can cause cerebral vasoconstriction. These tests can be skipped by confirming PPHNs by an echocardiogram.

5. **Chest X-ray** is useful in diagnosing the primary lung condition. Classic description of radiologic appearance of various neonatal respiratory disorders is given as follows:
   a. Grainy—often with low expansion: RDS (may be pneumonia)
   b. Patchy—pneumonia
   c. Fluffy—often with hyperexpansion: MAS
   d. Streaky—often with hyperexpansion: retained lung liquid or TTN
   e. Black–dark lung fields—primary or idiopathic PPHN or pulmonic stenosis (including tetralogy of Fallot); similar picture is also seen in pneumothorax
   f. White-out—collapse/atelectasis; severe RDS or pneumonia; also infradiaphragmatic TAPVR with obstruction
   g. Bubbly—pulmonary interstitial emphysema (PIE)
6. **Echocardiography** confirms the diagnosis of PPHN. The efficacy of therapeutic interventions can be assessed by serial echocardiograms [6]. Echocardiographic features suggestive of PPHN include the following:
   a. Absence of structural heart disease
   b. Dilated right ventricle (hypertrophy in long-standing PPHN)

c. Dilated right atrium
d. Septal bulge to left
e. TR and pulmonary insufficiency
f. Pulmonary pressures 30–60 mmHg. Pulmonary systolic pressure is similar to the right ventricular systolic pressure (RVSP) and is detected by the modified Bernoulli equation: RVSP = $4v^2$ TR + right atrial pressure (mmHg), where v is the velocity of TR in m/s.

7. **B-type natriuretic peptide (BNP)** is a peptide mainly released by the ventricle in response to strain and can be an early biomarker of PPHN [7–9]. Some centers obtain monthly echocardiograms with serial BNP levels in BPD patients to screen for PH.

Severity of PPHN and HRF

It is assessed by oxygenation index (OI), oxygenation saturation index (OSI), and alveolar–arterial oxygen difference ($AaDO_2$).

1. **OI** (Fig. 26.5) is the most commonly used index to assess severity of HRF during medical management of PPHN because it takes mean airway pressure into the consideration. OI = mean airway pressure (in cmH_2O) × FiO_2 × 100/PaO_2 (in mmHg).
   a. Based on OI, HRF can be classified into

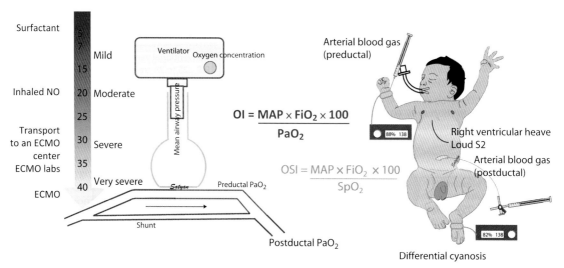

Fig. 26.5 Clinical Features and Assessment of Severity of PPHN With Oxygenation Index (OI) and Oxygen Saturation Index (OSI). Infants with PPHN present with labile hypoxemia with differential cyanosis (preductal oxygenation higher than postductal oxygenation, in the presence of a right-to-left shunt at the PDA level) and may have a loud second heart sound and a precordial right ventricular heave. Severity of PPHN can be assessed by calculating OI. Factors that influence oxygenation are in the numerator (mean airway pressure [MAP] and inspired oxygen) and oxygen level is in the denominator. OSI is similar to OI, but substitutes PaO_2 by SpO_2 as a measurement of oxygenation. OSI values are approximately half of OI (OI of 16 is approximately equal to OSI of 8). Copyright: Satyan Lakshminrusimha.

exception of diaphragmatic hernia) receive a dose of surfactant to improve lung recruitment.

d. *"Gentle" ventilation* with permissive hypercapnia (PaCO$_2$ 50–60 mmHg), avoiding hyperoxemia (PaO$_2$ 50–80 mmHg) with optimal mean airway pressure, PEEP, relatively low PIP, or tidal volume are recommended to ensure adequate lung recruitment while limiting barotrauma and volutrauma [17,23]. Low PEEP increases alveolar collapse and increases PVR by kinking alveolar pulmonary vasculature. Extremely high PEEP decreases venous return and causes overdistension and compresses extraalveolar vessels and increases PVR. Optimal PEEP maintains the lungs at FRC during expiration and results in lowest PVR. A tidal volume of 4–5 mL/kg is targeted (preferably using a volume guarantee mode).

e. *High-frequency ventilation:* PPHN secondary to severe parenchymal lung disease or lung hypoplasia may benefit from high-frequency jet ventilator (HFJV) or high-frequency oscillator ventilation (HFOV) to optimize lung inflation and minimize lung injury [24]. If an infant with PPHN on conventional mechanical ventilation requires a PIP of >28 cmH$_2$O or tidal volumes >6 mL/kg to maintain PaCO$_2$ <60 mmHg, we recommend switching to HFOV or HFJV.

f. **Oxygen** is a specific, selective, and potent pulmonary vasodilator. Increase in PaO$_2$ with ventilation with air reduces PVR following birth. Mechanical ventilation with high FiO$_2$ and supraphysiological PaO$_2$ used to be the traditional management of PPHN during the acute phase of illness. Fetal lamb studies have demonstrated that increased fetal PaO$_2$ and rhythmic distension of the lung augment endogenous NO release [25,26]. However, the using of high FiO$_2$ (especially 100% oxygen) can lead to oxygen toxicity. Studies in newborn lambs showed that brief (30 min) exposure to 100% O$_2$ resulted in increased contractility of pulmonary arteries [27]. In lambs with PPHN, a similar exposure at birth reduced subsequent response to acetylcholine and iNO [28,29] and increased the potential for oxidative stress [30]. Reactive oxygen species (ROS) can increase phosphodiesterase (PDE5) activity, and decrease endothelial nitric oxide synthase (eNOS) and soluble guanylate cyclase (sGC) activity, resulting in decreased cGMP. In the ovine ductal ligation model of PPHN, maintaining SpO$_2$ in the 90%–97% range resulted in low PVR [29]. Based on studies in lambs with PPHN, we recommend preductal SpO$_2$ in the 90%–97% range with PaO$_2$ between 50 and 80 mmHg in PPHN.

Inhaled nitric oxide

It is a selective pulmonary vasodilator with minimal effects on systemic blood pressure [31]. Endothelial NO is produced from L-arginine by the enzyme eNOS [31]. As an inhaled agent, iNO induced pulmonary vasodilation but does not significantly alter SVR (*selective effect of iNO*; Fig. 26.7) [32]. Inhaled NO is distributed to the well-ventilated lung segments leading to increased blood

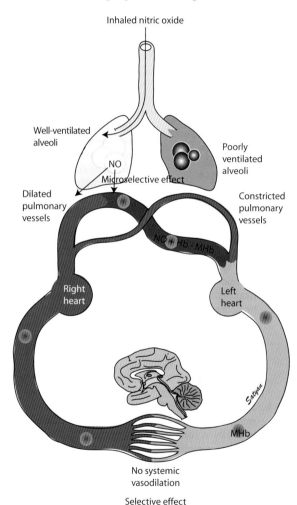

Fig. 26.7 Selective and Microselective Action of Inhaled Nitric Oxide (NO). Inhaled NO is a selective dilator of the pulmonary circulation without any significant systemic vasodilation as it combines with hemoglobin to form methemoglobin (MHb). As it is an inhaled vasodilator, it selectively goes to the well-ventilated alveoli and improves blood flow to these alveoli and reduces V/Q mismatch (microselective effect). Copyright: Satyan Lakshminrusimha.

flow to these segments, optimizing ventilation–perfusion match (*microselective effect of iNO*) [32]. Inhaled NO causes marked improvement in PaO_2 in later preterm and term newborn infants with PPHN [33]. Inhaled NO reduces the need for ECMO in late-preterm and term neonates (>34 weeks of gestation) with HRF [34–36].

1. *Optimal OI at initiation of iNO* in PPHN is not known. Konduri et al. demonstrated that early iNO with an OI of 15–25 did not reduce the need for ECMO but reduced the progression to severe HRF [37]. Post hoc analysis of this study suggested that surfactant therapy prior to randomization and initiation of therapy with iNO at an OI of ≤20 was associated with reduced use of ECMO or death [22]. We recommend initiation of iNO at OI ≥15 to 20 if there is clinical (labile oxygenation with pre–post SpO_2 difference) or echocardiographic evidence of PPHN.

2. *Starting dose of iNO*: The ideal starting dose of iNO in PPHN is not known. A common starting dose for iNO in many clinical trials is 20 ppm with

some trials evaluating doses between 5 and 20 ppm [38]. Doses >20 ppm did not add to the efficacy of iNO, but were associated with more adverse effects [35] such as methemoglobinemia and elevated nitrogen dioxide (NO_2) (>3 ppm) and are no longer recommended [33]. A dose of 5 ppm resulted in improved oxygenation without a significant decrease in pulmonary arterial pressure. A dose of 20 ppm improved oxygenation *and* decreased pulmonary arterial pressure [39]. In summary, we recommend the **20-20-20-20 rule** for initiation of iNO (Fig. 26.8)— start iNO if OI is ~15 to **20** at a dose of **20** ppm. A complete response to iNO is defined as an increase in PaO_2/FiO_2 ratio of ≥**20** mmHg in **20–30** min [40,41].

3. *Monitoring during iNO therapy*: Methemoglobin levels are monitored 8–12 h after initiation of iNO and then once a day, especially if iNO dose is ≥20 ppm. High FiO_2 and high cumulative iNO dose increase the risk for methemoglobinemia [42]. Levels should be maintained <5%. Some providers stop checking daily

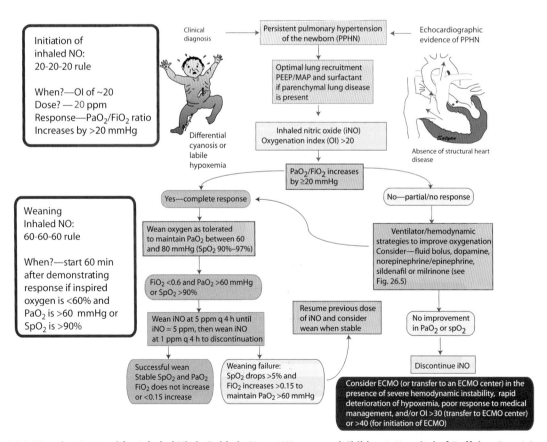

Fig. 26.8 Weaning Protocol for Inhaled Nitric Oxide in Use at Women and Children's Hospital of Buffalo. Copyright: Satyan Lakshminrusimha.

- Systemic hypotension is a common side effect of sildenafil and can increase morbidity in PPHN by worsening right-to-left shunt. Long-term therapy with sildenafil in children (1–17 years) has been associated with increased mortality (a black-box warning from FDA). However, similar information is not available in neonates.
- **b.** *Milrinone* (PDE 3 inhibitor):
  - Pulmonary arterial smooth muscle cells and cardiac myocytes have cAMP-specific phosphodiesterase type 3 (PDE 3), an enzyme that promotes degradation of cAMP.
  - Milrinone is an inodilator (inotrope + vasodilator) and acts by inhibiting PDE3 and increases cAMP in pulmonary arterial smooth muscle, systemic arterial smooth muscle cells, and cardiac myocytes.
  - IV milrinone has been shown to be effective in iNO-resistant PPHN in case series [59–61]. No randomized controlled trials have been performed evaluating milrinone in PPHN.
  - An optional loading dose of 50 mcg/kg over 30–60 min is used in some centers, but is associated with a higher incidence of systemic hypotension. The maintenance dose is 0.33–0.5 mcg/kg/min. In the absence of systemic hypotension, the dose can be escalated to 0.66–1 mcg/kg/min.
  - Systemic hypotension is a major clinical concern with the use of milrinone. A fluid bolus (10 mL/kg of lactated Ringer's solution or normal saline) prior to loading dose is used in some centers prior to a loading dose of milrinone.
  - One case series described intracranial hemorrhage in two neonates associated with the use of milrinone in PPHN [60]. A head ultrasound to rule out intracranial hemorrhage is recommended in critically ill patients with PPHN.
  - Milrinone is preferred in the presence of PPHN with left ventricular dysfunction without severe systemic hypotension (Fig. 26.9).
- **4. Bosentan** (endothelin-1 receptor blocker): Endothelin is a strong vasoconstrictor, and endothelin receptor antagonists are commonly used in adult patients with pulmonary arterial hypertension [62] and anecdotally in neonates with PPHN [63].
  - **a. Dose**—2 mg/kg/dose BID PO.
  - **b.** A multicenter, randomized, double-blind, placebo-controlled trial of bosentan in PPHN did not show any additive effect with iNO in term neonates with PPHN [64].
  - **c.** Bosentan is occasionally used in CDH or BPD with chronic PH.
  - **d.** Liver function tests must be monitored during bosentan therapy.
- **5. Steroids**: Glucocorticoids increase oxygenation in animal models of MAS [65] and decrease the duration of oxygen use and length of hospital stay and in infants with meconium aspiration [66,67]. Hydrocortisone decreases production of superoxide anions and inhibits PDE 5 [68]. Routine use of glucocorticoids in patients with PPHN is not recommended especially if there is suspicion of viral or bacterial sepsis. Stress dose hydrocortisone is occasionally used in iNO-resistant PPHN associated with systemic hypotension [68,69].

Extracorporeal membrane oxygenation

ECMO is a technique of modified cardiopulmonary bypass used to support heart and lung function. It is only available in select tertiary centers. It is an invasive procedure requiring cannulation of major vessels and anticoagulation. General accepted criteria to start ECMO are as follows:
- $AaDO_2$: >605 to 620 mmHg for 4–12 h;
- OI: >40 for 4 h;
- refractory HRF: preductal PaO_2 <40 mmHg; and/or
- hemodynamic compromise with high inotrope requirement and/or persistent acidosis (pH <7.15).

Asphyxia, hypothermia, and management of PPHN

Asphyxia and hypoxic ischemic encephalopathy (HIE) are associated with hypoxemia and acidosis. Infants with asphyxia commonly suffer from parenchymal lung disease associated with surfactant deficiency and/or MAS [70]. Hypothermia (33.5°C for 72 h) is standard of care for moderate-to-severe HIE [71]. However, case reports indicate that patients with HRF with high inspired oxygen need prior to cooling [72], may suffer from exacerbation of PPHN during hypothermia and/or rewarming [73].

Reporting of blood gases during hypothermia is also controversial. The solubility of gas within liquid increases with a decrease in temperature (Henry's law). With decreasing temperature, more gas is dissolved in plasma, and the partial pressure of CO_2 and O_2 decreases [74]. Maintenance of the same PCO_2 or PO_2 under hypothermic conditions will require greater CO_2 or O_2 content. Two acid-base management approaches during hypothermia are described in the literature for pediatric cardiac anesthesia management during profound hypothermia (usually 18–20°C) [75].

No studies have evaluated the optimal approach during PPHN management associated with mild hypothermia (33–34 °C) for HIE [76].

Management by the *α-stat technique* is focused on maintaining a normal pH and $PaCO_2$ at 37 °C and not at the current body temperature. As the temperature falls during induced hypothermia, $PaCO_2$ measured at the patient's temperature decreases and pH increases. Ventilation is adjusted to maintain a normal $PaCO_2$ at 37 °C. This approach is based on the fact that as temperature decreases, blood and tissue pH rise but the dissociative state of α-imidazole, and thus protein function, remains close to normal.

In the *pH-stat technique*, $PaCO_2$ in the blood gas drawn from a hypothermic patient is measured after warming the blood to 37 °C, but is mathematically corrected to the actual patient's temperature. Ventilation is adjusted to achieve a normal pH and $PaCO_2$ at patient's temperature. This results in higher CO_2 content (as compared to the α-stat method), and leads to concurrent cerebral vasodilation and pulmonary vasoconstriction, resulting in higher cerebral blood flow and more effective and homogenous brain cooling [75]. Thus, most studies evaluating hypothermia for HIE have adapted pH-stat method for acid-base management [71,77,78]. In addition, animal studies with hypothermia demonstrate better suppression of cerebral metabolic rate with pH-stat method [75]. Maintaining high $PaCO_2$ values (>50 mmHg, when corrected for body temperature) can theoretically be associated with high dissolved CO_2 levels and exacerbate pulmonary vasoconstriction.

The optimal range of $PaCO_2$ and PaO_2 during whole-body hypothermia for HIE is not known. The cerebral and pulmonary circulations respond to changes in pH, PCO_2, and PO_2 in opposite ways. Low $PaCO_2$ (<35 mmHg) [79] and high PaO_2 (>100 mmHg) [80] during the immediate postnatal period are associated with adverse outcomes in neonates with HIE undergoing whole-body hypothermia [81]. In contrast, animal studies have demonstrated that hypercarbia, acidosis (pH <7.25), and hypoxemia (PaO_2 <50 mmHg) increase PVR [18], leading to PPHN. Hence, we recommend adopting the pH-stat method and maintaining corrected $PaCO_2$ in the mid-40s and corrected PaO_2 in the 50–80 mmHg range to optimize hemodynamics

of the cerebral and pulmonary circulations [82]. These guidelines for corrected $PaCO_2$ are similar to those recommended by Chakkarapani and Thoresen [83].

In addition to pulmonary vasoconstriction, HIE can be associated with cardiac dysfunction [84,85]. Myocardial dysfunction can lead to secondary pulmonary venous hypertension. Cardiac dysfunction can be multifactorial—myocardial ischemic injury during asphyxia, increased right ventricular afterload due to PPHN, and reduced venous return secondary to high pressure from the ventilator may play a role [70]. We speculate that systemic hypotension coupled with PH increases right-to-left shunting observed in patients with PPHN. Cardiac function, systemic blood pressure, and blood gases should be closely monitored in patients with PPHN associated with HIE undergoing hypothermia.

Long-term outcome of PPHN

Most patients with PPHN improve their oxygenation, and the pulmonary vascular disease resolves with time with no long-term sequelae. However, some patients with PPHN (especially those associated with CDH and BPD) have significant long-term morbidity, irrespective of the treatment modality. Long-term neurodevelopmental follow-up including hearing screens should be provided to all infants with PPHN.

Conclusion

The incidence of severe PPHN requiring ECMO has decreased over the last 2 decades in developed countries. In contrast, PPHN, commonly secondary to sepsis, asphyxia, and meconium aspiration, continues to cause high mortality and morbidity in settings with limited resources. Further research to establish early diagnosis, prevent hypoxemia, and develop specific and potent pulmonary vasodilator therapy is required.

References

[1] Walsh-Sukys MC, Tyson JE, Wright LL, Bauer CR, Korones SB, Stevenson DK, et al. Persistent pulmonary hypertension of the newborn in the era before nitric oxide: practice variation and outcomes. Pediatrics 2000;105(1 Pt. 1): 14–20.

[2] Steurer MA, Jelliffe-Pawlowski LL, Baer RJ, Partridge JC, Rogers EE, Keller RL. Persistent pulmonary hypertension of the newborn in late preterm and term infants in California. Pediatrics 2017;139(1). pii: e20161165.

[3] Yoder BA, Kirsch EA, Barth WH, Gordon MC. Changing obstetric practices associated with decreasing incidence of meconium aspiration syndrome. Obstet Gynecol 2002;99 (5 Pt. 1):731–739.

[4] Sehgal A, Athikarisamy SE, Adamopoulos M. Global myocardial function is compromised in infants with pulmonary hypertension.

Acta paediatr 2012;101(4): 410–413.

[5] Van Meurs KP, Wright LL, Ehrenkranz RA, Lemons JA, Ball MB, Poole WK, et al. Inhaled nitric oxide for premature infants with severe respiratory failure. N Engl J Med 2005;353(1):13–22.

[6] D'Alto M, Romeo E, Argiento P, Di Salvo G, Badagliacca R, Cirillo AP, et al. Pulmonary arterial hypertension: the key role of echocardiography. Echocardiography 2014;32(Suppl. 1):S23–S27.

[7] Abassi Z, Karram T, Ellaham S, Winaver J, Hoffman A. Implications of the natriuretic peptide system in the pathogenesis of heart failure: diagnostic and therapeutic importance. Pharmacol Ther 2004;102(3):223–241.

[8] Reynolds EW, Ellington JG, Vranicar M, Bada HS. Brain-type natriuretic peptide in the diagnosis and management of persistent pulmonary hypertension of the newborn. Pediatrics 2004;114(5):1297–1304.

[9] Vijlbrief DC, Benders MJ, Kemperman H, van Bel F, de Vries WB. B-type natriuretic peptide and rebound during treatment for persistent pulmonary hypertension. J Pediatr 2012;160(1):111–115.e1.

[10] Golombek SG, Young JN. Efficacy of inhaled nitric oxide for hypoxic respiratory failure in term and late preterm infants by baseline severity of illness: a pooled analysis of three clinical trials. Clin Ther 2010;32(5):939–948.

[11] Thomas NJ, Shaffer ML, Willson DF, Shih MC, Curley MA. Defining acute lung disease in children with the oxygenation saturation index. Pediatr Crit Care Med 2010;11(1):12–17.

[12] Rawat M, Chandrasekharan PK, Williams A, Gugino S, Koenigsknecht C, Swartz D, et al. Oxygen saturation index and severity of hypoxic respiratory failure. Neonatology 2015;107(3):161–166.

[13] Benumof JL, Wahrenbrock EA. Dependency of hypoxic pulmonary vasoconstriction on temperature. J Appl Physiol 1977;42(1):56–58.

[14] Bifano EM, Pfannenstiel A. Duration of hyperventilation and outcome in infants with persistent pulmonary hypertension. Pediatrics 1988;81(5):657–661.

[15] Hendricks-Munoz KD, Walton JP. Hearing loss in infants with persistent fetal circulation. Pediatrics 1988;81(5):650–656.

[16] Dworetz AR, Moya FR, Sabo B, Gladstone I, Gross I. Survival of infants with persistent pulmonary hypertension without extracorporeal membrane oxygenation [comment]. Pediatrics 1989;84(1):1–6.

[17] Wung JT, James LS, Kilchevsky E, James E. Management of infants with severe respiratory failure and persistence of the fetal circulation, without hyperventilation. Pediatrics 1985;76(4):488–494.

[18] Rudolph AM, Yuan S. Response of the pulmonary vasculature to hypoxia and H+ ion concentration changes. J Clin Invest 1966;45(3):399–411.

[19] Kinsella JP, Abman SH. Recent developments in the pathophysiology and treatment of persistent pulmonary hypertension of the newborn. J Pediatr 1995;126(6):853–864.

[20] Antunes M, Greenspan J, Holt W, Vallieu D, Spitzer A. Assessment of lung-function pre-nitric oxide therapy—a predictor of response. Pediatr Res 1994;35:212A.

[21] Lotze A, Mitchell BR, Bulas DI, Zola EM, Shalwitz RA, Gunkel JH. Multicenter study of surfactant (beractant) use in the treatment of term infants with severe respiratory failure. Survanta in Term Infants Study Group. J Pediatr 1998;132(1):40–47.

[22] Konduri GG, Sokol GM, Van Meurs KP, Singer J, Ambalavanan N, Lee T, et al. Impact of early surfactant and inhaled nitric oxide therapies on outcomes in term/late preterm neonates with moderate hypoxic respiratory failure. J Perinatol 2013;33(12):944–949.

[23] Gupta A, Rastogi S, Sahni R, Bhutada A, Bateman D, Rastogi D, et al. Inhaled nitric oxide and gentle ventilation in the treatment of pulmonary hypertension of the newborn—a single-center, 5-year experience. J Perinatol 2002;22(6):435–441.

[24] Kinsella JP, Abman SH. Clinical approaches to the use of high-frequency oscillatory ventilation in neonatal respiratory failure. J Perinatol 1996;16(2 Pt. 2 Su):S52–S55.

[25] Tiktinsky MH, Morin FC 3rd. Increasing oxygen tension dilates fetal pulmonary circulation via endothelium-derived relaxing factor. Am J Physiol 1993;265(1 Pt. 2):H376–H380.

[26] Cornfield DN, Chatfield BA, McQueston JA, McMurtry IF, Abman SH. Effects of birth-related stimuli on L-arginine-dependent pulmonary vasodilation in ovine fetus. Am J Physiol 1992;262(5 Pt. 2):H1474–H1481.

[27] Lakshminrusimha S, Russell JA, Steinhorn RH, Ryan RM, Gugino SF, Morin FC 3rd, et al. Pulmonary arterial contractility in neonatal lambs increases with 100% oxygen resuscitation. Pediatr Res 2006;59(1):137–141.

[28] Lakshminrusimha S, Russell JA, Steinhorn RH, Swartz DD, Ryan RM, Gugino SF, et al. Pulmonary hemodynamics in neonatal lambs resuscitated with 21%, 50%, and 100% oxygen. Pediatr Res 2007;62(3):313–318.

[29] Lakshminrusimha S, Swartz DD, Gugino SF, Ma CX, Wynn KA, Ryan RM, et al. Oxygen concentration and pulmonary hemodynamics in newborn lambs with pulmonary hypertension. Pediatr Res 2009;66(5):539–544.

[30] Farrow KN, Groh BS, Schumacker PT, Lakshminrusimha S, Czech L, Gugino SF, et al. Hyperoxia increases phosphodiesterase 5 expression and activity in ovine fetal pulmonary artery smooth muscle cells. Circ Res 2008;102(2):226–233.

[31] Moncada S, Palmer RM, Higgs EA. Nitric oxide: physiology, pathophysiology, and pharmacology. Pharmacol Rev 1991;43(2):109–142.

[32] Lakshminrusimha S. The pulmonary circulation in neonatal respiratory failure. Clin Perinatol 2012;39(3):655–683.

[33] Davidson D, Barefield ES, Kattwinkel J, Dudell G, Damask M, Straube R, et al. Inhaled nitric oxide for the early treatment of persistent pulmonary hypertension of the term newborn: a randomized, double-masked, placebo-controlled, dose-response, multicenter study. The I-NO/PPHN Study Group. Pediatrics 1998;101(3 Pt. 1):325–334.

[34] Clark RH, Kueser TJ, Walker MW, Southgate WM, Huckaby JL, Perez JA, et al. Low-dose nitric oxide therapy for persistent pulmonary hypertension of the newborn. Clinical Inhaled Nitric Oxide Research Group. N Engl J Med 2000;342(7):469–474.

[35] Neonatal Inhaled Nitric Oxide Study Group. Inhaled nitric oxide in full-term and nearly full-term infants with hypoxic respiratory failure. N Engl J Med 1997;336(9):597–604.

[36] Roberts JD Jr, Fineman JR, Morin FC 3rd, Shaul PW, Rimar S, Schreiber

MD, et al. Inhaled nitric oxide and persistent pulmonary hypertension of the newborn. The Inhaled Nitric Oxide Study Group. N Engl J Med 1997;336(9):605–610.

[37] Konduri GG, Kim UO. Advances in the diagnosis and management of persistent pulmonary hypertension of the newborn. Pediatr Clin North Am 2009;56(3):579–600.

[38] Konduri GG, Solimano A, Sokol GM, Singer J, Ehrenkranz RA, Singhal N, et al. A randomized trial of early versus standard inhaled nitric oxide therapy in term and near-term newborn infants with hypoxic respiratory failure. Pediatrics 2004;113(3 Pt. 1):559–564.

[39] Tworetzky W, Bristow J, Moore P, Brook MM, Segal MR, Brasch RC, et al. Inhaled nitric oxide in neonates with persistent pulmonary hypertension. Lancet 2001;357(9250):118–120.

[40] Lakshminrusimha S, Keszler M. Persistent pulmonary hypertension of the newborn. NeoReviews 2015;16(12):e680–e692.

[41] Sharma V, Berkelhamer S, Lakshminrusimha S. Persistent pulmonary hypertension of the newborn. Matern Health Neonatol Perinatol 2015;1(1):1–18.

[42] Hamon I, Gauthier-Moulinier H, Grelet-Dessioux E, Storme L, Fresson J, Hascoet JM. Methaemoglobinaemia risk factors with inhaled nitric oxide therapy in newborn infants. Acta Paediatr 2010;99(10):1467–1473.

[43] Aly H, Sahni R, Wung JT. Weaning strategy with inhaled nitric oxide treatment in persistent pulmonary hypertension of the newborn. Arch Dis Child Fetal Neonatal Ed 1997;76(2):F118–F122.

[44] Sokol GM, Fineberg NS, Wright LL, Ehrenkranz RA. Changes in arterial oxygen tension when weaning neonates from inhaled nitric oxide. Pediatr Pulmonol 2001;32(1):14–19.

[45] Lakshminrusimha S, Wynn RJ, Youssfi M, Pabalan MJ, Bommaraju M, Kirmani K, et al. Use of CT angiography in the diagnosis of total anomalous venous return. J Perinatol 2009;29(6):458–461.

[46] Sood BG, Delaney-Black V, Aranda JV, Shankaran S. Aerosolized PGE1: a selective pulmonary vasodilator in neonatal hypoxemic respiratory failure results of a Phase I/II open label clinical trial. Pediatr Res 2004;56(4):579–585.

[47] Sood BG, Keszler M, Garg M, Klein JM, Ohls R, Ambalavanan N, et al. Inhaled PGE1 in neonates with hypoxemic respiratory failure: two pilot feasibility randomized clinical trials. Trials 2014;15(1):486.

[48] Kelly LK, Porta NF, Goodman DM, Carroll CL, Steinhorn RH. Inhaled prostacyclin for term infants with persistent pulmonary hypertension refractory to inhaled nitric oxide. J Pediatr 2002;141(6):830–832.

[49] Shiyanagi S, Okazaki T, Shoji H, Shimizu T, Tanaka T, Takeda S, et al. Management of pulmonary hypertension in congenital diaphragmatic hernia: nitric oxide with prostaglandin-E1 versus nitric oxide alone. Pediatr Surg Int 2008;24(10):1101–1104.

[50] Chotigeat U, Jaratwashirakul S. Inhaled iloprost for severe persistent pulmonary hypertension of the newborn. J Med Assoc Thai 2007;90(1):167–170.

[51] Ehlen M, Wiebe B. Iloprost in persistent pulmonary hypertension of the newborn. Cardiol Young 2003;13(4):361–363.

[52] Rimensberger PC, Spahr-Schopfer I, Berner M, Jaeggi E, Kalangos A, Friedli B, et al. Inhaled nitric oxide versus aerosolized iloprost in secondary pulmonary hypertension in children with congenital heart disease: vasodilator capacity and cellular mechanisms. Circulation 2001;103(4):544–548.

[53] Yilmaz O, Kahveci H, Zeybek C, Ciftel M, Kilic O. Inhaled iloprost in preterm infants with severe respiratory distress syndrome and pulmonary hypertension. Am J Perinatol 2014;31(4):321–326.

[54] Baquero H, Soliz A, Neira F, Venegas ME, Sola A. Oral sildenafil in infants with persistent pulmonary hypertension of the newborn: a pilot randomized blinded study. Pediatrics 2006;117(4):1077–1083.

[55] Vargas-Origel A, Gomez-Rodriguez G, Aldana-Valenzuela C, Vela-Huerta MM, Alarcon-Santos SB, Amador-Licona N. The use of sildenafil in persistent pulmonary hypertension of the newborn. Am J Perinatol 2010;27(3):225–230.

[56] Steinhorn RH, Kinsella JP, Butrous G, Dilleen M, Oakes M, Wessel DL. Intravenous sildenafil in the treatment of neonates with persistent pulmonary hypertension of the newborn. J Pediatr 2009;155(6):841–847.

[57] Juliana AE, Abbad FC. Severe persistent pulmonary hypertension of the newborn in a setting where limited resources exclude the use of inhaled nitric oxide: successful treatment with sildenafil. Eur J Pediatr 2005;164(10):626–629.

[58] Steiner M, Salzer U, Baumgartner S, Waldhoer T, Klebermass-Schrehof K, Wald M, et al. Intravenous sildenafil i.v. as rescue treatment for refractory pulmonary hypertension in extremely preterm infants. Klin Padiatr 2014;226(4):211–215.

[59] McNamara PJ, Shivananda SP, Sahni M, Freeman D, Taddio A. Pharmacology of milrinone in neonates with persistent pulmonary hypertension of the newborn and suboptimal response to inhaled nitric oxide. Pediatr Crit Care Med 2013;14(1):74–84.

[60] Bassler D, Choong K, McNamara P, Kirpalani H. Neonatal persistent pulmonary hypertension treated with milrinone: four case reports. Biol Neonate 2006;89(1):1–5.

[61] McNamara PJ, Laique F, Muang-In S, Whyte HE. Milrinone improves oxygenation in neonates with severe persistent pulmonary hypertension of the newborn. J Crit Care 2006;21(2):217–222.

[62] Rubin LJ, Badesch DB, Barst RJ, Galie N, Black CM, Keogh A, et al. Bosentan therapy for pulmonary arterial hypertension. N Engl J Med 2002;346(12):896–903.

[63] Mohamed WA, Ismail M. A randomized, double-blind, placebo-controlled, prospective study of bosentan for the treatment of persistent pulmonary hypertension of the newborn. J Perinatol 2012;32(8):608–613.

[64] Steinhorn RH, Fineman J, Kusic-Pajic A, Cornelisse P, Gehin M, Nowbakht P, et al. Bosentan as adjunctive therapy for persistent pulmonary hypertension of the newborn: results of the randomized multicenter placebo-controlled exploratory trial. J Pediatr 2016;177. 90-96.e3.

[65] Soukka H, Halkola L, Aho H, Rautanen M, Kero P, Kaapa P. Methylprednisolone attenuates the pulmonary hypertensive response in porcine meconium aspiration. Pediatr Res 1997;42(2):145–150.

[66] Tripathi S, Saili A. The effect of steroids on the clinical course and outcome of neonates with meconium aspiration syndrome. J Trop Pediatr 2007;53(1):8–12.

[67] Ward M, Sinn J. Steroid therapy for meconium aspiration syndrome in newborn infants. Cochrane Database Syst Rev 2003;4:Cd003485.

[68] Perez M, Wedgwood S, Lakshminrusimha S, Farrow KN, Steinhorn RH. Hydrocortisone normalizes phosphodiesterase-5 activity in pulmonary artery smooth muscle cells from lambs with persistent pulmonary hypertension of the newborn. Pulm Circ 2014;4(1):71–81.

[69] Perez M, Lakshminrusimha S, Wedgwood S, Czech L, Gugino SF, Russell JA, et al. Hydrocortisone normalizes oxygenation and cgmp regulation in lambs with persistent pulmonary hypertension of the newborn. Am J Physiol Lung Cell Mol Physiol 2012;302(6):L595–L603.

[70] Lapointe A, Barrington KJ. Pulmonary hypertension and the asphyxiated newborn. J Pediatr 2011;158(2 Suppl.):e19–e24.

[71] Shankaran S, Laptook AR, Ehrenkranz RA, Tyson JE, McDonald SA, Donovan EF, et al. Whole-body hypothermia for neonates with hypoxic-ischemic encephalopathy. N Engl J Med 2005;353(15):1574–1584.

[72] Thoresen M, Whitelaw A. Cardiovascular changes during mild therapeutic hypothermia and rewarming in infants with hypoxic-ischemic encephalopathy. Pediatrics 2000;106(1 Pt. 1):92–99.

[73] Shah SK, Khan AM, Cox CS Jr. Pulmonary hypertensive crisis requiring ECMO associated with re-warming from whole body hypothermia for hypoxic ischemic encephalopathy: clinical observations from a case series. Eur J Pediatr Surg 2010;20(3):205–206.

[74] Lumb AB. Nunn's Applied Respiratory Physiology. Philadelphia, PA, USA: Elsevier Health Sciences; 2016.

[75] Lake CL, Booker PD. Pediatric Cardiac Anesthesia. Riverwoods, IL: Lippincott Williams & Wilkins; 2005.

[76] Groenendaal F, De Vooght KM, van Bel F. Blood gas values during hypothermia in asphyxiated term neonates. Pediatrics 2009;123(1):170–172.

[77] Gluckman PD, Wyatt JS, Azzopardi D, Ballard R, Edwards AD, Ferriero DM, et al. Selective head cooling with mild systemic hypothermia after neonatal encephalopathy: multicentre randomised trial. Lancet 2005;365(9460):663–670.

[78] Shankaran S, Laptook AR, Pappas A, McDonald SA, Das A, Tyson JE, et al. Effect of depth and duration of cooling on deaths in the NICU among neonates with hypoxic ischemic encephalopathy: a randomized clinical trial. JAMA 2014;312(24):2629–2639.

[79] Pappas A, Shankaran S, Laptook AR, Langer JC, Bara R, Ehrenkranz RA, et al. Hypocarbia and adverse outcome in neonatal hypoxic-ischemic encephalopathy. J Pediatr 2011;158(5). 752-758.e1.

[80] Kapadia VS, Chalak LF, DuPont TL, Rollins NK, Brion LP, Wyckoff MH. Perinatal asphyxia with hyperoxemia within the first hour of life is associated with moderate to severe hypoxic-ischemic encephalopathy. J Pediatr 2013;163(4):949–954.

[81] Klinger G, Beyene J, Shah P, Perlman M. Do hyperoxaemia and hypocapnia add to the risk of brain injury after intrapartum asphyxia? Arch Dis Child Fetal Neonatal Ed 2005;90(1):F49–F52.

[82] Peeters LL, Sheldon RE, Jones MD Jr, Makowski EL, Meschia G. Blood flow to fetal organs as a function of arterial oxygen content. Am J Obstet Gynecol 1979;135(5):637–646.

[83] Chakkarapani E, Thoresen M. Use of hypothermia in the asphyxiated infant. Perinatology 2010;3:20–29.

[84] Van Bel F, Walther FJ. Myocardial dysfunction and cerebral blood flow velocity following birth asphyxia. Acta PaediatrScand 1990;79(8–9):756–762.

[85] Kabra SK, Saxena S, Sharma U. Myocardial dysfunction in birth asphyxia. Indian J Pediatr 1988;55(3):416–419.

Bronchopulmonary Dysplasia

Vineet Bhandari, MD, DNB, DM, Anita Bhandari, MD, P.K. Rajiv, DCH, MD

CHAPTER POINTS

- BPD is the most common chronic lung disease in infants
- An inherent genetic predisposition of an immature lung exposed to infection, hyperoxia, and ventilator-induced injury results in persistent inflammation, leading to impaired alveolarization and dysregulated vascularization, the pathologic hallmarks of BPD
- The management needs to be tailored to the clinical course during the early, evolving and established phases of BPD
- BPD is associated with long-term pulmonary and neurodevelopmental morbidities

Definition

The proposed criteria to define bronchopulmonary dysplasia (BPD) suggested in a National Institutes of Health (NIH) sponsored workshop in 1979 included a continued oxygen dependency during the first 28 days plus compatible clinical and radiographic changes.

In 2001, a workshop conducted by the NIH proposed a definition that divided BPD into three categories based on duration and level of supplemental oxygen therapy required [1,2].

Gestational age

Assessment	<32 weeks	>32 weeks
Time point of assessment	36 weeks post-menstrual age or discharge to home, whichever comes first	>28 days but <56 days postnatal age or discharge to home, whichever comes first

Treatment with oxygen >21% for at least 28 days plus

Mild BPD	Breathing room air	Breathing room air
Moderate BPD	Need for <30% oxygen	Need for <30% oxygen
Severe BPD*	Need for ≥30% oxygen or positive pressure ventilation or both	Need for ≥30% oxygen or positive pressure ventilation or both

*It has been proposed differentiating this group into two subgroups based on their respiratory disease phenotypes and define these as Type 1 and Type 2 severe BPD where Type 1 includes those requiring 30% or greater than 30% supplemental oxygen, high flow nasal cannula, or nasal CPAP at 36 weeks' PMA or at the time of discharge and Type 2 includes those on long-term mechanical ventilation at 36 weeks' PMA or the time of discharge [3].

Incidence

In developed countries, the majority of cases today ("new" BPD) are seen in infants <30 weeks' gestational age (GA) and ≤1200 g birth weight (BW). The incidence of BPD [using the 36 weeks' postmenstrual age (PMA) definition] was reported to be 42% (BW ≥ 501–750 g), 25% (BW ≥ 751–1000 g), 11% (BW ≥ 1001–1250 g), and 5% (BW ≥ 1251–1500 g) [4,5]. Infants with a BW of ≤1250 g account for 97% of all patients with BPD [6]. A physiologic definition based on an oxygen-reduction challenge at 36 weeks' PMA decreased the incidence of BPD by 10% [7]. A point prevalence of severe BPD has been reported to be 36.5% with a range of 11%–48% by the BPD collaborative group that comprised of eight US academic centers with an established BPD program [8].

Etiopathogenesis

Prematurity forms the foundation on which the etiopathogenesis of BPD rests. BPD is an end result of the gene–environmental interactions which cause a persistent inflammatory response in the lung leading to enhanced cell death [9]. Since the development of the lung is ongoing with the injurious response, if the healing process does not resolve the lung toward a normal phenotype, the reparative response leads to impaired alveolarization and dysregulated vascularization which are the characteristic pulmonary phenotypes of "new" BPD (Fig. 27.1) [10].

The complex processes and interaction of the environmental factors are explained in more detail in Fig. 27.2, with a focused explanation of the pathogenesis of ventilator-induced injury in Fig. 27.3.

Clinical course

Early phase (up to 1 postnatal week)

The infant may have severe respiratory distress syndrome (RDS) requiring intubation and one or more doses of surfactant administration. Infants with a hemodynamically significant patent ductus arteriosus (PDA) tend to remain intubated for the initial few days of life and have a high likelihood of failed extubation attempts in the first postnatal (PN) week.

Alternatively and less commonly, the infant may present with almost normal lung function requiring minimal respiratory support or minimal or no oxygen supplementation. These infants are usually managed with nasal continuous positive airway pressure (NCPAP) of 4–5 cm H_2O or even high-flow nasal cannula (>2 L/min). Such infants do reasonably well in the first few days of life; however, by day 5–7, they start showing evidence of worsening respiratory distress (increased work of breathing, tachypnea, and retractions) necessitating escalation of respiratory support and supplemental fraction of inspired oxygen (FiO_2). An illustrative scenario has been shown in Fig. 27.4, with progression of the disease to variable severity of BPD.

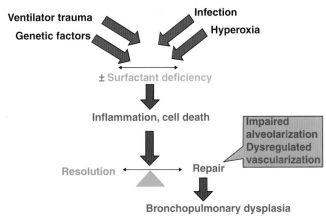

Fig. 27.1 Etiopathogenesis of BPD. BPD is the culmination of the interaction of genetic and environmental (ventilator-induced lung injury, hyperoxia, and ante- and postnatal infection) factors on the foundation of an immature (with/without surfactant deficiency) lung, resulting in a persistent inflammatory response in the lung leading to enhanced cell death. If there is inadequate resolution of lung injury (depending upon various factors, e.g., nutrition, stem cell secretome), the reparative process of the lung results in impaired alveolarization and dysregulated vascularization, the characteristic phenotypes of "new" BPD. Copyright: Vineet Bhandari.

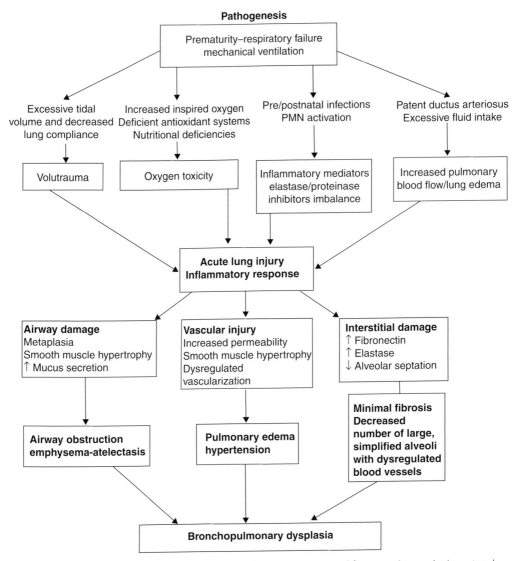

Fig. 27.2 Detailed Overview of the Pathogenesis of BPD. Multiple environmental factors acting on the immature lung leads to breakdown of the alveolar–capillary barrier (causing pulmonary edema) and release of inflammatory mediators. This, in turn, causes airway damage, vascular injury, and interstitial damage leading to the characteristic pathology of BPD. *PMN*, Polymorphonuclear neutrophils. Modified from http://www.drpkrajiv.net/bpd.html.

Evolving phase (>1 PN week to 36 weeks' PMA)

By the second week of PN life, these infants manifest increasing respiratory distress and FiO_2 requirements. They may get re-intubated, and the radiological picture is characterized by pulmonary edema, low volume lungs, and/or atelectasis. Fig. 27.5 shows the development of pulmonary and cardiac events in a complex background of suspected or proven sepsis

and the actions taken thereof. Each complication will be dealt subsequently in the chapter.

Established phase (>36 weeks' PMA)

Infants in this phase have tachypnea, dyspnea, crackles, and wheezing on physical examination. In infants with subglottic stenosis secondary to prolonged intubation, there may be presence of a stridor. Noisy breathing exacerbated

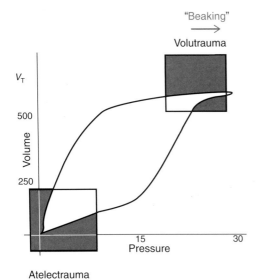

Fig. 27.3 Conceptual Model of Ventilator-Induced Lung Injury. Low positive end-expiratory pressure (PEEP) and high peak inspiratory pressure (PIP) to achieve higher mean airway pressure (MAP) to increase oxygenation contributes to the pathogenesis of BPD. Shearing stress of disproportionate high tidal volume facilitates the development of BPD. The deflation–inflation sequence leads primarily to capillary leakage and cytokine release into the alveolar compartment.

with high airflow activities, such as feeding and agitation may be heard in infants with tracheomalacia and bronchomalacia. Cardiac complications of severe BPD include pulmonary hypertension (PH) and cor pulmonale. Poor growth parameters may be related to undiagnosed hypoxia, cardiac disease, gastroesophageal reflux and swallow dysfunction, or recurrent aspiration. Osteopenia is common in extremely low BW infants. This is secondary to low calcium and Vitamin D intake, exacerbated by the calciuric effect of chronic diuretic therapy. "BPD spells," episodes of cyanosis, oxygen desaturations, and bradycardia, occur due to agitation, and are related to tracheomalacia and bronchomalacia.

Most cases of BPD are mild to moderate, characterized by an initial need for mechanical ventilation followed by days or weeks of O_2 supplementation. Mild BPD is clinically characterized by retractions, generally diminished breath sounds, and crepitant rales on auscultation. Moderate and severe disease is usually associated with significant respiratory and oxygen support (Fig. 27.6).

Acute episodes of respiratory deterioration

1. Infection
2. Pulmonary edema (secondary to PDA; possibly increased fluid administration or progression of disease)

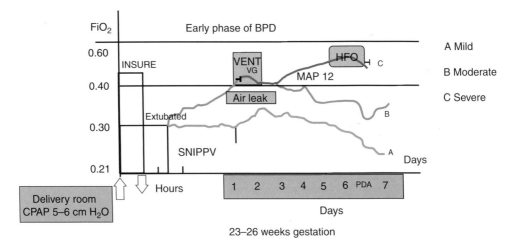

Fig. 27.4 Early Phase of BPD. After birth, either the infant is placed on CPAP of 5–6 cm H_2O or administered surfactant via the INSURE technique. If intubated, attempts are usually made to extubate to (S)NIPPV in the first 3 days of postnatal life. If kept successfully extubated over the first postnatal week, such infants usually do well and may have no or mild BPD (scenario depicted in A). However, if they are re-intubated and require high ventilator pressures (MAP ≥12 cm H_2O) and FiO_2 (≥0.50), they may progress to develop moderate–severe BPD (scenarios depicted in B and C). *CPAP,* Continuous positive airway pressure; *FiO_2,* fraction of inspired oxygen; *HFO,* high-frequency oscillator; *INSURE,* intubate, surfactant administration and extubate; *MAP,* mean airway pressure; *PDA,* patent ductus arteriosus; *SNIPPV,* synchronized nasal intermittent positive pressure ventilation; *VENT,* conventional ventilation; and *VG,* volume guarantee. Courtesy: P.K. Rajiv.

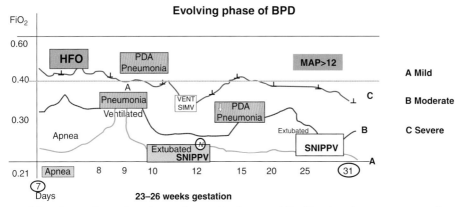

Fig. 27.5 Evolving Phase of BPD. Over the next few weeks of postnatal life, if intubated, attempts are usually made to extubate to (S)NIPPV. If kept successfully extubated, such infants usually do well and may have no or mild BPD (scenario depicted in A). Patients with complications, such as PDA or pneumonia, who require high ventilator pressures (MAP > 12 cm H_2O) and FiO_2 (≥ 0.50), are more likely to progress to moderate–severe BPD (scenarios depicted in B and C). FiO_2, Fraction of inspired oxygen; *HFO*, high-frequency oscillator; *MAP*, mean airway pressure; *PDA*, patent ductus arteriosus; *SIMV*, synchronized intermittent mandatory ventilation; *SNIPPV*, synchronized nasal intermittent positive pressure ventilation; and *VENT*, conventional ventilation. Courtesy: P.K. Rajiv.

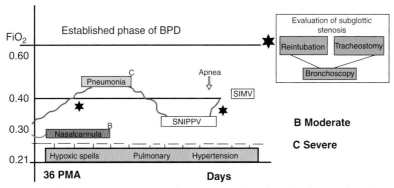

Fig. 27.6 Established Phase of BPD. Beyond 36 weeks of postmenstrual age (PMA), infants with mild BPD are on no support or minimal respiratory support (nasal cannula). If intubated, they continue to receive conventional SIMV. Attempts should be made to extubate to (S)NIPPV, if the ventilator settings can be weaned. Infants who have moderate-severe BPD (scenarios depicted in B and C) and are ventilator dependent may require tracheostomy. All infants with BPD should be screened for pulmonary hypertension. FiO_2, Fraction of inspired oxygen; *SIMV*, synchronized intermittent mandatory ventilation; *SNIPPV*, synchronized nasal intermittent positive pressure ventilation; and *VENT*, conventional ventilation. Courtesy: P.K. Rajiv.

3. Bronchospasm
4. Heart failure

Radiologic characteristics

Stage 1: Identical to RDS. Diffuse reticulogranular pattern with air bronchograms (Fig. 27.7).

Stage 2: Virtually homogenous opacification of lungs that obscures cardiac margins. The early radiographic changes seen in mild disease are replaced by coarse, irregularly shaped densities that are confluent and may contain vacuolar radiolucencies (Fig. 27.8).

Stage 3: Lucent vacuoles have expanded and are identifiable as air cysts among dense patches (Fig. 27.9).

Stage 4: Lungs appear bubbly on radiography as air cysts continue to enlarge. Opacities are reduced to strands, streaks, and small patches as cysts expand (Fig. 27.10).

Management

Antenatal interventions

1. **Prevention of BPD**: is ideal. Among antenatal factors, prevention of premature birth is the single most

infants further increases the degree of lung disease and mortality [25]. However, in patients with severe BPD and cor pulmonale, higher target oxygen saturation is recommended [25]. In established BPD, a slightly higher oxygen saturation of 88%–94% is recommended to prevent right-sided heart failure accompanying BPD. It has been difficult to establish a single oxygen saturation variable that can be effectively used to provide optimal management of BPD without major adverse effects. However, saturation around 90% seems to provide the best stability of both heart and lung function in older infants [26]. The appropriate level at which oxygen saturations should be maintained is controversial. While some have recently advocated use of 90%–95% SpO_2 as the target range [27], we and others have suggested maintaining SpO_2 ranges in the 87%–93% with alarm limits of 86% and 94%, respectively as these values are probably more physiological and have resulted in improved outcomes of BPD [28,29].

Recommended target ranges:

Recommended SpO_2 for improved neurological outcome	90%–95%
Suggested SpO_2 for decreased BPD outcome	87%–93%
Recommended CO_2 level	55–65 mmHg

Ventilator strategy

In an attempt to reduce ventilator-induced lung injury (VILI), it is important to extubate the infant in the first few days of PN life and provide noninvasive respiratory support utilizing the (S)NIPPV mode. If unsuccessful, and the child is intubated, consider using volume-targeted synchronized intermittent mandatory ventilation (SIMV) mode, along with pressure support. As noted earlier, efforts should continue to minimize (wean) invasive ventilation settings and extubate to noninvasive respiratory support. This has been summarized in Fig. 27.12.

Noninvasive ventilation: NCPAP. Management of infants at risk for or with established BPD should be directed at minimizing ventilator support and alveolar overdistention while supporting and maintaining adequate functional residual capacity (FRC) with end-expiratory pressure. These goals can be achieved with the use of nasal CPAP systems (variable-flow or bubble CPAP delivery) [30,31]. Although the primary use of nasal CPAP delivered with the bubble CPAP system is associated with lower rates of BPD [32], the multicenter COIN Trial did not show a significant benefit on the incidence of BPD at 36 weeks. Successful use of nasal CPAP requires tolerance of permissive hypercapnia (most centers usually limit this to 65 mmHg).

Conceptual model to reduce BPD

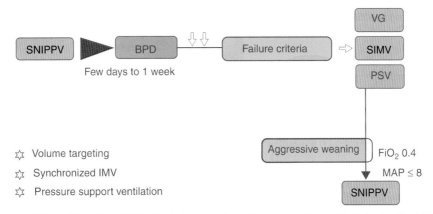

Fig. 27.12 Conceptual Model to Reduce BPD. Efforts to extubate and keep the infant extubated using the (S)NIPPV mode of noninvasive ventilation in the first few days of life should be made. If unsuccessful, use VG, SIMV or PSV modes of invasive ventilation. Aggressive weaning of the ventilator settings should be attempted in the first postnatal month of life in an effort to extubate the infant to (S)NIPPV mode. *BPD*, Bronchopulmonary dysplasia; *FiO₂*, fraction of inspired oxygen, *MAP*, mean airway pressure; *PSV*, pressure support ventilation; *SIMV*, synchronized intermittent mandatory ventilation; *SNIPPV*, synchronized nasal intermittent positive pressure ventilation; and *VG*, volume guarantee. Courtesy: P.K. Rajiv.

Nasal intermittent positive pressure ventilation. Noninvasive ventilation (NIV) with a set frequency, peak pressure, and PEEP has been used as an escalation technique to avoid invasive mechanical ventilation when CPAP alone is not sufficient. NIV is delivered through nasal prongs or mask interface, in the form of NIPPV through a ventilator, which can be synchronized (SNIPPV). The success of NIV is variable, depending on the device, the understanding and training of the caregiver applying it, and the settings and parameters applied. SNIPPV has been associated with greater TV delivery, reduced work of breathing, and a reduction in the need for intubation and BPD, especially in infants <30 weeks gestation [33–35]. Although potential complications of all noninvasive modes include gastric distention or rupture, damage to the nares or occiput by the interface, or apnea, the benefits of NIV are positive and in most cases outweigh the risks.

Once the infant is intubated, there are sufficient data to support the use of (S)NIPPV as the primary extubation mode for neonates, as this has been shown consistently to be more successful than NCPAP [36–39]. However, it is important to note that while smaller studies of NIPPV have shown a reduction in BPD [40], a large "pragmatic" trial did not confirm the earlier results [41]. However, significant concerns have been raised about the design of the "pragmatic" trial [40], and hence, additional large randomized controlled trials are necessary to confirm or refute the impact of (S)NIPPV on the incidence of BPD.

Invasive ventilation: IPPV or IMV. In spite of the development of numerous sophisticated ventilators for the newborn, there is still no clear advantage to any one approach to ventilating the preterm infant. The general approach should be one of preventing atelectasis, sustaining FRC, using a minimal TV (usually 4–6 mL/kg), and allowing the infant to trigger his or her own ventilation as much as possible.

There is currently no ideal strategy for mechanical ventilation that is optimal for minimizing the risks of pulmonary sequelae. There are also inconsistencies in determining what TV constitutes appropriate gas exchange without alveolar impairment. However, synchronized and patient-triggered modes of tidal ventilation with consistent TV delivery is preferred to prevent auto-triggering and increased work of breathing, especially in infants <1000 g [42]. The most commonly employed ventilation in early management of RDS include pressure-controlled continuous mandatory ventilation (CMV), pressure-controlled intermittent mandatory ventilation (IMV) (with mandatory breathing "synchronized" to patient inspiratory effort, commonly referred to as SIMV). Adaptive pressure controlled (i.e., volume-targeted pressure control) with CMV or IMV is becoming more popular. Pressure support (PSV) of spontaneous breaths is often used with IMV.

CMV is employed in the early management of RDS to decrease patient's work of breathing, especially during the period of surfactant replacement, while guaranteeing a set peak inspiratory pressure or TV. Adaptive pressure control provides consistent TV delivery, but no proven benefits for gas exchange [43].

Recommended TVs in management of BPD:

Recommendation	TV (mL/kg)
Early BPD	3.5–4
Evolving BPD	4–5
Established BPD	5–6

TV, Tidal volume.

Patient-triggered ventilation. Studies performed by using patient-triggered ventilation (PTV) have not shown any reduction in the incidence of BPD [44] although it has been suggested that it may be more beneficial for infants with a BW of <1000 g [42].

Volume-targeted ventilation versus pressure-limited ventilation. Preterm infants ventilated using volume-targeted ventilation (VTV) modes had reduced duration of mechanical ventilation, incidence of BPD, failure of primary mode of ventilation, hypocarbia, grade III/IV intraventricular hemorrhage (IVH), pneumothorax, and periventricular leukomalacia (PVL) compared with preterm infants ventilated using pressure-limited ventilation (PLV) modes. There was no evidence that infants ventilated with VTV modes had reduced death compared to infants ventilated using PLV modes [45].

In 2010, the Cochrane review of VTV versus PLV in the neonate concluded that although rates of death and BPD were not significantly different between the two ventilator strategies, statistically significant effects favoring volume targeting were shown for some clinically important outcomes. However, the numbers of trials and infants randomized were small and further studies are required to confirm the role of volume targeting in neonatal ventilation [46].

Mandatory minute ventilation. Mandatory minute ventilation (MMV) mode provides backup support of TV and/or a minimal respiratory rate, in the event the patient cannot meet the minute–volume target. However, the inconsistencies in breathing patterns and volumes in neonates have been a barrier for its long-term implementation [25].

High-frequency oscillatory ventilation. Indication for high-frequency oscillatory ventilation (HFOV): "Rescue" treatment only. Any evidence of air leak and/or mean airway pressure (MAP) >12 cm H_2O.

HFOV was introduced a few decades ago as an alternative strategy for mechanical ventilation. The initial goal of HFOV was focused on reducing the incidence of alveolar stretch and consequent VILI [47]. Many studies conducted over the past decade demonstrate variable outcomes. The practice of utilizing HFOV in neonatal intensive care units for the prevention of BPD remains unpredictable. Proactive strategies and HFOV, noted in a meta-analysis in low BW infants, revealed a minimal reduction in the development of BPD and no significant changes in neurologic outcomes [47]. Rescue strategies utilized in respiratory failure have not proven to affect or reduce the incidence of BPD in premature infants [48]. Neither tidal nor high-frequency ventilation strategies have been regarded as optimal for the prevention of BPD. In a number of studies comparing high-frequency and tidal ventilation, there were no significant differences in the development of BPD, and complications, such as air leak syndromes have been seen in high-frequency modes [25].

"Gentle ventilation": summary of approach. The strategies are focused on reducing the magnitude and duration of mechanical ventilatory support to the minimum possible to support cellular homeostasis, while achieving adequate gas exchange.
1. Redefining the goals for "adequate gas exchange" leading to reduced use of ventilatory support
   a. Targeting higher $PaCO_2$ (permissive hypercapnia)
   b. Tolerating a lower SpO_2 (permissive hypoxemia)
2. Refining the modes of mechanical ventilation
   a. Lower pressures, faster rates, shorter inspiratory times (Ti)
   b. VTV
   c. PTV
3. Pathophysiology in BPD and ventilatory strategy
   The constant alterations in lung mechanics are a critical feature of BPD. The reactive airways contribute to increased pulmonary resistance. Judicious adjustments, such as increasing PEEP and/or airway flow or by using a modality with variable inspiratory flow, such as pressure control or pressure support are reported to be superior to traditional fixed flow in time cycled pressure-limited ventilation (TCPLV). In addition, lung compliance may also show abnormalities. Ventilating the lung at optimal FRC (defined as the range in which incremental changes in pressure recruits the most lung volume) is the most difficult ventilatory endpoint to achieve. Assessing compliance at step by step changes in PEEP may be critical to reach this endpoint. Hence, alterations in resistance and compliance will change the time constant, and sufficient expiratory time to avoid gas trapping and inadvertent PEEP is imperative. Careful thought on the strategy, the best mode, or modality to ventilate a baby with BPD is best made on a case to case basis. Regarding strategy, if lung disease is homogeneous, pressure control ventilation may

offer an advantage, whereas heterogeneous lung disease may respond better to volume control ventilation because peak pressure and peak volume delivery occur at the end of inspiration, offering to make gas delivery more uniform throughout the lung.

Suggested ventilator settings and targets for infants with early, evolving, and established phases of BPD [10]
   Ventilatory parameters in phases of disease. Inspiratory time for each phase of BPD:
1. TV for each phase of BPD (minimum to maximum).
2. PEEP cutoffs for each phase of BPD—initial settings.
3. Pressure support for each phase of BPD (minimum to maximum).

	Early phase	Evolving phase	Established phase
Ti (s)	0.24–0.4	0.35–0.45	0.4–0.5
Tidal volume (mL/kg)	3–6	4–6	4–6
PEEP (cm H_2O)	4–6	4–6	5–7
PSV	6–8	6–10	6–18

Birth weight (g)	PSV levels (cm H_2O)
<1000	6–8
1000–1500	8–10
>1500	10–12

Monitoring of BPD patients
1. Pulse oximetry.
2. Transcutaneous O_2 and CO_2 monitoring.
3. Arterial blood gas monitoring.
4. Blood pressure monitoring.
5. Pulmonary graphics (see chapter on Ventilator Graphics) generally not reliable.
6. Near infrared spectroscopy (NIRS; see chapter on Monitroing of Gas Exchange.)

Early phase (up to 1 PN week) [10]
- Ensure antenatal steroid therapy and attempt to delay delivery for up to 48 h for optimal effect, as long as the there are no maternal/fetal contraindications to such an approach.
- Set initial FiO_2 at 0.3–0.4 for resuscitation.
- Follow recommendations for initial target SpO_2 in the first few minutes of life [22].

- Attempt to stabilize infant on NCPAP of ~6 cm H_2O.
- If infant exhibits increasing respiratory distress with FiO_2 >0.3–0.4 on NCPAP, give "early" surfactant, that is, within first 2 h of life.
- Once intubated, if possible, either use the INSURE or LISA techniques, and attempt to extubate to (S)NIPPV (settings as mentioned earlier).
- Administer loading dose of caffeine.
- If requiring long-term ventilation, use short inspiratory times (0.24–0.4 s), rapid rates (40–60 per min) and low PIP (14–20 cm H_2O), moderate PEEP (4–6 cm H_2O), and TVs (3–6 mL/kg).
- Wean PIP and rate, keeping the PEEP and Ti the same. The attempt should be to use the lowest MAP to maintain the blood gas targets, till the infant is ready to be extubated. For extubation settings, see chapter on Nasal Intermittent Positive Pressure Ventilation.
- Blood gas targets:

pH	7.25–7.35
PaO_2	40–60 mmHg
$PaCO_2$	45–55 mmHg

- High-frequency ventilation for "rescue" if conventional ventilation fails; usually, if MAP >12 cm H_2O or there is evidence of air leak.

Evolving phase (>1 PN week to 36 weeks' PMA) [10]
1. Avoid endotracheal tube ventilation; maximize NIV [(S)NIPPV/NCPAP] for respiratory support.
2. Wean PIP and rate, keeping the PEEP and Ti the same. The attempt should be to use the lowest MAP to maintain the blood gas targets, till the infant is ready to be extubated. For extubation settings, see chapter on Nasal intermittent positive pressure ventilation.
3. In the first few weeks of life, if the ventilator settings increase, rule out a PDA. If patient has PDA, manage with medical therapy. Consider at least two courses of medical therapy, before utilizing surgical ligation. (For additional detail, please refer to the chapter on Patent Ductus Arteriosus.)
4. If the increases in ventilator settings are not secondary to a PDA, consider diuretic therapy in an attempt to decrease ventilator settings and FiO_2 requirements.
5. Consider the possibility of ventilator-associated pneumonia (VAP). (For additional detail, please refer to the chapter on Ventilator-Associated Pneumonia and Infection Control.)
6. After PN week 3–4, consider a short course of dexamethasone therapy to attempt to extubate the infant to (S)NIPPV. For extubation settings, see chapter on Nasal Intermittent Positive Pressure Ventilation.
7. Blood gas targets:

pH	7.25–7.35
PaO_2	50–70 mmHg
$PaCO_2$	50–60 mmHg

Established phase (>36 weeks' PMA) [10]
1. If intubated, attempt to minimize ventilator settings (may need more FiO_2).
2. Maximize NIV [(S)NIPPV/NCPAP] for respiratory support.
3. Continue chronic diuretic therapy to attempt to minimize ventilator settings. The attempt should be to extubate and wean infant off O_2, if possible, prior to discharge home.
4. Screen for PH; if present, consider inhaled nitric oxide (iNO) trial to treat PH which may aid in lowering ventilator settings. Additional details are provided below in the Section: Complications.
5. Use of inhaled steroids and/or beta-agonists should be considered to decrease ventilator settings. The attempt should be to extubate and wean infant off O_2, if possible, prior to discharge home.
   A course of prednisolone might be helpful to wean O_2. Dose of prednisolone: 2 mg/kg/day orally divided twice per day for 5 days, then 1 mg/kg/dose orally daily for 3 days, and then 1 mg/kg/dose every other day for 3 doses [49].
6. Blood gas targets:

pH	7.25–7.35
PaO_2	50–70 mmHg
$PaCO_2$	50–65 mmHg

Management of severe BPD. If CXR shows uniform dense haziness, oxygenation is the basic problem. Aim to keep MAP relatively higher, with higher TV and Ti [3]. The addition of PSV reduces the work of breathing and facilitates uniform lung expansion in areas of atelectasis and facilitates weaning, but a close eye has to be kept on improved minute ventilation on lower settings, and higher PIP and MAP on higher settings [50]. This is used most often as a means to prepare the child for extubation. The levels mentioned are titrated based on the weight of the infant and severity of lung disease.

Initial settings:

PEEP	6–12 cm H_2O
TV	8–12 mL/kg
Ti	≥0.5 s
PSV	6–18 cm H_2O

Severe BPD is characterized by heterogeneous disease with different levels of airway resistance and lung compliance. Hence, management strategies have been recommended to utilize a prolonged Ti (0.5–0.8 s), slow

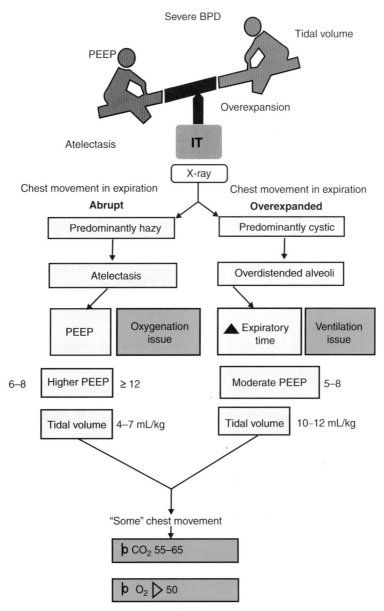

Fig. 27.13 Bedside Management of Severe BPD. This strategy for the two classical lung parenchymal abnormalities shows an algorithmic approach to each specific type of disease with bedside application. *IT*, inspiratory time; *PEEP*, positive end expiratory pressure. Courtesy: P.K. Rajiv.

ventilator rates (<20 per min), and high TV (8–12 mL/kg). The PEEP should be relatively high, too (>6–8 cm H_2O) [3]. SpO_2 targets in such infants should be kept at 92%–98%. Permissive hypercapnia with pCO_2 in the range of 55–65 mmHg, and pH ≥ 7.25 should be targeted to facilitate weaning of the ventilator in an effort to extubate to noninvasive support. With the predominant atelectatic type of severe BPD, if initial settings of PEEP

of >6–8 cm H_2O does not improve oxygenation, consider increasing it further from 8 to 10–12 cm H_2O and/or increasing the Ti to 0.6–0.8. For the predominant cystic (overexpanded) variety of severe BPD, where ventilation may be challenging, a larger TV (10–12 mL/kg) with slower ventilator rates (10–20 per min), with Ti ~0.5, may allow for improved CO_2 removal. This has been shown in Figs. 27.13 and 27.14. Use of bedside ventilator

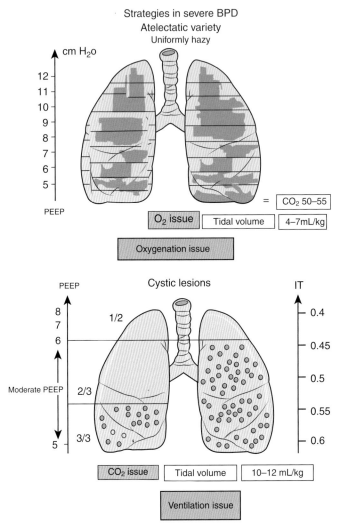

Fig. 27.14 Management of Severe BPD. The pictogram shows the key management control points in the bedside management of the two classical forms of the disease. *IT*, inspiratory time; *PEEP*, positive end expiratory pressure. Courtesy: P.K. Rajiv.

flow–volume loops can be used to titrate the PEEP levels to prevent airway collapse and gas trapping. It is important to note that while the previously mentioned guidelines are helpful, efforts have to be individualized to the infant to maintain FRC and allow for optimal gas exchange. For example, in Figs. 27.15 and 27.16, improvement was seen by increasing the PEEP, while in Figs. 27.17–27.20, ventilation was improved by decreasing Ti.

As examples for managing the atelectatic variety of severe BPD, Fig. 27.16 depicts the alteration in lung aeration after increasing the MAP which in this case was by increasing PIP, PEEP, and PS.

In Fig. 27.16, increasing the PEEP by 1 cm H_2O was sufficient to improve aeration.

In the cystic form of BPD, CO_2 retention tends to be the problem. The strategic focus on ventilation would be to keep lower MAPs, and increasing the expiratory phase to assist with CO_2 elimination. As examples for managing the cystic variety of severe BPD, Figs. 27.18–27.21 shows gradual resolution/improvement of the disease by decreasing the Ti.

Additional practical guidelines. **Early phase**: Extubation within the first 72 h of life is a priority. After surfactant administration in the first few hours of life (if

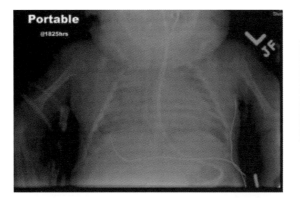

SIMV mode:
PIP 26 cm H_2O
PEEP 11 cm H_2O
Rate 40 per min
PS 13 cm H_2O
Ti 0.45 s
FiO_2 0.95

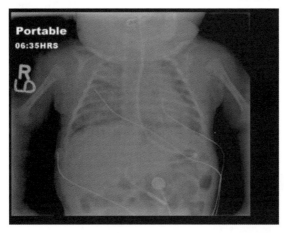

SIMV mode:
PIP 30 cm H_2O
PEEP 12 cm H_2O
Rate 40 per min
PS 17 cm H_2O
Ti 0.45 s
FiO_2 0.87

Fig. 27.15 Alteration in Lung Aeration in a Case of Severe Atelectatic BPD After Increasing MAP by Increasing PIP, PEEP, and PS. *FiO*$_2$, Fraction of inspired oxygen; *PEEP*, positive end expiratory pressure; *PIP*, peak inspiratory pressure; *PS*, pressure support; *SIMV*, synchronized intermittent mandatory ventilation; and *Ti*, inspiratory time.

required), try to wean PIP, keeping PEEP ~6 cm H_2O, and decreasing FiO_2, as long as the saturations are between 87% and 93% and blood gases are within the normal ranges (as specified in previous tables). Once the ventilator settings and FiO_2 have reached target values indicated, extubate to (S)NIPPV.

Extubation settings:

PIP	≤16 cm H_2O
PEEP	≤5 cm H_2O
Rate	15–25 per min
FiO_2	≤0.35

Evolving phase: Start with a PS appropriate for the weight of the infant and start weaning the PIP and FiO_2, as long as the saturations are between 87% and 93% and blood gases are within the acceptable ranges (as specified

in the tables). It is important to keep TV within the target range. Then start decreasing the ventilator PS level in increments of 2 cm H_2O, every 5–7 days allowing the infant to do most of the breathing till MAP/PIP/PEEP settings have reached the target values that will allow extubation to (S)NIPPV. Diuretics are added and short-course steroids (the latter after 3–4 weeks of PN life) given, if the weaning process is difficult. Once the ventilator settings and FiO_2 have reached target values, extubate to (S)NIPPV.

Established phase: Start with a PS appropriate for the weight of the infant, and start weaning the PIP and FiO_2, as long as the saturations are between 87% and 93% and blood gases are within the normal ranges (as specified in the tables). It is important to keep TV within the target range. The child is usually on chronic diuretics. PEEP can be increased to 7 cm H_2O. Then start decreasing PS level (over days to weeks in increments of 2 cm H_2O),

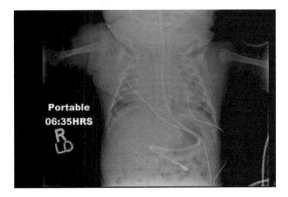

SIMV mode:
PIP 26 cm H_2O
PEEP 10 cm H_2O
Rate 40 per min
PS 13 cm H_2O
Ti 0.45 s
FiO_2 0.95

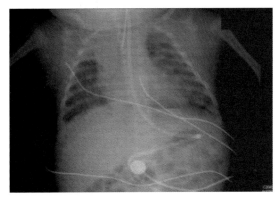

SIMV mode:
PIP 26 cm H_2O
PEEP 11 cm H_2O
Rate 40 per min
PS 13 cm H_2O
Ti 0.45 s
FiO_2 0.78

Fig. 27.16 Alteration in Lung Aeration in a Case of Severe Atelectatic BPD After Increasing Only PEEP. *FiO₂,* Fraction of inspired oxygen; *PEEP,* positive end expiratory pressure; *PIP,* peak inspiratory pressure; *PS,* pressure support; *SIMV,* synchronized intermittent mandatory ventilation; and *Ti,* inspiratory time.

allowing the infant to do most of the breathing till MAP/PIP/PEEP settings have reached the target values that will allow extubation attempt to (S)NIPPV. If not close to target settings for extubation, it may be helpful to give a short course of steroids to attempt to extubate to (S) NIPPV.

Surfactant replacement therapy

Surfactant replacement therapy is clearly associated with decreased severity of RDS and its associated mortality. Although there is not substantial evidence that survivors have a decreased incidence of BPD, survival without BPD appears to be improved in some of the meta-analyses that have been undertaken [51]. Use of synthetic surfactant (lucinactant) that contains the novel peptide sinapultide, a surfactant-associated protein B mimic revealed no statistically different differences in the outcomes of death and BPD, compared to animal-derived surfactants [52–55].

Newer minimally or less-invasive modes (using vascular catheters or feeding tubes) of surfactant delivery (LISA) that do not require endotracheal intubations have been/are being tested in multicenter randomized clinical trials in order to assess their impact on BPD [56,57]. Another attractive alternative, aerosol delivery, is waiting testing for clinical efficacy.

Nutrition

1. Fluid restriction: Nutrition and fluid management are important parts of maintaining and repairing injury caused by BPD. Caloric content must be increased to meet the high energy needs required to increase metabolic rate and oxygen consumption [58]. BPD energy requirements supersede standard infant caloric requirements by as much as 125% [58]. Fluid management must be pristine to prevent right-sided heart failure, a common complication of severe BPD. Fluid restriction may be accomplished by adding

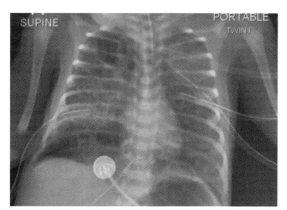

SIMV mode:
PIP 25 cm H₂O
PEEP 5 cm H₂O
Rate 45 per min
Ti 0.32 s
FiO₂ 0.65
TV 3.5 mL/kg

Fig. 27.17 Resolution/Improvement in a Case of Severe Cystic BPD After Manipulating the Ti. *FiO₂,* Fraction of inspired oxygen; *PEEP,* positive end expiratory pressure; *PIP,* peak inspiratory pressure; *PS,* pressure support; *SIMV,* synchronized intermittent mandatory ventilation; *Ti,* inspiratory time; and *TV,* tidal volume.

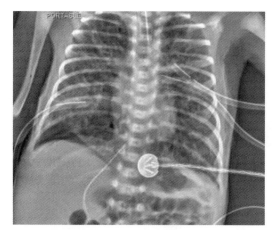

SIMV mode:
PIP 22 cm H₂O
PEEP 5 cm H₂O
Rate 45 per min
Ti 0.28 s
FiO₂ 0.45
TV   3–3.5 mL/kg

Fig. 27.18 Resolution/Improvement in a Case of Severe Cystic BPD After Manipulating the Ti. *FiO₂,* Fraction of inspired oxygen; *PEEP,* positive end expiratory pressure; *PIP,* peak inspiratory pressure; *PS,* pressure support; *SIMV,* synchronized intermittent mandatory ventilation; *Ti,* inspiratory time; and *TV,* tidal volume.

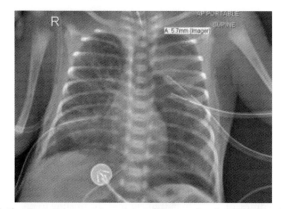

SIMV mode:
PIP 20 cm H₂O
PEEP 5 cm H₂O
Rate 40 per min
Ti 0.26 s
FiO₂ 0.4
TV 3–3.5 mL/kg

Fig. 27.19 Resolution/Improvement in a Case of Severe Cystic BPD After Manipulating the Ti. *FiO₂,* Fraction of inspired oxygen; *PEEP,* positive end expiratory pressure; *PIP,* peak inspiratory pressure; *PS,* pressure support; *SIMV,* synchronized intermittent mandatory ventilation; *Ti,* inspiratory time; and *TV,* tidal volume.

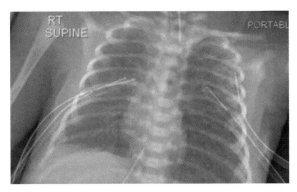

SIMV mode:
PIP 18 cm H_2O
PEEP 5 cm H_2O
Rate 40 per min
Ti 0.26 s
FiO_2 0.3
TV 3–3.5 mL/kg

Fig. 27.20 Resolution/Improvement in a Case of Severe Cystic BPD After Manipulating the Ti. *FiO₂*, Fraction of inspired oxygen; *PEEP*, positive end expiratory pressure; *PIP*, peak inspiratory pressure; *PS*, pressure support; *SIMV*, synchronized intermittent mandatory ventilation; *Ti*, inspiratory time; and *TV*, tidal volume.

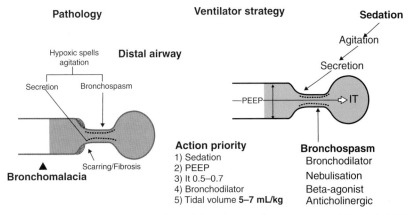

Fig. 27.21 Pictogram Showing the Pathological Basis and the Strategy for Treatment of Hypoxic "BPD Spells." *IT*, inspiratory time; and *PEEP*, positive end expiratory pressure. Courtesy: P.K. Rajiv.

diuretics, but electrolytes must be carefully monitored. Reducing lung fluid may improve lung function and decrease oxygen consumption and demand if cautiously implemented. Growth of BPD patients is dependent on adequate caloric intake and balance of protein, carbohydrates, fat, and key minerals, such as calcium, phosphorous, and iron that are essential for growth and repair. Parenteral nutrition implemented during the early phase of BPD, ideally on the first day, is later followed by enteral nutrition consisting of high-calorie formulas, up to 30 cal/oz. Carefully balancing the lipid to carbohydrate is essential to prevent increased CO_2 production Multiple studies suggest that fluid overload contributes to an increased risk of BPD [59] (refer to the chapter on Nutrition in the Preterm Neonate Requiring Respiratory Support for additional detail.) Recommendations for parenteral nutritional management of hospitalized very low BW infants:

	Initiation	Incre- ments	Mainte- nance
Fluids (mL/kg/day)	80–100	10–20	130–140
Calories (Kcal/kg/day)	40–60	10–15	120
Carbohydrate (glucose infusion rate) (mg/kg/min)	4–6	1	10–12
Protein (amino acids) (g/kg/day)	3	0.5–1	4
Lipids (g/kg/day)	0.5–1	0.5–1	3
Sodium (mEq./kg/day)	Minimal (first several days)	2 (4–6 days of life)	3 (after day 6)

2. Vitamin A: Supplementation by vitamin A demonstrated a significant decrease in BPD or death at 36 weeks' PMA following treatment with vitamin A (55% vs. 62%) [60]. A meta-analysis of all published trials revealed that vitamin A supplementation was associated with a modest reduction in death or BPD at 36 weeks, which was of borderline statistical significance (RR 0.91, 95% confidence interval 0.82, 1.00, NNT 17) [61].

> **If used, recommended dose: 5000 IU thrice weekly IM for 4 weeks**

3. Omega 3 fatty acids and BPD [62]: The critical fatty acids docosahexaenoic acid (DHA) and arachidonic acid (AA) decline in preterm infants within the first PN week and are associated with neonatal morbidities, including BPD. DHA and AA are precursors to downstream metabolites that terminate the inflammatory response. Treatment with Resolvin D1 and/or Lipoxin A4 could potentially prevent lung injury of BPD. This is currently under evaluation.

Patent ductus arteriosus [63]

Patients who developed a PDA or were at risk for right-heart failure were more likely to develop BPD. Fluid balance is interrupted by the presence of a PDA, but can be controlled by applying positive end expiratory pressure, invasively or noninvasively. Closure of the PDA is often accomplished by pharmacologic intervention with indomethacin or ibuprofen or acetaminophen. Surgical ligation of PDA has been associated with worse outcomes, and should be avoided [64].

Clinically significant PDA. A "symptomatic PDA" or clinically significant (csPDA) is defined when clinical manifestations of pulmonary, cardiovascular, or systemic compromise occur as a result of significant left-to-right shunting. Common signs and symptoms include:

Murmur (systolic or continuous)	Tachycardia
Hyperdynamic precordium	Wide pulse pressure >25 mmHg
Increasing ventilatory requirements	FiO_2 >0.4
Pulmonary edema	Acute pulmonary hemorrhage

The CXR shows evidence of cardiomegaly and increased pulmonary vascularity.

Echocardiogram: All patients with a suspected PDA should have an echocardiogram to confirm the diagnosis, establish the size of the shunt, and rule out ductal dependent congenital heart disease.

Hemodynamically significant PDA
1. Predominant left-to-right shunt through the ductus

2. Ductal diameter >1.5 mm
3. Enlarged left atrium (left atrial/aortic root or LA/Ao ratio >1.3)
4. Disturbed diastolic flow in the main pulmonary artery
5. Reverse end-diastolic flow in post ductal aorta

Medical management of PDA
1. Fluid restriction to ~120 mL/kg/day.
2. Consider diuretic therapy (furosemide 2 mg/kg/day).
3. Evaluate infant after 48–72 h of aforementioned management. If infant fulfills the criteria (as given next) for csPDA and hemodynamically significant PDA (hsPDA), consider pharmacologic management.
4. Indications for pharmacological treatment include the following:
   Presence of csPDA and hsPDA defined by:
   a. Presence of two or more clinical signs listed previously, *and*
   b. Presence of two or more echocardiographic findings noted earlier.

Drugs: Nonsteroidal anti-inflammatory agents: IV indomethacin or IV ibuprofen: While these are most effective if administered in the first 10–14 days of life, they may be used up to 4 weeks of life. A Cochrane database review showed no statistically significant difference in closure between ibuprofen and indomethacin. A decision to use one drug versus another should be based upon the infant's presentation and comorbidities. Acetaminophen may also be used.

Indication for surgical ligation for PDA: After 2–3 complete courses of indomethacin/ibuprofen. This can be attempted for up to 4 weeks of PN age, especially for extremely low BW (ELBW) infants.

(See chapter on Patent Ductus Arteriosus for more details.)

Inhaled nitric oxide (iNO) therapy

iNO may [65,66] or may not [67,68] be beneficial. More studies are needed to better identify potential benefits to the target population likely to develop BPD [69]. The use of iNO does seem to be safe in this population [69], although it does not seem to affect surfactant composition [70], or pulmonary function [71]. At present, routine use of iNO to decrease BPD in the preterm population is not recommended [72,73].

Caffeine administration

Caffeine stimulates the respiratory center of a premature infant and prevents severe cases of apnea that might otherwise result in intubation and invasive mechanical ventilation [74]. Minute ventilation, primarily by increasing TV, is increased as a result of caffeine administration. In premature infants, caffeine has been shown to prevent

BPD by reducing the need for additional respiratory support that may result in long-term sequelae. In a multicenter trial ($n = 2006$), infants <1250 g who received caffeine had lower BPD rates (36% compared to 47%) than infants who did not receive it. In addition, invasive ventilator days, need for CPAP, and supplemental oxygen were reduced by caffeine administration [74]. There is evidence supporting the benefits of routine caffeine use in infants <1250 g without long-term effects on gastrointestinal, neurodevelopmental, or other complications.

Use of caffeine has been associated with decreased incidence of BPD [75] and improved neurodevelopmental outcomes at 18–21 months corrected age [76]. However, improved survival without disability in infants who received caffeine was not sustained up to 5 years of age [77]. Early initiation (in the first 3 days of PN life) appears to be better [78]. All three methylxanthines (noted in the following table) have been shown to help with the management of apnea of prematurity and/or improve the chances of successful extubation in preterm neonates.

Methylxanthines

Drug	Loading dose (mg/kg)	Maintenance dose	Route	
Caffeine citrate	20–25	5–10 mg/kg every 24 h	IV/PO	Wide therapeutic range
Aminophylline	5–8	1.5–3 mg/kg/day divided every 8–12 h	IV/PO	Monitor levels
Theophylline	5–8	3–6 mg/kg/day divided every 6–8 h	PO	Monitor levels

These doses are used for management of apnea of prematurity. Changing aminophylline from IV to PO requires an increase in the dose by 20%. No need to adjust theophylline.

Diuretics [79–86]

Indications for initial diuretic therapy (usually, furosemide) include increasing ventilator support settings and FiO_2 requirements (>0.6), associated with pulmonary edema on the chest X-ray. This is usually seen at the end of first week of PN life in an intubated infant. The dose of furosemide is 2 mg/kg/dose IV given 1–2 times a day. We use this daily or every other day for the next 2–3 weeks, and/or till the infant reaches full feeds and then we replace with chronic diuretic therapy using spironolactone (2–4 mg/kg/day) and chlorothiazide (20–40 mg/kg/day). Hydrochlorothiazide (see table below for dose) may be used instead of chlorothiazide. Monitoring of electrolyte levels is required, with frequent supplementation with NaCl and/or KCl to maintain their levels within normal values.

Diuretics

Drug	Site of action	Route	Onset	Dose
Furosemide	Loop diuretic	IV	15–30 min	1 mg/kg/dose
		PO	30–60 min	1–3 mg/kg/dose
Hydrochlorothiazide	Distal tubule	PO	1–2 h	2–4 mg/kg/day
Spironolactone	Aldosterone antagonist	PO	3–5 days	1.5–3 mg/kg/day

Corticosteroids [87]

The use of dexamethasone may be considered in infants who are:

1. Requiring mechanical ventilation between 7 and 21 days of age,
2. In supplemental oxygen, and
3. At high risk of developing BPD.
4. The recommended course for use as used in the DART trial.

Time	Dose (mg/kg/dose)	Frequency (hourly)
Days 1–3	0.075	12
Days 4–6	0.050	12
Days 7 and 8	0.025	12
Days 9 and 10	0.01	12

1. Some individuals may receive subsequent doses of 0.01 mg/kg/day every 2–3 days if there is significant deterioration after the tapering of the dose on day 10.
2. Repeat courses may be indicated in selected infants with severe BPD, if still requiring invasive mechanical ventilation with FiO_2 requirements >0.6.

Hydrocortisone [88–92]: Hydrocortisone has been proposed as an alternative to dexamethasone because it is a less potent glucocorticoid and may mitigate against adrenal insufficiency experienced by some preterm infants and, thus, decrease the incidence of BPD.

Overall, although hydrocortisone may be a promising alternative to dexamethasone for treating babies with BPD or prolonged ventilator dependence, there is no evidence at this time to show that it is effective or safe.

Inhaled corticosteroids [93–99]: Inhaled corticosteroids have less systemic absorption than systemic corticosteroids and their use has been suggested as a strategy to minimize the short- and long-term adverse effects of systemic corticosteroids. There is currently little evidence to support the routine use of inhaled corticosteroids for the prevention or treatment of BPD (Level 1 evidence). Inhaled corticosteroids do not appear to offer significant benefits over systemic corticosteroids for the treatment of infants who remain ventilator-dependent (Level 1 evidence).

Bronchodilators and anticholinergics: [10] The commonly used bronchodilators and anticholinergics in clinical practice are summarized next. They are generally used for symptomatic relief.

Bronchodilators

Drug	Trade name	Preparation	Doses
Albuterol	Proventil Ventolin	Inhalation solution MDI, 90 mcg/puff oral	0.1–0.5 mg/kg every 2–6 h 1–2 Puffs every 4–6 h 0.1–0.3 mg/kg every 8 h
Levalbuterol	Xopenex	Inhalation solution MDI, 45 mcg/puff	0.31 mg every 8 h 1–2 Puffs every 4–6 h
Terbutaline	Brethaire	Inhalation solution MDI, 0.2 mcg/puff oral	0.1–0.3 mg/kg every 2–6 h 1–2 Puffs every 4–6 h 0.05–0.15 mg/kg every 8–12 h
Metaproterenol	Alupent	Inhalation solution MDI, 0.65 mg/puff	0.25–0.5 mg/kg every 2–4 h 1–2 Puffs every 4–6 h
Pirbuterol	Maxair	MDI, 200 mcg/puff	1–2 Puffs every 4–6 h Children over 12 years old

Anticholinergic

Drug	Trade name	Preparation	Doses
Atropine		Inhalation solution	0.05 mg/kg every 6–8 h
Ipratropium	Atrovent	Inhalation solution MDI 17 mcg/puff	75–175 mcg every 6–8 h 2–4 Puffs every 6–8 h
Triotropium	Spiriva	Inhalation, capsules, contain 18 mcg dry powder formulation	18 mcg once a day for adults (not used in children)

Summary of the pharmacological management of BPD

Drug	Treatment of	Effect	Side effects	Comments
Oxygen	Hypoxemia	Improved oxygenation	Longer hospital stay, home oxygen	Maintain saturations >89% and <95%

Drug	Treatment of	Effect	Side effects	Comments
Caffeine	Apnea of prematurity	Less apnea	Tachycardia, feeding intolerance	Initiate early (first 3 postnatal days)
Diuretics (loop, thiazides)	Pulmonary edema	Decreased pulmonary edema	Electrolyte imbalance, osteopenia, ototoxicity	Loop: use sparingly in early evolving BPD Thiazides: consider for judicious chronic use
Bronchodilators and anticholinergics (albuterol, ipratropium)	Bronchospasm	Bronchodilation	Tachycardia, arrhythmias	Limit use in infants with bronchospasm and acute clinical response
Steroids (early, moderately early, late, inhaled)	Inflammation	Improved oxygenation, earlier extubation	Short term: hyperglycemia, gastrointestinal perforation Long term: increased risk for cerebral palsy	Last resort therapy for rapidly deteriorating pulmonary status
Vitamin A	Impaired lung development	Small reduction in incidence of BPD	None reported	Used in some centers

Complications

1. **Pulmonary hypertension**: It has been recently recognized that PH occurs in some preterm infants as a complication of their BPD [100]. It has been reported to be more common in infants who are ELBW, have a history of oligohydramnios, and severe BPD and/or need for prolonged PPV [100]. In established BPD, the incidence of PH has been reported to be 25%–40% [101]. Diagnosis is usually made by echocardiography, but cardiac catheterization is considered the "gold standard" [101]. Routine echocardiography screening for all premature infants at 36 weeks' PMA has been suggested.

If evidence of PH is documented in an intubated and ventilated patient, iNO is given as a trial at 20 ppm to see if there is a response. If improvement is noted (decreasing FiO_2), keep on iNO for 1–2 weeks, and re-echo to see if there is any objective improvement in PH parameters. If present, add sildenafil (start with 0.5 mg/kg/dose q 6–8 h, titrate dose up by 0.5 mg/kg/dose every 24 h, as tolerated, to reach a maximum dose of 3 mg/kg/dose q6 in 2 weeks), in an attempt to wean off iNO, for chronic therapy. The main side effect is transient systemic hypotension [102,103]. Other pulmonary vasodilators that can be utilized include prostacyclins and bosentan [101]. BPD infants with PH are at higher risk for increased morbidity and mortality compared to BPD infants

without PH [100]. Infants with BPD-associated PH may be at increased risk for pulmonary vascular problems as they grow older [100].

2. **Airway Abnormalities**:
   a. Tracheomalacia: Usually managed with higher levels of PEEP and/or tracheostomy and/or aortopexy, based on severity.
   b. Bronchomalacia: Usually managed with higher levels of PEEP and/or tracheostomy, based on severity.
   c. Subglottic stenosis: May require surgical intervention. (For additional detail, please refer to the chapter on Airway Disorders.)
   d. Airway granulomas: May require surgical intervention.
   e. Pseudopolyps: May require surgical intervention.
   f. "BPD spells": These occur due to trachea-/bronchomalacia, as infants may have increased airway compliance. This may cause impaired clearance of secretions and tracheal collapse resulting in limitation of expiratory flow [104,105]. These infants clinically present with significant airway obstruction and severe cyanosis [104]. The spells are managed with sedation and/or muscle relaxants with increasing PEEP, depending upon severity. Morphine (0.05–0.1 mg/kg) or fentanyl (1–3 µg/kg) can be used for the short term. Side effects include respiratory depression. For chronic sedation, suggested to use lorazepam (0.05–0.1 mg/kg/dose q 4–6 hourly) or midazolam (0.05–0.1 mg/kg/dose q 2–4 hourly). For paralysis, consider using pancuronium bromide 0.1 mg/kg/dose; repeat as needed.

The primary strategy for managing "BPD spells" is sedation (morphine) and/or muscle relaxation. They generally do not respond well to ventilator changes of increasing PIP/PEEP or bronchodilators. Use of beta-agonists may increase large airway instability in infants with tracheomalacia and bronchomalacia. However, PEEP can be increased by 1–2 cm H_2O in the short term, along with an increase in Ti. See Fig. 27.21.

3. **Pneumonia**: It is difficult to diagnose "pneumonia" in neonates due to lack of a universally accepted definition. Bacterial tracheitis presents with respiratory deterioration (increasing ventilator settings and FiO_2 requirements) in an intubated infant, associated with increased and thick secretions. Tracheal aspirate culture usually has evidence of "many" (>2+) inflammatory cells with culture suggesting growth of a particular species. This may be treated with nebulized gentamicin or tobramycin, twice a day, for 5–7 days. Repeat tracheal aspirate cell counts/culture can be sent to confirm improvement. If treating systemically, first line treatment is ampicillin + gentamicin. The *second line* treatment should be as per the sensitivity pattern in the local NICU. (Refer to the chapter on Infection Control and Ventilator Associated Pneumonia Prevention for additional detail.)

4. **Necrotizing tracheobronchitis**: This is a rare complication of prolonged invasive mechanical ventilation. The exact etiology is not completely understood; however; impaired submucosal blood flow, inadequate humidification and/or exposure to high airway pressures have been suggested as contributing factors [106–108]. The clinical presentation is of acute obstructive respiratory failure with severe hypoxia. The diagnosis is usually made by tracheal endoscopy, which may also be therapeutic if tracheobronchial aspiration successfully relieves the obstruction [106,107].

5. **Electrolyte abnormalities due to diuretic use**: Hyponatremia, hypokalemia, and hypocalcemia and osteopenia (secondary to calciuria). This is most commonly seen with furosemide.

Bronchoscopy indications in an infant with established BPD

1. Airway evaluation in infants where repeated extubation attempts have been unsuccessful.
2. Persistent atelectasis.
3. Isolated or localized hyperinflation.
4. Anatomic evaluation of airway if congenital and/or acquired anomalies are suspected.

Tracheostomy indications

There are limited data for indications for tracheostomies in patients with BPD. Most are done for "severe BPD" indicated for chronic respiratory failure in infants unable to wean off ventilator support. Tracheostomy is usually considered in patients requiring prolonged mechanical ventilation usually in infants who are >100 days old. In one study, the average was 118 days and a weight of 2877 g [109]. The overall goal is to reduce the severity of respiratory distress including "BPD spells," perhaps an earlier discharge home, and improve long-term neurodevelopmental outcomes [3,109].

Pulmonary outcomes

It is important to keep in mind that many of the studies addressing pulmonary outcomes include preterm infants born before extensive use of antenatal steroids and surfactant and many survivors of BPD with neurological impairment may not be able to perform lung function tests.

Morbidity

Infants with BPD have higher rates of re-hospitalizations (up to 50%) in the first year of life [110,111]. Respiratory symptoms in patients with BPD persist beyond the first 2 years of life into the preschool years [112], adolescence, and early adulthood [113,114]. They are also more likely to have chest wall abnormalities [115]. It is unclear whether BPD severity or prematurity per se influences the persistence and severity of symptoms.

Radiologic findings

Chest radiograph and computed tomography (CT) scan abnormalities persist into adolescence and adulthood, with CT being more sensitive. Chest X-ray changes included mild hyperexpansion, blebs, interstitial thickening, peribronchial cuffing, and pleural thickening [116]. CT scan findings comprised of multifocal areas of hyperaeration, well-defined linear opacities, and triangular subpleural opacities [117–119]. A more severe clinical course correlates with greater radiologic abnormalities [118]. A CT scan scoring system has been proposed and may help with BPD prognosis [120].

Pulmonary function

Patients with BPD continue to have significant impairment and deterioration in lung function into late adolescence and adulthood [121–125]. This is particularly important as persistent airway obstruction in childhood has been correlated with development of chronic obstructive pulmonary disease in adulthood [126]. Studies have shown none to significant reduction in exercise capacity in children with BPD when compared with healthy term infants or preterm infants without lung disease [127,128], which may be improved with an exercise training program [129]. Lung abnormalities that may persist into adulthood include airway obstruction, airway hyper-reactivity, and emphysema [130,131].

Neurodevelopmental outcomes

Although preterm infants have an increased risk of neurodevelopmental impairment, BPD is an additional risk factor [132]. This is probably a result of multiple contributing factors including frequent episodes of hypoxia, poor growth, and, potentially, PN steroids [132]. Infants of <1500 g BW with BPD have greater fine and gross motor skill impairment as well as cognitive function and language delay compared with those without BPD [133,134]. Children with severe BPD have worse outcomes and require more interventions at 8 years of age than do children with mild or moderate BPD [135]. BPD does not seem to be associated with a specific neuropsychological but, rather, a global impairment. The spectrum of neurodevelopmental impairment seems to correlate well with BPD disease severity [111].

Summary of treatment

Therapeutic intervention	Current status
Early phase (up to 1 postnatal week)	
Oxygen supplementation	A wide variation in the acceptable oxygen saturation levels exists across centers but it is generally <95% (suggested: 87%–93%)
Ventilatory strategy	Avoid intubation; if intubated, give "early" surfactant Use short inspiratory times (0.24–0.4 s), rapid rates (40–60 per min) and low PIP (14–20 cm H_2O), moderate PEEP (4–6 cm H_2O), and tidal volumes (3–6 mL/kg) Extubate early to (S)NIPPV/nasal CPAP Blood gas targets: pH 7.25–7.35 PaO_2: 40–60 mmHg; $PaCO_2$: 45–55 mmHg High-frequency ventilation for "rescue" if conventional ventilation fails
Methylxanthines	Improves successful extubation rate Decreases BPD
Vitamin A	If considering use, dose is 5000 IU administered intramuscularly 3 times/week for 4 weeks; one additional infant survived without BPD for every 14–15 infants who received vitamin A
Fluids	Restrictive fluid intake may decrease BPD
Nutrition	Provide increased energy intake
Evolving phase (>1 PN week to 36 weeks PMA)	
Oxygen supplementation	Same as for early phase
Ventilatory strategy	Avoid endotracheal tube ventilation; maximize noninvasive ventilation [(S)NIPPV/nasal CPAP] for respiratory support Blood gas targets: pH 7.25–7.35; PaO_2: 50–70 mmHg; $PaCO_2$: 50–60 mmHg
Methylxanthines	Same as for early phase
Vitamin A	Same as for early phase; if using, continue for 4 postnatal weeks
Steroids	Dexamethasone is effective in weaning off mechanical ventilation when used "moderately early" and "delayed" Increased incidence of neurologic sequelae with early use (<96 h)
Diuretics	Furosemide: may use daily or every other day with transient improvement in lung function Spironolactone and thiazides: chronic therapy improves lung function, decreases oxygen requirement

Therapeutic intervention	Current status
Nutrition	Same as for early phase
Established phase (>36 weeks' PMA)	
Oxygen supplementation	For prevention of pulmonary hypertension and cor pulmonale; a wide variation in the acceptable oxygen saturation levels exists across centers, but it is generally ~95%
Ventilatory strategy	Blood gas targets: pH 7.25–7.35; PaO_2: 50–70 mmHg; $PaCO_2$: 50–65 mmHg
Steroids	Oral prednisolone may be helpful in weaning oxygen
Diuretics	Chronic therapy as for evolving phase; no clear duration of therapy
Beta-agonist	Transient relief: increased compliance and reduced pulmonary resistance; no significant effect on incidence or severity of BPD
Anticholinergics	Used in combination with beta-agonists in infants with bronchospasm; increased compliance and decreased respiratory system resistance
Nutrition	Same as for early phase
Immunization	Prophylaxis against RSV and influenza decreases incidence of hospital readmissions and morbidity

Criteria for discharge on oxygen:

Infants who remain oxygen dependent at time of discharge but are otherwise well may be eligible for discharge on home oxygen. Babies who are discharged on oxygen usually fit the following criteria:

1. At least 36 weeks post-conceptual age [136,137]
2. No acute medical problem
3. No apnea
4. Immunized [138]
5. Optimal weight gain [139]
6. Without aggressive retinopathy of prematurity: stabilized or in regression without continuous SpO_2 monitoring for at least 1 week prior to the expected date of discharge and stable on O_2 flow rate of 0.5 L/min [140,141]
7. With satisfactory intermittent SpO_2 spot check downloads 2–3 times/week.

Home therapy/follow-up management [142]

The target range for SpO_2 (functional) levels is 90%–95% [140,141]. The suggested parameters to wean oxygen flow are as follows.

If SpO_2 samples are 90%–95% more than 50% of the time, do not alter oxygen flow.

If SpO_2 samples are >95% more than 50% of the time, then decrease flow.

If SpO_2 samples are <90% more than 50% of the time, then increase flow.

Mild BPD

Baby girl Y was born at 27 weeks gestation to a 28-year-old G6P3L2 mother with h/o incompetent cervix who presented to the hospital in preterm labor. Mother delivered the baby precipitously via spontaneous vaginal delivery. Baby received positive pressure ventilation at delivery for primary apnea, to which she responded well. Apgars were 6 at 1 min of life and 8 at 5 min of life. She was transferred to the NICU on CPAP 5 0.3 FiO_2. Initial blood gas was 7.24/45/67/18/−5. Baby required increasing FiO_2 up to 0.4 and developed respiratory distress with tachypnea and retractions. She was intubated and given surfactant (Curosurf). Chest X-ray was done after surfactant administration and is shown in Fig. 27.22.

Baby remained intubated on low settings for 12 h and was extubated to CPAP 5 with FiO_2 of 0.25. Post-extubation capillary blood gas was 7.30/35/35/17/−8. She was loaded on caffeine 20 mg/kg and started on maintenance dose of 5 mg/kg/day. The baby remained nil per os (NPO) on TPN through the first week of life. She was started on trophic feeds with donor breast milk on day of life (DOL) 8 and reached full feeds by DOL 22 and TPN was discontinued at that time.

She continued to be on CPAP 5 for the first week of life. However, she developed worsening episodes of apnea with bradycardia and desaturations that required escalation of respiratory support to NIPPV. Her caffeine dose was also increased up to 7.5 mg/kg/day. She continued to be on NIPPV from DOL 7 to DOL 17 with FiO_2 ranging from 0.21 (room air) to 0.28. On DOL 17 she was weaned to CPAP 5 and then continued on it till DOL 30 with FiO_2 ranging from 0.22 to 0.3. Beyond that baby was weaned to nasal cannula 2 L/min at a FiO_2 of 0.21 (room air) and remained on it till

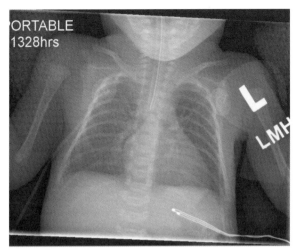

Fig. 27.22 **DOL 1.** Mild diffuse granular appearance of the lungs consistent with surfactant deficiency.

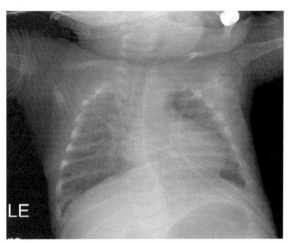

Fig. 27.23 **The 36 Weeks' PMA.** Diffuse granular opacities are again seen throughout the lungs consistent with chronic lung disease of prematurity. No focal consolidation, pleural effusion, or pneumothorax is identified. The cardiothymic silhouette remains within normal limits.

34 weeks PMA. Her caffeine was discontinued at 35 weeks' PMA. At 36 weeks' PMA baby was not on any respiratory support and was diagnosed with mild BPD. Chest X-ray at 36 weeks' PMA did show changes of BPD (Fig. 27.23). She received an echocardiogram at this time to evaluate for PH, which revealed normal cardiac function and anatomy.

Severe BPD

Baby boy R is a 24 + 4/7 week gestation male born to a 21-year-old G1P0 mother who presented to the hospital with preterm premature rupture of membranes and delivered via C section for non-reassuring fetal heart rate. Baby's Apgars were 1, 3, 4, and 7 at 1, 5, 10, and 15 min of life. He needed chest compressions and 3 doses of epinephrine during resuscitation and was intubated in the delivery room. Initial ventilator settings on SIMV were PIP/PEEP of 20/5, rate of 40, Ti 0.40 s, and a FiO_2 0.7. First ABG was 6.88/81.1/77.7/14.5/−20.7 and patient was given one dose of Survanta 4 mL/kg for significant RDS and FiO_2 requirement. Umbilical venous catheter was placed and X-ray obtained on DOL 1 is shown in Fig. 27.24.

For severe metabolic acidosis on the initial blood gas, baby received volume resuscitation and sodium bicarbonate correction. Capillary blood gas at 12 h of life was 7.31/43/44/20/−3. He was started on dopamine for hypotension, which was discontinued on DOL 2. He was also noted to be neutropenic on admission and was treated for presumed sepsis with antibiotics for 7 days. On DOL 3 echocardiogram was obtained which revealed a large PDA that did not respond to multiple courses of medical treatment over the next 2 weeks. Baby remained intubated and NPO during this period. Trophic feeds were

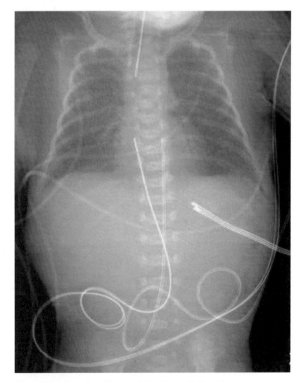

Fig. 27.24 **Patchy Bilateral Atelectasis in a Premature Infant Likely Secondary to Surfactant Deficiency.** Umbilical venous catheter is in the right atrium.

started on DOL 17 and baby reached full feeds on DOL 45. During this period baby was also diagnosed with necrotizing enterocolitis (NEC) Stage IIB and remained NPO with antibiotics for 10 days. On DOL 23 he was started on hydrochlorothiazide and received multiple doses of furosemide intermittently to help with fluid overload. He was also started on pulmicort on DOL 30 in the setting of evolving BPD. Baby continued to require ventilator support for 7 weeks of life with FiO_2 requirement as low as 0.25. On DOL 52 baby was extubated to NIPPV with settings of 22/6 and a rate of 30. Capillary blood gas obtained post extubation was 7.33/61/33/32/4. Baby remained on NIPPV till DOL 72 (35 weeks PMA) and was then weaned to CPAP 5 0.3 FiO_2.

At 36 weeks' PMA, baby continued to require CPAP with FiO_2 ranging from 0.3 to 0.4. Echocardiogram obtained for screening of PH at 36 weeks showed a small to moderate PDA, no PH, and normal function. Chest X-ray at 36 weeks' PMA is shown in Fig. 27.25.

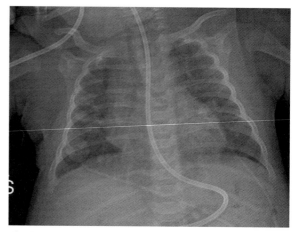

Fig. 27.25 Coarse Ground Glass Opacities Throughout Both Lungs Consistent With Chronic Lung Disease.

References

[1] Bancalari E, Claure N. Definitions and diagnostic criteria for bronchopulmonary dysplasia. Semin Perinatol 2006;30:164–170.

[2] Jobe AH, Bancalari E. Bronchopulmonary dysplasia. Am J Respir Crit Care Med 2001;163:1723–1729.

[3] Collaco JM, Shepherd EG, Keszler M, Cuevas-Guaman M, Welty SE, et al. Interdisciplinary care of children with severe bronchopulmonary dysplasia. J Pediatr 2017;181. 12–28.e1.

[4] Fanaroff AA, Hack M, Walsh MC. The NICHD neonatal research network: changes in practice and outcomes during the first 15 years. Semin Perinatol 2003;27:281–287.

[5] Fanaroff AA, Stoll BJ, Wright LL, Carlo WA, Ehrenkranz RA, Stark AR, et al. Trends in neonatal morbidity and mortality for very low birth weight infants. Am J Obstet Gynecol 2007;196:147.e1–147.e8.

[6] Walsh MC, Szefler S, Davis J, Allen M, Van Marter L, Abman S, et al. Summary proceedings from the bronchopulmonary dysplasia group. Pediatrics 2006;117:S52–S56.

[7] Walsh MC, Yao Q, Gettner P, Hale E, Collins M, Hensman A, et al. Impact of a physiologic definition on bronchopulmonary dysplasia rates. Pediatrics 2004;114:1305–1411.

[8] Guaman MC, Gien J, Baker CD, Zhang H, Austin ED, Collaco JM. Point

prevalence, clinical characteristics, and treatment variation for infants with severe bronchopulmonary dysplasia. Am J Perinatol 2015;32:960–997.

[9] Balany J, Bhandari V. Understanding the impact of infection, inflammation and their persistence in the pathogenesis of bronchopulmonary dysplasia. Front Med (Lausanne) 2015;21:2–90.

[10] Bhandari A, Bhandari V. Pitfalls, problems, and progress in bronchopulmonary dysplasia. Pediatrics 2009;123:1562–1573.

[11] Buhimschi CS, Weiner CP, Buhimschi IA. Clinical proteomics: a novel diagnostic tool for the new biology of preterm labor, part I: proteomics tools. Obstet Gynecol Surv 2006;61:481–486.

[12] Dodd JM, Crowther CA, Cincotta R, Flenady V, Robinson JS. Progesterone supplementation for preventing preterm birth: a systematic review and meta-analysis. Acta Obstet Gynecol Scand 2005;84:526–533.

[13] Feldman DM, Carbone J, Belden L, Borgida AF, Herson V. Betamethasone vs. dexamethasone for the prevention of morbidity in very-low-birth weight neonates. Am J Obstet Gynecol 2007;197:284.e1–284.e4.

[14] Lee BH, Stoll BJ, McDonald SA, Higgins RD. National Institute of Child Health and Human Development Neonatal Research

Network. Adverse neonatal outcomes associated with antenatal dexamethasone versus antenatal betamethasone. Pediatrics 2006;117:1503–1510.

[15] Bhandari V. Postnatal inflammation in the pathogenesis of bronchopulmonary dysplasia. Birth Defects Res A Clin Mol Teratol 2014;100:189–201.

[16] Fahey JO. Clinical management of intra-amniotic infection and chorioamnionitis: a review of the literature. J Midwifery Womens Health 2008;53:227–235.

[17] Watterberg K. Anti-inflammatory therapy in the neonatal intensive care unit: present and future. Semin Fetal Neonatal Med 2006;11:378–384.

[18] Sharek PJ, Baker R, Litman F, et al. Evaluation and development of potentially better practices to prevent chronic lung disease and reduce lung injury in neonates. Pediatrics 2003;111:e426–e431.

[19] Kattwinkel J. Textbook of neonatal resuscitation. 5th ed. Elk Grove Village, IL: American Academy of Pediatrics and the American Heart Association; 2006.

[20] Karlsen KA. The S.T.A.B.L.E. Program: pre-transport/post-resuscitation stabilization care of sick infants guidelines for neonatal healthcare providers. 5th ed. Park City, UT: S.T.A.B.L.E., Inc.; 2006.

[21] Keszler M. Golden first hour: newborn resuscitation. In: The contemporary management of neonatal pulmonary disorders conference in Tempe, AZ; 2010.

[22] Dawson JA, Kamlin CO, Vento M, Wong C, Cole TJ, Donath SM, et al. Defining the reference range for oxygen saturation for infants after birth. Pediatrics 2010;125: e1340–e1347.

[23] Cerny L, Torday JS, Rehan VK. Prevention and treatment of bronchopulmonary dysplasia: contemporary status and future outlook. Lung 2008;186:75–89.

[24] Sola A, Saldeno YP, Falvareto V. Clinical practices in neonatal oxygenation: where have we failed? What can we do? J Perinatol 2008;28:S28–S34.

[25] Ambalavanan N, Carlo WA. Ventilatory strategies in the prevention and management of bronchopulmonary dysplasia. Semin Perinatol 2006;30:192–199.

[26] Thomas W, Speer CP. Management of infants with bronchopulmonary dysplasia in Germany. Early Hum Dev 2005;81:155–163.

[27] Saugstad OD, Aune D. Optimal oxygenation of extremely low birth weight infants: a meta-analysis and systematic review of the oxygen saturation target studies. Neonatology 2014;105:55–63.

[28] Lakshminrusimha S, Manja V, Mathew B, Suresh GK. Oxygen targeting in preterm infants: a physiological interpretation. J Perinatol 2015;35: 8–15.

[29] Bizzarro MJ, Li FY, Katz K, Shabanova V, Ehrenkranz RA, Bhandari V. Temporal quantification of oxygen saturation ranges: an effort to reduce hyperoxia in the neonatal intensive care unit. J Perinatol 2014;34: 33–38.

[30] Courtney SE, Pyon KH, Saslow JG, Arnold GK, Pandit PB, Habib RH. Lung recruitment and breathing pattern during variable versus continuous flow nasal continuous positive airway pressure in premature infants: an evaluation of three devices. Pediatrics 2001;107:304–338.

[31] Pandit PB, Courtney SE, Pyon KH, Saslow JG, Habib RH. Work of breathing during constant- and variable-flow nasal continuous positive airway pressure in preterm neonates. Pediatrics 2001;108: 682–685.

[32] Aly H, Milner JD, Patel K, El-Mohandes AA. Does the experience with the use of nasal continuous positive airway pressure improve over time in extremely low birth weight infants? Pediatrics 2004;114:697–702.

[33] Greenhough A, Premkumar M, Patel D. Ventilatory strategies for the extremely premature infant. Paediatr Anaesth 2008;18:371–377.

[34] Baraldi E, Filippone M. Chronic lung disease after premature birth. N Engl J Med 2007;357:1946–1955.

[35] Ramanathan R. Optimal ventilatory strategies and surfactant to protect the preterm lungs. Neonatology 2008;93:302–308.

[36] Bhandari V. Nasal intermittent positive pressure ventilation in the newborn: review of literature and evidence-based guidelines. J Perinatol 2010;30:505–512.

[37] Meneses J, Bhandari V, Alves JG. Nasal intermittent positive-pressure ventilation vs. nasal continuous positive airway pressure for preterm infants with respiratory distress syndrome: a systematic review and meta-analysis. Arch Pediatr Adolesc Med 2012;166:372–376.

[38] Bhandari V. Noninvasive respiratory support in the preterm infant. Clin Perinatol 2012;39:497–511.

[39] Tang S, Zhao J, Shen J, Hu Z, Shi Y. Nasal intermittent positive pressure ventilation versus nasal continuous positive airway pressure in neonates: a systematic review and meta-analysis. Indian Pediatr 2013;50:371–376.

[40] Bhandari V. The potential of non-invasive ventilation to decrease BPD. Semin Perinatol 2013;37:108–114.

[41] Kirpalani H, Millar D, Lemyre B, Yoder BA, Chiu A, Roberts RS, et al. A trial comparing noninvasive ventilation strategies in preterm infants. N Engl J Med 2013;369:611–620.

[42] Claure N, Bancalari E. New modes of mechanical ventilation in the preterm newborn: evidence of benefit. Arch Dis Child Fetal Neonatal Ed 2007;92:F508–F512.

[43] Brown MK, DiBlasi RM. Mechanical ventilation of the premature neonate. Respir Care 2011;56:1298–1311.

[44] Greenough A, Rossor TE, Sundaresan A, Murthy V, Milner AD. Synchronized mechanical ventilation for respiratory support in newborn infants. Cochrane Database Syst Rev 2016;1–9:CD000456.

[45] Peng W, Zhu H, Shi H, Liu E. Volume-targeted ventilation is more suitable than pressure-limited ventilation for preterm infants: a systematic review and meta-analysis. Arch Dis Child Fetal Neonatal Ed 2014;99(2):F158–F165.

[46] Wheeler K, Klingenberg C, McCallion N, Morley CJ, Davis PG. Volume-targeted versus pressure-limited ventilation in the neonate. Cochrane Database Syst Rev 2010;11:CD003666.

[47] Greenough A, Sharma A. What is new in ventilation strategies for the neonate? Eur J Pediatr 2007;166:991–996.

[48] Gupta S, Sinha SK, Donn SM. Ventilatory management and bronchopulmonary dysplasia in preterm infants. Semin Fetal Neonatal Med 2009;14:367–373.

[49] Bhandari A, Schramm CM, Kimble C, Pappagallo M, Hussain N. Effect of a short course of prednisolone in infants with oxygen-dependent bronchopulmonary dysplasia. Pediatrics 2008;121:e344–e349.

[50] Gupta S, Sinha SK, Donn SM. The effect of two levels of pressure support ventilation on tidal volume delivery and minute ventilation in preterm infants. Arch Dis Child Fetal Neonatal Ed 2009;94:F80–F83.

[51] Engle WA. American Academy of Pediatrics Committee on Fetus and Newborn. Surfactant replacement therapy for respiratory distress in the preterm and term neonate. Pediatrics 2008;121:419–432.

[52] Donn SM. Lucinactant: a novel synthetic surfactant for the treatment of respiratory distress syndrome. Expert Opin Investig Drugs 2005;14:329–334.

[53] Sinha SK, Lacaze-Masmonteil T, Valls i Soler A, Wiswell TE, Gadzinowski J, Hajdu J, et al. A multicenter, randomized, controlled trial of lucinactant versus poractant alfa among very premature infants at high risk for respiratory distress syndrome. Pediatrics 2005;115:1030–1038.

[54] Moya FR, Gadzinowski J, Bancalari E, Salinas V, Kopelman B, Bancalari A, et al. A multicenter, randomized, masked, comparison trial of lucinactant, colfosceril palmitate, and beractant for the prevention of respiratory distress syndrome among very preterm infants. Pediatrics 2005;115:1018–1029.

[55] Pfister RH, Soll RF, Wiswell T. Protein containing synthetic surfactant versus animal derived surfactant extract for the prevention and treatment of respiratory distress syndrome.

Cochrane Database Syst Rev 2007;17:CD006069.

[56] Donn SM, Sinha SK. Aerosolized lucinactant: a potential alternative to intratracheal surfactant replacement therapy. Expert Opin Pharmacother 2008;9:475–478.

[57] Bhandari V. Making babies breathe better: hopeful signals? Pediatr Res 2008;64:123–124.

[58] Woolridge N. Pulmonary diseases. In: Samour PQ, editor. Handbook of pediatric nutrition. New York, NY: Jones & Bartlett Publishers; 2005. p. 307–349.

[59] Oh W, Poindexter BB, Perritt R, Lemons JA, Bauer CR, Ehrenkranz RA, et al. Association between fluid intake and weight loss during the first ten days of life and risk of bronchopulmonary dysplasia in extremely low birth weight infants. J Pediatr 2005;147:786–790.

[60] Kennedy KA, Stoll BJ, Ehrenkranz RA, Oh W, Wright LL, Stevenson DK, et al. Vitamin A to prevent bronchopulmonary dysplasia in very-low-birth-weight infants: has the dose been too low? The NICHD Neonatal Research Network. Early Hum Dev 1997;49:19–31.

[61] Darlow BA, Graham PJ. Vitamin A supplementation to prevent mortality and short- and long-term morbidity in very low birth weight infants. Cochrane Database Syst Rev 2011;5:CD000501.

[62] Martin CR, Zaman MM, Gilkey C, Salguero MV, Hasturk H, Kantarci A, et al. Resolvin D1 and lipoxin A4 improve alveolarization and normalize septal wall thickness in a neonatal murine model of hyperoxia-induced lung injury. PLoS One 2014;9:e98773.

[63] Heuchan AM, Clyman RI. Managing the patent ductus arteriosus: current treatment options. Arch Dis Child Fetal Neonatal Ed 2014;99:F431–F436.

[64] McNamara PJ, Sehgal A. Towards rational management of the patent ductus arteriosus: the need for disease staging. Arch Dis Child Fetal Neonatal Ed 2007;92:F424–F427.

[65] Mestan KK, Marks JD, Hecox K, Huo D, Schreiber MD. Neurodevelopmental outcomes of premature infants treated with inhaled nitric oxide. N Engl J Med 2005;353:23–32.

[66] Schreiber MD, Gin-Mestan K, Marks JD, Huo D, Lee G, Srisuparp P. Inhaled nitric oxide in premature infants with the respiratory distress syndrome. N Engl J Med 2003;349:2099–2107.

[67] Field D, Elbourne D, Truesdale A, Grieve R, Hardy P, Fenton AC, et al. Neonatal ventilation with inhaled nitric oxide versus ventilatory support without inhaled nitric oxide for preterm infants with severe respiratory failure: the INNOVO multicentre randomised controlled trial (ISRCTN 17821339). Pediatrics 2005;115:926–936.

[68] Hascoet JM, Fresson J, Claris O, Harmon I, Lombet J, Liska A, et al. The safety and efficacy of nitric oxide therapy in premature infants. J Pediatr 2005;146:318–323.

[69] Barrington KJ, Finer NN. Inhaled nitric oxide for preterm infants: a systematic review. Pediatrics 2007;120:1088–1099. [published correction appears in Pediatrics. 2008;121:451].

[70] Ballard PL, Truog WE, Merrill JD, Gow A, Posencheg M, Golombek SG, et al. Plasma biomarkers of oxidative stress: relationship to lung disease and inhaled nitric oxide therapy in premature infants. Pediatrics 2008;121:555–561.

[71] Ballard PL, Merrill JD, Truog WE, Godinez RI, Godinez MH, McDevitt TM, et al. Surfactant function and composition in premature infants treated with inhaled nitric oxide. Pediatrics 2007;120:346–353.

[72] Di Fiore JM, Hibbs AM, Zadell AE, Merrill JD, Eichenwald EC, Puri AR, et al. The effect of inhaled nitric oxide on pulmonary function in preterm infants. J Perinatol 2007;27:766–771.

[73] Dani C, Bertini G. Inhaled nitric oxide for the treatment of preterm infants with respiratory distress syndrome. Neonatology 2008;94:87–95.

[74] Schmidt B, Roberts RS, Davis P, Doyle LW, Barrington KJ, Ohlsson A, et al. Caffeine therapy for apnea of prematurity. N Engl J Med 2006;354:2112–2121.

[75] Tin W, Wiswell TE. Adjunctive therapies in chronic lung disease: examining the evidence. Semin Fetal Neonatal Med 2008;13:44–52.

[76] Schmidt B, Roberts RS, Davis P, Doyle LW, Barrington KJ, Ohlsson A, et al. Long-term effects of caffeine therapy for apnea of prematurity. N Engl J Med 2007;357:1893–1902.

[77] Schmidt B, Anderson PJ, Doyle LW, Dewey D, Grunau RE, Asztalos EV, et al. Survival without disability to age 5 years after neonatal caffeine therapy for apnea of prematurity. JAMA 2012;307:275–282.

[78] Davis PG, Schmidt B, Roberts RS, Doyle LW, Asztalos E, Haslam R, et al. Caffeine for apnea of prematurity trial: benefits may vary in subgroups. J Pediatr 2010;156:382–387.

[79] McCann EM, Lewis K, Deming DD, Donovan MJ, Brady JP. Controlled trial of furosemide therapy in infants with chronic lung disease. J Pediatr 1985;106:957–962.

[80] Kao LC, Durand DJ, McCrea RC, Birch M, Powers RJ, Nickerson BG. Randomized trial of long-term diuretic therapy for infants with oxygen-dependent bronchopulmonary dysplasia. J Pediatr 1994;124:772–781.

[81] Reiter PD, Makhlouf R, Stiles AD. Comparison of 6-hour infusion versus bolus furosemide in premature infants. Pharmacotherapy 1998;18:63–68.

[82] Rush MG, Engelhardt B, Parker RA, Hazinski TA. Double-blind, placebo-controlled trial of alternate-day furosemide therapy in infants with chronic bronchopulmonary dysplasia. J Pediatr 1990;117:112–118.

[83] Brion LP, Primhak RA, Yong W. Aerosolized diuretics for preterm infants with (or developing) chronic lung disease. Cochrane Database Syst Rev 2006;19:CD001694.

[84] Brion LP, Primhak RA, Ambrosio-Perez I. Diuretics acting on the distal renal tubule for preterm Infants with (or developing) chronic lung disease. Cochrane Database Syst Rev 2002;CD001817.

[85] Engelhardt B, Blalock WA, DonLevy S, Rush M, Hazinski TA. Effect of spironolactone-hydrochlorothiazide on lung function in infants with chronic bronchopulmonary dysplasia. J Pediatr 1989;114:619–624.

[86] Hoffman DJ, Gerdes JS, Abbasi S. Pulmonary function and electrolyte balance following spironolactone treatment in preterm infants with chronic lung disease: a double-blind, placebo-controlled, randomized trial. J Perinatol 2000;20:41–45.

[87] Jefferies AL. Postnatal corticosteroids to treat or prevent chronic lung disease in preterm infants. Paediatr Child Health 2012;17:573–574.

[88] Doyle LW, Ehrenkranz RA, Halliday HL. Postnatal hydrocortisone for preventing or treating bronchopulmonary dysplasia in preterm infants: a systematic review. Neonatology 2010;98:111–117.

[89] Watterberg KL, Gerdes JS, Cole CH, Aucott SW, Thilo EH, Mammel MC, et al. Prophylaxis of early adrenal insufficiency to prevent bronchopulmonary dysplasia: a multicenter trial. Pediatrics 2004;114:1649–1657.

[90] Peltoniemi O, Kari MA, Heinonen K, Saareia T, Nikolajev K, Andersson S, et al. Pretreatment cortisol values may predict responses to hydrocortisone administration for the prevention of bronchopulmonary dysplasia in high-risk infants. J Pediatr 2005;146: 632–637.

[91] van der Heide-Jalving M, Kamphuis PJ, van der Lann MJ, Bakker JM, Wiegant VM, Heijen CJ, et al. Short- and long-term effects of neonatal glucocorticoid therapy: is hydrocortisone an alternative to dexamethasone? Acta Paediatr 2003;92:827–835.

[92] Lodygensky GA, Rademaker K, Zimine A, Gex-Fabry M, Lieftink AF, Lazeyras F, et al. Structural and functional brain development after hydrocortisone treatment for neonatal chronic lung disease. Pediatrics 2005;116:1–7.

[93] Shah V, Ohlsson A, Halliday HL, Dunn MS. Early administration of inhaled corticosteroids for preventing chronic lung disease in ventilated very low birth weight neonates. Cochrane Database Syst Rev 2000;2:CD001969.

[94] Shah SS, Ohlsson A, Halliday H, Shah VS. Inhaled versus systemic corticosteroids for the treatment of chronic lung disease in ventilated very low birth weight preterm infants. Cochrane Database Syst Rev 2007;17:CD002057.

[95] Dimitriou G, Greenough A, Giffin FJ, Kavadis V. Inhaled versus systemic steroids in chronic oxygen dependency of preterm infants. Eur J Pediatr 1997;156:51–55.

[96] Nicholl RM, Greenough A, King M, Cheeseman P, Gamsu HR. Growth effects of systemic versus inhaled steroids in chronic lung disease. Arch Dis Child Fetal Neonatal Ed 2002;87:F59–F61.

[97] LaForce WR, Brudno DS. Controlled trial of beclomethasone dipropionate by nebulization in oxygen- and ventilator-dependent infants. J Pediatr 1993;122:285–288.

[98] Groneck P, Goetze-Speer B, Speer CP. Effects of inhaled beclomethasone compared to systemic dexamethasone on lung inflammation in preterm infants at risk of chronic lung disease. Pediatr Pulmonol 1999;27:383–387.

[99] Gupta GK, Cole CH, Abbasi S, Demissie S, Njinmbaum C, Nielsen HC, et al. Effects of early inhaled beclomethasone therapy on tracheal aspirate inflammatory mediators IL-8 and IL-1ra in ventilated preterm infants at risk for bronchopulmonary dysplasia. Pediatr Pulmonol 2000;30:275–281.

[100] Bhandari A, McGrath-Morrow S. Long-term pulmonary outcomes of patients with bronchopulmonary dysplasia. Semin Perinatol 2013;37:132–137.

[101] Berkelhamer SK, Mestan KK, Steinhorn RH. Pulmonary hypertension in bronchopulmonary dysplasia. Semin Perinatol 2013;37:124–131.

[102] Tan K, Krishnamurthy MB, O'Heney JL, Paul E, Sehgal A. Sildenafil therapy in bronchopulmonary dysplasia-associated pulmonary hypertension: a retrospective study of efficacy and safety. Eur J Pediatr 2015;174:1109–1115.

[103] Trottier-Boucher MN, Lapointe A, Malo J, Fournier A, Raboisson MJ, Martin B, et al. Sildenafil for the treatment of pulmonary arterial hypertension in infants with bronchopulmonary dysplasia. Pediatr Cardiol 2015;36:1255–1260.

[104] Bhandari A, Bhandari V. Bronchopulmonary dysplasia: an update. Indian J Pediatr 2007;74:73–77.

[105] Allen J, Zwerdling R, Ehrenkranz R, Gaultier C, Geggel R, Greenough A, et al. Statement on the care of the child with chronic lung disease of infancy and childhood. Am J Respir Crit Care Med 2003;168:356–396.

[106] Gaugler C, Astruc D, Donato L, Rivera S, Langlet C, Messer J. Neonatal necrotizing tracheobronchitis: three case reports. J Perinatol 2004;24:259–260.

[107] Bua J, Trappan A, Demarini S, Grasso D, Schleef J, Zennaro F. Neonatal necrotizing tracheobronchitis. J Pediatr 2011;159. 699–699.e1.

[108] Hasegawa H, Nagase Y, Sakai M, Henmi N, Tsuruta S. Tracheoplasty using the thymus against tracheo-esophageal fistula due to necrotizing tracheobronchitis in a very low birth weight infant. Pediatr Pulmonol 2014;49:E135–E139.

[109] Levit OL, Shabanova V, Bazzy-Asaad A, Bizzarro MJ, Bhandari V. Risk factors for tracheostomy requirement in extremely low birth weight infants. J Matern Fetal Neonatal Med 2018;31:447–452.

[110] Smith VC, Zupancic JA, McCormick MC, Croen LA, Green J, Escobar GJ, et al. Rehospitalization in the first year of life among infants with bronchopulmonary dysplasia. J Pediatr 2004;144:799–803.

[111] Jeng SF, Hsu CH, Tsao PN, Chou HC, Lee WT, Kao HA, et al. Bronchopulmonary dysplasia predicts adverse developmental and clinical outcomes in very-low-birthweight infants. Dev Med Child Neurol 2008;50:51–57.

[112] Vrijlandt EJ, Boezen HM, Gerritsen J, Stremmelaar EF, Duiverman EJ. Respiratory health in prematurely born preschool children with and without bronchopulmonary dysplasia. J Pediatr 2007;150:256–261.

[113] Halvorsen T, Skadberg BT, Eide GE, Roksund OD, Carlsen KH, Bakke P. Pulmonary outcome in adolescents of extreme preterm birth: a regional cohort study. Acta Paediatr 2004;93:1294–1300.

[114] Vrijlandt EJ, Gerritsen J, Boezen HM, Duiverman EJ. Dutch POPS-19 Collaborative Study Group. Gender differences in respiratory symptoms in 19-year-old adults born preterm. Respir Res 2005;6:117.

[115] Fawke J, Lum S, Kirkby J, Hennessy E, Marlow N, Rowell V, et al. Lung function and respiratory symptoms at 11 years in children born extremely preterm: the EPICure study. Am J Respir Crit Care Med 2010;182:237–245.

[116] Northway WH Jr, Moss RB, Carlisle KB, Parker BR, Popp RL, Pitlick PT, et al. Late pulmonary sequelae of bronchopulmonary dysplasia. N Engl J Med 1990;323:1793–1799.

[117] Oppenheim C, Mamou-Mani T, Sayegh N, de Blic J, Scheinmann P, Lallemand D. Bronchopulmonary dysplasia: value of CT in identifying pulmonary sequelae. AJR 1994;163:169–172.

[118] Mahut B, De Blic J, Emond S, Benoist MR, Jarreau PH, Lazaze-Masmonteil T, et al. Chest computed tomography findings in bronchopulmonary dysplasia and correlation with lung function. Arch Dis Child Fetal Neonatal Ed 2007;92: F459–F464.

[119] Simpson SJ, Logie KM, O'Dea CA, Banton GL, Murray C, Wilson AC,

489

et al. Altered lung structure and function in mid-childhood survivors of very preterm birth. Thorax 2017;72:702–711.

[120] Ochiai M, Hikino S, Yabuuchi H, Nakayama H, Sato K, Ohga S, et al. A new scoring system for computed tomography of the chest for assessing the clinical status of bronchopulmonary dysplasia. J Pediatr 2008;152:90–95.

[121] Doyle LW. Victorian Infant Collaborative Study Group. Respiratory function at age 8–9 years in extremely low birthweight/very preterm children born in Victoria in 1991–1992. Pediatr Pulmonol 2006;41:570–576.

[122] Doyle LW, Faber B, Callanan C, Freezer N, Ford GW, Davis NM. Bronchopulmonary dysplasia in very low birth weight subjects and lung function in late adolescence. Pediatrics 2006;118:108–113.

[123] Kennedy JD, Edward LJ, Bates DJ, Martin AG, Dip SN, Haslam RR, et al. Effects of birthweight and oxygen supplementation on lung function in late childhood in children of very low birth weight. Pediatr Pulmonol 2000;30:32–40.

[124] Kotecha SJ, Edwards MO, Watkins WJ, Henderson AJ, Paranjothy S, Dunstan FD, et al. Effect of preterm birth on later FEV1: a systematic review and meta-analysis. Thorax 2013;68:760–776.

[125] Gibson AM, Reddington C, McBride L, Callanan C, Robertson C, Doyle LW. Lung function in adult survivors of very low birth weight, with and without bronchopulmonary dysplasia. Pediatr Pulmonol 2015;50:987–994.

[126] Martinez FD. Early-life origins of chronic obstructive pulmonary disease. N Engl J Med 2016;375:871–878.

[127] Bhandari A, Panitch HB. Pulmonary outcomes in bronchopulmonary dysplasia. Semin Perinatol 2006;30:219–226.

[128] Vrijlandt EJ, Gerritsen J, Boezen HM, Grevink RG, Duiverman EJ. Lung function and exercise capacity in young adults born prematurely. Am J Respir Crit Care Med 2006;173:890–896.

[129] Smith LJ, van Asperen PP, McKay KO, Selvadurai H, Fitzgerald DA. Reduced exercise capacity in children born very preterm. Pediatrics 2008;122:e287–e293.

[130] Cutz E, Chiasson D. Chronic lung disease after premature birth. N Engl J Med 2008;358:743–745.

[131] Wong PM, Lees AN, Louw J, Lee FY, French N, Gain K, et al. Emphysema in young adult survivors of moderate-to-severe bronchopulmonary dysplasia. Eur Respir J 2008;32:321–328.

[132] Anderson PJ, Doyle LW. Neurodevelopmental outcome of bronchopulmonary dysplasia. Semin Perinatol 2006;30:227–232.

[133] Short EJ, Klein NK, Lewis BA, Fulton S, Eisengart S, Kercsmar C, et al. Cognitive and academic consequences of bronchopulmonary dysplasia and very low birth weight: 8-year-old outcomes. Pediatrics 2003;112:e359.

[134] Lewis BA, Singer LT, Fulton S, Salvator A, Short EJ, Klein N, et al. Speech and language outcomes of children with bronchopulmonary dysplasia. J Commun Disord 2002;35:393–406.

[135] Short EJ, Kirchner HL, Asaad GR, Fulton SE, Lewis BA, Klein N, et al. Developmental sequelae in preterm infants having a diagnosis of bronchopulmonary dysplasia: analysis using a severity-based classification system. Arch Pediatr Adolesc Med 2007;161:1082–1087.

[136] Greenough A, Hird MF, Gamsu HR. Home oxygen therapy following neonatal intensive care. Early Hum Dev 1991;26:29–35.

[137] Hudak BB, Allen MC, Hudak ML, Loughlin GM. Home oxygen therapy for chronic lung disease in extremely low-birth-weight infants. Am J Dis Child 1989;143:357–360.

[138] Austrian Technical Advisory Group on Immunisation (ATAGI) of the Commonwealth Department of Health and Aged Care. The Australian immunisation handbook. 7th ed. Canberra: National Health and Medical Research Council (NHMRC); 2000. https://vaccinateyourchildren.files.wordpress.com.

[139] Groothuis JR, Rosenberg AA. Home oxygen promotes weight gain in infants with bronchopulmonary dysplasia. Am J Dis Child 1987;141:992–995.

[140] Supplemental Therapeutic Oxygen for Prethreshold Retinopathy of Prematurity (STOP-ROP), a randomized, controlled trial, 1: primary outcomes. Pediatrics 2000;105:295–310.

[141] Askie LM, Henderson-Smart DJ, Irwig L, Simpson JM. Oxygen-saturation targets and outcomes in extremely preterm infants. N Engl J Med 2003;349:959–967.

[142] RPA Centre for Newborn Care Sydney. Guidelines, http://www.slhd.nsw.gov.au/rpa/neonatal/guidlines.html

Chapter 28

Congenital Diaphragmatic Hernia

Jayasree Nair, MD, Satyan Lakshminrusimha, MD

CHAPTER POINTS

- Pulmonary hypoplasia and pulmonary hypertension in varying degrees are usually seen in infants with CDH.
- Initial high PVR at birth subsides in the "honeymoon period" followed by worsening with pulmonary venous and arterial hypertension and cardiac dysfunction.
- Immediate intubation with "gentle ventilation," reduced oxygen exposure and judicious use of pulmonary vasodilators and vasopressors are the cornerstones in management of CDH
- As surgery tends to worsen PH, it is prudent to wait for relative stability with improving pulmonary and systemic hemodynamics prior to repairing the defect.
- Consider ECMO as a treatment option if there is failure to respond to optimal medical therapy with pulmonary vasodilators and vasopressors

Congenital diaphragmatic hernia (CDH) is an uncommon birth defect that occurs due to migration of intraabdominal contents to the chest through a defect in the diaphragm. Due to improving antenatal care, approximately two-thirds of these defects are recognized by antenatal imaging and referred to tertiary centers for delivery. The overall survival continues to be low at approximately 70% with long-term respiratory and nutritional morbidity such as pulmonary hypertension (PH) and gastroesophageal reflux (GER).

Demographics: The incidence of CDH varies in reports from 1.93 to 3.5/10,000 live births [1–3]. Although uncommon, it accounts for 8% of all major birth defects [4]. Male predominance and effects of ethnicity, higher maternal age, smoking, and alcohol use during pregnancy have also been observed [2]. About 40%–60% of CDH are associated with other abnormalities [5–7]. These include genetic syndromes as well as other nonsyndromic cardiac and noncardiac anomalies. Assessment of the extent of associated anomalies helps in planning postnatal management and prognostication as they may be associated with higher mortality rates [8].

Survival rates: Survival from CDH has improved to over 60%–80% depending on the level of care, availability of extracorporeal membrane oxygenation (ECMO), and the presence of associated anomalies, especially cardiac and genetic defects [9,10]. Population-based studies reporting regional outcomes without being confined to tertiary care centers, however, still report an overall survival close to 70% [11]. This may not include the "hidden mortality" from pregnancies that are terminated. A single-center review of fetal outcomes of prenatally diagnosed CDH before 24 weeks of gestation revealed that >70% of CDH associated with other anomalies underwent termination of pregnancy [12].

Pathophysiology

Depending on the location of the diaphragmatic defect, CDH is classified into *Bochdalek hernia* (posterolateral), Morgagni (anterolateral), or central. An anterior hernia can be associated with Pentalogy of Cantrell.

491

Bochdalek hernia accounts for ~70% of all CDH and has been extensively studied in animal models [13].

Morgagni hernias are anterior, retrosternal, or parasternal in location and are seen in less than 20%–25% of CDH. In these defects, abdominal viscera herniate through small foramen of Morgagni, which have been described as weak areas from an embryological perspective [14] adjacent to the lower end of the sternum. Infants with trisomy 21 have a higher likelihood of having a *Morgagni hernia* [15]. Another extremely rare type of CDH involves a *central tendon defect*, and accounts for <2% of CDH [16]. The extent of the defect varies from a small defect of the posterior rim to diaphragmatic agenesis. The size of the defect influences management especially the surgical technique that will be discussed in detail later in this chapter. Complete agenesis usually requires a patch to repair the defect [8].

Most CDH are unilateral with a left-sided preponderance (85%) [17]. Bilateral defects are very rare and usually fatal. Right-sided defects are associated with a poorer prognosis, usually related to migration of the liver into the thorax and complexities of repair.

Effects on lung and heart

Pulmonary hypoplasia, in varying degrees is a pathognomonic feature of CDH (Fig. 28.1). Bilateral pulmonary hypoplasia is seen in CDH with the lung on the ipsilateral side affected more severely than the contralateral side. Initially, hypoplasia was thought to be a response to the migration of intraabdominal contents into the thorax through the diaphragmatic defect leaving the left lung with very little space to grow. More recently, it is recognized that lung growth is also affected at the same time in embryogenesis, leading to pulmonary hypoplasia. A "dual hit" hypothesis in which abnormal development is followed by compression causing lung hypoplasia is widely accepted [18]. This would also explain why both lungs are hypoplastic in CDH. Other disruptions in lung structure and function that are also seen in association with CDH include hypoplasia and immaturity of the acinus [19] and surfactant abnormalities.

Pulmonary hypertension, often severe and resistant to conventional therapy, is almost always seen in infants with CDH. The lung vasculature undergoes significant remodeling with hypertrophy of the pulmonary arteries and reduced size of the pulmonary vascular bed, contributing to the "fixed" or irreversible component of PH. Altered vasoreactivity and "hyperresponsiveness" of the pulmonary arteries observed in this condition is thought to be mediated by endothelin-1 (ET-1) [20] and constitutes the "reversible" component of PH in CDH. Nitric oxide (NO) plays a role in influencing ET-1 action through the enzyme endothelial nitric oxide synthase (eNOS) in animal models as well as human studies [21].

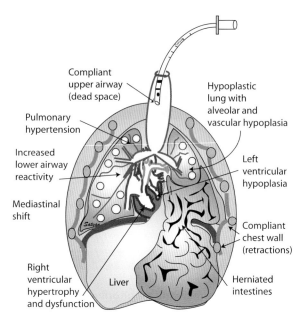

Fig. 28.1 Lung and Heart in CDH. Bilateral lung hypoplasia due to altered lung development and compression from the herniated contents is commonly seen in CDH. Pulmonary hypertension, with fixed and reversible components, is characteristic of CDH and is often resistant to conventional therapy. This contributes to RV dysfunction. Additionally, LV hypoplasia and dysfunction may be seen, which could influence management plans. Copyright: Satyan Lakshminrusimha.

Left ventricular (LV) structure and function: Reduced size and flow through the left heart are commonly seen in fetuses with CDH [22]. LV end-diastolic diameter in CDH fetuses was found to be 32% smaller than in controls (Fig. 28.1) [23]. Severity of LV hypoplasia may be correlated with severity and size of left-sided CDH [24]. Persistent PH of the newborn (PPHN) and pulmonary arterial hypertension observed in CDH is associated with impairment of right ventricular (RV) function. Pulmonary hypertension may be worsened by the presence of significant LV dysfunction. Diagnosis of this condition is important for prognosis as well as treatment options as inhaled NO may worsen postcapillary or pulmonary venous hypertension in infants with LV dysfunction [25].

Genetic basis

CDH may be seen as an isolated anomaly or as part of an identified genetic syndrome with other associated abnormalities. However in the majority of CDH (~80%), no definite causative factors are identified, suggesting that these infants may have a multifactorial or nongenetic etiology [26].

Chromosomal aneuploidies, copy number variants and cytogenetic rearrangements involving many chromosomes are identified in 10%–35% of all infants with CDH [26]. Infants with Trisomy 13 constitute 2%–5% of CDH cases while infants with trisomy 21 tend to have a higher incidence of *Morgagni hernia*.

Several syndromes are associated with CDH. These include Cornelia de Lange, Marfan's syndrome, Cutis laxa, Matthew-Wood, Pentalogy of Cantrell, Apert, Beckwith-Wiedemann, CHARGE, and Fryns syndromes.

Identification of a genetic cause may influence prognosis in an infant. Karyotype could identify chromosomal abnormalities; more recently whole exon sequencing (WES) of patient as well as parents is being evaluated. Genetic counseling and follow-up is essential for identifying risk in future pregnancies in the family.

Antenatal diagnosis and monitoring

In the last few decades, with improved antenatal surveillance, 50%–68% CDH are diagnosed on antenatal ultrasounds, especially those with associated anomalies [27,28]. However, some cases are diagnosed postnatally, either due to inadequate antenatal surveillance/limited ultrasound imaging or due to a "late" presentation of a CDH.

Antenatal prediction of outcome

Early detection during the antenatal period facilitates delivery at a tertiary center with pediatric surgical as well as neonatal intensive care expertise that can efficiently manage infants with this challenging condition. Identification of reliable prenatal prognostic factors is important for counseling the parents regarding possible outcomes and available treatments, including fetal therapies. Ultrasound is the commonest modality of diagnosis. Further investigational modalities include fetal echocardiography and fetal MRI that help in identification and quantification of individual prognostic markers as shown in Table 28.1. In the last decade, fetal MRI is being increasingly utilized to estimate liver position as well as total and relative lung volume. Commonly used antenatal prognostic factors are listed in Table 28.1 and have been studied more extensively with left-sided CDH (Fig. 28.2).

Lung-to-head ratio (LHR) (Fig. 28.3) was initially proposed in 1996, when Metkus et al. noted that survival rate was 100% for those infants with CDH whose right lung-to-head circumference ratio (LHR) was greater than 1.35 [31]. However, as lung and head grow with gestation, utility of this absolute ratio as proposed is limited by varying measurements at each gestational age. This drawback led to the modified ratio called *observed to expected lung-to-head ratio (O/E LHR)*, with several formulas proposed for calculation [32]. O/E LHR normalizes LHR to expected lung volumes

Table 28.1 Antenatal and postnatal factors associated with poor prognosis in CDH (Fig. 28.2)

Antenatal	Postnatal
Bilateral, right	Severity of pulmonary hypertension
Large size	Presence of LV dysfunction
Lower gestational age at diagnosis	Initial arterial blood gases with low PaO_2 and high $PaCO_2$
LHR, O/E LHR	Patch repair (size of the defect at surgery)
Liver in chest	Higher scores (scoring systems)*
Stomach position grades 3 and 4	
Associated anomalies esp. cardiac	
Low lung volume by fetal MRI	

*Multiple scoring systems have been described, most recently one by the Japanese CDH study group [29] based on APGAR score at 1 min and best OI ≥8. Based on these criteria, patients were classified into three risk categories. The 90-day survival rates in categories 1–3 were 10, 88, and 52%, respectively ($P < 0.001$). Another scoring system used very low birth weight, absent or low 5-min Apgar score, presence of chromosomal or major cardiac anomaly, and suprasystemic pulmonary hypertension as components to discriminate between a population at high risk of death (~50%) intermediate risk (~20%), or low risk (<10%) [30].

at that gestational age and values less than 25% have a poor predicted survival, while those more than 45% have a more than 75% survival [33].

Liver position

Another important factor in prognostication is the position of the liver. The presence of the *liver in the chest cavity* (liver-up) confers a poor prognosis with increased need for ECMO and decreased survival rates [35,36]. More recently, quantifying the amount of liver herniating into the chest is found to be superior to simply classifying it as liver-up or liver-down in predicting morbidity and mortality [37].

The *position of the stomach* in relation to thoracic structures has also been evaluated. A grading scale of 0–3 with multiple levels of progressively aberrant fetal stomach position was proposed by Kitano et al. who concluded that right thoracic stomach herniation was associated with a poor prognosis. In addition, a combination of these prognostic markers holds greater significance than a single marker alone. In infants with intrathoracic liver herniation, LHR

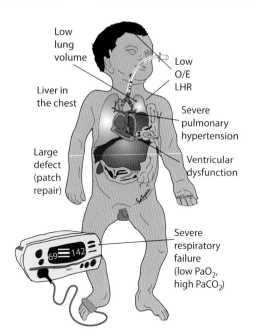

Fig. 28.2 Prognostic Factors in Left-Sided CDH. Extent of pulmonary hypoplasia, low LHR, the presence of liver in chest, and size of defect are some important prenatal predictors. Severe pulmonary hypertension, respiratory failure, and the presence of LV dysfunction are poor prognostic factors noted postnatally. Copyright: Satyan Lakshminrusimha.

at 22–28 weeks predicted postnatal survival better than in infants with no liver herniation [38].

MRI measurements of *total lung volume* and *observed-to-expected total fetal lung volume* (o/e TFLV) are reliable prognostic indicators of mortality and need for ECMO [39]. Improved MRI techniques have allowed increased accuracy in quantifying ipsilateral as well as contralateral lung volumes. MRI calculation of lung volumes also has the advantage of decreased interobserver variability and therefore greater accuracy [40]. In a meta-analysis, a threshold of o/e TFLV <25% predicted neonatal mortality [41]. Polyhydramnios is seen in many infants with CDH and a recent abstract suggested increased risk for intra uterine fetal demise and increased duration of hospital stay in CDH infants with antenatal polyhydramnios [42].

Predicting severity of PH in CDH

Besides predicting overall outcomes in CDH, these abovementioned prognostic markers have been useful in predicting pulmonary morbidities specifically fetal lung volumes and liver herniation. A recent study of ultrasound markers in CDH associated an LHR <1, thoracic liver, and aberrant stomach position with delayed time to

resolution of PPHN in infants with CDH [43]. Evaluation of fetal pulmonary vasculature by power Doppler imaging in infants with CDH has shown that infants with fewer than three pulmonary artery divisions had an increased risk of death than those with more pulmonary artery divisions [44]. The modified McGoon index (MGI)—calculated by the ratio of the diameters of pulmonary arteries and the descending aorta—is another echocardiographic measure of pulmonary vasculature that has been used in predicting neonatal outcomes and severity of PPHN. A value of 1.25 has been used as a cutoff to predict mortality in CDH [45]. Assessment of pulmonary vascular reactivity to oxygen using fractional moving blood volume has been evaluated in fetuses with normal lung development and pulmonary hypoplasia in CDH [46]. However, prenatal prediction of severity of PH is still not very well established.

Monitoring. Due to a risk of intrauterine demise (2%–8%) in infants with CDH [47], close monitoring is required with frequent visits to check fetal well-being. The risk of demise is higher if additional anomalies are detected.

Timing and mode of delivery. The CDH Study Group database retrospectively analyzed mode of delivery in 3906 infants with prenatally diagnosed CDH. They noted no differences in patient characteristics, requirement for ECMO, length of hospital stay or intubation, requirement for O_2 at 30 days or overall survival in the different groups of vaginal (induced or spontaneous) and cesarean sections (emergent or scheduled) [48]. However, outcomes were strongly associated with the GA at birth with lower GA having worse outcomes. Similar results were seen previously by Hutcheon et al. who noted decreased neonatal and infant mortality with advancing gestation, from 25 and 36% at 37 weeks of gestation, respectively, to 17 and 20% at 40 weeks of gestation [49]. Appropriate timing for delivery should be decided on a case-by-case basis, with an attempt to continue pregnancy until 38–39 weeks while ensuring fetal well-being.

Fetal surgery. Prenatal intervention in CDH has been attempted to improve pulmonary outcomes. Initial studies in fetal lambs prompted open repair in fetuses; however, these trials observed poorer outcomes and higher risk of prematurity in the infants who underwent fetal surgery. Further studies in the lamb CDH model demonstrated that tracheal occlusion led to improved lung growth as there was no egress of lung fluid. Initial attempts at tracheal occlusion used devices and sutures that had the potential for tracheal damage. In addition, higher risk of prematurity remained as the pregnant women underwent multiple surgeries, initially to place the occluder devices and later an EXIT procedure when they went into labor.

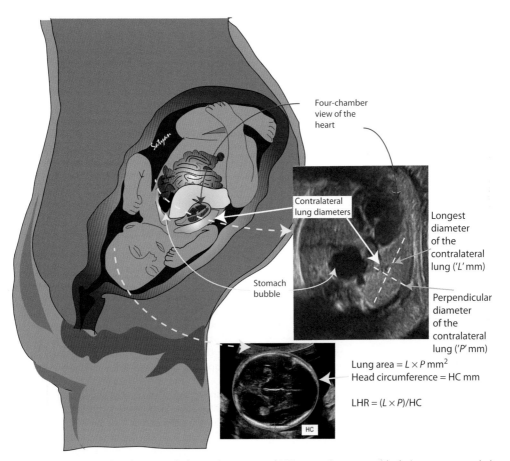

Fig. 28.3 Lung-to-Heart Ratio (LHR). LHR and observed-to-expected LHR are an important calculation on antenatal ultrasounds that helps in prognostication. Measurement of LHR is depicted in this figure. Adapted from Chandrasekharan PK, Rawat M, Madappa R, Rothstein DH, Lakshminrusimha S. Congenital Diaphragmatic hernia—a review. *Matern Health Neonatol Perinatol* 2017;3:6 [34]. Copyright: Satyan Lakshminrusimha.

More recently, the FETENDO and FETO trials have utilized fetal endoscopic tracheal occlusion, now being used as a percutaneous procedure under local anesthesia with minimum morbidity to the pregnant mother. Tracheal occlusion has been shown to reduce the number of type II pneumocytes and hence affect surfactant production. The use of tracheal balloons endoscopically to plug the trachea at about 27–30 weeks, followed by unplugging them endoscopically at around 34 weeks allows some surfactant generation prior to spontaneous onset of labor. In addition, prenatal steroids have also been used in conjunction with tracheal occlusion to accelerate fetal lung maturity. While the initial trials of tracheal occlusion did not show improved mortality and morbidity, more promising numbers with better and less invasive techniques are being reported by centers in Europe. Compared to expectant management, FETO increased survival in severe (O/E LHR <25%) CDH from

24% to 49% with left-sided lesions and from 0% to 35% in right-sided CDH [50].

In addition to the usual risks of fetal surgery such as premature rupture of membranes, bleeding, abruption, and preterm labor, infants undergoing tracheal occlusion also were noted to have local effects of tracheal occlusion including vocal cord paresis. In addition, almost all the infants undergoing tracheal occlusion are postnatally noted to have tracheomegaly, which does not seem to cause any significant long-term problems and improves over time [51].

Currently, there are two randomized clinical trials enrolling moderate and severe cases in multiple centers in Europe, Australia and North America (TOTAL trial and FETO trials with multiple NCT numbers). Although there is evidence of improving outcomes in severe cases, fetal tracheal occlusion therapy is currently not recommended outside a clinical trial [52].

Summary for antenatal management once a CDH is diagnosed

- Referral to a tertiary care center used to managing infants with this condition with facilities for pediatric surgery, high-frequency ventilation (HFV), pulmonary vasodilator therapy, and ECMO.
- Antenatal ultrasounds to assess severity of CDH based on O/E LHR, liver and stomach position, side of CDH, and so on. MRI, if available, may be of benefit to determine fetal lung volume.
- Diagnosis and evaluation for other associated anomalies, including cardiac anomalies with fetal echocardiograms.
- Genetic analysis/counseling.
- Antenatal steroids for fetuses with CDH at risk of delivery <34 weeks.
- Delivery once fetus is 38–39 weeks with appropriate mode of delivery depending on individual characteristics with cesarean sections reserved for standard obstetric indications.

Postnatal presentation of CDH

With improved antenatal screening, most CDH are usually born through a planned delivery under controlled situations. However, previously undiagnosed CDH may present with respiratory distress at or soon after birth. Milder cases may present later as infants with respiratory or gastrointestinal symptoms prompting a radiological evaluation. Very small defects may present later in life with respiratory issues.

Classical signs associated with CDH at birth are respiratory distress with difficulty in ventilation and signs of PPHN–cyanosis, labile oxygenation due to intracardiac shunting, and systemic hypotension. On examination, a scaphoid abdomen with bowel sounds auscultated in the chest and heart sounds displaced to the right (with a left-sided CDH) would usually make the clinician suspect CDH. Often, a chest X-ray is obtained in an infant with respiratory distress and a diagnosis is established. The severity of presenting symptoms depends on the severity of pulmonary hypoplasia and PH. Arterial blood gas analysis typically reveals hypoxemia and acidosis.

Hemodynamics in CDH and cardiac dysfunction

In infants with CDH and PH (CDH–PH), the physiological postnatal fall in pulmonary vascular resistance (PVR) does not occur. PVR remains high causing the thin-walled RV to dilate with the increased pressures. This leads to the classic echocardiographic signs of flattening of the interventricular septum and later to leftward displacement. Under chronic stress, the RV starts to undergo structural remodeling

leading to hypertrophy. RV diastolic dysfunction is common in CDH [53]. In addition, as previously mentioned, infants with CDH may already have a component of LV dysfunction. The combination of progressive RV enlargement and septal bowing along with decreased LV filling due to persistently high pulmonary pressures precipitates significant LV dysfunction [54]. This causes systemic hypotension due to reduced LV output and is one of the hallmark signs of severe PH in CDH. Recognition of left and right ventricular dysfunction helps direct treatment focusing on the specific pathology detected in each infant, especially in the choice of pulmonary vasodilator as well as inotropes. In fact, the presence of cardiac dysfunction could be a significant factor influencing prognosis and severity in CDH [53].

Natural course of CDH–PH (Fig. 28.4)

A review of over 3000 infants by the CDH study group revealed ~70% incidence of PH on an echocardiogram performed on the first day after birth [55]. Over 70% of infants in this study continued to demonstrate evidence of PH on a second echocardiogram at a median of 24 days after birth. A "honeymoon period" has also been reported in the initial 24 h when infants appear to have relatively better oxygenation. This period is commonly followed by a worsening of symptoms, onset of cardiac dysfunction and pulmonary venous and arterial hypertension [56]. Symptoms of PH are likely to worsen postoperatively, even in infants who are well controlled prior to surgery. In addition, many infants with CDH have a subacute or "late PH" that will be discussed in a later section. Later in childhood, these infants will require close follow-up for monitoring and detection of chronic PH.

Management

Over the last few decades, the focus of CDH management has shifted from immediate surgical intervention to postnatal stabilization and surgery when medically stable. Management of CDH–PH and cardiac dysfunction along with appropriate "lung protective" ventilator strategies form the cornerstones of treatment before and after surgery. This change in strategy has improved outcomes for infants with CDH managed with a combination of gentle ventilation, reduced oxygen exposure and appropriate inodilators (Fig. 28.5) [56].

Delivery room:

1. Immediate gastric decompression with an orogastric tube, endotracheal intubation and avoidance of bag mask ventilation are recommended for infants with known CDH presenting with respiratory distress. End-tidal CO_2 detector is used to confirm endotracheal tube placement. Recently, the CDH Euro consortium has

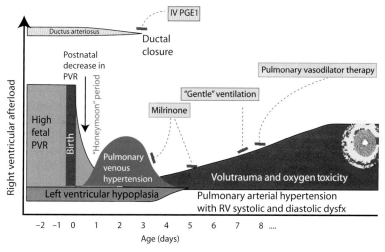

Fig. 28.4 Natural Course and Management Options in CDH. Initial high PVR at birth subsides in the "honeymoon period" followed by worsening with pulmonary venous and arterial hypertension and cardiac dysfunction. Later stages are characterized by a subacute or late PH along with effects of chronic ventilation and oxygen toxicity. IV PGE1 and Milrinone may be an option in infants with early evidence of LV dysfunction. Gentle ventilation should be practiced to minimize deleterious effects on the already hypoplastic lungs. Pulmonary vasodilator therapy remains the cornerstone of subacute or late PH management. Copyright: Satyan Lakshminrusimha.

suggested spontaneous breathing as an initial option at birth in infants without respiratory distress who have better predictive markers [52]. Use of adequate sedation has been suggested prior to intubation to reduce stress [52]; however, paralytics/neuromuscular agents have not shown any benefit and may further decrease lung compliance [57]. An orogastric tube placement and continuous suction is necessary in most infants.

2. Monitoring of heart rate as well as pre and postductal oxygen saturations are recommended. A preductal pulse oximeter probe is usually placed on the right upper limb and postductal on either of the lower limbs or the left upper limb. The CDH EURO consortium published an expert opinion in which they recommend preductal SpO_2 of 80%–95% in the delivery room [52] and avoiding hyperoxia. In fact, during the first 2 h after birth, preductal oxygen saturations >70% are acceptable as long as the infant is otherwise stable and improving [58].

3. There are no data or recommendation on the role of delayed cord clamping in CDH but this approach may be beneficial by increasing oxygen carrying capacity of blood. However, as most currently practiced protocols involve immediate endotracheal intubation, there may be logistic difficulties in delaying cord clamping and this approach needs to be investigated further.

Surfactant therapy in CDH: Currently, surfactant use is not recommended for infants with CDH [52,59]. A retrospective analysis by the CDH Study Group showed that infants who received surfactant therapy had a lower survival rate (57.3% vs. 70.0%, $P = 0.0033$) and had an increased likelihood of ECMO (69.8% vs. 50.6%, $P = 0.04$) and development of chronic lung disease [60]. However, if chest X-ray demonstrates lung fields consistent with surfactant deficiency, especially in preterm infants with CDH, surfactant may be considered.

Vascular access: Since infants with CDH are very likely to require ventilator support, it is prudent to obtain central vascular access. Preductal oxygenation is best assessed with blood gases drawn via a right radial arterial catheter. However, postductal/umbilical arterial catheters are acceptable if a preductal site is not available. Umbilical venous catheters may be placed for intravenous/inotrope delivery; however, repositioned anatomy of the umbilical vein in infants with CDH (liver-up) may cause difficulties in appropriate placement [61]. If an umbilical venous line is not placed, consider placement of a percutaneous intravenous central catheter (preferably a double-lumen) for nutrition and vasoactive medications.

Monitoring and general principles of care:
- An initial chest X-ray will confirm the diagnosis, position of the endotracheal tube and ensure adequate lung expansion (8–9 ribs expansion on contralateral side).
- Infants with CDH should have continuous invasive blood pressure monitoring through an indwelling arterial catheter or frequent noninvasive blood pressure measurements to detect systemic hypotension.
- Measures of adequate perfusion include pH >7.2, lactate <5 mmol/L, and a urine output of >1 mL/kg/h

Table 28.2 Suggested initial ventilator settings for infants with CDH (OI 15–25)

Ventilatory mode	PEEP	Tidal volume/Amp/PIP	Rate/Frequency	FiO$_2$
Conventional ventilator, volume guarantee	3–5 cmH$_2$O	4 mL/kg	40/min	Lowest FiO$_2$ to achieve preductal saturations of >70%
Conventional ventilator SIMV/PC PS	3–5 cmH$_2$O	20–25 cmH$_2$O	40/min	
HFOV	MAP 11–12 cmH$_2$O	24–28	8–10 Hz	

repair and stabilization of PH postoperatively by measures described below.

Appropriate oxygen exposure in CDH–PH. Hypoxia may increase PVR and worsen PH, while hyperoxia is known to induce production of free radicals that could also worsen PH and BPD. Appropriate oxygen saturation targets, pre and postductal as mentioned above, are a useful guide to the clinician in setting FiO$_2$ values. After stabilization, maintaining saturations in the mid-1990s and maintaining a preductal PaO$_2$ range of 55–80 mmHg on blood gases has been recommended [58]. Changing ventilation modes, appropriate management of PH using medications and ECMO should be considered if inadequate oxygenation is noted in these infants.

Summary of ventilator support based on OI and clinical course of disease

OI of 15–25

Initial stage. Currently in our unit, gentle ventilation with CV, volume guarantee mode is preferred with initial settings as shown in Table 28.2. Some units do admit these infants with prenatally diagnosed CDH on to high-frequency ventilation with HFOV, initial settings as described in Table 28.2. HFJV is a less commonly used, but usual settings include a low PEEP of 6–7 cmH$_2$O and MAP 10–11 cmH$_2$O and rate 360/min. In general for all modes, target preductal oxygen saturations >70% are acceptable as long as infant improving and stable, with a recommended initial FiO$_2$ of less than 1.0 to maintain preductal SpO$_2$. Additional tests done at this stage include a chest X-ray and an echocardiogram to detect presence and extent of PH and cardiac dysfunction.

Maintenance phase. Continued gentle ventilation on same mode as above with modifications targeted at maintaining appropriate expansion on chest X-ray, target saturations as mentioned below and permissive hypercapnia (Table 28.3).

Table 28.3 Ventilatory targets during maintenance phase for infants with CDH

Modality	Target
Chest X-ray	Contralateral expansion of 8–9 ribs
FiO$_2$	Target oxygen saturations of 80%–95% (preductal) and ≥70% (postductal)
Blood gas	PaCO$_2$ <65 mmHg and an arterial pH >7.2

Surgery is usually performed in this stage when PH is relatively stable or absent and infant is on stable ventilator settings. Usually a deterioration is anticipated after surgery, both in terms of ventilator requirements and PH. Echocardiogram and CXR should be repeated postop and management titrated based on similar targets of target expansion, SpO$_2$ targets and permissive hypercapnia. If OI increases above 25, please see management in the next section.

Weaning phase. If infant remains stable after surgery and settings can be weaned a general weaning protocol is shown in Table 28.4.

1. Targeting same SpO$_2$ and blood gas parameters (PaCO$_2$ 50–65) as above.
2. Noninvasive ventilator modes such as NIPPV and CPAP may play a role in the weaning process after surgery (nasal ventilation may increase stomach distension and compromise respiratory status before surgery).
3. Infants could also be extubated to high-flow nasal cannula or regular nasal cannula as tolerated.

OI 25–40

Initial phase. If infant appears sicker with a high OI, settings on the conventional ventilator can be increased as shown in Table 28.5. "Rescue" HFOV can be used to stabilize infant as well as described below.

- Infants with an OI in this range will most likely have evidence of PH on echocardiogram which is recommended early if there is clinical instability. iNO could be begun at this point, though definitive evidence

Table 28.4 Suggested ventilator weaning protocol for infants with CDH after surgical repair

Ventilatory mode	Order of weaning	PEEP	Tidal volume/ PIP/Amp	Rate/Frequency	FiO$_2$
Conventional ventilator	TV/PIP first, then PEEP and rate	3–5 cmH$_2$O	Wean to 4 mL/kg or PIP <25	40/min	Wean FiO$_2$ to 0.6, then attempt to wean iNO
HFOV	Amp first then MAP and frequency	MAP 11–12 cmH$_2$O	24–28	8–10 Hz	

Table 28.5 Suggested initial ventilator settings in CDH with severe disease (OI ≥ 40)

Ventilatory mode	PEEP	Tidal volume/Amp/PIP	Rate/Frequency	FiO$_2$
Conventional ventilator, volume guarantee	4–5 cmH$_2$O	4–6 mL/kg	40/min	Lowest FiO$_2$ to achieve preductal saturations of >70%
Conventional ventilator SIMV/PC PS	4–5 cmH$_2$O	20–25 cmH$_2$O	40/min	
Rescue HFOV indications		PIP > 25–28 cmH$_2$O to keep PCO$_2$ < 65	8–10 Hz	Not attaining preductal saturation targets
HFOV	11–17 cmH$_2$O	30–50 cmH$_2$O	10 Hz	Lowest FiO$_2$ to achieve preductal saturations of >70%

of benefit is lacking. If capability of administering other vasodilators exist, then sildenafil could be beneficial. Evidence of cardiac dysfunction would take the clinician toward PGE1/milrinone therapy. These are described later in this chapter as well as in a later chapter.

- Treatment of concomitant hypotension warrants treatment with agents such as Vasopressin as described below.
- Hydrocortisone therapy, especially with evidence of low blood pressures and/or low cortisol levels, could be considered.

Maintenance phase. With the ventilator management as described, most infants will stabilize, though some may show evidence of worsening OI. If OI >40, management is described in the following section.

Ventilation targets in this stage include those described in Table 28.3. Again, surgery may occur in this phase if there is hemodynamic stability without escalating support or worsening PH on serial echocardiograms. Worsening clinical condition leading to OI >40 is a possibility postoperatively and requires frequent blood gas monitoring and assessment of hemodynamic parameters.

Weaning phase. Once the infant has been stabilized, weaning is attempted following the same parameters as shown in Table 28.4.

OI >40

A high OI >40 reflects very severe disease and likely refractory PH. An OI ≥40 presents for at least 3 h is an indication for ECMO. Optimizing medical management at this time may help stabilize the infant's clinical condition significantly or could potentially provide time while arranging transfer to a regional ECMO center.

- Our usual practice would involve admitting these infants onto HFOV with similar settings as mentioned in Table 28.5. Volume guarantee CMV remains an alternative.
- Immediate echocardiogram would help direct PH treatment, iNO if available is started immediately and additional medications are added as warranted. Optimizing PH therapy is imperative especially in centers where ECMO is not available.
- Vasopressin, stress doses of hydrocortisone as well as other vasopressors such as milrinone and dopamine may be used. Specific indications in CDH are listed for each agent later in this chapter.

Surgery in these infants with high OI: There is no definitive optimal time of surgery–general consensus if to operate once infant is "relatively stable." If possible, infants with high OI >40 should be transferred to an ECMO center and surgery performed either on ECMO or after decannulation.

However, if ECMO is *unavailable or not an option*, optimal timing of surgery has to be decided on a case by case basis. Since most of the mortality from CDH occurs due to uncontrolled PH, management of PH takes priority. While there is no absolute contraindication to operating in a critical infant, this decision must be taken by the surgeon, neonatologist, and cardiologist after complete discussions with the infant's family.

Complications of mechanical ventilation in CDH

A general review of complications of mechanical ventilation is provided in another chapter in this book. Briefly, due to pulmonary hypoplasia, the risk of air leaks and pneumothoraces remains high, especially if high pressures are used during ventilation. However, less than optimal expansion will precipitate ventilation perfusion mismatch and worsening PH.

Hemodynamic support

Due to the high occurrence and risk of hypotension, these infants should have close monitoring of blood pressures in the range appropriate for gestational and postnatal age. Prior approaches included raising systemic blood pressure to reduce right-to-left shunting. While there is no evidence to support this, it is important to maintain "normal" or physiological systemic blood pressures. The presence of hypotension or markers of inadequate tissue perfusion should prompt the use of 1–2 volume boluses. Crystalloid solutions such as normal saline or ringer lactate can be used for this purpose. Anemia or abnormal coagulation profile should prompt use of packed red blood cells or fresh frozen plasma. An echocardiogram or sometimes a targeted neonatal echocardiogram should be obtained to assess ventricular filling, systolic and diastolic function, status of the ductus arteriosus, and extent of PH. Further management should involve use of appropriate inotropes and vasopressors. Use of a "targeted approach" to cardiovascular therapy has been suggested based on the presence of left, right, or biventricular dysfunction on ECHO [53]. Common agents used to manage hypotension in the NICU include dopamine, dobutamine, and norepinephrine. However, these agents increase both systemic and PVR and should be used with caution in infants with severe PH. Milrinone and vasopressin have been found to have specific advantages in infants with CDH and PH and are discussed in detail below.

Diagnosis and management of CDH–PH. Evidence of PH on echocardiogram includes demonstration of elevated right ventricular systolic pressures (RVSP) as indicated by

tricuspid regurgitation jet and its ratio to the systolic blood pressure. An RVSP that is more than 1/2 SBP indicates moderate and more than 2/3rd SBP indicates severe PH [70]. Other indicators of elevated pulmonary arterial pressure include right-to-left or bidirectional shunts through the patent ductus arteriosus and the patent foramen ovale. In addition, bowed position of the septum, dilation and hypertrophy of the RV also indicate PHT [70]. Details about echocardiography in persistent PPHN are described in another chapter in this book.

Pulmonary vasodilators

Inhaled nitric oxide (iNO)

The use of iNO in CDH–PH is controversial. The presence of PH on echocardiogram and failure to maintain target preductal saturations is an indication to begin therapy [52]. iNO is a potent "selective" pulmonary vasodilator that acts though the cyclic GMP pathway to cause pulmonary vascular smooth muscle relaxation. It works by selectively being delivered to aerated alveoli, hence it is important to ensure adequate lung recruitment for effective drug delivery. While the role of iNO is well established in PPHN, infants with CDH in the "acute" or early stage of PH may not respond to this medication. The "NINOS" trial in 1997 [71] randomized 53 infants with CDH to receive iNO or placebo. While there was no difference in the combined outcome of ECMO and/or death between the groups, there were a significantly larger number of infants in the iNO group who went on to ECMO [71]. This study published over 20 years ago suggested that infants with CDH do not respond well to iNO, unlike other neonatal populations with PH, such as idiopathic PPHN or meconium aspiration syndrome. Although this was a small study using treatment strategies such as hyperventilation and alkalization that are no longer used now, the results showing a lack of benefit from iNO have been replicated in other studies [72] as well as a Cochrane meta-analysis [73]. In spite of these results, iNO continues to be tried in infants with CDH–PH and its use has shown an increase in the United States [74]. This increase has not affected ECMO utilization or mortality rates in CDH [74].

Current CDH treatment recommendations include a trial of iNO at 20 ppm for a short period of time, following which it should be discontinued if no improvement is noted [52,64]. Infants with an OI of at least 15–25 with echocardiographic evidence of PH without postcapillary or pulmonary venous hypertension with left ventricular dysfunction are ideal candidates for a trial of iNO. The presence of left ventricular dysfunction and pulmonary venous hypertension can be determined with an echocardiogram [25]. Failure to respond to iNO is attributed to the presence of LV dysfunction suggested by a left-to-right shunt at the atrial level and a right-to-left shunt through the ductus [75]. Additionally, presence of pulmonary venous hypertension in some infants with CDH indicates that they may not improve saturations in response to iNO. In these suspected nonresponders, it may be prudent to evaluate other therapies to manage CDH–PH such as milrinone to treat LV dysfunction ± prostaglandin E1 infusion to maintain a patent ductus arteriosus to reduce preload on the right ventricle. Patients with isolated PPHN physiology without LV dysfunction with preductal desaturations with right-to-left shunts at the ductal and atrial level may benefit from iNO for improvement in oxygenation and/or pre-ECMO stabilization [75].

Dose: 10–20 ppm (usually 20 ppm).

Indications:

1. CDH with hypoxemic respiratory failure with OI >15–25
2. Evidence of PH with left to right (or bidirectional shunt) at atrial and ductal (if patent) level
3. Reduce right ventricular afterload

Relative contraindications:

1. Left ventricular dysfunction (with poor output and ductal dependent systemic circulation)
2. Pulmonary venous (postcapillary) PH

Other pulmonary vasodilators

Sildenafil, a PDE5 inhibitor that is widely used in management of PPHN and pediatric PH. Sildenafil has not been well studied in infants with CDH. Available literature in the form of case reports suggests a possible role in managing CDH–PH, both in IV [76] and enteral form [77], by decreasing PVR. Recently, the CDH EURO guidelines included IV sildenafil as an option in recommendations for treatment of CDH–PH [52]. During acute preoperative phase of CDH–PH, it is difficult to administer enteral pulmonary vasodilators as many patients are on continuous orogastric decompression. The FDA issued a black box warning against the use of Sildenafil in pediatric patients based on reports of higher mortality with chronic use; however, this was noted with high doses which are not used in the neonatal population.

Dose:

1. Intravenous—continuous infusion is preferred. The typical preferred dose is a load of 0.4 mg/kg over 3 h followed by a continuous infusion of 1.6 mg/kg/h. In infants with poor intravenous access, intermittent boluses of 0.25–0.5 mg/kg/dose infused over 30–60 min every 6–8 h can be used.
2. Enteral—preferred mode for chronic, postoperative CDH–PH. Initially, sildenafil can be started at 0.5 mg/dose every 6–8 h and gradually increased to a maximum of 3 mg/dose q 6–8 h.

Indications:

a. Adjunct therapy (usually IV) to inhaled NO for CDH–PH.
b. Primary therapy for CDH–PH—preferred drug for chronic therapy for postoperative CDH–PH.

Relative contraindications:

a. Systemic hypotension that is not responsive to inotropic therapy.
b. Prior history of untoward reactions including persistent priapism.
c. In some patients, sildenafil therapy is associated with severe GER; lowering the dose of sildenafil may be beneficial in some patients with CDH with severe reflux.
d. In preterm infants with CDH, some centers do not use sildenafil if severe retinopathy of prematurity (ROP) is present. However, there is no evidence to support this practice.

Bosentan is a nonselective endothelin receptor A and B antagonist that is being used as an adjuvant in treating infants with PPHN. The role of endothelin in pathogenesis of CDH–PH has been described earlier in this chapter. A recent Cochrane meta-analysis concluded that there is inadequate evidence to support the use of endothelin receptor antagonists either as stand-alone therapy or as adjuvant to iNO in PPHN in term and late preterm infants [78]. While there are no studies that have reported on use of Bosentan specifically in CDH, this remains a possible treatment option that needs further research [79] especially in the late or chronic PHT seen in these infants. Use of this medication in acute stages of PHT would be difficult as it is only available in oral form and liver toxicity remains a concern. At present, its use is restricted by the manufacturers and requires a special informed consent to be obtained from the physician as well as the parent.

Dose—1–2 mg/kg/dose usually twice a day.

Indications—it is used in the management of persistent, chronic PH as adjuvant therapy to sildenafil.

Contraindications—liver dysfunction.

Prostacyclin (PGI_2) analogues in various formulations (iloprost, epoprostenol, treprostinil, and beraprost) and delivery routes (oral, IV, subcutaneous, and inhaled) are being evaluated in treatment of pediatric PHT [79]. This drug acts by activating the enzyme adenylate cyclase, increasing production of cyclic AMP (cAMP) producing vasodilation. A small study in nine patients with CDH from 1993 found that prostacyclin was an effective pulmonary vasodilator and improved OI without affecting overall outcome [80]. They suggested that it could be used as a "bridge" to ECMO in CDH with severe PHT.

Dose: Epoprostenol—IV 1–3 ng/kg/min initial dose followed by maintenance of 50–80 ng/kg/min.

Inhaled 50 ng/kg/min initial dose followed by maintenance of 25–50 ng/kg/min.

Inhalation therapy has the advantages of reduced systemic side effects. Inhaled iloprost used alone or as combination therapy in acute PH has shown promising results [81].

Dose: 2.5–5 μg/breath.

Subcutanous and IV: Trepostinil have been well studied in adults with PH. In young children, subcutaneous treprostinil is well tolerated and has the additional advantage of not requiring IV access during chronic therapy. Some centers are using this medication in combination therapy to treat late PH.

Treprostinil: SQ or IV initial dose of 1.25–2 ng/kg/min followed by maintenance of 50–80 ng/kg/min.

Indication for prostacyclins—It can be used in the management of persistent, chronic PH as an adjuvant therapy to sildenafil.

Precautions: Systemic hypotension may be seen with IV route and BP must be monitored while administering these medications. While the inhaled route has fewer systemic effects, drug delivery by this route remains variable, increasing the risk of rebound PH [82].

Prostaglandin E1: The American Thoracic Society Guidelines on pediatric PHT recommend Prostaglandin E1 as an option to maintain patency of the ductus arteriosus and improve cardiac output in CDH with PH or RV failure [64]. By maintaining a PDA, it facilitates a "pop off" for the overloaded RV in cases of severe PHT [83]. It has potential for use with milrinone in targeting CDH infants with LV dysfunction and RV-dependent systemic circulation [75]. It is available in IV as well as inhaled routes.

Dose: Continuous IV infusion: Initial dose of 0.05–0.1 mcg/kg/min; maintenance: 0.01–0.4 mcg/kg/min.

Indications: To maintain ductal patency especially in infants with PH and RV failure.

Precautions: This drug can cause apnea, especially in infants <2 kg at birth. This effect is usually seen within the first hour of infusion and is rare at doses <0.15 mcg/kg/min.

Milrinone

Milrinone, a phosphodiesterase 3 (PDE3) inhibitor, has been found to be beneficial in treating infants and neonates with PHT. It acts by increased cAMP to cause systemic vasodilation but also has inotropic and lusitropic effects [53]. It has been suggested as first-line therapy in infants with CDH who have echocardiographic evidence of LV dysfunction and hypotension [53]. However, it does have the potential to worsen hypotension in the initial period and hence is titrated up to a steady state. A volume bolus has sometimes been recommended prior to beginning a milrinone infusion [34]. A case series by Patel et al. evaluated use of this medication in CDH and noted significant improvement in RV function and OI, without any demonstrable decrease in PA pressures [84]. While

several studies and case reports have shown improvement in severe PPHN with milrinone therapy, there are no other studies published in CDH. Yet, its use in the United States in term and preterm infants continues to rise [85]. A phase 2 multicenter RCT evaluating milrinone in CDH is currently approved and about to begin enrolment (NCT02951130).

Dose: About 0.25–0.75 mcg/kg/min as a continuous infusion with an optional load of 30–75 mcg/kg. The commonest side effect is systemic hypotension.

Vasopressin

Recently, vasopressin is being evaluated for its role in managing hemodynamics in infants with CDH who have refractory hypotension. Besides acting as a systemic vasoconstrictor and raising the blood pressure, vasopressin simultaneously vasodilates the pulmonary circulation. These dual actions suggest that vasopressin may have a unique role in management of sick neonates with CDH but requires further evaluation in larger studies. A retrospective analysis in 13 patients with CDH at a single center who met ECMO criteria, concluded that 6 infants no longer required ECMO after vasopressin initiation [86]. Use of a vasopressin analogue terlipressin in treating infants with CDH has also been described in case reports [87,88].

Dose: Very limited data available: GA ≥37 weeks: Continuous IV infusion: Initial: 0.1 milliunits/kg/min, increase in 0.1 milliunits/kg/min increments every hour as needed for clinical response to a maximum dose of 1.2 milliunits/kg/min [89].

Indication: Refractory PH and hypotension.

Precautions: Hyponatremia is commonly noted and requires close monitoring and correction. Unrecognized water intoxication and hyponatremia could lead to altered sensorium and seizures. Additionally, extravasation of this drug may lead to severe vasoconstriction and localized tissue necrosis; hence, appropriate needle/IV placement must be ensured prior to starting this therapy.

Role of hydrocortisone supplementation/adrenal insufficiency in CDH

In a retrospective study, Kamath et al. noted that low random cortisol levels (≤15 μg/dL) were associated with increased severity of illness [90]. They recommended that infants with CDH should be evaluated for adrenal insufficiency and steroid supplementation, while an option needs further evaluation with larger studies. In infants with CDH who have resistant hypotension, hydrocortisone should be considered [52].

Extracorporeal membrane oxygenation

CDH is one of the three commonest indications for neonatal respiratory ECMO in the ELSO registry. CDH also has the worst prognosis and survival among them (51%) [91]. Failure to respond to optimal medical therapy with pulmonary vasodilators and vasopressors leads the clinician to consider ECMO as a treatment option.

Indications for ECMO:

The following indications are commonly used for initiation of ECMO in CDH:

1. Severe hypoxemia: An OI >40 for 3 h, high-pressure settings on the ventilator (PIP >28 cmH$_2$O), inability to maintain saturation targets (<85% preductal and <70% postductal)
2. Inability to ventilate in spite of optimal ventilator settings: Acidosis (pH <7.15) and hypercapnia (PaCO$_2$ >65–70 mmHg)
3. Signs of hypoperfusion: Serum lactate >5 mM/L and systemic hypotension with evidence of low urine output (<0.5 mL/kg/h for 12–24 h) unresponsive to fluid and vasopressor therapy

These are general indications for ECMO use in the CDH Euro consortium guidelines [52]. However, center-specific guidelines vary and would determine individual treatment based on additional criteria such as weight (typically birth weight >2 kg) and gestational age (typically >34 weeks of gestation) as well.

Type of ECMO: There is considerable debate on the type of ECMO that is optimal in treating infants with CDH. Both veno-arterial (VA) and veno-venous (VV) ECMO use has been described, with each one having some benefits and some disadvantageous. VA ECMO is more commonly used, relatively "simpler" to perform using a carotid artery and a jugular vein and helps to stabilize hemodynamics rapidly by supporting the failing heart as is often seen in sick infants with CDH. VV ECMO has the advantages of sparing ligation of the carotid artery and maintaining a pulsatile flow with additional advantages of pulmonary vasodilation and improved coronary artery perfusion [92]. It may also filter microemboli in the ECMO circuit. Direct comparison of VA and VV ECMO have shown no difference in outcome measures such as mortality [92,93]; however, VV ECMO had lower neurological and increased renal complications [93]. While infants on VV ECMO were also noted to require more inotropes, a recent case report suggests utilizing a combination of PGE1 for ductal patency and optimal lung recruitment strategy on VV ECMO as a new therapeutic approach [94]. The American Pediatric Surgery Association guidelines conclude that while VA ECMO remains the preferred option, there is no difference in survival between the two modes and VV ECMO is preferable in selected cases due to lower neurological complications [67].

Duration of ECMO: Average time on ECMO for neonates with CDH is 10 days [91]; however, infants with this condition constituted the majority of ECMO runs over 21 days [95]. It is generally recognized that optimal time on ECMO is <2 weeks and longer ECMO runs are associated with worse outcomes and risk of complications [96,97].

Surgical management of CDH

Optimal timing of surgery in infants with CDH remains a topic of debate. While no longer "emergent," surgery is required for repairing the defect, allowing space for ipsilateral lung expansion and for establishing enteral nutrition. As surgery tends to worsen PH, the neonatologist and the surgeon wait for relative stability/improving pulmonary and systemic hemodynamics prior to repairing the defect. Unfortunately, this may not always be possible in the sick infant with CDH and surgery in the initial few days, surgery on ECMO as well as after decannulation have been described. The focus now is on individualizing care based on the clinical status of each infant. Studies evaluating "early" vs. "delayed" surgery have not shown any difference in ECMO/death [98,99]. CDH study group data suggest that a majority of infants are repaired after 48 h [100]. On ECMO, surgery may have the additional risk of excessive bleeding. While no consensus exists on preferred timing of repair in patients who are placed on ECMO, a review by APSA recommends early repair on ECMO as it may improve survival [67]. However, a recent study found better outcomes with higher survival and fewer complications in CDH patient who underwent surgery after decannulation [101].

Type of surgery: Traditionally, surgical repair of diaphragmatic hernia was done by an open surgery through a subcostal incision. Thoracic as well as abdominal approaches have been described [102]. Size of the defect as well as clinical condition of the infant plays a major role in determining whether the surgeon performs a primary closure or uses a synthetic patch (e.g., GORE-TEX) to close the defect. Large defects usually undergo a patch repair. Infants on ECMO or those who are on multiple vasodilators and pressors tend to have larger defects and may also predominantly require patch repair. Additionally, use of muscle flaps to close the defect instead of synthetic patches has been described [102]. Patch repair is associated with a significant risk of reherniation as compared to primary anastomosis. Thoracoscopic techniques are now being used more frequently due to advantages of decreased recovery time [103] and smaller scars [34]. Some of them may need to be converted to open repair during surgery [104]. Additionally, reports suggest an increased risk of recurrence following the use of minimally invasive techniques for repair [67,103,104]. Infants who undergo this procedure should have careful

505

monitoring of blood gases and $ETCO_2$ as there is a risk of hypercarbia and acidosis [102,105].

Late PH in CDH

A significant number of infants with CDH are noted to have persistence of PH after the initial acute period. In fact, presence of PH at 2 weeks predicted poorer short-term pulmonary outcomes and death [106]. Many of these infants continue to require mechanical ventilation. Treatment modalities for these infants include all the therapies mentioned earlier including iNO and other pulmonary vasodilators. Treprostinil has also showed promise in case reports of late PH in CDH [107]. However, further research is needed in this field to enhance outcomes.

Follow-up of infants with CDH complications and morbidities

General follow-up guidelines

Over the last few decades, there has been a better understanding of the complex needs of CDH survivors. This recognition comes as decades of research have identified several long-term complications and morbidities in infants who have survived to discharge. These infants may be followed up in multidisciplinary CDH clinics or incorporated into a hospital's "high-risk" multidisciplinary follow-up clinic [108]. Follow-up for these infants usually requires a pediatric surgeon, pediatric cardiologist, pulmonologist, a developmental pediatrician and a gastroenterologist along with therapists and nutritionists [108]. The American Academy of Pediatrics has published guidelines for postdischarge follow-up of infants with CDH through 16 years of age [109] which can be individualized to each patient based on their specific needs. Observations on long-term follow-up from these clinics also facilitate research on benefits of specific neonatal interventions and ultimately lead to better clinical practices. System-wise, the common morbidities encountered by survivors with CDH are listed below.

Respiratory complications

With better ventilation strategies and advances in care, more neonates with CDH are surviving the initial neonatal period. These infants, besides having some pulmonary hypoplasia and pulmonary vascular abnormalities are also likely to suffer from effects of prolonged mechanical ventilation. Both obstructive and restrictive lung disease may occur. Panitch et al. in their study of CDH survivors concluded that their lung function remained abnormal in first 3 years [110]. Recurrent respiratory infections remains a

common morbidity causing readmissions and infants with CDH are often placed on palivizumab prophylaxis for RSV [108]. While studies specifically evaluating use of palivizumab in this patient population are lacking, moderate-to-severe PH and ECMO use are qualifying conditions in the AAP guidelines for use of palivizumab. Liver involvement, patch repair, need for pulmonary vasodilators and ECMO, and prolonged duration of ventilation were also identified as risk factors for poorer respiratory outcomes.

Chronic PH

Infants with CDH continue to have pulmonary vascular abnormalities and hypertension persisting after hospital discharge. Cardiac catheterization has revealed pulmonary arterial as well as venous stenosis [25]. Chronic vasodilator therapy remains the mainstay of treatment; however, these infants have a high mortality and morbidity rate [75].

Gastrointestinal outcomes

Anatomical and functional abnormalities of the GI tract in CDH may lead to the significant gastroesophageal reflux seen in infants, older children, and adults with this condition. The CDH EURO consortium recommends prophylactic antireflux medication along with enteral feed initiation [52]. GERD treatment can be maximized with medical therapy and multiple medications, but for infants with persistent symptoms, decreased growth and feed aversions, surgical treatment with fundoplication and/or gastrostomy tube (GT) insertion may be considered. Failure to thrive remains a major concern for these infants in the first year and there seems to be a trend toward earlier placement of GT [111].

Surgical issues

Recurrence or reherniation may be seen in up to 15% of CDH survivors postdischarge [112,113]. Infants with patch repair for large hernias have a higher recurrence risk, especially in the first year. Bowel obstruction remains another complication that may be encountered in these infants, potentially as a result of intestinal adhesions.

Chest wall deformities and scoliosis are recognized in this population [112], likely arising as a result of abnormalities during development. Some may be severe enough to require surgical correction later.

Neurodevelopmental morbidities and outcomes

Abnormalities in neurodevelopment including neurocognitive and functional delays and behavioral issues are frequently observed in CDH survivors [108], necessitating frequent follow-up with a developmental pediatrician. Longer duration of mechanical ventilation may predispose the infant to motor abnormalities at 1 year [114]. As in other high-risk conditions, early intervention programs, appropriate developmental therapies, and identification of specific problems during close follow-up in the first 5 years are essential to enhance neurodevelopmental outcomes. The AAP follow-up guidelines also include recommendations for neuroimaging prior to discharge and then as needed [109]. Neurological morbidities such as infarctions and hemorrhages are more common in infants who have undergone ECMO, placing them at higher risk for adverse neurodevelopmental outcomes. Incidence of sensorineural hearing loss (SNHL) was high in CDH survivors but of late has been decreasing [115,116], likely reflecting improved respiratory practices and judicious antibiotic use. Besides the use of ototoxic medications, need for ECMO, prolonged ventilation and reflux have been associated with SNHL in CDH. A subset of patients may also have conductive hearing loss [116] or develop late SNHL [117] in later childhood. Hence, close follow-up of all CDH survivors for hearing loss is essential.

Future directions and therapies

Antenatal

Stem cells in CDH: Amniotic fluid-based stem cells have been studied in experimental models of CDH. These multipotent cells are postulated to cause lung growth by direct differentiation into different alveolar and vascular cell types as well as immune modulation [118,119]. However, these remain in the experimental stage and would need additional research and safety studies prior to being applied in practice [120].

Sildenafil, used antenatally in a nitrofen rat model of CDH, decreased the extent of PH and altered lung microstructure without causing adverse effects on retina or brain of the rat pups [21]. Increased VEGF and eNOS as well as enhanced vasodilation were noted in the pups with CDH. Additionally, another recent study investigating timing of administration concluded that when given at a gestational age corresponding to 20 weeks of gestation in humans, antenatal sildenafil use attenuated vascular remodeling by decreased muscularization of smaller arteries in the lung [121]. These encouraging results warrant further research and evaluation of antenatal sildenafil as a therapeutic management in infants with prenatally diagnosed CDH [120].

Vitamin A: The role of retinoic acid in normal diaphragm development has been described earlier in this chapter. In addition, deficiencies in retinoic acid receptors [122] can be seen in CDH. Most studies showing benefits from vitamin A administration have been done in the nitrofen model of CDH, which involves changes in the retinoic acid pathway. Although some advantages in lung structure and maturation are seen [123], inconsistent results are obtained in nonnitrofen animal models. While decreased vitamin A levels can be seen in infants with CDH [124], no human studies are available to review on this topic. Currently, it remains an experimental therapy.

Antioxidants like vitamin E and *n*-acetyl cysteine have shown some promise in the nitrofen rodent model of CDH [125]; however, these also have not been studied in humans.

Postnatal

Several medications are being investigated in adult phase II and III trials for PH. These include newer medications targeting the endothelin (Macitentan), NO (Riociguat), and prostacyclin (Selexipag) pathways [70]. A tyrosine-kinase inhibitor imatinib has been found to improve hemodynamics in adults with PH. While there are no large studies evaluation its benefits in CDH, it has been studied antenatally in a nitrofen model of CDH [126] and postnatally in an infant with CDH and intractable PHT [127,128]. More clinical trials are needed to improve management of this orphan disease.

References

[1] McGivern MR, Best KE, Rankin J, et al. Epidemiology of congenital diaphragmatic hernia in Europe: a register-based study. Arch Dis Child Fetal Neonatal Ed 2015;100(2): F137–F144.

[2] Balayla J, Abenhaim HA. Incidence, predictors and outcomes of congenital diaphragmatic hernia: a population-based study of 32 million births in the United States. J Matern Fetal Neonatal Med 2014;27(14):1438–1444.

[3] Wright JC, Budd JL, Field DJ, Draper ES. Epidemiology and outcome of congenital diaphragmatic hernia: a 9-year experience. Paediatr Perinat Epidemiol 2011;25(2):144–149.

[4] Doyle NM, Lally KP. The CDH study group and advances in the clinical care of the patient with congenital diaphragmatic hernia. Semin Perinatol 2004;28(3):174–184.

[5] Grizelj R, Bojanic K, Vukovic J, Weingarten TN, Schroeder DR, Sprung

J. Congenital diaphragmatic hernia: the side of diaphragmatic defect and associated nondiaphragmatic malformations. Am J Perinatol 2017;34(9):895–904.

[6] Stoll C, Alembik Y, Dott B, Roth MP. Associated malformations in cases with congenital diaphragmatic hernia. Genet Couns 2008;19(3): 331–339.

[7] Zaiss I, Kehl S, Link K, et al. Associated malformations in congenital

diaphragmatic hernia. Am J Perinatol 2011;28(3):211–218.

[8] Lally KP, Lally PA, Congenital Diaphragmatic Hernia Study Group. et al. Defect size determines survival in infants with congenital diaphragmatic hernia. Pediatrics 2007;120(3): e651–e657.

[9] Bojanic K, Woodbury JM, Cavalcante AN, et al. Congenital diaphragmatic hernia: outcomes of neonates treated at Mayo Clinic with and without extracorporeal membrane oxygenation. Paediatr Anaesth 2017;27(3):314–321.

[10] Gray BW, Fifer CG, Hirsch JC, et al. Contemporary outcomes in infants with congenital heart disease and bochdalek diaphragmatic hernia. Ann Thorac Surg 2013;95(3):929–934.

[11] Grizelj R, Bojanic K, Vukovic J, et al. Epidemiology and outcomes of congenital diaphragmatic hernia in Croatia: a population-based study. Paediatr Perinat Epidemiol 2016;30(4):336–345.

[12] Oh T, Chan S, Kieffer S, Delisle MF. Fetal outcomes of prenatally diagnosed congenital diaphragmatic hernia: nine years of clinical experience in a Canadian tertiary hospital. J Obstet Gynaecol Can 2016;38(1):17–22.

[13] Keijzer R, Puri P. Congenital diaphragmatic hernia. Semin Pediatr Surg 2010;19(3):180–185.

[14] Skandalakis J, Grey S. Embryology for surgeons: the embryological basis for the treatment of congenital anomalies, vol. 387. Baltimore, MD: Williams & Wilkins; 1994. 366.

[15] Honoré LH, Torfs CP, Curry CJ. Possible association between the hernia of Morgagni and trisomy 21. Am J Med Genet 1993;47(2):255–256.

[16] Clugston RD, Greer JJ. Diaphragm development and congenital diaphragmatic hernia. Semin Pediatr Surg 2007;16(2):94–100.

[17] McHoney M. Congenital diaphragmatic hernia. Early Hum Dev 2014;90(12):941–946.

[18] Keijzer R, Liu J, Deimling J, Tibboel D, Post M. Dual-hit hypothesis explains pulmonary hypoplasia in the nitrofen model of congenital diaphragmatic hernia. Am J Pathol 2000;156(4):1299–1306.

[19] George DK, Cooney TP, Chiu BK, Thurlbeck WM. Hypoplasia and immaturity of the terminal lung unit (acinus) in congenital diaphragmatic hernia. Am Rev Respir Dis 1987;136(4):947–950.

[20] Keller RL, Tacy TA, Hendricks-Munoz K, et al. Congenital diaphragmatic hernia: endothelin-1, pulmonary hypertension, and disease severity. Am J Respir Crit Care Med 2010;182(4):555–561.

[21] Luong C, Rey-Perra J, Vadivel A, et al. Antenatal sildenafil treatment attenuates pulmonary hypertension in experimental congenital diaphragmatic hernia. Circulation 2011;123(19):2120–2131.

[22] Vogel M, McElhinney DB, Marcus E, Morash D, Jennings RW, Tworetzky W. Significance and outcome of left heart hypoplasia in fetal congenital diaphragmatic hernia. Ultrasound Obstet Gynecol 2010;35(3):310–317.

[23] Van Mieghem T, Gucciardo L, Done E, et al. Left ventricular cardiac function in fetuses with congenital diaphragmatic hernia and the effect of fetal endoscopic tracheal occlusion. Ultrasound Obstet Gynecol 2009;34(4):424–429.

[24] Byrne FA, Keller RL, Meadows J, et al. Severe left diaphragmatic hernia limits size of fetal left heart more than does right diaphragmatic hernia. Ultrasound Obstetr Gynecol 2015;46(6):688–694.

[25] Kinsella JP, Ivy DD, Abman SH. Pulmonary vasodilator therapy in congenital diaphragmatic hernia: acute, late, and chronic pulmonary hypertension. Semin Perinatol 2005;29(2):123–128.

[26] Wynn J, Yu L, Chung WK. Genetic causes of congenital diaphragmatic hernia. Semin Fetal Neonatal Med 2014;19(6):324–330.

[27] Garne E, Haeusler M, Barisic I, et al. Congenital diaphragmatic hernia: evaluation of prenatal diagnosis in 20 European regions. Ultrasound Obstet Gynecol 2002;19(4):329–333.

[28] Gallot D, Coste K, Francannet C, et al. Antenatal detection and impact on outcome of congenital diaphragmatic hernia: a 12-year experience in Auvergne, France. Eur J Obstet Gynecol Reprod Biol 2006;125(2):202–205.

[29] Terui K, Nagata K, Kanamori Y, et al. Risk stratification for congenital diaphragmatic hernia by factors within 24 h after birth. J Perinatol 2017;37(7):805–808.

[30] Brindle ME, Cook EF, Tibboel D, Lally PA, Lally KP. Congenital Diaphragmatic Hernia Study Group. A clinical prediction rule for the severity of congenital diaphragmatic hernias in newborns. Pediatrics 2014;134(2):e413–e419.

[31] Metkus AP, Filly RA, Stringer MD, Harrison MR, Adzick NS. Sonographic predictors of survival in fetal diaphragmatic hernia. J Pediatr Surg 1996;31(1):148–151.

[32] Benachi A, Cordier AG, Cannie M, Jani J. Advances in prenatal diagnosis of congenital diaphragmatic hernia. Semin Fetal Neonatal Med 2014;19(6):331–337.

[33] Shue EH, Miniati D, Lee H. Advances in prenatal diagnosis and treatment of congenital diaphragmatic hernia. Clin Perinatol 2012;39(2):289–300.

[34] Chandrasekharan PK, Rawat M, Madappa R, Rothstein DH, Lakshminrusimha S. Congenital Diaphragmatic hernia—a review. Matern Health, Neonatol Perinatol 2017;3:6.

[35] Albanese CT, Lopoo J, Goldstein RB, et al. Fetal liver position and perinatal outcome for congenital diaphragmatic hernia. Prenat Diagn 1998;18(11):1138–1142.

[36] Kitano Y, Nakagawa S, Kuroda T, et al. Liver position in fetal congenital diaphragmatic hernia retains a prognostic value in the era of lung-protective strategy. J Pediatr Surg 2005;40(12):1827–1832.

[37] Lazar DA, Ruano R, Cass DL, et al. Defining "liver-up": does the volume of liver herniation predict outcome for fetuses with isolated left-sided congenital diaphragmatic hernia? J Pediatr Surg 2012;47(6): 1058–1062.

[38] Jani J, Keller RL, Benachi A, et al. Prenatal prediction of survival in isolated left-sided diaphragmatic hernia. Ultrasound Obstet Gynecol 2006;27(1):18–22.

[39] Büsing KA, Kilian AK, Schaible T, Endler C, Schaffelder R, Neff KW. MR relative fetal lung volume in congenital diaphragmatic hernia: survival and need for extracorporeal membrane oxygenation. Radiology 2008;248(1):240–246.

[40] Strizek B, Cos Sanchez T, Khalife J, Jani J, Cannie M. Impact of operator experience on the variability of fetal lung volume estimation by 3D-ultrasound (VOCAL) and magnetic resonance imaging in fetuses with congenital diaphragmatic hernia. J Matern Fetal Neonatal Med 2015;28(7):858–864.

[41] Oluyomi-Obi T, Kuret V, Puligandla P, et al. Antenatal predictors of outcome in prenatally diagnosed congenital diaphragmatic hernia (CDH). J Pediatr Surg 2017;52(5):881–888.

[42] Berger V, Sparks T, Gosnell K, Farrell J, Velez JG, Norton ME. Does polyhydramnios predict adverse perinatal outcome in congenital diaphragmatic hernia? [10P]. Obstetr Gynecol 2017;129(Suppl. 1):S166.

[43] Lusk LA, Wai KC, Moon-Grady AJ, Basta AM, Filly R, Keller RL. Fetal ultrasound markers of severity predict resolution of pulmonary hypertension in congenital diaphragmatic hernia. Am J Obstet Gynecol 2015;213(2). 216.e211–218.e211.

[44] Mahieu-Caputo D, Aubry MC, El Sayed M, Joubin L, Thalabard JC, Dommergues M. Evaluation of fetal pulmonary vasculature by power Doppler imaging in congenital diaphragmatic hernia. J Ultrasound Med 2004;23(8):1011–1017.

[45] Casaccia G, Crescenzi F, Dotta A, et al. Birth weight and McGoon Index predict mortality in newborn infants with congenital diaphragmatic hernia. J Pediatr Surg 2006;41(1):25–28.

[46] DeKoninck P, Jimenez J, Russo FM, Hodges R, Gratacos E, Deprest J. Assessment of pulmonary vascular reactivity to oxygen using fractional moving blood volume in fetuses with normal lung development and pulmonary hypoplasia in congenital diaphragmatic hernia. Prenat Diagn 2014;34(10):977–981.

[47] Harrison MR, Bjordal RI, Langmark F, Knutrud O. Congenital diaphragmatic hernia: the hidden mortality. J Pediatr Surg 1978;13(3):227–230.

[48] Burgos CM, Frenckner B, Luco M, Harting MT, Lally PA, Lally KP. Prenatally diagnosed congenital diaphragmatic hernia: optimal mode of delivery? J Perinatol 2017;37(2):134–138.

[49] Hutcheon JA, Butler B, Lisonkova S, et al. Timing of delivery for pregnancies with congenital diaphragmatic hernia. BJOG 2010;117(13):1658–1662.

[50] Jani JC, Nicolaides KH, Gratacos E, et al. Severe diaphragmatic hernia treated by fetal endoscopic tracheal occlusion. Ultrasound Obstet Gynecol 2009;34(3):304–310.

[51] Jani J, Valencia C, Cannie M, Vuckovic A, Sellars M, Nicolaides KH. Tracheal diameter at birth in severe congenital diaphragmatic hernia treated by fetal endoscopic tracheal occlusion. Prenat Diagn 2011;31(7):699–704.

[52] Snoek KG, Reiss IK, Greenough A, et al. Standardized postnatal management of infants with congenital diaphragmatic hernia in Europe: the CDH EURO Consortium Consensus—2015 Update. Neonatology 2016;110(1):66–74.

[53] Patel N, Kipfmueller F. Cardiac dysfunction in congenital diaphragmatic hernia: pathophysiology, clinical assessment, and management. Semin Pediatr Surg 2017;26(3):154–158.

[54] Baumgart S, Paul JJ, Huhta JC, et al. Cardiac malposition, redistribution of fetal cardiac output, and left heart hypoplasia reduce survival in neonates with congenital diaphragmatic hernia requiring extracorporeal membrane oxygenation. J Pediatr 1998;133(1):57–62.

[55] Putnam LR, Tsao K, Morini F, et al. Evaluation of variability in inhaled nitric oxide use and pulmonary hypertension in patients with congenital diaphragmatic hernia. JAMA Pediatr 2016;170(12):1188–1194.

[56] Nair J, Lakshminrusimha S. Update on PPHN: mechanisms and treatment. Semin Perinatol 2014;38(2):78–91.

[57] Murthy V, D'Costa W, Nicolaides K, et al. Neuromuscular blockade and lung function during resuscitation of infants with congenital diaphragmatic hernia. Neonatology 2013;103(2): 112–117.

[58] Morini F, Capolupo I, van Weteringen W, Reiss I. Ventilation modalities in infants with congenital diaphragmatic hernia. Semin Pediatr Surg 2017;26(3):159–165.

[59] Logan JW, Rice HE, Goldberg RN, Cotten CM. Congenital diaphragmatic hernia: a systematic review and summary of best-evidence practice strategies. J Perinatol 2007;27(9): 535–549.

[60] Van Meurs K. the Congenital Diaphragmatic Hernia Study Group. Is surfactant therapy beneficial in the treatment of the term newborn infant with congenital diaphragmatic hernia? J Pediatr 2004;145(3):312–316.

[61] Raisanen P, Cassel I, Martin G, Graziano K. Umbilical venous catheter complication in an infant with left-sided congenital diaphragmatic hernia: extravasation owing to hepatic vein catheterization. J Pediatr Surg 2010;45(12):e33–e35.

[62] Rawat M, Chandrasekharan PK, Williams A, et al. Oxygen saturation index and severity of hypoxic respiratory failure. Neonatology 2015;107(3):161–166.

[63] Walsh-Sukys MC, Tyson JE, Wright LL, et al. Persistent pulmonary hypertension of the newborn in the era before nitric oxide: practice variation and outcomes. Pediatrics 2000;105(1 Pt. 1):14–20.

[64] Abman SH, Hansmann G, Archer SL, et al. Pediatric pulmonary hypertension: guidelines from the American Heart Association and American Thoracic Society. Circulation 2015;132(21):2037–2099.

[65] Snoek KG, Capolupo I, van Rosmalen J, et al. Conventional mechanical ventilation versus high-frequency oscillatory ventilation for congenital diaphragmatic hernia: a randomized clinical trial (the VICI-trial). Ann Surg 2016;263(5):867–874.

[66] Wung JT, James LS, Kilchevsky E, James E. Management of infants with severe respiratory failure and persistence of the fetal circulation, without hyperventilation. Pediatrics 1985;76(4):488–494.

[67] Puligandla PS, Grabowski J, Austin M, et al. Management of congenital diaphragmatic hernia: a systematic review from the APSA outcomes and evidence based practice committee. J Pediatr Surg 2015;50(11): 1958–1970.

[68] Wheeler K, Klingenberg C, McCallion N, Morley CJ, Davis PG. Volume-targeted versus pressure-limited ventilation in the neonate. Cochrane Database Syst Rev 2010;11: CD003666.

[69] Nair J, Orie J, Lakshminrusimha S. Successful treatment of a neonate with idiopathic persistent pulmonary hypertension with inhaled nitric oxide via nasal cannula without mechanical ventilation. AJP Rep 2012;2(1): 29–32.

[70] Harting MT. Congenital diaphragmatic hernia-associated pulmonary hypertension. Semin Pediatr Surg 2017;26(3):147–153.

[71] The Neonatal Inhaled Nitric Oxide Study Group (NINOS). Inhaled nitric oxide and hypoxic respiratory failure in infants with congenital diaphragmatic hernia. Pediatrics 1997;99(6):838–845.

[72] Clark RH, Kueser TJ, Walker MW, et al. Low-dose nitric oxide therapy for persistent pulmonary hypertension of

the newborn. Clinical Inhaled Nitric Oxide Research Group. N Engl J Med 2000;342(7):469–474.

[73] Finer NN, Barrington KJ. Nitric oxide for respiratory failure in infants born at or near term. Cochrane Database Syst Rev 2006;4:CD000399.

[74] Campbell BT, Herbst KW, Briden KE, Neff S, Ruscher KA, Hagadorn JI. Inhaled nitric oxide use in neonates with congenital diaphragmatic hernia. Pediatrics 2014;134(2):e420–e426.

[75] Gien J, Kinsella JP. Management of pulmonary hypertension in infants with congenital diaphragmatic hernia. J Perinatol 2016;36(Suppl. 2):S28–S31.

[76] Bialkowski A, Moenkemeyer F, Patel N. Intravenous sildenafil in the management of pulmonary hypertension associated with congenital diaphragmatic hernia. Eur J Pediatr Surg 2015;25(2):171–176.

[77] Noori S, Friedlich P, Wong P, Garingo A, Seri I. Cardiovascular effects of sildenafil in neonates and infants with congenital diaphragmatic hernia and pulmonary hypertension. Neonatology 2007;91(2):92–100.

[78] More K, Athalye-Jape GK, Rao SC, Patole SK. Endothelin receptor antagonists for persistent pulmonary hypertension in term and late preterm infants. Cochrane Database Syst Rev 2016;8:CD010531.

[79] Lakshminrusimha S, Mathew B, Leach CL. Pharmacologic strategies in neonatal pulmonary hypertension other than nitric oxide. Semin Perinatol 2016;40(3):160–173.

[80] Bos AP, Tibboel D, Koot VC, Hazebroek FW, Molenaar JC. Persistent pulmonary hypertension in high-risk congenital diaphragmatic hernia patients: incidence and vasodilator therapy. J Pediatr Surg 1993;28(11):1463–1465.

[81] Mulligan C, Beghetti M. Inhaled iloprost for the control of acute pulmonary hypertension in children: a systematic review. Pediatr Crit Care Med 2012;13(4):472–480.

[82] Cosa N, Costa E Jr. Inhaled pulmonary vasodilators for persistent pulmonary hypertension of the newborn: safety issues relating to drug administration and delivery devices. Med Dev 2016;9:45–51.

[83] Gupta N, Kamlin CO, Cheung M, Stewart M, Patel N. Prostaglandin E1 use during neonatal transfer: potential beneficial role in persistent pulmonary hypertension of the newborn. Arch Dis Child Fetal Neonatal Ed 2013;98(2):F186–F188.

[84] Patel N. Use of milrinone to treat cardiac dysfunction in infants with pulmonary hypertension secondary to congenital diaphragmatic hernia: a review of six patients. Neonatology 2012;102(2):130–136.

[85] Hagadorn JI, Brownell EA, Herbst KW, Trzaski JM, Neff S, Campbell BT. Trends in treatment and in-hospital mortality for neonates with congenital diaphragmatic hernia. J Perinatol 2015;35(9):748–754.

[86] Acker SN, Kinsella JP, Abman SH, Gien J. Vasopressin improves hemodynamic status in infants with congenital diaphragmatic hernia. J Pediatr 2014;165(1). 53.e51–58.e51.

[87] Stathopoulos L, Nicaise C, Michel F, et al. Terlipressin as rescue therapy for refractory pulmonary hypertension in a neonate with a congenital diaphragmatic hernia. J Pediatr Surg 2011;46(2):e19–e21.

[88] Papoff P, Caresta E, Versacci P, Grossi R, Midulla F, Moretti C. The role of terlipressin in the management of severe pulmonary hypertension in congenital diaphragmatic hernia. Paediatr Anaesth 2009;19(8):805–806.

[89] Mohamed A, Nasef N, Shah V, McNamara PJ. Vasopressin as a rescue therapy for refractory pulmonary hypertension in neonates: case series. Pediatr Crit Care Med 2014;15(2):148–154.

[90] Kamath BD, Fashaw L, Kinsella JP. Adrenal insufficiency in newborns with congenital diaphragmatic hernia. J Pediatr 2010;156(3). 495.e491–497.e491.

[91] Paden ML, Rycus PT, Thiagarajan RR, Registry E. Update and outcomes in extracorporeal life support. Semin Perinatol 2014;38(2):65–70.

[92] Kugelman A, Gangitano E, Pincros J, Tantivit P, Taschuk R, Durand M. Venovenous versus venoarterial extracorporeal membrane oxygenation in congenital diaphragmatic hernia. J Pediatr Surg 2003;38(8):1131–1136.

[93] Guner YS, Khemani RG, Qureshi FG, et al. Outcome analysis of neonates with congenital diaphragmatic hernia treated with venovenous vs venoarterial extracorporeal membrane oxygenation. J Pediatr Surg 2009;44(9):1691–1701.

[94] Moscatelli A, Pezzato S, Lista G, et al. Venovenous ECMO for congenital diaphragmatic hernia: role of ductal patency and lung recruitment. Pediatrics 2016;138(5).

[95] Prodhan P, Stroud M, El-Hassan N, et al. Prolonged extracorporeal membrane oxygenator support among neonates with acute respiratory failure: a review of the Extracorporeal Life Support Organization registry. ASAIO J 2014;60(1):63–69.

[96] Seetharamaiah R, Younger JG, Bartlett RH, Hirschl RB. Congenital Diaphragmatic Hernia Study Group. Factors associated with survival in infants with congenital diaphragmatic hernia requiring extracorporeal membrane oxygenation: a report from the Congenital Diaphragmatic Hernia Study Group. J Pediatr Surg 2009;44(7):1315–1321.

[97] Tiruvoipati R, Vinogradova Y, Faulkner G, Sosnowski AW, Firmin RK, Peek GJ. Predictors of outcome in patients with congenital diaphragmatic hernia requiring extracorporeal membrane oxygenation. J Pediatr Surg 2007;42(8):1345–1350.

[98] Hollinger LE, Lally PA, Tsao K, Wray CJ, Lally KP. Congenital Diaphragmatic Hernia Study Group. A risk-stratified analysis of delayed congenital diaphragmatic hernia repair: does timing of operation matter? Surgery 2014;156(2):475–482.

[99] Rozmiarek AJ, Qureshi FG, Cassidy L, Ford HR, Hackam DJ. Factors influencing survival in newborns with congenital diaphragmatic hernia: the relative role of timing of surgery. J Pediatr Surg 2004;39(6):821–824.

[100] Kotecha S, Barbato A, Bush A, et al. Congenital diaphragmatic hernia. Eur Respir J 2012;39(4):820–829.

[101] Partridge EA, Peranteau WH, Rintoul NE, et al. Timing of repair of congenital diaphragmatic hernia in patients supported by extracorporeal membrane oxygenation (ECMO). J Pediatr Surg 2015;50(2):260–262.

[102] Zani A, Zani-Ruttenstock E, Pierro A. Advances in the surgical approach to congenital diaphragmatic hernia. Semin Fetal Neonatal Med 2014;19(6):364–369.

[103] Vijfhuize S, Deden AC, Costerus SA, Sloots CE, Wijnen RM. Minimal access surgery for repair of congenital

diaphragmatic hernia: is it advantageous? An open review. Eur J Pediatr Surg 2012;22(5):364–373.

[104] Gander JW, Fisher JC, Gross ER, et al. Early recurrence of congenital diaphragmatic hernia is higher after thoracoscopic than open repair: a single institutional study. J Pediatr Surg 2011;46(7):1303–1308.

[105] McHoney M, Giacomello L, Nah SA, et al. Thoracoscopic repair of congenital diaphragmatic hernia: intraoperative ventilation and recurrence. J Pediatr Surg 2010;45(2):355–359.

[106] Lusk LA, Wai KC, Moon-Grady AJ, Steurer MA, Keller RL. Persistence of pulmonary hypertension by echocardiography predicts short-term outcomes in congenital diaphragmatic hernia. J Pediatr 2015;166(2). 251.e251–256.e251.

[107] Olson E, Lusk LA, Fineman JR, Robertson L, Keller RL. Short-term treprostinil use in infants with congenital diaphragmatic hernia following repair. J Pediatr 2015;167(3):762–764.

[108] Tracy S, Chen C. Multidisciplinary long-term follow-up of congenital diaphragmatic hernia: a growing trend. Semin Fetal Neonatal Med 2014;19(6):385–391.

[109] Lally KP, Engle W. American Academy of Pediatrics Committee. Post-discharge follow-up of infants with congenital diaphragmatic hernia. Pediatrics 2008;121(3):627–632.

[110] Panitch HB, Weiner DJ, Feng R, et al. Lung function over the first 3 years of life in children with congenital diaphragmatic hernia. Pediatr Pulmonol 2015;50(9):896–907.

[111] Chiu PP, Sauer C, Mihailovic A, et al. The price of success in the management of congenital diaphragmatic hernia: is improved survival accompanied by an increase in long-term morbidity? J Pediatr Surg 2006;41(5):888–892.

[112] Jancelewicz T, Chiang M, Oliveira C, Chiu PP. Late surgical outcomes among congenital diaphragmatic hernia (CDH) patients: why long-

term follow-up with surgeons is recommended. J Pediatr Surg 2013;48(5):935–941.

[113] Jancelewicz T, Vu LT, Keller RL, et al. Long-term surgical outcomes in congenital diaphragmatic hernia: observations from a single institution. J Pediatr Surg 2010;45(1):155–160.

[114] Friedman S, Chen C, Chapman JS, et al. Neurodevelopmental outcomes of congenital diaphragmatic hernia survivors followed in a multidisciplinary clinic at ages 1 and 3. J Pediatr Surg 2008;43(6):1035–1043.

[115] Wilson MG, Riley P, Hurteau AM, Baird R, Puligandla PS. Hearing loss in congenital diaphragmatic hernia (CDH) survivors: is it as prevalent as we think? J Pediatr Surg 2013;48(5):942–945.

[116] Partridge EA, Bridge C, Donaher JG, et al. Incidence and factors associated with sensorineural and conductive hearing loss among survivors of congenital diaphragmatic hernia. J Pediatr Surg 2014;49(6):890–894.

[117] Robertson CM, Cheung PY, Haluschak MM, Elliott CA, Leonard NJ. High prevalence of sensorineural hearing loss among survivors of neonatal congenital diaphragmatic hernia. Western Canadian ECMO Follow-up Group. Am J Otol 1998;19(6):730–736.

[118] Pederiva F, Ghionzoli M, Pierro A, De Coppi P, Tovar JA. Amniotic fluid stem cells rescue both in vitro and in vivo growth, innervation, and motility in nitrofen-exposed hypoplastic rat lungs through paracrine effects. Cell Transplant 2013;22(9):1683–1694.

[119] Di Bernardo J, Maiden MM, Hershenson MB, Kunisaki SM. Amniotic fluid derived mesenchymal stromal cells augment fetal lung growth in a nitrofen explant model. J Pediatr Surg 2014;49(6):859–864.

[120] Jeanty C, Kunisaki SM, MacKenzie TC. Novel non-surgical prenatal approaches to treating congenital diaphragmatic hernia. Semin Fetal

Neonatal Med 2014;19(6):349–356.

[121] Mous DS, Kool HM, Buscop-van Kempen MJ, et al. Clinically relevant timing of antenatal sildenafil treatment reduces pulmonary vascular remodeling in congenital diaphragmatic hernia. Am J Physiol: Lung Cell Mol Physiol 2016;311(4):L734–L742.

[122] Mendelsohn C, Lohnes D, Decimo D, et al. Function of the retinoic acid receptors (RARs) during development (II). Multiple abnormalities at various stages of organogenesis in RAR double mutants. Development 1994;120(10):2749–2771.

[123] Gallot D, Coste K, Jani J, et al. Effects of maternal retinoic acid administration in a congenital diaphragmatic hernia rabbit model. Pediatr Pulmonol 2008;43(6):594–603.

[124] Beurskens LW, Tibboel D, Lindemans J, et al. Retinol status of newborn infants is associated with congenital diaphragmatic hernia. Pediatrics 2010;126(4):712–720.

[125] Gonzalez-Reyes S, Martinez L, Martinez-Calonge W, Fernandez-Dumont V, Tovar JA. Effects of antioxidant vitamins on molecular regulators involved in lung hypoplasia induced by nitrofen. J Pediatr Surg 2006;41(8):1446–1452.

[126] Chang YT, Ringman Uggla A, Osterholm C, et al. Antenatal imatinib treatment reduces pulmonary vascular remodeling in a rat model of congenital diaphragmatic hernia. Am J Physiol Lung Cell Mol Physiol 2012;302(11):L1159–L1166.

[127] Frenckner B, Broome M, Lindstrom M, Radell P. Platelet-derived growth factor inhibition—a new treatment of pulmonary hypertension in congenital diaphragmatic hernia? J Pediatr Surg 2008;43(10):1928–1931.

[128] Ghofrani HA, Morrell NW, Hoeper MM, et al. Imatinib in pulmonary arterial hypertension patients with inadequate response to established therapy. Am J Respir Crit Care Med 2010;182(9):1171–1177.

Chapter | **29** |

Care of Extremely Low Birth Weight Infants

Narendra Dereddy, MD, Kirtikumar Upadhyay, MD, Ramasubbareddy Dhanireddy, MD

CHAPTER POINTS

- Care of the ELBW infant in the first hour of life (The Golden hour) is very important in improving their survival and outcomes.
- Prenatal corticosteroids, early surfactant use, and optimal ventilation strategies to avoid both volutrauma and atelectrauma reduce the severity of RDS and duration of mechanical ventilation.
- Early and aggressive nutrition with adequate provision of calories and protein to mimic intrauterine growth, improves both short term outcomes and long term neurodevelopment.

Introduction

Infants born with a birth weight less than 1000 g are defined as extremely low birth weight (ELBW) and are typically born at gestational age of 27 weeks or younger. With recent advances in neonatal care, survival of these extremely preterm infants has improved and with it the challenges of management of associated morbidities have also increased. In the mid-1960s, ELBW infants had a survival rate of ~5%

(i.e., mortality rate was 95%) [1]. In 1960, infants who were born at 28 weeks of gestation were considered "previable," whereas the survival rate for ELBW infants born between 23 and 28 weeks of gestational age in the United States today is ~75% [2]. Age of viability is considered to be 23 weeks of gestation currently with a survival rate of about 30% [3]. There are reports of survival with intensive care even at 22 weeks of gestation, but the reported survival at this gestation is extremely low (<5%) and the neurodevelopmental outcomes are poor. The rate of preterm deliveries at the edge of viability is increasing; often because of the increased use of artificial reproductive technologies (Table 29.1).

The management of ELBW infants is a multidisciplinary team effort and outcomes are dependent on the quality of evidence-based care provided by this team comprising the nurses, respiratory therapists, dieticians, pharmacists, physical/occupational therapists, social worker, and physicians with support from many other departments of the hospital. In this chapter, we present the current evidenced-based practices to help improve the outcomes of these extremely preterm infants.

Prenatal management

Prenatal consultation

Parents anticipating preterm delivery should be met by the neonatologist and provided counseling. When delivery is expected at extremely preterm gestations (22–25 weeks of gestation), the obstetrician and the neonatologist should meet with the parents together when possible and should explain the expected course of their premature infant. In the United States, National Institute of Child Health and Development (NICHD) calculator can be used to give guidance to the family on the outcomes at various gestational ages based on the gender, expected birth weight, singleton or multiple pregnancy, and receipt of antenatal corticosteroids (CSs) [4]

Table 29.1 Evolution of neonatal–perinatal medicine	
1940–50	Infants <1 kg were classified as stillborn
1950s	Introduction of Apgar scores made these infants live-born but previable and allowed to die without technologic intervention
1960s	1 kg limit persisted until the widespread use of mechanical ventilation in the late 1960s
1970s	Limit of viability started rolling back
1980s	Survivors with GA of 24 weeks and BW of 500–600 g were rare
1990s	Introduction of Surfactant/antenatal steroids Survivors with GAs of 24 weeks and BWs of 500–600 g were common
2000s	Limit of viability rolled back further up to 24 weeks of gestational age and 500 g birth weight
2010s	Pushing the edge of viability to 22 weeks.

BW, Birth weight; GA, gestational age.

(at https://www.nichd.nih.gov/epbo-calculator/Pages/epbo_case.aspx). When available, local survival and developmental outcome data should be provided to the parents to help them make decisions.

Prenatal steroids

Prenatal CS before anticipated preterm birth is an important antenatal therapy that had improved the outcomes of preterm infants. Either betamethasone (two 12-mg doses given intramuscularly 24 h apart) or dexamethasone (four 6-mg doses intramuscularly every 12 h) should be used. A single repeat course should be considered if more than 14 days have elapsed since the first course and delivery is expected within the next 7 days in women who are at less than 34 0/7 weeks of gestation. Rescue course could be provided as early as 7 days from the prior dose based on the clinical scenario. There are robust data to support their use for anticipated preterm delivery between 24 0/7 and 33 6/7 weeks of gestation. Some observational studies and data from the NICHD Neonatal Research Network showed reduction in death, intraventricular hemorrhage (IVH), periventricular leukomalacia (PVL), and neurodevelopmental impairment (NDI) at 18–22 months for infants who had been exposed to antenatal CSs and born at 23 0/7 through 23 6/7 weeks of gestation [5–8]. At 22 0/7 through 22 6/7 weeks of gestation, no significant difference in these outcomes was noted (90.2% vs. 93.1%). Hence, prenatal CS may be considered for pregnant women starting at 23 0/7 weeks of gestation who are at risk of preterm delivery within 7 days, based on a family's decision regarding resuscitation.

Magnesium for neuroprotection

Several clinical trials have evaluated the use of intravenous magnesium sulfate for neuroprotection in preterm births [9–12]. Although none of the individual trials found evidence of improvement in the primary outcome of death or cerebral palsy, meta-analysis showed that prenatal administration of magnesium sulfate reduces the occurrence of cerebral palsy when given with neuroprotective intent (relative risk [RR], 0.71; 95% confidence interval [CI], 0.55–0.91) [13]. American College of Obstetricians and Gynecologists (ACOG) recommends individual institutions should develop specific guidelines regarding whom to treat, treatment regimens, and monitoring in accordance with one of the larger trials [14]. At our institution, we use $MgSO_4$ for neuroprotection for 30 weeks and lower gestational ages and preterm delivery is expected within 24 h. The doses used are a loading dose of 4 g followed by a maintenance dose of 2 g/h for up to 12 h.

Delivery room care of the ELBW neonate (Fig. 29.1)

Temperature maintenance

Hypothermia after delivery is common, particularly in ELBW infants and is associated with increased mortality and morbidity, including respiratory distress syndrome (RDS), metabolic derangements, and IVH [15–18]. ELBW infants have a tendency to become hypothermic due to high surface area to volume ratio, lack of subcutaneous fat, poorly keratinized immature epidermis, and lack of brown adipose tissue. Maintaining appropriate body temperature (36.5–37.5°C) in the delivery room (DR) is one of the important supportive therapies for ELBW infants that can improve their outcomes using minimal resources. With each fall in axillary temperature by 1°C, there is 28% increase in neonatal mortality [19].

DR temperature should be maintained at 77–79°F (25–26°C) prior to the infant's delivery and during resuscitation. Radiant warmer should be turned on to 100% power prior to delivery and all the surfaces that the infant is going to come in contact with should be warm to prevent conductive heat losses. Chemical warming blankets/mattresses should be used when available. Infant's head should be covered with a prewarmed double cap soon after birth. They should also be covered with polyurethane sheet or bag up to the neck without prior drying to prevent evaporative heat and maintain humidity [20–22]. This measure will have the added benefit of preventing insensible water losses. Commercially available materials like neowraps (Fisher and Paykel, USA) are commonly used in the United States, but any transparent polyurethane material or bag can be used for this purpose.

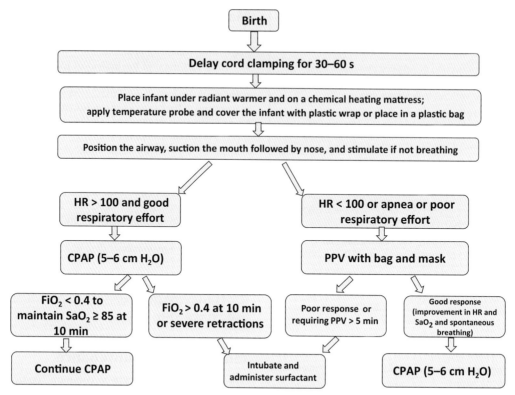

Fig. 29.1 Delivery Room Management of ELBW Infants.

Prewarmed transport incubators should be used to transport the infant to the NICU. Once in the NICU, these infants should be cared in an incubator with 70%–80% humidity for the first week of life and 40%–50% afterward.

Placental transfusion after birth

Allowing extra blood transfusion soon after birth from placenta increases the neonate's blood volume, improves left ventricular (LV) contractility, and hence hemodynamic stability [23–25]. The two methods employed for placental transfusion after birth are delayed umbilical cord clamping and umbilical cord milking, with the former being well-studied and commonly used.

Delayed umbilical cord clamping

A recent systematic review indicates that delaying cord clamping (DCC) up to 3 min in vigorous preterm babies significantly reduces hemodynamic instability, improves cerebral circulation, reduces IVH all grades, necrotizing enterocolitis (NEC), and the need for transfusions, although peak serum bilirubin was higher in the transfused group. However, no clear differences were found in the primary

outcome of death, severe IVH or PVL [26]. International Liaison Committee on Resuscitation (ILCOR) and ACOG have recently recommended delaying umbilical cord clamping in vigorous term and preterm infants for at least 30–60 s after birth [27]. Infant should be held at or below the level of the placenta although a recent trial in term infants born vaginally and placed on the maternal chest or abdomen did not find any difference in the volume of placental transfusion. Hence, skin-to-skin contact soon after delivery is appropriate while waiting for delayed cord clamping. In case of C-section, infant can be laid on the maternal abdomen or the legs or can be held by the obstetrician close to the level of the placenta. While waiting for cord clamping, the neonatal and obstetric teams should evaluate the baby's tone and breathing and initial steps of resuscitation such as drying, clearing the airway, and stimulating the infant should be performed. Infant should be wrapped in a clear polyethylene plastic sheet or placed in a plastic bag to prevent hypothermia. Current recommendations are to proceed with immediate cord clamping if the infant needs further resuscitation, but a recent study by Katheria et al. showed that ventilation while awaiting DCC was feasible without any adverse effects [28]. If the placental perfusion is impaired in conditions such as placental abruption, cord clamping should not be delayed.

Umbilical cord milking

Umbilical cord milking or stripping achieves placental transfusion in a rapid time frame, usually less than 10–15 s compared to DCC [29–31]. It may have advantages when the infant is depressed at birth and needs immediate resuscitation. However, umbilical cord milking has not been studied as rigorously as delayed umbilical cord clamping. A recent meta-analysis involving 501 preterm infants comparing umbilical cord milking with immediate cord clamping found that infants in the umbilical cord-milking groups had higher hemoglobin levels and decreased incidence of IVH with no increase in adverse effects [32]. The method of umbilical cord milking varied considerably in the trials in terms of the number of times the cord was milked, the length of milked cord, and whether the cord was clamped before or after milking. Another recent trial evaluating infants born before 32 weeks of gestation found that among those infants born by cesarean delivery, umbilical cord milking was associated with higher hemoglobin levels and improved blood pressure compared with those in the delayed umbilical cord clamping group, but the differences were not seen among those born vaginally [33]. Currently, there is insufficient evidence to either support or refute umbilical cord milking in term or preterm infants but should be considered in preterm infants who needs resuscitation and cord clamping cannot be delayed.

Respiratory support in the DR

ELBW neonates frequently require respiratory support in the DR due to poor respiratory drive, poor muscle strength, and structurally and functionally immature lungs. Goal of respiratory support in the DR should be to maintain airway patency, establish and maintain an adequate functional residual capacity (FRC) and adequate ventilation. They are frequently intubated and given positive pressure ventilation (PPV) through an endotracheal tube (ETT). Although it helps in the DR stabilization, PPV, more so invasive mechanical ventilation can result in lung injury from barotrauma, volutrauma, and predispose these infants to chronic lung disease [34,35]. Noninvasive modes of respiratory support (nasal CPAP) in a spontaneously breathing infant can avoid lung damage and are being increasingly used in extremely preterm infants.

CPAP

CPAP should be the initial respiratory support to all ELBW infants with respiratory distress. It helps the spontaneously breathing preterm infant by several mechanisms: (1) it maintains airway patency by splinting and dilating the upper airway, thereby preventing obstructive apnea; (2) reduces the work of breathing by decreasing airway resistance and by stenting the compliant chest wall of the preterm infant; and (3) improves ventilation perfusion matching by maintaining FRC and by preventing repeated alveolar collapse and expansion; it reduces protein leak and hyaline membrane formation [36,37]. CPAP should be maintained at all times in nonintubated infant including during transport from the DR. Several large randomized controlled trials (COIN, SUPPORT, and VON DR management trials) compared the early CPAP strategy with immediate intubation and surfactant administration [38–40]. In all these trials, early CPAP use with selective intubation and surfactant administration had similar outcomes compared to early intubation with surfactant administration and mechanical ventilation. In a pooled analysis of RCTs, early CPAP use was associated with a small but statistically significant reduction in BPD or death compared to early-intubated group. There was increase in the incidence of air leaks in the CPAP group in the COIN trial where a PEEP of 8 cmH_2O was used; hence, we recommend an initial PEEP of 5 cmH_2O and increase up to 6 cmH_2O if there is poor response.

PPV in the DR

In infants requiring PPV due to either apnea or poor response to CPAP, use of T-piece resuscitator is recommended to be able to monitor the pressures being delivered [41]. A starting PIP of 16–18 cmH_2O is recommended and can be adjusted based on response. When self-inflating or flow inflating bags are used for delivering PPV, a manometer should be used to monitor the pressures being delivered [42,43]. Visible chest rise is not always seen in ELBW infants and excessive pressures may be used if chest rise is used as criteria for effective PPV. A second resuscitator should listen for breath sounds to evaluate for effective PPV. If prolonged PPV is required (greater than 5 min) or if the infant is not responding to mask PPV, infant should be intubated and once stable, surfactant should be administered.

Suggested initial settings for PPV in the delivery room

	FiO$_2$	PEEP (cmH$_2$O)	T_i (s)	PIP (cmH$_2$O)	Rate
Initial settings	0.3	5	0.3	18*	40–60
Escalate if no response	In increments of 0.1 (increase to 1.0 if needing chest compressions)	6–7	0.35	Increase if there is no adequate air entry increments of 2 up to 25	40–60

*For infants below 25 weeks of gestation, consider lower PIP.

Sustained lung inflation

Sustained lung inflation (SLI) is a lung recruitment strategy in the DR where high inflation pressure is maintained for a prolonged period soon after birth to clear the lung fluid and establish a FRC [44]. RCTs comparing SLI to intermittent PPV (IPPV) in extremely preterm infants have used inspiratory pressures between 20 and 30 cmH$_2$O sustained for 10–15 s and used for one to three breaths [45–49]. The results of these trials are mixed with some showing a short-term improvement, while others did not find any difference. A meta-analysis of these trials did not show a significant difference in the rates of BPD or death between the SLI and the IPPV groups [50]. Till further data are available, we do not recommend SLI for lung recruitment and advocate early use of CPAP for this purpose.

Sustained lung inflation parameters

PIP	Duration	Breaths
20 cmH$_2$O	15 s	1–3

Use of oxygen and pulse oximeter in the delivery room

Oxygen should be judiciously used in ELBW infants as they have poor antioxidant defense mechanisms. Free radicals from excess O$_2$ can cause lung damage by inflammation and subsequent fibrosis [51,52]. FiO$_2$ should be titrated based on the preductal pulse oximetry to target saturation goals in the reference range based on the study by Dawson and coworkers and recommended by ILCOR [53–55]. Pulse oximetry is now widely employed in the DR to objectively evaluate newborn postnatal arterial oxygen saturation and is recommended by ILCOR. The sensor is preferably put on the right hand or wrist to evaluate oxygenation of preductal blood. Sensor should be protected from intense light to avoid false readings. Reliable readings can be mostly achieved within 60–90 s after birth. Extremely preterm infants may take longer to achieve the target O$_2$ saturation as the reference values are based on term infants and moderately preterm infants. As long as the heart rate is improving, we suggest using oxygen conservatively. Meta-analysis of RCTs comparing initial administration of low (0.21–0.3) versus high FiO$_2$ (0.65–1.0) showed no significant difference in the BPD rates or mortality rates between the two groups [56–60]. The 2015 ILCOR recommends starting resuscitation for preterm infants with a low FiO$_2$ concentration between 0.21 and 0.30 and titrating based on preductal oxygen saturations. Oxygen should be titrated up to 100% before escalating the infant's resuscitation to chest compressions and/or epinephrine administration [27].

Preductal O$_2$ saturation targets in the first 10 min of life [27]

Time after birth (min)	Target SpO$_2$ range
1	60%–65%
2	65%–70%
3	70%–75%
4	75%–80%
5	80%–85%
10	85%–95%

Surfactant administration

Introduction of surfactant as an efficient therapy for RDS in the early 1990s resulted in a significant reduction in neonatal mortality and early respiratory morbidity [61]. Surfactant administration in extremely premature infants with inadequate endogenous surfactant reduces the alveolar surface tension, prevents atelectasis and hyaline membrane formation. Both animal-derived and synthetic surfactants are available. Animal-derived surfactants are superior to synthetic ones but some of the second-generation synthetic surfactants are at least not inferior to the animal-derived surfactants [62]. Porcine-derived surfactant showed better outcomes compared to the bovine minced lung surfactant, likely because of the higher initial dose of surfactant protein B used in porcine-derived surfactant studies [63]. Newer synthetic surfactants containing peptide analogs of surfactant protein B and C are currently being studied [64,65]. The timing of surfactant administration for the prevention and/or treatment of RDS are controversial. It can be administered prophylactically within minutes after birth, or as a rescue treatment after the signs and symptoms of RDS manifest. Both prophylactic and early rescue treatments (within 2 h after birth) have comparable outcomes [66]. Recent studies have supported initial CPAP therapy without prophylactic surfactant administration in managing RDS in ELBW infants [67]. There is a high CPAP failure rate in these infants, especially those born at or below 26 weeks of gestation. If the infant needs endotracheal intubation for resuscitation or due to respiratory failure, surfactant should be administered. Despite the early use of surfactant, the incidence of BPD has not changed. This might be due to structural immaturity of the premature lungs and the lung injury caused by PPV. To minimize mechanical ventilation and hence lung injury leading to BPD, INSURE technique (intubation, surfactant, and rapid extubation to CPAP) has been proposed [68]. But ELBW infants have a high failure rate with INSURE and may need continued invasive mechanical ventilation. To completely avoid ET intubation and PPV, recently studies have used a thin catheter or a feeding tube inserted into the trachea under direct visualization and administering surfactant in the spontaneously breathing infant. These minimally invasive surfactant treatment or less invasive surfactant administration techniques (MIST and LISA) have shown improved short-term outcomes, but no difference in the long-term outcome of BPD [69–73].

Golden hour (Fig. 29.2). The phrase "The Golden Hour" is a term borrowed from emergency and cardiovascular medicine and refers to the first hour of an infant's life following delivery. During this time period of an infant's life, there is a profound and critical transition period of adaptation that takes place. Analyses of videotaped resuscitations suggest that management during this period of transition in very low birth-weight infants may impact long-term outcomes, and that care during this time frame should be optimized. Components of "Golden hour" for ELBW infants should include thermoregulation, respiratory management (judicious oxygen use, establish and maintain FRC: CPAP and early surfactant administration), early intravenous access for initiation of glucose and amino acid infusions and early administration of antibiotics where indicated. Quality improvement initiatives following the golden hour approach have shown improvements in outcomes such as admission temperature, BPD, and ROP in ELBW infants [74–76].

Management of RDS

ELBW infants with RDS may require respiratory support ranging from nasal cannula oxygen to high-frequency ventilation. The following strategies in ELBW infants will help minimize volutrauma from mechanical ventilation and decrease the incidence of bronchopulmonary dysplasia.

Early caffeine therapy

Inadequate respiratory effort and drive can contribute to failure of noninvasive ventilator strategies in ELBW infants. A loading dose of caffeine (10 mg/kg of caffeine base) should be administered as soon as possible (within an hour of birth preferably). The caffeine for apnea of prematurity trial showed a significantly less BPD in the caffeine group and is probably attributable to the less PPV in the infants in the caffeine group [77]. Two small RCTs showed caffeine administration with in first few minutes compared to first 2 h showed improved short-term respiratory outcomes in the early caffeine group [78,79].

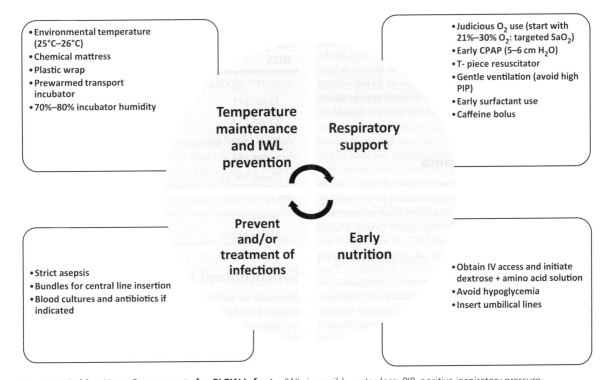

- Environmental temperature (25°C–26°C)
- Chemical mattress
- Plastic wrap
- Prewarmed transport incubator
- 70%–80% incubator humidity

Temperature maintenance and IWL prevention

- Judicious O_2 use (start with 21%–30% O_2: targeted SaO_2)
- Early CPAP (5–6 cm H_2O)
- T- piece resuscitator
- Gentle ventilation (avoid high PIP)
- Early surfactant use
- Caffeine bolus

Respiratory support

Prevent and/or treatment of infections

- Strict asepsis
- Bundles for central line insertion
- Blood cultures and antibiotics if indicated

Early nutrition

- Obtain IV access and initiate dextrose + amino acid solution
- Avoid hypoglycemia
- Insert umbilical lines

Fig. 29.2 **Golden Hour Components for ELBW Infants.** *IWL*, insensible water loss; *PIP*, positive inspiratory pressure.

only if the infant is having frequent apneas or if respiratory acidosis worsens. We start with NIPPV rate of 40 breaths/min and peak inspiratory pressure of 20–24 cmH$_2$O and wean based on blood gases. As most of the currently available NIPPV devices are nonsynchronized, we recommend weaning the rate and attempt CPAP once the infant has been stable on a rate of 20 breaths/min.

Neurally adjusted ventilatory assist. Neurally adjusted ventilatory assist (NAVA) is a newer mode of synchronized ventilation that can be applied for both invasive and noninvasive forms of ventilation. NAVA delivers ventilatory assistance proportional to the respiratory effort and in synchrony to the patient's effort [97]. A catheter inserted in the esophagus measures the electrical activity of the diaphragm (Edi) and relays it to the ventilator. Ventilator then delivers synchronous breath with the electrical activity (once the Edi crosses the trigger level) and proportional to the Edi. The pressure delivered is derived by the formula: NAVA level × (Edi signal − Edi min) + PEEP. When the Edi signal has fallen to 70% of its peak value, the patient is allowed to exhale and the ventilator no longer offers any assist until the next breath is initiated and the trigger level is again reached. Hence the delivered pressure, inspiratory time and respiratory rate are determined by the infant. Studies have shown that NAVA improved patient–ventilator synchrony and improved short-term

outcomes (lower FiO$_2$, decreased frequency and duration of desaturations, lower PIP), but studies on long-term outcomes are lacking [98–100].

Management/prevention of nonrespiratory complications in ELBW infants

Preterm and acutely ill infants are at risk of stress from overstimulation in the NICU. Repeated handling for procedures and assessments/interventions can decrease hemodynamic stability and result in significant physiologic consequences such as blood pressure changes, alterations in cerebral blood flow, hypoxia, and other stress behaviors. Rest periods of less than 60 min duration are ineffective and insufficient for the infant to complete a normal sleep cycle. Biorhythmic balance and physiologic homeostasis is essential for optimal outcome. The goal of a NICU caregiver is to alter the environment and caregiver stressors that interfere with physiologic stability, promote individual neurobehavioral organization and maturation, conserve energy, teach parents to interpret infant behavior, and identify stressors and promote infant–parent interaction and caregiving.

We use following general guidelines in our unit for management of ELBW infants

Daily bedside care	Guidelines
General care	• All patients ≤1000 g should have a stop sign placed on a porthole of isolette to remind staff about minimum stimulation and hand hygiene • Gloves after hand hygiene are to be used prior to any patient or line contact • All care should be clustered and done twice a shift unless medically necessary to intervene otherwise. All other disciplines involved in the care of the infant (respiratory therapist, physical therapist) should be informed at the beginning of the shift of the touch times to coordinate care • All labs (heel sticks, peripheral sticks) should be coordinated • Monitor blood loss from labs • Monitor total daily intake (consider flushes and medications) • Monitor urine output closely • Monitor for hypernatremia, hyponatremia, and hyperkalemia (Target Na$^+$ levels: 135–145 meq/L: Target K$^+$ levels: 3.5–5.5 meq/L) • Monitor for labile blood glucose (target glucose levels 60–150 mg/dL) • Weigh infant daily • Maintaining thermoregulation should be done safely and consistently • Kangaroo care is encouraged and should be part of care • Infants should only be bathed every 4 days. Use only sterile water to clean skin • Oral care • Isolettes will be changed out once a week and reservoir cleaned. Filter to be changed when isolettes are cleaned

Daily bedside care	Guidelines
Skin care	Prevent or minimize skin breakdown by • Use water-based gel leads • Protect skin with a pectin-based barrier for taping intravenous lines, endotracheal tubes and temperature probes • Minimize tape use • Avoid adhesives and adhesive enhancements • Avoid using alcohol
Temperature	Minimize insensible water loss and maintain a thermoneutral environment by • Use of a prewarmed, double-walled isolette • Place the temperature probe on the lateral side of the abdomen (visible at all times) so that it can be repositioned without being removed • Set servo control on 36.5°C For hypothermic or extremely premature infants, the servo temperature may need to be increased above 36.5°C to rewarm the infant then weaned to standard range when normal skin temperature is obtained Use of a saran-wrap blanket or plastic tent for infant less than 1000 g if needed. Avoid saran-wrap contact with skin • Use humidity 80% and wean daily by 5%–10% • Prewarm linens, hands, and anything else that may touch the infant • Use portholes to provide care and to access infant instead of opening the top or side of the isolette • Room temperatures should be kept at 22–26°C (72–76°F) • Recommend using clear drapes when under a radiant heat source (heat can penetrate most clear drapes, but, not cloth or opaque drapes)
Respiratory support	• Protect the infant's airway and use caution when repositioning to avoid dislodgement. Always use "two for tubes rule" when turning patient or when providing kangaroo care (two caregivers to be present while changing infant's position or while moving the infant) • Wean oxygen, as tolerated, to avoid hyperoxia. Maintain SpO_2 between the prescribed target range • Humidify respiratory gases to minimize insensible water loss (37°C with 100% relative humidity) • Use consistent positioning during chest X-ray for tube placement • Minimize suctioning to only when indicated clinically • Monitor closely for changes in breathing, oxygenation, and ventilation (by observing chest wall movement and auscultating breath sounds) • Oxygen monitoring Target oxygen saturations 90%–95% with pulse ox alarm settings 85%–95%
Supportive care	• Mimic fetal positioning, provide close boundaries, facilitate hand to mouth movements, avoid rapid position changes for cerebral blood flow, turning slowly and gently • Consult physical therapist for help with positioning • Ensure only minimal handling and stimulation (use bed scale and clustered care), maintain low environmental noise levels (<45 dBA), maintain low light in the environment and protect eyes when lights are used, incorporate cycled lighting after 32 weeks, avoid strong scented items such as lotions and wipes • Teach parents how to use gentle touch and containment • Assess and treat pain. Provide comfort measures for mild–moderate procedures such as heel sticks

Neutral thermal environmental temperatures for ELBW infants

Age	Temperature	
	At start (°C)	Range (°C)
0–24 h	35.0	34.0–35.4
24–96 h	34.0	34.0–35.0
4–12 days	33.5	33.0–34.0
12–14 days	33.5	32.6–34.0
2–3 weeks	33.1	32.2–34
3–4 weeks	32.6	31.6–33.6

Smaller gestational age and younger infants require temperature at the higher end of the range within each category. Use humidity of 70%–80% in the first week of life and wean daily by 5%–10% after the first week to 40%.

Hemodynamic instability and neonatal shock

Shock is defined as a physiologic state characterized by tissue hypoxia due to reduced oxygen delivery and/or increased oxygen consumption or inadequate oxygen utilization. It is manifested by tissue hypoperfusion (e.g., cold extremities, acrocyanosis, and poor capillary refill), hypotension, and metabolic acidosis. Shock is often initially reversible but must be recognized and treated immediately to prevent progression to irreversible organ dysfunction. The etiology of neonatal shock can be organized based on the underlying pathogenesis: hypovolemic, distributive, cardiogenic, and obstructive shock. However, these processes are not mutually exclusive, and neonates with circulatory failure may have a combination of more than one form of shock.

Defining hypotension

There is no widely accepted definition of hypotension in extremely preterm infants. The wide range of observed BP values based on GA and postnatal age makes it challenging to determine hypotension based on a specific value. The graph below suggests blood pressure values for extremely preterm infants (<28 weeks of gestation) for the first 72 h of life (Fig. 29.4).

In our clinical practice, there is not a strict numerical threshold for defining hypotension. Antihypotensive therapy is considered for infants in whom a reliable BP trend is **inconsistent**

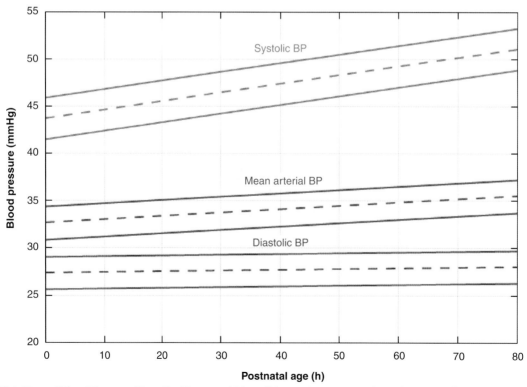

Fig. 29.4 Normal Blood Pressure (Systolic, Mean, and Diastolic) Based on Postnatal Age in ELBW Infants. The *dotted line* represents median and the solid lines represent 5th and 95th percentiles.

with expected physiological changes, or when the infant develops clinical or laboratory evidence of poor perfusion. As a result, BP values are monitored frequently (either continuously through a UAC or hourly with a BP cuff) in conjunction with ongoing assessment of peripheral perfusion.

Management of neonatal shock

Initial stabilization	Guidelines
Airway/ breathing	• Neonates in shock generally are in respiratory distress or are apneic and almost always require positive pressure ventilation, endotracheal intubation, and mechanical ventilation
Vascular access	• Vascular access should be established and blood samples obtained for initial testing • Central lines for frequent blood drawing and consistent vascular access should be considered
Fluid resuscitation	• Isotonic crystalloid infusion of 20 mL/ kg over 10–15 min • Further aggressive fluid resuscitation is generally needed for patients with hypovolemic or distributive shock • Excessive isotonic fluid administration (>30 mL/kg) in preterm infants is associated with an increased risk of death and intraventricular hemorrhage. As a result, assessing the response to the initial fluid bolus is important to determine if further fluid resuscitation is warranted
Other evaluation and measures	• A brief review of the history, physical examination • Basic laboratory tests (electrolytes, blood gas, complete blood count, lactate, blood culture, renal and liver function tests, and type and cross) • Chest radiograph, electrocardiogram, or echocardiography as necessary based on history and physician evaluation • Start empiric antibiotics after obtaining blood culture • Correct underlying hypothermia, electrolyte abnormalities, acidosis, and altered glucose homeostasis • Initiate appropriate therapies if suspected congenital heart disease, pneumothorax/tamponade, acute blood loss, suspected arrhythmias, etc.

Subsequent therapy. For patients who remain hypotensive despite adequate fluid resuscitation, vasoactive agents may be useful in restoring adequate tissue perfusion. Vasopressor therapy has little role in the management of patients with purely hemorrhagic or hypovolemic shock. Following table describes commonly used vasoactive agents in management of shock in ELBW infants. The pharmacokinetics of the various vasopressor agents are considerably more variable in neonates compared with older patients and it is challenging to accurately predict the effects of these medications on myocardial contractility, heart rate, and systemic vascular resistance. There are no definitive data demonstrating that one agent is more efficacious over another.

Vasopressor agents	Guidelines
Dopamine	• Dose dependent effect: 5–20 mcg/ kg/min • Infants with distributive shock who do not respond adequately to fluid resuscitation, dopamine should be infused beginning at a rate of 5 mcg/kg/min with titration up to a maximum of 20 mcg/kg/min • Dopamine can also be used for the management of cardiogenic shock • Dopamine clearance is much lower in patients with renal or hepatic failure, and careful titration is necessary
Dobutamine	• Dose: 5–20 mcg/kg/min • Increases cardiac output via improved myocardial contractility and increased HR • More useful for neonates with cardiogenic shock refractory to dopamine or epinephrine
Epinephrine	• Dose: 0.1–1 mcg/kg/min • Increases myocardial contractility and is a potent vasoconstrictor • Sometimes used for distributive shock that is refractory to dopamine or as a first-line vasoactive therapy for cardiogenic shock. • There are limited safety and efficacy data on epinephrine in neonates • Higher dose can increase myocardial oxygen consumption and worsen the outcomes

Vasopressor agents	Guidelines
Milrinone	• Dose: 0.25–0.75 mcg/kg/min • Safety and efficacy is not established in ELBW infants • Phosphodiesterase enzyme inhibitor which improves myocardial contractility and reduces afterload through systemic vasodilation • May be useful for some causes of cardiogenic shock and right ventricular dysfunction • Always use after ECHO and in consultation with pediatric cardiologist
Hydrocortisone	Dose: 0.5–1 mg/kg every 6–8 h Useful for neonates with distributive (particularly septic) or cardiogenic shock that is refractory to fluid resuscitation and vasoactive therapy May be useful for infants with known or suspected adrenal insufficiency Dose should be gradually tapered over a period of at least 7–10 days

Intraventricular hemorrhage

IVH in preterm infants has decreased in recent years in most neonatal centers. The incidence ranges from 20% to 30% of VLBW infants [101] and more frequently (~45%) seen in ELBW infants [102]. Majority of IVH occurs in the first 3 days after birth while more than 50% of them within first 24 h of life. The exact etiology remains unknown although poor cerebral autoregulation, germinal matrix with poor vascular support and increased fibrinolytic activity has been implicated. IVH is graded from 1 through 4. A grade 1 represents a subependymal hemorrhage while a grade 2 involves IVH without ventricular dilatation. A grade 3 IVH has blood in the ventricle but with concomitant ventricular dilatation. The most severe is a grade 4 IVH in which there is extension of the bleed into the brain parenchyma [103]. Premature infants with moderate-to-severe IVH (grade 3–4) are at high risk of posthemorrhagic hydrocephalus, cerebral palsy, and mental retardation, while infants with mild IVH (grade 1–2) are at risk of developmental disabilities [104]. The use of antenatal steroids has reduced the incidence of severe grade 3 or grade 4 IVH. IVH prevention bundles comprising transport in utero, use of antenatal steroids, temperature regulation, midline head positioning for the first week of life, minimal handling of the infant, avoiding rapid fluid infusion, bicarbonate infusion, and fluctuations in blood pressures and PCO_2 have been implemented with success in some recent studies [105,106]. Grade 1 and 2 IVH can be monitored clinically, whereas grade 3/4 IVH should be monitored closely with daily head circumference measurements and weekly to biweekly neurosonograms. Once significant hydrocephalus develops (defined as bifrontal index of >0.6 on head ultrasound), our practice is to place either a subgaleal shunt or ventricular access device for intermittent CSF removal. If the hydrocephalus does not resolve with these procedures, a ventricular-peritoneal shunt procedure is performed when the infant weights greater than 2 kg.

Retinopathy of prematurity

ROP is a developmental disease, which can be viewed as an arrest of normal retinal neuronal and vascular development in the preterm infant; this results in pathological compensatory mechanisms that result in aberrant vascularization of the retina and can progress to retinal detachment. Prematurity is the most important risk factor for ROP [107]. The incidence of ROP is over 80% in infants less than 1000 g. The incidence of blindness approaches 10% [108]. The international classification of ROP defines the location by zones, the extent by clock hours, and the severity by stages. Special pathologic features are defined by the terms plus disease and threshold disease [109]. The risk factors such as prematurity, hyperoxemia, hyperglycemia, sepsis, low IGF-1, blood transfusions, and poor postnatal weight gain have been implicated in development of ROP. The only effective prophylaxis for ROP is the prevention of prematurity. Meticulous oxygen monitoring has not provided a complete solution and various supplements such as vitamin E and selenium therapy have not proven effective [110]. All infants born less than 31 weeks of gestation should have an eye examination regardless of oxygen requirement. The first eye exam occurs at 31 weeks postmenstrual age or at 4 weeks chronologic age, whichever is later. Frequency of eye examinations depends on the severity and rate of progression of retinopathy [111].

Retinopathy of prematurity screening protocol [111]

Gestational age at birth (weeks)	Age at initial examination (weeks)	
	Postmenstrual	Chronologic
22	31	9
23	31	8
24	31	7
25	31	6
26	31	5
27	31	4

Gestational age at birth (weeks)	Age at initial examination (weeks)	
	Postmenstrual	Chronologic
28	32	4
29	33	4
30	34	4
Older gestational age, high-risk factors		4

Patent ductus arteriosus

Patent ductus arteriosus (PDA) is another common complication of ELBW infants. The ductus arteriosus represents an embryological connection between the aorta and pulmonary artery. This duct remains open after the first 5 days of life in 50% of all ELBW infants, often with increasing oxygen requirements and acidosis [112]. Infants can present with bounding pulses, wide pulse pressure, and a classic machinery-type murmur due to augmentation of a left-to-right shunt resulting in increased pulmonary blood flow [113]. Prostaglandin inhibitors such as indomethacin and ibuprofen are mainstay of medical management. These medications constrict the smooth muscle of the ductus arteriosus. However, dilemma in selecting appropriate patients with clinically significant PDA continues due to lack of evidence and potential adverse effects of current treatment [114,115]. The efficacy of this treatment is greater when initiated within 10 days of life. As with many medications, complications with prostaglandin inhibitors include thrombocytopenia and impaired renal function. Prostaglandin inhibitors may further decrease blood flow to the bowel and some studies have reported a higher incidence of spontaneous intestinal perforations and other GI symptoms with this treatment, especially when used in conjunction with corticosteroids [116,117]. Surgical closure of hemodynamically significant PDA is reserved for those infants who did not respond or would not be a candidate for medical management with deteriorating clinical status often with increasing ventilator requirements because of increased pulmonary blood flow. Adverse effects include left vocal cord paralysis [118] and postcardiac ligation syndrome of unknown etiology, causing myocardial dysfunction, and systemic hypotension requiring inotropic support in the immediate postoperative period [119,120]. Less invasive interventional catheter closure of PDA techniques have been showing promise in management of ELBW infants with better tolerance of procedure, less likelihood of postcardiac ligation syndrome and

improved postop respiratory outcomes; however, safety and efficacy of these procedures are not well established in ELBW infants [121,122]. Our NICU does not have a fixed protocol for the management of PDA. Our general principle is to treat PDA medically, preferably after 7 days of life (to allow for spontaneous closure), if it is moderate to large in size and is symptomatic (e.g., mechanical ventilator dependency, pulmonary edema, pulmonary hemorrhage, impaired renal function). We do not treat PDA regardless of the size or echocardiogram findings, if the infant is asymptomatic.

Sepsis (Fig. 29.5)

Sepsis remains one of the most common causes of neonatal morbidity and mortality in the preterm population. It is defined as any bacterial infection with systemic manifestations, documented by a positive blood culture. Neonatal sepsis can be classified into two categories based on postnatal age at onset: Early onset less than 7 days and late onset greater than 7 days. The incidence of sepsis varies between 1 and 8 cases per thousand live births. Prevalence increases inversely with lower gestational age affecting 25–40% of ELBW infants. Mortality rates are 10%–30%. Currently, group B streptococcus, gram-negative bacilli and *Listeria monocytogenes* are most commonly associated with early onset sepsis, whereas enterococcus, coagulase-negative staphylococcus, and gram-negative bacilli are more frequently responsible for late onset sepsis. Most episodes of early onset sepsis are caused by an ascending infection or acquired during vaginal delivery from bacteria colonizing the mother's genital tract. The bacteria causing late onset disease may be transmitted either vertically during the peripartum period or horizontally from colonized caregivers [123]. Inadequate handwashing can be a major source for the spread of microorganisms from one patient to another [124]. The use of ETs, central venous, and arterial lines and Foley catheters also significantly increase the risk for neonatal infection. Leucopenia/leukocytosis, band/segmented neutrophil ratio of >0.2, low absolute neutrophil count, thrombocytopenia, or elevation of acute phase reactants such as CRP, procalcitonin, IL-6 could suggest an infectious process [125,126]. A blood culture is the gold standard to diagnose neonatal sepsis. If the clinical signs and symptoms are suggesting meningitis or if the blood cultures are positive, a lumbar puncture should always be performed. When the clinical suspicion of sepsis is high, empiric antimicrobial therapy should be started immediately after obtaining the appropriate culture specimens. The choice of empiric therapy is based on several factors including time and setting of the disease, microorganism frequency and susceptibility in NICU, the site of the suspected infection and penetration of the specific antibiotic to that site, and hepatic and/or renal dysfunction. In the United States,

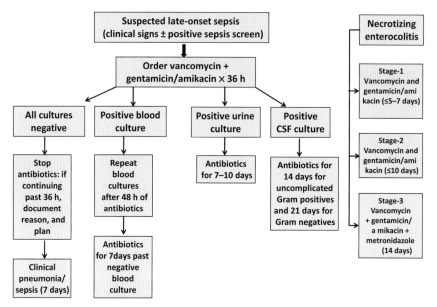

Fig. 29.5 Antibiotic Algorithm for Suspected Late-Onset Sepsis in ELBW Infants.

the most common pathogens responsible for early-onset neonatal sepsis are GBS and *Escherichia coli* [127]. A combination of ampicillin and an aminoglycoside (usually gentamicin) is generally used as initial therapy, and this combination of antimicrobial agents also has synergistic activity against GBS and *L. monocytogenes* [128,129]. Third-generation cephalosporins such as cefotaxime represent a reasonable alternative to an aminoglycoside. However, several studies have reported rapid development of resistance when cefotaxime has been used routinely for the treatment of early-onset neonatal sepsis [130] and extensive/prolonged use of third-generation cephalosporins is a risk factor for invasive candidiasis [131]. Because of its excellent CSF penetration, empirical or therapeutic use of cefotaxime should be restricted for use in infants with meningitis attributable to gram-negative organisms [132]. Evidence-based data has demonstrated a strong relationship between antenatal/postnatal infection and subsequent brain damage in both preterm and term infants. Through a cytokine-mediated pathway, white matter is especially vulnerable in the infant exposed to infection. PVL can result in spastic diplegia and other significant neurodevelopmental disabilities [133]. Figure 29.5 shows our algorithm for suspected late-onset sepsis. Each unit should develop their own algorithm based on local epidemiology and antibiograms. We do not routinely use antifungal prophylaxis in our extremely premature neonates, as the incidence of fungal infections is very low in our NICU. Antifungal prophylaxis with fluconazole may have a role in units with high incidence of systemic fungal infections.

Necrotizing enterocolitis

NEC is an inflammatory process resulting from a complex interaction of multiple factors in preterm infants that results in mucosal injury caused by ischemia, necrosis, and the host response to that injury [134]. The loss of mucosal integrity allows passage of bacteria and their toxins into the bowel wall and then into the systemic circulation, resulting in a generalized inflammatory response and overwhelming sepsis in the severe forms of NEC [135,136]. The incidence of NEC is approximately 10% of all NICU admissions [137]. The onset of NEC symptoms usually present around 3 weeks of life, [138]. Mortality can be as high as 40% despite vigorous therapy. Gut immaturity, infection, inflammatory mediators, ischemia, and enteral feeds have all been associated with NEC, although the etiology remains elusive despite significant research [134]. Breast milk feeding reduces the incidence of NEC; however, exclusively breastfed infants have occasionally developed NEC. Bell et al. used a combination of clinical and radiographic diagnostic bedside criteria, which could be used to gauge the severity of NEC [139]. Modified Bell's criteria have extensively been used to describe various stages of NEC [140]. Stage 1 includes nonspecific symptoms such as lethargy, hypothermia, irritability, vomiting, abdominal distention, apnea, bile stain residuals, and bloody stools. Peritoneal signs such as abdominal distention, tenderness, and guarding are frequently observed. Hallmark of stage 2 is pneumatosis intestinalis appearing as soap bubbles or linear intramural streaks on X-ray, especially in the right lower quadrant of preterm infants and is pathognomonic of NEC. Stage 3 denotes free abdominal air secondary to intestinal perforation. Portal air, which represents tracking of air through the bowel wall along the mesenteric vessels and into the portal system, can be associated with NEC. The presence of thrombocytopenia and metabolic acidosis is highly suggestive of necrotic bowel. Definitive NEC may require medical or surgical management based on the clinical presentation. Medical intervention typically includes abdominal decompression, bowel rest, broad-spectrum intravenous antibiotics, and parenteral nutrition. We typically give bowel rest for 2–5 days for stage 1 NEC and 10 days for stage 2 NEC. Surgical interventions are generally required in patients with intestinal perforation, fixed dilated bowel loop, or deteriorating clinical or biochemical status (e.g., shock or a decreasing platelet count, neutrophil count, or both). Surgical procedures may involve drain placement, exploratory laparotomy with resection of diseased bowel, and enterostomy with creation of a stoma. Surgical management has changed over the last decade [141]. More often than not peritoneal drain placement is preferred to stabilize these critically ill infants before considering surgery [142]. Late complications of NEC include intestinal strictures, bowel obstruction, and malabsorption. A certain amount of small intestine is necessary for survival. Short-gut syndrome is not uncommon and full recovery can take months to years.

Fluids, electrolytes, and nutrition management

Premature ELBW infants require careful fluid, electrolyte, and nutritional management. Excess fluid intake in the first few days of life increases the incidence of BPD and PDA, whereas inadequate fluid intake results in hypovolemia, hypersomolarity, metabolic abnormalities, and renal failure. The following are the general principles we recommend in ELBW infants.

Fluids

We suggest an initial fluid intake for ELBW infants cared in humidified incubator between 80 and 100 mL/kg/day. For extremely immature infant born at 23–24 weeks of gestation and infants exposed to radiant heat for extended periods, fluids may be initiated at 120 mL/kg/day. Fluids should be adjusted based on daily weights and serum sodium changes. Increase the fluid intake in increments of 10–20 mL/kg/day for hypernatremia (serum Na > 145 meq/L) or rapidly raising serum sodium. The table shows our suggested initial and

subsequent parenteral nutrition initiation and advancement guidelines.

Initial fluid goals by birth weight (g)	Fluid (mL/kg/day)	Dextrose solution	Glucose infusion rate (mg/kg/min)
<600	140	D5W	4.9
601–800*	120	D7.5W	6.25
801–1200	100	D7.5W	5.2
1201–1800	100	D10W	6.75
1801–2500	90	D10W	6.25
>2500	80	D10W	5.5

Parenteral nutrition initiation and advancement guidelines

Glucose	Initial GIR of 4–6 mg/kg/min and advance by 1–2 mg/kg/min/day to a goal of 12 mg/kg/min. Serum glucose goal 60–150 mg%
Protein	Initiate at 3 g/kg/day and advance by 0.5–1 g/kg/day to a goal of 3.5 g/kg/day
Lipids	Start at 0.5–1 g/kg/day and advance by 1 g/kg/day to a goal of 3 g/kg/day. Goal serum TG < 200 mg%
Sodium (Na)	Do not add Na to fluids on the first day; wait until 48 h when Na begins to fall. Na⁺ is usually given as NaCl, but sodium acetate may be used to decrease metabolic acidosis from renal bicarbonate wasting in ELBW infants. Usual maintenance for Na⁺ is 2–4 mEq/kg/day
Potassium (K)	Do not add K to IV fluids for the first 1–2 days after birth, until urine output is well established and serum K level starts to decline. K may be given as KCl or K-acetate. Usual maintenance for K is 1–3 mEq/kg/day
Calcium	Start at 2 meq/kg: advance to goal of 3 meq/kg/day
Phosphorous	Start at 1 mmol/kg. Advance to 1.5 mmol/kg: Ca:P molar ratio of 1.3
Goal parenteral calories	95–100 kcal/kg/day

Enteral feeding guidelines

Birth weight (g)	Beginning enteral feeds (first feed by 6–48 h)	Feeding method	Beginning volume	Increase by (increments)
<750	HM (EBM/DBM*) or preterm formula 24 cal	Enteral feeding q4 h (3 h continuous and 1 h off)	Trophic feeds 10 mL/kg/day for 3 days—bolus as small volumes for pump	10 mL/kg/day everyday up to a full enteral volume of 150 mL/kg/day
751–1000	HM (EBM/DBM) or preterm formula 24 cal**		10 mL/kg/day	10 mL/kg/day everyday up to a full enteral volume of 150 mL/kg/day
1001–1500	HM (EBM/DBM) or Preterm formula 24 cal		15 mL/kg/day	15 mL/kg/day everyday to a full enteral volume of 150 mL/kg/day

*Use of DBM needs consent from mother or legal guardian.
**High protein preterm formula should be considered for infants <1000 g.

- All human milk feeds to be fortified when enteral feeding volume reaches 40 mL/kg/day.
- Add liquid protein to target enteral protein goal of 4–4.5 gm/kg/day, when off TPN.
- *Do not* check for residuals between feeds unless clinical signs of abdominal distension/emesis/discoloration/tenderness. Keep feeding tube vented to air between feeds when on continuous feeds (3 h on and 1 h off).
- When restarting feeds after brief period of NPO status (<48 h), try to resume feeds at last stopped volume.
- Use minimal enteral feeding (MEF) as much as possible, even if on pressor low dose, PDA treatment, blood transfusion, and so on. Physician discretion recommended.

Water and electrolyte homeostasis in newborn infants is influenced by physiologic adaptations following birth and developmental effects on the distribution of total body water and water loss. Fluid and electrolyte therapy must account for these factors in determining maintenance requirements and correction of any abnormalities.

Hypokalemia

Hypokalemia is defined as a serum potassium level of less than 3.5 mEq/L. It rarely a cause for concern until the serum potassium level is less than 3.0 mEq/L. It usually results from excessive losses of potassium. Common contributing factors include chronic diuretic use, renal tubular defects, or significant output from a nasogastric tube or ileostomy. It is usually asymptomatic; however, it can cause weakness and paralysis, ileus, urinary retention, and conduction defects detected on the electrocardiogram (Fig. 29.6—e.g., ST segment depression, low-voltage T waves, and U waves). It should be corrected by increasing potassium supplementation by 1–2 mEq/kg/day. In severe or symptomatic hypokalemia, KCl (0.5–1 mEq/kg) is infused intravenously over 1 h with continuous ECG monitoring. Rapid administration of potassium chloride is not recommended, because it is associated with life-threatening cardiac dysfunction.

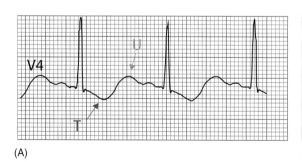

(A)

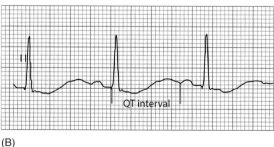

(B)

Fig. 29.6 Changes in EKG Associated With Hypokalemia in Lead V4 (A) and Lead II (B).

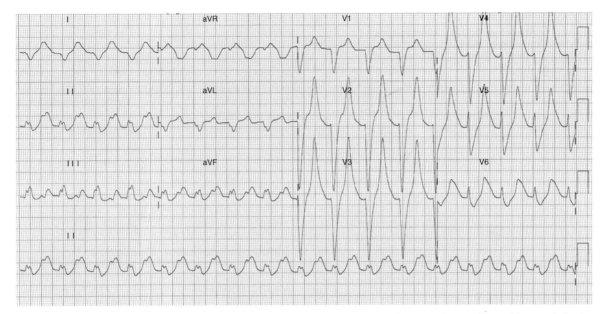

Fig. 29.7 **EKG Showing Prolonged PR Interval, Broad QRS Complexes, and Peaked T Waves in an Infant With Hyperkalemia.**

Hyperkalemia (Fig. 29.7)

Hyperkalemia is defined as a serum potassium level of greater than 6 mEq/L measured in a nonhemolyzed specimen. Hyperkalemia is a potentially life threatening condition that is most commonly seen in the first few days of life in ELBW infants or infants with impaired renal functions. The risk factors need to be identified early and prompt treatment should be offered to aviod rapid deterioration in clinical status, cardiac arrhythmias, and/or death.

Risk factors for hyperkalemia in the neonate include: extreme prematurity (<27 weeks of gestation), low systemic blood flow, acute renal failure (most commonly perinatal asphyxia), sepsis, IVH, hemolysis secondary to ABO/Rh incompatibilities, excessive skin bruising, postblood transfusion, severe metabolic acidosis, type IV RTA, and so on. Suggestions to account for this phenomenon include potassium shifts from the intracellular to extracellular phase, oliguria, immaturity of the renal tubular mechanisms for potassium secretion and a reduced glomerular filtration rate.

EKG changes in hyperkalemia

Hyperkalemia severity	EKG changes
Mild (5.5–6.6 meq/L)	Peaked T wave Prolonged PR interval
Moderate (6.5–8 meq/L)	Loss of P wave Prolonged QRS complex S–T segment elevation

Hyperkalemia severity	EKG changes
Severe (>8 meq/L)	Progressive widening of QRS complexes High-grade AV block, bundle branch blocks and fascicular blocks Sine wave Ventricular tachycardia and fibrillation

In nonhemolyzed blood, potassium level	Management
Serum potassium > 5.5 meq/L but <6 meq/L without ECG changes and infant is asymptomatic	Monitor clinically; correct acidosis; stop all potassium supplementation; stop all medications causing hyperkalemia; cardiac monitoring
Serum potassium > 6 meq/L but <7 meq/L without ECG changes and infant is asymptomatic	Same as above. In addition, monitor K^+ 1–2 hourly using blood gas analyzer

In nonhemolyzed blood, potassium level	Management
Serum potassium > 7 meq/L with normal ECG	Same as above In addition: administration of intravenous glucose and insulin (0.05 units/kg human regular insulin with 2 mL/kg 10% dextrose in water), followed by a continuous infusion of insulin (0.1 units/kg/h with 2–4 mL/kg/h 10% dextrose in water) If K$^+$ rise persists: albuterol nebulization over 20 min (repeat as necessary) Increase urinary excretion with intravenous administration of furosemide (1 mg/kg/dose) in infants with adequate renal function
Arrhythmias	Same as above In addition, give immediately IV 10% calcium gluconate (100 mg/kg/dose) as a push over 1–2 min with EKG monitoring Correct acidosis: give bicarbonate (4.2% NaHCO$_3$) (0.5 meq/mL) Dose (meq) = weight [kg] × base deficit × 0.3 (typical dose 1–2 mEq/kg over 30–60 min) Give calcium gluconate before bicarbonate
Refractory hyperkalemia	Same as above Organize transfer to tertiary center Discuss peritoneal dialysis Pediatric nephrology consult

Neonatal hyperglycemia

It is often defined as blood glucose >125 mg/dL (6.9 mmol/L) or plasma glucose >150 mg/dL (8.3 mmol/L). However, these levels are frequently observed and may not require intervention. Most clinicians become concerned about hyperglycemia when plasma glucose concentration exceeds 180–200 mg/dL (10–11.1 mmol/L). However, higher levels of hyperglycemia are required to produce the hyperosmolality and osmotic diuresis that may be clinically important. Plasma osmolality increases by 1 mosmol/L for each 18 mg/dL increase in plasma glucose concentration. Hyperglycemia typically occurs when a newborn cannot adapt to parenteral glucose infusion by decreasing endogenous glucose production or increasing peripheral glucose uptake. This is usually related to an associated clinical condition such as extreme prematurity or sepsis.

Our management guideline for hyperglycemia in ELBW infants is described below.

Blood glucose levels	Management
If blood glucose level is >10 mmol/L (180 mg/dL)	Check urine for glucose (very low birth weight infants may have a lower renal threshold for glucose and are at an increased risk of osmotic diuresis related to hyperglycemia so checking for glycosuria at a lower glucose level may be prudent in these infants) Document the glucose intake in mg/kg/min Draw a lab sample to confirm hyperglycemia, but do not delay treatment
If the blood glucose level is 1. persistently (minimum of 2 samples 4 h apart) ≥ 11.1 mmol/L (200 mg/dL), or 2. persistently (minimum of 2 samples 4 h apart) ≥ 10 mmol/L (180 mg/dL) with persistent (2 samples) glycosuria	Consider decreasing glucose infusion rate (GIR) to 4–6 mg/kg/min by decreasing volume and/or concentration. We do not recommend to infuse lower concentration fluid than D5W due to potential for hypoosmolarity and cerebral edema Consider starting Insulin treatment Initial therapy: bolus of insulin via a syringe pump over 15 min as a dose between 0.05 and 0.1 units/kg The blood glucose level is monitored every 30–60 min, and if it remains elevated, the insulin dose is repeated as a bolus every 4–6 h

Blood glucose levels Management

If the glucose level remains elevated after three bolus doses, a continuous infusion is considered

Continuous infusion: 0.01 and 0.05 units/kg/h

Adjust in small increments up to a maximum rate of 0.1 units/kg/hour to maintain glucose levels of 150–200 mg/dL (8.3–11 mmol/L)

The blood glucose concentration should be monitored within 30 min–1 h of the start of the infusion and after any change in the rate of glucose or insulin infusion. Glucose concentration should be monitored hourly until stable, and then less frequently.

Infusion rates are decreased in increments of 0.01–0.05 units/kg/hour in response to glucose levels < 150 mg/dL (8.33 mmol/L). Insulin infusion can be discontinued when the glucose level remains stable below 150 mg/dL (8.33 mmol/L) at the lowest infusion rate.

Plastic tubing used for infusion should be primed with insulin for at least 20 min before treatment because insulin nonspecifically binds to the tubing, resulting in decreased availability to the patient.

Outcomes of ELBW infants

The mortality of ELBW infants has dramatically declined over the last 50 years due to medical innovations in the management of neonates, particularly those born preterm. However, we are still struggling to achieve optimal respiratory and neurological outcomes in tiniest babies compared to their term counterparts [143,144]. Even though survival rates have reached a plateau in developed countries with significantly improved short-term morbidities in these infants [145]; a high prevalence of behavioral, emotional, and cognitive problems continue. Most outcome studies point to an inverse correlation with gestational age and birth weight. Other factors with negative correlations to outcome include intrauterine growth restriction, perinatal infections, BPD, severe IVH, PVL, posthemorrhagic ventricular dilatation, surgical NEC, PDA, low socioeconomic status, and low level of maternal education and schooling.

The incidence of sudden infant death syndrome (SIDS) is 3 times higher in ELBW infants compared to term infants. This is more prevalent in infants with severe BPD [146,147]. Fifty percent of ELBW infants require readmission to hospital within the first 2 years and continue to need home health services for a decade [148]. Respiratory symptoms, such as wheezing, are common in childhood and airway obstructive limitations are observable to adulthood. Hypertension, gastroesophageal reflux and growth problems are prevalent in the first years. Though most ELBW do achieve normal growth and even approximate their genetic potential, their overall physical stature will be toward the lower range for height and weight [149,150]. The prevalence of cerebral palsy is estimated at 8.5%, with 4.4% nonambulatory at 18–24 months. Hypotonia, minor motor incoordination, language, and developmental delays are common diagnoses impacting on mobility, function, and participation in social activities. A 20-year review of extremely preterm infants with birth weight less than 500 g at our center, showed survival of 28.7%. Severe disability defined by the presence of at least one of the following was observed in 34% of surviving infants at 24 months: bilateral blindness, hearing impairment requiring amplification, cerebral palsy, or a mental developmental index (MDI) or psychomotor developmental index (PDI) score of less than 70 using the Bayley Scales of Infant Development II (BSID-II) and/or gross motor functional classification system $\geq$ III [151]. Subtle and nonspecific neurocognitive disorders have been observed in 50%–70% of nondisabled ELBW with normal intelligence, often emerging after starting school. These include disorders with language, visual processing, attention and executive functions, autism-spectrum disorders, attention deficit/hyperactivity disorders, and emotional disorders [149,152].

In summary, the take-home message regarding ELBW infants remains cautious optimism. We have come a long way in last few years and outcomes have significantly improved for these extremely preterm infants at the edge of viability. It is very heartening to know that more and more ELBW infants continue to survive today and participate in society alongside their term-born peers. Their indescribable struggle and sheer exhibition of resilience toward productive and meaningful life deserve our standing ovation.

Clinical cases

Case 1

A 22-year-old G1 P0 mother presented with preterm labor with cervical dilation of 4 cm at 25 weeks of gestation. She received good prenatal care and pregnancy was uneventful. She was started on a betamethasone course, magnesium sulfate for neuroprotection and tocolytics. Labor progressed and a 650-g female infant was delivered by vaginal route 3 days later. NICU team was present in the delivery room. Delivery room temperature was increased prior to delivery to 26°C, radiant warmer was turned on, and all equipment were checked. Infant cried immediately after birth. She was covered with a prewarmed blanket and cord clamping was delayed for 1 min while monitoring heart rate. After the cord was clamped, she was brought to the radiant warmer and placed on a chemical warming mattress and covered with a polythene wrap. Airway was positioned (slight neck extension-sniffing position) and cleared with a suction catheter. Simultaneously, temperature probe and pulse oximeter probe were placed. After these initial steps, infant's heart rate was >100/min, she was spontaneously breathing, but with severe subcostal and intercostal retractions. CPAP of 5 cmH$_2$O was applied via mask and infant's preductal SpO$_2$ and heart rate were monitored. Supplemental O$_2$ was started at 30% and gradually increased to 60% to achieve target SpO$_2$. Infant's work of breathing slowly improved but still was requiring 60% O$_2$ and had significant retractions at 10 min of life. Infant was electively intubated and surfactant was administered. After surfactant administration, FiO$_2$ improved to 0.3. PPV was continued with PIP of 16 cmH$_2$O, PEEP of 5 cmH$_2$O, and a rate of 40/min. Infant was transported to the NICU in a prewarmed transport incubator. In the NICU, infant was placed in an incubator with humidity of 80% and on conventional ventilator, assist control, volume guarantee mode. Initial settings were tidal volume of 3.2 mL (5 mL/kg), PEEP: 5 cmH$_2$O, rate: 40/min, T_i: 0.35 s, and a peak pressure limit of 22 cmH$_2$O. Umbilical venous and arterial lines were placed and labs including blood culture were drawn. D5W starter TPN (3 g% trophamine and 10 meq/L of calcium) was started at 100 mL/kg/day along with intralipids at 0.5 g/kg/day. Initial blood glucose was 50 mg% and the first blood gas was 7.30/50/70/−3. Infant was given a loading dose of caffeine (20 mg/kg) and started on maintenance caffeine (8 mg/kg/day). Blood gases were repeated every 8 h and rate was weaned to 30 and further down to 20/min. Peak pressure remained below 16 cmH$_2$O, MAP measured on the ventilator was about 9 cmH$_2$O and FiO$_2$ requirements were <0.3. At about 24 h of life, infant was extubated to CPAP of 5 cmH$_2$O. Infant remained on CPAP for another 2 weeks. PEEP was increased to 6 on D3 of life for increasing FiO$_2$ requirements, which was later weaned slowly down to 4 cmH$_2$O. Infant was weaned to room air from CPAP and remained on room air till discharge. TPN was optimized to deliver calories of 100 kcal/kg/day. Feeds were started on Day 2 with mother's expressed breast milk at 10 mL/kg/day. Trophic feeds were continued for 2 days and then gradually advanced to a volume of 150 mL/kg/day. Human milk fortifier was added at feeding volume of 40 mL/kg/day. Bottle feeds were started at 33 weeks of corrected gestational age and infant was able to take all oral feeds by 37 weeks. Head ultrasound on day 7 of life showed a right grade 1 IVH and the one at 36 weeks of corrected gestational age was normal. ROP screening started at 31 weeks corrected gestational age and followed every 2 weeks showed stage 1 disease in Zone 2 at its worst, but normalized later. Infant was discharged home with parents at 37 weeks corrected gestational age.

Case 2

A 35-year-old G3 P2 mother presents to the emergency department in preterm labor at 24 weeks of gestation and delivers a 520-g male infant precipitously. The neonatal team was called emergently to the ED. Infant was delivered limp and was apneic. After initial steps of resuscitation, infant continued to be apneic and bradycardic (HR < 60/min). PPV was delivered with bag and mask (PIP: 18 cmH$_2$O, PEEP: 5 cmH$_2$O, and FiO$_2$: 0.3). Infant did not respond to increase in pressures and FiO$_2$. He was intubated with a 2.5-Fr ET and PPV continued via ETT. Heart rate and SpO$_2$ slowly improved, but infant was still requiring >80% O$_2$ (Fig. 29.8). He was brought to the NICU and placed on conventional ventilator: SIMV mode, PIP: 18 cmH$_2$O; PEEP: 5 cmH$_2$O, T_i: 0.35 s, and rate of 40/min. He required about 80% O$_2$ to maintain target O$_2$ saturations. Surfactant was administered with improvement in O$_2$ requirements to 30% (Fig. 29.9).

Initial blood gas showed respiratory acidosis (7.15/65/55/−4). After adjustments in respiratory rate and PIP, respiratory acidosis improved. FiO$_2$ gradually increased again to about 50% at 24 h of life and infant was given a second dose of surfactant. At around 3 days of life, infant's respiratory acidosis worsened (7.15/70/+4) and did not improve with escalation in PIP up to 24 cmH$_2$O and pressure volume loop on the ventilator graphics showed plateauing beyond PIP of 20 cmH$_2$O (Fig. 29.10).

Infant was switched to high-frequency oscillator (HFOV) with MAP of 14 cmH$_2$O, amplitude 30 and 14 Hz with

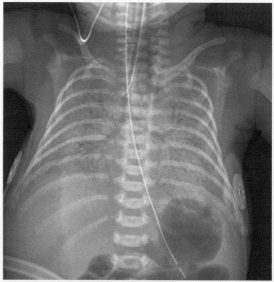

Fig. 29.8 Chest X-ray Showing Severe RDS With Air Broinchograms (Presurfactant Administration).

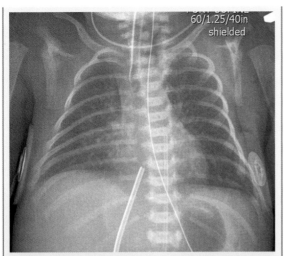

Fig. 29.9 Chest X-ray Showing Improved Aeration Postsurfactant Administration.

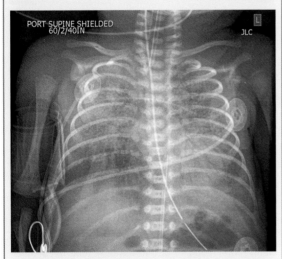

Fig. 29.10 Worsening of Lung Disease Necessitating Switching to High-Frequency Ventilation.

improvement in ventilation. HFOV settings were adjusted to achieve adequate lung expansion (8–10 ribs lung expansion) and target PCO_2. Infant remained on the HFOV at 3 weeks of life and ventilatory settings were unable to be weaned. He was on a MAP of 16 cmH_2O, amplitude of 40, frequency of 13 Hz, and 40% O_2. Based on the NICHD Neonatal Research Network BPD outcome calculator (https://neonatal.rti.org/index.cfm?fuseaction=bpdcalculator.start), this infant had a 70% probability of developing moderate-to-severe BPD. Hence, he was started on dexamethasone.

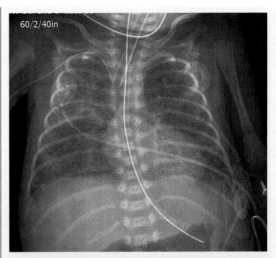

Fig. 29.11 Chest X-ray Showing Improved Aeration and Decreased Opacities After Starting Dexamethasone.

Neonatal BPD outcome estimator infants with GA 23–30 weeks and birth weight 501–1249 g

Time period	Ventilator type	FiO₂	Death	Severe BPD	Moderate BPD	Mild BPD	No BPD
Day 21	HF vent	40	20.2	29.1	42.6	7.5	0.6

Probability of outcome (expressed as a percent).

After starting steroids, ventilation and oxygenation improved and infant was extubated to NIPPV (PIP: 20 cmH_2O; PEEP: 7 cmH_2O; T_i: 0.5 s; rate: 40/min) after 5 days (Fig. 29.11). Over the next 4 weeks, infant was slowly weaned from NIPPV (rate was weaned by 5 every 2–3 days as tolerated to a rate of 10) to CPAP and subsequently to nasal cannula O_2 (starting at 4 L/min and weaned to 1 L) and room air. Infant was discharge home at 39 weeks corrected gestational age without any respiratory support.

Case 3

A 27-year-old G2 P1 mother presents with preterm premature rupture of membranes at 22 weeks of gestation. NICU team counseled the mother on the mortality, morbidity, and adverse neurodevelopmental outcomes associated with extreme prematurity. She wanted everything to be done for her infant if the she reaches 23 weeks of gestation. She developed chorioamnionitis at 23 weeks of gestation, went into preterm labor, and delivered a female infant weighing 420 g. Infant was resuscitated by the neonatal team with APGARs of 2 and 5 at 1 and 5 min of life. She was intubated

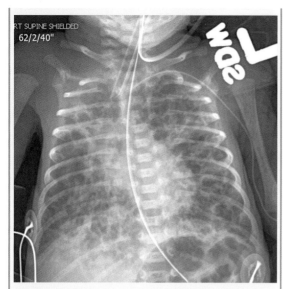

Fig. 29.12 **Chest X-ray Showing Severe Pulmonary Interstitial Emphysema in a 23-Week Preterm Infant.**

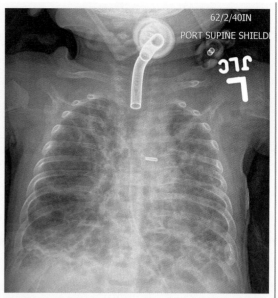

Fig. 29.13 **Chest X-ray Showing Changes of BPD With Areas of Atelectasis and Cystic Change.**

and given surfactant in the DR. She was brought to the NICU and placed on conventional ventilator: SIMV mode, PIP: 16 cmH$_2$O, PEEP: 5 cmH$_2$O, T_i: 0.3 s, and rate of 40. He required about 80% O$_2$ to maintain target O$_2$ saturations and was given 2 additional doses of surfactant (Poractant alfa) at 12 h intervals. After 24 h of life, infant could not be ventilated well on conventional ventilator and hence was transitioned to high-frequency oscillator (PCO$_2$ > 70 even at PIP of 25 cmH$_2$O and rate of 60/min). On the HFOV, she required high amplitude (>40) and lower frequency (12 Hz) for adequate ventilation. Oxygen requirement remained high at about 60%. Chest X-ray on D4 showed severe PIE (Fig. 29.12).

Infant was switched to HFJV and was maintained on the jet ventilator for 3 weeks with slight improvement in the PIE changes, but she remained on high pressures. She was given a course of dexamethasone (see the table for our unit protocol) with some improvement in ventilation, but still could not be weaned to extubation.

Dexamethasone course for BPD

Time	Dose	Frequency
Days 1–3	0.075 mg/kg/dose	12-hourly
Days 4–6	0.050 mg/kg/dose	12-hourly

Time	Dose	Frequency
Days 7 and 8	0.025 mg/kg/dose	12-hourly
Days 9 and 10	0.01 mg/kg/dose	12-hourly

At 8 weeks of life, infant was switched back to conventional ventilator, as she was uncomfortable on the jet ventilator. Despite good nutritional support and a second course of dexamethasone (6 weeks after the initial course), infant could not be weaned off mechanical ventilation. At 40 weeks corrected gestational age, tracheostomy and gastrostomy tube placements were performed (Fig. 29.13). Infant remained in the NICU on mechanical ventilation through the tracheostomy tube for another 2 months and was discharged home on home ventilation via tracheostomy (maximum ventilator settings after tracheostomy: PIP: 34 cmH$_2$O, PEEP: 7 cmH$_2$O, T_i: 0.45 s, rate: 30/min) (home ventilator settings: PIP: 26 cmH$_2$O, PEEP: 6 cmH$_2$O, T_i: 0.4 s, rate: 25/min, pressure support: 14 cmH$_2$O). Over the next several months, home ventilator pressures were gradually weaned and infant eventually came off mechanical ventilation at the age of 14 months.

References

[1] Behrman RE, Babson GS, Lessel R. Fetal and neonatal mortality in white middle class infants: mortality risks by gestational age and weight. Am J Dis Child 1971;121:486–489.

[2] Patel RM, Kandefer S, Walsh MC, Bell EF, Carlo WA, Laptook AR, et al. Causes and timing of death in extremely premature infants from 2000 through 2011. N Engl J Med 2015;372(4):331–340. (22).

[3] American College of Obstetricians and Gynecologists. Periviable birth. Obstetric care consensus no. 4. Obstet Gynecol 2016;127:e157–e169.

[4] Available from: https://www.nichd.nih.gov/about/org/der/branches/ppb/programs/epbo/pages/epbo_case.aspx.

[5] Carlo WA, McDonald SA, Fanaroff AA, Vohr BR, Stoll BJ, Ehrenkranz RA, et al. Association of antenatal corticosteroids with mortality and neurodevelopmental outcomes among infants born at 22 to 25 weeks' gestation. Eunice Kennedy Shriver National Institute of Child Health and Human Development Neonatal Research Network. JAMA 2011;306:2348–2358.

[6] Mori R, Kusuda S, Fujimura M. Antenatal corticosteroids promote survival of extremely preterm infants born at 22 to 23 weeks of gestation. Neonatal Research Network Japan. J Pediatr 2011;159. 110.e1–114.e1.

[7] Chawla S, Bapat R, Pappas A, Bara R, Zidan M, Natarajan G. Neurodevelopmental outcome of extremely premature infants exposed to incomplete, no or complete antenatal steroids. J Matern Fetal Neonatal Med 2013;26:1542–1547.

[8] Abbasi S, Oxford C, Gerdes J, Sehdev H, Ludmir J. Antenatal corticosteroids prior to 24 weeks' gestation and neonatal outcome of extremely low birth weight infants [published erratum appears in Am J Perinatol 2011;28:87–8]. Am J Perinatol 2010;27:61–66.

[9] Crowther CA, Hiller JE, Doyle LW, Haslam RR. Effect of magnesium sulfate given for neuroprotection before preterm birth: a randomized controlled trial. Australasian Collaborative Trial of Magnesium Sulphate (ACTOMg SO$_4$) Collaborative Group. JAMA 2003;290:2669–2676.

[10] Marret S, Marpeau L, Zupan-Simunek V, Eurin D, Leveque C, Hellot MF, et al. Magnesium sulphate given before very-preterm birth to protect infant brain: the randomized controlled PREMAG trial. PREMAG Trial Group. BJOG 2007;114:310–318.

[11] Rouse DJ, Hirtz DG, Thom E, Varner MW, Spong CY, Mercer BM, et al. A randomized, controlled trial of magnesium sulfate for the prevention of cerebral palsy. Eunice Kennedy Shriver NICHD Maternal-Fetal Medicine Units Network. N Engl J Med 2008;359:895–905.

[12] Marret S, Marpeau L, Follet-Bouhamed C, Cambonie G, Astruc D, Delaporte B, et al. Effect of magnesium sulphate on mortality and neurologic morbidity of the very-preterm newborn (of less than 33 weeks) with two-year neurological outcome: results of the prospective PREMAG trial. le groupe PREMAG [French]. Gynecol Obstet Fertil 2008;36:278–288.

[13] Doyle LW, Crowther CA, Middleton P, Marret S, Rouse D. Magnesium sulphate for women at risk of preterm birth for neuroprotection of the fetus. Cochrane Database Syst Rev 2009;1. CD004661.

[14] American College of Obstetricians and Gynecologists. Magnesium sulfate before anticipated preterm birth for neuroprotection. Committee opinion no. 455. Obstet Gynecol 2010;115:669–671.

[15] Silverman WA, Fertig JW, Berger A. The influence of the thermal environment upon the survival of newly born premature infants. Pediatrics 1958;22(5):876–886.

[16] Chang H-Y, Sung Y-H, Wang S-M, Lung H-L, Chang J-H, Hsu C-H, et al. Short- and long-term outcomes in very low birth weight infants with admission hypothermia. PLoS ONE 2015;10(7):e0131976.

[17] Gandy GM, Adamsons K Jr, Cunningham N, Silverman WA, James LS. Thermal environment and acid base homeostasis in human infants during the first few hours of life. J Clin Invest 1964;43:751–758.

[18] Lyon AJ, Freer Y. Goals and options in keeping preterm babies warm. Arch Dis Child Fetal Neonatal Ed 2011;96(1):F71–F74.

[19] Laptook AR, Salhab W, Bhaskar B. Neonatal Research Network. Admission temperature of low birth weight infants: predictors and associated morbidities. Pediatrics 2007;119(3).

[20] Vohra S, Frent G, Campbell V, Abbott M, Whyte R. Effect of polyethylene occlusive skin wrapping on heat loss in very low birth weight infants at delivery: a randomized trial. J Pediatr 1999;134(5):547–551.

[21] Laptook AR, Watkinson M. Temperature management in the delivery room. Semin Fetal Neonatal Med 2008;13:383–391.

[22] McCall EM, Alderdice FA, Halliday HL, Jenkins JG, Vohra S. Interventions to prevent hypothermia at birth in preterm and/or low birth weight infants. Cochrane Database Syst Rev 2010;(3). CD004210.

[23] Bhatt S, Alison BJ, Wallace EM, Crossley KJ, Gill AW, Kluckow M, et al. Delaying cord clamping until ventilation onset improves cardiovascular function at birth in preterm lambs. J Physiol 2013;591:2113–2126.

[24] Niermeyer S, Velaphi S. Promoting physiologic transition at birth: re-examining resuscitation and the timing of cord clamping. Semin Fetal Neonatal Med 2013;18:385–392.

[25] Raju TNK. Timing of umbilical cord clamping after birth for optimizing placental transfusion. Curr Opin Pediatr 2013;25:180–187.

[26] Rabe H, Diaz-Rossello JL, Duley L, Dowswell T. Effect of timing of umbilical cord clamping and other strategies to influence placental transfusion at preterm birth on maternal and infant outcomes. Cochrane Database Syst Rev 2012;(8). CD003248.

[27] Perlman JM, Wyllie J, Kattwinkel J, Wyckoff MH, Aziz K, Guinsburg R, et al. Part 7: Neonatal resuscitation: 2015 international consensus on cardiopulmonary resuscitation and emergency cardiovascular care science with treatment recommendations. Circulation 2015;132:S204–S241.

[28] Katheria AC, Brown MK, Faksh A, Hassen KO, Rich W, Lazarus D, et al. Delayed cord clamping in newborns born at term at risk for resuscitation: a feasibility randomized clinical trial. J Pediatr 2017;187:313–317.

[29] Rabe H, Jewison A, Alvarez RF, Crook D, Stilton D, Bradley R, et al. Milking

compared with delayed cord clamping to increase placental transfusion in preterm neonates: a randomized controlled trial. Obstetr Gynecol 2011;117(2 Pt 1):205–211.

[30] Upadhyay A, Gothwal S, Parihar R, Garg A, Gupta A, Chawla D, et al. Effect of umbilical cord milking in term and near term infants: randomized control trial. Am J Obstet Gynecol 2013;208(2):120.e1–120.e6.

[31] Katheria A, Blank D, Rich W, Finer N. Umbilical cord milking improves transition in premature infants at birth. PLoS ONE 2014;9:e94085.

[32] Dang D, Zhang C, Shi S, Mu X, Lv X, Wu H. Umbilical cord milking reduces need for red cell transfusions and improves neonatal adaptation in preterm infants: meta-analysis. J Obstet Gynaecol Res 2015;41(6):890–895.

[33] Katheria AC, Truong G, Cousins L, Oshiro B, Finer NN. Umbilical cord milking versus delayed cord clamping in preterm infants. Pediatrics 2015;136(1):61–69.

[34] Björklund LJ, Ingimarsson J, Curstedt T, John J, Robertson B, Werner O, et al. Manual ventilation with a few large breaths at birth compromises the therapeutic effect of subsequent surfactant replacement in immature lambs. Pediatr Res 1997;42:348–355.

[35] Hillman NH, Moss TJM, Kallapur SG, Bachurski C, Pillow JJ, Polglase GR, et al. Brief, large tidal volume ventilation initiates lung injury and a systemic response in fetal sheep. Am J Respir Crit Care Med 2007;176:575–581.

[36] Heldt GP, McIlroy MB. Distortion of chest wall and work of diaphragm in preterm infants. J Appl Physiol 1987;62:164–169. (1985).

[37] Heldt GP, McIlroy MB. Dynamics of chest wall in preterm infants. J Appl Physiol 1987;62:170–174.

[38] Morley CJ, Davis PG, Doyle LW, Brion LP, Hascoet JM, Carlin JB, et al. Nasal CPAP or intubation at birth for very preterm infants. N Engl J Med 2008;358(7):700–708.

[39] Finer NN, Carlo WA, Walsh MC, Rich W, Gantz MG, Laptook AR, et al. Early CPAP versus surfactant in extremely preterm infants. N Engl J Med 2010;362:1970–1979.

[40] Dunn MS, Kaempf J, de Klerk A, de Klerk R, Reilly M, Howard D, et al. Randomized trial comparing 3 approaches to the initial respiratory management of preterm neonates. Pediatrics 2011;128:e1069–e1076.

[41] Subramaniam P, Ho JJ, Davis PG. Prophylactic nasal continuous positive airway pressure for preventing morbidity and mortality in very preterm infants. Cochrane Database Syst Rev 2016;6. CD001243.

[42] Committee on Fetus and Newborn. Respiratory support in preterm infants at birth. Pediatrics 2014;133:171–174.

[43] Hooper SB, Siew ML, Kitchen MJ, te Pas AB. Establishing functional residual capacity in the non-breathing infants. Semin Fetal Neonatal Med 2013;18:336–343.

[44] Schmolzer GM, Te Pas AB, Davis PG, Morley CJ. Reducing lung injury during neonatal resuscitation of preterm infants. J Pediatr 2008;153:741–745.

[45] Tingay DG, Bhatia R, Schmölzer GM, Wallace MJ, Zahra VA, Davis PG. Effect of sustained inflation vs. stepwise PEEP strategy at birth on gas exchange and lung mechanics in preterm lambs. Pediatr Res 2014;75(2):288–94.

[46] Harling AE, Beresford MW, Vince GS, Bates M, Yoxall CW. Does sustained lung inflation at resuscitation reduce lung injury in the preterm infant? Arch Dis Child Fetal Neonatal Ed 2005;90:F406–F410.

[47] Lindner W, Högel J, Pohlandt F. Sustained pressure—controlled inflation or intermittent mandatory ventilation in preterm infants in the delivery room? A randomized, controlled trial on initial respiratory support via nasopharyngeal tube. Acta Paediatr 2005;94:303–309.

[48] te Pas AB, Walther FJ. A randomized, controlled trial of delivery-room respiratory management in very preterm infants. Pediatrics 2007;120:322–329.

[49] Lista G, Boni L, Scopesi F, Mosca F, Trevisanuto D, Messner H, et al. Sustained lung inflation at birth for preterm infants: a randomized clinical trial. Pediatrics 2015;135:e457–e464.

[50] Jiravisitkul P, Rattanasiri S, Nuntnarumit P. Randomised controlled trial of sustained lung inflation for resuscitation of preterm infants in the delivery room. Resuscitation 2017;111:68–73.

[51] Schmölzer GM, Kumar M, Aziz K, Pichler G, O'Reilly M, Lista G, et al. Sustained inflation versus positive pressure ventilation at birth: a systematic review and meta-analysis.

Arch Dis Child Fetal Neonatal Ed 2014;100:F361–F368.

[52] Vento M, Moro M, Escrig R, Arruza L, Villar G, Izquierdo I, et al. Preterm resuscitation with low oxygen causes less oxidative stress, inflammation, and chronic lung disease. Pediatrics 2009;124:e439–e449.

[53] Tataranno ML, Oei JL, Perrone S, Wright IM, Smyth JP, Lui K, et al. Resuscitating preterm infants with 100% oxygen is associated with higher oxidative stress than room air. Acta Paediatr 2015;104:759–765.

[54] Dawson JA, Kamlin CO, Vento M, Wong C, Cole TJ, Donath SM, et al. Defining the reference range for oxygen saturation for infants after birth. Pediatrics 2010;125:e1340–e1347.

[55] Rabi Y, Dawson JA. Oxygen therapy and oximetry in the delivery room. Semin Fetal Neonatal Med 2013;18:330–335.

[56] Dawson JA, Vento M, Finer NN, Rich W, Saugstad OD, Morley CJ, et al. Managing oxygen therapy during delivery room stabilization of preterm infants. J Pediatr 2012;160:158–161.

[57] Rabi Y, Singhal N, Nettel-Aguirre A. Room-air versus oxygen administration for resuscitation of preterm infants: the ROAR study. Pediatrics 2011;128:e374–e381.

[58] Kapadia VS, Chalak LF, Sparks JE, Allen JR, Savani RC, Wyckoff MH. Resuscitation of preterm neonates with limited versus high oxygen strategy. Pediatrics 2013;132:e1488–e1496.

[59] Rook D, Schierbeek H, Vento M, Vlaardingbroek H, van der Eijk AC, Longini M, et al. Resuscitation of preterm infants with different inspired oxygen fractions. J Pediatr 2014;164:1322–1326.

[60] Oei JL, Saugstad OD, Lui K, Wright IM, Smyth JP, Craven P, et al. Targeted oxygen in the resuscitation of preterm infants, a randomized clinical trial. Pediatrics 2017;139:e20161452.

[61] Oei JL, Vento M, Rabi Y, Wright I, Finer N, Rich W, et al. Higher or lower oxygen for delivery room resuscitation of preterm infants below 28 completed weeks gestation: a meta-analysis. Arch Dis Child Fetal Neonatal Ed 2017;102:F24–F30.

[62] Soll RF. Prophylactic natural surfactant extract for preventing morbidity and mortality in preterm infants. Cochrane Database Syst Rev 2000;2. CD000511.

[63] Ardell S, Pfister RH, Soll R. Animal derived surfactant extract versus protein free synthetic surfactant for the prevention and treatment of respiratory distress syndrome. Cochrane Database Syst Rev 2015;5. CD000144.

[64] Singh N, Halliday HL, Stevens TP, Suresh G, Soll R, Rojas-Reyes MX. Comparison of animal-derived surfactants for the prevention and treatment of respiratory distress syndrome in preterm infants. Cochrane Database Syst Rev 2015;12. CD010249.

[65] Ricci F, Murgia X, Razzetti R, Pelizzi N, Salomone F. In vitro and in vivo comparison between porctant alfa and the new generation synthetic surfactant CHF5633. Pediatr Res 2017;81(2):369–375.

[66] Rey-Santano C, Mielgo VE, Murgia X, Gomez-Solaetxe MA, Salomone F, Bianco F, et al. Cerebral and lung effects of a new generation synthetic surfactant with SP-B and SP-C analogs in preterm lambs. Pediatr Pulmonol 2017;52(7):929–938.

[67] Bahadue FL, Soll R. Early versus delayed selective surfactant treatment for neonatal respiratory distress syndrome. Cochrane Database Syst Rev 2012;11. CD001456.

[68] Isayama T, Chai-Adisaksopha C, McDonald SD. Noninvasive ventilation with vs without early surfactant to prevent chronic lung disease in preterm infants: a systematic review and meta-analysis. JAMA Pediatr 2015;169:731–739.

[69] More K, Sakhuja P, Shah PS. Minimally invasive surfactant administration in preterm infants: a meta-narrative review. JAMA Pediatr 2014;168:901–908.

[70] Göpel W, Kribs A, Härtel C, Avenarius S, Teig N, Groneck P, et al. Less invasive surfactant administration is associated with improved pulmonary outcomes in spontaneously breathing preterm infants. Acta Paediatr 2015;104:241–246.

[71] Kanmaz HG, Erdeve O, Canpolat FE, Mutlu B, Dilmen U. Surfactant administration via thin catheter during spontaneous breathing: randomized controlled trial. Pediatrics 2013;131:e502–e509.

[72] Kribs A, Roll C, Göpel W, Wieg C, Groneck P, Laux R, et al. Nonintubated surfactant application vs conventional therapy in extremely preterm infants: a randomized clinical trial. JAMA Pediatr 2015;169:723–730.

[73] Aldana-Aguirre JC, Pinto M, Featherstone RM, Kumar M. Less invasive surfactant administration versus intubation for surfactant delivery in preterm infants with respiratory distress syndrome: a systematic review and meta-analysis. Arch Dis Child Fetal Neonatal Ed 2017;102:F17–F23.

[74] Vento M, Cheung P-Y, Aguar M. The first golden minutes of the extremely-low-gestational-age neonate: a gentle approach. Neonatology 2009;95(4):286–298.

[75] Ashmeade TL, Haubner L, Collins S, Miladinovic B, Fugate K. Outcomes of a neonatal golden hour implementation project. Am J Med Qual 2016;31(1):73–80.

[76] Lambeth TM, Rojas MA, Holmes AP, Dail RB. First golden hour of life: a quality improvement initiative. Adv Neonatal Care 2016;16(4):264–272.

[77] Schmidt B, Roberts RS, Davis P, Doyle LW, Barrington KJ, Ohlsson A, et al. Caffeine therapy for apnea of prematurity. N Engl J Med 2006;354(20):2112–2121.

[78] Dekker J, Hooper SB, van Vonderen JJ, Witlox R, Lopriore E, te Pas AB. Caffeine to improve breathing effort of preterm infants at birth: a randomized controlled trial. Pediatr Res 2017;82(2):290–296.

[79] Sauberan J, Akotia D, Rich W, Durham J, Finer N, Katheria A. A pilot randomized controlled trial of early versus routine caffeine in extremely premature infants. Am J Perinatol 2015;32:879–886.

[80] Mariani G, Cifuentes J, Carlo WA. Randomized trial of permissive hypercapnia in preterm infants. Pediatrics 1999;104(5 Pt 1):1082–1088.

[81] Thome UH, Genzel-Boroviczeny O, Bohnhorst B, Schmid M, Fuchs H, Rohde O, et al. Neurodevelopmental outcomes of extremely low birthweight infants randomised to different PCO_2 targets: the PHELBI follow-up study. Arch Dis Child Fetal Neonatal Ed 2017;102(5):F376–F382.

[82] Ma J, Ye H. Effects of permissive hypercapnia on pulmonary and neurodevelopmental sequelae in extremely low birth weight infants: a meta-analysis. SpringerPlus 2016;5(1):764.

[83] Amitay M, Etches PC, Finer NN, Maidens JK. Synchronous mechanical ventilation of the neonate with respiratory disease. Crit Care Med 1993;21:118–124.

[84] Bernstein G, Heldt GP, Mannino FL. Increased and more consistent tidal volumes during synchronized intermittent mandatory ventilation in newborn infants. Am J Respir Crit Care Med 1994;150:1444–1448.

[85] Cleary JP, Bernstein G, Mannino FL, Heldt GP. Improved oxygenation during synchronized intermittent mandatory ventilation in neonates with respiratory distress syndrome: a randomized, crossover study. J Pediatr 1995;126:407–411.

[86] Jarreau PH, Moriette G, Mussat P, Mariette C, Mohanna A, Harf, et al. Patient-triggered ventilation decreases the work of breathing in neonates. Am J Respir Crit Care Med 1996;153:1176–1181.

[87] Shefali-Patel D, Murthy V, Hannam S, Lee S, Rafferty GF, Greenough A. Randomised weaning trial comparing assist control to pressure support ventilation. Arch Dis Child Fetal Neonatal Ed 2012;97(6):F429–F433.

[88] Peng W, Zhu H, Shi H, Liu E. Volume-targeted ventilation is more suitable than pressure-limited ventilation for preterm infants: a systematic review and meta-analysis. Arch Dis Child Fetal Neonatal Ed 2014;99(2):F158–F165.

[89] Cools F, Offrings M, Askie LM. Elective high frequency ventilation versus conventional ventilation for acute pulmonary dysfunction in preterm infants. Cochrane Database Syst Rev 2015;3:CD000104.

[90] Moriette G, Paris-Llado J, Walti H, Escande B, Magny JF, Cambonie G, et al. Prospective randomized multicenter comparison of high-frequency oscillatory ventilation and conventional ventilation in preterm infants of less than 30 weeks with respiratory distress syndrome. Pediatrics 2001;107(2):363–372.

[91] Sun H, Cheng R, Kang W, Xiong H, Zhou C, Zhang Y, et al. High-frequency oscillatory ventilation versus synchronized intermittent mandatory ventilation plus pressure support in preterm infants with severe respiratory distress syndrome. Resp Care 2014;59(2):159–169.

[92] Marlow N, Greenough A, Peacock JL, Marston L, Limb ES, Johnos AH. Randomized trial of high frequency oscillatory ventilation or conventional ventilation in babies of gestational age 28 weeks or less. Respiratory and neurological outcomes at two years. Arch Dis Child Fetal Neonatal Ed 2006;91(5):F320–F326.

[93] Truffert P, Paris-Liado J, Escande B, Magny JF, Cambonie G, Saliba E. Neuromotor outcome at 2 years of very preterm infants who were treated with high-frequency oscillatory ventilation or conventional ventilation for neonatal respiratory distress syndrome. Pediatrics 2007;1994(4): e860–e865.

[94] Zivanovic S, Peacock J, Alcazar-Paris M, Lo JW, Lunt A, MarlowN, for the United Kingdom Oscillatory Study Group. et al. Late outcomes of a randomized trial of high-frequency oscillation in neonates. N Engl J Med 2014;370:1121–1130.

[95] Keszler M, Donn SM, Bucciarelli RL, Alverson DC, Hart M, Lunyong V, et al. Multicenter controlled trial comparing high-frequency jet ventilation and conventional mechanical ventilation in newborn infants with pulmonary interstitial emphysema. J Pediatr 1991;119(1 Pt 1):85–93.

[96] Keszler M, Modanlou HD, Brudno DS, Clark FI, Cohen RS, Ryan RM, et al. Multicenter controlled clinical trial of high-frequency jet ventilation in preterm infants with uncomplicated respiratory distress syndrome. Pediatrics 1997;100(4):593–599.

[97] Stein H, Firestone K. Application of neurally adjusted ventilatory assist in neonates. Semin Fetal Neonatal Med 2014;19(1):60–69. (Firestone KS, Beck J, Stein H. Neurally adjusted ventilatory assist for noninvasive support in neonates. Clin Perinatol 2016;43(4):707–724.).

[98] Lee J, Kim HS, Jung YH, Shin SH, Choi CW, Kim EK, et al. Non-invasive neurally adjusted ventilatory assist in preterm infants: a randomised phase II crossover trial. Arch Dis Child Fetal Neonatal Ed 2015;100(6):F507–F513.

[99] Gibu CK, Cheng PY, Ward RJ, Castro B, Heldt GP. Feasibility and physiological effects of noninvasive neurally adjusted ventilatory assist in preterm infants. J Pediatr Res 2017;. [Epub ahead of print].

[100] Kallio M, Koskela U, Peltoniemi O, Kontiokari T, Pokka T, Suo-Palosaari M, et al. Neurally adjusted ventilatory assist (NAVA) in preterm newborn infants with respiratory distress syndrome—a randomized controlled trial. Eur J Pediatr 2016;175(9):1175–1183.

[101] Jain NJ, Kruse LK, Demissie K, Khandelwal M. Impact of mode of delivery on neonatal complications: trends between 1997 and 2005. J Matern Fetal Neonatal Med 2009;22(6):491–500.

[102] Wilson-Costello D, Friedman H, Minich N, Fanaroff AA, Hack M. Improved survival rates with increased neurodevelopmental disability for extremely low birth weight infants in the 1990s. Pediatrics 2005;115:997–1003.

[103] Volpe JJ. Intracranial hemorrhage: germinal matrix hemorrhage. In: Volpe JJ, editor. Neurology of the newborn. Philadelphia, PA: Saunders Elsevier; 2008. 517–288.

[104] Murphy BP, Inder TE, Rooks V, Taylor GA, Anderson NJ, Mogridge N, et al. Post hemorrhagic ventricular dilatation in the premature infant: natural history and predictors of outcome. Arch Dis Child Fetal Neonatal Ed 2002;87:F37–F41.

[105] Wells JT, Ment LR. Prevention of intraventricular hemorrhage in preterm infants. Early Hum Dev 1995;42:209–233.

[106] Shankaran S, Bauer CR, Bain R, et al. Prenatal and perinatal risk and protective factors for neonatal intracranial hemorrhage. Arch Pediatr Adolesc Med 1996;150:491–497.

[107] Heidary G, Vanderveen D, Smith LE. Retinopathy of prematurity: current concepts in molecular pathogenesis. Semin Ophthalmol 2009;24:77–81.

[108] Chen J, Smith LE. Retinopathy of prematurity. Angiogenesis 2007;10(2):133–140.

[109] Leviton A, Dammann O, Engelke S, et al. The clustering of disorders in infants born before the 28th week of gestation. Acta Paediatr 2010;99:1795–1800.

[110] Hellström A, Smith LE, Dammann O. Retinopathy of prematurity. Lancet 2013;382(9902):1445–1457.

[111] American Academy of Ophthalmology; American Association for Pediatric Ophthalmology and Strabismus; American Association of Certified Orthoptists. Screening examination of premature infants for retinopathy of prematurity. Pediatrics 2013;131(1):189–195.

[112] Koch J, Hensley G, Roy L, Brown S, Ramaciotti C, Rosenfeld CR. Prevalence of spontaneous closure of the ductus arteriosus in neonates at a birth weight of 1000 grams or less. Pediatrics 2006;117:1113–1121.

[113] Hermes-DeSantis ER, Clyman RI. Patent ductus arteriosus: pathophysiology and management. J Perinatol 2006;26:S14–S18.

[114] Bose CL, Laughon MM. Patent ductus arteriosus: lack of evidence for common treatments. Arch Dis Child Fetal Neonatal Ed 2007;92:F498–F502.

[115] Noori S, Seri I. Treatment of the patent ductus arteriosus: when, how and for how long? J Pediatr 2009;155:774–776.

[116] Paquette L, Friedlich P, Ramanathan R, Seri I. Concurrent use of indomethacin and dexamethasone increases the risk of spontaneous intestinal perforation in very low birth weight neonates. J Perinatol 2006;26(8):486–492.

[117] Attridge JT, Clark R, Walker MW, Gordon PV. New insights into spontaneous intestinal perforation using a national data set: (1) SIP is associated with early indomethacin exposure. J Perinatol 2006;26(2): 93–99.

[118] Zbar RI, Chen AH, Behrendt DM, Bell EF, Smith RJ. Incidence of vocal fold paralysis in infants undergoing ligation of patent ductus arteriosus. Ann Thorac Surg 1996;61: 814–816.

[119] Moin F, Kennedy KA, Moya FR. Risk factors predicting vasopressor use after patent ductus arteriosus ligation. Am J Perinatol 2003;20:313–320.

[120] Noori S, Friedlich P, Seri I, Wong P. Changes in myocardial function and hemodynamics after ligation of the ductus arteriosus in preterm infants. J Pediatr 2007;150: 597–602.

[121] Philip R, Waller BR, Agrawal V, Wright D, Arevalo A, Zurakowski D, et al. Morphologic characterization of the patent ductus arteriosus in the premature infant and the choice of transcatheter occlusion device. Catheter Cardiovasc Interv 2016;87(2):310–317.

[122] Backes CH, Cheatham SL, Deyo GM, Leopold S. Percutaneous patent ductus arteriosus (PDA) closure in very preterm infants: feasibility and complications. J Am Heart Assoc 2016;5(2):e002923.

[123] Polin RA, St Geme JW III. Neonatal sepsis. Adv Pediatr Infect Dis 1992;7:25–61.

[124] Larson EL. APIC guideline for handwashing and hand antisepsis in health care settings. Am J Infect Control 1995;23:251–269.

[125] Benitz WE. Adjunct laboratory tests in the diagnosis of early-onset neonatal sepsis. Clin Perinatol 2010;37(2):421–438.

[126] Gabay C, Kushner I. Acute-phase proteins and other systemic responses to inflammation. N Engl J Med 1999;340(6):448–454.

[127] Stoll BJ, Hansen NI, Sánchez PJ, Eunice Kennedy Shriver National Institute of Child Health and Human Development Neonatal Research Network. et al. Early onset neonatal sepsis: the burden of group B Streptococcal and E. coli disease continues. Pediatrics 2011;127(5):817–826.

[128] Baker CN, Thornsberry C, Facklam RR. Synergism, killing kinetics, and antimicrobial susceptibility of group A and B streptococci. Antimicrob Agents Chemother 1981;19(5):716–725.

[129] MacGowan A, Wootton M, Bowker K, Holt HA, Reeves D. Ampicillin-aminoglycoside interaction studies using Listeria monocytogenes. J Antimicrob Chemother 1998;41(3):417–418.

[130] Bryan CS, John JF Jr, Pai MS, Austin TL. Gentamicin vs cefotaxime for therapy of neonatal sepsis. Relationship to drug resistance. Am J Dis Child 1985;139(11):1086–1089.

[131] Manzoni P, Farina D, Leonessa M, et al. Risk factors for progression to invasive fungal infection in preterm neonates with fungal colonization. Pediatrics 2006;118(6):2359–2364.

[132] Bégué P, Floret D, Mallet E, et al. Pharmacokinetics and clinical evaluation of cefotaxime in children suffering with purulent meningitis. J Antimicrob Chemother 1984;14:161–165.

[133] Volpe J. Postnatal sepsis, necrotizing enterolitis, and the critical role of systemic inflammation in white matter injury in premature infants. J Pediatr 2008;153(2):160–163.

[134] Lee JS, Polin RA. Treatment and prevention of necrotizing enterocolitis. Semin Neonatol 2003;8:449–459. (594).

[135] Nowicki PT. Ischemia and necrotizing enterocolitis: where, when and how. Semin Pediatr Surg 2005;14:152–158.

[136] Caplan MS, MacKendrick W. Inflammatory mediators and intestinal injury. Clin Perinatol 1994;21:235–246.

[137] Stoll BJ. Epidemiology of necrotizing enterocolitis. Clin Perinatol 1994;21:205–218.

[138] Hsueh W, Caplan MS, Tan X, MacKendrick W, Gonzalez-Crussi F. Necrotizing enterocolitis of the newborn: pathogenetic concepts in perspective. Pediatr Dev Pathol 1998;1:2–16.

[139] Bell MJ, Ternberg JL, Feigin RD, Keating JP, Marshall R, Barton L, et al. Neonatal necrotizing enterocolitis: therapeutic decisions based upon clinical staging. Ann Surg 1978;187:1–7.

[140] Kliegman RM, Walsh MC. Neonatal necrotizing enterocolitis: pathogenesis, classification, and spectrum of disease. Curr Probl Pediatr 1987;17(4):243–288.

[141] Moss RL, Dimmitt RA, Barnhart DC, et al. Laparotomy versus peritoneal drainage for necrotizing enterocolitis and perforation. N Engl J Med 2006;354:2225–2234.

[142] Sola JE, Tepas JJ III, Koniaris LG. Peritoneal drainage versus laparotomy for necrotizing enterocolitis and intestinal perforation: a meta-analysis. J Surg Res 2010;161:95–100.

[143] Rees S, Inder T. Fetal and neonatal origins of altered brain development. Early Hum Dev 2005;81:753–761.

[144] Jobe AH, Bancalari E. Bronchopulmonary dysplasia. Am J Respir Crit Care Med 2001;163:1723–1729.

[145] Saigal S, Doyle LW. An overview of mortality and sequelae of preterm birth from infancy to adulthood. Lancet 2008;371(9608):261–269.

[146] Carroll JL, Loughlin GM. Sudden infant death syndrome. Pediatr Rev 1993;14:83–93.

[147] Malloy MH. Prematurity and sudden infant death syndrome: United States 2005–2007. J Perinatol 2013;33(6):470–475.

[148] Morris BH, Gard CC, Kennedy K. NICHD Neonatal Research Network. Rehospitalization of extremely low birth weight (ELBW) infants: are there racial/ethnic disparities? J Perinatol 2005;25(10):656–663.

[149] Saigal S, Doyle LW. An overview of mortality and sequelae of preterm birth from infancy to adulthood. Lancet 2008;371:261–269.

[150] Doyle LW, Anderson P. Adult outcomes of extremely preterm infants. Pediatrics 2010;126:342–351.

[151] Upadhyay K, Pourcyrous M, Dhanireddy R, Talati AJ. Outcomes of neonates with birth weight <500 g: a 20 year experience. J Perinatol 2015;35(9):768–772.

[152] Johnson S, Wolke D. Behavioural outcomes and psychopathology during adolescence. Early Hum Dev 2013;89:199–207.

Further reading

[153] Leone F, Trevisanuto D, Cavallin F, Parotto M, Zanardo V. Efficacy of INSURE during nasal CPAP in preterm infants with respiratory distress syndrome. Minerva Pediatr 2013;65(2):187–192.

[154] Kirsten GF, Kirsten CL, Henning PA, Smith J, Holgate SL, Bekker A, et al. The outcome of ELBW infants treated with NCPAP and InSurE in a resource-limited institution. Pediatrics 2012;129(4):e952–e959.

[155] Greenough A, Murthy A, Milner AD, Rossor TE, Sundaresa A. Synchronized mechanical ventilation for respiratory support in newborn. Cochrane Database Syst 2016;8. CD00456.

Section | VI |

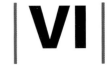

Cardiac Issues in Neonatal Respiratory Care

Chapter | 30A |

Echocardiography and Hemodynamics

Regan E. Giesinger, MD, Maura H.F. Resende, MD, Elaine Neary, MD, PhD, Patrick J. McNamara, MB, MSc

CHAPTER POINTS

- The cardiovascular and respiratory systems are intricately connected. Assessment and management should include integration of factors that influence the performance of both systems.
- Assessment of circulatory adequacy should be based on a comprehensive evaluation and not limited to blood pressure.
- The use of targeted neonatal echocardiography provides valuable insight and may enable therapy tailored to specific physiology.

The cardiovascular and respiratory systems are intricately interwoven from the earliest stages of fetal development. Synergy between these two systems is essential to ensure that the complex processes involved in delivery of oxygenated blood is adequate to maintain cellular metabolism (Fig. 30A.1). Disease states may interrupt this process at any point and it may be difficult to identify the underlying pathophysiology. Both lung parenchymal disease and acute pulmonary hypertension present with hypoxemic respiratory failure in the perinatal period. Because of the close relationship between lung recruitment and aeration and pulmonary blood flow, many infants have a component of both pathologies contributing to their clinical presentation making it difficult to identify the magnitude of each component. Additionally, after identification of a presumptive or definitive diagnosis, treatment aimed at one system may have significant impact on the other. Clinical assessment may be challenging as there is significant overlap between disease phenotypes. The current technology used for bedside monitoring is limited compared to those widely used in adults. Echocardiography may be an important adjunctive tool. In this chapter, we aim to illustrate the intricate relationship between the respiratory and cardiovascular systems, present a physiologically driven approach to understanding how disease pathology and treatment of cardiorespiratory disease interact and illustrate how echocardiography may be used to enhance physiologic definition and individualize therapy.

Cardiopulmonary interdependence

The transition

The transitional period is characterized by a dramatic change in both cardiovascular and respiratory function that must occur over a period of minutes to achieve survival. The combination of high pulmonary vascular resistance (PVR), low-resistance placental circuit, and presence of shunts results in a complex fetal circulatory pattern. Due to high-downstream PVR, most of the fetal right ventricular output (90%) is diverted across the ductus arteriosus into the systemic circulation to be oxygenated by the placenta. Low pulmonary blood flow contributes little to left atrial pressure and this, when combined with high PVR, produces a significant pressure gradient between the right and left atrium. The result is that a large proportion of highly oxygenated placental return flows right to left across the foramen ovale and makes a major contribution to left ventricular output (LVO), hence cerebral and coronary flow. After birth,

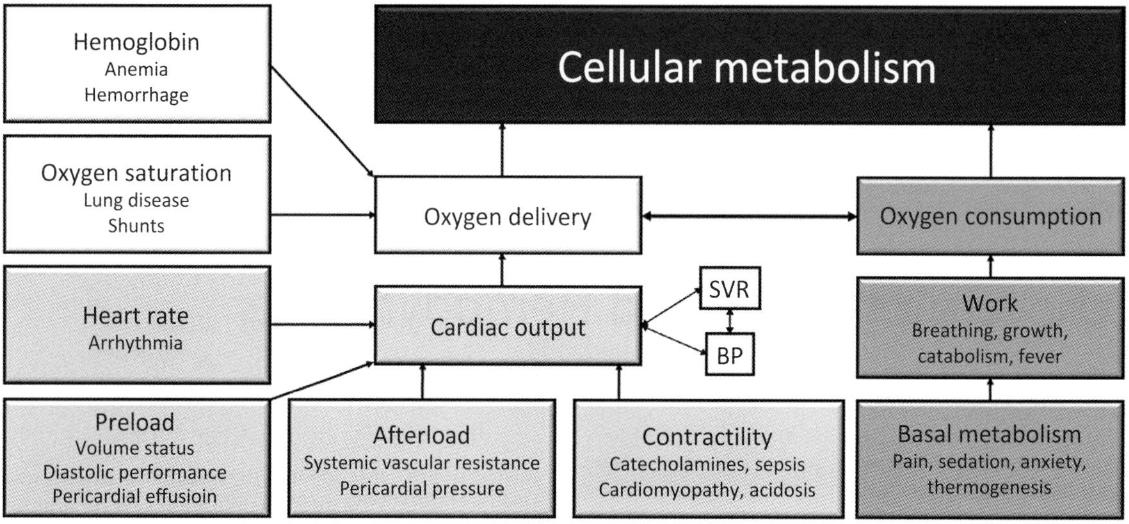

Fig. 30A.1 **Factors That Contribute to Metabolic Homeostasis.**

separation of the placenta leads to a simultaneous increase in systemic vascular resistance (SVC), reduction in right atrial preload and therefore a dramatic reduction in right ventricular output, which may impact the systemic circulation. If sustained, this may result in cerebral and myocardial ischemia. The augmentation in pulmonary blood flow, secondary to postnatal lung recruitment, and the resultant escalation of pulmonary venous return replaces umbilical flow as the major contributor to delivery of oxygenated blood to the left atrium and hence, the primary contributor to LVO. For infants in whom this does not occur successfully, there may be significant consequences.

The contribution of lung aeration and pulmonary mechanics to successful transition cannot be underestimated. Several factors are thought to result in the immediate postnatal augmentation of pulmonary blood flow that is required to offset the hemodynamic effects of placental separation. First, high-negative intrathoracic pressure due to lung inflation with sustained peak end-expiratory pressure results in an increase in alveolar-capillary transmural pressure gradient and therefore an increase in capillary size in aerated regions. Second, as fetal lung fluid dissipates, an increasing proportion of the alveoli become oxygenated. Fetal lamb studies have shown that administration and withdrawal of oxygen independently mediates reduction and increase in pulmonary vascular tone, respectively, and therefore modulates pulmonary blood flow.

Though technically challenging due to limitations of cord length, maternal needs and the requirement for equipment and personnel to be in close shared proximity with the obstetrical staff, ventilation prior to cord clamping is an area of active research [1,2]. Initiation of ventilation, with the resultant increase in pulmonary blood flow, prior

to the removal of the placental source of left atrial preload may limit the duration of low cardiac output immediately following cord clamping. A period of placental transfusion immediately following delivery prior to clamping of the cord is recommended by both neonatal and obstetric guidelines for otherwise stable preterm infants not requiring resuscitation [3,4]. The associated reduced risk of intraventricular hemorrhage may relate to improved cardiovascular stability with onset of spontaneous respiration prior to cord clamping. The value of delayed cord clamping for neonates requiring resuscitation and mechanical ventilation has not been demonstrated, though theoretically these neonates may have an even greater need due to a delay in establishing pulmonary blood flow [1].

Impaired transition

When pulmonary blood flow fails to increase to a level sufficient to provide adequate delivery of oxygenated blood to the systemic circulation the neonate may develop the clinical phenotype of acute pulmonary hypertension. There are significant cardiovascular consequences. High PVR contributes to high right ventricular afterload to which the neonatal myocardium, especially the right ventricle, is poorly adapted. This may directly result in RV dilation and impaired RV systolic performance. The impact on the LV is equally important but more complex. Poor pulmonary blood flow leads to impaired LV preload which may result in low cardiac output, particularly if atrial right-to-left shunt is small or absent. Further, poor preload may impair LV contractility by the Frank–Starling mechanism. Right ventricular changes may also have a significant impact on LV performance. The right and left ventricles are interlinked with multiple shared fibers which results in ventricular interdependence [5]. Similarly, left ventricular contractility is dependent on its conformation and leftward deviation of the septum due to RV dilation and high right ventricular pressure results in impaired LV performance. Hypoxemia and low cardiac output may also contribute to impaired coronary artery flow and myocardial hypoperfusion. The end result may be poor systemic blood flow and shock which, if not promptly corrected, may be fatal.

Preterm infants, in particular, may be at increased risk of acute pulmonary hypertension early in their postnatal course. Both a higher frequency of lung disease which results in reduced alveolar recruitment and oxygenation and immaturity of biochemical pathways and enzyme systems may predispose premature infants to failure of transition. The cardiovascular consequences are similar to term infants, and additionally, the preterm myocardium presents unique challenges. Premature infants have less compliant ventricles due to a higher proportion of noncontractile tissue, disorganized orientation of myofibrils, and immature calcium handling. This may lead to exaggerated impact of afterload on the RV. Dramatic changes in cardiac loading conditions such as a rapid drop in PVR with surfactant administration may be poorly tolerated by the LV and may precipitate acute systolic dysfunction. This may have important implications for outcomes because there is evidence that a period of low cerebral blood flow may precede intraventricular hemorrhage, suggesting that ischemia–reperfusion injury may be a contributor. The mortality for preterm infants with pulmonary hypertension is significantly higher than matched patients who transition smoothly.

The impact of ventilation on the cardiovascular system

Unsupported inspiratory breathing occurs due to contraction of respiratory muscles to expand the lung and produce negative intrathoracic pressure. A gradient develops between the atmospheric pressure and the respiratory units and air flows down the pressure gradient into the lung. Negative pleural pressure transmits to the right atrium and an increase in abdominal pressure due to diaphragmatic contraction occurs. The result is an increase in the systemic venous to right atrial pressure gradient, hence an increase in venous return. This process is responsible for the variation in stroke volume that occurs with the respiratory cycle. The initiation of positive pressure ventilation significantly changes these relationships.

Impact on right heart filling

Ventilated breaths distend alveoli using positive intrathoracic pressure, the peak of which occurs which is at end-inspiration. Stretching of the alveoli is associated with increased transpleural pressure which transmits to the right atrium. Right atrial filling is preserved at moderate levels due to a concurrent increase in abdominal pressure [6]. At extremes of inflation, transpleural pressure, and therefore pericardial pressure, may be sufficiently high to compromise atrial preload by limiting the ability of the chambers to distend [7]. The application of positive end-expiratory pressure reduces the tidal volume and peak inspiratory pressure required to ventilate the lung while maintaining mean airway pressure. Fewer areas of localized overexpansion, which may contribute to transpleural pressure, may occur due to homogenous lung recruitment. Though transpleural pressure remains above atmospheric throughout the respiratory cycle, there is less overall impact on hemodynamics. Changes in airway pressure, mediated both by changing peak end-expiratory pressure and manipulation of mean airway pressure on high-frequency modes, is associated with an inverse change in right ventricular output in neonates [8–10]. This is particularly important in patients with right ventricular dysfunction in whom pulmonary blood flow may be dependent on maintaining a high gradient between right atrial and pulmonary artery pressure. Significant overdistension may be associated with low cardiac output in some neonates and the use of excessive mean airway pressure should be avoided, particularly in hemodynamically compromised patients.

Impact on PVR

Throughout the lung of healthy newborn pulmonary venous pressure is greater than the intraalveolar pressure in areas of appropriate ventilation-perfusion matching. Alveolar distension beyond pulmonary venous pressure leads to impaired flow through the adjacent pulmonary capillary bed and produces an increase in PVR. High-tidal volume ventilation in which alveoli are overdistended is associated with a sharp increase in pulmonary artery acceleration time due to increased resistance and is associated with increased right ventricular afterload [6]. At levels below functional residual capacity, derecruitment results in areas of localized alveolar hypoxia which is associated with hypoxic pulmonary vasoconstriction. Additionally, small vessels become tortuous and may collapse resulting in further increase in PVR [11]. Right ventricular performance is particularly vulnerable to elevated afterload [12] and dramatic over or underrecruitment may cause negative impact. For patients who have preexisting pulmonary hypertension, myocardial dysfunction or significant lung disease with associated gas trapping or impaired gas exchange, changes in lung volume may also have an important impact on pulmonary blood flow, therefore cardiac output. The impact of augmented intrathoracic pressure on hemodynamics in critically ill neonates may be even greater.

Impact on left ventricular performance

Given the dependence of pulmonary blood flow on airway pressure, an impact on left ventricular preload may be anticipated. Reduced left ventricular end-diastolic volume [13], stroke volume [13], and impaired systemic perfusion [14] have been associated with excessive lung volumes. When PVR is sufficiently high to result in right ventricular dilation and dysfunction, left ventricular function may also be impaired. Abnormal left ventricular shape due to septal flattening or paradoxical septal motion has a negative impact on myocardial performance [15] and may impair left ventricular filling [16,17]. Though the right ventricular effects predominate, right ventricular dysfunction may contribute to left ventricular dysfunction due to interdependent fibers [18] and changes in transpleural pressure may have an independent impact on left ventricular afterload. This may be particularly important for patients with preexisting conditions that make them especially vulnerable, such as severe left ventricular dysfunction. Negative pressure inspiration is associated with increased aortic transluminal pressure because the pleural pressure declines more significantly that the aortic pressure. The associated increase in left ventricular wall stress may be relieved with the application of positive pressure [19].

Cardiovascular assessment

Clinical assessment

Making a distinction whether the etiology of hypoxia relates primarily to parenchymal versus cardiovascular etiology may be complex but is important. Treatments for cardiovascular disease such as inhaled nitric oxide (iNO) are unlikely to have maximum efficacy in the setting of uncorrected atelectasis and therefore optimization of recruitment and carbon dioxide clearance are important primary therapies for hypoxia. The presence of work of breathing suggests inadequate lung recruitment and is an important clinical clue. Arterial carbon dioxide, which is less susceptible to local effects due to poor tissue perfusion than capillary or venous samples, in the normal range in the presence of significant hypoxia suggests inadequate pulmonary blood flow and should trigger investigation for pulmonary hypertension or congenital heart disease. Chest radiography is important to assess for alternate etiologies (e.g., pneumothorax) and assess cardiac size and silhouette. All of these investigations, however, are nonspecific; comprehensive echocardiography may be invaluable in establishing a definitive diagnosis and delineating the actual physiology. The role of neonatologists in performing comprehensive echocardiography and integrating

hemodynamic information in critically ill neonates is a crucial component of refining the care.

Ensuring appropriate lung recruitment, minute ventilation, pulmonary and systemic blood flow require careful attention to detail in the preterm or sick-term infant. With increased emphasis on lung protection, low tidal volume ventilation, the "open lung" strategy has become an important part of modern neonatal care. The focus of this approach is to attain and maintain lung volume above functional residual capacity using sustained inflation after a recruitment maneuver to open atelectatic lung units. Clinicians may use a target fraction of inspired oxygen (FiO_2) of less than 0.3 to indicate adequate lung recruitment based on animal [20] and neonatal data suggesting this as an appropriate target [21,22]. This presumes, however, that ventilation and perfusion matching may be accomplished using recruitment alone which may not be accurate for neonates with concurrent abnormalities of pulmonary blood flow. Overdistension in an attempt to reduce FiO_2 to below 0.3 in patients with pulmonary hypertension is a danger when using this parameter in isolation. Additionally, though lung volume and mean airway pressure are strongly associated, compliance may be highly variable depending on the degree of intrinsic lung disease and other dynamic patient factors such as infant position [23]. Reduction in right ventricular output has been associated with increasing lung volume; however, serial measurements are required to determine the clinical relevance. Changes may significantly impact on pulmonary blood flow and frequent reassessment is recommended. Diaphragm position in relation to posterior ribs on chest radiography, though a commonly used diagnostic test, lacks precision for assessment of lung volume [24]. Flow and pressure volume loops available on modern neonatal ventilators may provide valuable information on recruitment and compliance, however, are not available on high-frequency modes. Determination of lung volume using magnetic resonance imaging (MRI) is widely used in prognostication for fetal patients with congenital diaphragmatic hernia, lung masses [25], and congenital heart disease [26]. Postnatal lung volume assessment using MRI has been explored in patients with diaphragmatic hernia [27] and patients with bronchopulmonary dysplasia [28]; however, limited availability and experience and the need for transport restrict its clinical relevance to assess dynamic states of recruitment. Changes in echocardiography measurements, a tool which is available in real time and at the bedside, may be useful.

The utilization of echocardiography in the neonatal intensive care unit

Echocardiography by the neonatologist is increasingly practiced in intensive care units across the world. Although the program name changes between regions (targeted neonatal echocardiography [Pan-American region], clinician performed ultrasound [Australasia], neonatologist performed echocardiography [Europe]), the fundamental principles which define the field are similar. In this chapter, we will refer to American Society of Echocardiography Guidelines for Targeted Neonatal Echocardiography (TnECHO), as it is the terminology our group is most familiar with, although either term would be appropriate. Distinct from echocardiography practiced by cardiologists in which the focus is on the diagnosis and management of major and minor structural heart disease, echocardiography by the neonatologist is utilized in conjunction with clinical assessment to identify and guide the intensive care treatment of deranged cardiovascular physiology. It is of paramount importance to emphasize that neonates with impaired oxygenation and/or systemic blood flow may have structural heart disease and therefore a full anatomic assessment should be performed and reviewed by a pediatric cardiologist either at the time of or before first echocardiography assessment by the neonatologist. There are several advantages, however, of the model in which the intensive care physician performs bedside echocardiography. First, the in-depth knowledge of transitional and neonatal physiology which is fundamental to neonatal intensive care practice is also important in the interpretation of echocardiography imaging. Particularly during the transitional period, the evaluation of echocardiography in isolation of the clinical status may be difficult and inaccurate. PVR may decline slowly after birth and, in the absence of hypoxemia, this may represent a variation of normal whereas in the hypoxic neonate this may represent a pathological state. Second, the ability to make rapid, real-time assessment in acutely ill patients allows the titration of intensive care therapies with changes in physiology. Longitudinal monitoring is difficult within the current model of pediatric cardiology practice. Finally, the neonatologist is uniquely positioned to understand the disease states given the nature of their training and clinical expertise. This allows echocardiography to be used optimally to understand the natural history of longer term conditions such as patent ductus arteriosus (PDA) or chronic pulmonary hypertension and to conduct research focused on understanding the normal variation in neonatal physiology and how this is modified by disease.

Standards for training and operating procedures are established in many areas of the world [29–31]. There is no published scientific evidence to support-specific requirements for number, type or frequency of imaging to constitute proficiency, hence there is significant heterogeneity in training programs. High-quality cardiac image acquisition, however, is difficult given the anatomic complexity, dynamic nature, and the importance of precise measurements to interpretation. This is particularly true in preterm and sick-term neonates given the restrictions of size, air interference from invasive ventilation, and often

patient lability. Hence, it is important that neonatologists performing echocardiography be highly experienced and diligent. Comprehensive assessment including measurements in multiple imaging planes is recommended given the intrinsic operator and measurement error that may occur when relying on a single value for decision-making. The TnECHO specify essential and disease-specific imaging sequences and measurements which are recommended in all studies [31]. Each measurement has advantages and limitations which must be understood by TnECHO practitioners in order to avoid misinterpretation (Table 30A.1). In isolation, individual measurements have a variety of contributing factors including operator dependency and changes in loading conditions. When clinical assessment and a series of corroborating measurements are used to create a pattern, TnECHO may provide valuable insight into pathophysiology.

The use of TnECHO as a tool for serial monitoring of changes in an individual patient allows comparison between measurements with therapy and over time. To apply TnECHO broadly and make determinations about deviation from normal on the first assessment, it is important to define the reference ranges for each measurement over different gestational ages. The neonatal, and particularly the preterm, cardiovascular system is unique due to its transitional state, immaturity, and the persistence of fetal shunts. It is, therefore, difficult to extrapolate pediatric or adult data to the neonatal heart. Published normative data for indices of right and left ventricular function and cardiac output of healthy term neonates in the transitional period is available [39,40]. For preterm infants, an additional layer of complexity relates to the lack of clear definition of what constitutes a "healthy" preterm. Some data describing changes in left and right ventricular functional indices have been published; however, continued work in this area is required.

Assessment of pulmonary pressure

Echocardiography evaluation of pulmonary hypertension should include (1) estimation of pulmonary pressure and PVR, (2) appraisal of the impact on right ventricular function, and (3) any impact on systemic circulation (Table 30A.2). Several techniques are recommended for evaluation of pulmonary arterial pressure. *First*, the estimation, using the modified Bernoulli equation, of right ventricular systolic pressure (RVSp) using peak velocity of the tricuspid regurgitant jet if measurable and complete is commonly considered the most robust echocardiography measure of pulmonary pressure. This measure may not be reliable, however, if there is inadequate regurgitation or in the presence of RV dysfunction. It is important that the Doppler measurement of velocity is taken from a line of insonation parallel to regurgitant flow; poor Doppler

Table 30A.1 Advantages and limitations of TnECHO measurements used in the assessment of pulmonary hemodynamics [32]

Assessment	Measurement	Advantages	Limitations
Established in clinical practice			
RV systolic pressure	Peak velocity of TR jet	• Calculation of RVSp (modified Bernoulli equation)	• Incomplete or inadequate TR [33] • Underestimated by RV dysfunction [33] • Assumes RA pressure
	Septal wall motion (eccentricity index [34])	• Direct assessment of relative LVSp and RVSp over the duration of the cardiac cycle	• Relative to systemic pressure; systemic hypertension may underestimate RVSp
	PDA shunt direction	• Direct assessment of relative systemic and pulmonary pressure over the duration of the cardiac cycle	• Absence of PDA
RV systolic performance	RV output	• Reflects volume of PBF in the absence of pulmonary to aortic shunt	• Angle dependent • Precise annulus measurement may be technically difficult due to suboptimal visualization of PA
Systemic blood flow	LV output	• Reflects volume of SBF • If PDA open, only preductal (CNS, coronary) SBF	• Angle dependent; requires precise placement of sample volume • Precise annulus measurement dependent on alignment of PLx plane
	Qualitative assessment of LV filling; mid-cavity flow acceleration	• Easily visualized, rapid	• Imprecise • Detects abnormalities only at the extremes of filling
Evidence of utility in other populations (limited normative data, consider for longitudinal assessment)			
Pulmonary vascular resistance	RVET:PAAT ratio	• Predictive of PH [35] • Easily measured, not angle dependent	• Influenced by poor RV performance • Confounded by concurrent TR, PA dilation, PDA shunt
	Mid-systolic notching of PA Doppler waveform	• Associated with PH [35] • Easily measured, not angle dependent	• Influenced by poor RV performance • Confounded by TR, PA dilation, PDA shunt • May occur in high flow states [35]
RV systolic performance	RV fractional area change	• Reflective of RV ejection fraction on MRI [36] (adult data)	• Dependent on high-quality imaging windows for endocardial definition [37] • Apical four-chamber FAC influenced by septal motion [36]
	TAPSE (tricuspid annular plane systolic excursion)	• Highly reproducible measure (longitudinal motion) [37] • Feasible in most patients [38]	• Reflects displacement of tricuspid annulus at a single point; ≠ septal or outlet motion; ≠ RWM abnormalities [38] • Angle and possibly load dependent [38]
	Tissue Doppler imaging	• Highly reproducible measure of longitudinal RV performance [38] • Feasible in most patients	• Reflects displacement of tricuspid annulus at a single point; ≠ septal or outlet motion; ≠ RWM abnormalities • Affected by overall motion of the heart, angle and load [36]
Research/investigational use			
	RV peak systolic strain	• Allows segmental assessment of RWM abnormalities	• Influenced by image quality • Limited normative data

CNS, Central nervous system; FAC, fractional area change; LV, left ventricle; LVSp, left ventricular systolic pressure; MRI, magnetic resonance imaging; PA, pulmonary artery; PAAT, pulmonary artery acceleration time; PBF, pulmonary blood flow; PDA, patent ductus arteriosus; PH, pulmonary hypertension; PLx, parasternal long axis; RV, right ventricle; RVET, right ventricular ejection time; RVSp, right ventricular systolic pressure; RWMA, regional wall motion; TR, tricuspid regurgitation.

Table 30A.2 Targeted neonatal echocardiography measurements for neonates with acute pulmonary hypertension

Evaluation of pulmonary hemodynamics	Impact on systemic circulation	Impact on RV performance
Quantitative:	**LV preload:**	**Subjective**:
Tricuspid regurgitation	PV Doppler	2D assessment of contractility
Transductal Doppler	Transmitral Doppler	Dilatation of ventricular cavity
Semiquantitative:	**LV contractility:**	and RVOT
PAAT:RVET	Fractional shortening	**Objective:**
Interventricular septal motion	Ejection fraction	RVO/MPA stroke distance
Pattern of shunt across PDA and PFO	mVCFc	TAPSE
	Systemic flow:	Fractional area change
	LVO	

LVO, Left ventricular output; *MPA*, main pulmonary artery; *mVCFc*, mean velocity of circumferential fiber shortening; *PAAT*, pulmonary artery acceleration time; *PDA*, patent ductus arteriosus; *PFO*, patent foramen ovale; *PV*, pulmonary valve; *RVET*, right ventricular ejection time; *RVO*, right ventricular output; *RVOT*, right ventricular outflow tract; *TAPSE*, tricuspid annular plane systolic excursion.
Adapted from Jain A, McNamara PJ. Persistent pulmonary hypertension of the newborn: physiology, hemodynamic assessment and novel therapies. Curr Pediatr Rev 2013;9:55–66 [44].

alignment will underestimate true RVSp. *Second*, assessment of directionality of ductal shunt may provide valuable information. Right-to-left ductal shunt will only occur if the pressure at the pulmonary end of the ductus is higher than the pressure at the aortic end at a designated portion of the cardiac cycle. Pulmonary pressure may be considered suprasystemic if right-to-left ductal shunt is present for greater than 30% of systole [41]. *Third*, qualitative assessment of septal flattening may be a subjective way to quantify the relative pressure difference between the left and right ventricles at various points in the cardiac cycle. Subjective assessment however, has low interrater reliability and objective measurements such as eccentricity index [42] may be superior. Finally, the duration of acceleration of systolic flow in the pulmonary artery may be used to estimate the downstream resistance because blood is expected to reach its peak velocity more quickly in a rigid circuit [43]. Indexing the pulmonary artery acceleration time to right ventricular ejection time (RVET) accounts for the impact of variable heart rate.

Assessment of right ventricular systolic performance

Assessment of RV function may be difficult due to (1) its complex geometry and highly trabeculated surface which makes it difficult to identify the endocardial boarders and (2) its anterior position in the chest which may impact imaging windows. Qualitative assessment is unreliable and therefore quantitative measures utilizing a standardized approach may improve reliability and validity. There are limited data comparing echocardiography measurements of myocardial performance to the emerging gold

standard technique of cardiac MRI. In adult patients, several measurements including fractional area change, peak systolic velocity as measured by tissue Doppler imaging, tricuspid annular plane systolic excursion (TAPSE), and peak longitudinal strain are predictive of low RV ejection fraction measured using cardiac MRI. The majority of this data are collected using echocardiography imaging from the apical four-chamber view. Fractional area change, measured by tracing the endocardial boarder at end-diastole and end-systole and calculating the percentage difference, may have superior reliability in the neonatal population when measured from the apical three-chamber view (Fig. 30A.2). In patients with pulmonary hypertension, a low TAPSE, which is a measure of longitudinal RV systolic performance, has been associated with risk of death or extracorporeal membrane oxygenation [45] (Fig. 30A.3). Similar data are emerging for neonates with perinatal asphyxia, in whom TAPSE is associated with risk of death or abnormal brain MRI despite therapeutic hypothermia [46].

Assessment of LV systolic performance

Shortening fraction and ejection fraction as measured by M-mode echocardiography in either the parasternal long or short axis plane are often used to assess left ventricular systolic performance in neonates. The utilization of M-mode echocardiography includes several assumptions; first, the measurement change in diameter in the plane of insonation is representative of global myocardial function and second, that the left ventricle is spherical in shape. Regional wall motion abnormalities cannot be accounted for using this technique, and particularly for neonates with

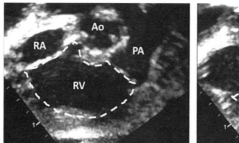
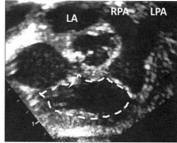

Fig. 30A.2 **Right Ventricular Three-Chamber View.** The right atrium (RA), right ventricle (RV), pulmonary artery (PA), and aorta (Ao) can be seen from a medial apical position. This view may be used to calculate fractional area change by tracing the diastolic and systolic areas and using the formula: [(diastolic area) − (systolic area)]/(diastolic area). *LA*, Left atrium; *LPA*, left pulmonary artery; *RPA*, right pulmonary artery.

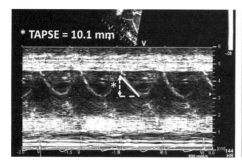
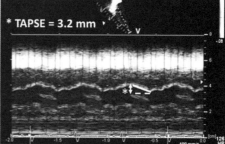

Fig. 30A.3 **Tricuspid Annular Plane Systolic Excursion (TAPSE) in the Normal Range for a Term Infant on the Tight.** The left panel demonstrates a very low TAPSE in a 24-h-old infant with pulmonary hypertension, right ventricular dysfunction, and hypoxic ischemic encephalopathy.

septal flattening in the setting of pulmonary hypertension, the assumption of a spherical LV shape is inaccurate. The left ventricular shape of preterm neonates is distorted for up to several weeks following delivery, limiting the applicability of fractional shortening, and particularly M-mode ejection fraction in which diameter measurements are cubed and therefore the potential for inaccuracy is exponentially increased [47]. The Simpson's biplane method of estimating LV volume is more accurate due to the separation of the cavity into discrete disks and the measurement of diameter in two planes which facilitates the assumption of a conical shape. LVO may be calculated using the following: velocity time integral (VTI) measured by pulsed-wave Doppler with the angle of insonation parallel to the direction of flow and the sample volume at the level of the hinge points of the aortic valve, the heart rate, and the radius of the aortic valve annulus measured in the parasternal long-axis plane [48]. Cardiac MRI data suggest that LVO measurement by echocardiography is a robust measure of systemic blood flow [49] and normative data exists in the neonatal population [40,50].

Novel modalities

As the availability of high-frequency, high-resolution technology becomes increasingly available, techniques that are in widespread use in adult patients are becoming more practical for neonatal assessment and are increasingly used, particularly as research tools. The use of tissue Doppler imaging to assess myocardial velocity has been used as an adjunct measurement to assess systolic and diastolic performance in neonates undergoing PDA ligation [51], patients with acute [52] and chronic pulmonary hypertension [53] and other hemodynamic conditions. Reproducibility is high [52] and normative data has been published for some populations during the transitional period [39,40,54]. Measurement of peak strain and strain rate using speckle tracking echocardiography are feasible in term and preterm infants [55]. The use of this technique makes quantification of regional wall motion abnormalities possible and may, therefore, allow more detailed appraisal of heart function. Measurement of LV rotational mechanics using assessment of torsion has been explored; however, the published evidence is limited [56,57].

Hemodynamic assessment in specific situations

Detailed clinical assessment is the cornerstone of intensive care management and the evolution and response to treatment are important. The assessment of circulatory adequacy is complex and should not be limited to blood pressure. Optimizing tissue oxygenation to satisfy the metabolic needs of the tissue represents the goal of cardiovascular care (Fig. 30A.1). It is important to recognize that, while, mean arterial pressure is a symptom of neonatal cardiovascular health it does not predict cardiac output. Neonates with low cardiac output may vasoconstrict their less essential vascular beds (e.g., skin) to maintain perfusion pressure to more vulnerable organs; hence, normal blood pressure in an otherwise unwell appearing neonate should not be used to rule out poor perfusion. The use of systolic and diastolic pressure may provide added insight into pathophysiology because disorders that reduce cardiac output (e.g., pulmonary hypertension, myocardial dysfunction) may be reflected in declining systolic arterial pressure, whereas those that cause peripheral vasodilation (e.g., sepsis) may start out as predominantly diastolic hypotension. All infants if left untreated, however, may develop profound hypotension when adaptive mechanisms fail. TnECHO assessment may modify clinical impression in a significant proportion of neonates [58]. When performing echocardiography, a comprehensive study according to the American Society of Echocardiography guidelines [31] is recommended; however, particular attention to predictable features associated with specific disease phenotypes is sensible.

Classic pulmonary hypertension in the term/preterm neonate

As previously described, acute pulmonary hypertension is characterized by high RV afterload, impaired LV preload and biventricular systolic dysfunction. The transitional shunts may play an important modulator role in supporting systemic perfusion, albeit at the expense of a marginally lower PaO$_2$. Monitoring pre and postductal oxygen saturation may provide an indicator of right-to-left ductal shunt in the presence of suprasystemic level pulmonary artery pressure. The absence of a gradient, however, does not rule out pulmonary hypertension. If the ductus arteriosus is very small or absent or if the flow is bidirectional, there may be insufficient deoxygenated blood flowing to the systemic circulation to have a clinically apparent impact on postductal oxygen saturation. Clinical assessment should consider markers of circulatory adequacy and tissue oxygenation. Oxygenation index is

one tool used to standardize therapy; however, the location of arterial blood gas measurement is an important consideration. As most arterial lines are placed in the postductal umbilical artery, the implications on monitoring need to be considered. Significant right-to-left ductal shunt may modify both the arterial oxygen content and potentially systolic arterial pressure. In the presence of a high-volume right-to-left ductal shunt, postductal systolic arterial pressure may be higher leading to underestimation of preductal perfusion pressure. It is therefore recommended to monitor both pre and postductal blood pressure concurrently, particularly in neonates with a gradient in oxygenation.

Echocardiography assessment of pulmonary hypertension should always include, in addition to estimation of pulmonary pressure, measures of RV health and the adequacy of systemic blood flow as changes in these parameters are direct consequences of high-PVR. The presence and direction of ductal and atrial shunt are of particular importance and patency of fetal shunts may be lifesaving (Fig. 30A.4). In the presence of very low pulmonary blood flow, right-to-left atrial shunt may support LVO and provide an important source of perfusion to preductal organs such as the coronaries and the brain. In the presence of very low LVO, right-to-left ductal shunt may also support cerebral perfusion through retrograde flow into the proximal branches of the aortic arch. Additionally, right-to-left ductal shunt may provide supplemental systemic flow which, though the oxygen content is lower than optimal, may be adequate to prevent organ ischemia. Finally, afterload reduction via the provision of an alternate, lower resistance pathway to right ventricular output may be an important protective mechanism against RV failure.

Acute pulmonary hypertension and structural congenital heart disease

Recognition is of fundamental importance to the management of acute pulmonary hypertension in neonates with congenital heart disease. A neonate with unrestrictive pulmonary blood flow in the setting of cyanotic congenital heart disease should have a baseline saturation in the range of 75%–80%. Saturation lower than this level may suggest inadequate mixing of pulmonary and systemic circulations (e.g., due to restrictive atrial defect or ductus arteriosus in neonates with transposition of the great arteries) or concurrent acute pulmonary hypertension and critical hypoxemia (e.g., PaO$_2$ <25 mmHg or SpO$_2$ <60%) should prompt urgent attention [59]. Acute pulmonary hypertension may occur due to pulmonary hypoplasia (e.g., related to cardiomegaly in Ebstein's anomaly [60]), pulmonary interstitial glycogenosis [61], pulmonary lymphangectasia [62], or due to remodeling in the setting of abnormal in utero flow

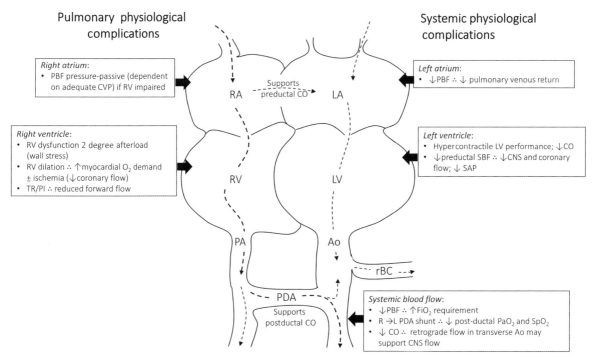

Pulmonary physiological complications

Systemic physiological complications

Right atrium:
• PBF pressure-passive (dependent on adequate CVP) if RV impaired

RA · · · Supports preductal CO · · → LA

Left atrium:
• ↓PBF ∴ ↓ pulmonary venous return

Right ventricle:
• RV dysfunction 2 degree afterload (wall stress)
• RV dilation ∴ ↑myocardial O_2 demand ± ischemia (↓coronary flow)
• TR/PI ∴ reduced forward flow

RV   LV

Left ventricle:
• Hypercontractile LV performance; ↓CO
• ↓preductal SBF ∴ ↓CNS and coronary flow; ↓ SAP

PA   Ao

· · · rBC · · →

· · · PDA · · ·

Supports postductal CO

Systemic blood flow:
• ↓PBF ∴ ↑FiO_2 requirement
• R →L PDA shunt ∴ ↓ post-ductal PaO_2 and SpO_2
• ↓ CO ∴ retrograde flow in transverse Ao may support CNS flow

Fig. 30A.4 Cardiovascular Consequences of Acute Pulmonary Hypertension [32]. *Ao,* Aorta; *CNS,* central nervous system; *CO,* cardiac output; *LA,* left atrium; *LV,* left ventricle; *PA,* pulmonary artery; *PBF,* pulmonary blood flow; *PDA,* patent ductus arteriosus; *PI,* pulmonary insufficiency; *RA,* right atrium; *rBC,* right brachiocephalic; *RV,* right ventricle; *SAP,* systolic arterial pressure; *SBF,* systemic blood flow; *TR,* tricuspid regurgitation.

patterns and the risk may be higher in early term or preterm infants [63].

Other causes of pulmonary hypertension that may complicate the course of neonates with congenital heart disease include pulmonary arterial disease in the setting of chronic left-to-right shunt and pulmonary venous disease due to left atrial hypertension [64]. Progressive pulmonary arterial hypertension may occur in simple (e.g., ventricular or atrioventricular septal defects, PDA) or more complex (e.g., anomalous venous drainage, single ventricle with unobstructed pulmonary blood flow) lesions [65]. A high volume of pulmonary blood flow may initially be tolerated because the healthy pulmonary vascular bed is compliant; however, over time the pulmonary vasculature becomes more muscular and undergoes remodeling which increases PVR [66]. This may be further compounded by exposure of the pulmonary circulation to higher than normal SpO_2. Pulmonary vascular disease associated with progressive pulmonary vasculature alterations may later present as Eisenmenger's syndrome and may be lethal. These changes typically take prolonged exposure; however, the impact of simultaneous lung parenchymal disease due to

prematurity, concurrent inflammatory changes with infection, and the impact of chronic ventilation and oxygen exposure on the development of shunt-related pulmonary hypertension in the medically complex or preterm neonate is unclear. Pulmonary venous hypertension due to high left atrial pressure may lead to the development of pulmonary edema and therefore impaired oxygenation and ventilation. It is important to differentiate these two entities as their management significantly differs. Neonates with anatomic heart disease which results in restrictive pulmonary venous drainage, such as hypoplastic left heart with a restrictive atrial septal defect, have an increased likelihood of abnormal development of pulmonary veins, arterioles, and lymphatics during fetal and neonatal life. The latter may predispose these babies to abnormalities of pulmonary blood flow and may require modification of treatment approach [67].

Congenital diaphragmatic hernia

Congenital diaphragmatic hernia (CDH) affects approximately one in every 3000 babies [68]. Depending on the severity of the herniation of abdominal organs into the chest, the lungs growth can be affected by its compression, leading to pulmonary hypoplasia and acute pulmonary hypertension. Poor prognostic markers include diagnosis prior to 25 weeks gestation, herniation of the liver and low lung-to-head ratio [69,70]. The use of biomarkers has been suggested to predict severity of pulmonary vascular disease and cardiac impact, such as growth factors (vascular endothelial growth factor A (VEGF-A), placental growth factor (PGF)) and brain-type natriuretic peptide levels [71–73].

The postnatal course may be complicated by both parenchymal and cardiovascular disease. Lung branching is reduced due to compression by abdominal contents and interference in normal signaling results in lung immaturity. Particularly if delivered preterm, surfactant deficiency may result in reduced functional residual capacity and may predispose to acute pulmonary hypertension. In addition, infants with CDH may have a reduced pulmonary vascular bed with vascular muscular hypertrophy and exaggerated pulmonary vasoreactivity to stimuli such as hypoxemia [74,75]. The associated impairment in pulmonary blood flow may exacerbate hypoxia and contribute to hypercapnia. The ratio of pulmonary artery flow acceleration time (or time-to-peak velocity (TPV)) indexed to RVET as a measurement of PVR may be used to predict disease severity. TPV/RVET ratio equal or less than 0.29 was associated with a 61.9% risk of death or extracorporeal membrane oxygenation (ECMO) on postnatal day 1 as compared to 100% survival of infants with higher ratios in one study [76] and may be associated with a greater respiratory illness severity.

The growth of the heart may be impacted by altered flow patterns related to abnormal position of the inferior vena cava resulting and due to compression by abdominal organs resulting in impaired filling. The result is small left heart structures which may contribute to left atrial hypertension and pulmonary edema. Postnatal factors contributing to ongoing impairment in LV filling may include RV conformational change due to PH, poor pulmonary blood flow, and external compression by gas filled intrathoracic organs. Smaller left heart diastolic diameter and increased right heart diastolic diameter have been associated with poor prognosis [77,78]. Both right and left ventricular function may be impaired in this population, and the presence of systolic dysfunction may be a more important predictor of outcome than absolute pulmonary pressure [79,80]. For fetuses with early evidence of poor prognosis, balloon tracheal occlusion may be used to improve lung growth, though the impact of this new technique on the cardiovascular system remains to be explored [81]. Antenatal therapy with sildenafil is associated with improved lung growth and pulmonary vascular responsiveness in animal models and may be an avenue for future investigation in human studies [82–84].

Hypoxic ischemic encephalopathy

Cardiovascular dysfunction in patients with hypoxic ischemic encephalopathy (HIE) is common and often multifactorial [85]. Both the asphyxial insult and therapeutic hypothermia modulate the cardiovascular system and the effect of temperature may reduce the sensitivity and specificity of commonly used clinical parameters for detecting impaired circulatory function. Asphyxia is associated with failed transition which commonly results in acute pulmonary hypertension and with transient myocardial ischemia which occurs in approximately 29%–38% of asphyxiated neonates [86,87]. As a result, hypotension and poor perfusion with or without hypoxic respiratory failure may occur. Hypothermia is associated with thermoregulatory vasoconstriction which has been shown to increase systemic arterial pressure and exacerbate oxygenation failure in neonates with HIE [88]. The effect on PVR is less well understood. Though there was no difference in clinically apparent pulmonary hypertension between treated and untreated neonates in the randomized trials of whole body cooling, the majority of trials excluded neonates with significant hypoxemic respiratory failure [89]. In animal models, a 1° change in temperature produces a 1% change in PVR [90] suggesting that neonates who already have high PVR due to failed transition are at the highest risk of hypoxemia when therapeutic hypothermia is initiated. Optimal medical management of pulmonary hypertension is recommended prior to initiating therapeutic hypothermia and caution is advised.

Both the primary insult, via myocardial ischemia and pulmonary hypertension, and therapeutic hypothermia may contribute to low cardiac output in asphyxiated newborns (Fig. 30A.5). Whole body cooling is associated with a 67% reduction in cardiac output, which is primarily related to sinus bradycardia [85]. Whether this contributes to neuroprotection via reduction in reperfusion injury is unknown; however, redistribution of blood flow toward the cerebral circulation in cooled patients has been associated with worse neurodevelopmental outcome [91]. The clinical significance of this observation is uncertain and highlights the difficulty of determining "optimum" cerebral blood flow in asphyxiated neonates. The ability to assess whether systemic blood flow is adequate may also be compromised by the coexistence of tissue injury. Anuria or oliguria may result from acute kidney injury. Metabolic acidosis and elevated lactate are common, which may be related to the initial insult [92] and may take up to 75 h to normalize after birth [93], making it more difficult to identify poor tissue perfusion. Hypocapnea is independently associated with increased risk of poor outcome, whether this is a reflection of more severe metabolic acidosis, a surrogate marker for tissue injury, and low metabolism, or is a modulator of outcome via cerebral vasoconstriction is

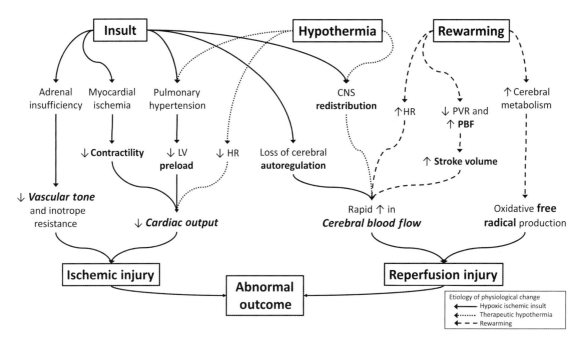

Fig. 30A.5 Putative schematic of the factors that may contribute to changes in central nervous system perfusion and oxygenation, and may therefore influence brain outcomes, during the therapeutic hypothermia and rewarming phases following hypoxic ischemic encephalopathy [96]. *HR*, Heart rate; *LV*, left ventricle; *PBF*, pulmonary blood flow; *PVR*, pulmonary vascular resistance.

unknown [94]. Echocardiography may provide valuable adjunctive information about myocardial performance and pulmonary pressure and serial scans may facilitate better physiologic definition of response to therapy. Measurements, particularly ventricular output, however, should be interpreted in the context of temperature in light of data associating high cerebral blood flow with increased illness severity prior to the cooling era [95].

Rewarming reverses many of the temperature-induced changes and may be a period of vulnerability for neonates with brain injury. Changes in drug metabolism, temperature-induced increase in cardiac output and reversal of hypoxic pulmonary vasoconstriction may theoretically precipitate dramatic changes in cerebral blood flow and oxygen delivery, the effects of which are unknown.

The infant of a diabetic mother

Maternal hyperglycemia, and consequent fetal hyperinsulinemia, has been shown to retard production and secretion of surfactant, leading to an increased risk for respiratory distress syndrome which may increase the risk of acute pulmonary hypertension [97,98]. Independent of lung disease, accelerated muscularization of pulmonary arteries, demonstrated in an animal model [99], and other conditions associated with maternal diabetes such as chronic fetal hypoxia and polycythemia may increase risk of pulmonary hypertension in this population. Exposure to a high-fat diet during gestation is also associated with a higher incidence of acute pulmonary hypertension, reduced surfactant production, and fewer pulmonary vessels at birth in a rat model [100].

Importantly, fetal hyperinsulinism is also associated with hypertrophic cardiomyopathy characterized by generalized cardiomegaly [101]. Asymmetric septal hypertrophy due to regional differences in insulin receptor density may cause left ventricular outflow tract (LVOT) obstruction in up to 5% of all IDM infants [102–104] (Fig. 30A.6). Recent studies have correlated elevated levels of biomarkers, such as cardiac-specific troponin I (cTnI) and N-terminal pro-brain natriuretic peptide (NT-pro BNP), in IDM patients with echocardiogram parameters to predict hypertrophic cardiomyopathy and left ventricular dysfunction [105,106]. cTnI is an inhibitory protein involved in cardiac muscle relaxation and released in settings of myocardial injury. Serum levels are correlated with degree of septal hypertrophy, which may be due to suboptimal coronary artery oxygen delivery to compensate for high myocardial oxygen demand [105].

Echocardiography may demonstrate increased interventricular septum/posterior wall thickness and corresponding impaired left ventricular diastolic function [107,108].

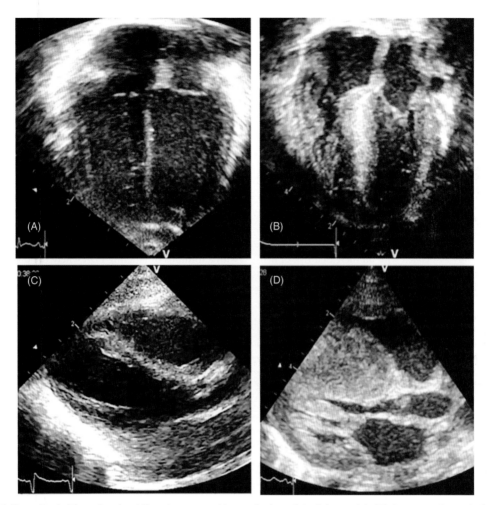

Fig. 30A.6 Normal apical four chamber (A) and parasternal long axis view of the left ventricle (C) demonstrating typical wall thickness for a term neonate. Hypertrophic heart, with asymmetric septal hypertrophy as seen from the apex (B) and the parasternal long axis (D). The mitral valve may move paradoxically into the left ventricular outflow tract (LVOT) during systole (systolic anterior motion of the mitral valve, SAM) due to a combination of the venturi effect and/or abnormal placement of the papillary muscles to create dynamic LVOT obstruction.

Hyperdynamic left ventricular systolic function is the norm as evidenced by both conventional and novel echocardiography measurements [108,109], though myocardial strain and torsion may show subtle abnormalities [110]. The dominant physiological concern for neonates with HOCM is one of impaired left heart filling and consequently impaired cardiac output. Compensatory tachycardia reduces diastolic duration and therefore further compromises stroke volume. Pulmonary hypertension with limited left atrial preload in this setting may be particularly problematic as high left atrial pressure is essential for forward flow into the poorly compliant hypertrophic ventricle; however, right-to-left ductal shunt may maintain systemic blood flow in situations where LVOT obstruction is severe. Low cardiac output in these patients is associated with lower cerebral resistance to compensate the low flow through carotid arteries [111,112].

Patent ductus arteriosus

Persistence of the ductus arteriosus after the immediate transitional period is common in premature infants born at extremely low gestational age. The architecture of the ductal wall [113,114], its blood supply, and response to vasoactive substances such as oxygen [114,115], prostaglandin, and nitric oxide [116] favor ductal patency. The role of the

PDA may either be transitional, supportive, or pathological depending on the specific pathophysiology. For some neonates, such as those with significant pulmonary hypertension, patency may be advantageous; specifically, the PDA may provide an avenue for right-to-left shunt to support systemic blood flow in situations where pulmonary venous return to the left atrium is poor while simultaneously reducing RV wall stress. In healthy neonates during a normal transition, the ductal shunt may be negligible and patency may be of no clinical consequence. For many preterm infants, however, ductal patency allows diversion of a portion of the systemic cardiac output to recirculate through the pulmonary vascular bed which may lead to pulmonary edema and impaired lung compliance [117]. The pathological role of the PDA in neonates remains contentious, despite several decades of study and over 50 randomized trials of therapy [118]. Nevertheless, PDA has been consistently associated with an increased risk of neonatal morbidities such as BPD, NEC, impaired neurodevelopmental outcome and mortality.

One of the potential contributors to failure of interventional trials to modify outcomes may relate to heterogeneity of the definition of hemodynamic significance. Though ductal diameter prior to 36 h of life is predictive of need for later intervention [119], reliance on a single metric is not without limitations. These include operator or equipment-related measurement error, assumptions regarding ductal geometry, potential vasoactive responsiveness of the PDA, and evidence that diameter alone does not explain variance in indicators of shunt volume (Fig. 30A.7). Shunt volume is governed by Pouiselle's Law in which the flow in a conduit is related to radius and length, viscosity of the fluid, and the relative pressure at either end. Though size is important, its use in isolation represents a physiological oversimplification. Pulsed-wave Doppler flow pattern may provide some information regarding the relative pressure differences between the systemic and pulmonary circulation. High-velocity flow in the presence of a pulsatile pattern may be associated with a significant pressure gradient, whereas low velocity flow is more likely to suggest elevated pulmonary artery pressure. Although elevated peak systolic velocity may suggest a closing ductus (continuous flow), high shunt volume or marginal vessel restriction may also lead to higher velocity (pulsatile). Additionally, in patients with a tortuous or tapering PDA where the diameter varies across its length, the precise position of the pulsed-wave Doppler sample gate may influence measured velocity. These factors emphasize the importance of a more comprehensive assessment based not only on estimates of diameter or transductal flow patterns, but surrogate indicators of shunt volume (Table 30A.3). The ratio of left atrial to aortic annulus diameter is commonly used and in the presence of a diagnosis of PDA has good specificity, however, has low interrater reliability, and limited sensitivity.

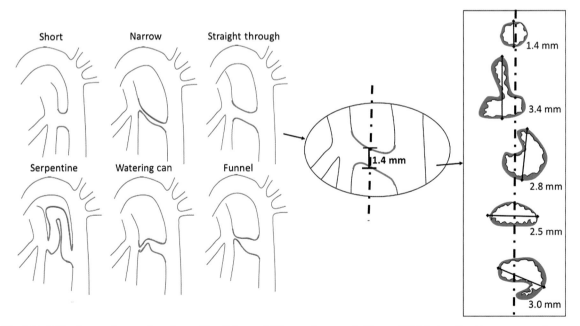

Fig. 30A.7 The Patent Ductus Arteriosus May Take on Different Geometric Shapes Which Are Not Homogenous in Diameter and Length. These differences may have important implications for measurement in different planes. A PDA which is 1.4 mm in the plane of insonation may be nontubular and therefore its largest diameter may vary widely.

Table 30A.3 Modified staging system for determining the magnitude of the hemodynamically significant ductus arteriosus (HSDA) based on clinical and echocardiography criteria

C1 asymptomatic	E1 no evidence of ductal flow (2D or Doppler interrogation)
C2 mild • Oxygenation difficulty (OI < 6) • Need for respiratory support (nCPAP) or mechanical ventilation (MAP < 8) • Feeding intolerance (>20% gastric aspirates) • Radiologic evidence of increased pulmonary vascularity	**E2 small nonsignificant ductus arteriosus** • Transductal diameter < 1.5 mm • Continuous transductal flow (V_{max} > 2.5 m/s) • Left heart nondilated (LA:Ao < 1.5) • No left heart pressure loading (EA < 1.0, IVRT > 45) consistent with preterm pattern • Forward end-organ diastolic flow (celiac, middle cerebral) • No retrograde descending aorta diastolic flow
C3 moderate • Oxygenation difficulty (OI 7–14) • Need for NIPPV or increasing ventilation requirements (MAP 9–12) • Not feeding 2° abdominal distension/emesis • Oliguria with mild elevation in creatinine • Systemic hypotension (low mean or diastolic pressure) • Radiologic evidence of cardiomegaly or pulmonary edema • Mild metabolic acidosis (pH 7.1–7.21 and/or base deficit −7 to −12)	**E3 moderate hsDA** • Transductal diameter 1.5–2.5 mm • Pulsatile transductal flow V_{max} 1.5–2.5 m/s) • Mild-to-mod left heart dilation (LA:Ao 1.5–2) • Mild-to-mod left heart pressure loading (EA ≥ 1 or IVRT 30–45 ms) • Decreased or absent diastolic flow in end-organ vessels (celiac, middle cerebral artery) • Retrograde diastolic flow descending aorta
C4 severe • Oxygenation difficulty (OI > 15) • High ventilation requirements (MAP > 12) • Profound or recurrent pulmonary hemorrhage • "NEC-like" abdominal distension (tenderness, erythema) • Acute renal failure • Hemodynamic instability requiring cardiotropic agent • Moderate–severe metabolic acidosis (pH < 7.1 or base deficit ≥ −12)	**E4 large hsDA** • Transductal diameter > 2.5 mm • Pulsatile transductal flow (V_{max} < 2.5 m/s) • Severe left heart dilation (LA:Ao > 2) • Severe left heart volume loading (EA ≥ 1 or IVRT < 30 ms) • Retrograde diastolic flow in end-organ vessels (celiac, middle cerebral artery) • Retrograde diastolic flow descending aorta

EA, Ratio of early to active phase transmitral flow; *IVRT*, isovolumic relaxation time; *LA:Ao*, left atrium to aorta ration; *MAP*, mean airway pressure; *mod*, moderate; *nCPAP*, nasal continuous positive airway pressure; *NEC*, necrotizing enterocolitis; *NIPPV*, noninvasive positive pressure ventilation; *OI*, oxygenation index; V_{max}, peak velocity.
Adapted from McNamara PJ, Sehgal A. Towards rational management of the patent ductus arteriosus: the need for disease staging. Arch Dis Childhood Fetal Neonatal Ed 2007;92:F424–F427 [120].

Importantly, the presence of left atrial dilation should not be used in isolation for the diagnosis of hemodynamically significant ductus arteriosus as other serious disorders (e.g., coarctation of the aorta) may result in atrial enlargement due to high LV afterload or diastolic dysfunction. The presence of diastolic flow reversal in the descending thoracic aorta has been shown to have superior ability to predict shunt volume as compared to other markers using assessment of shunt volume by cardiac MRI [117]. Assessment of shunt volume should include measures of left heart size and flow, the adequacy of systemic blood flow and should rule out the presence of contraindications to therapy such as significant LV dysfunction or coarctation of the aorta (Table 30A.4).

Post-PDA ligation cardiorespiratory considerations

The immediate postoperative period after ligation of a hemodynamically significant PDA is a period of physiological stress to the cardiorespiratory system.

1. **Early considerations (0–6 h):** The presence of a hemodynamically significant left-to-right shunt leads to pulmonary edema and reduced lung compliance [121,122]. Escalation of mean airway pressure may promote an open lung strategy. After ductal ligation, pulmonary overcirculation is immediately alleviated resulting in a reduction in left atrial preload and restoration of cardiac output to the

Table 30A.4 Echocardiography features suggesting moderate-to-large volume left-to-right PDA shunt

Assessment	Measurement
Evidence of ductal flow	Ductal diameter > 1.5 mm
	Pulsatile flow pattern
	Turbulent diastolic flow at the PA annulus
	LPA diastolic flow velocity > 50 cm/s
Pulmonary overcirculation	Pulmonary vein D wave > 50 cm/s
	Mitral valve E wave > 80 cm/s
	Mitral valve EA ratio > 1
	Isovolumic relaxation time < 40 ms
	Left ventricular output > 320 mL/min/kg
Left heart dilation	Left atrial to aortic root ratio > 1.6
	Large left-to-right PFO shunt
	LV dilation > 2SD above the normal for size (kg)
Evidence of abnormal systemic diastolic flow	Diastolic flow reversal in postductal aorta
	Diastolic flow absence or reversal celiac artery, SMA
	Diastolic flow absence or reversal MCA

MCA, Middle cerebral artery; *PA*, pulmonary artery; *PFO*, patent foramen ovale; *SMA*, superior mesenteric artery.

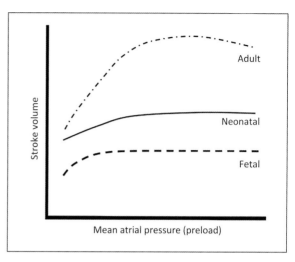

Fig. 30A.8 The Shape of the Frank–Starling Relationship Varies Based on Properties of the Myocardium [126]. In the fetal and neonatal period, the relationship between atrial filling and stroke volume is relatively flat as compared to the normal adult.

normal range [123]. Though preload and stroke volume have a proportional relationship [124,125] according to the Frank–Starling law, unless filling pressure are subphysiological, the reduction in atrial preload is unlikely to have any measureable impact on contractility [126] (Fig. 30A.8). Ligation simultaneously reduces pulmonary edema, which is associated with improved lung compliance [127,128] and overdistension caused by excessive mean airway pressure if the postoperative neonate remains on preoperative settings may contribute to low cardiac output. Finally, ligation is associated with an immediate augmentation in left ventricular afterload, the magnitude of which is dependent on the relative difference between preligation PVR and SVR. In patients with lower PVR the magnitude of the increase is higher. The clinical impact of this augmentation in LV afterload is negligible in the immediate postoperative period, although echocardiography may reveal lower cardiac output and changes in LV function using strain analysis in patients who have later cardiorespiratory deterioration. A small proportion of patients with impaired adrenal gland responsiveness may develop early systolic and diastolic hypotension which is poorly responsive to any cardiovascular agent.

2. **Delayed cardiorespiratory decompensation (6–12 h):** Preterm neonates who undergo ductal ligation are at risk for postligation cardiac syndrome which is characterized by systolic hypotension requiring cardiotropic support and progressive impairment in ventilation and oxygenation. Research to date suggests this decompensation is mediated by impaired left ventricular systolic and diastolic function secondary to sustained exposure to elevated LV afterload [129]. A steep inverse relationship between afterload and myocardial contractility has been demonstrated in both preterm animal and human studies [130–132]. Impaired forward flow due to either impaired myocardial contractility [123] or ventricular filling due to high afterload and diastolic dysfunction [133] may be associated with later onset of progressive pulmonary edema and need for escalation of mean airway pressure and oxygen (Fig. 30A.9).

3. **Short-term surgical complications:** Thoracotomy is associated with risk of surgical complications such as pneumothorax and pericardial effusion which should be considered in the differential diagnosis of any neonate with early postoperative decompensation.

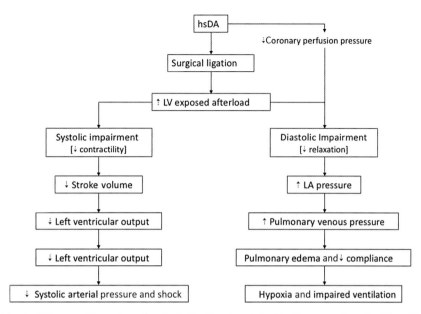

Fig. 30A.9 Physiological Changes Occurring after PDA Ligation Mediated by Exposure to a Sustained Increase in Afterload. Left ventricular (LV) systolic dysfunction contributes to the development of impaired systemic perfusion and shock while LV diastolic dysfunction produces pulmonary edema resulting in oxygenation and ventilation failure.

Additional rare but important considerations may include clip migration with impingement on the aorta or branch pulmonary artery, vascular rupture, or chylothorax. Though intraoperative assessment of arterial pressure and systemic perfusion are the norm prior to closure of the surgical site, it may be difficult to appropriately position the clip or ligature, particularly for a large ductus, and echocardiography may be beneficial in a compatible clinical situation such as the development of an arm-leg arterial pressure gradient.

4. **The role of echocardiography in the prevention of PLCS:** Echocardiography assessment in the immediate postoperative period may facilitate the anticipation of postoperative cardiorespiratory instability. LVO < 198 mL/min/kg at 1 h postligation is highly sensitive for the prediction of need for cardiotropic therapy for delayed cardiorespiratory deterioration at 8–12 h [134]. Other echocardiography measures, such as myocardial velocity using tissue Doppler imaging and peak longitudinal strain using speckle tracking are reduced following ligation, particularly in neonates with low cardiac output [51].

Chronic pulmonary hypertension in the preterm infant

Bronchopulmonary dysplasia and associated chronic pulmonary hypertension are common in extreme preterm infants. Among infants with severe BPD, the reported incidence of PH is between 15% and 58% [135–137]. Younger gestation, growth restriction, and multiple gestation infants may be at particular risk [138]. In a recent single-center study, 18% of a cohort of 145 extremely low birth weight infants screened with echocardiography at 4 weeks of age were diagnosed with pulmonary hypertension. A rate of 50% in the subpopulation of infants on oxygen at 36 weeks was identified [136]. Though bronchopulmonary dysplasia is the most frequent association in preterm infants, pulmonary hypertension may also occur in the context of congenital cardiac or respiratory anomalies, congenital diaphragmatic hernia, and lung hypoplasia [139,140]. Genetic predisposition may also play a role. The mechanisms responsible for the development of elevated PVR and altered reactivity are not completely understood. Intermittent hypoxic episodes [135], impaired alveolar development with dysregulated angiogenesis of the pulmonary circulation [141], vascular remodeling [33], and pulmonary venous congestion secondary to left heart disease, systemic hypertension and aortic stiffness [138] have been suggested as possible contributors.

Though the gold standard for diagnosis of pulmonary hypertension in adults, cardiac catheterization is rarely performed in this population in favor of noninvasive testing. Echocardiography is the most widely used modality and has been found to be 80%–88% sensitive as a diagnostic test [34,138], though it is important to remember that, unlike catheter-based measurements echocardiography measurements are relative and depend on interpretation in context (Table 30A.1). For example, the presence of systemic hypertension, a common comorbidity in patients with bronchopulmonary dysplasia may cause elevated left-ventricular end systolic pressure which may result in underestimation of a diagnosis of pulmonary hypertension made solely on the basis of assessment of septal flattening. Cardiac MRI, high-resolution CT [35,36], and the use of biomarkers such as BNP [37] have been proposed as alternative investigative tools, though neither CT nor MRI are practical for serial monitoring and BNP has not been sufficiently evaluated.

The optimum approach to neonates at risk of chronic pulmonary hypertension remains a controversy. The features of chronic pulmonary hypertension are often subtle and may be difficult to isolate from symptoms caused by concomitant parenchymal lung disease. The onset is insidious and the timing is likely variable. Echocardiography evidence may be present as early as 28 weeks gestation [136]. Though the presence of pulmonary vascular disease at day 7 of life has been associated with a higher risk of bronchopulmonary dysplasia and chronic pulmonary hypertension [138], late presentation may occur after previously negative evaluations at term corrected gestation [136]. The optimum approach to diagnosis and screening is not established and the role screening may play in modulating health outcomes is not certain [38]. A high index of suspicion is required. Though there is insufficient evidence to recommend a specific screening algorithm, consideration of echocardiography for neonates diagnosed with bronchopulmonary dysplasia to rule out chronic pulmonary hypertension is recommended. The echocardiography assessment should be comprehensive and include anatomic reappraisal due to the potential of pulmonary vein stenosis masquerading as chronic pulmonary hypertension. Close collaboration with a pediatric cardiologist in these situations is warranted.

Role of targeted neonatal echocardiography in guiding cardiorespiratory care

Historically, the approach to low arterial pressure has been based on an arbitrary numerical definition of hypotension based on the infants mean arterial pressure less than their gestational age in weeks which was popularized by a consensus statement published on the treatment of respiratory distress syndrome and based on expert opinion without cited evidence [142]. The goal of ensuring adequate arterial pressure is to ensure that the perfusion pressure and flow to the organs, particularly the brain, is sufficient to provide enough oxygen to meet the metabolic demands of

the tissue and prevent ischemia. Many investigators have explored the "minimum required" arterial pressure to prevent brain injury throughout the history of modern neonatology, and there remains no conclusion. This is likely related to several factors. First, there is no standardization of methodology and therefore the duration of "hypotension" required to be considered exposed, the mechanism by which arterial pressure is measured (e.g., cuff, arterial line) and the definition of hypotension are variable. Second, many studies are small and therefore underpowered to detect a relevant endpoint. Third, none of the published literature takes etiology of low mean arterial pressure into consideration. Important changes in systolic and diastolic pressure may be missed by using a calculated composite. Finally, arterial pressure is only one component of the determinates of oxygen delivery, sufficient to meet metabolic demands, and is also an imprecise surrogate for cardiac output [143]. There may be many infants in whom low mean arterial pressure does not equate to any change in delivery of oxygen to the brain. Fluctuations in mean arterial pressure to numbers considered "hypotensive" are frequent in the otherwise well preterm infant during the on postnatal day 1 and have no influence on tissue oxygen extraction as measured by NIRS [144].

Though there is some variation between practitioners, the most common practice for the treatment of hypotension is to utilize an algorithmic escalation of therapy which is universally applied to all neonates [145]. One danger of this approach is that it fails to consider variation between patients. Dopamine, for example, at doses of 6–8 mcg/kg/min has been shown to have a predominantly vasoconstrictive effect in some preterm neonates and a predominant inotropic effect in others of similar gestation [146]. Second, the variable contributors to low mean arterial pressure may require different therapeutic strategies. The components of systolic and diastolic arterial pressure may provide greater diagnostic insights than looking at the composite of mean; for example, systolic arterial pressure is generated by the force of cardiac contraction and may be reflective of cardiac output. The diastolic, on the other hand, reflects the resting pressure of blood against the arterial wall between contractions and may be more related to vascular tone (Fig. 30A.10).

The utilization of echocardiography in combination with clinical assessment may improve the precision of pathophysiological appraisal and aid in the selection of therapy ("right drug" for "right patient" at "right time"). Recent evidence highlights the potential benefits of comprehensive echocardiography assessments performed by trained neonatologists in multiple areas of neonatal care. First, the introduction of a targeted neonatal echocardiography-based triaging algorithm for neonates referred for PDA ligation has contributed to reduction in unnecessary intervention. The use of a comprehensive preoperative assessment of shunt volume to guide decision-making

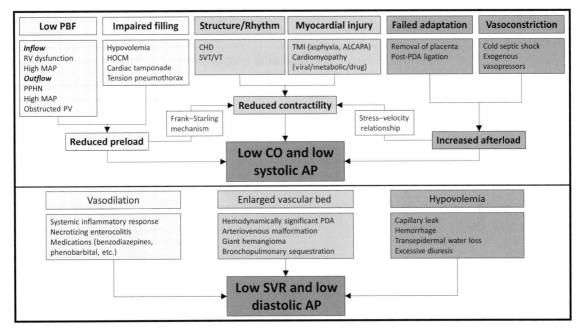

Fig. 30A.10 Differential Diagnosis of Low Systolic Arterial Pressure (Low Cardiac Output) and Low Diastolic Arterial Pressure (Low Systemic Vascular Resistance). Adapted from Giesinger RE, McNamara PJ. Hemodynamic instability in the critically ill neonate: an approach to cardiovascular support based on disease pathophysiology. Semin Perinatol 2016;40(3): 174–188 [147].

reduced the frequency of PDA ligation with no increase in short-term morbidities [148]. Second, routine utilization of TnECHO to assess preterm infants with hypoxic respiratory failure has improved timeliness of diagnosis and was associated with earlier and more targeted use of nitric oxide in preterm infants with pulmonary hypertension [149]. Third, TnECHO may be a more accurate diagnostic method compared to current gold standards for routine daily tasks such as umbilical line positioning. Chest radiography has poor sensitivity and specificity for predicting the location of the tip position of umbilical venous lines [150]. Trained pediatric house staff are able to reliably identify catheters which, though appropriately positioned on radiography, have their tip within either the right or left atrium, placing the neonate at increased risk of serious complications (e.g., pericardial tamponade, arrhythmia) [151]. Finally, TnECHO assessment may be useful for prognostication and defining populations of interest, who are at greatest risk of predetermined outcomes. For example, a TnECHO-based scoring system utilizing a composite of five measurements derived on postnatal day 2 has been developed which may be useful in the prediction of BPD in infants with PDA. Though there is limited evidence describing the impact of targeted therapy on outcomes, the development of enhanced monitoring and directed therapy has potential to improve the quality of care as our understanding of neonatal pathophysiology develops. Study of the pharmacologic and biologic properties of cardiovascular therapeutic agents in the neonatal population is an emerging field.

Acute pulmonary hypertension in the term neonate

Historically, the treatment of shock in the infant with acute PH has included the administration of potent systemic vasoconstricting agents in an effort to increase SVC and therefore reverse the ductal shunt and push blood into the pulmonary circulation. Though this may be effective in some patients, there are a variety of problems with this approach. First, most of the agents used to induce systemic vasoconstriction also have vasoconstrictor effects in the pulmonary vasculature which may be counter-effective and potentially harmful. Dopamine, in particular, has been shown to increase pulmonary artery pressure to a greater extent than systemic arterial pressure in a piglet model [152]. Second, pulmonary hypertension is associated with myocardial dysfunction and the augmentation in afterload which occurs using this approach may be poorly tolerated. Third, the impact of the resultant systemic hypertension on cerebral blood flow is unknown. As an alternative, a

Table 30A.5 Suggested therapies for treatment of systemic hypotension and/or low cardiac output for neonates with acute pulmonary hypertension

Type of hypotension	Pathophysiology	Additional TnECHO findings	Therapeutic interventions
Normal SAP Normal DAP	↓ PBF ↓ LV preload LV compensates by increasing contractility and/or heart rate to maintain SBF	**Critical:** ↓ RVO ↑EF, normal LVO **Other:** ↓ PV, transmitral flow ± mild ↓ RV contractility	**First line:** iNO, volume Optimize sedation **Second line:** Milrinone
↓ SAP Normal DAP	↓ PBF ↓ LV preload LV unable to compensate causing ↓ SBF	**Critical:** ↓ RVO with normal EF, ↓ LVO **Other:** ↓ PV, transmitral flow ± mild ↓ RV contractility	**First line:** iNO, volume MAP, optimize sedation **Second line:** Milrinone Vasopressin Dobutamine
↓↓ SAP Normal DAP	Very ↓ PBF Very ↓ LV preload ↓↓LV systolic function with ↓↓ SBF and RV failure	**Critical:** ↓↓ RVO ↓ EF, ↓ LVO Moderate – severely ↓ RV contractility **Other:** ↓↓ PV and transmitral flow	**First line:** iNO, volume MAP, optimize sedation **Second line:** Vasopressin Dobutamine **Third line:** Prostaglandin Epinephrine Steroids
↓↓ SAP ↓DAP	Very ↓ PBF Very ↓ LV preload LV and RV failure ↓↓ SBF Impending cardiac arrest	**Critical:** ↓↓ RVO ↓ EF, ↓↓ LVO Severe ↓ RV contractility **Other:** ↓↓ PV and transmitral flow TR often absent	**First line:** iNO, volume, MAP **Second line:** Vasopressin Prostaglandin Epinephrine Steroids (early ECMO referral)

DAP, Diastolic arterial pressure; ECMO, extracorporeal membrane oxygenation; EF, ejection fraction; iNO, inhaled nitric oxide; LV/RV, left and right ventricle; LVO/RVO, left and right ventricular output; MAP, mean airway pressure; PBF, pulmonary blood flow; PV, pulmonary vein; SAP, systolic arterial pressure; SBF, systemic blood flow; TR, tricuspid regurgitation.
Adapted from Jain A, McNamara PJ. Persistent pulmonary hypertension of the newborn: physiology, hemodynamic assessment and novel therapies. Curr Pediatr Rev 2013;9:55–66 [44].

strategy employing support of myocardial performance and maintenance of fetal circulatory patterns to augment systemic perfusion may be used while instituting pulmonary vasodilator therapy.

Empiric cardiotropic management in a neonate with acute PH should focus first on optimization of pulmonary blood flow (Table 30A.5). Appropriate lung recruitment and administration of iNO may improve left heart filling and heart function sufficiently to correct mild-to-moderate systolic hypotension. Echocardiography is recommended in all neonates with suspected acute pulmonary hypertension and evidence of poor systemic blood flow to confirm the diagnosis and assess myocardial function (Fig. 30A.11). For infants with impaired right ventricular performance first-line therapies include drugs with positive inotropic properties and favorable effects in the peripheral circulation.

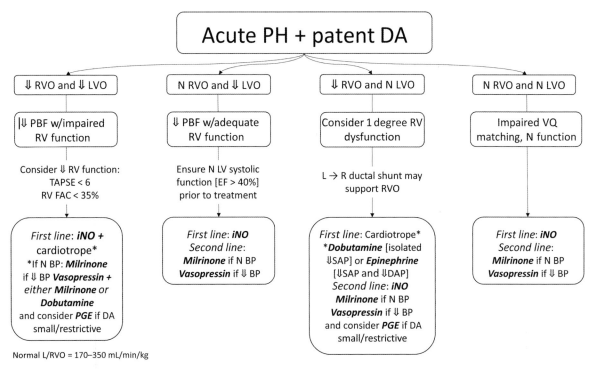

Fig. 30A.11 An Approach to Echocardiography Guided Therapy for Acute Pulmonary Hypertension in the Term Neonate without Hypoxic Ischemic Encephalopathy. *BP*, Blood pressure; *DA*, ductus arteriosus; *DAP*, diastolic arterial pressure; *EF*, ejection fraction; *FAC*, fractional area change; *iNO*, inhaled nitric oxide; *L*, left; *LV*, left ventricle; *N*, normal; *PBF*, pulmonary blood flow; *PGE*, prostaglandin; *PH*, pulmonary hypertension; *R*, right; *R/LVO*, right and left ventricular output; *RV*, right ventricle; *SAP*, systolic arterial pressure; *TAPSE*, tricuspid annular plane systolic excursion.

Dobutamine, a catecholamine agonist with action at myocardial α1 and β1 receptors and possible mild pulmonary and systemic vasodilator effects, has been shown to increase cardiac output in term [153] and preterm [154] infants and may provide benefit as first-line therapy. Milrinone, a phosphodiesterase 3 inhibitor, has been shown to improve cardiac output and reduce PVR in neonates with acute pulmonary hypertension [155]. Caution is advised, however, as the systemic vasodilator properties may exacerbate diastolic or severe hypotension to the detriment of coronary and cerebral perfusion pressure, and therefore, milrinone is not recommended for infants with existing diastolic hypotension. For infants with low diastolic or severely low arterial pressure in whom a systemic vasopressor is required, vasopressin, an endogenous hormone, has a favorable pharmacologic profile. It is a potent constrictor in the systemic circulation which has nitric-oxide-mediated vasodilator properties in the pulmonary vascular bed and has been utilized as an effective therapy for hypotension and oxygenation failure in term neonates with acute PH [156]. For infants with acute PH and RV dysfunction with a restrictive PDA, prostaglandin has beneficial properties.

As previously described, right-to-left ductal shunt may support systemic circulation and provide afterload reduction for the RV; however, in addition, PGE1 is a nonselective vasodilator and may therefore reduce PVR.

Acute pulmonary hypertension in the preterm neonate

The treatment of acute PH in the preterm infant is an area of considerable clinical controversy. As in term infants, the principles of optimal ventilation and lung recruitment are fundamental. The administration of surfactant is associated with improved PVR in preterms with reduced FRC secondary to respiratory distress syndrome. Adequate treatment of lung disease in these patients may be sufficient to improve ventilation/perfusion matching and correct pulmonary hypertension. The utilization of iNO, which is standard of care in term infants, is contentious in preterms. Multiple randomized trials have been done with highly varied methodology and primary outcome measures to answer the question of whether iNO has benefit for the preterm infant with hypoxic respiratory failure (Table 30A.6). It is

Table 30A.6 Characteristics of randomized controlled trials of nitric oxide for early rescue therapy of hypoxic respiratory failure in preterm infants [32]

Identifier	GA/wt, n	Inclusion criteria	Intervention/duration	Primary outcome	PH on echo (n, %)
Mercier et al. [86]	<33/40, n = 85	• OI 12.5–30 • ≤7 days of life	• 10–20 ppm (based on OI) • Duration unclear	Reduction in OI after 2 h	Not reported
Srisuparp et al. [38]	<2 kg, n = 34	• Clinical RDS, surfactant • OI varied by BW (min 4, max 12) • ≤72 h of life	• 20 ppm • Max of 7 days	Effects of iNO on oxygenation	Not reported
Su et al. [83]	≤31/40 and ≤1.5 kg n = 65	• OI ≥ 25	• 5–20 ppm • ↓ by 1 ppm Q6 h as dictated by FiO$_2$	Effects of iNO on oxygenation	Not reported
Wei et al. [84]	≤34/40, n = 60	• MV, 2 h after surfactant • OI ≥ 11 • <7 days of life	• 5 ppm starting • At least 7 days or when extubated	OI before and during treatment	Not reported

a/AO$_2$, Alveolar-arterial oxygen gradient; *BPD*, bronchopulmonary dysplasia; *BW*, birth weight; *FiO$_2$*, fraction of inspired oxygen; *MAP*, mean airway pressure; *MV*, mechanical ventilation; *OI*, oxygenation index; *ppm*, parts per million.

important to differentiate between the primary end-points of acute improvement in oxygenation and the outcomes of morbidities such as BPD and mortality.

1. **Efficacy of iNO as rescue therapy for HRF:** Improved oxygenation and increased pulmonary blood flow with administration of exogenous nitric oxide have been documented in animal and laboratory studies as early as 2/3 completed gestation [157,158]. Similarly, observational studies in human preterm infants at high risk of pulmonary hypertension (e.g., prolonged oligohydramnios, pulmonary hypoplasia) have demonstrated a high rate of improved oxygenation with iNO administration regardless of gestational age [159–161]. Of the infants enrolled in clinical trials with oxygenation as an outcome measure, response was identified in just over 50% of cases [162]. This may not, however, truly reflect the proportion of appropriately selected neonates with iNO responsive disease. The severity of oxygenation failure in the trials varied from an oxygenation index of 11–25 and echocardiography was neither used as an entry criterion nor frequently reported and therefore, the relative contribution of pulmonary hypertension to the disease physiology in included infants is unknown and likely variable [163–166]. Emerging data suggest that preterm infants in the transitional period with documented pulmonary hypertension have a similar response rate to iNO as term infants [167]. iNO is recommended for acute rescue therapy of hypoxic preterms with suspected or proven pulmonary

hypertension, particularly in the context of prolonged oligohydramnios [168]. The optimum starting dose, duration, and weaning strategy are not well studied in preterm infants, though strategies utilized for term neonates may require modification due to the unique considerations of the preterm circulation. Ischemia–reperfusion injury due to rapid augmentation in cerebral blood flow may be a contributing factor for IVH and excessive reduction in PVR in the presence of a PDA may contribute to pulmonary edema and/or pulmonary hemorrhage. Further study is required.

2. **Impact of iNO on neonatal outcomes:** iNO use has not been demonstrated to improve neonatal outcomes in several randomized trials; however, there are methodologic considerations that make the current body of literature incomplete. First, neonates selected for inclusion were highly variable between trials, and the definition of physiological contributors to respiratory disease was incomplete. The administration of iNO to a preterm infant with pulmonary hypertension as the primary physiological determinant of hypoxemia is likely to have a significantly different impact on outcome as compared to those neonates in whom hypoxia is caused by parenchymal lung disease or pulmonary edema in the setting of left-to-right PDA shunt, for example. Observational studies suggest improved oxygenation and lower mortality for those infants presumed to be high risk of pulmonary hypertension, such as those with prolonged oligohydramnios, when treated with

iNO; however, limited data are available for neonates without pulmonary hypoplasia [159,160]. Second, iNO responsiveness may be an important predictor of outcome in hypoxic preterms [169] and the response rate to iNO in the clinical trials was low at 51%–55% [162]. This suggests that those patients with the greatest likelihood of benefit may not have been targeted appropriately by the selection process.

3. **Treatment of shock:** There is limited published evidence specific to the use of cardiotropic agents for preterm infants with acute PH and therefore extrapolation from term data may be required. The choice of agent should take into consideration the disease pathophysiology both in identifying therapeutic strategies for intervention and in monitoring for side effects because many agents impact on both the systemic and pulmonary circulation. Similar strategies as in term neonates are recommended (Fig. 30A.12). Milrinone has been associated with improved RV function and reduced pulmonary artery pressure in preterm neonates, though particular caution when using milrinone is suggested as the half-life in preterm infants is approximately 10 h as compared to 4 h and milrinone has been suggested to be a negative inotrope in an experimental animal model [170]. In addition, caution is advised when used in the setting of neonatal hypoxia-ischemia or borderline hypotension. Vasopressin may be efficacious in the correction of systemic hypotension in the setting of acute PH without provoking pulmonary vasoconstriction [171]. Though not evidence based, prostaglandin may also confer the same benefits as in term infants; caution is advised, however, as reduction of PVR associated with improving PH in the presence of a wide open ductus may result in replacement of PH-related hypoxia with hypoxia due to pulmonary edema and ductal physiology.

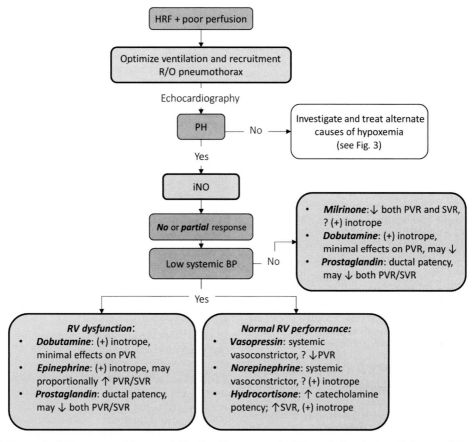

Fig. 30A.12 Suggested Management Approach for the Management of Hypoxic Respiratory Failure and Shock in the Preterm Infant With Acute Pulmonary Hypertension [32].

Structural congenital heart disease

The treatment of acute pulmonary hypertension in the neonate with congenital heart disease includes the use of sedation, muscle relaxation, and judicious use of iNO. Mortality is high in these patients despite ECMO [63] and both specific cardiac anatomy and associated conditions (e.g., genetic abnormalities) likely play a role. Milrinone may have particular benefit in this population because it is independent of beta-adrenergic receptors which may be downregulated in the presence of congestive heart failure and has pulmonary vasodilator properties. The use of milrinone both augments cardiac output and reduces PVR. In addition to its role in ensuring ductal patency, prostaglandin E1 is a nonspecific vasodilator and may, therefore, also be advantageous in the treatment of pulmonary hypertension.

For those survivors with long-term pulmonary hypertension, some medical therapies have been explored, particularly in adult survivors of childhood congenital heart disease both before and after surgical repair. Anticoagulation may be required to prevent pulmonary artery thrombosis due to the higher risk of coagulation abnormalities in the setting of an abnormal pulmonary vascular bed [172]. Diuretic therapy may be useful, particularly in the setting of right ventricular volume and pressure overload. Calcium channel blockers, antiarrythmics, and iron supplementation are used in adult patients with Eisenmenger Syndrome and may be areas for further study in the pediatric population, though their use in neonates has not been evaluated. Novel pulmonary vasodilator therapies have been explored, again in adult populations, and may include endothelin receptor antagonists (e.g., bosentan [173], ambrisentan [174]), prostacyclins (e.g., iloprost, treprostinil), and phosphodiesterase 5 inhibitors (e.g., sildenafil, tadalafil). In some patients, lung–heart transplantation may be a treatment alternative. Bosentan is a competitive dual endothelin receptor antagonist that acts as a vasodilator and neurohormonal blocker to improve LV function and diminish cardiac remodeling. In one trial (FUTURE), using Bosentan in neonates with acute pulmonary hypertension, there were minimal side effects; however, there was no improvement in oxygenation or other outcomes in severe cases [175]. Sildenafil, a phosphodiesterase inhibitor which acts on vascular smooth muscle, may have synergistic effect when used with iNO [176,177]. Sildenafil administration prior to VSD repair may prevent postsurgical pulmonary hypertension and pulmonary hypertensive crisis, diminish duration of intubation and shorten length of ICU stay and may also be useful in long-term therapy [178–180].

Congenital diaphragmatic hernia

Neonates with CDH have small lung volumes and ventilation targets should take this into consideration, though no one specific mode of ventilation has proven advantage over another. Overexpansion may be detrimental as preexisting pulmonary hypertension may be compounded by exogenous compression of the capillary bed. Intubation without bag mask ventilation and attention to gastric decompression are important as intestinal gas may compromise not only lung expansion but also may limit pulmonary blood flow, impair left heart filling and produce shock. iNO is commonly used to treat hypoxic respiratory failure [181,182]. Though some neonates do have improved short-term indicators of response with improved oxygenation, iNO has not been shown to reduce the overall risk of death or ECMO in the CDH population and there are likely several contributing factors [183]. First, there are multiple contributing factors to impaired pulmonary blood flow in this population of which pulmonary arterial hypertension is only one. Second, some patients, such as those with severe LV dysfunction may actually have harm from pulmonary vasodilator therapy if systemic blood flow is dependent on right-to-left ductal shunt, and therefore the potential improvement in patients with pulmonary arterial hypertension as the primary cause of hypoxemia may be diluted in the larger population. Because the etiology of impaired pulmonary blood flow may be multifactorial, detailed physiological characterization may aid management. Echocardiography assessment of LV function and atrial shunt direction may be invaluable tools to decision-making. The presence of right-to-left shunt at both the atrial and the ductal level suggest that pulmonary arterial hypertension is a more important contributor to impaired pulmonary blood flow. If left-to-right atrial shunt is present in the setting of right-to-left ductal shunt, this suggests that the left atrial pressure is high and pulmonary venous hypertension may be a significant contributor to disease. In this setting, pulmonary vasodilator therapy may be less effective and may, in fact, be detrimental.

Pulmonary vasodilator therapy has limited evidence specific to the CDH population, though medications such as sildenafil and milrinone are used in clinical practice [184,185]. Milrinone may be advantageous both for infants with pulmonary arterial and pulmonary venous hypertension. Systemic afterload reduction improves left heart filling and may therefore improve stroke volume in the setting of LV diastolic dysfunction. Caution is advised in the setting of systemic hypotension or severe HIE where therapeutic hypothermia is in progress given the vasodilator effect of milrinone [186]. Treatment of systemic hypotension may include the use of systemic vasoconstricting agents such as vasopressin or norepinephrine for neonates with normal LV function and acute pulmonary hypertension. For neonates with LV dysfunction and systemic hypotension, epinephrine is recommended. A combined approach using epinephrine to stabilize arterial pressure and milrinone for neonates with LV dysfunction or vasopressin and milrinone for neonates with pulmonary arterial hypertension is physiologically advantageous; however, there is limited specific evidence for the use of any particular approach to cardiovascular care in neonates with CDH. Prostaglandin therapy may be important to provide afterload reduction to the RV and systemic blood flow in the case of LV dysfunction [187].

Hypoxic ischemic encephalopathy

The treatment of pulmonary hypertension and shock with concurrent HIE requires consideration of the goals of therapy. Hypoxia secondary to pulmonary hypertension is likely to have a negative impact on neurological outcome, and it has been suggested that neonates with PH are more likely to have abnormal postrewarming brain MRI [188]. It is not known whether this association is related to a common pathophysiology, in which the severity of PH may be a marker of the severity of brain injury, or whether hypoxia and low cardiac output followed by dramatic cardiovascular changes with their treatment may result in ischemia–reperfusion and exacerbate brain injury. Treatment aimed at gradual restoration of oxygenated systemic blood flow, avoidance of systemic hypertension, and careful monitoring during periods of high vulnerability, such as rewarming, are recommended. Therapy for pulmonary hypertension includes iNO and, if refractory, may require modulation of target temperature although given the proven benefits of therapeutic hypothermia for brain outcomes, early rewarming should only be considered as a last resort if the perceived disadvantages of severe or prolonged hypoxia out way the benefits of continued cooling.

Echocardiography assessment may be particularly useful in this patient population due to the relatively high risk of myocardial dysfunction. Ventricular dysfunction may be treated with positive inotropes such as dobutamine or epinephrine and the combined inotrope/vasopressor action of epinephrine may be particularly useful in situations of myocardial dysfunction with diastolic or severe hypotension. Right ventricular dysfunction may benefit from afterload reduction using iNO, though the role of iNO in the nonhypoxic patient has not been studied. Vasopressin may be a useful adjunct for neonates with systemic hypotension and RV dysfunction. Pulmonary blood flow is pressure passive in the setting of severe RV dysfunction and therefore depends on a pressure gradient between right atrium and pulmonary circulation. Splanchnic vasoconstriction due to vasopressin administration may result in greater blood return to the right atrium sufficient to augment right atrial pressure and may improve pulmonary blood flow. Severe left ventricular dysfunction in patients with critically low cardiac output may require a strategy in which PVR is kept high and ductal patency is maintained to promote right-to-left ductal shunt. A parallel is drawn to the treatment of hypoplastic left heart syndrome; this approach assumes a functional inactivity of the left ventricle and requires the right ventricle to become the source of systemic blood flow. Adrenal insufficiency should be suspected when neonates are presenting with vasopressor-resistant shock and empiric hydrocortisone treatment is recommended.

Careful consideration of the impact of organ injury on drug metabolism is recommended. This is particularly important during the rewarming period when reversal of cooling-mediated cardiovascular changes may significantly modulate blood flow and oxygenation. Little is known about the impact of these changes on neurological outcomes and close monitoring with weaning to avoid hypertension or hyperoxia is prudent.

Infant of a diabetic mother

The management of acute pulmonary hypertension and/or shock in the infant of a diabetic mother requires modification from routine neonatal intensive care strategies if significant septal hypertrophy is identified, particularly in the presence of LVOT obstruction. The most appropriate approach depends on the degree of obstruction to left heart outflow (Fig. 30A.13). If the dominant clinical concern is hypoxia and LVOT obstruction is mild or absent, treatment of pulmonary hypertension with strategies that reduce PVR such as iNO is the most appropriate. Adequate lung recruitment is important; however, avoidance of high-mean airway pressure is relevant in this population because cardiac output may be dependent on maintaining high left atrial pressure to overcome high left ventricular end-diastolic pressure secondary to impaired ventricular compliance and restrictive filling. Situations that compromise left heart preload, including vasodilator drugs such as milrinone, should be avoided. Conditions in which the left heart is preload compromised result in closer approximation of the septum and the mitral valve and therefore may exacerbate obstruction. Positive inotropes (epinephrine, dobutamine, and dopamine) are contraindicated as more forceful contraction may worsen obstruction and tachycardia should be avoided as it reduces diastolic time, hence limits filling.

Vasopressin has a favorable biological profile for several reasons. First, increased SVR may increase left-to-right ductal shunt which may be beneficial in this population because the resultant increase in pulmonary blood flow may contribute to left atrial filling and therefore, to cardiac output. Second, higher afterload results in reduced velocity of fiber shortening. Since ejection time is limited, this results in incomplete emptying of the LV, hence greater end-systolic volume which adds to preload to improve cardiac output. Third, the antidiuretic effect of vasopressin

```
                              ┌──────────┐
                              │  Volume  │
                              └──────────┘
                                   │
          ┌────── No ──────┬───────────────────────┬────── Yes ──────┐
          │                │ Is the LVOT severely  │                 │
          │                │      obstructed?      │                 │
          ▼                └───────────────────────┘                 ▼
  Augment LV filling                                          R → L shunt to support SBF*
```

Augment LV filling

| **Optimize LV preload:** avoid hyperinflation, consider iNO (only if concurrent acute PH and hypoxemia) |

R → L shunt to support SBF*

| Maintain **ductal patency :** Prostaglandin infusion |

| ↑ **Afterload** (e.g., vasopressin) |———————| ↑ **PVR** with lower target saturations (e.g., target SpO₂ preductal > 85%) |

| ↑ Diastole by ↓ **heart rate** |

Preductal blood flow depends on retrograde flow in the aortic arch [not ideal for brain and coronary circulation]

| ↓ Systole by **negative inotropy** |

Fig. 30A.13 Suggested Approach to Management of Shock for Infants With Hypertrophic Obstructive Cardiomyopathy Depending on Whether There is Severe Left Ventricular Outflow Tract (LVOT) Obstruction. *iNO,* Inhaled nitric oxide; *LV,* left ventricle; *SBF,* systemic blood flow.

may increase circulating volume and this may be beneficial in the acute phases of treatment. Norepinephrine has some β1 activity, however, may be a reasonable alternative and phenylephrine is used in adults and in anesthetic practice for treatment of shock due to obstructive cardiomyopathy, though there is limited experience with this agent in most neonatal intensive care units.

For neonates with hypotension and moderate or severe LVOT obstruction in whom adequate augmentation of left ventricular filling is not possible, a strategy in which the PVR is kept high and the right heart, via right-to-left ductal shunt, is temporarily used to supply systemic circulation may be the only way to accomplish adequate systemic blood flow. In this case, prostaglandin to maintain ductal patency and avoidance of pulmonary vasodilators is warranted. Extracorporeal membrane oxygenation may be an alternative for neonates with refractory shock, though there is limited published evidence [189,190].

Long-term management may be required, though hypertrophic cardiomyopathy in infants of a diabetic mother is transient and typically resolves over 3–6 months. Beta-blockers may improve left heart filling based on their ability to reduce heart rate and for their negative inotropic properties. Calcium channel blockers (e.g., verapamil, diltiazem) may also be used to reduce myocardial stiffness. Drugs which reduce systemic afterload (e.g., nitrates, angiotensin-converting enzyme inhibitors, milrinone) should be avoided in this population as they may worsen LVOT obstruction. Diuretics should be used with caution when hypertrophic cardiomyopathy is severe enough to cause pulmonary edema as dehydration may compromise LV filling.

Patent ductus arteriosus

The optimal management strategy and timing of PDA closure are controversial. Regardless of specific approach, however, the aim of treatment is to minimize overcirculation and support systemic blood flow. Intensive care strategies to minimize shunt include maintaining PVR high via modulation of CO_2 and oxygen. Permissive hypercapnia with a target CO_2 of 50–60 mmHg, arterial pH 7.25–7.35 and target oxygen saturations in the 88%–93% range to minimize the provision of exogenous oxygen may be associated with higher PVR and therefore mitigate shunt. The application of optimum PEEP may reduce atelectasis associated lung injury and is associated with reduced LV afterload which may promote flow into the systemic circulation [191,192]. Maintenance of adequate hemoglobin may have several benefits. First, maintaining optimum oxygen carrying capacity is important to ensure adequate delivery of oxygen to tissues in a situation where perfusion may be compromised. Second, reduced delivery of oxygen in the anemic patient may result in a compensatory increase in cardiac output which may exacerbate pulmonary overcirculation and cause declining respiratory status. Third, according to Poiseuille's Law, flow is inversely related to viscosity and anemia may be associated with lower viscosity blood in some patients [193]. Fluid restriction, though historically a cornerstone of management, is not recommended except in special circumstances because depletion of intravascular volume may lead to further compromise in postductal organ perfusion without improvement in ductal shunt [194]. Reduction in exogenous fluid administration in response to oliguria and associated hyponatremia with the administration of nonsteroidal antiinflammatory medications (NSAIDs) should be considered. The routine use of diuretics, particularly furosemide, is also questionable [195,196] and a systematic review concluded that there was insufficient evidence to support its routine administration [197]. Furosemide is linked with increased production of prostaglandin E_2 in the kidney and may be associated with prolonged ductal patency [198]. Judicious use of these strategies may be reasonable for symptom management in the preterm infant with established shunt who is awaiting surgical ligation.

The timing of intervention differs between centers and individual practitioners. There are three accepted strategies, each of which have both merit and disadvantages. Prophylactic therapy within the first 6 h of life has been shown to reduce the risk of severe IVH [199]. Though causality has not been proven, this may relate to modulation of ductal shunt in the early transitional period because the likelihood of PDA was reduced from 50% to 24% in the treated group. A prophylactic approach, however, results in exposure of many infants who would not otherwise have required therapy to an intervention and potentially harm in the situation where the ductal shunt is physiologically important, such as those with aortic coarctation, significant left ventricular dysfunction or pulmonary hypertension. Early targeted therapy, in which echocardiography assessment of ductal patency is conducted early on the first day of life, may be preferable in centers in which imaging is widely available. This approach has been associated with reduced frequency of pulmonary hemorrhage and a lower likelihood of symptomatic PDA [200]. Finally, the decision to treat a symptomatic PDA on the basis of the presence of clinical and echocardiography evidence of left-to-right shunt may be made at any time during the course of a premature infant, though earlier treatment is preferable as the risks of necrotizing enterocolitis, pulmonary morbidity, and surgical ligation are lower [201]. Comprehensive TnECHO evaluation of shunt volume may facilitate enhanced selection of candidates for treatment.

Specific therapies aimed at ductal closure include the use of NSAIDs, acetaminophen, surgical ligation, and in some centers, the use of percutaneous catheter closure techniques (Fig. 30A.14). Indomethacin, a cyclooxygenase inhibitor, at a dose of 0.2 mg/kg every 12–24 h is the most established treatment to promote ductal closure. A course of three doses of treatment is effective in approximately 50% of cases [202]. A second course of indomethacin is often given and may be efficacious, particularly with partial success or complete success with remanifestation following of the first course [203]. Ibuprofen has been suggested as an alternative NSAID based on a reported lower risk of adverse effects [204], although whether efficacy is equivalent remains uncertain [205]. The use of acetaminophen as a primary strategy or following failure of NSAIDs has

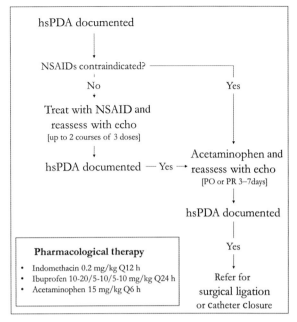

Fig. 30A.14 Management Alternatives for Treatment of a Hemodynamically Significant PDA (hsPDA). One possible treatment algorithm includes the use of an NSAID × two courses followed by treatment with 3–7 days of acetaminophen and then, if the ductus remains hemodynamically significant, consideration for surgical ligation or percutaneous catheter closure if performed. *NSAID,* Nonsteroidal antiinflammatory drug; *PO,* per os; *PR,* per rectum.

been reported and may be effective at avoiding surgical ligation in almost half of treated neonates [206]. Minimal side effects have been reported, although the total number of treated infants reported in the literature is low and the optimal route of delivery is uncertain. Surgical ligation for closure of the symptomatic ductus is a controversial topic, though remains a common procedure in many neonatal practices. Surgical PDA closure has been associated in some literature with a higher risk of impaired neurodevelopment [207,208]; however, when analysis is adjusted for the presence of postnatal confounders which occur prior to the time of ligation, this association is no longer evident suggesting that ligation is a marker of a sicker cohort and not causal of poor outcome [209]. Surgical morbidities including air leak, reexpansion pulmonary edema [210], and recurrent laryngeal nerve palsy occur with variable frequency [211,212]. A possible alternative in some centers, which may reduce the risks of surgical complications related to thoracotomy, is percutaneous catheter closure via a transvenous route which is becoming increasingly possible due to the availability of appropriate device sizes and pioneering of new, safer image guided techniques [213,214].

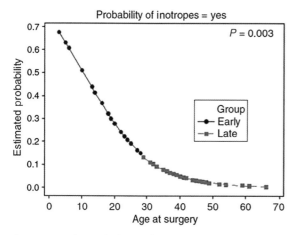

Fig. 30A.15 The Probability of Developing Post-Ligation Cardiac Syndrome (PLCS) by Postnatal Age at the Time of Surgery [215].

PDA ligation postoperative management

Perioperative assessment includes the assessment of PLCS risk based on the postnatal age and weight with younger, smaller babies (age < 28 days, weight < 1 kg) at greater risk of postoperative LV decompensation [215] (Fig. 30A.15). The chronically volume overloaded cardiovascular system adapts by LV dilation and hypertrophy [216], undergoes extensive remodeling of the vascular endothelium with associated changes in secretion of vasoactive substances [217] and increases sympathetic activation with higher levels of circulating norepinephrine and other catecholamines [218]. There is limited study specific to the adaptation of the preterm infant to chronic PDA shunt; however, changes in myocardial architecture may provide relative protection against wall stress and increasing SVR which may alter the degree of change in exposed vascular resistance from pre to postligation. Neonates with concurrent pulmonary hypertension, too, are theoretically at a reduced risk of PLCS due to higher resistance in the pulmonary vascular bed preoperatively. Preoperative adrenal function testing may inform postoperative management. Though perioperative steroids have not been shown to improve postoperative stability overall [219], in a subset of neonates with documented adrenal insufficiency who develop postoperative cardiorespiratory decompensation, hydrocortisone may be beneficial.

The postoperative management of neonates following PDA ligation may vary depending on the availability of early postoperative echocardiography. If available, echocardiography measurement of LVO 1 h postoperatively may be used to guide targeted prophylaxis using milrinone. Neonates with LVO < 198 mL/min/kg may be candidates and milrinone may be given at a starting dose of 0.33 mcg/kg/min with a concurrent bolus of saline over 1 h to ensure adequate LV preload and avoid hypotension due to vasodilation. The administration of prophylactic milrinone is associated with a reduced risk for postligation cardiac syndrome [148], likely by mitigating the effects of augmented systemic afterload on LV systolic function. If echocardiography is not readily available, universal milrinone prophylaxis or prophylaxis of patients at high risk on clinical grounds may be an option, though this approach has not been studied.

Symptomatic treatment of postligation cardiac syndrome should be focused on agents that have positive inotropic properties. The treatment of systolic hypotension should include dobutamine or epinephrine as a first-line agent depending on the severity of the clinical presentation. The combined inotrope–vasopressor activity of epinephrine makes it a desirable agent for advanced disease or severe hypotension. Drugs with a predominant vasopressor profile (dopamine, vasopressin, norepinephrine) should be avoided as the primary pathophysiological concern is one of LV failure in the face of afterload. Hydrocortisone should be considered for inotrope resistant hypotension, particularly if the infant has a documented failed ACTH stimulation test. Despite milrinone prophylaxis, and in patients in who milrinone is not indicated, the postoperative course may be complicated by pulmonary edema resulting in ventilation and oxygenation issues without systemic hypotension. This may be related to diastolic dysfunction of the LV in the presence of afterload the specific risk factors remain to be delineated.

Chronic pulmonary hypertension

BPD associated PH is a slowly progressive chronic disease requiring long-term therapy. Parents must be trained to administer medications and therefore practical, safe and ideally, nonintravenous options are required. The evidence for sildenafil, the most widely studied option, as one component of a beneficial long-term strategy is slowly emerging [220–223]; monotherapy has been suggested to reduce echocardiography markers of chronic PH, PVR, and O_2 requirement after 1 month of therapy on a small scale [224]. Many of the neonates with chronic PH in these trials received concurrent therapy with other agents (e.g., corticosteroids, Bosentan, diuretics); there are no published studies comparing sildenafil to control in this population. While off-label use of this medication is increasing [225], caution is warranted. High-dose sildenafil was associated with mortality in one pediatric study randomizing a heterogeneous group to low, medium or high-dose ranges [226] leading the US Food and Drug Administration (FDA) to issue a warning against its use in children [227]. No specific recommendation was made for neonates; infants with BPD associated PH were not included in this study.

PGI$_2$ analogues are being increasingly used. Epoprostenol and treprostinil IV are associated with improved oxygenation and reduced PAP, however systemic delivery is impractical and may be complicated by hypotension and significant bleeding due to the antiplatelet effect of PGI$_2$. Case reports of use of inhaled iloprost alone [228] or in combination with sildenafil [229,230] have demonstrated reduced FiO$_2$ and echocardiography markers of PH. Treprostinil is a subcutaneous preparation, delivered continuously via in an indwelling catheter, that may offer advantages over inhaled preparations including continuous delivery in an outpatient setting and avoidance of common airway complications (e.g., cough, wheeze) [231]. It has been used successfully in a diaphragmatic hernia patient with infrequent catheter changes that were done by parents [232]. PGI$_2$ analogues are promising; however, current evidence is limited. Bosentan is used sporadically; outside of occasional case reports [220,233], however, there is very little evidence to support this practice. Finally, diuretic therapy, widely used for RV failure in the setting of pulmonary hypertension for adults [234], may have a role in the treatment of neonatal chronic PH. Some neonates with BPD have improved lung mechanics with combination thiazide/spironolactone therapy [235], though there is limited data to direct diuretic therapy specific to preterm infants with chronic PH.

Respiratory morbidity is important, with far-reaching implications, but understanding the outcome for these neonates is challenging. Preterms with acute PH are a difficult group to study as they have a high incidence of confounding comorbidities (e.g., IVH, infection, IUGR). BPD too is complex, multifactorial, and poorly understood with an inconsistent definition [236]. Improved management has changed the preterm respiratory course substantially and altered the clinical phenotype of BPD [237]. In the present era, chronic PH is associated with a two-year mortality rate of up to 47% with 75% of those deaths occurring in the first 6 months of life [135]. Survivors may have a prolonged course of cardiorespiratory morbidity that may persist for years [238]. Early studies suggest that long-term survivors may have RV dilation and hypertrophy [238,239], which may be an important contributor to late morbidity and mortality. Intercurrent infection may precipitate acute decompensation, which may be fatal [240]. It is unclear whether the course of disease may be modified by early recognition and therapy, though this has been suggested [224], and prevention is an attractive alternative if possible.

Animal evidence suggests that iNO may promote growth [241,242], improve alveolar architecture [243] and may be protective of inflammatory [244] and hyperoxic [245] stress. Large-scale trials, however, failed to demonstrate reduction in lung disease [246] and prolonged exposure of preterm infants to iNO is not recommended. This may be, in part, because BPD is a complex disease which is influenced by a variety of genetic, antenatal and postnatal factors that result in a diverse pathophysiology with a similar phenotype [236]. Failure to define an appropriate population for a preventative therapy may result in subclinical harm. For example, chronic exposure to iNO in neonates with a PDA may reduce PVR and increase shunt volume. Progressive pulmonary edema and oxidative stress may worsen lung disease in a subset of patients and thus mask positive effects in others. Free radical production may also play a role. Reactive oxygen species (ROS) are constitutively produced by cellular sources however, when combined with oxygen, NO creates supra-physiologic levels of nitrogen dioxide (NO$_2$) and peroxynitrite which may be toxic [247]. For acutely unwell neonates, reduction in toxic ROS due to reduction in required FiO$_2$ may offset NO$_2$ effects. Excessive or prolonged exposure in combination with other free radicals, however, may cause cellular injury and compromise cell growth [247]. Despite extensive study, there is insufficient evidence to support the use of iNO to prevent BPD or associated chronic PH and its use is not recommended.

Online supplementary material

Please visit MedEnact to access the videos on LV hypertrophy; PDA Assessment; Pulmonary Hypertension on Echocardiography; RV Dysfunction

References

[1] Bhatt S, Alison BJ, Wallace EM, Crossley KJ, Gill AW, Kluckow M, et al. Delaying cord clamping until ventilation onset improves cardiovascular function at birth in preterm lambs. J Physiol 2013;591(8):2113–2126.

[2] Polglase GR, Morley CJ, Crossley KJ, Dargaville P, Harding R, Morgan DL, et al. Positive end-expiratory pressure differentially alters pulmonary hemodynamics and oxygenation in ventilated, very premature lambs. J Appl Physiol (1985) 2005;99(4):1453–1461.

[3] Committee Opinion No. 684. Delayed umbilical cord clamping after birth. Obstetr Gynecol 2017;129(1):e5–e10.

[4] American Academy of Pediatrics and American Heart Association. In: Zaichkin J, editor. Textbook

of neonatal resuscitation (NRP). 7th ed. Elk Grove Village, IL USA: American Academy of Pediatrics and American Heart Association; 2016.

[5] Jouk PS, Usson Y, Michalowicz G, Grossi L. Three-dimensional cartography of the pattern of the myofibres in the second trimester fetal human heart. Anat Embryol 2000;202(2):103–118.

[6] Jardin F, Vieillard-Baron A. Right ventricular function and positive pressure ventilation in clinical practice: from hemodynamic subsets to respirator settings. Intensive Care Med 2003;29(9):1426–1434.

[7] Katira BH, Giesinger RE, Engelberts D, Zabini D, Kornecki A, Otulakowski G, et al. Adverse heart–lung interactions in ventilator-induced lung injury. Am J Respir Crit Care Med 2017;196(11):1411–1421.

[8] Gullberg N, Winberg P, Sellden H. Changes in stroke volume cause change in cardiac output in neonates and infants when mean airway pressure is altered. Acta Anaesthesiol Scand 1999;43(10):999–1004.

[9] de Waal K, Evans N, van der Lee J, van Kaam A. Effect of lung recruitment on pulmonary, systemic, and ductal blood flow in preterm infants. J Pediatr 2009;154(5):651–655.

[10] Hsu HS, Chen W, Wang NK. Effect of continuous positive airway pressure on cardiac output in neonates. Zhonghua Minguo Xiaoerke Yixuehui Zazhi 1996;37(5):353–356.

[11] Creamer KM, McCloud LL, Fisher LE, Ehrhart IC. Ventilation above closing volume reduces pulmonary vascular resistance hysteresis. Am J Respir Crit Care Med 1998;158(4):1114–1119.

[12] Thornburg KL, Morton MJ. Filling and arterial pressures as determinants of RV stroke volume in the sheep fetus. Am J Physiol 1983;244(5):H656–H6563.

[13] Reller MD, Donovan EF, Kotagal UR. Influence of airway pressure waveform on cardiac output during positive pressure ventilation of healthy newborn dogs. Pediatr Res 1985;19(4):337–341.

[14] Tana M, Polglase GR, Cota F, Tirone C, Aurilia C, Lio A, et al. Determination of lung volume and hemodynamic changes during high-frequency ventilation recruitment in preterm neonates with respiratory distress syndrome. Crit Care Med 2015;43(8):1685–1691.

[15] Milstein JM, Glantz SA. Mechanically increased right ventricular afterload alters left ventricular configuration, not contractility, in neonatal lambs. Pediatr Res 1993;33(4 Pt. 1):359–364.

[16] Whittenberger JL, Mc GM, Berglund E, Borst HG. Influence of state of inflation of the lung on pulmonary vascular resistance. J Appl Physiol 1960;15:878–882.

[17] Kelly DT, Spotnitz HM, Beiser GD, Pierce JE, Epstein SE. Effects of chronic right ventricular volume and pressure loading on left ventricular performance. Circulation 1971;44(3):403–412.

[18] Poveda F, Gil D, Marti E, Andaluz A, Ballester M, Carreras F. Helical structure of the cardiac ventricular anatomy assessed by diffusion tensor magnetic resonance imaging with multiresolution tractography. Rev Esp Cardiol (Engl Ed) 2013;66(10):782–790.

[19] Shekerdemian L, Bohn D. Cardiovascular effects of mechanical ventilation. Arch Dis Childhood 1999;80(5):475–480.

[20] Suzuki H, Papazoglou K, Bryan AC. Relationship between PaO_2 and lung volume during high frequency oscillatory ventilation. Acta Paediatr Jpn 1992;34(5):494–500.

[21] Tana M, Zecca E, Tirone C, Aurilia C, Cota F, Lio A, et al. Target fraction of inspired oxygen during open lung strategy in neonatal high frequency oscillatory ventilation: a retrospective study. Minerva Anestesiol 2012;78(2):151–159.

[22] De Jaegere A, van Veenendaal MB, Michiels A, van Kaam AH. Lung recruitment using oxygenation during open lung high-frequency ventilation in preterm infants. Am J Respir Crit Care Med 2006;174(6):639–645.

[23] Thome U, Topfer A, Schaller P, Pohlandt F. Effects of mean airway pressure on lung volume during high-frequency oscillatory ventilation of preterm infants. Am J Respir Crit Care Med 1998;157(4 Pt. 1):1213–1218.

[24] Thome U, Topfer A, Schaller P, Pohlandt F. Comparison of lung volume measurements by antero-posterior chest X-ray and the SF6 washout technique in mechanically ventilated infants. Pediatr Pulmonol 1998;26(4):265–272.

[25] Zamora IJ, Sheikh F, Cassady CI, Olutoye OO, Mehollin-Ray AR, Ruano R, et al. Fetal MRI lung volumes are predictive of perinatal outcomes in fetuses with congenital lung masses. J Pediatr Surg 2014;49(6):853–858.

[26] Berger-Kulemann V, Berger R, Mlczoch E, Sternal D, Mailath-Pokorny M, Hachemian N, et al. The effects of hemodynamic alterations on lung volumes in fetuses with tetralogy of Fallot: an MRI study. Pediatr Cardiol 2015;36(6):1287–1293.

[27] Schopper MA, Walkup LL, Tkach JA, Higano NS, Lim FY, Haberman B, et al. Evaluation of neonatal lung volume growth by pulmonary magnetic resonance imaging in patients with congenital diaphragmatic hernia. J Pediatr 2017;188. 96.e1–102.e1.

[28] Walkup LL, Tkach JA, Higano NS, Thomen RP, Fain SB, Merhar SL, et al. Quantitative magnetic resonance imaging of bronchopulmonary dysplasia in the neonatal intensive care unit environment. Am J Respir Crit Care Med 2015;192(10): 1215–1222.

[29] de Boode WP, Singh Y, Gupta S, Austin T, Bohlin K, Dempsey E, et al. Recommendations for neonatologist performed echocardiography in Europe: Consensus Statement endorsed by European Society for Paediatric Research (ESPR) and European Society for Neonatology (ESN). Pediatr Res 2016;80(4): 465–471.

[30] Singh Y, Gupta S, Groves AM, Gandhi A, Thomson J, Qureshi S, et al. Expert consensus statement 'Neonatologist-performed Echocardiography (NoPE)'-training and accreditation in UK. Eur J Pediatr 2016;175(2): 281–287.

[31] Mertens L, Seri I, Marek J, Arlettaz R, Barker P, McNamara P, et al. Targeted Neonatal Echocardiography in the Neonatal Intensive Care Unit: practice guidelines and recommendations for training. Writing Group of the American Society of Echocardiography (ASE) in collaboration with the European Association of Echocardiography (EAE) and the Association for European Pediatric Cardiologists (AEPC). J Am Soc Echocardiogr 2011;24(10):1057–1078.

[32] Giesinger RE, More K, Odame J, Jain A, Jankov RP, McNamara PJ. Controversies in the identification and management of acute pulmonary hypertension in preterm neonates. Pediatr Res 2017;82(6):901–914.

[33] Mourani PM, Ivy DD, Gao D, Abman SH. Pulmonary vascular effects of inhaled nitric oxide and oxygen

tension in bronchopulmonary dysplasia. Am J Respir Crit Care Med 2004;170(9):1006–1013.

[34] Mourani PM, Sontag MK, Younoszai A, Ivy DD, Abman SH. Clinical utility of echocardiography for the diagnosis and management of pulmonary vascular disease in young children with chronic lung disease. Pediatrics 2008;121(2):317–325.

[35] Ambalavanan N, Mourani P. Pulmonary hypertension in bronchopulmonary dysplasia. Birth Defects Res A Clin Mol Teratol 2014;100(3):240–246.

[36] del Cerro MJ, Sabate Rotes A, Carton A, Deiros L, Bret M, Cordeiro M, et al. Pulmonary hypertension in bronchopulmonary dysplasia: clinical findings, cardiovascular anomalies and outcomes. Pediatr Pulmonol 2014;49(1):49–59.

[37] Kim GB. Pulmonary hypertension in infants with bronchopulmonary dysplasia. Kor J Pediatr 2010;53(6):688–693.

[38] Al-Ghanem G, Shah P, Thomas S, Banfield L, El Helou S, Fusch C, et al. Bronchopulmonary dysplasia and pulmonary hypertension: a meta-analysis. J Perinatol 2017;37(4): 414–419.

[39] Jain A, Mohamed A, El-Khuffash A, Connelly KA, Dallaire F, Jankov RP, et al. A comprehensive echocardiographic protocol for assessing neonatal right ventricular dimensions and function in the transitional period: normative data and z scores. J Am Soc Echocardiogr 2014;27(12):1293–1304.

[40] Jain A, El-Khuffash AF, Kuipers BC, Mohamed A, Connelly KA, McNamara PJ, et al. Left ventricular function in healthy term neonates during the transitional period. J Pediatr 2017;182. 197.e2–203.e2.

[41] Musewe NN, Poppe D, Smallhorn JF, Hellman J, Whyte H, Smith B, et al. Doppler echocardiographic measurement of pulmonary artery pressure from ductal Doppler velocities in the newborn. J Am Coll Cardiol 1990;15(2):446–456.

[42] Ryan T, Petrovic O, Dillon JC, Feigenbaum H, Conley MJ, Armstrong WF. An echocardiographic index for separation of right ventricular volume and pressure overload. J Am Coll Cardiol 1985;5(4):918–927.

[43] Kitabatake A, Inoue M, Asao M, Masuyama T, Tanouchi J, Morita T, et al. Noninvasive evaluation of

pulmonary hypertension by a pulsed Doppler technique. Circulation 1983;68(2):302–309.

[44] Jain A, McNamara PJ. Persistent pulmonary hypertension of the newborn: physiology, hemodynamic assessment and novel therapies. Curr Pediatr Rev 2013;9:55–66.

[45] Malowitz JR, Forsha DE, Smith PB, Cotten CM, Barker PC, Tatum GH. Right ventricular echocardiographic indices predict poor outcomes in infants with persistent pulmonary hypertension of the newborn. Eur Heart J Cardiovasc Imaging 2015;16(11):1224–1231.

[46] Giesinger RE, El Shahed AE, Castaldo MP, Jain A, Whyte HE, Mertens L, et al. Right ventricular function in neonates with hypoxic ischemic encephalopathy undergoing therapeutic hypothermia and rewarming. San Francisco, CA: Pediatric Academic Society; 2017.

[47] Lee LA, Kimball TR, Daniels SR, Khoury P, Meyer RA. Left ventricular mechanics in the preterm infant and their effect on the measurement of cardiac performance. J Pediatr 1992;120(1):114–119.

[48] Slama M, Susic D, Varagic J, Ahn J, Frohlich ED. Echocardiographic measurement of cardiac output in rats. Am J Physiol Heart Circ Physiol 2003;284(2):H691–H697.

[49] Ficial B, Finnemore AE, Cox DJ, Broadhouse KM, Price AN, Durighel G, et al. Validation study of the accuracy of echocardiographic measurements of systemic blood flow volume in newborn infants. J Am Soc Echocardiogr 2013;26(12):1365–1371.

[50] Winberg P, Jansson M, Marions L, Lundell BP. Left ventricular output during postnatal circulatory adaptation in healthy infants born at full term. Arch Dis Childhood 1989;64(10 Spec No.):1374–1378.

[51] El-Khuffash AF, Jain A, Weisz D, Mertens L, McNamara PJ. Assessment and treatment of post patent ductus arteriosus ligation syndrome. J Pediatr 2014;165(1). 46.e1–52.e1.

[52] Richardson C, Amirtharaj C, Gruber D, Hayes DA. Assessing myocardial function in infants with pulmonary hypertension: the role of tissue Doppler imaging and tricuspid annular plane systolic excursion. Pediatr Cardiol 2017;38(3):558–565.

[53] Bokiniec R, Wlasienko P, Borszewska-Kornacka M, Szymkiewicz-Dangel J. Evaluation of left ventricular

function in preterm infants with bronchopulmonary dysplasia using various echocardiographic techniques. Echocardiography 2017;34(4): 567–576.

[54] James AT, Corcoran JD, Jain A, McNamara PJ, Mertens L, Franklin O, et al. Assessment of myocardial performance in preterm infants less than 29 weeks gestation during the transitional period. Early Hum Dev 2014;90(12):829–835.

[55] de Waal K, Lakkundi A, Othman F. Speckle tracking echocardiography in very preterm infants: feasibility and reference values. Early Hum Dev 2014;90(6):275–279.

[56] Breatnach CR, Forman E, Foran A, Monteith C, McSweeney L, Malone F, et al. Left ventricular rotational mechanics in infants with hypoxic ischemic encephalopathy and preterm infants at 36 weeks postmenstrual age: a comparison with healthy term controls. Echocardiography 2017;34(2):232–239.

[57] James A, Corcoran JD, Mertens L, Franklin O, El-Khuffash A. Left ventricular rotational mechanics in preterm infants less than 29 weeks' gestation over the first week after birth. J Am Soc Echocardiogr 2015;28(7). 808.e1–817.e1.

[58] El-Khuffash A, Herbozo C, Jain A, Lapointe A, McNamara PJ. Targeted neonatal echocardiography (TnECHO) service in a Canadian neonatal intensive care unit: a 4-year experience. J Perinatol 2013;33(9):687–690.

[59] Jouannic JM, Gavard L, Fermont L, Le Bidois J, Parat S, Vouhe PR, et al. Sensitivity and specificity of prenatal features of physiological shunts to predict neonatal clinical status in transposition of the great arteries. Circulation 2004;110(13):1743–1746.

[60] Barre E, Durand I, Hazelzet T, David N. Ebstein's anomaly and tricuspid valve dysplasia: prognosis after diagnosis in utero. Pediatr Cardiol 2012;33(8):1391–1396.

[61] Radman MR, Goldhoff P, Jones KD, Azakie A, Datar S, Adatia I, et al. Pulmonary interstitial glycogenosis: an unrecognized etiology of persistent pulmonary hypertension of the newborn in congenital heart disease? Pediatr Cardiol 2013;34(5):1254–1257.

[62] Saul D, Degenhardt K, Iyoob SD, Surrey LF, Johnson AM, Johnson MP, et al. Hypoplastic left heart syndrome and the nutmeg lung pattern in utero:

a cause and effect relationship or prognostic indicator? Pediatr Radiol 2016;46(4):483–489.

[63] Sallaam S, Natarajan G, Aggarwal S. Persistent pulmonary hypertension of the newborn with D-transposition of the great arteries: management and prognosis. Congenit Heart Dis 2016;11(3):239–244.

[64] Ivy DD, Abman SH, Barst RJ, Berger RM, Bonnet D, Fleming TR, et al. Pediatric pulmonary hypertension. J Am Coll Cardiol 2013;62(25 Suppl.):D117–D126.

[65] Chen IC, Dai ZK. Insight into pulmonary arterial hypertension associated with congenital heart disease (PAH-CHD): classification and pharmacological management from a pediatric cardiological point of view. Acta Cardiol Sin 2015;31(6):507–515.

[66] Neema PK. Eisenmenger syndrome: an unsolved malady. Ann Card Anaesth 2012;15(4):257–258.

[67] Graziano JN, Heidelberger KP, Ensing GJ, Gomez CA, Ludomirsky A. The influence of a restrictive atrial septal defect on pulmonary vascular morphology in patients with hypoplastic left heart syndrome. Pediatr Cardiol 2002;23(2):146–151.

[68] Stege G, Fenton A, Jaffray B. Nihilism in the 1990s: the true mortality of congenital diaphragmatic hernia. Pediatrics 2003;112(3 Pt. 1):532–535.

[69] Lusk LA, Wai KC, Moon-Grady AJ, Basta AM, Filly R, Keller RL. Fetal ultrasound markers of severity predict resolution of pulmonary hypertension in congenital diaphragmatic hernia. Am J Obstetr Gynecol 2015;213(2). 216.e1–218.e1.

[70] Spaggiari E, Stirnemann JJ, Sonigo P, Khen-Dunlop N, De Saint Blanquat L, Ville Y. Prenatal prediction of pulmonary arterial hypertension in congenital diaphragmatic hernia. Ultrasound Obstet Gynecol 2015;45(5):572–577.

[71] Baptista MJ, Rocha G, Clemente F, Azevedo LF, Tibboel D, Leite-Moreira AF, et al. N-terminal-pro-B type natriuretic peptide as a useful tool to evaluate pulmonary hypertension and cardiac function in CDH infants. Neonatology 2008;94(1):22–30.

[72] Partridge EA, Hanna BD, Rintoul NE, Herkert L, Flake AW, Adzick NS, et al. Brain-type natriuretic peptide levels correlate with pulmonary hypertension and requirement for extracorporeal membrane oxygenation in congenital

diaphragmatic hernia. J Pediatr Surg 2015;50(2):263–266.

[73] Patel N, Moenkemeyer F, Germano S, Cheung MM. Plasma vascular endothelial growth factor A and placental growth factor: novel biomarkers of pulmonary hypertension in congenital diaphragmatic hernia. Am J Physiol Lung Cell Mol Physiol 2015;308(4):L378–L383.

[74] O'Toole SJ, Irish MS, Holm BA, Glick PL. Pulmonary vascular abnormalities in congenital diaphragmatic hernia. Clin Perinatol 1996;23(4):781–794.

[75] Yamataka T, Puri P. Pulmonary artery structural changes in pulmonary hypertension complicating congenital diaphragmatic hernia. J Pediatr Surg 1997;32(3):387–390.

[76] Kipfmueller F, Heindel K, Schroeder L, Berg C, Dewald O, Reutter H, et al. Early postnatal echocardiographic assessment of pulmonary blood flow in newborns with congenital diaphragmatic hernia. J Perinat Med 2018;46(7):735–743.

[77] Yamoto M, Inamura N, Terui K, Nagata K, Kanamori Y, Hayakawa M, et al. Echocardiographic predictors of poor prognosis in congenital diaphragmatic hernia. J Pediatr Surg 2016;51(12):1926–1930.

[78] Manso PH, Figueira RL, Prado CM, Goncalves FL, Simoes AL, Ramos SG, et al. Early neonatal echocardiographic findings in an experimental rabbit model of congenital diaphragmatic hernia. Braz J Med Biol Res 2015;48(3):234–239.

[79] Altit G, Bhombal S, Van Meurs K, Tacy TA. Ventricular performance is associated with need for extracorporeal membrane oxygenation in newborns with congenital diaphragmatic hernia. J Pediatr 2017;191:28–34.e1.

[80] Aggarwal S, Stockmann P, Klein MD, Natarajan G. Echocardiographic measures of ventricular function and pulmonary artery size: prognostic markers of congenital diaphragmatic hernia? J Perinatol 2011;31(8): 561–566.

[81] Harrison MR, Mychaliska GB, Albanese CT, Jennings RW, Farrell JA, Hawgood S, et al. Correction of congenital diaphragmatic hernia in utero IX: fetuses with poor prognosis (liver herniation and low lung-to-head ratio) can be saved by fetoscopic temporary tracheal occlusion. J Pediatr Surg 1998;33(7):1017–1022.

[82] Mous DS, Kool HM, Buscop-van Kempen MJ, Koning AH, Dzyubachyk O, Wijnen RM, et al. Clinically relevant timing of antenatal sildenafil treatment reduces pulmonary vascular remodeling in congenital diaphragmatic hernia. Am J Physiol Lung Cell Mol Physiol 2016;311(4):L734–L742.

[83] Russo FM, Toelen J, Eastwood MP, Jimenez J, Miyague AH, Vande Velde G, et al. Transplacental sildenafil rescues lung abnormalities in the rabbit model of diaphragmatic hernia. Thorax 2016;71(6):517–525.

[84] Yamamoto Y, Thebaud B, Vadivel A, Eaton F, Jain V, Hornberger LK. Doppler parameters of fetal lung hypoplasia and impact of sildenafil. Am J Obstetr Gynecol 2014;211(3). 263.e1–268.e1.

[85] Armstrong K, Franklin O, Sweetman D, Molloy EJ. Cardiovascular dysfunction in infants with neonatal encephalopathy. Arch Dis Childhood 2012;97(4):372–375.

[86] Martin-Ancel A, Garcia-Alix A, Gaya F, Cabanas F, Burgueros M, Quero J. Multiple organ involvement in perinatal asphyxia. J Pediatr 1995;127(5):786–793.

[87] Kanik E, Ozer EA, Bakiler AR, Aydinlioglu H, Dorak C, Dogrusoz B, et al. Assessment of myocardial dysfunction in neonates with hypoxic–ischemic encephalopathy: is it a significant predictor of mortality? J Matern Fetal Neonatal Med 2009;22(3):239–242.

[88] Thoresen M, Whitelaw A. Cardiovascular changes during mild therapeutic hypothermia and rewarming in infants with hypoxic–ischemic encephalopathy. Pediatrics 2000;106(1 Pt. 1):92–99.

[89] Jacobs SE, Berg M, Hunt R, Tarnow-Mordi WO, Inder TE, Davis PG. Cooling for newborns with hypoxic ischaemic encephalopathy. Cochrane Database Syst Rev 2013;1:CD003311.

[90] Rubini A. Effect of perfusate temperature on pulmonary vascular resistance and compliance by arterial and venous occlusion in the rat. Eur J Appl Physiol 2005;93(4):435–439.

[91] Hochwald O, Jabr M, Osiovich H, Miller SP, McNamara PJ, Lavoie PM. Preferential cephalic redistribution of left ventricular cardiac output during therapeutic hypothermia for perinatal hypoxic–ischemic encephalopathy. J Pediatr 2014;164(5). 999.e1–1004.e1.

[92] Allanson ER, Waqar T, White C, Tuncalp O, Dickinson JE. Umbilical lactate as a measure of acidosis and predictor of neonatal risk: a systematic review. BJOG 2017;124(4):584–594.

[93] Shah S, Tracy M, Smyth J. Postnatal lactate as an early predictor of short-term outcome after intrapartum asphyxia. J Perinatol 2004;24(1):16–20.

[94] Lingappan K, Kaiser JR, Srinivasan C, Gunn AJ. Relationship between PCO$_2$ and unfavorable outcome in infants with moderate-to-severe hypoxic ischemic encephalopathy. Pediatr Res 2016;80(2):204–208.

[95] Nishimaki S, Iwasaki S, Minamisawa S, Seki K, Yokota S. Blood flow velocities in the anterior cerebral artery and basilar artery in asphyxiated infants. J Ultrasound Med 2008;27(6):955–960.

[96] Giesinger RE, Bailey LJ, Deshpande P, McNamara PJ. Hypoxic–ischemic encephalopathy and therapeutic hypothermia: the hemodynamic perspective. J Pediatr 2017;180:22–30.

[97] Gewolb IH, O'Brien J. Surfactant secretion by type II pneumocytes is inhibited by high glucose concentrations. Exp Lung Res 1997;23(3):245–255.

[98] Morriss FH Jr. Infants of diabetic mothers: fetal and neonatal pathophysiology. Perspect Pediatr Pathol 1984;8(3):223–234.

[99] Colpaert C, Hogan J, Stark AR, Genest DR, Roberts D, Reid L, et al. Increased muscularization of small pulmonary arteries in preterm infants of diabetic mothers: a morphometric study in noninflated, noninjected, routinely fixed lungs. Pediatr Pathol Lab Med 1995;15(5):689–705.

[100] Baack ML, Forred BJ, Larsen TD, Jensen DN, Wachal AL, Khan MA, et al. Consequences of a maternal high-fat diet and late gestation diabetes on the developing rat lung. PLoS One 2016;11(8):e0160818.

[101] Mehta A, Hussain K. Transient hyperinsulinism associated with macrosomia, hypertrophic obstructive cardiomyopathy, hepatomegaly, and nephromegaly. Arch Dis Childhood 2003;88(9):822–824.

[102] Elmekkawi SF, Mansour GM, Elsafty MS, Hassanin AS, Laban M, Elsayed HM. Prediction of fetal hypertrophic cardiomyopathy in diabetic pregnancies compared with postnatal outcome. Clin Med Insights Womens Health 2015;8:39–43.

[103] Maron BJ, Towbin JA, Thiene G, Antzelevitch C, Corrado D, Arnett D, et al. Contemporary definitions and classification of the cardiomyopathies: an American Heart Association Scientific Statement from the Council on Clinical Cardiology, Heart Failure and Transplantation Committee; Quality of Care and Outcomes Research and Functional Genomics and Translational Biology Interdisciplinary Working Groups; and Council on Epidemiology and Prevention. Circulation 2006;113(14):1807–1816.

[104] Thorsson AV, Hintz RL. Insulin receptors in the newborn. Increase in receptor affinity and number. N Engl J Med 1977;297(17):908–912.

[105] Korraa A, Ezzat MH, Bastawy M, Aly H, El-Mazary AA, Abd El-Aziz L. Cardiac troponin I levels and its relation to echocardiographic findings in infants of diabetic mothers. Ital J Pediatr 2012;38:39.

[106] Mert MK, Satar M, Ozbarlas N, Yaman A, Ozgunen FT, Asker HS, et al. Troponin T and NT proBNP levels in gestational, type 1 and type 2 diabetic mothers and macrosomic infants. Pediatr Cardiol 2016;37(1):76–83.

[107] Cimen D, Karaaslan S. Evaluation of cardiac functions of infants of diabetic mothers using tissue Doppler echocardiography. Turk Pediatr Arsivi 2014;49(1):25–29.

[108] Kozak-Barany A, Jokinen E, Kero P, Tuominen J, Ronnemaa T, Valimaki I. Impaired left ventricular diastolic function in newborn infants of mothers with pregestational or gestational diabetes with good glycemic control. Early Hum Dev 2004;77(1–2):13–22.

[109] Demiroren K, Cam L, Oran B, Koc H, Baspinar O, Baysal T, et al. Echocardiographic measurements in infants of diabetic mothers and macrosomic infants of nondiabetic mothers. J Perinat Med 2005;33(3):232–235.

[110] Al-Biltagi M, Tolba OA, Rowisha MA, Mahfouz Ael S, Elewa MA. Speckle tracking and myocardial tissue imaging in infant of diabetic mother with gestational and pregestational diabetes. Pediatr Cardiol 2015;36(2):445–453.

[111] Kojo M, Ogawa T, Yamada K, Sonoda H, Saito K. Multivariate autoregressive analysis of carotid artery blood flow waveform in an infant of a diabetic mother with cardiomyopathy. Acta Paediatr Jpn 1995;37(5):588–593.

[112] Van Bel F, Van de Bor M, Walther FJ. Cerebral blood flow velocity and cardiac output in infants of insulin-dependent diabetic mothers. Acta Paediatr Scand 1991;80(10):905–910.

[113] Clyman RI, Chan CY, Mauray F, Chen YQ, Cox W, Seidner SR, et al. Permanent anatomic closure of the ductus arteriosus in newborn baboons: the roles of postnatal constriction, hypoxia, and gestation. Pediatr Res 1999;45(1):19–29.

[114] Clyman RI, Mauray F, Wong L, Heymann MA, Rudolph AM. The developmental response of the ductus arteriosus to oxygen. Biol Neonate 1978;34(3–4):177–181.

[115] Kajino H, Chen YQ, Seidner SR, Waleh N, Mauray F, Roman C, et al. Factors that increase the contractile tone of the ductus arteriosus also regulate its anatomic remodeling. Am J Physiol 2001;281(1):R291–R301.

[116] Clyman RI, Waleh N, Black SM, Riemer RK, Mauray F, Chen YQ. Regulation of ductus arteriosus patency by nitric oxide in fetal lambs: the role of gestation, oxygen tension, and vasa vasorum. Pediatr Res 1998;43(5):633–644.

[117] Broadhouse KM, Price AN, Durighel G, Cox DJ, Finnemore AE, Edwards AD, et al. Assessment of PDA shunt and systemic blood flow in newborns using cardiac MRI. NMR Biomed 2013;26(9):1135–1141.

[118] Benitz WE. Treatment of persistent patent ductus arteriosus in preterm infants: time to accept the null hypothesis? J Perinatol 2010;30(4):241–252.

[119] Kluckow M, Evans N. Early echocardiographic prediction of symptomatic patent ductus arteriosus in preterm infants undergoing mechanical ventilation. J Pediatr 1995;127(5):774–779.

[120] McNamara PJ, Sehgal A. Towards rational management of the patent ductus arteriosus: the need for disease staging. Arch Dis Childhood Fetal Neonatal Ed 2007;92:F424–F427.

[121] Balsan MJ, Jones JG, Guthrie RD. Effects of a clinically detectable PDA on pulmonary mechanics measures

in VLBW infants with RDS. Pediatr Pulmonol 1991;11(2):161–165.

[122] Chang LY, McCurnin D, Yoder B, Shaul PW, Clyman RI. Ductus arteriosus ligation and alveolar growth in preterm baboons with a patent ductus arteriosus. Pediatr Res 2008;63(3):299–302.

[123] McNamara PJ, Stewart L, Shivananda SP, Stephens D, Sehgal A. Patent ductus arteriosus ligation is associated with impaired left ventricular systolic performance in premature infants weighing less than 1000 g. J Thorac Cardiovasc Surg 2010;140(1):150–157.

[124] Takahashi Y, Harada K, Ishida A, Tamura M, Takada G. Left ventricular preload reserve in preterm infants with patent ductus arteriosus. Arch Dis Childhood 1994;71(2):F118–F121.

[125] Takahashi Y, Harada K, Ishida A, Tamura M, Tanaka T, Takada G. Changes in left ventricular volume and systolic function before and after the closure of ductus arteriosus in full-term infants. Early Hum Dev 1996;44(1):77–85.

[126] Van Hare GF, Hawkins JA, Schmidt KG, Rudolph AM. The effects of increasing mean arterial pressure on left ventricular output in newborn lambs. Circ Res 1990;67(1):78–83.

[127] Gerhardt T, Bancalari E. Lung compliance in newborns with patent ductus arteriosus before and after surgical ligation. Biol Neonate 1980;38(1–2):96–105.

[128] Szymankiewicz M, Hodgman JE, Siassi B, Gadzinowski J. Mechanics of breathing after surgical ligation of patent ductus arteriosus in newborns with respiratory distress syndrome. Biol Neonate 2004;85(1):32–36.

[129] El-Khuffash AF, Jain A, McNamara PJ. Ligation of the patent ductus arteriosus in preterm infants: understanding the physiology. J Pediatr 2013;162(6):1100–1106.

[130] Reller MD, Morton MJ, Reid DL, Thornburg KL. Fetal lamb ventricles respond differently to filling and arterial pressures and to in utero ventilation. Pediatr Res 1987;22(6):621–626.

[131] Romero TE, Friedman WF. Limited left ventricular response to volume overload in the neonatal period: a comparative study with the adult animal. Pediatr Res 1979;13(8):910–915.

[132] Igarashi H, Shiraishi H, Endoh H, Yanagisawa M. Left ventricular contractile state in preterm infants: relation between wall stress and velocity of circumferential fiber shortening. Am Heart J 1994;127(5):1336–1340.

[133] Ting JY, Resende M, More K, Nicholls D, Weisz DE, El-Khuffash A, et al. Predictors of respiratory instability in neonates undergoing patent ductus arteriosus ligation after the introduction of targeted milrinone treatment. J Thorac Cardiovasc Surg 2016;152(2):498–504.

[134] Jain A, Sahni M, El-Khuffash A, Khadawardi E, Sehgal A, McNamara PJ. Use of targeted neonatal echocardiography to prevent postoperative cardiorespiratory instability after patent ductus arteriosus ligation. J Pediatr 2012;160(4). 584.e1–589.e1.

[135] Khemani E, McElhinney DB, Rhein L, Andrade O, Lacro RV, Thomas KC, et al. Pulmonary artery hypertension in formerly premature infants with bronchopulmonary dysplasia: clinical features and outcomes in the surfactant era. Pediatrics 2007;120(6):1260–1269.

[136] Bhat R, Salas AA, Foster C, Carlo WA, Ambalavanan N. Prospective analysis of pulmonary hypertension in extremely low birth weight infants. Pediatrics 2012;129(3):e682–e689.

[137] An HS, Bae EJ, Kim GB, Kwon BS, Beak JS, Kim EK, et al. Pulmonary hypertension in preterm infants with bronchopulmonary dysplasia. Korean Circ J 2010;40(3):131–136.

[138] Mourani PM, Sontag MK, Younoszai A, Miller JI, Kinsella JP, Baker CD, et al. Early pulmonary vascular disease in preterm infants at risk for bronchopulmonary dysplasia. Am J Respir Crit Care Med 2015;191(1):87–95.

[139] Cerro MJ, Abman S, Diaz G, Freudenthal AH, Freudenthal F, Harikrishnan S, et al. A consensus approach to the classification of pediatric pulmonary hypertensive vascular disease: Report from the PVRI Pediatric Taskforce, Panama 2011. Pulm Circ 2011;1(2):286–298.

[140] Lammers AE, Adatia I, Cerro MJ, Diaz G, Freudenthal AH, Freudenthal F, et al. Functional classification of pulmonary hypertension in children: report from the PVRI pediatric taskforce, Panama 2011. Pulm Circ 2011;1(2):280–285.

[141] Poon CY, Edwards MO, Kotecha S. Long term cardiovascular consequences of chronic lung disease of prematurity. Paediatr Respir Rev 2013;14(4):242–249.

[142] British Association of Perinatal Medicine, Royal college of Physicians. Development of Audit Measures and Guidelines for Good Practice in the Management of Neonatal Respiratory Distress Syndrome. Report of a Joint Working Group of the British Association of Perinatal Medicine and the Research Unit of the Royal College of Physicians. Arch Dis Childhood. 1992;67(10 Spec No.): 1221–1227

[143] Kluckow M, Evans N. Low superior vena cava flow and intraventricular haemorrhage in preterm infants. Arch Dis Childhood Fetal Neonatal Ed 2000;82(3):F188–F194.

[144] Binder-Heschl C, Urlesberger B, Schwaberger B, Koestenberger M, Pichler G. Borderline hypotension: how does it influence cerebral regional tissue oxygenation in preterm infants? J Matern Fetal Neonatal Med 2016;29(14):2341–2346.

[145] Dasgupta SJ, Gill AB. Hypotension in the very low birthweight infant: the old, the new, and the uncertain. Arch Dis Childhood Fetal Neonatal Ed. 2003;88(6):F450–F454.

[146] Zhang J, Penny DJ, Kim NS, Yu VY, Smolich JJ. Mechanisms of blood pressure increase induced by dopamine in hypotensive preterm neonates. Arch Dis Childhood Fetal Neonatal Ed 1999;81(2):F99–F104.

[147] Giesinger RE, McNamara PJ. Hemodynamic instability in the critically ill neonate: an approach to cardiovascular support based on disease pathophysiology. Semin Perinatol 2016;40(3):174–188.

[148] Resende MH, More K, Nicholls D, Ting J, Jain A, McNamara PJ. The impact of a dedicated patent ductus arteriosus ligation team on neonatal health-care outcomes. J Perinatol 2016;36(6):463–468.

[149] Cheng DR, Peart S, Tan K, Sehgal A. Nitric therapy in preterm infants: rationalised approach based on functional neonatal echocardiography. Acta Paediatr 2016;105(2):165–171.

[150] Ades A, Sable C, Cummings S, Cross R, Markle B, Martin G. Echocardiographic evaluation of umbilical venous catheter placement. J Perinatol 2003;23(1):24–28.

[151] Pulickal AS, Charlagorla PK, Tume SC, Chhabra M, Narula P, Nadroo AM. Superiority of targeted neonatal

echocardiography for umbilical venous catheter tip localization: accuracy of a clinician performance model. J Perinatol 2013;33(12): 950–953.

[152] Cheung PY, Barrington KJ, Pearson RJ, Bigam DL, Finer NN, Van Aerde JE. Systemic, pulmonary and mesenteric perfusion and oxygenation effects of dopamine and epinephrine. Am J Respir Crit Care Med 1997;155(1):32–37.

[153] Martinez AM, Padbury JF, Thio S. Dobutamine pharmacokinetics and cardiovascular responses in critically ill neonates. Pediatrics 1992;89(1):47–51.

[154] Osborn D, Evans N, Kluckow M. Randomized trial of dobutamine versus dopamine in preterm infants with low systemic blood flow. J Pediatr 2002;140(2):183–191.

[155] McNamara PJ, Laique F, Muang-In S, Whyte HE. Milrinone improves oxygenation in neonates with severe persistent pulmonary hypertension of the newborn. J Crit Care 2006;21(2):217–222.

[156] Mohamed A, Nasef N, Shah V, McNamara PJ. Vasopressin as a rescue therapy for refractory pulmonary hypertension in neonates: case series. Pediatr Crit Care Med 2014;15(2):148–154.

[157] Liu YA, Theis JG, Coceani F. Contractile and relaxing mechanisms in pulmonary resistance arteries of the preterm fetal lamb. Biol Neonate 2000;77(4):253–260.

[158] Skimming JW, DeMarco VG, Cassin S. The effects of nitric oxide inhalation on the pulmonary circulation of preterm lambs. Pediatr Res 1995;37(1):35–40.

[159] Uga N, Ishii T, Kawase Y, Arai H, Tada H. Nitric oxide inhalation therapy in very low-birthweight infants with hypoplastic lung due to oligohydramnios. Pediatr Int 2004;46(1):10–14.

[160] Chock VY, Van Meurs KP, Hintz SR, Ehrenkranz RA, Lemons JA, Kendrick DE, et al. Inhaled nitric oxide for preterm premature rupture of membranes, oligohydramnios, and pulmonary hypoplasia. Am J Perinatol 2009;26(4):317–322.

[161] Semberova J, O'Donnell SM, Franta J, Miletin J. Inhaled nitric oxide in preterm infants with prolonged preterm rupture of the membranes: a case series. J Perinatol 2015;35(4):304–306.

[162] Barrington KJ, Finer N, Pennaforte T. Inhaled nitric oxide for respiratory failure in preterm infants. Cochrane Database Syst Rev 2017;1:CD000509.

[163] Su PH, Chen JY. Inhaled nitric oxide in the management of preterm infants with severe respiratory failure. J Perinatol 2008;28(2):112–116.

[164] Srisuparp P, Heitschmidt M, Schreiber MD. Inhaled nitric oxide therapy in premature infants with mild to moderate respiratory distress syndrome. J Med Assoc Thai 2002;85(Suppl. 2):S469–S478.

[165] The Franco-Belgium Collaborative NO Trial Group. Early compared with delayed inhaled nitric oxide in moderately hypoxaemic neonates with respiratory failure: a randomised controlled trial. The Franco-Belgium Collaborative NO Trial Group. Lancet. 1999;354(9184): 1066–1071.

[166] Wei QF, Pan XN, Li Y, Feng L, Yao LP, Liu GL, et al. [Efficacy of inhaled nitric oxide in premature infants with hypoxic respiratory failure]. Zhongguo Dang Dai Er Ke Za Zhi 2014;16(8):805–809.

[167] Mohamed AS, Mohamed I, Baczynski M, Louis D, McNamara KP, Jain A, et al. Echocardiography predictors of response to inhaled nitric oxide therapy in hypoxic preterm neonates. Pediatric Academic Society Meeting (Accepted as abstract); 2017.

[168] Abman SH, Hansmann G, Archer SL, Ivy DD, Adatia I, Chung WK, et al. Pediatric pulmonary hypertension: guidelines grom the American Heart Association and American Thoracic Society. Circulation 2015;132(21):2037–2099.

[169] Baczynski M, Ginty S, Weisz D, McNamara P, Kelly E, Shah P, et al. Short and long term clinical outcomes of preterm neonates with refractory hypoxic respiratory failure following rescue treatment trial with inhaled nitric oxide. Arch Dis Child Fetal Neonatal Ed 2017;102(6): F508–F514.

[170] James AT, Bee C, Corcoran JD, McNamara PJ, Franklin O, El-Khuffash AF. Treatment of premature infants with pulmonary hypertension and right ventricular dysfunction with milrinone: a case series. J Perinatol 2015;35(4): 268–273.

[171] Bidegain M, Greenberg R, Simmons C, Dang C, Cotten CM, Smith PB. Vasopressin for refractory

hypotension in extremely low birth weight infants. J Pediatr 2010;157(3):502–504.

[172] Silversides CK, Granton JT, Konen E, Hart MA, Webb GD, Therrien J. Pulmonary thrombosis in adults with Eisenmenger syndrome. J Am Coll Cardiol 2003;42(11):1982–1987.

[173] Galie N, Beghetti M, Gatzoulis MA, Granton J, Berger RM, Lauer A, et al. Bosentan therapy in patients with Eisenmenger syndrome: a multicenter, double-blind, randomized, placebo-controlled study. Circulation 2006;114(1): 48–54.

[174] Zuckerman WA, Leaderer D, Rowan CA, Mituniewicz JD, Rosenzweig EB. Ambrisentan for pulmonary arterial hypertension due to congenital heart disease. Am J Cardiol 2011;107(9):1381–1385.

[175] Steinhorn RH, Fineman J, Kusic-Pajic A, Cornelisse P, Gehin M, Nowbakht P, et al. Bosentan as adjunctive therapy for persistent pulmonary hypertension of the newborn: results of the randomized multicenter placebo-controlled exploratory trial. J Pediatr 2016;177. 90.e3–96.e3.

[176] Huddleston AJ, Knoderer CA, Morris JL, Ebenroth ES. Sildenafil for the treatment of pulmonary hypertension in pediatric patients. Pediatr Cardiol 2009;30(7):871–882.

[177] Milger K, Felix JF, Voswinckel R, Sommer N, Franco OH, Grimminger F, et al. Sildenafil versus nitric oxide for acute vasodilator testing in pulmonary arterial hypertension. Pulm Circ 2015;5(2):305–312.

[178] Bigdelian H, Sedighi M. The role of preoperative sildenafil therapy in controlling of postoperative pulmonary hypertension in children with ventricular septal defects. J Cardiovasc Thorac Res 2017;9(3):179–182.

[179] El Midany AA, Mostafa EA, Azab S, Hassan GA. Perioperative sildenafil therapy for pulmonary hypertension in infants undergoing congenital cardiac defect closure. Interact Cardiovasc Thorac Surg 2013;17(6):963–968.

[180] Peiravian F, Amirghofran AA, Borzouee M, Ajami GH, Sabri MR, Kolaee S. Oral sildenafil to control pulmonary hypertension after congenital heart surgery. Asian Cardiovasc Thorac Ann 2007;15(2):113–117.

[181] Putnam LR, Tsao K, Morini F, Lally PA, Miller CC, Lally KP, et al. Evaluation of variability in inhaled nitric oxide use and pulmonary hypertension in patients with congenital diaphragmatic hernia. JAMA Pediatr 2016;170(12): 1188–1194.

[182] Campbell BT, Herbst KW, Briden KE, Neff S, Ruscher KA, Hagadorn JI. Inhaled nitric oxide use in neonates with congenital diaphragmatic hernia. Pediatrics 2014;134(2): e420–e426.

[183] The Neonatal Inhaled Nitric Oxide Study Group. Inhaled nitric oxide and hypoxic respiratory failure in infants with congenital diaphragmatic hernia. The Neonatal Inhaled Nitric Oxide Study Group (NINOS). Pediatrics. 1997;99(6): 838–845.

[184] Noori S, Friedlich P, Wong P, Garingo A, Seri I. Cardiovascular effects of sildenafil in neonates and infants with congenital diaphragmatic hernia and pulmonary hypertension. Neonatology 2007;91(2):92–100.

[185] Patel N. Use of milrinone to treat cardiac dysfunction in infants with pulmonary hypertension secondary to congenital diaphragmatic hernia: a review of six patients. Neonatology 2012;102(2):130–136.

[186] Bailey JM, Hoffman TM, Wessel DL, Nelson DP, Atz AM, Chang AC, et al. A population pharmacokinetic analysis of milrinone in pediatric patients after cardiac surgery. J Pharmacokinet Pharmacodyn 2004;31(1):43–59.

[187] Hofmann SR, Stadler K, Heilmann A, Hausler HJ, Fitze G, Kamin G, et al. Stabilisation of cardiopulmonary function in newborns with congenital diaphragmatic hernia using lung function parameters and hemodynamic management. Klinisc Padiatr 2012;224(4):e1–e10.

[188] More KS, Sakhuja P, Giesinger RE, Ting JY, Keyzers M, Sheth JN, Lapointe A, Jain A, Moore AM, Miller SP, McNamara PJ. Cardiovascular associations with abnormal brain magnetic resonance imaging in neonates with hypoxic ischemic encephalopathy undergoing therapeutic hypothermia and rewarming. Am J Perinatol. 2018;35(10):979–989.

[189] Goldberg JF, Mery CM, Griffiths PS, Parekh DR, Welty SE, Bronicki RA, et al. Extracorporeal membrane oxygenation support

[190] Arzuaga BH, Groner A. Utilization of extracorporeal membrane oxygenation in congenital hypertrophic cardiomyopathy caused by maternal diabetes. J Neonatal Perinatal Med 2013;6(4):345–348.

[191] Berger TM, Stocker M. [Ventilation of newborns and infants]. Der Anaesth 2004;53(8):690–701.

[192] Carter RS, Snyder JV, Pinsky MR. LV filling pressure during PEEP measured by nadir wedge pressure after airway disconnection. Am J Physiol 1985;249(4 Pt. 2): H770–H776.

[193] Salazar Vazquez BY, Martini J, Chavez Negrete A, Cabrales P, Tsai AG, Intaglietta M. Microvascular benefits of increasing plasma viscosity and maintaining blood viscosity: counterintuitive experimental findings. Biorheology 2009;46(3):167–179.

[194] De Buyst J, Rakza T, Pennaforte T, Johansson AB, Storme L. Hemodynamic effects of fluid restriction in preterm infants with significant patent ductus arteriosus. J Pediatr 2012;161(3):404–408.

[195] Green TP, Thompson TR, Johnson DE, Lock JE. Diuresis and pulmonary function in premature infants with respiratory distress syndrome. J Pediatr 1983;103(4):618–623.

[196] Green TP, Thompson TR, Johnson DE, Lock JE. Furosemide promotes patent ductus arteriosus in premature infants with the respiratory-distress syndrome. N Engl J Med 1983;308(13):743–778.

[197] Brion LP, Campbell DE. Furosemide in indomethacin-treated infants—systematic review and meta-analysis. Pediatr Nephrol 1999;13(3):212–218.

[198] Wong R. Maintenance diet and the effects of furosemide on hamsters. Am J Psychol 1981;94(2):339–354.

[199] Schmidt B, Davis P, Moddemann D, Ohlsson A, Roberts RS, Saigal S, et al. Long-term effects of indomethacin prophylaxis in extremely-low-birth-weight infants. N Engl J Med 2001;344(26):1966–1972.

[200] Kluckow M, Jeffery M, Gill A, Evans N. A randomised placebo-controlled trial of early treatment of

the patent ductus arteriosus. Arch Dis Childhood Fetal Neonatal Ed 2014;99(2):F99–F104.

[201] Clyman RI. Recommendations for the postnatal use of indomethacin: an analysis of four separate treatment strategies. J Pediatr 1996;128(5 Pt. 1):601–607.

[202] Trus T, Winthrop AL, Pipe S, Shah J, Langer JC, Lau GY. Optimal management of patent ductus arteriosus in the neonate weighing less than 800 g. J Pediatr Surg 1993;28(9):1137–1139.

[203] Louis D, Wong C, Ye XY, McNamara PJ, Jain A. Factors associated with non-response to second course indomethacin for PDA treatment in preterm neonates. J Matern Fetal Neonatal Med 2018;31(11):1407–1411.

[204] Ohlsson A, Shah SS. Ibuprofen for the prevention of patent ductus arteriosus in preterm and/or low birth weight infants. Cochrane Database Syst Rev 2011;7:CD004213.

[205] Lin YJ, Chen CM, Rehan VK, Florens A, Wu SY, Tsai ML, et al. Randomized trial to compare renal function and ductal response between indomethacin and ibuprofen treatment in extremely low birth weight infants. Neonatology 2017;111(3):195–202.

[206] Weisz DE, Martins FF, Nield LE, El-Khuffash A, Jain A, McNamara PJ. Acetaminophen to avoid surgical ligation in extremely low gestational age neonates with persistent hemodynamically significant patent ductus arteriosus. J Perinatol 2016;36(8):649–653.

[207] Kabra NS, Schmidt B, Roberts RS, Doyle LW, Papile L, Fanaroff A. Neurosensory impairment after surgical closure of patent ductus arteriosus in extremely low birth weight infants: results from the Trial of Indomethacin Prophylaxis in Preterms. J Pediatr 2007;150(3). 229. e1–234.e1.

[208] Madan JC, Kendrick D, Hagadorn JI, Frantz ID 3rd. Patent ductus arteriosus therapy: impact on neonatal and 18-month outcome. Pediatrics 2009;123(2):674–681.

[209] Weisz DE, Mirea L, Rosenberg E, Jang M, Ly L, Church PT, et al. Association of patent ductus arteriosus ligation with death or neurodevelopmental impairment among extremely preterm infants. JAMA Pediatr 2017;171(5):443–449.

[210] Chiang MC, Lin WS, Lien R, Chou YH. Reexpansion pulmonary edema following patent ductus arteriosus ligation in a preterm infant. J Perinat Med 2004;32(4):365–367.

[211] Pharande P, Karthigeyan S, Walker K, D'Cruz D, Badawi N, Luig M, et al. Unilateral vocal cord paralysis after surgical closure of a patent ductus arteriosus in extremely preterm infants. J Paediatr Child Health 2017;53(12):1192–1198.

[212] Rukholm G, Farrokhyar F, Reid D. Vocal cord paralysis post patent ductus arteriosus ligation surgery: risks and co-morbidities. Int J Pediatr Otorhinolaryngol 2012;76(11):1637–1641.

[213] Zahn EM, Nevin P, Simmons C, Garg R. A novel technique for transcatheter patent ductus arteriosus closure in extremely preterm infants using commercially available technology. Catheter Cardiovasc Interv 2015;85(2):240–248.

[214] Zahn EM, Peck D, Phillips A, Nevin P, Basaker K, Simmons C, et al. Transcatheter closure of patent ductus arteriosus in extremely premature newborns: early results and midterm follow-up. JACC Cardiovasc Interv 2016;9(23):2429–2437.

[215] Teixeira LS, Shivananda SP, Stephens D, Van Arsdell G, McNamara PJ. Postoperative cardiorespiratory instability following ligation of the preterm ductus arteriosus is related to early need for intervention. J Perinatol 2008;28(12):803–810.

[216] Noma K, Brandle M, Rupp H, Jacob R. Left ventricular performance in rats with chronic cardiac overload due to arterio-venous shunt. Heart Vessels 1990;5(2):65–70.

[217] Nadaud S, Philippe M, Arnal JF, Michel JB, Soubrier F. Sustained increase in aortic endothelial nitric oxide synthase expression in vivo in a model of chronic high blood flow. Circ Res 1996;79(4):857–863.

[218] Flaim SF, Minteer WJ, Nellis SH, Clark DP. Chronic arteriovenous shunt: evaluation of a model for heart failure in rat. Am J Physiol 1979;236(5):H698–H704.

[219] Satpute MD, Donohue PK, Vricella L, Aucott SW. Cardiovascular instability after patent ductus arteriosus ligation in preterm infants: the role of hydrocortisone. J Perinatol 2012;32(9):685–689.

[220] Mourani PM, Sontag MK, Ivy DD, Abman SH. Effects of long-term sildenafil treatment for pulmonary hypertension in infants with chronic lung disease. J Pediatr 2009;154(3).379.e1–384.e2.

[221] Hon KL, Cheung KL, Siu KL, Leung TF, Yam MC, Fok TF, et al. Oral sildenafil for treatment of severe pulmonary hypertension in an infant. Biol Neonate 2005;88(2):109–112.

[222] Caputo S, Furcolo G, Rabuano R, Basilicata AM, Pilla LM, De Simone A, et al. Severe pulmonary arterial hypertension in a very premature baby with bronchopulmonary dysplasia: normalization with long-term sildenafil. J Cardiovasc Med (Hagerstown) 2010;11(9):704–706.

[223] Kadmon G, Schiller O, Dagan T, Bruckheimer E, Birk E, Schonfeld T. Pulmonary hypertension specific treatment in infants with bronchopulmonary dysplasia. Pediatr Pulmonol 2017;52(1):77–83.

[224] Tan K, Krishnamurthy MB, O'Heney JL, Paul E, Sehgal A. Sildenafil therapy in bronchopulmonary dysplasia-associated pulmonary hypertension: a retrospective study of efficacy and safety. Eur J Pediatr 2015;174(8):1109–1115.

[225] Baker CD, Abman SH, Mourani PM. Pulmonary hypertension in preterm infants with bronchopulmonary dysplasia. Pediatr Allergy Immunol 2014;27(1):8–16.

[226] Barst RJ, Ivy DD, Gaitan G, Szatmari A, Rudzinski A, Garcia AE, et al. A randomized, double-blind, placebo-controlled, dose-ranging study of oral sildenafil citrate in treatment-naive children with pulmonary arterial hypertension. Circulation 2012;125(2):324–334.

[227] USFaD Administration. Revatio (sildenafil): drug safety communication—recommendation against use in children; 2012Available from: http://www.fda.gov/Drugs/DrugSafety/ucm317123.htm.

[228] Piastra M, De Luca D, De Carolis MP, Tempera A, Stival E, Caliandro F, et al. Nebulized iloprost and noninvasive respiratory support for impending hypoxaemic respiratory failure in formerly preterm infants: a case series. Pediatr Pulmonol 2012;47(8):757–762.

[229] Gurakan B, Kayiran P, Ozturk N, Kayiran SM, Dindar A. Therapeutic combination of sildenafil and iloprost in a preterm neonate with pulmonary hypertension. Pediatr Pulmonol 2011;46(6):617–620.

[230] Hwang SK, O YC, Kim NS, Park HK, Yum MK. Use of inhaled iloprost in an infant with bronchopulmonary dysplasia and pulmonary artery hypertension. Korean Circ J 2009;39(8):343–345.

[231] Hill NS, Preston IR, Roberts KE. Inhaled therapies for pulmonary hypertension. Respir Care 2015;60(6):794–802.

[232] Olson E, Lusk LA, Fineman JR, Robertson L, Keller RL. Short-term treprostinil use in infants with congenital diaphragmatic hernia following repair. J Pediatr 2015;167(3):762–764.

[233] Rugolotto S, Errico G, Beghini R, Ilic S, Richelli C, Padovani EM. Weaning of epoprostenol in a small infant receiving concomitant bosentan for severe pulmonary arterial hypertension secondary to bronchopulmonary dysplasia. Minerva Pediatr 2006;58(5):491–494.

[234] Westerhof BE, Saouti N, van der Laarse WJ, Westerhof N, Vonk Noordegraaf A. Treatment strategies for the right heart in pulmonary hypertension. Cardiovasc Res 2017;113(12):1465–1473.

[235] Stewart A, Brion LP, Ambrosio-Perez I. Diuretics acting on the distal renal tubule for preterm infants with (or developing) chronic lung disease. Cochrane Database Syst Rev 2011;9:CD001817.

[236] Aschner JL, Gien J, Ambalavanan N, Kinsella JP, Konduri GG, Lakshminrusimha S, et al. Challenges, priorities and novel therapies for hypoxemic respiratory failure and pulmonary hypertension in the neonate. J Perinatol 2016;36(Suppl. 2):S32–S36.

[237] Jobe AJ. The new BPD: an arrest of lung development. Pediatr Res 1999;46(6):641–643.

[238] Fouron JC, Le Guennec JC, Villemant D, Perreault G, Davignon A. Value of echocardiography in assessing the outcome of bronchopulmonary dysplasia of the newborn. Pediatrics 1980;65(3):529–535.

[239] Bush A, Busst CM, Knight WB, Hislop AA, Haworth SG, Shinebourne EA. Changes in pulmonary circulation in severe bronchopulmonary dysplasia. Arch Dis Childhood 1990;65(7):739–745.

[240] McIntyre CM, Hanna BD, Rintoul N, Ramsey EZ. Safety of epoprostenol

and treprostinil in children less than 12 months of age. Pulm Circ 2013;3(4):862–869.

[241] Tang JR, Markham NE, Lin YJ, McMurtry IF, Maxey A, Kinsella JP, et al. Inhaled nitric oxide attenuates pulmonary hypertension and improves lung growth in infant rats after neonatal treatment with a VEGF receptor inhibitor. Am J Physiol Lung Cell Mol Physiol 2004;287(2): L344–L351.

[242] Tang JR, Seedorf G, Balasubramaniam V, Maxey A, Markham N, Abman SH. Early inhaled nitric oxide treatment decreases apoptosis of endothelial cells in neonatal rat lungs after vascular endothelial growth factor inhibition. Am J Physiol Lung

Cell Mol Physiol 2007;293(5): L1271–L1280.

[243] Tourneux P, Markham N, Seedorf G, Balasubramaniam V, Abman SH. Inhaled nitric oxide improves lung structure and pulmonary hypertension in a model of bleomycin-induced bronchopulmonary dysplasia in neonatal rats. Am J Physiol Lung Cell Mol Physiol 2009;297(6):L1103–L1111.

[244] Wright CJ, Agboke F, Chen F, La P, Yang G, Dennery PA. NO inhibits hyperoxia-induced NF-kappaB activation in neonatal pulmonary microvascular endothelial cells. Pediatr Res 2010;68(6):484–489.

[245] ter Horst SA, Walther FJ, Poorthuis BJ, Hiemstra PS, Wagenaar GT.

Inhaled nitric oxide attenuates pulmonary inflammation and fibrin deposition and prolongs survival in neonatal hyperoxic lung injury. Am J Physiol Lung Cell Mol Physiol 2007;293(1):L35–L44.

[246] Mercier JC, Hummler H, Durrmeyer X, Sanchez-Luna M, Carnielli V, Field D, et al. Inhaled nitric oxide for prevention of bronchopulmonary dysplasia in premature babies (EUNO): a randomised controlled trial. Lancet 2010;376(9738):346–354.

[247] Berkelhamer SK, Farrow KN. Developmental regulation of antioxidant enzymes and their impact on neonatal lung disease. Antioxid Redox Signal 2014;21(13):1837–1848.

Chapter | **30B**

Patent Ductus Arteriosus

Durga P. Naidu, MD, John P. Breinholt III, MD, P. Syamasundar Rao, MD

CHAPTER POINTS

- In the fetal circulation ductus arteriosus (DA) diverts less oxygenated blood from the pulmonary artery into the descending aorta and placenta for oxygenation.
- Spontaneous closure of DA occurs soon after birth, but persistence beyond 72 hours of life is defined as a patent DA (PDA).
- The prevalence of isolated PDA is approximately 0.05% of full-term infants but is very high (up to 80%) in the premature; the earlier the gestational age the higher the incidence.
- Medium to large PDAs in the premature babies result in left to right shunt causing pulmonary and cardiac compromise.

- While clinical signs and serum brain natriuretic peptide (BNP) levels may identify a hemodynamically significant (hs) PDA, it is best diagnosed and quantified by echo-Doppler studies.
- Prophylactic pharmacological or surgical closure of PDAs in all premature infants is no longer recommended.
- All hsPDA are initially treated with conservative management (fluid restriction, diuretic therapy and respiratory and other supportive measures) to allow for spontaneous PDA closure. Should this fail, pharmacologic therapy with indomethacin or ibuprofen is instituted (Ibuprofen is currently preferred). Should two courses of pharmacologic therapy fail to close the PDA, surgical (conventional, bedside or video-assisted) or percutaneous closure of the PDA, depending upon the institutional expertise, may have to be undertaken.

Introduction

The ductus arteriosus (DA) is a vascular muscular structure that usually connects the main pulmonary artery (PA) (at its junction with the left pulmonary artery [LPA]) with the descending thoracic aorta at the level of left subclavian artery. The configuration of the patent DA (PDA) varies considerably, but most often has a conical or funnel shape with a wider aortic end (ampulla) and smaller pulmonary end. The DA develops from the sixth aortic arch and is completely functional by the eighth week of gestation [1,2]. Patency of the DA in the fetus is primarily maintained by continuous exposure to low partial pressure of oxygen and local and circulating prostaglandins along with constant blood flow from the main PA to the descending aorta, largely secondary to high pulmonary vascular resistance induced by relative hypoxemia and nonfunctional lungs [2–4].

PDA is defined as the persistence of DA patency beyond 72 h of postnatal age [1,5,6]. The incidence and prevalence of PDA depend on the gestational age at birth [1,5,7,8], associated congenital heart defects, exposure to high altitude with consequent low partial pressure of oxygen [9], prenatal exposure to certain infectious agents [10], and some associated genetic disorders [11]. Incidence of isolated PDA is approximately 0.05% of term live births and constitutes up to 5%–10% of patients with congenital heart defects [1,2]. Incidence may be higher (up to 0.2%) if one includes children with silent PDA (no murmur but diagnosed by echocardiogram performed for other indications) [2,12]. Incidence of PDA may be very high (up to 80%) in babies born premature, earlier the gestational age higher the incidence [1,5,7,8]. There is a female preponderance with female-to-male ratio of nearly 2 to 1 [2].

The objective of this chapter is to discuss the influence of isolated PDA in neonates with particular attention to premature infants. In this review, we will discuss the role of the DA in the fetus, physiology of natural ductal closure, etiology of persistent DA, hemodynamic changes resulting from PDA, and the implications of PDA for neonatal respiratory care. We will also discuss the clinical findings and diagnosis of PDA, its clinical and anatomical classification, and finally a review of available options for management of the PDA in infants including describing our own institutional experience with transcatheter occlusion of PDA in the premature infants. Discussion of issues related to PDA in the diagnosis and management of cyanotic congenital heart defects is beyond the scope of this chapter.

Ductus arteriosus in the fetus

Exchange of respiratory gases and metabolites in the fetus is through utero-placental connection, while the lungs are utilized for exchange of respiratory gases in the postnatal circulation. Consequently, the cardiovascular and pulmonary circulations are altered in the fetus (Fig. 30B.1) to accommodate such a requirement [3,13–16]. The DA is a vascular conduit that usually connects the PA to the descending thoracic aorta (Fig. 30B.1), which in fetal circulation directs the deoxygenated blood from the PA into the descending aorta for oxygenation [3,4,15,16]. The blood from the superior vena cava and coronary sinus and a portion of inferior vena caval blood that did not enter the left atrium traverses through the tricuspid valve into the right ventricle. This less oxygenated blood is ejected into the main PA by the right ventricle. The flow to the lungs versus descending aorta depends upon the relative vascular resistance of distal vasculature. The placenta in the normal fetus, which is connected to the descending aorta via umbilical arteries, is a low resistance circuit while the pulmonary circulation is a high resistance circuit. Consequently, most

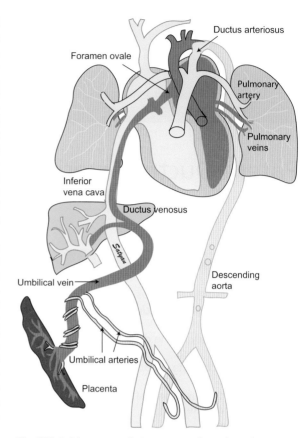

Fig. 30B.1 Diagrammatic Representation of Fetal Circulation. The intensity of blue color represents the degree of oxygen desaturation. The ductus arteriosus shunts deoxygenated blood from the pulmonary artery to aorta. The venous return from the placenta is transported by the umbilical vein and the ductus venosus into the inferior vena cava. From there, a substantial proportion is shunted into the left atrium via the foramen ovale. The residual portion goes into the right ventricle. The blood getting into the left atrium via the foramen ovale is directed into the left ventricle and from there, pumped into the ascending aorta. Thus, the oxygenated blood reaches the brain via the brachiocephalic vessels and the coronary arteries. The reaming blood goes into the right ventricle. The right ventricular blood is propelled into the pulmonary artery. Since the resistance in the pulmonary circuit is high, the majority of the blood is forced via the ductus arteriosus into the descending aorta. From the descending aorta, the desaturated blood goes into placenta via the umbilical arteries. Copyright: Satyan Lakshminrusimha, MD.

of the blood from the main PA is diverted into the descending aorta via the DA with only a small portion (7% of combined ventricular output) delivered to the lungs. From the descending aorta, the blood is transported via the umbilical arteries into the placenta for exchange of gases, transport of nutritive

Table 30B.1 Factors influencing prenatal ductal patency and postnatal ductal closure (Fig. 30B.2) [3,14,16,17]

Factors influencing ductal patency (prenatal—Fig. 30B.2A)	Factors influencing ductal closure (postnatal—Fig. 30B.2B)
Low partial pressure of oxygen (PO$_2$)	Increase in the partial pressure of oxygen (functional closure)
High levels of cyclooxygenase-mediated metabolic products (PGE$_2$ and PGI$_2$)	Decrease in circulating cyclooxygenase-mediated metabolic products (PGE$_2$ and PGI$_2$) (functional closure)
Kept open because of constant flow	No anterograde flow following drop in pulmonary vascular resistance
High circulating adenosine levels	Programmed cell death (anatomic closure)

substrates, and excretion of waste products of metabolism. Factors influencing prenatal ductal patency and postnatal ductal closure are described in Table 30B.1; Fig. 30B.2 [3,14,16,17].

Pathophysiology of ductal closure after birth

In term neonates, closure of the DA is a two-stage process. The first stage involves functional ductal closure resulting from muscular constriction and the second stage is an anatomical closure of the DA. Functional closure of the DA happens within 10–15 h of life, which is mediated by an increase in the partial pressure of oxygen in the blood and a decrease in circulating cyclooxygenase-mediated metabolic products (PGE$_2$, PGI$_2$, etc.) [1,18–22]. An increase in oxygen tension inhibits smooth muscle voltage-dependent potassium channels which facilitates influx of calcium into the cells of ductal tissue causing ductal constriction, resulting in functional occlusion of the DA [1,23–25]. Ductal constriction leads to insufficient dispersion of nutrients to ductal smooth muscle and ultimate progression to programmed cell death [20,26,27]. Anatomic closure of the DA involves conversion of a constricted and functionally occluded DA into a noncontractile atretic ligamentum arteriosus. Following functional closure of the DA, progressive nutritional deprivation leads to hypoxia-induced cell death with simultaneous remodeling of ductal connective tissue for another 2–3 weeks. Ductal tissue remodeling by formation of new noncontractile connective tissue is mediated by vascular endothelial growth factor and transforming growth factor beta.

Etiology of patency of the ductus arteriosus

Multiple risk factors have been identified possibly contributing to the etiology and pathogenesis of the PDA.

Prematurity

Prevalence of PDA is extremely high in the premature and low birth weight infants. Neonates delivered at 24 weeks of gestation have an incidence of PDA up to 85% and infants born between 25 and 28 weeks of gestation have an incidence of PDA up to 65% [28,29]. Newborns weighing less than 1200 g at birth have nearly 80% risk of ductal patency while those weighing 2000 g have nearly 40% risk of having a PDA [1,30,31]. In premature neonates, the etiopathogenesis of PDA is mainly secondary to developmental immaturity. Poor ductal muscular tissue response to the natural mechanisms of ductal closure (poor constrictor response to oxygen and poor dilator effect of prostaglandins) as described earlier is an equally contributing factor [2]. In the majority of preterm infants, the DA fails to constrict and even those infants who achieve ductal constriction fail to have significant ischemia-induced remodeling of ductal tissue [6]. Additional risk factors reported are respiratory distress syndrome and thrombocytopenia within 24 h of life [32]. All other etiological factors associated with PDA in term infants contribute an additional risk in preterm infants.

Genetic factors

Several genetic conditions are associated with higher incidence of PDA, but no specific genetic abnormality has been linked to PDA. Also, no clear genetic mechanism has been defined for development of PDA [2,33,34]. The etiology may be explained based on multifactorial inheritance [11], similar to other congenital heart defects. There is nearly a 3%–5% recurrence risk of PDA in siblings, presumably related to multifactorial inheritance pattern [2,11]. Higher incidence of PDA has been noted in chromosomal abnormalities such as trisomy 21 and 18, in single gene mutations such as Holt–Oram syndrome and Carpenter's syndrome, deletion syndromes such as 4q, 16p13.3 (Rubinstein–Taybi), and 9p (CHARGE), and in X-linked mutations such as incontenia pigmenti [2]. Another association is in Char syndrome, an autosomal dominant inherited disorder with a mutation in the transcription factor AP-2 β (TFAP2B) gene

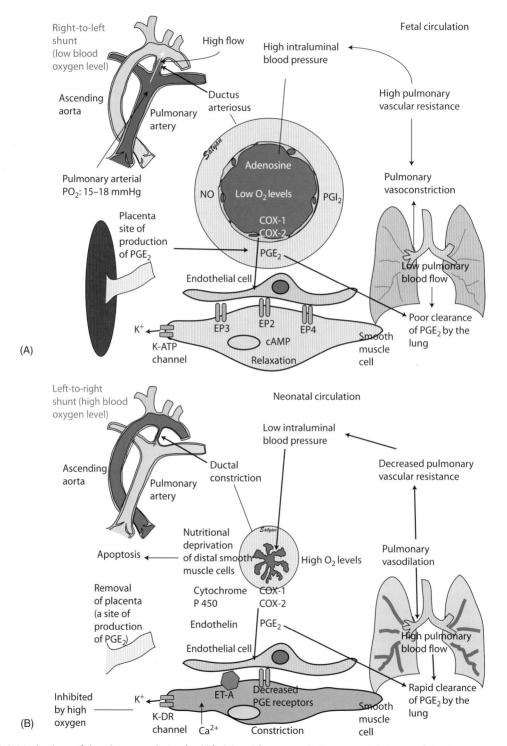

Fig. 30B.2 Mechanisms of ductal patency during fetal life (A) and factors mediating postnatal closure of the ductus arteriosus (B). *PGE₂*, Prostaglandin E₂; *PGI₂*, prostacyclin; *NO*, nitric oxide; *COX*, cyclooxygenase; *EP*, prostaglandin E receptors (see Table 30B.1 and text for complete details). Copyright: Satyan Lakshminrusimha, MD.

and maps to chromosome 6p12-21. Char syndrome is characterized by PDA, facial dysmorphism, and hand abnormalities (mostly commonly an abnormal fifth finger) [33].

Environment factors

High altitude results in low environmental oxygen tension which leads to low dissolved oxygen and consequent increased risk for PDA [9]. Maternal exposure to antiepileptic medications such as valproate and phenytoin is associated with higher incidence of PDA [30,35]. Maternal usage of cocaine [36] or amphetamines [31] also confers a higher incidence of congenital heart defects including PDA. Fetal alcohol syndrome [37] and maternal smoking [38] also have a higher incidence of PDA.

On the contrary, the prevalence of ductal patency is lower in neonates whose mothers were treated with prenatal steroids at least 24 h prior to delivery. This is probably related to inhibition of prostaglandin production, augmented ductal responsiveness to the ductal constricting effect of oxygen and reduced sensitivity to dilating effects of prostaglandins, or a combination thereof [39].

Infectious

Congenital rubella infection, especially during first trimester, leads to congenital rubella syndrome and a higher incidence of PDA [2,40,41]. Ductal tissue in congenital rubella syndrome resembles that of an immature ductus with extensive subendothelial elastic lamina [10].

Hemodynamic changes associated with PDA

Usually, the PDA produces a left-to-right shunt (aorta to PA) because the aortic pressures, both systolic and diastolic, are higher than those in the PA. The extent of the shunt is directly proportional to the minimal ductal diameter and inversely related to the length of the ductus. In a large, nonrestrictive ductus, the shunt is related to the ratio of the pulmonary-to-systemic vascular resistance; the lower the ratio, the greater the shunt. In a term infant, the ductal shunt is minimal at birth because of high pulmonary vascular resistance at the beginning.

Term infant

A normal physiological drop in pulmonary vascular resistance will increase the left-to-right shunt and pulmonary blood flow. In babies with moderate-to-large PDAs, the left atrium and left ventricle dilate; these changes are similar to those seen in patients with ventricular septal defects. Increased left atrial

(LA) pressure may produce pulmonary edema with resultant decreased lung compliance. LA dilatation may sometimes result in opening of the patent foramen ovale (PFO), causing additional left-to-right shunt. With large shunts, compensatory mechanisms ensue: left ventricular (LV) dilatation increases LV stroke volume with normalization of cardiac output. The left ventricle, with time, hypertrophies. Neuroendocrine adaptation increases sympathetic activity and circulating catecholamines [42–44]; these may result in tachycardia and increased sweating as seen in some of these babies. The diastolic runoff due to ductal shunting decreases diastolic blood pressure. A combination of increased intramyocardial tension secondary to LV dilatation with resultant increase in myocardial oxygen demand, tachycardia, and low aortic diastolic pressure may produce subendocardial ischemia [45].

Preterm infant

In the premature infant, because of relatively underdeveloped pulmonary vasculature, the shunt may take place even prior to physiologic reduction of PA pressure/resistance. In addition, the compensatory mechanisms are not well developed (immature myocardium with less contractile elements, less sympathetic innervation, and less well developed Frank–Starling mechanisms and a less compliant left ventricle [46–48]) in the premature neonate and consequently the premature baby may not be able to handle the shunting across the ductus as effectively as a full-term baby.

Impact of PDA on lung function

The adverse effects of PDA are pulmonary overcirculation and systemic hypoperfusion. Excessive blood flow to the lungs may produce pulmonary edema, decreased lung compliance, and may even result in pulmonary hemorrhage. The increased capillary permeability leading to leakage of serum proteins into the pulmonary tissue may lead to inactivation of surfactant. These changes may precipitate respiratory failure and an increased need for mechanical ventilation [1,6,49]. Prolonged duration of pulmonary overcirculation and persistent pulmonary edema decrease lung compliance and may accelerate the inflammatory process and predispose the premature neonate to develop bronchopulmonary dysplasia (BPD) [49,50].

Persistent symptomatic PDA has traditionally been considered a risk factor for BPD. Increased pulmonary blood flow and inflammatory response to prolonged ventilation as mentioned previously were considered to increase the risk of BPD. However, this association has been questioned recently. Retrospective reviews have suggested that while both BPD and PDA are strongly associated with lower gestational age at birth, PDA and the decision to treat a PDA were not associated with an increased incidence of BPD [51]. In infants with BPD, pruning and remodeling of pulmonary vasculature lead to pulmonary hypertension (PH). Reduced vascular growth in BPD limits vascular surface area over time, causing further elevations of pulmonary vascular resistance, especially in response to high cardiac output. Reduced vascular surface area in BPD implies that relatively small increases in left-to-right shunting through a PFO, ASD, or PDA may induce a far greater hemodynamic injury compared to neonates with normal lungs [52].

Impact of PDA on systemic hemodynamics

The left-to-right shunt across the PDA leads to a decrease in systemic blood pressure (systolic, diastolic, and mean arterial pressures) with resultant systemic hypoperfusion to organs such as intestine, kidneys, skin, brain, and muscle. Systemic hypoperfusion may cause necrotizing enterocolitis (NEC), renal insufficiency, intraventricular hemorrhage (IVH), and significant metabolic acidosis [1,6]. In the cerebral circulation, hypoperfusion followed by reperfusion may cause postperfusion injury leading to increased risk of IVH [53–55].

A large PDA may delay the physiological drop in PA pressure or even can lead to the development of significant PH [1,54].

Influence of PDA on neonatal respiratory care and management

Impact of PDA on neonatal respiratory care depends on the hemodynamic effect of the PDA and the patient's ability to compensate for the hemodynamic changes [56]. The hemodynamic impact depends on the size (minimal ductal diameter) of the DA and the degree of the shunt. A large PDA with left-to-right shunt (aorta to PA) results in increased pulmonary blood flow and increased interstitial edema, causing a decrease in pulmonary compliance and a need for higher respiratory support. Elevated PCO_2 on blood gases is commonly observed in premature patients with PDA. In order to meet the ventilator requirements of these infants, an increase in ventilator rate or positive inspiratory pressure (PIP) may be necessary. Due to decreased lung compliance, increased positive end expiratory pressure (PEEP), PIP and/or mean airway pressure may be necessary in preterm infants on mechanical ventilation. The A-a gradient may be elevated in some patients. Pulmonary hemorrhage is often associated with rapid respiratory deterioration.

Prolonged need for mechanical ventilation and respiratory support will increase the risk of BPD [57,58]. Left-to-right shunt for a prolonged period is likely to increase the size of the left ventricle which may lead to LV dysfunction. This will in turn increase the LA pressure leading to further worsening of pulmonary vascular congestion. Pulmonary venous hypertension may further complicate PH associated with BPD. Large ducti may even produce signs of systemic shock [46].

Clinical features

Signs and symptoms of an infant with a PDA depend on the size of the DA and effective left-to-right shunting, which in turn depends on the relative vascular resistances in systemic and pulmonary circulations. Term neonates with a small PDA usually have no significant hemodynamic abnormality and remain asymptomatic. Medium-to-large PDAs will show increasing left-to-right shunt as the normal regression of pulmonary vascular resistance occurs and at that time may develop signs of heart failure. Some term neonates with a large PDA may have persistence of high pulmonary vascular resistance limiting the left-to-right shunt and pulmonary blood flow and do not develop the usual signs and symptoms of a PDA. In such neonates, continuous exposure of the pulmonary vasculature to elevated pressures delays normal regression of the pulmonary arteriolar resistance.

In preterm infants, symptoms of excessive blood flow may develop early because of an underdeveloped pulmonary vasculature and poor compensatory mechanisms [54] as mentioned earlier. A progressive increase in the need for ventilator support, an increased oxygen requirement, signs of systemic hypoperfusion, and/or development of shock in a preterm baby who is a few days old should prompt the investigation for a PDA [56]. The clinical presentation is also influenced by whether the baby has no lung disease, is recovering from lung disease (idiopathic respiratory distress syndrome), or has BPD. Signs and symptoms of PDA are described in Table 30B.2.

As mentioned earlier, the clinical findings depend upon whether the baby has no pulmonary disease, is recovering from lung disease, or has active lung disease. The classical clinical signs of PDA (hyperdynamic precordium, murmur, and bounding pulses) can easily be identified in babies without lung disease and in those that recovered from lung disease. In babies with significant lung disease, these clinical features may be masked and echo-Doppler studies are necessary to detect the ductus. In addition, the findings of hyperdynamic precordium, murmur suggestive of PDA (continuous murmur is usually not present), and bounding pulses of moderate-to-large PDAs are commonly seen in babies who are not on ventilator. Some of these signs become less obvious when the baby is ventilated, particularly with positive pressure ventilation. Consequently, it is our practice to disconnect the baby from the ventilator for brief periods during cardiac evaluation. Even simple continuous positive airway pressure (CPAP) may obscure some of the clinical signs alluded to earlier.

A baby who is requiring progressively increased respiratory support or failing to tolerate normal respiratory weaning process should arise the suspicion of PDA and call for echo-Doppler study to exclude/confirm PDA.

Table 30B.2 Signs and symptoms of PDA

Increased pulmonary blood flow	Decreased systemic blood flow	Increased volume load on heart leading to congestive heart failure
Systolic murmur at the left upper sternal border (classic continuous machinery murmur of PDA is not usually heard in the neonates)	Systolic and diastolic hypotension	Hyperactive (hyperdynamic) cardiac impulse
Accentuated pulmonary component of the second heart sound	Increased pulse pressure (bounding peripheral pulses)	Tachycardia
Loud third heart sound Mid-diastolic flow murmur at the apex	Signs of systemic hypoperfusion	Cardiomegaly
Hyperactive precordium Increased pulse volume (bounding pulses) (wide pulse pressure may be documented via umbilical arterial catheter)	Metabolic acidosis	Hepatomegaly
Palmar pulses		Left and/or right ventricular enlargement
Tachypnea at baseline with episodes of apnea		Rales in the lung fields
Increased work of breathing (respiratory distress)		Poor weight gain
Need for assisted ventilation		Difficulty with oral feeds

Diagnosis and work-up

Radiology

Chest X-ray shows enlarged cardiac size (cardiomegaly) and increased pulmonary vascular markings [1]. Pulmonary venous congestion may be seen and some of these changes may be in addition to or confused with pulmonary changes associated with respiratory distress syndrome or other pulmonary parenchymal disease.

Electrocardiogram

Electrocardiogram (ECG) in a patient with PDA is normal in early postnatal period. In the presence of significant left-to-right shunt for prolonged periods, signs of LA enlargement and/or LV enlargement will manifest on the ECG, but these findings are nonspecific [1]. LA enlargement is suspected when broad, bifid P waves in lead II and a prolonged terminal negative portion of the P wave in lead V_1 are observed [59].

Echocardiography

Echocardiogram along with Doppler interrogation (echo-Doppler) is indicated whenever there is a clinical suspicion for PDA, and indeed, it is the investigative procedure of choice for the diagnosis of a PDA as well as for its quantification. The echo-Doppler study is also helpful in excluding

any congenital cardiac defects, particularly in excluding aortopulmonary window, truncus arteriosus, or other lesions causing left-to-right shunt. Occasionally, a question of coarctation of the aorta may arise; a careful review of the 2-dimensional (2D) and color, pulsed and continuous wave Doppler findings may help to clarify the issue. Rarely, it may be difficult to exclude aortic coarctation in the presence of a large PDA and may require angiography to confirm/exclude such a diagnosis [44]. Echo-Doppler findings in conjunction with clinical findings help in classifying the severity of the PDA and aid in the management [1,60–62]. McNamara and Sehgal proposed a staging system for determining the magnitude and severity of hemodynamically significant patent ductus arteriosus (hsPDA) [62].

Echo-Doppler studies in parasternal long and short axis, apical four- and two-chamber, subcostal and suprasternal notch views should be performed to define the hemodynamic effects and the size of the ductus. Color Doppler-guided continuous wave Doppler interrogation of the ductal flow in multiple views, recording the maximal Doppler flow velocity magnitudes, should also be performed. Estimation of pulmonary arterial pressures should also be undertaken during the echo-Doppler study. Finally, the diastolic flow pattern in the descending aorta (anterograde diastolic flow [normal], absent diastolic flow or retrograde diastolic flow) should also be scrutinized. Defining the shape and configuration of the PDA is of importance to the interventional cardiologist in planning ductal closure.

As alluded to in the "Hemodynamic changes associated with PDA" section, moderate-to-large PDAs result in

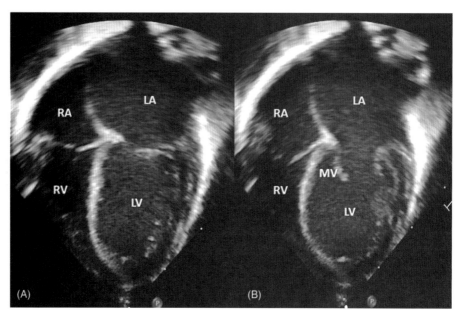

Fig. 30B.3 Selected echocardiographic frames from an apical four-chamber view with the closed (A) and open (B) mitral valve (MV) demonstrating enlarged left atrium (LA) and left ventricle (LV), but this is subjective. *RA*, Right atrium; *RV*, right ventricle.

LA and LV dilatation, while in a small PDA, these cardiac chambers are likely to be normal in size.

Left atrium

Visual estimate of the LA size is very subjective (Fig. 30B.3) and quantitatively measured on M-mode tracing in the parasternal short axis view (Fig. 30B.4) as LA to the aortic root (LA/Ao ratio) and compared with normal values [63]. However, the normal standards for many weight categories in the premature infant have not been adequately established. In a normal infant, this ratio is less than 1.2:1. LA/Ao ratios between 1.2:1 and 1.4:1 suggest that the PDA is small. In moderate-sized PDA, the ratio may be between 1.4:1 and 1.6:1, and in large PDA the ratio is likely be ≥ 1.6. While these ratios are generally reliable, false positives may occur in infants with mitral valve regurgitation and false negative results may be seen in babies who have been fluid restricted.

Similarly, the LA area may be mapped in apical four-chamber (Fig. 30B.5) and apical two-chamber views to estimate LA volume using biplane area length method, but again normal values are nonexistent for many weight categories in the preterm babies.

Left ventricle

The LV internal dimension in end-diastole (LVIDd) and end-systole (LVIDs) may be recorded in parasternal long

and short (Fig. 30B.6) axis views; the recordings are made at the tips of the mitral valve. For some low weight categories, normal values have not been established, and in such situation visual estimate (Fig. 30B.3) is all that we have.

Left ventricular function

Several echocardiographic techniques have been used in the past to evaluate LV function, as reviewed elsewhere [64–66]. Practical and easily used techniques in both term and premature neonates are LV fractional shortening using M-mode echo (Fig. 30B.6) and Simpson's LV area shortening on 2D echocardiogram (Fig. 30B.7).

LV fractional shortening. LV fractional shortening or shortening fraction (SF) (Fig. 30B.6) was one of the earliest described echo techniques for the assessment of LV function [67]. It is the most commonly utilized and easy to use technique for quick estimation of global LV systolic function. It may be derived as follows:

$$SF = \left[\frac{(LVIDd - LVIDs)}{LVIDd} \right] 100$$

where SF is shortening fraction, LVIDd is left ventricular internal dimension in end-diastole, and LVIDs is left ventricular end-systolic dimension.

The normal value is 33% ± 5%. The SF is age and heart rate independent. However, it is load-dependent. In babies,

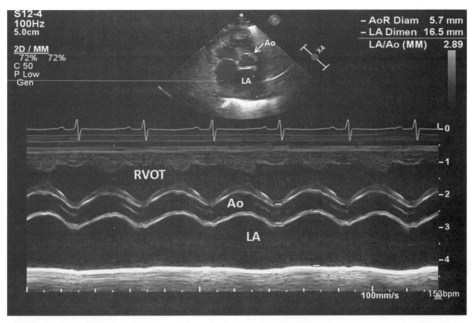

Fig. 30B.4 A selected echocardiographic frame from M-mode tracing in the parasternal short axis view demonstrating measurements of the aorta (Ao) and left atrium (LA). Note the increased LA/Ao ratio. *RVOT*, Right ventricular outflow tract.

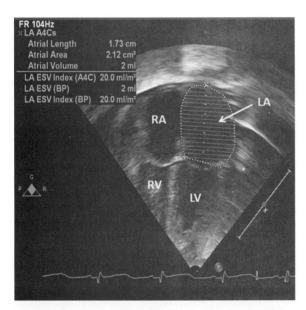

Fig. 30B.5 Selected echocardiographic frames in an apical four-chamber view showing mapping of the left atrial (LA) area. While the calculations can be made (inset to the left upper part), normal values for several premature baby groups have not been established. Apical two-chamber view is not shown. *LV*, Left ventricle; *RA*, right atrium; *RV*, right ventricle.

less than 5 days old and those with elevated right ventricular (RV) pressure, interventricular septal flattening may be present which makes the SF less reliable.

LV area shortening. Area shortening of the LV utilizing Simpson's rule (Fig. 30B.7) is particularly valuable in the term and premature neonates [68]. The LV area shortening is calculated as follows:

$$AS = \frac{(LVAd - LVAs)}{LVAd}$$

where AS is area shortening, LVAd is LV area in diastole, and LVAs is LV area in systole.

The normal values are 50%–60%. This method of evaluation of LV function is useful even when LV dysynergy or flat to paradoxical ventricular septal motion is present. However, it is also load-dependent.

Pulmonary artery pressure

Echo-Doppler studies are useful in estimating the PA pressures in most babies. Several techniques have been used in the past as reviewed elsewhere [66]. Attempts to record Doppler jets in multiple views in the right heart should be made in all subjects. The Doppler jet velocity (V in m/s) may be utilized to calculate pressure difference (ΔP

593

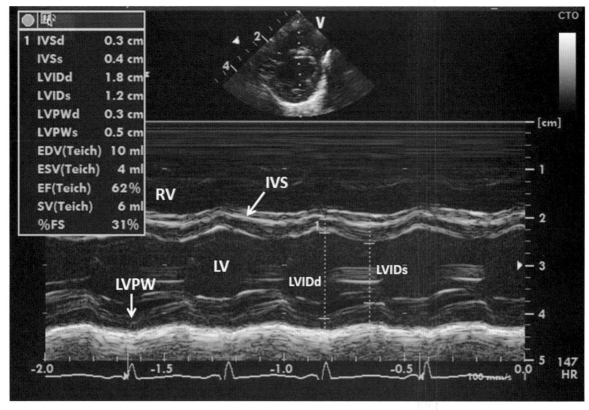

Fig. 30B.6 Selected echocardiographic frames from the parasternal short axis view showing the left ventricular (LV) internal dimension in end-diastole (LVIDd) and systole (LVIDs) which may be used to calculate fractional shortening (%FS) as well as others as indicated in the inset. *IVS*, Interventricular septum; *LVPW*, left ventricular posterior wall; *RV*; right ventricle.

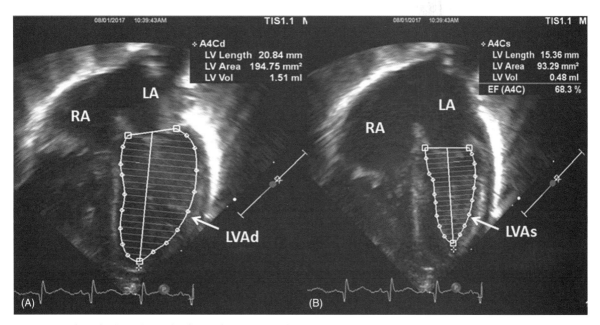

Fig. 30B.7 Selected echocardiographic frames from an apical four-chamber view of the left ventricle measuring left ventricular area in diastole (LVAd) in (A) and in end-systole (LVAs) in (B) demonstrating calculation of area shortening of the LV using Simpson's rule. The LV area shortening is 68% (see inset in B); normal values are 50%–60%. *LA*, Left atrium; *RA*, right atrium.

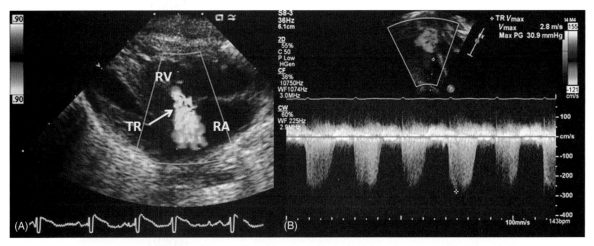

Fig. 30B.8 (A) Parasternal two-dimensional and color Doppler recording to demonstrate tricuspid regurgitent (TR) jet. (B) Continuous wave Doppler recording of TR jet is shown. This is utilized in calculating pulmonary artery systolic pressure: peak velocity of 2.8 indicates 31 mmHg gradient (by modified Bernoulli equation) across the tricuspid valve; to this, an assumed right atrial (RA) pressure of 5 mmHg is added to calculate the pulmonary artery pressure (see the text). *RV*, Right ventricle.

in mmHg) between the two cardiac chambers by using a modified Bernoulli equation:

$$Gradient\ (\Delta P) = 4V^2$$

Measuring arm systolic blood pressure simultaneously is helpful in quantifying the level of the PA pressure by comparing to the systemic blood pressure.

Tricuspid insufficiency jet. If an adequate tricuspid insufficiency jet can be recorded, the RV outflow tract is scrutinized initially to exclude pulmonary stenosis. If there is no evidence for RV outflow tract obstruction, peak velocity of the tricuspid regurgitant jet (V) may be used to estimate PA systolic pressure (Fig. 30B.8):

$$PAP = RVP = 4V^2 + 5\ mmHg$$

where PAP is pulmonary artery systolic pressure, RVP is right ventricular systolic pressure, and V is regurgitant tricuspid jet velocity. The right atrial pressure is assumed to be 5 mmHg. A good envelope of the tricuspid insufficiency jet is important to give credence to this method of PA pressure estimation (Fig. 30B.9).

Pulmonary insufficiency jet. In the presence of pulmonary insufficiency jet (Fig. 30B.10), PA diastolic pressure may be predicted:

$$PA\ diastolic\ pressure = 4V^2 + 5\ mmHg$$

where PA is pulmonary artery and V is pulmonary insufficiency jet velocity. The 5 mmHg is the assumed RV end-diastolic pressure.

Patent ductus arteriosus jet. PDA Doppler velocity should be recorded in multiple views which helps in estimating the PA diastolic pressure (Figs. 30B.11–30B.14):

$$PA\ pressure = BP - 4V^2$$

where PA is pulmonary artery, BP is arm blood pressure (or pressure recorded via an indwelling umbilical artery catheter), and V is PDA peak flow velocity.

A high PDA Doppler velocity (Figs. 30B.11 and 30B.12) indicates low PA pressure while a low PDA velocity (Fig. 30B.14) suggests high PA pressure. Mild elevation of PA pressure is demonstrated in Fig. 30B.13.

If no adequate Doppler jets could be recorded in the right heart, indirect signs such as right atrial and RV dilatation, RV hypertrophy, PA dilatation, and flattening of the interventricular septum may suggest elevated PA pressures, but the magnitude of increase may not be quantified. Shorter acceleration times (<100 ms) and "spike and dome" appearance of the PA flow velocity curve may also indicate increased PA pressure.

PDA diameter

Color flow Doppler is a very useful method for identifying the PDA and may be used to determine its size and estimate the degree of ductal shunting. The color Doppler signal is extremely sensitive and may detect even a tiny PDA with a color flow signal appearing in the main PA close to the origin of LPA. Since the magnitude of left-to-right shunt across the PDA is largely determined by its narrowest diameter, minimal ductal diameter determined by angiography [69] has been used to classify the ductal sizes (Table 30B.3).

595

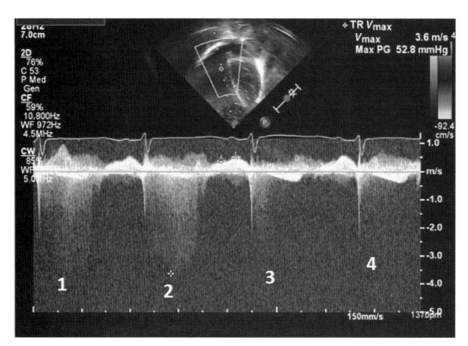

Fig. 30B.9 An Example of Importance of Recording the Tricuspid Insufficiency Jet With a Complete Envelope is Shown. Tricuspid insufficiency recordings marked 1 and 2 are satisfactory while those labeled 3 and 4 are not satisfactory. It is a good practice to have tricuspid insufficiency jets in all cycles as illustrated in Fig. 30B.6B to give credence to this method of PA pressure estimation.

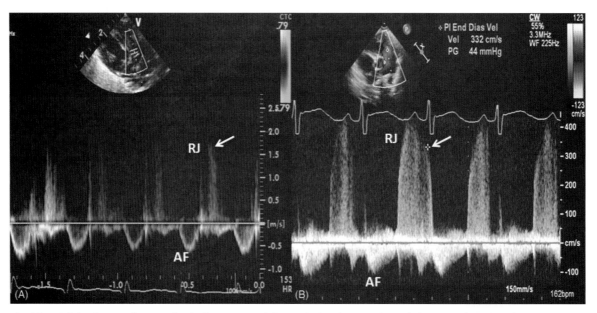

Fig. 30B.10 (A) Pulse Doppler recording in the parasternal short axis view (inset at the top) showing pulmonary valve regurgitant jet (RJ) which is low (arrow pointing to end-diastolic velocity) (1.6 m/s); this would suggest low pulmonary artery pressure (see the text for details). (B) Continuous wave Doppler recording in the parasternal short axis view (inset at the top) illustrating high pulmonary valve RJ *(arrow)* (3.3 m/s). This would suggest high-pulmonary artery pressure (see the text for details). *AF,* Anterograde pulmonary flow.

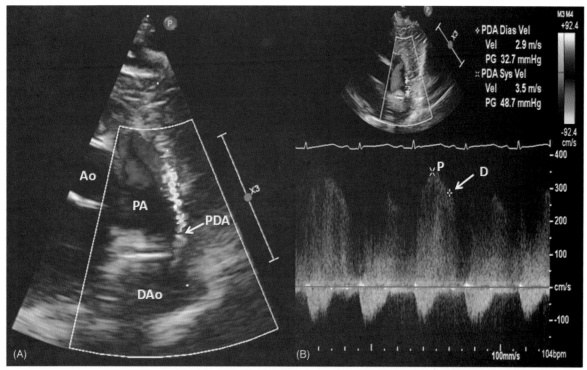

Fig. 30B.11 (A) Selected echocardiographic frame from the parasternal short axis two-dimensional and color Doppler recording demonstrating patent ductus arteriosus (PDA) with left-to-right shunt. (B) High Doppler velocity across the PDA suggests relatively low pulmonary artery pressure. Pulmonary artery (PA) diastolic (D) *(arrow)* velocity (2.9 m/s) may be used to calculate PA diastolic pressure (see the text for details). *Ao*, Aorta; *DAo*, descending aorta; *P*, peak velocity.

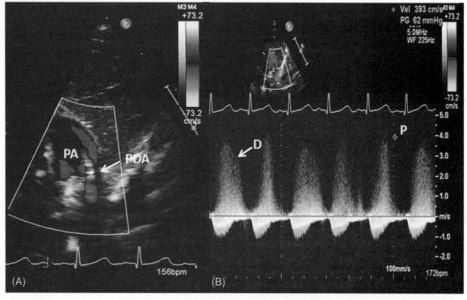

Fig. 30B.12 This figure is similar to Fig. 30B.11, but from a different premature baby illustrating a small patent ductus arteriosus (PDA) and estimation of pulmonary artery (PA) diastolic (D) *(arrow)* pressure. *P*, Peak velocity.

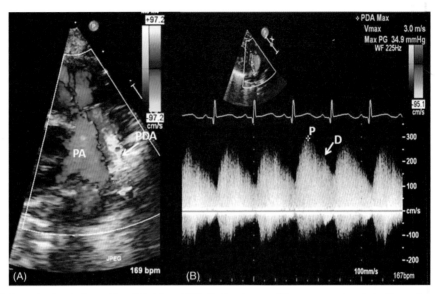

Fig. 30B.13 This figure is also similar to Figs. 30B.11 and 30B.12, but from a different premature baby illustrating a moderate patent ductus arteriosus (PDA) and estimation of pulmonary artery (PA) diastolic (D) *(arrow)* pressure. The estimated PA pressure is likely to be higher than those illustrated in Figs. 30B.10 and 30B.11. *P*, Peak velocity.

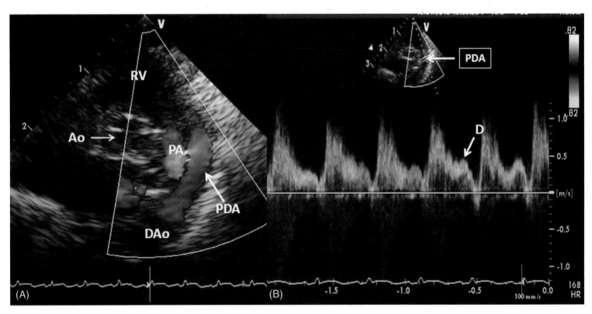

Fig. 30B.14 This figure is also similar to Figs. 30B.11–30B.13, but from a different premature baby illustrating a large patent ductus arteriosus (PDA) and estimation of pulmonary artery (PA) diastolic (D) *(arrow)* pressure. The estimated PA pressure is likely to be higher than those illustrated in Figs. 30B.11–30B.13. Apart from low Doppler velocity (<0.5 m/s), note laminar flow across the PDA; both these characteristics suggest near systemic PA pressures. *Ao*, Aorta; *DAo*, descending aorta; *P*, peak velocity; *RV*, right ventricle.

Table 30B.3 Classification of sizes of the patent
ductus arteriosus [69]

Type	Description
Silent PDA	Less than 1.5 mm and no murmur
Very small PDA	≤1.5 mm with audible murmur
Small PDA	1.5–3 mm
Moderate PDA	3–5 mm
Large PDA	>5 mm

Echocardiographic estimation of angiographic minimal
ductal diameter is not very accurate [70]; however, echo is
the method of clinical relevance for the premature babies.
Color flow imaging of the ductus in multiple views is performed to identify the narrowest diameter; the color is
deleted and 2D diameter determined. Both the color and
2D diameters are used to measure the size of the ductus
(Figs. 30B.15 and 30B.16). Examples of small (Figs. 30B.11

and 30B.12), medium (Fig. 30B.13), and large (Figs. 30B.14
and 30B.17) PDAs are shown.
    Early studies indicated that a narrowest PDA diameter
>1.5 mm is associated with the need of PDA treatment
with a sensitivity of 81% and a specificity of 85% [71,72].
In a 2013 study, the PDA diameter >1.5 mm was also
found to be predictive of the development of symptoms
with a sensitivity of 91% and a specificity of 100% [73].
A more recent study suggested that PDA size ≥2 mm and
peak-systolic-to-end-diastolic Doppler velocity ratio ≥2
on days 3 and 7 are associated with the requirement for
PDA treatment at a future date [74]. Since the patients'
sizes and the degree of maturation vary, ductal diameter
may not, by itself, be a reliable indicator of its size. Some
degree of normalization (mm/kg or mm/BSA [body surface area]) may help resolve this issue. In one study [75],
a PDA diameter of 1.4 mm/kg was found to be suggestive of significant ductus, although the number of subjects
investigated in this study was small. The ratio of minimal
ductal diameter to the origin of the LPA (PDA:LPA ratio)
was suggested as a method of quantification of the size of
the ductus [76]. This investigator suggested that the ratio

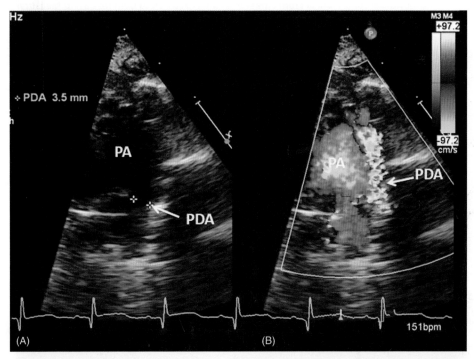

Fig. 30B.15 Selected Echocardiographic Frames From the Parasternal Short Axis View Demonstrating Measurement of Minimal Ductal Diameter. The color signal in (B) is deleted and 2-dimensional (2D) diameter measured (A). *PA*, Pulmonary artery; *PDA*, patent ductus arteriosus.

599

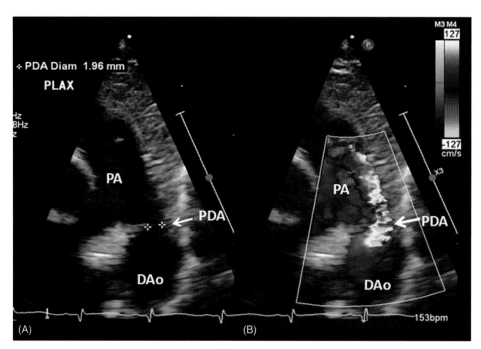

Fig. 30B.16 Selected Echocardiographic Frames From Parasternal Short Axis View Demonstrating Measurement of Minimal Ductal Diameter in a Different Premature Baby. The color signal in (B) is deleted and 2-dimensional (2D) diameter measured (A). *DAo*, Descending aorta; *PA*, pulmonary artery; *PDA*, patent ductus arteriosus.

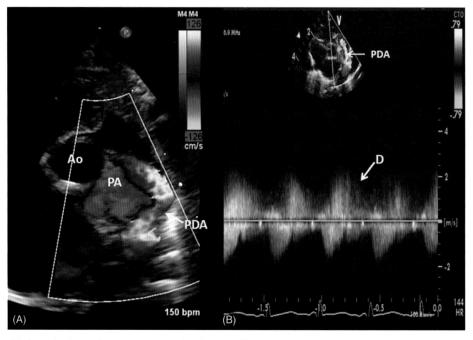

Fig. 30B.17 This figure is also similar to Fig. 30B.11, but from a different premature baby illustrating a moderate-to-large patent ductus arteriosus (PDA) and estimation of pulmonary artery (PA) diastolic (D) *(arrow)* pressure. The estimated PA pressure is likely to be higher than those illustrated in Figs. 30B.11 and 30B.12.

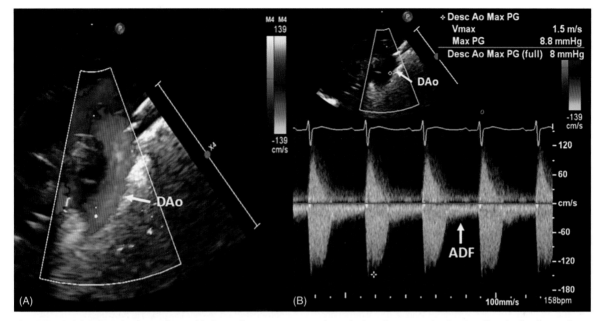

Fig. 30B.18 (A) Selected echocardiographic frame from a suprasternal notch view demonstrating laminar flow in the descending aorta (DAo) in a premature infant with a small ductus. (B) Continuous wave Doppler recording shows normal anterograde diastolic flow (ADF) in the DAo in the same infant shown in (A). The diastolic flow oscillates around zero baseline.

is <0.5 in small PDAs, between 0.5 and 1.0 in moderate PDAs, and ≥1.0 in large PDAs.

Descending aortic flow pattern

In the early 1980s, the finding of retrograde descending aortic flow in early diastole that continued throughout diastole was described in babies with aortic runoff lesions including PDA [77]. Absent anterograde diastolic or presence of retrograde diastolic flow in the descending aorta in a baby with a minimal PDA diameter ≥1.5 mm may indicate a hsPDA [78]. The descending aortic diastolic flow pattern may also estimate the degree of left-to-right shunt [76], normal anterograde diastolic flow—ratio of pulmonary-to-systemic blood flow (Qp:Qs) of 1, absent diastolic flow—Qp:Qs of 1.3, and retrograde diastolic flow—Qp:Qs of 1.7 or larger. Normal anterograde and abnormal retrograde diastolic flow patterns are illustrated in Figs. 30B.18 and 30B.19, respectively.

Summary of echo-Doppler findings of the PDA

In small PDAs, the LA (LA:Ao ratio <1.4:1) and LV are likely to be normal in size and the LV function is normal. In moderate-to-large PDAs, the LA (LA:Ao ratio >1.4:1) and

LV are dilated. At the beginning, the LV function is normal; hyperdynamic LV may be observed and with time, LV function becomes poor with resultant increased LV end-diastolic and LA pressures with consequent worsening of the respiratory status. In small PDAs, the minimal ductal diameter is small with high Doppler velocity across the PDA (Figs. 30B.11 and 30B.12), while in large PDAs, the minimal ductal diameter is larger with a low Doppler velocity across the ductus (Figs. 30B.14 and 30B.17). In moderate-sized PDAs, these values are in the middle (Fig. 30B.13). The PA pressures are usually normal in small PDAs while they may be high in large PDAs. The PA pressures may also reflect the degree of pulmonary parenchymal disease. In very low birth weight infants, the PA pressures may not increase in proportion to the severity of pulmonary parenchymal disease because of the underdeveloped pulmonary vasculature. Finally, anterograde descending aortic diastolic flow is present in small PDAs (Fig. 30B.18) while in large PDAs, the descending aortic diastolic flow is retrograde (Fig. 30B.19). Table 30B.4 lists characteristics of various PDA sizes.

Comments

No single parameter discussed earlier is likely to be accurate by itself. A combination of the aforementioned parameters

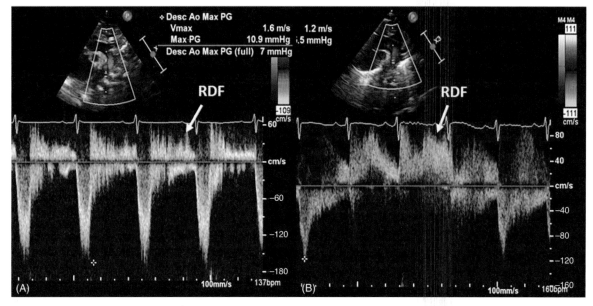

Fig. 30B.19 Pulse Doppler recordings from a suprasternal notch view demonstrating retrograde diastolic flow (RDF) in the DAo in two different premature babies (A and B) with large PDAs signifying that there is likely be an hsPDA.

Table 30B.4 Echocardiographic characterization of the PDA in the premature infants

Parameter	Small PDA	Moderate PDA*	Large PDA*
Left atrial size	Normal	Mildly dilated	Moderate-to-severely dilated
LA:Ao ratio	≤1.4:1	1.4–1.6	≥1.6
Left ventricular (LV) size	Normal	Mildly dilated	Moderate-to-severely dilated
LV systolic function	Normal	Normal	Normal, hypercontractile or diminished function
Minimal ductal diameter	≤1.4 mm	1.4–2.0 mm	≥2.0 mm
PDA Doppler velocity	High (3.0–4.0 m/s)	~2.0 m/s	Low (~1.0 m/s)
Estimated PA pressure	Normal	Mildly elevated	Moderate-to-severely elevated
Descending aortic Doppler flow velocity pattern	Normal anterograde flow (Fig. 30B.18)	Normal anterograde flow (Fig. 30B.18)	Normal or absent anterograde flow or presence of retrograde flow (Fig. 30B.19)

Ao, Aorta; *LA*, left atrium; *LV*, left ventricle; *PDA*, patent ductus arteriosus; *PA*, pulmonary artery.
*May be considered hemodynamically significant patent ductus arteriosus (hsPDA) if associated with clinical deterioration.

is more likely to be helpful in quantifying the ductal significance. The PDA may be classified as small when the minimal PDA diameter is ≤1.4 mm, LA:Ao ratio ≤1.4:1, and the descending aortic diastolic flow is anterograde, while a PDA diameter ≥2.0 mm and LA:Ao ratio ≥1.6 along with retrograde descending aortic diastolic flow may indicate a large or hsPDA (Table 30B.4). Values in between suggest moderate PDA (Table 30B.4).

Ductal aneurysm

Another interesting echocardiographic finding related to the DA is ductal aneurysm. Ductal aneurysms are found in late trimester fetuses and young infants with incidence of up to 8% [79]. Spontaneous resolution of ductal aneurysm occurs because of thrombosis and even if it persists has no clinical significance in infants [79–81] but may lead to symptoms warranting surgical management in adults [2]. As many as one-fourth of infants with a ductal aneurysm have an underlying disorder such as trisomy 13, trisomy 21, Ehlers–Danlos syndrome, Marfan's syndrome, or Smith–Lemli–Opitz syndrome [80].

Cardiac catheterization

Given the echo-Doppler studies are reasonably accurate in diagnosing the PDA, cardiac catheterization is not necessary for diagnosis and is only performed as a part of percutaneous occlusion of PDA, as discussed in a latter section of this chapter.

Biomarkers

Levels of cardiac biomarkers (natriuretic peptides) are elevated in congestive heart failure (CHF). Different types of cardiac biomarkers have been studied in premature neonates with PDA; these include atrial natriuretic peptides (ANPs) with its inactive fragment mid-regional pro-ANP (MR-proANP) and brain natriuretic peptide (BNP) with its inactive fragment N-terminal pro-BNP (NTpBNP) [82]. Increased levels of ANPs are produced in response to increased transmural pressure from the stretch of atrial wall [83] while increased BNPs are produced in response to increased volume and pressure overload on LV myocardium [84].

Level of biomarkers peak at around 48 h of life in both term and preterm healthy neonates and these values continue to decrease until 1 month of life [84,85]. Healthy preterm neonates have higher levels of biomarkers compared to term neonates but follow the same trend [85,86]. It is further noted that the levels of biomarkers are increased in preterm infants with hsPDA [87]. Several other studies examined BNP levels in preterm infants during the first week of life; these studies involve small number of subjects and used different cutoff levels as markers of hsPDA [88–92]. Marked variability found in these studies may be related to variable daily fluid intake, differences in magnitude of left-to-right shunt, and variable ductal constrictive response to treatment. In preterm (gestational age of 28–30 weeks) neonates, plasma levels of NTpBNP on day 3 of life were reported to have excellent sensitivity (95%–100%) but variable specificity (58%–95%) in estimating hsPDA requiring future treatment [93,94]. hsPDA is associated with a rise of B-type natriuretic peptide (sensitivity of 92.9% and specificity of 73.3%); these levels normalize after successful ductal closure [1,90,95]. Even in term neonates with hsPDA, levels of BNP are elevated when compared to those without PDA, hemodynamically insignificant PDA and with cyanotic heart disease [96]. Further detailed review of biomarkers in hsPDA in preterm infants is outside the scope of this chapter but can be found elsewhere [11,90].

Table 30B.5 Angiographic classification of the patent ductus arteriosus [97]

Type A	(Conical) ductus, with well-defined aortic ampulla and constriction of the PDA near the pulmonary artery end
Type B	Very large (window) ductus, with very short length
Type C	(Tubular) ductus, which is without constrictions
Type D	(Complex) ductus, which has multiple constrictions
Type E	(Elongated) ductus, with the constriction remote from the anterior edge of the trachea

Classification of the PDA

Angiographic classification of PDA was proposed by Krichenko et al. [97] and has been in use since that time with a positive influence in percutaneous closure of PDA. The proposed classification includes types A–E (Table 30B.5) and is based on the angiographic appearance of the PDA in the lateral view. Types A and B have subtypes 1, 2, and 3 based on the relationship of ductal insertion into the PA to the tracheal position.

Angiography is presently considered as gold standard for precise delineation of the ductus prior to percutaneous closure [98]. Careful use of echocardiographic data is likely to minimize the radiation and aid in successful ductal closure [99]. In comparison to angiographic data, echo tends to overestimate the narrowest ductal diameter [70,99] but has a reasonably good correlation with estimation of ductal length [72].

Echocardiographic classification of the PDA in the premature infant is useful in the management of preterm infants and was detailed in Table 30B.4.

Severity of the PDA (hemodynamically significant)

Definitions of hsPDA have varied; the published studies used different criteria to define hsPDA which makes it difficult to compare outcomes of one study to the next [1,50,60,62]. Hemodynamic significance of the PDA is mainly defined based on the clinical and diagnostic markers and was tabulated by McNamara and Sehgal [62]; this complex table is presented in a simplified form in Table 30B.6.

Studies that attempt to characterize hsPDA will be briefly reviewed. Neonates weighing less than 1500 g requiring

Table 30B.6 Clinical and diagnostic markers of hemodynamically significant PDA

Clinical markers	Diagnostic markers
Oxygenation difficulty	Cardiomegaly and increased pulmonary vascular markings on chest radiogram
Need for prolonged respiratory support	Minimal ductal diameter ≥1.5 mm
Presence of bradycardia or apnea	Characteristics of Doppler flow across the ductus (low velocity)
Feeding intolerance	Left atrium to aorta (LA:Ao) ratio ≥1.6
Systemic hypotension	Dilated and poor left ventricular function
Oliguria with elevation of plasma creatinine	Flow pattern in the descending aorta (reversal of diastolic flow)
Requirement of cardiotropic agent(s) and others	Elevated cardiac biomarkers (no specific criteria as of now)

mechanical ventilation in their first 30 h of life and a PDA measuring 1.5 mm or more are likely to require management for PDA (83% sensitivity and 90% specificity) [72]. Another recent retrospective study of 29 infants <29 weeks of gestation suggested that babies with a minimal PDA diameter >1.5 mm between 6 and 48 h of age are likely to develop hsPDA with a sensitivity of 91% and a specificity of 100% [72]. Another feature of echocardiography determining hsPDA is LA:Ao ratio greater than 1.5 after the first day of life (88% sensitivity and 95% specificity) [60,61]. Absence of anterograde diastolic or presence of retrograde diastolic descending aortic flow may indicate hsPDA, especially if the minimal PDA diameter is ≥1.5 mm [78]. High levels of BNP (above 70 pg/mL) suggest hsPDA with a sensitivity of 92.9% and a specificity of 73.3%; the BNP values normalize following successful treatment [90]. Perfusion index (PI) of ≤1.57% and ≤1.32% on days 1 and 3, respectively, may identify hsPDA with a sensitivity of 66.7% and a specificity of 100% [100]; lower PI indicated diminished perfusion to lower extremities secondary to large left-to-right shunt across the PDA.

Management

Over the last 4 decades, there have been substantial changes in thinking regarding the management of PDA in the premature infant [101,102]. Early on, closure of the PDA in all preterm infants was advocated [103,104] while

others suggested that no PDA needs closure in premature babies [105,106]. Prophylactic, early asymptomatic, early symptomatic, and late symptomatic treatment options to address the PDA have been considered over time. Comparison of surgical with pharmacologic (indomethacin or ibuprofen) closure did not reveal any differences in outcomes [107] although the surgical approach was associated with significant morbidity [108,109]. Eventually, treatment of the PDA based on the magnitude of left-to-right shunt across the ductus came into vogue [62]. While there is a general consensus that babies with hsPDA should be closed, it is not clear if such closures should be performed when the PDA shunt becomes clinically significant or closure should be done early on, prior to the clinical manifestation of the shunt. Conservative management is advocated by some clinicians given the relatively high prevalence of spontaneous closure of the ductus (closure rates: infants with birth weights of 1000–1500 g—67%–94% [110]; infants with birth weights <1000 g—31%–34% [110,111]); the conservative approach might provide an opportunity for spontaneous closure of the PDA. Symptoms of pulmonary overcirculation are usually treated with fluid restriction and/or diuretics. If these efforts fail, and the infant demonstrates evidence of a worsening respiratory status or fails to progress in efforts to wean off respiratory support, PDA closure is sought. In asymptomatic infants, closure of PDA is indicated at a later age to prevent long-term complications from progressive left heart dilatation [112] and to minimize risk of endarteritis [113]. Currently available treatment modalities for addressing PDA in premature infants will be reviewed.

Conservative or expectant management

Conservative approach involves watchful waiting along with fluid restriction [114] and appropriate respiratory support (CPAP or endotracheal ventilation), as indicated by the clinical scenario. Maintenance of adequate levels of hematocrit (>45%) by appropriate blood transfusion to optimize cardiac output and oxygen delivery to tissues should be undertaken. Provision of electrolytes, glucose, and sufficient calories should be incorporated into the treatment regimen as per the standard-of-care guidelines for the premature infants. Discussion of issues related to intravenous (IV) hyperalimentation versus enteral feeding is beyond the scope of this presentation. Enteral feeding while watching for feed intolerance and signs of NEC seems to be a reasonable approach in a clinically asymptomatic premature infant. Studies in the past [110,111] have shown spontaneous closure of PDAs in a substantial proportion of premature babies as mentioned earlier. Thus, the conservative approach provides opportunity for spontaneous closure of PDA to manifest.

Early randomized clinical trials suggested that liberal fluid intake (170 mL/kg/day) may be associated with higher prevalence of PDA in the premature neonate [115,116]. More recent analysis of multiple randomized clinical trials indicates that restricted fluid intake (50–80 mL/kg/day) resulted in lower risk for PDA when compared to liberal fluid administration (80–170 mL/kg/day) [117].

Very low birth weight infants may receive 70–80 mL/kg/day which may be adjusted depending upon weight gain/loss, need for phototherapy, and serum electrolytes [114]. In babies with significant ductal shunt and/or signs of CHF, treatment of CHF should be instituted along with better ventilatory support and restriction of fluid intake (no more than 120–130 mL/kg/day). Use of digoxin, a drug commonly used in the past, is no longer in vogue to treat CHF in the premature neonate because of low effectiveness and potential toxicity. However, diuretics such as chlorothiozide (10–20 mg/kg/dose NG, every 12 h) and/or furosemide (1 mg/kg/dose IV, every 12–24 h) may be used. Because of concern that furosemide may increase PGE_2 synthesis [118] (which in turn may promote ductal patency), furosemide is not generally used during the first week of life.

Advantages of the conservative approach include avoidance of pharmacologic agents (indomethacin or ibuprofen) and procedures (surgical or percutaneous closure) to treat PDA both of which carry inherent risk [1]. The disadvantage of the conservative approach is decreased efficacy for subsequent pharmacological therapy, thus increasing the risk of treatment failure [1,6,26].

Respiratory management of hsPDA

Respiratory management of hsPDA is dependent on patient's status. Respiratory acidosis may be managed by noninvasive ventilation either using a nasal CPAP device or a high-flow nasal cannula. Persistent respiratory distress may require intubation and mechanical ventilation. Presence of pulmonary edema and increasing inspiratory oxygen requirement may be managed by increasing PEEP or mean airway pressure. Occasionally, persistent respiratory distress may necessitate a switch to high frequency ventilation. Pulmonary hemorrhage and hemorrhagic pulmonary edema may be managed by increased mean airway pressure. Blood in the alveoli may result in surfactant deficiency. There are no randomized trials evaluating the use of surfactant in pulmonary hemorrhage [119], but anecdotal reports suggest benefit in some preterm infants [120].

Pharmacological management of the PDA

Since the initial description more than 40 years ago [121,122], pharmacological agents (nonselective cyclooxygenase inhibitors) have been recognized as effective alternatives to surgical ligation in the management for PDA in the premature neonate; the overall success rate appears high. Four agents, namely, indomethacin, ibuprofen, mefenamic acid (MA), and paracetamol (acetaminophen), have been used in clinical trials; only indomethacin and ibuprofen are currently approved by the US Food and Drug Administration (FDA) for clinical use. Since the mechanism of action is nonselective cyclooxygenase inhibition, the response to therapy decreases with increasing postnatal age of the infant [1,102,123].

Prophylactic use of Indomethacin

The effect of prophylactic IV indomethacin in randomized control trials (RCTs) was studied (19 RCTs consisting of a total of 2872 premature infants with weight ranges from 500 to 1750 g) [124]. The dosages administered are listed in Table 30B.7. The prevalence of symptomatic PDA, the requirement for surgical ligation of PDA, and severe IVH were lower in the indomethacin group when compared to the placebo group. However, there was no difference in overall mortality rate or neurodevelopmental outcome. In addition, oliguria, reduced weight loss, and greater need for oxygen were seen with prophylactic use of indomethacin [123]. In another RCT studying indomethacin prophylaxis (0.1 mg per kg body weight, IV) involving 1202 extremely low birth weight infants (birth weights of 500–999 g), the prevalence of PDA and severity of IVH were lower in the indomethacin group compared to the placebo group but did not have any favorable effect on survival rate without neurosensory impairment at 18 months [125].

Prophylactic use of ibuprofen

Prophylactic use of ibuprofen has also been studied [127]. The results of four RCTs consisting of 672 premature infants were examined. The dosages of ibuprofen used are also listed in Table 30B.7. The prevalence of PDA and the requirement for surgical ligation or rescue treatment with cyclooxygenase inhibitors to treat PDA were lower in the ibuprofen group when compared to the placebo group. These effects were similar to those seen with indomethacin. However, there was no difference in mortality, IVH, BPD, NEC, gastrointestinal hemorrhage, and intestinal perforation. There was a significant reduction in urine output and increase in the serum creatinine levels in patients receiving ibuprofen. It should also be noted that spontaneous closure of the ductus occurred in 60% of the control group babies.

Prophylactic use of indomethacin or ibuprofen

Based on the above and other studies, the prophylactic therapy appears to expose the premature infants to

Table 30B.7 Dosages for pharmacological closure of patent ductus arteriosus

Name of the drug	Age at initiation of therapy	Dose of the drug	Frequency*
Indomethacin (prophylactic)	<48 h	1st dose 0.1–0.2 mg/kg (NG or IV**) 2nd dose 0.1–0.2 mg/kg (NG or IV) 3rd dose 0.1–0.2 mg/kg (NG or IV)	Every 12–24 h[#]
Indomethacin (therapeutic or rescue)	2–7 days	All three doses 0.2 mg/kg (NG or IV)	Every 12–24 h
Indomethacin (therapeutic or rescue)	>7 days	All three doses 0.25 mg/kg (NG or IV)	Every 12–24 h
Ibuprofen (prophylactic and therapeutic)	<6 h (Prophylactic) >2 days (Therapeutic)	1st dose 10 mg/kg (NG or IV) 2nd dose 5 mg/kg (NG or IV) 3rd dose 5 mg/kg (NG or IV)	Every 24 h
Paracetamol	≤14 days	60 mg (oral or IV)[##]	Every day for 3 days

IV, Intravenous; *NG*, nasogastric; *RCT*, randomized controlled trial.
*Depending upon urine output.
**Intravenous (IV) infusion over 30 min. Because of unreliable gastrointestinal absorption, many neonatologists prefer IV administration.
[#]In a few studies, the drug was administered daily for 6 days.
[##]Oral in four RCTs and IV in one RCT [126].

unfavorable effects of drug treatment without any evidence for long-term benefit, and therefore, prophylactic treatment with cyclooxygenase inhibitors is not recommended [101].

Pharmacologic treatment of symptomatic PDA

Following the diagnosis of significant ductus, cyclooxygenase inhibitors may be used. The term hemodynamically significant or hsPDA has been used to signify clinically important ductus, but unfortunately, as mentioned earlier, definitions of hsPDA have varied [1,50,60]. As mentioned in the "Echocardiography" section, we do not use a single parameter to decide if a hsPDA is present; however, a combination of factors, namely, minimal ductal diameter ≥1.4 mm, LA:Ao ratio ≥1.6, and absent anterograde or presence of retrograde descending aortic diastolic flow, will lead us to conclude a large and hsPDA. This, of course, must be associated with clinical deterioration.

To address such PDAs, initially orally administered indomethacin was used (aspirin was tried in a few babies but was subsequently discontinued) [121,122]. However, because of poor absorption and low closure rates, oral therapy was switched to the IV preparation, once it was

available. Ibuprofen became available 20 years later; both oral and IV preparations were obtainable. Multicenter RCTs suggested equal efficacy of indomethacin and ibuprofen in pharmacologic closure of the ductus [107,128]. Gastrointestinal and renal adverse effects were also similar as was the prevalence of NEC, retinopathy of prematurity (ROP), and neurodevelopmental outcome. Some studies indicated that IV ibuprofen has lower renal toxicity [129] and less adverse effects on cerebral [130] and mesenteric [131] blood flow when compared to IV indomethacin. Addition of a nitric oxide synthase inhibitor, N(G)-monomethyl-L-arginine (L-NMMA) to indomethacin, improved the ductal closure rate (92% vs. 42%), but at the expense of elevating creatinine levels and increasing the blood pressure, and therefore, such therapy is not recommended [44].

Other cyclooxygenase inhibitors

Two other cyclooxygenase inhibitors, namely, MA and paracetamol, have been investigated in the treatment of PDA.

Mefenamic acid. There are limited data on the use of MA [132]. The drug (2 mg/kg/dose ×3, at 12-h intervals) was administered to 16 premature babies (mean gestational age—30.1 weeks; mean weight—1320 g) with PDA and the results were compared with their prior experience in 30 premature babies receiving indomethacin. The PDA closure rate with indomethacin was 70% while that with MA was 93.3% ($P < 0.05$). Feeding intolerance was observed in two babies in each group. The authors recommend MA for ductal closure in babies that do not tolerate indomethacin therapy [132]. To our knowledge, there are no other studies examining the role of MA in treating PDA.

Paracetamol. Initial experience with paracetamol (15 mg/kg per dose every 6 h) in five premature babies (gestational age of 26–32 weeks; at 3–35 days of age) who either have contraindications for or failed therapy with ibuprofen was attractive in that ductal closure was achieved in all five babies within 48 h of paracetamol administration [133]. In another retrospective study involving 105 premature babies (all <32 weeks of gestation), the prevalence of PDA (14% vs. 28%) and requirement for surgery for ductus (2.9% vs. 8.0%) were lower in the paracetamol group when compared with historical controls [134]. The results of other studies using IV and oral paracetamol are also appealing [126,135–137]. A recently published meta-analysis of comparison between paracetamol (dosages are given in Table 30B.7) and ibuprofen from five RCTs consisting of 677 patients suggested that the PDA closure rates were comparable between the 2 groups as was prevalence of NEC, IVH, BPD, ROP, risk of sepsis, and death [138]. However, paracetamol group had a lower incidence of renal failure ($P < 0.07$) and gastrointestinal hemorrhage ($P < 0.009$). The authors concluded that paracetamol has a comparable efficacy, but with lower incidence of some of the adverse events associated with ibuprofen [138]. While the reported experience with paracetamol is encouraging, FDA approval for its use is necessary for adopting paracetamol for routine use in the United States. Outside the United States, it may be used as per the local regulations.

Approach to pharmacological therapy

Following the diagnosis of a significant or hsPDA, usually based on clinical and echocardiographic criteria, conservative therapy, including fluid restriction and/or diuretics (and other measures) as mentioned earlier, should be instituted. Should there be deterioration in clinical status, needing more intense ventilatory management and requiring more frequent diuretic administration, or fails to progress in efforts to wean off respiratory support, therapy with IV indomethacin or ibuprofen may be started. The suggested dosages are listed in Table 30B.7.

Some physicians prefer ibuprofen over indomethacin because of reported favorable gastrointestinal and renal effects [129–131], as reviewed earlier. Treatment with indomethacin or ibuprofen is contraindicated in babies with renal dysfunction (creatinine >1.6 mg/dL), bleeding,

NEC, and thrombocytopenia. PDA closure rates after the first course of indomethacin or ibuprofen is approximately 60%–70%; also, the ductus may reopen in 20%–25% and a second course may be required [114]. Although some neonatologists use as many as three to four courses of indomethacin or ibuprofen, most neonatologists limit the drug therapy to two courses. For nonresponsive babies, surgical or catheter interventional management, as discussed in the next section, may have to be instituted.

Conventional surgical closure of the PDA

Successful surgical ligation of the PDA was first performed by Gross and Hubbard in 1939 [139]. Thereafter, surgery became the treatment of choice for the PDA until the development of less invasive percutaneous approaches. The surgical approach was adopted to the premature infant with PDA in the early 1960s [140,141]. Surgery is usually performed via a limited posterolateral thoracotomy; the ductus is identified and ligated with nonabsorbable sutures or occluded by placement of metallic clips. Ligation and division may also be undertaken, but not usually performed in premature neonates. Because of the risks of transportation, bedside ligation of the PDA was advocated at some institutions [142–145].

The timing and indications for surgical intervention are not clearly established. The utility of prophylactic surgical ligation (RCT) has been studied [146]; the incidence of NEC was lower than in control subjects (8% vs. 30%), but the overall mortality, IVH, BPD, and ROP were comparable. Similar to prophylactic pharmacologic closure, prophylactic surgical closure is not recommended. Most neonatologists and cardiologists would recommend surgical closure after unsuccessful pharmacological closure attempts [111] or if the infant is deemed not to be a candidate for indomethacin/ibuprofen therapy because of comorbidities such as thrombocytopenia, NEC, and renal dysfunction. If the ductus remains open for more than 2 weeks, there is a greater than fourfold increase in mortality [147,148]. Therefore, the ductus should be closed. Early surgical ligation resulted in earlier extubation and a decreased requirement for digoxin and diuretics, and full feeds could be established earlier when compared with the control group [149]. Comparison of surgical and pharmacologic closure revealed no differences in mortality [150], but the surgery group may have a higher risk for development of BPD, neurosensory impairment, and ROP [150,151]. In addition, surgery is associated with higher hospital costs and complications such as hypotension, pneumothorax, laryngeal, or phrenic nerve palsy (resulting in vocal cord paralysis and diaphragmatic paralysis, respectively), hemodynamic decompensation, erroneous closure of blood vessels other than PDA (e.g., LPA), chylothorax, scoliosis, and infection [1,152–157].

Video-assisted thoracoscopic surgical closure of the PDA

Video-assisted thoracoscopic surgical (VATS) technique for interruption of the PDA was initially described by Laborde and et al. [158] and subsequently modified by them [159] and others [160,161]. While it has been in use since the early 1990s, the procedure is available only in a limited number of institutions. The infant is positioned in the right lateral decubitus position and three to four thoracostomies, depending upon the patient's size, are created. The thoracostomies are used for the camera, the lung retractor (anteriorly), electrocautery/dissectors, and the clip [162]. Once the thoracostomy ports are in place, the pleural reflection over the aorta is cut open and the ductus identified. After careful blunt dissection, a plane is created both above and below the ductus and a clip is placed occluding the ductus. For a detailed description of the procedure, the reader is referred elsewhere [162].

Most of the early studies [158–161,163] included patients of all ages with only few premature babies. In one relatively recent study, the results of VATS interruption of PDA in 99 premature babies (gestational age—23–31 weeks; weight—420 g to 1.5 kg) were examined [164]; the procedure was successful in all but three babies whose procedure had to be converted to open PDA ligation. Fifteen patients died of complications of prematurity. In another VATS-PDA closure study [165], 70 of the 200 subjects were low birth weight infants; the results were good although there were 2 hospital deaths. In general, interruption of the PDA by the VATS procedure has been thought to be safe with smaller incisions, less recurrent laryngeal nerve injury, no chest tube requirement, less pain medication need but with equal efficacy when compared with conventional surgery. Additionally, less morbidity, decreased hospital length of stay, increased cost-effectiveness, and better esthetic results were ascribed to VATS when compared with conventional surgical ligation. Even in extremely low birth weight infants, VATS closure of the PDA performed by an experienced person is thought to be superior to conventional surgical ligation [162,164]. Potential long-term complications, namely, scoliosis, decreased shoulder mobility, and chest wall pain syndrome that are seen with conventional thoracotomy approach, are not observed with VATS [160]. Complications associated VATS include pneumothorax, pleural effusion, recurrent laryngeal nerve injury, chylothorax, and residual shunts but are rare [159,161,164,165]. While not yet widely available, the VATS closure of PDA has been known to be safe and is applicable to most infants including extremely low birth weight down to 420 g [162].

Percutaneous closure of the PDA

As mentioned earlier, successful surgical closure of the PDA was first described by Gross and Hubbard in 1939 [139]

and remained as therapy of choice for the PDA until percutaneous methods came into vogue. Transcatheter PDA closure was first described by Porstmann et al. [166]. This was followed by additional device development, described by Rashkind and Cuaso in the late 1970s [167]. These initial attempts paved the way for the advancement of several other PDA occluding devices which were reviewed elsewhere [168–171]. The discussion of which PDAs should be closed and what devices should be used has, in the past, centered around the closure of PDAs in older infants, children, and adults [69,172–178]. Only recently, the issue of percutaneous closure of PDAs in the premature infants is being tackled [179–183]. Ductal closure is contraindicated in patients with severe PH and those with ductal-dependent congenital cardiac abnormalities [178].

Devices available for closure of PDAs in term infants

Devices approved by the US FDA include the Gianturco coil, the Gianturco-Grifka vascular occlusion device (GGVOD), the Amplatzer duct occluder (ADO) [178], and more recently the ADO II and Nit-Occlud. The Gianturco coil is composed of stainless-steel wire with Dacron fibers to increase thrombogenicity [184] and has been in use for PDA occlusion since 1992 [178,185]. The advantage of the Gianturco coil is the feasibility of its use for small PDAs without causing occlusion of the vessels on either end of ductus, but the disadvantages are the lack of controlled coil delivery, potential for embolization, and the inability to reposition [178]. The GGVOD is a nylon sac with a long occluding wire and has been in use since 1996 [186]. Use of this device is very limited because of need for larger size delivery sheath, difficulty in the retrieval of a malpositioned device, and the potential for development of descending aortic obstruction [178,187,188]. It is no longer manufactured. The ADO is composed of a Nitinol wire mesh with polyester fibers and is self-expandable [189,190]. The ADO device has been in use since 1997 and is available in various sizes [178]. The Amplatzer ductal occluder II (ADO II) is a newer device which is a fabric free Nitinol wire mesh articulated into two low profile disks; the device can be deployed through smaller delivery sheaths [191,192]. The Nit-Occlud device is a Nitinol coil with a reverse cone configuration and is implanted utilizing a controlled delivery system [193].

Devices available for closure of PDAs in premature infants

Transcatheter PDA closure in the preterm infant has been largely excluded from the evolution of PDA devices due to catheter and introducer size constraints, as well as the limitations inherent to the devices manufactured for this defect. Over the last decade, devices and their delivery mechanisms have improved and implants are now

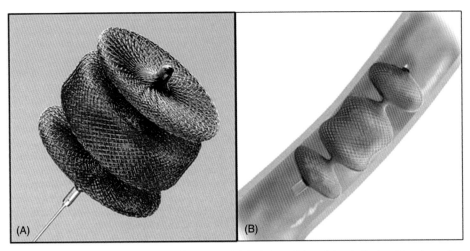

Fig. 30B.20 (A) Photograph of Amplatzer Vascular Plug Type II. (B) Artist's rendition of the device in a blood vessel.

produced that can successfully close the PDAs in preterm infants. However, there are no devices manufactured in the United States specifically for the PDAs in preterm babies. The Amplatzer Ductal Occluder II Additional Sizes (ADOII-AS) has been available overseas with CE Mark approval since 2012 [194]. In 2017, an FDA trial for this device has started. Nevertheless, closure of PDAs in preterm neonates has been reported using existing products developed for other vessel targets. These include detachable coils [181,195], the ADO II (St. Jude Medical,

Minneapolis, MN) [195], the Amplatzer Vascular Plug II (Fig. 30B.20) [183,196], the Medtronic Micro Vascular Plug (Medtronic, Minneapolis, MN) [197] (Fig. 30B.21), and ADOII-AS [198].

Indications and selection for percutaneous closure of PDA in premature infants

The systemic-to-pulmonary shunt resulting from a large PDA results in congestive cardiac failure, which manifests

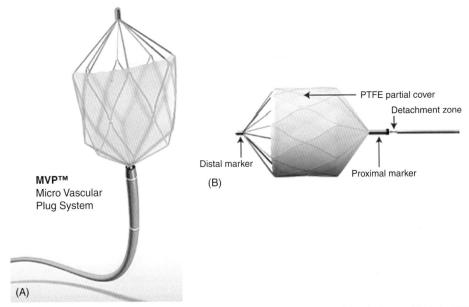

Fig. 30B.21 (A) Photograph of Medtronic Micro Vascular Plug. (B) Various components of the device are labeled. *PTFE,* Polytetrafluoroethylene.

clinically with a wide pulse pressure and bounding pulses. The pulmonary overcirculation caused by the PDA leads to pulmonary edema which predisposes the neonate to BPD. Blood flow to the kidney and gastrointestinal tract is compromised predisposing to acute renal failure (ARF) and NEC. Hypoperfusion followed by reperfusion increases the risk of IVH. These potential outcomes factor prominently in the decision to seek PDA closure. Conservative management is typically observed. Symptoms of pulmonary overcirculation are often treated with fluid restriction and/or diuretics. The opportunity for spontaneous closure is provided and is then frequently followed by medical management with indomethacin or ibuprofen. If these efforts fail, and the patient demonstrates evidence of a worsening respiratory status, or fails to progress in efforts to wean off support, PDA closure is sought. At this point, PDA closure by surgical versus percutaneous methods become available options; recently, percutaneous techniques are increasingly being considered.

Method of percutaneous closure of PDA in the premature infant

The primary location for closure has been in the catheterization laboratory, although bedside implantation using echocardiographic guidance alone has been described [195]. Bedside approaches have largely employed the femoral artery [195]. However, femoral artery occlusion or insufficiency remains an important concern, particularly in the smaller patients. To mitigate this concern, efforts to avoid arterial access have been made [183,196,197]. Using the femoral artery to perform guidance angiography has

been avoided by means of careful echocardiographic evaluation of the PDA to determine its diameter and length as well as by anterograde (via the femoral vein) angiography (Fig. 30B.22 and Video 30B.1).

A 4 French sheath is placed in a femoral vein, and a 4 French catheter is used to traverse the right heart and cross the PDA into the descending aorta. Either a 4 French wedge catheter or a 4 French angled catheter may be used and manipulated with wire guidance into position and angiography performed (Fig. 30B.22 and Video 30B.1). The diameter and the length of the ductus are measured (Fig. 30B.22). Depending on the device chosen, a 4 French catheter is used to deliver the Medtronic Micro Vascular Plug device directly, or the catheter is exchanged over a guidewire for a 4 French delivery sheath with the intent of using an Amplatzer Vascular Plug II. The selection of the device size for implantation largely depends upon the echocardiographic and angiographic (Fig. 30B.22) minimal PDA diameter and length. Once the device is deployed within the PDA, a low volume hand injection of contrast is made to confirm the position of the device relative to the pulmonary origin of the PDA (Videos 30B.2 and 30B.3). Echocardiography is performed prior to device release to exclude any obstruction to blood flow in the descending aorta or the branch pulmonary arteries. The Micro Vascular Plug is challenging to image with ultrasound, making the contrast injection (Video 30B.2) of particular importance in the procedure. Device releases are shown in Videos 30B.4 and 30B.5. We believe that this procedure represents a major step forward by avoiding the potential complications of surgical ligation, including pneumothorax, phrenic nerve injury, and scoliosis.

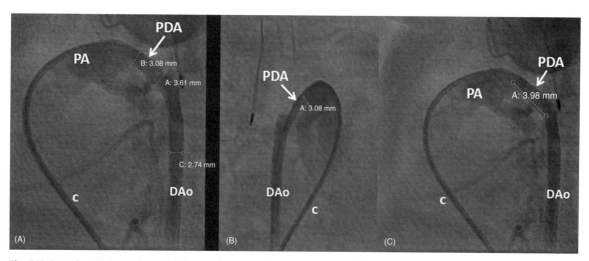

Fig. 30B.22 Selected cineangiographic frames demonstrating measurements of the patent ductus arteriosus (PDA) in left anterior oblique (A and C) and right anterior oblique (B) views. The measurements of the diameter (A and B) and the length (C) of the ductus are shown. *c*, Catheter; *DAo*, descending aorta; *PA*, pulmonary artery.

Reported experience with percutaneous closure of the PDA

Initial experience with closure of the PDA in the premature babies consisted of single case reports [179,180]. The first case series reported includes 10 premature babies (gestational age 24–30 weeks) with weights of 1600–2650 g at the time of the procedure [181]. The PDAs measured 2–3.6 mm. The investigators used Flipper coils with successful closure in 9 of the 10 babies. Evidence of immediate improvement was observed in two infants, but no benefit was seen immediately in the remaining babies. In another study [182], eight infants (gestational age 27–32 weeks) weighing 930–1800 g with PDAs measuring 2–3.5 mm had PDA closure by three French bioptome-assisted coil delivery. Complete occlusion was demonstrated in seven of the eight infants while one baby had a small residual shunt. Five patients were discharged shortly after the procedure while the remaining three required prolonged ventilation. In a study involving 24 premature babies weighing 755–2380 g, echocardiographically guided closure of the PDA with the Amplatzer Vascular Plug II was performed [183]; there was minimal procedural morbidity and survival to discharge occurred in 96% cases with one late death unrelated to PDA occlusion. In a recent study [198], the ADOII-AS was used to occlude PDAs measuring 2.2–4 mm in 32 premature babies (gestational age 24–36 weeks) weighing 680–2480 g. Complete occlusion was achieved in 31 infants. Four deaths related to prematurity and one death related to the procedure occurred.

Percutaneous PDA closure experience at our institution

Percutaneous closure of PDAs in premature infants was introduced in our institution in late 2015. In the first 18 months, 34 premature infants under 3 kg at the time of the procedure underwent device closure. All procedures were performed as described above, with either the Medtronic Micro Vascular Plug (n = 29) or Amplatzer Vascular Plug II (n = 5). These devices were selected largely due to the ability to implant the devices entirely within the DA, with no protruding disk within the descending aorta or PA. The microvascular plug has the advantage of delivery via a 4 French catheter, or even a 3 French catheter with the smaller sized devices. The Amplatzer Vascular Plug II requires a stiffer delivery sheath that is more likely to cause hemodynamic instability by propping open the tricuspid and pulmonary valves.

Complete closure was achieved in all patients. There were no procedural complications, with no escalation of respiratory management. One trans-catheter device embolized 9 days after deployment and was successfully retrieved and another device implanted. There were no long-term sequelae, and the patient was stable at the time of device retrieval. Patients were extubated in a median of 3.5 days (0–29 days) and were weaned off all respiratory support and oxygen in a median of 16 days (0–153). Of the 24 patients discharged at the time of this report, two were discharged on oxygen therapy. An example of follow-up echo-Doppler study is shown in Figs. 30B.23–30B.25.

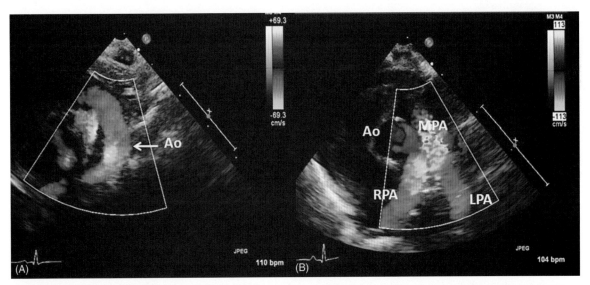

Fig. 30B.23 Selected echocardiographic frames from suprasternal notch (A) and parasternal short axis (B) views demonstrating laminar flow in the aorta (Ao) (A) and branch pulmonary arteries (B) in a premature baby who had percutaneous occlusion of the ductus occluded with a Medtronic Micro Vascular Plug a month earlier. *MPA*, Main pulmonary artery; *LPA*, left pulmonary artery; *RPA*, right pulmonary artery.

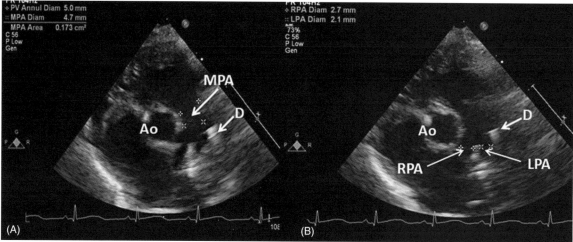

Fig. 30B.24 Selected echocardiographic frames from the parasternal short axis views showing wide-open main (MPA) (A) and branch (B) pulmonary arteries in the premature baby shown in Fig. 30B.21. The device (D) is in the ductal structure without encroaching on to the left pulmonary artery (LPA). *Ao*, Aorta; *RPA*, right pulmonary artery.

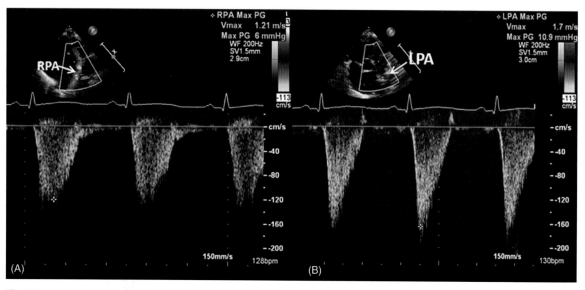

Fig. 30B.25 Selected echocardiographic frames from parasternal short axis views showing pulse Doppler velocity tracings in the right (RPA) (A) and the left (LPA) (B) pulmonary arteries in the premature baby shown in Figs. 30B.21 and 30B.22. The Doppler flow velocities are within normal range without evidence for obstruction.

Percutaneous closure of PDA in the premature has become the modality of choice to treat this disease in our institution. Continued development and availability of devices suitable for this application will be important to improve outcomes in this vulnerable population.

Which procedure

In case of failure of pharmacological closure of PDA, multiple options, namely, conventional surgical closure, bedside surgical occlusion, VATS interruption, and percutaneous closure, are available. To the best of our knowledge, there are no RCTs comparing one procedure to the next. Consequently, our recommendation is that the decision to select one of these procedures should be based on the availability of a given expertise at a given time at a given institution. During the last 15 years of the senior author's experience, we exclusively used conventional surgical closure during the first 5 years [157], VATS closure during the next 5 years [162], and currently percutaneous closure [197]; this has largely depended upon the availability of that particular expertise at that time. Multiinstitutional RCTs should be undertaken in the future to determine the best option for the premature neonate with PDA who is unresponsive to pharmacologic therapy.

Summary and conclusions

The DA is a muscular structure that connects the main PA with the descending thoracic aorta and is useful in the fetal circulation to divert less oxygenated blood from the PA into the descending aorta and placenta for oxygenation. It closes spontaneously after birth, but persistence beyond 72 h of life is defined as a PDA. It is much more frequent in the premature than in the term infants; the earlier the gestational age, the higher the incidence. Antenatal steroid use decreases the incidence and respiratory distress syndrome increases the persistent patency of the ductus. The PDA produces a left-to-right shunt, largely proportional to the minimal ductal diameter and may cause pulmonary and cardiac compromise. Clinical signs and serum BNP levels may assist in identifying a significant ductus. hsPDAs may be best diagnosed and quantified by echo-Doppler studies using multiple criteria, including minimal ductal diameter and LA:Ao ratio, among others.

A summary of management of preterm infants with PDA is outlined in Table 30B.8. Management strategies used in the past, such as to completely ignore the ductus or administer prophylactic pharmacological or surgical treatment

Table 30B.8 Summary of management of the PDA in premature infants

PDA status	Management recommendations
No PDA or small PDA on echo-Doppler study	1. Routine preterm infant care as per the institutional standard-of-care protocol 2. May receive 70–80 mL/kg/day of fluid which may be adjusted depending upon weight gain/loss, need for phototherapy, and serum electrolytes 3. Prophylactic pharmacological closure of the PDA is not recommended 4. Prophylactic surgical/transcatheter interruption of the PDA is not recommended
Moderate-to-large PDA on echo-Doppler study ± clinical signs of congestive heart failure	**A. Conservative management** 1. Restrict fluid intake (120–130 mL/kg/day) 2. Administer diuretics such as chlorothiozide (10–20 mg/kg/dose NG, every 12 h) and/or furosemide (1 mg/kg/dose IV, every 12–24 h)* 3. Appropriate respiratory support (CPAP or endotracheal ventilation), as per the pulmonary status 4. Maintain adequate levels of hematocrit (>45%) and provide electrolytes, glucose, and sufficient calories as per the standard-of-care guidelines for premature infants **B. Pharmacological closure of the PDA** 1. If the baby needs for more intense ventilatory management, requires more frequent diuretic administration, or fails to progress in efforts to wean off respiratory support despite the above described conservative management, pharmacological closure with cyclooxygenase inhibitors is indicated 2. Indomethacin or ibuprofen may be given. See Table 30B.4 for dosages, route, and frequency of drug administration** **C. Surgical or percutaneous closure** 1. For babies nonresponsive to two courses of pharmacological therapy, surgical or catheter interventional management, may be indicated 2. For these babies conventional surgical closure, bedside surgical occlusion, VATS interruption and percutaneous closure are available options 3. Since there are no RCTs comparing one procedure with the other, the current recommendation is to select one of these procedures based on the availability of a given expertise at a given time at a given institution

IV, Intravenous; *CPAP*, continuous positive airway pressure; *PDA*, patent ductus arteriosus; *NG*, nasogastric; *RCTs*, randomized controlled studies; *VATS*, video-assisted thoracoscopic surgical.
*Because of concern that furosemide may increase PGE$_2$ synthesis [118], furosemide is not usually administered during the first week of life.
**Contraindications for indomethacin and ibuprofen administration: creatinine > 1.6 mg/dL, bleeding, necrotizing enterocolitis, and thrombocytopenia.

to all premature babies with PDA, are no longer recommended. The latter is because of (1) prevalence of BPD and long-term outcomes are not altered, (2) spontaneous closure benefit is not realized, and (3) exposes many infants to the adverse effects of such prophylactic therapy. When a significant or hsPDA is detected, conservative management with fluid restriction, diuretic therapy, and respiratory and other supportive measures is first provided, as needed. If no improvement is found, pharmacologic therapy with indomethacin or ibuprofen (IV or PO) should be instituted. Ibuprofen is preferred by some because of less renal toxicity. Paracetamol is used in some countries outside the United States. Failure after two courses of pharmacologic therapy calls for surgical (conventional, bedside, or VATS) or percutaneous closure of the ductus depending upon the institutional expertise.

Online supplementary materials

Please visit MedEnact to access the following videos:

▶ **Video 30B.1** Cineangiogram in left anterior oblique view with the catheter positioned in the distal part of patent ductus arteriosus to demonstrate the ductus and to perform measurements as indicated in Fig. 30B.22.

▶ **Video 30B.2** Cineangiogram in left anterior oblique view prior to device (Medtronic Micro Vascular Plug) release demonstrating the position of the devise in the ductus without evidence for residual shunt or obstruction to the pulmonary arteries.

▶ **Video 30B.3** Cineangiogram in left anterior oblique view prior to device (Amplatzer Vascular Plug II) release demonstrating the position of the devise in the ductus without evidence for residual shunt or obstruction to the pulmonary arteries.

▶ **Video 30B.4** Cineradiogram in left anterior oblique view demonstrating release of Medtronic Micro Vascular Plug device.

▶ **Video 30B.5** Cineradiogram in left anterior oblique view demonstrating release of Amplatzer Vascular Plug type II device.

References

[1] Dice JE, Bhatia J. Patent ductus arteriosus: an overview. J Pediatr Pharmacol Ther 2007;12:138–146.

[2] Schneider DJ, Moore JW. Patent ductus arteriosus. Circulation 2006;114:1873–1882.

[3] Rao PS. Perinatal circulatory physiology. Indian J Pediatr 1991;58:441–451.

[4] Rao PS. Fetal and neonatal circulation. In: Kambam J, editor. Cardiac anesthesia for infants and children. St. Louis, MO: Mosby-Year Book; 1994. p. 10–19.

[5] Clyman RI. Ibuprofen and patent ductus arteriosus. N Engl J Med 2000;343:728–730.

[6] Hermes-DeSantis ER, Clyman RI. Patent ductus arteriosus: pathophysiology and management. J Perinatol 2006;26(Suppl. 1):S14–S18.

[7] Hammerman C. Patent ductus arteriosus. Clinical relevance of prostaglandins and prostaglandin inhibitors in PDA pathophysiology and treatment. Clin Perinatol 1995;22:457–479.

[8] Smith GC. The pharmacology of the ductus arteriosus. Pharmacol Rev 1998;50:35–58.

[9] Miao CY, Zuberbuhler JS, Zuberbuhler JR. Prevalence of congenital cardiac anomalies at high altitude. J Am Coll Cardiol 1990;12:224–228.

[10] Gittenberger-de Groot AC, Moulaert AJ, Hitchcock JF. Histology of the persistent ductus arteriosus in cases of congenital rubella. Circulation 1980;62:183–186.

[11] Nora JJ. Multifactorial inheritance hypothesis for the etiology of congenital heart diseases: the genetic environmental interaction. Circulation 1968;38:604–617.

[12] Lloyd TR, Beekman RH III. Clinically silent patent ductus arteriosus. Am Heart J 1994;127:1664–1665.

[13] Rudolph AM. Congenital diseases of the heart. Chicago, IL: Year Book Medical Publishers, Inc.; 1974. p. 1–41.

[14] Rudolph AM. Congenital diseases of the heart. Oxford: Wiley-Blackwell; 2009. 265.

[15] Rao PS. Perinatal circulatory physiology: it's influence on clinical manifestations of neonatal heart disease—Part I. Neonatol Today 2008;3(2):6–12.

[16] Rao PS. Perinatal circulatory physiology. In: Rao PS, Vidyasagar D, editors. Perinatal cardiology: a multidisciplinary approach. Minneapolis, MN: Cardiotext Publishing; 2015.

[17] Mentzer RM, Ely SW, Lasley RD, et al. Hormonal role of adenosine in maintaining patency of the ductus arteriosus in the fetal lambs. Ann Surg 1985;202:223–230.

[18] Rudolph AM. Fetal and neonatal pulmonary circulation. Ann Rev Physiol 1979;41:383–395.

[19] Dawes GS. Foetal and neonatal physiology. Chicago, IL: Year Book Medical; 1968.

[20] Christie A. Normal closing time of the foramen ovale and the ductus arteriosus: an anatomic and statistical study. Am J Dis Child 1930;40:323–326.

[21] Moss AJ, Emmanouilides GC, Duffie ER Jr. Closure of ductus arteriosus. Lancet 1963;1:703–704.

[22] Coceani F, Olley PM. Prostaglandins and the ductus arteriosus. Pediatr Cardiol 1983;4(Suppl. II):33–37.

[23] Kennedy JA, Clark SL. Observations on the physiologic reactions of the

ductus arteriosus. Am J Physiol 1942;136:140–147.

[24] Heymann MA, Rudolph AM. Control of ductus arteriosus. Physiol Rev 1975;55:62–78.

[25] Thébaud B, Michelakis ED, Wu XC, et al. Oxygen-sensitive Kv channel gene transfer confers oxygen responsiveness to preterm rabbit and remodeled human ductus arteriosus: implications for infants with patent ductus arteriosus. Circulation 2004;110:1372–1379.

[26] Levin M, McCurnin D, Seidner SR, et al. Postnatal constriction, ATP depletion, and cell death in the mature and immature ductus arteriosus. Am J Physiol Regul Integr Comp Physiol 2006;290:R359–R364.

[27] Kajino H, Goldbarg S, Roman C, et al. Vasa vasorum hypoperfusion is responsible for medial hypoxia and anatomic remodeling in the newborn lamb ductus arteriosus. Pediatr Res 2002;51:228–235.

[28] Echtler K, Stark K, Lorenz M, et al. Platelets contribute to postnatal occlusion of the ductus arteriosus. Nat Med 2010;16:75–82.

[29] Benitz WE. Committee on Fetus and Newborn. Patent ductus arteriosus in preterm infants. Pediatrics 2016;137:1–6.

[30] Anoop P, Sasidharan CK. Patent ductus arteriosus in fetal valproate syndrome. Indian J Pediatr 2003;70:681–682.

[31] Zierler S. Maternal drugs and congenital heart disease. Obstet Gynecol 1985;65:155–165.

[32] Du JF, Liu TT, Wu H. Risk factors for patent ductus arteriosus in early preterm infants: a case-control study. Zhongguo Dang Dai Er Ke Za Zhi 2016;18:15–19.

[33] Satoda M, Pierpont ME, Diaz GA, et al. Char syndrome, an inherited disorder with patent ductus arteriosus, maps to chromosome 6p12-p21. Circulation 1999;99:3036–3042.

[34] Bruneau BG. The developmental genetics of congenital heart disease. Nature 2008;451:943–948.

[35] Thomas SV, Ajaykumar B, Sindhu K, et al. Cardiac malformations are increased in infants of mothers with epilepsy. Pediatr Cardiol 2008;29:604–608.

[36] Lipshultz SE, Frassica JJ, Orav EJ. Cardiovascular abnormalities in infants prenatally exposed to cocaine. J Pediatr 1991;118:44–51.

[37] Sardor GG, Smith DF, MacLeod PM. Cardiac malformations in the

fetal alcohol syndrome. J Pediatr 1981;98:771–773.

[38] Woods SE, Raju U. Maternal smoking and the risk of congenital birth defects: a cohort study. J Am Board Fam Pract 2001;14:330–334.

[39] Eronen M, Kari A, Pesonen E, et al. The effect of antenatal dexamethasone administration on fetal and neonatal ductus arteriosus: a randomized double blind study. Am J Dis Child 1993;147:187–192.

[40] Gibson S, Lewis K. Congenital heart disease following maternal rubella during pregnancy. Am J Dis Child 1952;83:117–119.

[41] Swan C, Tostevin AL, Black GHB. Final observations on congenital defects in infants following infectious disease during pregnancy with special reference to rubella. Med J Aust 1946;2:889–908.

[42] Friedman WF. The intrinsic physiologic properties of the developing heart. In: Friedman WF, Lesch M, Sonnenblick EH, editors. Neonatal heart disease. New York, NY: Grune and Stratton; 1973. p. 21–41.

[43] Rudolph AM. The ductus arteriosus and persistent patency of the ductus arteriosus. In: Rudolph AM, editor. Congenital diseases of the heart: clinical–physiological considerations. 3rd ed. Chichester, UK: John Wiley and Sons; 2009. p. 115–147.

[44] Moore P, Brook MM, Heyman MA. Patent ductus arteriosus and aortopulmonary window. In: Allen HD, Driscoll DJ, Shaddy RE, Felts TF, editors. Moss & Adams' heart disease in infants, children, and adolescents: including the fetus and young adult. 7th ed. Philadelphia, PA: Wolters Kluwer/Lippincott Williams & Wilkins; 2008. p. 683–702.

[45] Hoffman JIE, Buckberg GD. Regional myocardial ischemia: causes, prediction, and prevention. Vasc Surg 1974;8:115–131.

[46] Baylen BG, Ogata H, Oguchi K, et al. The contractility and performance of the preterm left ventricle before and after early patent ductus arteriosus occlusion in surfactant-treated lambs. Pediatr Res 1985;19:1053–1058.

[47] Friedman WF. The intrinsic physiologic properties of the developing heart. Prog Cardiovasc Dis 1972;15:87–111.

[48] Appleton RS, Graham TP Jr, Cotton RB, et al. Altered early left ventricular diastolic cardiac function in the

premature infant. Am J Cardiol 1987;59:1391–1394.

[49] Chang LY, McCurnin D, Yoder B, et al. Ductus arteriosus ligation and alveolar growth in preterm baboons with a patent ductus arteriosus. Pediatr Res 2008;63:299–302.

[50] Zonnenberg I, de Waal K. The definition of a haemodynamic significant duct in randomized controlled trials: a systematic literature review. Acta Paediatr 2012;101:247–251.

[51] Chock VY, Punn R, Oza A, Benitz WE, et al. Predictors of bronchopulmonary dysplasia or death in premature infants with a patent ductus arteriosus. Pediatr Res 2014;75(4):570–575.

[52] Abman SH, Hansmann G, Archer SL, et al. Pediatric pulmonary hypertension: guidelines from the American Heart Association and American Thoracic Society. Circulation 2015;132(21):2037–2099.

[53] Mohamed MA, El-Dib M, Alqahtani S, et al. Patent ductus arteriosus in premature infants: to treat or not to treat? J Perinatol 2017;37:652–657.

[54] Mann D, Qu JZ, Mehta V. Congenital heart diseases with left-to-right shunts. Int Anesthesiol Clin 2004;42:45–58.

[55] Jim WT, Chiu NC, Chen MR, et al. Cerebral hemodynamic change and intraventricular hemorrhage in very low birth weight infants with patent ductus arteriosus. Ultrasound Med Biol 2005;31:197–202.

[56] Teixeira LS, McNamara PJ. Enhanced intensive care for the neonatal ductus arteriosus. Acta Paediatr 2006;95:394–403.

[57] Rojas MA, Gonzalez A, Bancalari E, et al. Changing trends in the epidemiology and pathogenesis of neonatal chronic lung disease. J Pediatr 1995;126:605–610.

[58] van de BM, Verloove-Vanhorick SP, Brand R, Ruys JH. Patent ductus arteriosus in a cohort of 1338 preterm infants: a collaborative study. Paediatr Perinat Epidemiol 1988;2:328–336.

[59] Edhouse J, Thakur RK, Khalil JM. ABC of clinical electrocardiography. Conditions affecting the left side of the heart. BMJ 2002;324:1264–1267.

[60] Skinner J. Patent ductus arteriosus. Semin Neonatol 2001;6:49–61.

[61] Iyer P, Evans N. Re-evaluation of the left atrial to aortic root ratio as a marker of patent ductus arteriosus. Arch Dis Child Fetal Neonatal Ed 1994;70:F112–F117.

[62] McNamara PJ, Sehgal A. Towards rational management of the patent ductus arteriosus: the need for disease staging. Arch Dis Child Fetal Neonatal Ed 2007;92:F424–F427.

[63] Johnson GL, Bret GL, Gewitz MH, et al. Echocardiographic characteristics of premature infants with patent ductus arteriosus. Pediatrics 1983;72:864–871.

[64] Rao PS, Kulangara RJ. Echocardiographic evaluation of global left ventricular performance in infants and children. Indian Pediatr 1982;19:21–32.

[65] Rao PS. Non-invasive evaluation of left ventricular function in infants and children. Saudi Med J 1983;4:195–209.

[66] Rao PS. Echocardiographic evaluation of neonates with suspected heart disease. In: Rao PS, Vidyasagar D, editors. Perinatal cardiology: a multidisciplinary approach. Minneapolis, MN: Cardiotext Publishing; 2015.

[67] Belenkie I, Nutter DO, Clark DW, et al. Assessment of left ventricular dimensions and function by echocardiography. Am J Cardiol 1973;31:755–762.

[68] Lee LA, Kimball TR, Daniels SR, et al. Left ventricular mechanics in the preterm infant and their effect on the measurement of cardiac performance. J Pediatr 1992;120:114–119.

[69] Rao PS. Percutaneous closure of patent ductus arteriosus—current status. J Invasive Cardiol 2011;23:517–520.

[70] Subramanian U, Hamzeh RK, Sharma SK, Rao PS. Reliability of echocardiographic estimation of angiographic minimal ductal diameter. Poster presentation at the 30th Annual Scientific Session of Society for Cardiac Angiography and Interventions, Orlando, FL, May 9–12, 2007. Cath Cardiovasc Intervent 2007;69:S87.

[71] Evans N, Iyer P. Longitudinal changes in the diameter of the ductus arteriosus in ventilated preterm infants: correlation with respiratory outcomes. Arch Dis Child Fetal Neonatal Ed 1995;72:F156–F161.

[72] Kluckow M, Evans N. Early echocardiographic prediction of symptomatic patent ductus arteriosus in preterm infants undergoing mechanical ventilation. J Pediatr 1995;127:774–779.

[73] Heuchan AM, Young D. Early color Doppler duct diameter and symptomatic patent ductus arteriosus in cyclo-oxygenase inhibitor naïve population. Acta Pediatr 2013;102:254–257.

[74] Yum SK, Moon CJ, Youn YA, et al. Echocardiographic assessment of patent ductus arteriosus in very low birth weight infants over time: prospective observational study. J Matern Fetal Neonatal Med 2017;23:1–12.

[75] El Hajjar M, Vaksmann G, Rakza T, et al. Severity of the ductal shunt: a comparison of different markers. Arch Dis Child Fetal Neonatal Ed 2005;90:F419–F422.

[76] Evans N. Diagnosis of the preterm patent ductus arteriosus: clinical signs, biomarkers, or ultrasound? Semin Perinatol 2012;36:114–122.

[77] Serwer GA, Armstrong BE, Anderson PA. Noninvasive detection of retrograde descending aortic flow in infants using continuous wave Doppler ultrasonography. Implications for diagnosis of aortic run-off lesions. J Pediatr 1980;97:394–400.

[78] Agarwal R, Deorari AK, Paul VK. Patent ductus arteriosus in preterm neonates. Indian J Pediatr 2008;75:277–280.

[79] Rutishauser M, Ronen G, Wyler F. Aneurysm of the nonpatent ductus arteriosus in the newborn. Acta Pediatr Scand 1977;66:649–651.

[80] Dyamenahalli U, Smallhorn JF, Geva T, et al. Isolated ductus arteriosus aneurysm in the fetus and infant: a multi-institutional experience. J Am Coll Cardiol 2000;36:262–269.

[81] Cruickshank B, Marquis RM. Spontaneous aneurysm of the ductus arteriosus. Am J Med 1958;25:140–149.

[82] Weisz DE, McNamara PJ, El Khuffash A. Cardiac biomarkers and haemodynamically significant patent ductus arteriosus in preterm infants. Early Hum Dev 2017;105:41–47.

[83] Edwards BS, Zimmerman RS, Schwab TR, et al. Atrial stretch, not pressure, is the principal determinant controlling the acute release of atrial natriuretic factor. Circ Res 1988;62:191–195.

[84] Sundsfjord JA, Thibault G, Larochelle P, Cantin PM. Identification and plasma concentrations of the N-terminal fragment of proatrial natriuretic factor in man. J Clin Endocrinol Metab 1988;66:605–610.

[85] Mannarino S, Garofoli F, Cerbo RM, et al. Cord blood, perinatal BNP values in term and preterm newborns. Arch Dis Child Fetal Neonatal Ed 2010;95:F74.

[86] El-Khuffash A, Davis PG, Walsh K, Molloy EJ. Cardiac troponin T and N-terminalpro-B type natriuretic peptide reflect myocardial function in preterm infants. J Perinatol 2008;28:482–486.

[87] da Graca RL, Hassinger DC, Flynn PA, et al. Longitudinal changes of brain-type natriuretic peptide in preterm neonates. Pediatrics 2006;117: 2183–2189.

[88] Puddy VF, Mirmansour C, Williams AF, et al. Plasma brain natriuretic peptide as a predictor of hemodynamically significant patent ductus arteriosus in preterm infants. Clin Sci 2002;103:75–77.

[89] Choi BM, Lee KH, Eun BL, et al. Utility of rapid B-natriuretic peptide assay for diagnosis of symptomatic patent ductus arteriosus in preterm infants. Pediatrics 2005;115: e255–e261.

[90] Sanjeev S, Pettersen M, Lua J, et al. Role of plasma B-type natriuretic peptide in screening for hemodynamically significant patent ductus arteriosus in preterm neonates. J Perinatol 2005;25: 709–713.

[91] Czernik C, Lemmer J, Metze B, et al. B-Type natriuretic peptide to predict ductus intervention in infants <28 weeks. Pediatr Res 2008;64:286–290.

[92] Chen S, Tacy T, Clyman R. How useful are B-type natriuretic peptide measurements for monitoring changes in patent ductus arteriosus shunt magnitude. J Perinatol 2010;30:780–785.

[93] Nuntnarumit P, Khositset A, Thanomsingh P. N-terminal probrain natriuretic peptide and patent ductus arteriosus in preterm infants. J Perinatol 2009;29:137–142.

[94] Ramakrishnan S, Heung TM, Round J, et al. Early N-terminal pro-brain natriuretic peptide measurements predict clinically significant ductus arteriosus in preterm infants. Acta Paediatr 2009;98:1254–1259.

[95] El-Kuffash A, Molloy EJ. Are B-type natriuretic peptide (BNP) and N-terminal-pro-BNP useful in neonates? Arch Dis Child Fetal Neonatal Ed 2007;92:320–324.

[96] Davlouros PA, Karatza AA, Xanthopoulou I, et al. Diagnostic role of plasma BNP levels in neonates with signs of congenital heart disease. Int J Cardiol 2011;147:42–46.

[97] Krichenko A, Benson LN, Burrows P, et al. Angiographic classification of the isolated, persistently patent ductus arteriosus and implications for percutaneous catheter occlusion. Am J Cardiol 1989;63:877–879.

[98] Carmo Mendes I, Heard H, Peacock K, et al. Echocardiographic versus angiographic assessment of patent arterial duct in percutaneous closure: towards X-ray free duct occlusion? Pediatr Cardiol 2017;38:302–307.

[99] Smith BG, Tibby SM, Qureshi SA, et al. Quantification of temporal, procedural, and hardware-related factors influencing radiation exposure during pediatric cardiac catheterization. Catheter Cardiovasc Interv 2012;80:931–936.

[100] Khositseth A, Muangyod N, Nuntnarumit P. Perfusion Index as a diagnostic tool for patent ductus arteriosus in preterm infants. Neonatology 2013;104:250–254.

[101] Bhat R. Patent ductus arteriosus in the premature infant. In: Rao PS, Vidyasagar D, editors. Perinatal cardiology: a multidisciplinary approach. Minneapolis, MN: Cardiotext Publishing; 2015.

[102] El-Khuffash A, Weisz DE, McNamara PJ. Reflections of the changes in patent ductus arteriosus management during the last 10 years. Arch Dis Child Fetal Neonatal Ed 2016;101:F474–F478.

[103] Mahony L, Carnero V, Brett C, et al. Prophylactic indomethacin therapy for patent ductus arteriosus in very-low-birth-weight infants. N Engl J Med 1982;306:506–510.

[104] Cassady G, Crouse DT, Kirklin JW, et al. A randomized, controlled trial of very early prophylactic ligation of the ductus arteriosus in babies who weighed 1000 g or less at birth. N Engl J Med 1989;320:1511–1516.

[105] Cotton RB, Stahlman MT, Kovar I, et al. Medical management of small preterm infants with symptomatic patent ductus arteriosus. J Pediatr 1978;92:467–473.

[106] Benitz WE. Treatment of persistent patent ductus arteriosus in preterm infants: time to accept the null hypothesis? J Perinatol 2010;30:241–252.

[107] Gersony WM, Peckham GJ, Ellison RC, et al. Effects of indomethacin in premature infants with patent ductus arteriosus: results of a national collaborative study. J Pediatr 1983;102:895–906.

[108] Mikhail M, Lee W, Toews W, et al. Surgical and medical experience with 734 premature infants with patent ductus arteriosus. J Thorac Cardiovasc Surg 1982;83:349–357.

[109] El-Khuffash AF, Jain A, McNamara PJ. Ligation of the patent ductus arteriosus in preterm infants: understanding the physiology. J Pediatr 2013;162:1100–1106.

[110] Nemerofsky SL, Parravicini E, Batemean D, et al. The ductus arteriosus rarely requires treatment in infants > 1000 grams. Am J Perinatol 2008;25:661–666.

[111] Koch J, Hensley G, Roy L, et al. Prevalence of spontaneous closure of the ductus arteriosus in neonates at a birth weight of 1000 grams or less. Pediatrics 2006;117:1113–1121.

[112] Fisher RG, Moodie DS, Sterba R, Gill CC. Patent ductus arteriosus in adults—long term follow-up: nonsurgical vs. surgical treatment. J Am Coll Cardiol 1986;8:280–284.

[113] Campbell M. Natural history of patent ductus arteriosus. Br Heart J 1968;30:4–13.

[114] Bhat R, Fisher E, Raju TNK, Vidyasagar D. Patent ductus arteriosus: recent advances in diagnosis and management. Pediatr Clin North Am 1982;29:1117–1136.

[115] Bell EF, Warburton D, Stonestreet BS, et al. Effect of fluid administration on the development of symptomatic patent ductus arteriosus and congestive heart failure in premature infants. N Engl J Med 1980;302:598–604.

[116] Stonestreet BS, Bell EF, Warburton D, et al. Renal response in low birth weight neonates. Results of prolonged intake of two different amounts of fluid and sodium. Am J Dis Child 1983;137:215–219.

[117] Bell EF, Acarregui MJ. Restricted versus liberal water intake for preventing morbidity and mortality in preterm infants. Cochrane Rev Cochrane Library 2001;3:CD000503.

[118] Green TP, Thompson TR, Johnson DE, et al. Furosemide promotes patent ductus arteriosus in premature infants with respiratory distress syndrome. N Engl J Med 1983;308:743–748.

[119] Aziz A, Ohlsson A. Surfactant for pulmonary haemorrhage in neonates. Cochrane Database Syst Rev 2012;7:CD005254.

[120] Yen TA, Wang CC, Hsieh WS, et al. Short-term outcome of pulmonary hemorrhage in very-low-birth-weight preterm infants. Pediatr Neonatol 2013;54(5):330–334.

[121] Friedman WF, Herschklan MJ, Printz MP, et al. Pharmacologic closure of patent ductus arteriosus in the premature infant. N Engl J Med 1976;295:526–529.

[122] Heymann MA, Rudolph AM, Siverman NH. Closure of the ductus arteriosus in premature infants by inhibition of prostaglandin synthesis. N Engl J Med 1976;295:530–533.

[123] Van Overmeire B, Chemtob S. The pharmacologic closure of the patent ductus arteriosus. Semin Fetal Neonatal Med 2005;10:177–184.

[124] Fowlie PW, Davis PG. Prophylactic intravenous indomethacin for preventing mortality and morbidity in preterm infants. Evid Based Child Health 2010;5:416–471.

[125] Schmidt B, Davis P, Moddemann D, et al. Trial of indomethacin prophylaxis in preterms investigators. Long-term effects of indomethacin prophylaxis in extremely-low-birth-weight infants. N Engl J Med 2001;344:1966–1972.

[126] Sinha R, Negi V, Dalal SS. an interesting observation of PDA closure with oral paracetamol in preterm neonates. J Clin Neonatol 2013;2:30–32.

[127] Shah SS, Ohlsson A. Ibuprofen for the prevention of patent ductus arteriosus in preterm and/or low birth weight infants. Cochrane Database Syst Rev 2006;1:CD004213.

[128] Van Overmeire B, Smets K, Lecoutere D, et al. Comparison of ibuprofen and indomethacin for the closure of patent ductus arteriosus. N Engl J Med 2000;343:674–681.

[129] Ohlsson A, Walia R, Shah SS. Ibuprofen for the treatment of patent ductus arteriosus in preterm and/or low birth weight infants. Cochrane Database Syst Rev 2010;4:CD003481.

[130] Mosca F, Bray M, Lattanzio M, et al. Comparative evaluation of the effects of indomethacin and ibuprofen on cerebral perfusion and oxygenation in preterm infants with patent ductus arteriosus. J Pediatr 1997;131:549–555.

[131] Pezzati M, Vagni V, Biagiotti R, et al. Effects of indomethacin and ibuprofen on mesenteric and renal

blood flow in preterm infants with patent ductus arteriosus. J Pediatr 1999;135:733–738.

[132] Sakhalkar VS, Merchant RH. Therapy of symptomatic patent ductus arteriosus in preterms using mefenamic acid and indomethacin. Indian Pediatr 1992;29:313–318.

[133] Hammerman C, Bin-Nun A, Markovitch E, et al. Ductal closure with paracetamol: a surprising new approach to patent ductus arteriosus treatment. Pediatrics 2011;128:e1618–e1621.

[134] Aikio O, Harkin P, Saarela T, et al. Early paracetamol treatment associated with lowered risk of persistent ductus arteriosus in very preterm infants. J Matern Fetal Neonat Med 2014;27:1252–1256.

[135] Oncel MY, Yurttutan S, Degirmencioglu H, et al. Intravenous paracetamol treatment in the management of patent ductus arteriosus in extremely low birth weight infants. Neonatology 2013;103:166–169.

[136] Oncel MY, Yurttutan S, Erdeve O, et al. Oral paracetamol versus oral ibuprofen in the management of patent ductus arteriosus in preterm infants: a randomized controlled trial. J Pediatr 2014;164. 510. e1–514.e1.

[137] Valerio E, Valente MR, Salvadori S, et al. Intravenous paracetamol for PDA closure in the preterm: a single-center experience. Eur J Pediatr 2016;175:953–966.

[138] Huang X, Wang F, Wang K. Paracetamol versus ibuprofen for the treatment of patent ductus arteriosus in preterm neonates: a meta-analysis of randomized controlled trials. J Matern Fetal Neonatal Med 2018;31:2216–2222.

[139] Gross RE, Hubbard JP. Surgical ligation of patent ductus arteriosus: a report of first successful case. J Am Med Assoc 1939;112:729–731.

[140] Powell ML. Patent ductus arteriosus in premature infants. Med J Aust 1963;2:58–60.

[141] Decancq HG Jr. Repair of patent ductus arteriosus in a 1,417 gm infant. Am J Dis Child 1963;106:402–410.

[142] Eggert LD, Jung AJ, McGough EC, et al. Surgical treatment of patent

ductus arteriosus in preterm infants—four year experience with ligation in the newborn intensive care unit. Pediatr Cardiol 1982;2:15–18.

[143] Ko YC, Chang CI, Chiu IS, et al. Surgical ligation of patent ductus arteriosus in very-low-birth-weight premature infants in the neonatal intensive care unit. J Formos Med Assoc 2009;108:69–71.

[144] Metin K, Maltepe F, Kır M, Bilen Ç, et al. Ligation of patent ductus arteriosus in low birth weight premature infants: timing for intervention and effectiveness of bed-side surgery. J Cardiothorac Surg 2012;7:129–134.

[145] Avsar MK, Demir T, Celiksular C, Zeybek C. Bedside PDA ligation in premature infants less than 28 weeks and 1000 grams. J Cardiothorac Surg 2016;11:146–151.

[146] Cassady G, Crouse DT, Kirklin JW, et al. A randomized controlled trial of very early prophylactic ligation of the ductus arteriosus in babies who weighed 1000 g or less. N Engl J Med 1989;320:1511–1516.

[147] Brooks JM, Travadi JN, Patole SK, et al. Is surgical ligation of patent ductus arteriosus necessary? The Western Australia experience of conservative management. Arch Dis Child Fetal Neonatal Ed 2005;90:F235–F239.

[148] Noori S, Mc Coy M, Friedlich P, et al. Failure of ductus arteriosus closure is associated with increased mortality in preterm infants. Pediatr 2009;123:e138–e144.

[149] Cotton RB, Stahlman MT, Bender HW, et al. Randomized trial of early closure of symptomatic patent ductus arteriosus in small preterm infants. J Pediatr 1978;93:647–651.

[150] Malviya M, Ohlsson A, Shah S. Surgical versus medical treatment with cyclooxygenase inhibitors for symptomatic patent ductus arteriosus in preterm infants. Cochrane Database Syst Rev 2003;1:CD003951.

[151] Kabra NS, Schmidt B, Roberts RS. Neurosensory impairment after surgical closure of patent ductus arteriosus in extremely low birth weight infants: results from the Trial of Indomethacin Prophylaxis in Preterms. J Pediatr 2007;150:229–234.

[152] Chorne N, Leonard C, Piecuch R, et al. Patent ductus arteriosus and its treatment as risk factors for neonatal

and neurodevelopmental morbidity. Pediatrics 2007;119:1165–1171.

[153] Koehne PS, Bein G, Alexi-Meskhishvili V. Patent ductus arteriosus in very low birth weight infants: complications of pharmacological and surgical treatment. J Perinat Med 2001;29:327–334.

[154] Moin F, Kennedy KA, Moya FR. Risk factors predicting vasopressor use after patent ductus arteriosus ligation. Am J Perinatol 2003;20:313–320.

[155] Shelton JE, Julian R, Walburgh E, et al. Functional scoliosis as a long term complication of surgical ligation of patent ductus arteriosus in premature infants. J Pediatr Surg 1986;21:855–857.

[156] Raval MV, Laughon MM, Bose CL, et al. Patent ductus arteriosus ligation in premature infants: who really benefits and at what cost? J Pediatr Surg 2007;42:69–75.

[157] Harting MT, Blakely ML, Cox CS Jr, et al. Acute hemodynamic decompensation following patent ductus arteriosus ligation in premature infants. J Invest Surg 2008;21:133–138.

[158] Laborde F, Noirhomme P, Karam J, et al. A new video-assisted thoracoscopic surgical technique for interruption of patent ductus arteriosus in infants and children. J Thorac Cardiovasc Surg 1993;105:278–280.

[159] Laborde F, Folliguet TA, Etienne PY, Carbognani D, Batisssa A, Petrie J. Video-thorascopic surgical interruption of patent ductus arteriosus: routine experience in 332 pediatric cases. Eur J Cardiothorac Surg 1997;11:1052–1055.

[160] Burke RP, Wernovsky G, van der Velde M, et al. Video-assisted thoracoscopic surgery for congenital heart disease. J Thorac Cardiovasc Surg 1995;109:499–508.

[161] Hines MH, Bensky AS, Hammon JW, Pennington DG. Video-assisted thoracoscopic ligation of patent ductus arteriosus: safe and outpatient. Ann Thorac Surg 1998;66:853–859.

[162] Hines MH. Video assisted thoracoscopic surgical (VATS) closure of the patent ductus arteriosus in premature and term newborn infants. In: Rao PS, Vidyasagar D, editors. Perinatal cardiology:

a multidisciplinary approach. Minneapolis, MN: Cardiotext Publishing; 2015.

[163] Bensky AS, Raines KH, Hines MH. Late follow-up after thoracoscopic ductal ligation. Am J Cardiol 2000;86:360–361.

[164] Hines MH, Raines KH, Payne RM, et al. Video-assisted ductal ligation in preterm infants. Ann Thorac Surg 2003;76:1417–1420.

[165] Miyaji K. Video-assisted thoracoscopic interruption of patent ductus arteriosus. Kyobu Geka 2016;69:622–625.

[166] Porstmann W, Wierny L, Warnke H. Der Verschluß des Ductus arteriosus persistens ohne Thorakotomie (Vorläufige, Mitteilung). Thoraxchirurgie 1967;15:199–203.

[167] Rashkind WJ, Cuaso CC. Transcatheter closure of a patent ductus arteriosus: successful use in a 3.5 kg infant. Pediatr Cardiol 1979;1:3–7.

[168] Rao PS. Summary and comparison of patent ductus arteriosus closure devices. Curr Intervent Cardiol Rep 2001;3:268–274.

[169] Rao PS. History of transcatheter patent ductus arteriosus closure devices. In: Rao PS, Kern MJ, editors. Catheter based devices for the treatment of noncoronary cardiovascular disease in adults and children. Philadelphia, PA: Lippincott, Williams & Wilkins; 2003. p. 145–153.

[170] Rao PS. Historical aspects of transcatheter treatment of heart disease in children. Pediatr Therapeut 2012;S5:002.

[171] Rao PS. History of transcatheter interventions in pediatric cardiology. In: Vijayalakshmi IB, editor. Cardiac catheterization and imaging (from pediatrics to geriatrics). New Delhi, India: Jaypee Publications; 2015. p. 3–20.

[172] Rao PS. Which method to use for transcatheter occlusion of patent ductus arteriosus? Cathet Cardiovasc Diagn 1996;39:49–51.

[173] Rao PS. Transcatheter occlusion of patent ductus arteriosus: which method to use and which ductus to close? Am Heart J 1996;132:905–907.

[174] Rao PS, Sideris EB. Transcatheter occlusion of patent ductus arteriosus: state of the art. J Invasive Cardiol 1996;8:278–288.

[175] Rao PS. Transcatheter occlusion of patent ductus arteriosus: which method to use and which ductus to close? Am Heart J 1996;132:905–909.

[176] Rao PS. Transcatheter closure of moderate-to-large patent ductus arteriosus. J Invasive Cardiol 2001;13:303–306.

[177] Rao PS. Percutaneous closure of patent ductus arteriosus: state of the art. J Invasive Cardiol 2007;19:299–302.

[178] Yarrabolu TR, Rao PS. Transcatheter closure of patent ductus arteriosus. Pediatr Therapeut 2012;S5:005.

[179] Haneda N, Masue M, Tasaka M, et al. Transcatheter closure of patent ductus arteriosus in an infant weighing 1180 g. Pediatr Int 2001;43:176–178.

[180] Thukaram R, Suarez WA, Sundararaghavan S. Transcatheter closure of the patent arterial duct using the Flipper coil in a premature infant weighing 1400 g: a case report. Catheter Cardiovasc Interv 2005;66:18–20.

[181] Roberts P, Adwani S, Archer N, Wilson N. Catheter closure of the arterial duct in preterm infants. Arch Dis Child Fetal Neonatal 2007;92:248–250.

[182] Francis E, Singhi AK, Lakshmivenkateshaiah S, Kumar RK. Transcatheter occlusion of patent ductus arteriosus in pre-term infants. JACC Cardiovasc Interv 2010;3:550–555.

[183] Zahn EM, Peck D, Phillips A, et al. Transcatheter closure of patent ductus arteriosus in extremely premature newborns: early results and midterm follow-up. J Am Coll Cardiol Intv 2016;9:2429–2437.

[184] Gianturco C, Anderson JH, Wallace S. Mechanical device for arterial occlusion. Am J Roentgenol 1975;124:428–435.

[185] Cambier PA, Kirby WC, Wortham DC, Moore JW. Percutaneous closure of the small (less than 2.5 mm) patent ductus arteriosus using coil embolization. Am J Cardiol 1992;69:815–816.

[186] Grifka RG, Vincent JA, Nihill MR, et al. Transcatheter patent ductus arteriosus closure in an infant using the Gianturco-Grifka vascular occlusion device. Am J Cardiol 1996;78:721–723.

[187] Grifka RG. Transcatheter PDA closure using the Gianturco-Grifka vascular occlusion device. Curr Intervent Cardiol Rep 2001;3:174–182.

[188] Doshi AR, Rao PS. Development of aortic coarctation following device closure of patent ductus arteriosus. J Invasive Cardiol 2013;25:464–467.

[189] Sharafuddin MJ, Gu X, Titus JL, et al. Experimental evaluation of a new self-expanding patent ductus arteriosus occluder in a canine model. J Vasc Interv Radiol 1996;7:877–887.

[190] Masura J, Walsh KP, Thanopoulous B, et al. Catheter closure of moderate- to large-sized patent ductus arteriosus using the new Amplatzer duct occluder: immediate and short-term results. J Am Coll Cardiol 1998;31:878–882.

[191] Thanopoulous B, Eleftherakis N, Tzannos K, Stefanadis C. Transcatheter closure of the patent ductus arteriosus using the new Amplatzer duct occluder: initial clinical applications in children. Am Heart J 2008;156:917.e1–917.e6.

[192] Venczelova Z, et al. The new Amplatzer duct occluder II: when is its use advantageous? Cardiol Young 2011;21:495–504.

[193] Moore JW, Greene J, Palomares S, et al. Pivotal and Continuing Access Studies of the Nit Occlud PDA Investigators. Results of the combined U.S. Multicenter Pivotal Study and the Continuing Access Study of the Nit-Occlud PDA device for percutaneous closure of patent ductus arteriosus. JACC Cardiovasc Interv 2014;7:1430–1436.

[194] Kenny D, Morgan GJ, Bentham JR, Wilson N, Martin R, Tometzki A, Oslizlok P, Walsh KP. Early clinical experience with a modified Amplatzer ductal occluder for transcatheter arterial duct occlusion in infants and small children. Catheter Cardiovasc Interv 2013;82:534–540.

[195] Bentham J, Meur S, Hudsmith L, Archer N, Wilson N. Echocardiographically guided catheter closure of arterial ducts in small preterm infants on the neonatal intensive care unit. Catheter Cardiovasc Interv 2011;77:409–415.

[196] Delaney JW, Fletcher SE. Patent ductus arteriosus closure using the Amplatzer® vascular plug II for all anatomic variants.

619

Catheter Cardiovasc Interv 2013;81:
820–824.

[197] Wang-Giuffre EW, Breinholt JP. Novel
use of the medtronic micro vascular
plug for PDA closure in preterm

infants. Catheter Cardiovasc Interv
2017;89:1059–1065.

[198] Morville P, Akhavi A. Transcatheter
closure of hemodynamic significant
patent ductus arteriosus in 32

premature infants by Amplatzer
ductal occluder additional size-
ADOIIAS. Catheter Cardiovasc Interv
2017;90:612–617.

Further reading

[199] Kajino H, Chen Y, Chemtob S, et al.
Tissue hypoxia inhibits prostaglandin and nitric oxide production and
prevents ductus arteriosus reopen-

ing. Am J Physiol Regul Integr Comp
Physiol 2000;279:R278–R286.

[200] Farombi-Oghuvbu I, Matthews T,
Mayne PD, et al. N-terminal pro-B-

type natriuretic peptide: a measure of
significant patent ductus arteriosus.
Arch Dis Child Fetal Neonatal Ed
2008;93:F257–F260.

Chapter |30C|

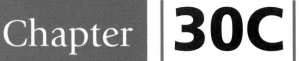

Cyanotic Heart Disease in a Neonate

Rakhi Balachandran, MD, Karunakar Vadlamudi, MD, Raman Krishna Kumar, DM

CHAPTER POINTS

- Newborns with critical congenital heart defects may require mechanical ventilation as a part of the stabilization process.
- Ventilation strategies are largely dictated by the physiology of the congenital heart condition because pulmonary vascular resistance is very sensitive to small changes in gas exchange.
- It is important to have a basic understanding of the physiology of common critical heart diseases in the newborn in order to provide the most appropriate ventilation settings.
- Overzealous ventilation is an important cause of systemic hypoperfusion in neonates with duct dependent circulation and single ventricle physiology.

This chapter will present essential information for the neonatologist on congenital cyanotic heart disease (CCHD) in a newborn. In the last 2 decades, dramatic advancements have enabled a very high survival rate in newborns with cyanotic heart defects even in resource-limited environments [1]. Some form of therapy is now feasible for most defects. The role of the neonatologist is to suspect heart disease, ensure initial stabilization, and organize secure transportation. The first section of the chapter will seek to provide the necessary background information regarding CCHD. The second section will discuss the principles of mechanical ventilation in neonates with CCHD.

Background information

Heart diseases that manifest during newborn period very often require urgent attention. Prompt treatment can often yield gratifying results and in many instances excellent long-term event-free survival can be expected. Today, some form of palliative or definitive treatment is feasible for most newborns with congenital heart disease (CHD). The list of cardiac emergencies at birth includes cyanotic heart disease that can present anytime after birth with severe cyanosis, hypoxemia, impaired systemic perfusion or shock, and occasionally respiratory distress. Recently, many infants with CCHD that were not detected prenatally are diagnosed by pulse oximetry-based CCHD screening at birth.

Disease categories

A classification of congenital heart defects associated with severe cyanosis in the newborns is shown in Table 30C.1.

Duct-dependent pulmonary circulation

The following lesions are listed as duct-dependent.
1. Anatomical (severe stenosis to atresia of the pulmonary valve)
   a. With intact ventricular septum: Critical pulmonary valve stenosis or pulmonary atresia with intact ventricular septum
   b. With interventricular communication: Examples include—tetralogy of Fallot (TOF) with critical pulmonic stenosis (PS), TOF with pulmonary atresia, single ventricle, corrected transposition, transposition with ventricular septal defect (VSD) and severe PS

Table 30C.1 Cyanotic congenital heart defects in newborns

Physiologic categories	Conditions	Manifestation
Duct-dependent pulmonary blood flow	Pulmonary atresia, critical pulmonary stenosis, Ebstein's anomaly	Cyanosis, hypoxia
Duct-dependent systemic blood flow	Hypoplastic left heart syndrome	Heart failure, shock, circulatory failure, acidosis and cyanosis is often minimal unless the atrial septum is restrictive
Obstruction of pulmonary venous return	Obstructed TAPVR, mitral atresia with a restrictive patent foramen ovale	Cyanosis, hypoxia, heart failure
Parallel circulation with poor mixing	D-Transposition with intact ventricular septum	Cyanosis, hypoxia
Admixture lesions	Persistent truncus arteriosus, unobstructed TAPVR, Double outlet right ventricle with subpulmonic VSD (Taussig–Bing anomaly), single ventricle with increased blood flow	Cyanosis is often mild, heart failure is the dominant symptom

TAPVR, Total anomalous pulmonary venous return; *VSD*, ventricular septal defect.

2. Functional (pulmonary valve is patent but forward flow is restricted)
   a. Example: Severe Ebstein's anomaly. These neonates usually present with cyanosis correlating with closure of the duct postnatally and acidosis due to hypoxia. In transposition, severe cyanosis may occur in the presence of an open duct if the atrial septal communication is severely restrictive

Admixture lesion causing cyanosis in newborn period

These are the lesions where mixing occurs in one of the chamber of heart and the final systemic saturation depends upon this admixture and flow streaming into pulmonary and aortic circulation. Here severity of cyanosis is dependent of the severity of pulmonary stenosis. If PS is severe or if there is pulmonary atresia in association with any of these defects, the presentation is that of duct-dependent pulmonary atresia.

In absence of PS, the cyanosis is often mild and may not be clinically apparent. For example, in persistent truncus arteriosus or single ventricle with no PS the saturations are often in the 90s. These lesions present with increased pulmonary flow and heart failure.

Examples include persistent truncus arteriosus, unobstructed total anomalous pulmonary venous return (TAPVR), double outlet right ventricle with subpulmonic VSD (Taussig–Bing anomaly), and single ventricle with increased blood flow.

Parallel circulation

Transposition with great arteries (TGA)—considered to be the commonest cyanotic heart disease of the newborn in this group. Normally, both systemic and pulmonary circulation are in series, but in TGA due to ventricular arterial (VA) discordance, circulation becomes parallel; and hence to maintain hemodynamics it depends on adequate mixing either at atrial, ventricular, or great arteries level.

Obstructed pulmonary venous return

Obstruction of pulmonary venous return typically occurs in the obstructed form of TAPVR. The presentation is dramatic. Severe cyanosis results from a marked reduction in effective pulmonary blood flow (PBF). Pulmonary vascular resistance (PVR) is severely elevated with right to left shunting at the patent foramen ovale/ASD and PDA. The X-ray appearance (ground glass appearance) is characteristic.

Diagnostic evaluation

One of the major reasons for delay in referral of infants with critical CHD is failure to suspect heart disease in a newborn baby at initial clinical evaluation. Clinical diagnosis of heart disease in a newborn can be quite challenging. Manifestations of potentially life-threatening CHD are often subtle and can be confused with noncardiac conditions. For instance, low cardiac output states resulting from critical aortic stenosis or other left-sided obstructive lesions may be mistaken for sepsis. Unfortunately, the cost of failure to recognize CHD is, not infrequently, death. This is because many forms of CHD that manifest in the early neonatal period are fatal without specific interventions. It is possible to recognize CHD through careful clinical evaluation using the principles outlined later and a few additional tests. The diagnostic strategy for suspected CHD in a newborn is largely dictated by the condition of a newborn.

The main purpose of evaluation of cyanosis in a newborn is to arrive at an accurate and comprehensive diagnosis of the cardiac condition in the shortest possible time. This enables timely initiation of life-saving therapy. For all duct-dependent circulation and selected cases of transposition, prostaglandin E_1 (PGE$_1$) infusion needs to be started as soon as possible. For obstructed TAPVR, immediate surgery is often the only option. While clinical evaluation is helpful, accurate diagnosis mandates thorough echocardiography.

Initial resuscitation and stabilization of a newborn with suspected heart disease

This section presents the basic principles of initial stabilization of a newborn with CCHD.

Airway and respiratory support

Like in any other emergency situation, a stable airway needs to be established first. Newborns with severe respiratory distress should immediately receive a bag and mask ventilation and supplemental oxygen to target preductal SpO$_2$ in the 85%–95% range (although, later the oxygen concentration may need to be reduced in some cases of ductal-dependent circulation).

If respiratory distress continues to be profound after the initial resuscitation, the newborn should be intubated and mechanical ventilation should be initiated. Analgesia, sedation, and atropine are recommended prior to nonemergent intubation with optional paralysis. Even in the most emergent situations, sufficient time is often available to organize the requirements for performing intubation. The decision to intubate a newborn and initiate mechanical ventilation electively prior to transport requires consideration of the following variables: condition of the newborn in terms of severity of cyanosis, hemodynamic stability, gestational age, transport distance, and risk of apnea with PGE$_1$ infusion.

Access

A secure peripheral or central intravenous access is very essential. Inotropic agents with vasoconstrictor properties, such as Dopamine and Epinephrine, can only be administered via a reliable central access. Umbilical arterial and venous lines are the first choice for vascular access. If central access is unavailable and an inotrope needs to be infused, dobutamine may be a reasonable choice.

If an umbilical arterial line cannot be placed, it may be impractical to obtain arterial access prior to transport; and unnecessary arterial punctures for blood gas sampling should be avoided because these sites will be required for placement of an arterial line prior to definitive surgery. An arterial sample is, however, necessary for ABG analysis.

Oxygen

The potential dangers of excessive oxygen in a newborn with suspected heart disease include acceleration of closure of the ductus arteriosus and unacceptable decline in the PVR. Both these situations can have catastrophic consequences (Fig. 30C.1A). Duct closure is fatal in duct-dependent lesions. A marked decline in PVR translates into excessive PBF, often at the cost of reduced systemic blood flow. This is particularly likely to happen in duct-dependent conditions. For these reasons, the FiO$_2$ needs to be titrated to maintain an oxygen saturation of 85 ± 5%. In most situations this allows a reasonable balance between pulmonary and systemic blood flows (Fig. 30C.1B).

Prostaglandin

PGE$_1$ is a very essential drug and should be available in every newborn nursery. It can restore ductal patency in most newborns with closing ducts and is therefore lifesaving in duct-dependent situations. Its effect is usually confirmed by improving saturations in newborns with duct-dependent pulmonary circulation and resolution of the circulatory failure and acidosis in newborns with duct-dependent systemic circulation. Its efficacy declines somewhat with increasing age particularly after 15 days, and it is usually not effective in opening a closed duct after 30 days. The initial dose of prostaglandin is 0.05–0.1 mcg/kg/min. Once the duct has opened up (this can be confirmed by the clinical response or by echocardiography), the dose may be reduced to as low as 0.01 mcg/kg/min. This allows maintenance of ductal patency with minimal adverse effects. Adverse effects of PGE$_1$ infusion include apnea (12%), bradycardia (7%), flushing (10%), tachycardia (3%), hypotension (4%), fever (14%), diarrhea (2%), gastric distension (1%), and seizures (4%). Leukocytosis frequently accompanies prostaglandin use. Administration over several days may result in increased lung and body water from capillary leak, thrombocytopenia, gastric outlet obstruction, and cortical hyperostosis.

Transportation

The decision to transport a newborn to a tertiary referral center with facilities of specialized care for neonates and infants with heart disease should be a joint one involving

(A)

(B)

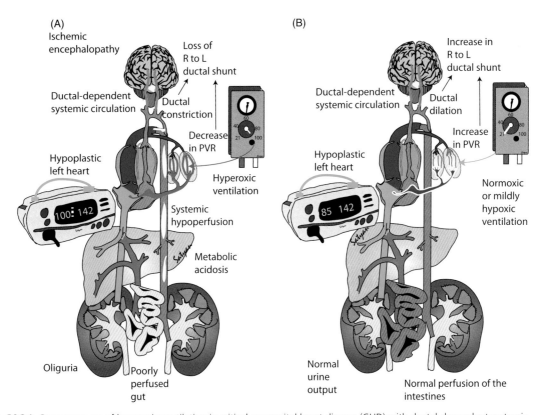

Fig. 30C.1 Consequences of hyperoxic ventilation in critical congenital heart disease (CHD) with ductal-dependent systemic circulation (A). Ductal constriction and drop in pulmonary vascular resistance (PVR) result in "systemic steal" with hypoperfusion of the brain, gut, and kidneys. Maintaining SpO_2 around 85% and increasing positive end expiratory pressure (PEEP) (B) increases PVR and maintains ductal patency and supports right to left shunt to sustain systemic circulation. Copyright: Satyan Lakshminrusimha.

the referring pediatrician and the pediatric cardiology team. A thorough communication of important information that is obtained at the referring center helps reduce problems during transport and also helps to prepare the pediatric cardiac center to receive the newborn. Emergency procedures can be planned on arrival with minimal delay. The following list could serve as a checklist of points to be communicated by a pediatrician or a neonatologist to the pediatric cardiology center prior to transportation of a newborn with suspected heart disease.

Communication checklist for transportation

1. **Prenatal background**: Term or preterm, birth order, age of mother, important maternal conditions.
2. **Birth**: Mode of delivery, relevant antenatal issues, Apgar scores, birth weight, significant postnatal events if any?
3. **Clinical presentation**: Why was heart disease suspected? Are there associated anomalies or abnormal facies?

4. **Current condition**: Vitals (heart rate, respiratory rate, oxygen saturation, peripheral circulation), lab tests (a baseline arterial blood gas analysis report is valuable, if available), feeding.
5. **Preliminary diagnosis of the cardiovascular condition**: Results of the physical examination, chest X-ray, ECG, and echocardiogram.
6. **What has been done so far to resuscitate the newborn?** What access has been obtained? Is the child ventilated or breathing spontaneously? What medications have been given (specifically, inotropes, prostaglandin)?
7. **Relevant socioeconomic issues**: What is the social and economic background of the family? Which family members are likely to accompany the child? How much has been communicated to them?
8. **Logistics**: Transport distance, mode of transport, and transporting personnel? Expected time of departure and arrival?

Personnel for neonatal transport

Whenever feasible, the newborn should be accompanied by the resident neonatologist or pediatrician taking care of the baby and a nurse. Both the team members should be familiar with the underlying condition and should be aware of the potential problems the newborn may face during transport. Periodic communication with the pediatric heart center regarding patient's status is important.

Monitoring during transport

Ideally, it is necessary to continuously monitor ECG, blood pressure (NIBP/IBP), and oxygen saturations during transportation. When the newborn reaches the referral center, it is necessary to summarize the condition during transport and indicate important events, if any that occurred during transport.

Care of the newborn during transport

A secure airway and an intravenous access are vital. Newborns on prostaglandin can have periods of apnea. For this reason a number of units in the West would routinely intubate and mechanically ventilate a newborn on prostaglandin infusion during transport. Transporting a newborn with CHD on prostaglandin infusion often amounts to taking a calculated risk in low resource environments. The physician involved with the transport should be alert to this possibility for apnea and be ready to support respiration with assisted ventilation.

Excessive oxygen (>2 L/min; $FiO_2 > 0.4$) should be avoided during transport of most newborns with heart disease. This is advisable even if PGE_1 is used to keep the duct open. High FiO_2 reduces PVR and can result in excessive PBF at the cost of systemic circulation. This is particularly dangerous in hypoplastic left heart syndrome (Fig. 30C.1A).

Attention to other basic details, such as temperature control, fluid balance, avoidance of hypoglycemia, and hypocalcemia, are all mandatory as in any neonatal transport situations.

Sepsis frequently complicates the management of newborns with heart disease. The potential for nosocomial sepsis is particularly high for sick newborns that are being transported. Meticulous attention to aseptic precautions is extremely important.

Definitive management of congenital heart disease

Specific treatment options in the tertiary center are largely dictated by the precise diagnosis and are listed in Table 30C.2.

Mechanical ventilation in newborns with congenital heart disease

Why does ventilation become necessary? How does it alter hemodynamics?

A critically ill neonate might require mechanical ventilation in the emergency room or intensive care unit for impaired oxygenation, impaired ventilation, apnea

Table 30C.2 Definitive treatment of cyanotic congenital heart disease in newborns

Conditions	Specific treatments	Comments
D-Transposition with intact ventricular septum	Balloon septostomy followed by arterial switch operation	Arterial switch needs to be performed within the first few weeks
Pulmonary atresia—intact ventricular septum	Wire perforation of atretic pulmonary valve followed by balloon dilation or surgical restoration by RVOT patch, stenting of the patent arterial duct may also be required in addition	Treatment dictated by precise anatomic issues (extent of RV hypoplasia and tricuspid valve annulus dimension, presence of right ventricle-dependent coronary circulation) and experience of the center
Pulmonary atresia with VSD or other defects, "severe" TOF	Emergency BT shunt or stenting of the arterial duct	Definitive procedure later in life dictated by precise anatomy
Critical pulmonary stenosis	Balloon valvotomy	Excellent long-term outcomes, 5%–10% immediate mortality
Obstructed TAPVR	Emergency surgical repair	Good long-term outcome, immediate surgical mortality of 5%–20%

TOF, Tetralogy of Fallot.

of the newborn, protection of airway, or for facilitating optimal transport to a specialized center. In neonates with CHD the commonest indication for mechanical ventilation include respiratory distress, profound cyanosis due to a right heart obstructive lesion, or severe systemic hypoperfusion due to a left heart obstructive lesion. A neonate undergoing repair of CHD also requires a variable period of mechanical ventilation in the operating room for provision of anesthetic, protection of airway, and stabilization of cardiorespiratory function throughout the perioperative period. The commonest presenting signs that aid the clinician in diagnosing CHD in a neonate are the presence of a murmur, cyanosis, respiratory distress, heart failure, and shock [2]. Mechanical ventilation decreases the work of breathing, decreases myocardial oxygen consumption, and facilitates manipulation of PVR by influencing the arterial blood gases.

Heart and lungs work synergistically to facilitate optimal tissue oxygen delivery, and intervention in one system can significantly impact the other [3]. Mechanical ventilation by changing lung volumes and intrathoracic pressure can affect the key determinants of cardiac performance, namely, atrial filling or the preload and the impedance to ventricular emptying or the afterload. The cardiopulmonary interactions can be quite significant in a critically ill neonate requiring mechanical ventilation and an understanding of this phenomenon is necessary for optimal hemodynamic and respiratory management in the intensive care unit (Fig. 30C.2). Systemic venous return depends on the pressure gradient between the extrathoracic veins and right atrial pressure. Spontaneous respiration decreases the intrathoracic pressure, increases the intraabdominal pressure with inspiratory diaphragmatic descent, and thus increases the venous return by increasing the gradient for right atrial filling. Positive pressure

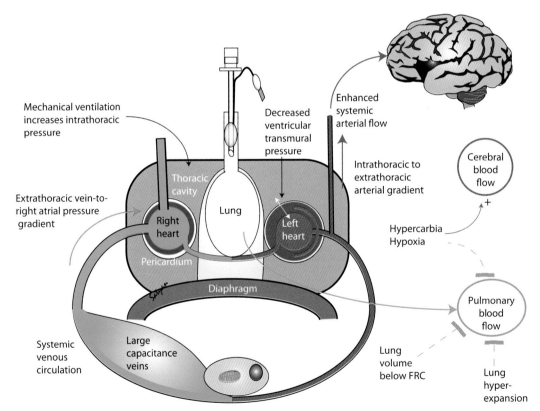

Fig. 30C.2 Impact of Mechanical Ventilation and Increased Intrathoracic Pressure on Hemodynamics—Cardiopulmonary Interactions. Increased intrathoracic pressure from mechanical ventilation reduces the gradient between extrathoracic vein to right atrium leading to impaired venous return. However, intrathoracic pressure also decreases left ventricular transmural pressure and enhances systemic arterial flow. Hypercarbia (respiratory acidosis) and to a lesser extent hypoxia enhance cerebral blood flow. Hypo- or hyperexpansion of the lung (below or above FRC), hypercarbia and hypoxia reduce pulmonary blood flow (PBF). FRC, Functional residual capacity; PVR, pulmonary vascular resistance. Copyright: Satyan Lakshminrusimha.

ventilation reduces this gradient by directly increasing intrathoracic pressure and causes a reduction in right ventricular preload. Hypovolemia, septic shock, and gas trapping with obstructive airway disease can exaggerate this ventilation-induced reduction in preload causing significant hemodynamic compromise. Mechanical ventilation can also impact right ventricular afterload by influencing PVR through changes in lung volume (Fig. 30C.3). PVR depends on the balance in vascular tone of alveolar and extraalveolar vessels. When lung is inflated above functional residual capacity (FRC) the compression of alveolar vessels can increase PVR. When the inflating volumes are too minimal the increase in PVR is facilitated by the collapse of extraalveolar vessels, which become tortuous as a result of the loss of alveolar volume. Additionally, terminal airway collapse at low lung volumes can result in alveolar hypoxia. This hypoxia can result in pulmonary vasoconstriction. Hence, maintenance of lungs at FRC without producing large shifts in lung volume is essential for optimal hemodynamic performance by maintaining a stable PVR. Effect of mechanical ventilation on the left ventricle is predominant by affecting the afterload [4]. The primary determinant of left ventricular afterload is myocardial wall stress, which is a function of left ventricular transmural pressure (the difference between left ventricular systolic pressure and intrathoracic pressure). Positive pressure ventilation reduces transmural pressure by increasing the intrathoracic pressure, and hence the pressure differential across the left ventricular wall. This is the basis for beneficial effects of mechanical ventilation in off-loading the left ventricle in patients with ventricular dysfunction.

Specific considerations in neonatal population with CHD

This section will discuss the specific considerations in each of the CHD categories. Table 30C.3 summarizes the broad principles that dictate ventilatory management.

It is important to recognize that there are no strict guidelines with respect to a fixed respiratory rate for each cardiac lesion. In our clinical experience, the average respiratory rate required to maintain target CO_2 depends on the type of ventilator and the individual lung compliance for each patient given the cardiac condition, the PBF, presence of pulmonary venous obstruction, associated respiratory infection, if any, and other specific considerations. It may vary from as low as 20/min in a neonate with good lung compliance to as high as 45/min in a patient with poor lung compliance. The standard inspiratory time that is used is between 0.40 and 0.44 for all neonates irrespective of the type of lesion. The positive end expiratory pressure (PEEP) is never escalated beyond 7 due to the impact of higher PEEP on these critically ill neonates with a substrate of low cardiac output. The tidal volume settings are usually between 6 and 8 mL/kg in all cases.

Duct-dependent lesions. The ductus arteriosus is a fetal vascular channel, which can be a lifesaving conduit in the critically ill neonate with CHD for maintaining PBF or systemic perfusion. Duct-dependent pulmonary circulation includes right heart obstructive lesions, such as pulmonary atresia, severe pulmonary stenosis, or tricuspid atresia. The duct-dependent systemic circulation include left heart

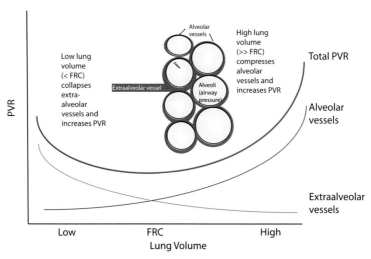

Fig. 30C.3 Lung Volume (LV) and Pulmonary Vascular Resistance (PVR). Low LV collapses extraalveolar pulmonary vessels and increases PVR. High LV compresses alveolar pulmonary vessels and increases PVR. PVR is lowest at functional residual capacity (FRC). Copyright: Satyan Lakshminrusimha.

Table 30C.3 Recommended ventilatory settings for typical intensive care situations in neonates with congenital heart disease

Lesions	Broad goals	Saturation targets	Typical FiO$_2$	Other ventilator settings
Duct-dependent systemic circulation	• Maintain ductal patency • Avoid decrease in PVR so as to prevent pulmonary overcirculation and maintain systemic blood flow	80%–85%	0.21	Respiratory rate to target PaCO$_2$ of 45–50 mmHg
Duct-dependent pulmonary circulation	• Maintain ductal patency • Identify pulmonary overcirculation and underperfusion in a given clinical setting • Manipulation of PVR to avoid pulmonary overcirculation	75%–85%	0.21–0.4	Respiratory rate to target PaCO$_2$ of 40 mmHg
TGA with IVS	• Maintain adequate mixing at the atrial level • Ventilatory measures have less impact on oxygen saturation	70%–80%	0.21–0.5	Respiratory rate to target PaCO$_2$ of 40 mmHg
CHD with increased Q_p (e.g., truncus, TGA VSD), single ventricle, and no PS	• Decrease pulmonary overcirculation • Maintain somewhat high PVR	Target SpO$_2$ 75%–90%	0.21	Respiratory rate to target PaCO$_2$ of 45–50 mmHg
Postoperative pulmonary hypertension	• Avoid increase in PVR • Avoid triggers of high PVR, namely, hypoxia, hypercarbia, and acidosis	Target SpO$_2$ >90%	>0.4	Respiratory rate to target PaCO$_2$ of 30–35 mmHg

CHD, Cyanotic heart disease; *PS*, pulmonic stenosis; *PVR*, pulmonary vascular resistance; *TGA with IVS*, transposition with intact ventricular septum; *VSD*, ventricular septal defect.

obstructive lesions like severe coarctation of aorta, aortic arch interruption, or hypoplastic left heart syndrome. Although initiation of PGE$_1$ is a critical pharmacological intervention that restores ductal patency, mechanical ventilation and regulation of arterial blood gases play a key role in balancing systemic and pulmonary circulations.

Duct-dependent systemic circulation (Fig. 30C.4). These infants present with profound hypotension and impending circulatory collapse. Mechanical ventilation is required as a part of cardiorespiratory resuscitation along with emergent initiation of PGE1 infusion. Ventilator settings should target maintaining a low fraction of inspired oxygen (FiO$_2$) preferably room air (21%) and maintaining mild respiratory acidosis (PaCO$_2$, 45–50 mmHg) to increase PVR. Hypercarbia can also improve cerebral blood flow (Fig. 30C.2) and prevent adverse neurological outcomes [5]. In a randomized crossover study that evaluated the response of hypoxia and hypercarbia on oxygen delivery and ratio of pulmonary to systemic blood flow (Q_p:Q_s) in 10 infants with

hypoplastic left heart syndrome, hypercarbia was associated with better oxygen delivery, whereas both measures reduced Q_p/Q_s ratio [6].

Duct-dependent pulmonary circulation. These patients present with severe cyanosis and metabolic acidosis secondary to decreased PBF and profound hypoxemia. Initiation of mechanical ventilation to decrease work of breathing and ventilator adjustments to optimize PVR can be lifesaving along with prostaglandin therapy to maintain ductal patency. Target SpO$_2$ should be around 75%–85% to obtain a Q_p/Q_s ratio of 1.0. An increase in oxygen saturation >90% indicates pulmonary overcirculation due to increased shunting across the ductus, and subsequent ventilator strategy should aim at reducing FiO$_2$ and increasing PaCO$_2$ to around 40 mmHg. In patients who have developed pulmonary edema following increased PBF a diuretic infusion is a reasonable adjunct to treatment. Systemic vasodilators like milrinone can be considered to improve tissue perfusion and correct lactic acidosis in patients who have compromised systemic perfusion.

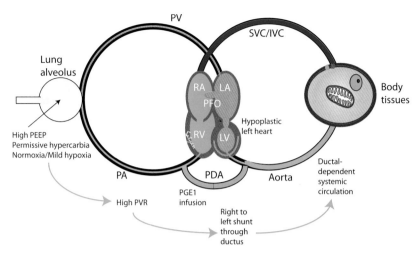

Fig. 30C.4 Ductal-Dependent Systemic Circulation in Hypoplastic Left Heart Syndrome. Maintaining ductal patency with prostaglandin E$_1$ (PGE$_1$) infusion and avoiding hyperoxia and preventing fall in pulmonary vascular resistance (PVR) by permissive hypercarbia (PaCO$_2$ in the 55–65 mmHg range), avoiding hyperoxia (SpO$_2$ of around 85%) and high PEEP (6–8 cmH$_2$O) will increase systemic blood flow. *PFO*, Patent foramen ovale. Copyright: Satyan Lakshminrusimha.

Transposition of great arteries with intact ventricular septum (Fig. 30C.5A)

Transposition of great arteries with intact ventricular septum is characterized by atrioventricular concordance with ventriculoarterial discordance. The systemic and pulmonary circulation is parallel and this condition is incompatible with life unless there is intercirculatory mixing through an atrial septal defect (ASD) or a PDA. In neonates with closing ductus severe hypoxia ensues due to poor intercirculatory mixing and decreased PBF. Maintaining patency of ductus with PGE$_1$ will facilitate mixing and increased PBF if the PVR is less than systemic vascular resistance (SVR).

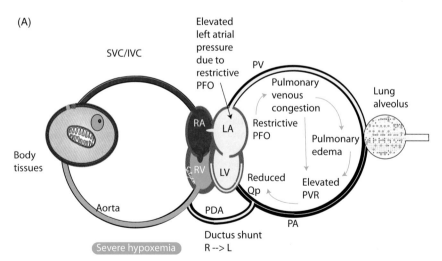

Fig. 30C.5 (A) Transposition of great arteries (TGA) without ventricular septal defect (VSD) and restrictive patent foramen ovale (PFO). High left atrial (LA) pressure may lead to pulmonary congestion and further decrease gas exchange. Elevated pulmonary vascular resistance (PVR) limits pulmonary blood flow (Q_p) and contributes to hypoxemia. Maintaining the patency of the ductus arteriosus may not improve oxygenation because of the right-to-left shunt across PDA. (B) Balloon atrial septostomy (BAS) improves oxygenation in this patient by improving admixture at the atrial level and reducing pulmonary venous congestion. Copyright: Satyan Lakshminrusimha.

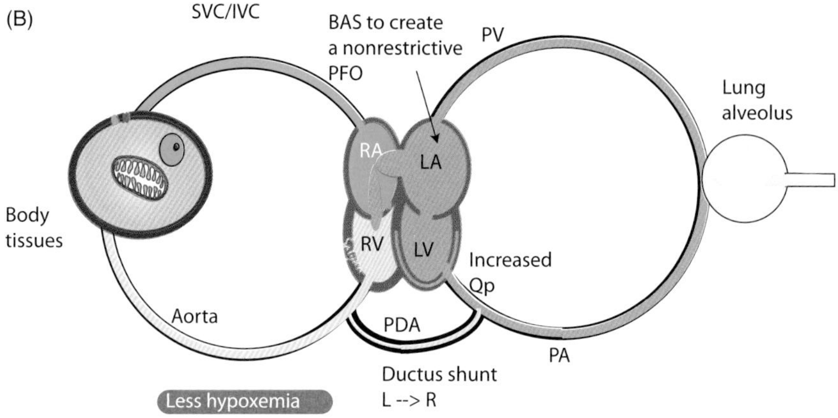

Fig. 30C.5 (cont.)

Patients who do not respond to PGE$_1$ may require emergent balloon atrial septostomy (BAS) for facilitating mixing at atrial level. A potentially dangerous situation is when the PVR is high due to a restrictive foramen ovale with elevated left atrial pressures, and the shunting across the ductus occurs from pulmonary artery to aorta decreasing effective PBF and leading to severe hypoxemia. Ventilatory maneuvers to decrease PVR may not be effective unless a BAS is performed to decompress the LA (Fig. 30C.5B).

Complex CHD with increased pulmonary blood flow

These lesions include truncus arteriosus, TGA–VSD, and single ventricle variants without pulmonary obstruction and are characterized by increased PBF. In transposition physiology with a significant VSD, anatomic right to left shunt provides effective PBF, that is, volume of systemic venous blood that reaches pulmonary circulation; and anatomic left to right shunt provides effective systemic blood flow, that is, volume of pulmonary venous blood that reaches the systemic circulation. The intercirculatory mixing through VSD depends on the relationship between SVR and PVR. If PVR is low, increased right to left shunt at the VSD further increases PBF and hastens the development of pulmonary vascular occlusive disease. Reducing PVR will not greatly influence systemic oxygenation but will only augment the recirculating volume in the pulmonary circuit. This might decrease the effective systemic blood flow and can precipitate a low cardiac output state. In other single ventricle lesions with increased PBF, mechanical ventilation should aim at preventing fall in PVR. This is achieved by avoiding high concentrations of oxygen and permitting hypoventilation to increase PCO$_2$ to 45–50 mmHg. Keeping a higher PEEP will also help to minimize pulmonary overcirculation by its incremental effects on PVR. Metabolic

acidosis resulting from systemic hypo perfusion should be corrected appropriately. Temporary medical management should be followed by appropriate surgical palliation or correction.

Ventricular dysfunction

Mechanical ventilation can affect right and left ventricular function by impacting the key determinants of ventricular performance, namely, preload, afterload, and contractility.

Right ventricular dysfunction. This can occur in neonates with Ebstein's anomaly or severe pulmonary artery hypertension (PAH) or impaired myocardial protection after cardiopulmonary bypass (CPB). Positive pressure ventilation decreases the right ventricular preload by affecting the systemic venous return. The ventilator strategies should aim at minimizing the mean airway pressures, decreasing inspiratory times, and facilitating lower tidal volumes. LVs above and below FRC can increase PVR (Fig. 30C.2). Avoiding alveolar hyperinflation by choosing lower tidal volumes of 6–8 mL/kg and minimizing atelectasis by judicious use of PEEP can prevent dramatic alterations in PVR produced by surges in the LVs.

Left ventricular dysfunction. Institution of positive pressure ventilation improves left ventricular function by decreasing LV afterload. This effect is primarily brought about by a rise in intrathoracic pressure, which in turn reduces ventricular transmural pressure (the chief determinant of left ventricular wall stress). Additionally, adjunctive use of PEEP facilitates alveolar recruitment in patients with left ventricular failure and pulmonary edema who are prone to develop pulmonary atelectasis. Mechanical ventilation also provides hemodynamic support in critically ill neonates with left ventricular dysfunction by reducing

630

the work of breathing by respiratory muscle unloading and decreasing myocardial oxygen consumption.

Pulmonary hypertension

Ventilatory management in patients with pulmonary hypertension should aim to mitigate the factors that increase PVR, namely, hypoxia, hypercarbia, acidosis, atelectasis, and extreme swings in LV. Arterial blood gas management should target PaO_2 of 80–100 mmHg, $PaCO_2$ between 30–35mmHg and maintenance of mild respiratory alkalosis. Patients on mechanical ventilation should also receive adequate sedation and pain relief, as increased sympathetic response to pain can precipitate increase in PVR. Patients particularly at the risk of perioperative pulmonary hypertension include obstructed infracardiac total anomalous pulmonary venous connection (TAPVC), complete atrioventricular canal defects, and patients with CHD and Down's syndromes. Pulmonary hypertensive crisis is a potential complication, which can develop in the postoperative period after repair of obstructed TAPVC. This should receive emergent attention by ventilation with 100% oxygen, sedation, and institution of pulmonary vasodilators like inhaled nitric oxide (iNO) or sildenafil.

Postoperative ventilation: general principles

Neonates undergoing corrective or palliative procedures for CHD require a variable period of ventilation in the postoperative intensive care unit. Preoperative lung disease, fluid overload, alterations in lung compliance after CPB, and anesthesia or unstable postoperative hemodynamics might prolong the requirement for ventilator support. The target of mechanical ventilation should be to obtain adequate oxygenation (with minimal FiO_2) and ventilation, as well as to optimize the postoperative cardiorespiratory function till recovery.

Though traditionally pressure-controlled ventilation strategies have been favored in neonates, the advent of newer generation ventilators with advanced microprocessor technology has allowed delivery of volume-targeted breaths in neonates. Variable tidal volumes, which occur in pressure-controlled modes due to changes in lung compliance, can lead to repeated alveolar derecruitment and atelectrauma [7]. Volume-targeted ventilation modes allow better control of peak inspiratory pressure (PIP) and delivery of a target tidal volume (V_t) at a limited pressure [8]. The volume-targeted ventilatory modes that are frequently used in pediatric cardiac surgical population include pressure-regulated volume control (PRVC) mode, pressure-controlled ventilation with volume guarantee (PCV-VG) and volume-assured pressure support (VAPS). All these modes utilize the potential advantages of a decelerating form of inspiratory flow pattern of pressure control ventilation that facilitates uniform distribution of gases and delivery of a target tidal volume at a favorable inspiratory pressure. In PRVC mode, the PIP for delivering the target V_t is optimized by the ventilator after measuring the compliance and average tidal volume of the previous 3–5 breaths.

All patients on mechanical ventilation should have continuous SpO_2 monitoring, end tidal carbon dioxide ($ETCO_2$) monitoring, and frequent assessment of gas exchange by arterial blood gas analysis. The pressure, flow, and volume waveforms on the ventilator interface should be constantly observed for gaining an insight into lung mechanics. Patients should be provided adequate pain relief and sedation in the postoperative period to facilitate patient–ventilator synchrony and to avoid sympathetic overactivity. Though there is an increasing trend toward fast tracking and early extubation in pediatric cardiac surgery, neonates have been recognized as a vulnerable population. Extubation is generally attempted when effective independent respiration seems likely, oxygen and ventilation requirements are sufficiently low and postoperative evaluation shows adequate cardiac recovery. Factors that contribute to delayed extubation include younger age, lung disease, prolonged CPB time, presence of genetic syndrome, need for surgical reintervention, delayed sternal closure, and pulmonary hypertension [9–11]. The weaning practices vary from institution to institution and till date a clear-cut criteria has not been established. However, the general guidelines for weaning after surgery of CHD include the following:

1. Mean airway pressure 8–9 cmH_2O (for neonates generally)
2. FiO_2 less than/or equal to 0.5
3. Hemodynamic stability with minimal inotropic support
4. Reliable rhythm (sinus or paced)
5. Absent or minimal drainage from chest drains
6. Absence of pulmonary artery hypertensive crisis
7. Appropriate neurological status to ensure airway protection
8. Chest radiograph without significant lung pathology
9. Appropriate blood gases given the underlying physiology
10. Absence of any major residual cardiac defect.

Successful extubation of most neonates is likely to occur when a low rate of mechanical ventilation is well tolerated with pressure support of spontaneous breaths. The decrease in respiratory rate is best accomplished by limiting the inspiratory time to around 0.45–0.5 s and gradually increasing expiratory time. One suggested criteria that may be followed to guide extubation include: FiO_2 <0.5, intermittent ventilation rate <10 breaths/min, PIP $\leq$ 25 cmH_2O, spontaneous effective tidal volume $\geq$6 mL/kg, and pressure support $\leq$10 cm H_2O. A course of dexamethasone, typically around 24 h in duration, around the time of extubation may expedite successful extubation by reducing airway inflammation and edema in patients who are at high risk for postextubation stridor. Prophylactic steroids have been known to reduce postextubation stridor in adults and children with airway anomalies; however, the benefits in neonatal population are unclear [12].

Extubation failure is a potential complication after neonatal cardiac surgery. This can lead to prolonged intensive care unit stay, increase complications, and increased mortality. Extubation is challenging in neonates primarily due to immature respiratory function, small caliber of the airways, and the potential for apnea and atelectasis. In a recent analysis of 156 neonates undergoing congenital heart surgery, extubation failure occurred in 16% patients. Airway diseases and mechanical ventilation longer than 7 days are significant risk factors predisposing to extubation failure in the postoperative period [13].

Conclusions

Advances in early diagnosis and improved cardiac surgical techniques have resulted in increasing number of neonates presented to the emergency department and operating room for treatment. Mechanical ventilation plays a key role in stabilizing these patients in the intensive care unit and during the perioperative period. Volume-targeted ventilator modes are being increasingly used in neonates with CHD. Given the wide diversity of CHD, an understanding of individualized pathophysiology is imperative for choosing optimum ventilatory strategy in each clinical scenario for favorable outcomes.

References

[1] Reddy SN, Kappanayil M, Balachandran R, Sudhakar A, Sunil GS, Raj BR, et al. Preoperative determinants of outcomes of infant heart surgery in a limited-resource setting. Semin Thorac Cardiovasc Surg 2015;27:331–338.

[2] Strobel AM, Lu LN. The critically ill infant with congenital heart disease. Emerg Med Clin N Am 2015;33:501–518.

[3] Shekerdemian L, Bohn D. Cardiovascular effects of mechanical ventilation. Arch Dis Child 1999;80:475–480.

[4] Pinsky MR, Summer WR. Cardiac augmentation by phasic high intrathoracic pressure support in man. Chest 1983;84:370–375.

[5] Silvestre C, Vyas H. Is permissive hypercapnia helpful or harmful? Paediatr Child Health 2014;25:192–195.

[6] Tabbutt S, Ramamoorthy C, Montenegro LM, et al. Impact of inspired gas mixtures on preoperative infants with hypoplastic left heart syndrome during controlled ventilation. Circulation 2001;104:I159–I164.

[7] Arca MJ, Uhing M, Wakeham M. Current concepts in acute respiratory support for neonates and children. Semin Pediatr Surg 2015;24:2–7.

[8] Habre W. Neonatal ventilation. Best Pract Res Clin Anaesthesiol 2010;24:353–364.

[9] Manrique AM, Feingold B, Filippo SD, et al. Extubation after cardiothoracic surgery in neonates, children and adults; one year of institutional experience. Pediatr Crit Care Med 2007;8:552–555.

[10] Harrison AM, Cox AC, Davis S, et al. Failed extubation after cardiac surgery in children; prevalence, pathogenesis and risk factors. Pediatr Crit Care Med 2002;3:148–152.

[11] Polito A, Patorno E, Costello M, et al. Peri-operative factors associated with prolonged mechanical ventilation after complex congenital heart surgery. Pediatrc Crit Care Med 2011;12:e122–126.

[12] Khemani RG, Randolph A, Markowitz B. Corticosteroids for the prevention and treatment of post extubation stridorinneonates, children and adults. Cochrane Database Syst Rev 2009;3:CD001000.

[13] Miura S, Hamamoto N, Osaki M, et al. Extubation failure in neonates after cardiac surgery: prevalence, etiology and risk factors. Ann Thorac Surg 2017;103:1293–1299.

Further reading

[14] Ewer AK, Furmston AT, Middleton LJ, Deeks JJ, Daniels JP, Pattison HM, et al. Pulse oximetry as a screening test for congenital heart defects in newborn infants: a test accuracy study with evaluation of acceptability and cost-effectiveness. Health Technol Assess 2012;16:1–184.

Chapter **30D**

Neonatal Arrhythmias

Sudeep Verma, MD, FNB, Karunakar Vadlamudi, MD, Mathew Kripail, MD, Hariram Malakunte, MD, DCH

CHAPTER POINTS

- Diagnosis of arrhythmias in neonates needs high index of suspicion as signs and symptoms are nonspecific.
- Document the rhythm disturbance by standard 12 lead plus V3R, V4R, V7 electrocardiogram.
- Decision to treat an arrhythmia should be based on hemodynamic instability not merely making the rhythm appear normal.
- Understanding the mechanism of arrhythmias is vital for appropriate management.
- Arrhythmias that present with hemodynamic comprise should be managed aggressively as per NRP/PALS guidelines.

Abbreviations

ABG	Arterial blood gas
AET	Atrial ectopic tachycardia
AF	Atrial fibrillation
AFL	Atrial flutter
ASD	Atrial septal defect
AVCD	Atrioventricular canal defect
AVRT	Atrioventricular reentrant tachycardia
AVN	Atrioventricular node
AVNRT	Atrioventricular nodal reentrant tachycardia
AVR	Accelerated ventricular rhythm
AV synchrony	Atrioventricular synchrony
AV dissociation	Atrioventricular dissociation
BPM	Beats per minute
CCTGA	Congenitally corrected transposition of great arteries
CHF	Congestive heart failure
DC	Direct current
DORV	Double outlet right ventricle
EAT	Ectopic atrial tachycardia
ECG	Electrocardiogram
ECHO	Echocardiogram
IV	Intravenous
JET	Junctional ectopic tachycardia
LBBB	Left bundle branch block
MAT	Multifocal atrial tachycardia
PAC	Premature atrial contractions
PJRT	Paroxysmal junctional reciprocating tachycardia
PSVT	Paroxysmal supraventricular tachycardia
PVC	Premature ventricular complex
RBBB	Right bundle branch block
RFA	Radiofrequency ablation
RV	Right ventricle
SVT	Supraventricular tachycardia
TAPVC	Total anomalous pulmonary venous connection
TEP	Temporary esophageal pacing
VF	Ventricular fibrillation
WPW	Wolff–Parkinson–White

Electrocardiogram (ECG) in neonates differs significantly from the normal adult pattern due to change in the hemo-dynamics and physiology after birth along with changes in position and size of the heart in relation with the body. Similarly, difference exists between term and preterm ECG, but the basic principles of interpretation remain same (Table 30D.1). The normal values of ECG from birth to 3 months of age adapted from European Society of Cardiology is given in the Table 30D.2. Incidence of arrhythmias in neonates is 1% during first 10 days of life. Fifteen percent of neonates with arrhythmia have congenital heart disease. Common arrhythmias in neonate associated with structurally normal hearts are as follows:

1. Premature atrial contractions (PAC)
2. Atrial flutter (AFL)
3. Atrioventricular reentrant tachycardia (AVRT)
4. Permanent junctional reciprocating tachycardia (PJRT)
5. Ventricular tachycardia (VT)
6. Heart block

Types of rhythm disturbances

12-lead ECG with rhythm strip is the single most important test to determine the type of arrhythmia. During the emergency situations at least rhythm strip from defibrillator should be recorded to diagnose the abnormality and to assess response to treatment (as shown in Fig. 30D.1).

In neonates the rhythm abnormalities are divided mainly into the following four groups:
1. Tachyarrhythmia: Rhythm disturbances with fast heart rate
2. Bradyarrhythmia: Rhythm disturbances with slow heart rate
3. Irregular rhythm/premature beats/(ectopics)
4. Others like bundle branch blocks (BBB), long QT syndrome (LQTS)
5. **Some normal variations**: Sinus arrhythmia, short periods of junctional rhythm, sinus pauses <2 s, atrial ectopics

---

Table 30D.1 Differences in ECG pattern of preterm and term neonates

Preterm versus term
- Shorter QRS
- Shorter PR and QT intervals
- Less RV dominance at birth
- QRS axis: 65–175 degree in preterm versus 55–200 degree in term
- Lower precordial voltages

Steps to consider in interpretation of ECG

- Rate and its variation
- QRS type (narrow or broad)
- Regular or irregular QRS
- Presence of P wave and P axis,
- P–QRS relation, AV dissociation
- Measurement of RP interval (Fig. 30D.2)
- Response to adenosine

Tachyarrhythmia: rhythm disturbances with fast heart rate

- **Increased activity of normal sinus node**: Sinus tachycardia, relative tachycardia
- **Reentrant tachycardia**: Pathway between atria and ventricles/within AV node/locally with atria/ventricle—AVRT, atrioventricular nodal reciprocating tachycardia (AVNRT), AFL or atrial fibrillation (AF)
- **Ectopic automatic focus**: Nonreciprocating tachycardia from single abnormal focus—ectopic atrial tachycardia (EAT), junctional ectopic tachycardia (JET), VT
- **Triggered activity**: Due to digoxin activity, electrolyte disturbances, and excess catecholamines

---

Rhythm	Characteristics	Conditions	Treatments
Sinus tachycardia	• Rate more than 98th percentile for that age. In the 1st week of life upper limit is 166/min while 179/min in the 1st month. But always <230/min • Regular narrow QRS, normal P-wave axis and PR interval • Begins and ends slowly • Waxing and waning present	• Pain, fever, hypovolemia, anemia • Congestive heart failure, cardiac tamponade	Identify the cause and treat the underlying etiology

Table 30D.2 Normal values for waves and intervals of ECG from birth to 3 months

Age group	Heart rate (beats/min)	Frontal plane QRS axis (degree)*	P-wave amplitude (mm)	PR interval (s)*	QRS duration V5*	Q III (mm)†	Q V6 (mm)†	R V1 (mm)‡	SV1 (mm)‡	R/S V1†	RV 6 (mm)‡	S V6 (mm)‡	R/S V6†	SV1 + RV6 (mm)†	R + SV4 (mm)†
0–1 days	93–154 (123)	+59 to +192 (135)	2.8	0.08–016 (0.11)	0.02–0.08 (0.05)	5.2	1.7	5–26	0–22.5	9.8	0–11	0–9.8	10	28	52
1–3 days	91–159 (123)	+64 to +197 (134)	2.8	0.08–0.14 (0.11)	0.02–0.07 (0.05)	5.2	2.1	5–27	0–21	6	0–12	0–9.5	11	29	52
3–7 days	90–166 (129)	+77 to +187 (132)	2.9	0.08–0.14 (0.10)	0.02–0.07 (0.05)	4.8	2.8	3–24	0–17	9.7	0.5–12	0–9.8	10	25	48
7–30 days	107–182 (149)	+65 to +160 (110)	3.0	0.07–0.14 (0.10)	0.02–0.08 (0.05)	5.6	2.8	3–21.5	0–11	7	2.5–16	0–9.5	12	22	47
1–3 months	121–179 (150)	+31 to +114 (75)	2.6	0.07–0.13 (0.10)	0.02–0.08 (0.05)	5.4	2.7	3–18.5	0–12.5	7.4	5–21	0–7.2	12	29	53

*2nd–98th percentile (mean).
†98th percentile (1 mm = 100 µV).
‡2nd–98th percentile (1 mm = 100 µV).

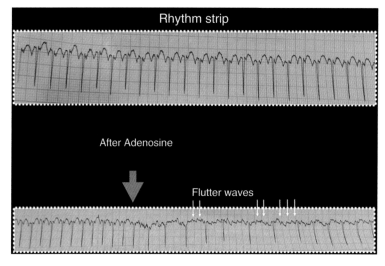

Fig. 30D.1 Rhythm strip showing SVT (above). Flutter waves are evident after Adenosine administration (below).

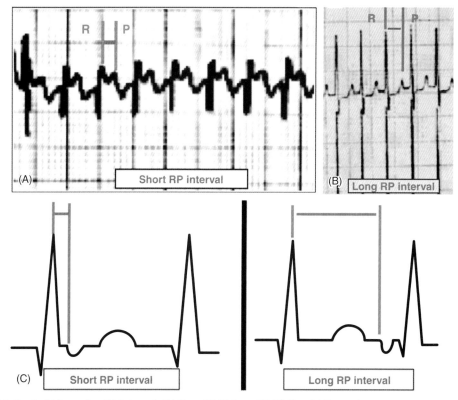

Fig. 30D.2 Method of Measuring RP Interval. (A) Short RP (B) Long RP (C) Pictorial Illustration.

Rhythm	Characteristics	Conditions	Treatments
Sinus arrhythmia	• Irregularly irregular rate with normal QRS, normal P axis	• Usually less pronounced in neonates due to fast heart rate	• No treatment required
Supraventricular tachycardia (SVT) (blanket term) Typical paroxysmal supraventricular tachycardia (PSVT)	Origin above bundle of HIS. Two ways are as follows: • **Reentrant circuits** • Abrupt onset and termination, typically referred as typical paroxysmal supraventricular tachycardia (PSVT) • 1:1 AV relationship • **Automated focus** No. 1:1 AV relationship • Rapid regular tachycardia (constant RR interval) • Rate usually 230/min • Begins and ends abruptly • Abnormal P axis or absent P-wave (in 40% cases), QRS complexes narrow in most of the SVT (90%) • AVRT: RP interval >70 ms • Atrioventricular nodal reciprocating tachycardia (AVNRT): RP interval <70 s	**Between atria and ventricles**: • Most common is atrioventricular reciprocating tachycardia (AVRT) **Others**: • AVNRT • Paroxysmal junctional reciprocating tachycardia (PJRT) **Within atria**: • Atrial flutter (AFL) • Atrial fibrillation (AF) • Atrial ectopic tachycardia (AET) • Junctional ectopic tachycardia (JET) • Most common pathological tachycardia in neonate (abnormal rhythm arises from atria, AV junction or accessory pathways)	**Stable**: • Vagal maneuvers • Adenosine • Propranolol • Digoxin **Refractory**: • Procainamide or flecainide **Unstable**: • Cardioversion • Transesophageal pacing
Wolff–Parkinson–White (WPW) syndrome (accessory pathway between atria and ventricle mediated tachycardia) (Fig. 30D.3)	• PR interval <100 ms • QRS complex duration ≥80 ms • Absence of Q waves in V6 • Left axis deviation Two of the four aforementioned criteria required for diagnosis Delta wave seen on surface ECG	• Mostly seen in structurally normal heart • Other causes: Ebstein's anomaly, CCTGA, hypertrophied cardiomyopathy and cardiac tumors	
AVNRT (Fig. 30D.4)	• Atrioventricular node reentry, P wave usually not visible, superimposed on QRS complex • AV block usually terminates tachycardia • P waves are usually obscured by QRS due to short RP interval 70 ms	• AVNRT is less common in healthy newborns • Usually associated with cardiorespiratory disorders such as congenital diaphragmatic hernia, congenital heart disease or sepsis	• Adenosine
PJRT	• Long RP tachycardia • Inverted P waves in II, III, AVF leads with P wave proceeds QRS • AV block always terminates tachycardia • Unusually slow conduction occurs over the accessory pathway, resulting in incessant behavior and a characteristically short PR interval • Can lead to tachycardia-induced cardiomyopathy if uncontrolled	• Restarts typically after cardioversion or Adenosine	**Stable**: • Beta-blocker • Amiodarone • Flecainide **Incessant/Unstable**: • Radiofrequency ablation **Maintenance**: • Flecainide

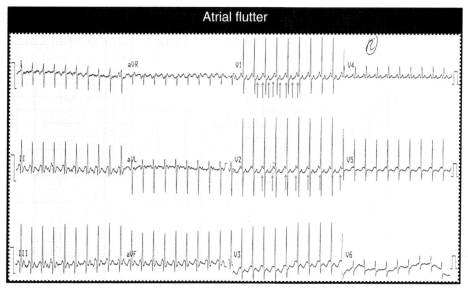

Fig. 30D.5 **ECG Showing Narrow Complex Tachycardia With Flutter Waves (Sawtooth Pattern) 2:1 Conduction Best Seen in Precordial Leads V1, V2, V4.**

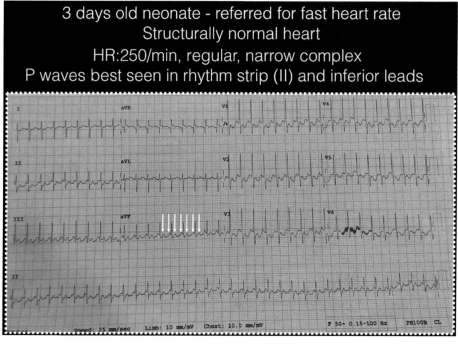

Fig. 30D.6 **ECG Showing Atrial Flutter With 2:1 Conduction.** Note: the P waves are best seen in limb leads II, III, and AVF (*arrow*), regular RR intervals, narrow QRS complexes.

(A)

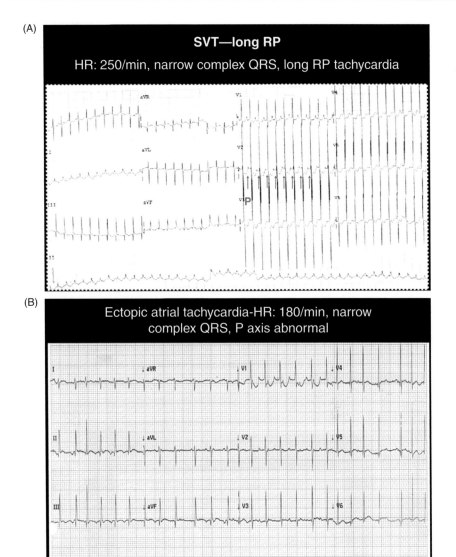

SVT—long RP

HR: 250/min, narrow complex QRS, long RP tachycardia

(B)

Ectopic atrial tachycardia-HR: 180/min, narrow complex QRS, P axis abnormal

Fig. 30D.7 (A–B) ECG showing supraventricular tachycardia (SVT)—long RP tachycardia. Ectopic atrial tachycardia (EAT). Note: the abnormal P wave and axis (*arrow*) with narrow QRS complexes.

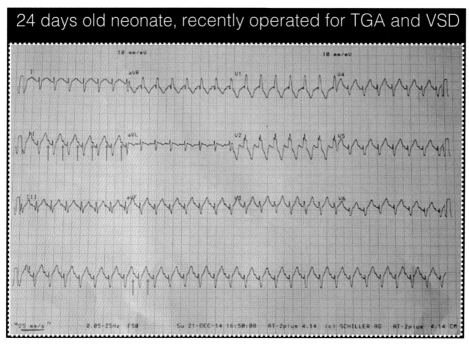

Fig. 30D.8 Postoperative ECG of a Neonate With Junctional Ectopic Tachycardia (JET) Operated for Transposition of Great Arteries (TGA) With Ventricular Septal Defect (VSD). Note: the P waves (*arrow*) inverted in limb lead II and P waves dissociated from QRS with atrial rate less than the ventricular rate.

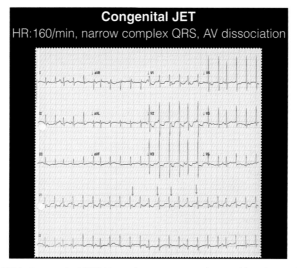

Fig. 30D.9 ECG of a Neonate With Congenital JET. Note: the narrow complexes with atrioventricular dissociation (AV dissociation).

Rhythm	Characteristics	Conditions	Treatments
Ventricular tachycardia (VT) (Fig. 30D.10)	• Rate between 200 and 500 beats/min • Abnormal QRS (not like sinus and may not be necessarily wide) • AV dissociation • T waves typically opposite to QRS polarity • At slower rate atria may be depolarized in a retrograde manner with 1:1 ventricular to atrial association • Capture beats • Narrow QRS than other beats, fusion beats • More than three ventricular complexes comprise VT	• Uncommon • The most common form of neonatal VT is an automatic mechanism arising from the right ventricular outflow tract • Myocarditis • Rare cardiac tumors (hamartomas and rhabdomyomas) • Electrolyte and metabolic abnormalities • Cardiac channelopathies such as long QT syndrome (LQTS) and Brugada syndrome	**Stable**: • Lidocaine, Procainamide **Chronic therapy**: • Beta-blocker and antiarrhythmic drugs—class IA, IB, IC, and III • Digoxin and adenosine not useful **Unstable**: • Electrical cardioversion
Polymorphic ventricular tachycardia (Fig. 30D.11)	• QRS complexes change its polarity and amplitude to appear rotating around the ECG baseline (to turn on a point) • It can deteriorate to ventricular fibrillation (VF) if not treated promptly	• LQTS—hypomagnesemia • Antiarrhythmic drug toxicity	• Correct electrolyte disturbances • Magnesium sulfate • Chronic therapy—beta-blocker
Accelerated ventricular rhythm (AVR)	• Regular wide QRS with rate (sustained/nonsustained) • <20% of the sinus rate	• Uncommon, benign rhythm in otherwise healthy neonates	• Usually no hemodynamic compromise and resolves with time
VF	• Complete chaotic rhythm—rapid and irregular rhythm with hemodynamic instability	• Consider LQTS or Brugada syndrome	• Asynchronous cardioversion • Lidocaine + Asynchronous cardioversion.

Important points for tachycardia

- Undetected prolonged tachycardia can lead to cardiac dysfunction followed by circulatory Collapse.
- Tachycardia is considered wide if QRS duration is more than 0.09 s.
- Common signs and symptoms of SVT in infants include vomiting, pale or blue skin, restless ness, irritability, unusual sleepiness, feeding difficultly and fast breathing.

- SVT is considered sustained if persists more than 30 s. Sustained SVT leads to CHF in 50% of neonates after 48 h.
- P waves may be difficult to recognize both in sinus tachycardia or SVT once the rate exceeds >200/min.
- All broad complexes in neonate should be considered as VT until proven otherwise.
- SVTs like AF and MAT are rare in neonates. AF is often associated with cardiac abnormalities, especially with LA enlargement.
- Approach to the various tachycardia is given in Figs. 30D.12–30D.14.

(A)

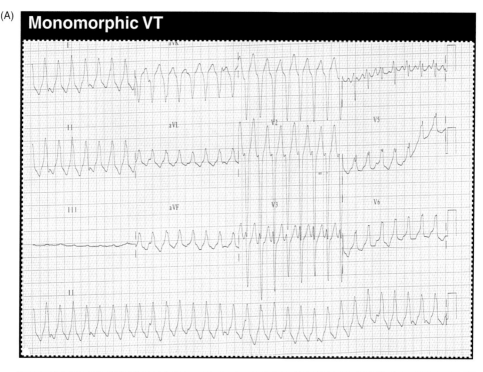

(B)

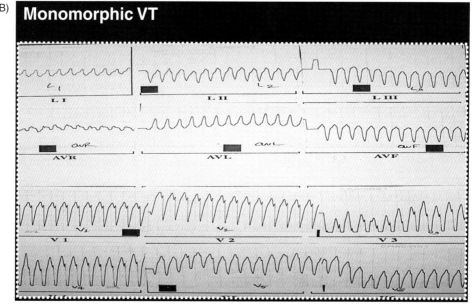

Fig. 30D.10 (A–B) ECG showing broad, uniform QRS complexes within each lead and AV dissociation suggestive of monomorphic ventricular tachycardia (VT).

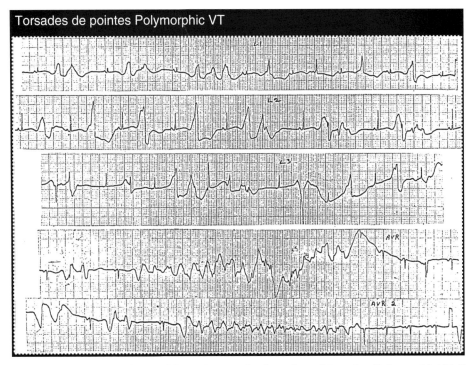

Fig. 30D.11 ECG Showing QRS Complexes With Varying Amplitude, Axis, and Duration (Polymorphic VT). Note: the QRS complexes twist around the isoelectric line (Torsades de pointes).

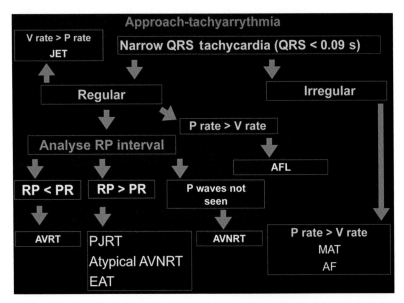

Fig. 30D.12 An Approach to Tachyarrhythmias. *AF*, Atrial fibrillation; *AFL*, atrial flutter; *AVNRT*, atrioventricular nodal reentrant tachycardia; *AVRT*, atrioventricular reentrant tachycardia; *EAT*, ectopic atrial tachycardia; *JET*, junctional ectopic tachycardia; *MAT*, multifocal atrial tachycardia; *PJRT*, paroxysmal junctional reciprocating tachycardia; *P rate*, atrial rate; *V rate*, ventricular rate.

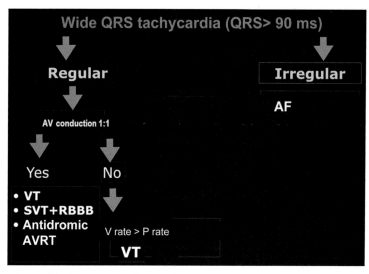

Fig. 30D.13 An Approach to Wide QRS Tachycardia. *AVRT*, Atrioventricular reentrant tachycardia; *P rate*, atrial rate; *RBBB*, right bundle branch block; *SVT*, supraventricular tachycardia; *V rate*, ventricular rate; *VT*, ventricular tachycardia.

Tachycardia	Nature	RP interval	Adenosine response	Mechanism
AVRT	Paroxysmal/ Incessant	Short	Terminate	Reentrant
AVNRT	Paroxysmal	Short	Terminate	Reentrant
WPW	Paroxysmal/ Incessant	Short	Terminate	Reentrant
PJRT	Incessant	Long	Terminate	Reentrant
EAT	Paroxysmal/ Incessant	Long	None/ Terminate	Automatic
MAT	Paroxysmal	Long	None/ Terminate	Automatic
JET	Incessant	AV dissociation	None/slow down	Automatic
AFL	Paroxysmal/ Incessant	Long	AV block	Reentrant

Fig. 30D.14 Features of Various Tachycardias. *AVNRT*, Atrioventricular nodal reentrant tachycardia; *AVRT*, atrioventricular reentrant tachycardia; *EAT*, ectopic atrial tachycardia; *JET*, junctional ectopic tachycardia; *MAT*, multifocal atrial tachycardia; *PJRT*, paroxysmal junctional reciprocating tachycardia; *WPW*, Wolff–Parkinson–White.

Premature beats and pauses

Rhythm	Characteristics	Causes	Treatments
Sinus pauses (Fig. 30D.15)	• Sinus pauses are usually followed by escape beats from the atria or the atrioventricular (AV) junction • Pauses of more than 2 s are considered abnormal	• May occur in healthy newborns	• Usually no treatment is needed • Long pause may indicate LQTS
Atrial ectopics (Fig. 30D.16)	• Premature P wave having different morphology and axis compared to sinus P wave • May or may not conduct to ventricles with or without block • If significant number of PAC's are blocked it produces bradycardia • Can initiate or terminate SVT	• Common in neonates • Mostly benign in nature and tend to decline within few postnatal weeks • Can occur with digitalis toxicity • PACs are the most common type of arrhythmias in neonates	• Benign no treatment is required • Digitalis toxicity management
Ventricular ectopics (Fig. 30D.17)	• Usually abnormal QRS with normal/prolonged QRS duration (up to 0.08 ms) not similar to sinus rhythm without preceding P wave • Usually followed by a full compensatory pause	• Isolated PVC's are normally seen in healthy neonates • Frequent and sustained PVC's rarely denotes diseased heart • When occur in groups of two or three (couplets or triplets) may denote myocardial dysfunction	• Address underlying cause • Usually no treatment is required • More worrisome if underlying heart disease present or due to myocardial dysfunction or in couplets
Premature junctional complexes	• Premature origin of beats from AV node or proximal bundle of HIS • Narrow normal QRS complexes with usually absent P or P seen after QRS	• Isolated junctional ectopics are seen with normal hearts	• If not due to underlying structural heart disease—no treatment is required

Important points about premature/ectopic beats

• Ectopic beats are commonly seen in 30% of healthy preterm and term infants.
• It may be unifocal (uniform PVC's) or multifocal (different QRS complexes).
• PAC's are the most common rhythm abnormalities in the neonate.

Bradyarrhythmia: rhythm disturbances with low heart rate

Primary: Due to depolarization of pacemaker cells or decrease conduction through the cardiac conduction system. Example: myocarditis, surgical heart block

Secondary: Due to alteration of normal functioning of the heart causing slowing down of sinus node pacemaker or conduction through AV node. Example: hypoxia

Symptomatic bradycardia: Cardinal signs of unstable hemodynamics with bradycardia like shock with hypotension, poor end organ perfusion, altered consciousness, respiratory failure, and sudden collapse

(A)

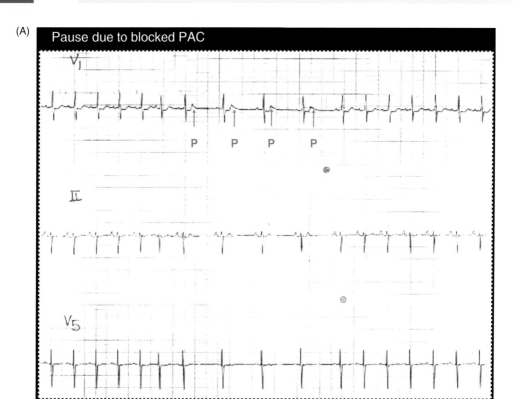

(B)

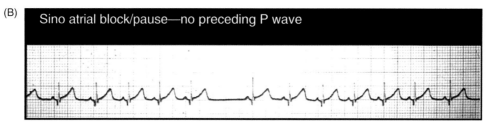

Fig. 30D.15 (A–B) ECG displaying the typical pattern of frequent premature atrial contractions (PAC) (*arrows*) followed by pause (blocked PAC). Note: the prolonged RR interval.

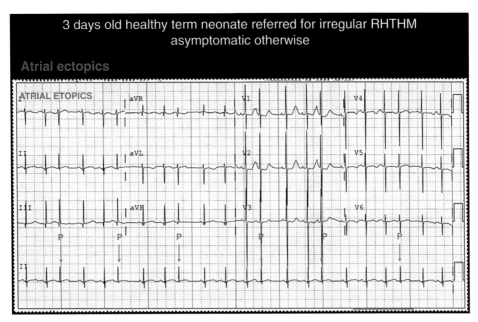

Fig. 30D.16 Atrial Ectopic Beats.

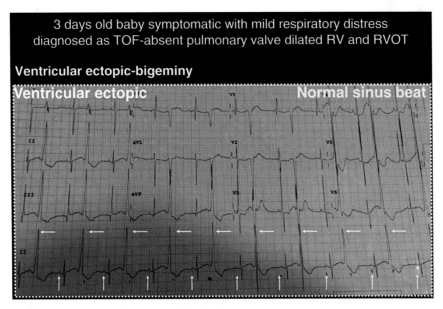

Fig. 30D.17 Ventricular ectopics (*horizontal arrows*) with bigeminy.

Rhythm	Characteristics	Causes	Treatments
Sinus bradycardia	• Heart rate lower than normal for age • During 1st week lower limit is 91/min (2nd percentile) while it is 107/min at 2nd percentile during 1st month of life	• Usually secondary to underlying systemic illness—hypothermia, hypothyroidism, acidosis, hypoxia, hypoglycemia, etc. • Most common pathological cause is hypoxia • Propranolol or digoxin may be the causative mechanism • 20%–90% of healthy neonates may show features of transient bradycardia like sinus bradycardia, sinus pauses, and junctional escape • May be result of stressful labor	• Treat underlying cause • If symptomatic and heart rate less than 60/min and poor perfusion, then begin CPR • If not improved Epinephrine (0.01–0.03 mg/kg/dose) • Atropine (0.02 mg/kg) minimum dose 0.1 mg/dose and maximum 2 mg/dose) • Isoprenaline (0.02 mcg/kg/min, maximum dose of 0.5 mcg/kg/min) • Temporary transvenous cardiac pacing
First-degree heart block (Fig. 30D.18)	• Slowed conduction through the AV node resulting in PR interval prolongation • Usually not associated with diseased conduction system	• Electrolyte disturbances and associated with some CHD such as DORV, ASD, AVCD, CCTGA, Ebstein's anomaly • Drugs that prolong the PR interval. Example: Digoxin	• Treat underlying cause, otherwise no treatment required
Second-degree heart block (Mobitz type I) (Fig. 30D.18)	• Intermittent block of conduction of atrial beats to the ventricle resulting in dropped QRS complexes • Progressive lengthening of the PR interval until a QRS is dropped and the cycle starts again with a shorter PR interval that progressively lengthens • Usually indicates block in the AV node	• Wenckebach conduction occurs in healthy neonates	• Address underlying cause otherwise no treatment needed
Second-degree heart block (Mobitz type II) (Fig. 30D.18)	• Patterned dropping of QRS complex with a fixed ratio of atrial depolarization's (P waves) to conducted beats with a consistent PR interval throughout • Higher risk than Mobitz I • Variation in the RR interval distinguishes second-degree from third-degree AV block	• May progress to complete heart block • Occasionally, infants who have congenital LQTS present with bradycardia due to second-degree AV block	• Treat underlying cause • If symptomatic with low ventricular rate, then may need pacemaker
Third-degree heart block (complete heart block) (Fig. 30D.19)	• Complete block of AV node resulting in AV dissociation between atrial and ventricular events • No relationship between the P waves and QRS complexes with regular RR intervals and regular PP intervals. • Atrial rate > ventricular rate.	• Neonatal heart block is associated with maternal autoimmune disease, that is, systemic lupus • Complex CHD or rarely infective causes like myocarditis	• Emergency pacing is indicated in all symptomatic neonates, wide complex escape rhythm, asymptotic neonates with rate <55/bpm and cardiomegaly

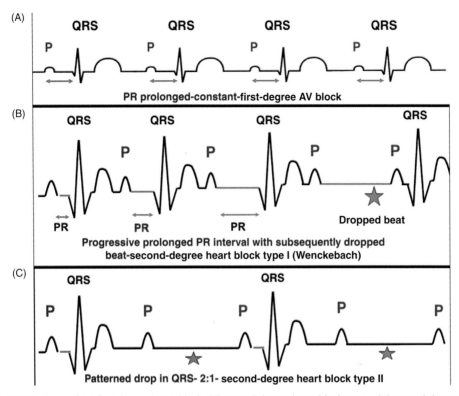

Fig. 30D.18 ECG features of (A) first-degree heart block, (B) second-degree heart block-type I, (C) second-degree heart block type II.

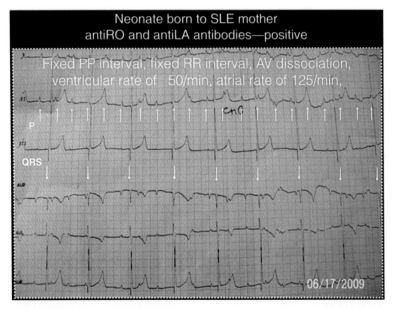

Fig. 30D.19 Complete Heart Block.

Others

Long QT syndrome

If QT interval is greater than 50% of RR interval, then diagnosis of LQTS is evident. Otherwise in a suspected case of LQTS or positive family history, Adrenaline test is required to diagnose it (Figs. 30D.20 and 30D.21).

Bundle branch block

- RBBB/LBBB very rare in neonates, usually associated with structural heart disease like RBBB with prolonged PR seen with Ebstein's/postcardiac surgery.
- LBBB is seen with myocarditis/severe cardiomyopathy. Hereditary BBB is an autosomal dominant inherited disease. Left anterior fascicular block are seen with AVCD, tricuspid atresia.

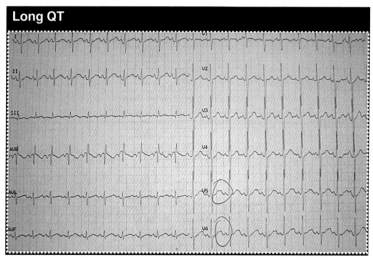

Fig. 30D.20 ECG showing long QT interval (depicted in *circles*).

Evaluation and management protocol

1. To assess hemodynamic status of the neonate
2. Support airway, breathing, maintain temperature
3. IV access, intubation if needed
4. Emergency treatment for unstable arrhythmia (DC shock) and later to assess type and nature
5. If stable, then 12-lead ECG to decide type and nature of rhythm disturbance
6. Risk factor for arrhythmia—to rule out secondary causes like 7H, 5Ts (see later)
7. Antenatal and drug history
8. Assessment with serum electrolytes, ECHO (to rule out associated structural heart disease, ventricular function), arterial/venous blood gas
9. Management of rhythm disturbances—acute and long term
10. Requirement of inotropes and diuretics
11. Need for invasive therapy, radiofrequency ablation
12. Follow-up and chronic therapy

Management of arrhythmia in neonates

General points

- Most important decision in managing neonatal rhythm disturbances is to assess first hemodynamic instability.
- If baby have no signs of circulation/pulseless or having signs of poor perfusion, then consider it as impending arrest and act according to Pediatric and Neonatal Advanced Life Support (PALS and NALS) guidelines.
- With hemodynamic compromise, immediate treatment is to perform synchronized cardioversion for SVT and defibrillation—DC shock for VT.
- During every step of management, maintain airways, oxygenation, and circulation.
- Always try to identify the reversible causes (7H)—hypovolemia, hypoxia, hydrogen ion (acidosis), hypothermia, hypoglycemia, hypokalemia/hyperkalemia, hypomagnesemia, and 5T—toxins/drugs, tamponade, tension pneumothorax, thrombosis, trauma (Fig. 30D.22).

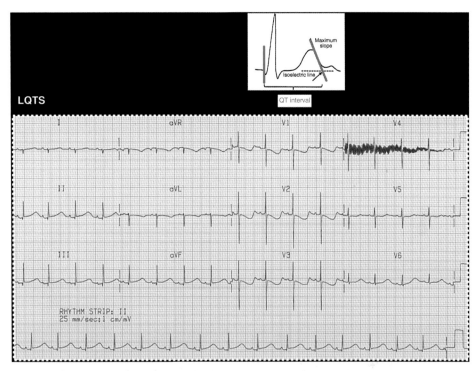

Fig. 30D.21 **Method of Measuring QT Interval and ECG Showing Long QT Interval.**

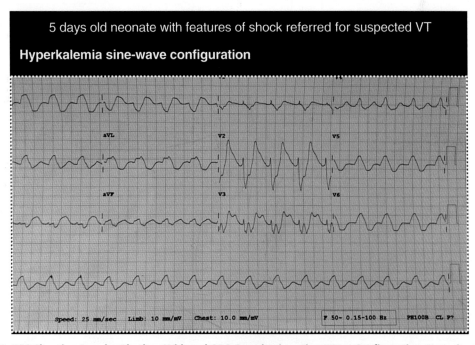

Fig. 30D.22 **ECG Showing Regular Rhythm, Widened QRS Complex in a Sine-Wave Configuration.** Note: there are no discernible P waves. The T waves fused with the widened QRS complexes.

Specific treatment

1. **Vagal maneuvers**: Initiate diving reflex by placing bagged iced over the nasal bridge for 10 s to maximum of 30 s.
2. **Cardioversion**: Usually, reentry tachycardias respond well to DC cardioversion, while tachycardias due to abnormal focus (JET/EAT/PJRT) do not respond. Paddle size for neonates and up to 10 kg is 4.5 cm.
   a. **Synchronized**: Used for unstable patients with SVT, VT with pulses, and AFL who have a perfusing rhythm with evidence of cardiovascular compromise. Used electively for selected stable SVT, AFL, or VT. Start with dose of 0.25–0.5 J/kg for SVT/VT with a pulse with cardiovascular instability. Augment every time by 50%–100% with maximum dose is 2 J/kg. If no response, then reevaluate the diagnosis of SVT and check the reversible causes.
   b. **Unsynchronized/Defibrillation**: Pulseless arrest with VT/VF (shockable rhythm). It is used in

between CPR but not for asystole or pulseless electrical activity. Initiate with dose of 1–2 J/kg followed by 4 J/kg. If still arrhythmia persists, then again use 4 J/kg.

3. **Adenosine**: Drug of choice for SVT. To be administered as fast as possible in view of short half-life of 10 s. It acts by producing transient AV conduction block. Dose required 0.1 mg/kg followed by 0.2 mg/kg. It should be given using two syringes connected to a stopcock or three-way T-connector followed by rapid normal saline bolus flush (Fig. 30D.1).
4. **Antiarrhythmic drugs**: If vagal maneuver or adenosine fails in a stable patient, then consult pediatric cardiologist. Usually, digoxin and/or beta-blocker are the first line agents. Other drugs that can be used are Amiodarone, Flecainide, Procainamide, Sotalol, Quinidine, etc. Verapamil should not be used in infants, as it has been associated with irreversible electromechanical dissociation and sudden death. Flecainide and Sotalol were proved to be effective in

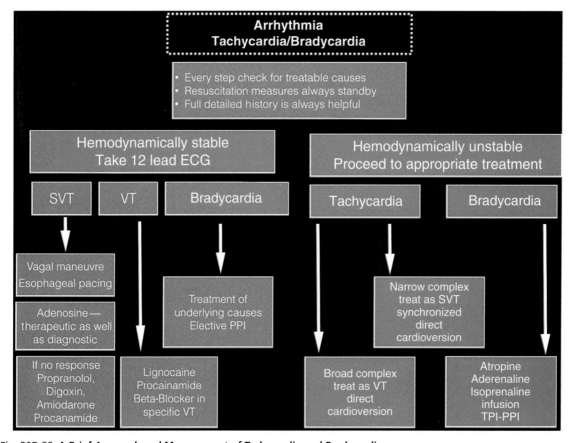

Fig. 30D.23 **A Brief Approach and Management of Tachycardia and Bradycardia.**

case of refractory SVT either alone or in combination. In case of unstable SVT not responded with two doses of shock, then consider Amiodarone or Procainamide.

5. **Transoesophageal pacing (TEP)**: Whenever available or feasible TEP is effective in terminating tachyarrhythmias. Burst pacing through TEP may help in terminating reentrant type of SVT.

6. **Maintenance therapy**: In an easily reverted Adenosine reentrant tachycardia, drug of choice is long-acting Beta-blocker. If status is not known or in case of WPW syndrome: Propranolol, 0.5 mg/kg/dose should be given by oral route in divided doses. Neonate

presenting with shock or in patients where tachycardia was difficult to control or patients who required intravenous Amiodarone, more potent drugs like Sotalol/Amiodarone/Flecainide is required alone or in combination. Digoxin should be used in combination with beta-blocker/Flecainide. Digoxin dose should be reduced to half when given along with Amiodarone.

7. **Radiofrequency ablation**: Reserved for difficult arrhythmia unable to control with medications like PJRT.

8. Approach to the treatment of various rhythm disturbances is given in the Fig. 30D.23.

Further reading

[1] White AJ. Washington manual of pediatrics. 2nd ed. Wolters Kluwer; 2016.

[2] Gleason C, Devaskar S. Avery diseases of the newborn. 9th ed. Elsevier Health Sciences; 2012.

[3] Cloherty JP, Eichenwald EC, Hansen AR, Stark AR. Manual of neonatal care. 7th ed. Wolters Kluwer Health/Lippincott Williams and Wilkins; 2012.

[4] Killen SAS, Fish FA. Fetal and neonatal arrhythmias. Neoreviews 2008;9: e242–e252.

[5] Allen H, Gutgesell H, Clark E, Driscoll D. 6th ed. Moss and Adams'

Heart disease in infants, children and adolescents including the fetus and the young, vol. 1. Philadelphia: Lippincott Williams and Wilkins; 2001.

[6] Kothari S, Skinner JR. Neonatal tachycardias: an update. Arch Dis Child Fetal Neonatal Ed 2006;91: F136–F144.

[7] Schwartz PJ, Garson A, Paul T, Stramba-Badiale M, Vetter VL, Villain E, et al. A Task Force of the European Society of Cardiology. Guidelines for the interpretation of the neonatal

electrocardiogram. Eur Heart J 2002;23: 1329–1344.

[8] Andre D, Rautahariu P, Boisselle E, Soumis F, Megelas M, Choquette A. Normal ECG standards for infants and children. Pediatr Cardiol 1979–80;1: 123–152.

[9] Kleinman ME, Chameides L, Schexnayder SM, et al. Pediatric Advanced Life Support. 2010 American Heart Association Guidelines for cardiopulmonary resuscitation and emergency cardiovascular care. Circulation 2010;122:S876–S908.

Chapter | 31A |

Neonatal Shock Management

Abbas Hyderi, MD, FRCPC, FAAP, R.V. Jeya Balaji MD, Karunakar Vadlamudi, MD

CHAPTER POINTS

- Pathophysiology of shock in newborns is unique since it is associated with physiologic transition from fetal circulation to neonatal circulation at birth.
- The key to the management of shock in the newborn period is early identification and determination of etiology to provide appropriate care.
- Frequent reassessment and close monitoring are essential to prevent progression to irreversible shock
- Selecting an inotrope or vasopressor is determined by the cause of shock and the desired therapeutic activity targeting the underlying pathogenesis.
- Vasopressors should be initiated in refractory hypotension despite adequate fluid resuscitation.

Introduction

Hypotension in a newborn has been traditionally used interchangeably as neonatal shock erroneously. Neonatal shock is a more complex cellular phenomenon and usually an end result of homeostasis and disequilibrium due to interplay between cardiovascular (CV), respiratory, and neurohumoral systems among others. What makes this pathophysiologic state even more dramatic and challenging is the fact that neonate is in the process of "adaptation" of circulations especially in the extremely premature and prone to multiple disease states while critically ill.

Definition

Shock can be defined in many ways, but a commonly known definition is that shock is a state of cellular and tissue hypoxia due to reduced oxygen delivery and/or increased oxygen consumption or inadequate oxygen utilization. In other words, shock is simply a state of "mismatch" of metabolic supply and demand at the cellular level, but not merely a numerical low value of blood pressure (BP) as may be often mistaken.

Stages of shock

Classically, shock "phases" are usually classified as follows:
1. Compensated (vital organ function maintained by compensatory mechanisms).
2. Uncompensated (failure of compensatory mechanisms, clinically presents with features systemic hypoperfusion [e.g., low BP, lactic acidosis, oliguria, poor cap refill time, and so on]).
3. Irreversible (in the event of persistence of aforementioned, progresses to irreparable cell damage and cell death/tissue necrosis).

Types of shock

Classically, shock "types" are usually denoted as hypovolemic shock, cardiogenic, and distributive shock. However, certain subtypes exist depending on clinical situation and age groups, including septic shock, anaphylactic shock, or neurogenic shock.

Shock pathophysiology

To understand the pathophysiology it may be important to review some hemodynamic terms in context of the cardiac cycle. Details of fetal, transitional, and postnatal circulation are well-detailed elsewhere in the book and reader is thus referred. Some hemodynamic concepts are as follows:

- Ideally hemodynamic equilibrium → $(VO_2 = DO_2)$ where VO_2, oxygen consumption and DO_2 is oxygen delivery to the tissue. Loss of this equilibrium leads to shock
- BP: Force exerted by circulating blood on the walls of arterial vessels
- Pulse pressure (PP) = Systolic – Diastolic BP and Mean BP (MBP) = DBP + one-third PP
- Cardiac output (CO) = Stroke volume (SV) × Heart rate (HR)
- SV is volume blood ejected with each beat effected by preload, contractility and afterload
- BP = CO × Systemic vascular resistance (SVR) or SVR = BP/CO (used in estimating SVR)
- Systemic flow = Velocity (v) × Cross-sectional area (CSA)
- Cerebral perfusion pressure (CPP) = MBP − Intracranial pressure (ICP)
- DO_2 (in mL/min) = Blood flow (Q) × Arterial oxygen content (CaO_2)
- CaO_2 = Arterial O_2 content depends on O_2 bound to hemoglobin (Hb) + Dissolved O_2
- CaO_2 content calculated as = [1.34 × Hb (g/dL) × SaO_2] + [0.0031 × PaO_2 (mmHg)] and expressed as mL/dL
- CvO_2 = Venous oxygen content = [1.34 × Hb (g/dL) × SvO_2] + [0.0031 × PvO_2 (mmHg)] and expressed as mL/dL
- Tissue oxygen extraction is estimated as CaO_2 − CvO_2 or SaO_2 − SvO_2 if further simplified
- VO_2 = (O_2 consumption) − VO_2 (initially not effected by decrease in flow until tissues capacity to extract O_2 is exhausted, at this point VO_2 becomes directly flow-dependent) [1]
- Regional tissue saturation (rSO_2)* of vital organs like brain, renal, intestine, and so on.
- FOE* = (Fractional oxygen extraction) fraction of tissue O_2 consumed (0.15–0.33) [2,3]
- TOI* = Tissue oxygen index is the ratio of oxygenated HbO_2 to total Hb (55%–85%) [2,3]
- V/Q ratio = Ventilation perfusion ratio is currently being able to be estimated (>0.8–1)

*Derived by near infrared spectroscopy (NIRS). For example, if SaO_2 is 92% and SvO_2 is 77%. Then FOE is 15 or 0.15% (normal range).

Lastly, to summarize from above, **shock is a state where delivery of oxygen (DO_2) not able to meet the cellular oxygen demand/consumption in tissue (VO_2).** Hence, to reverse chock the six prominent variables of shock in the CaO_2 equation need to be manipulated to regain hemodynamic equilibrium/*clinical reversal of shock*. Key factors are HR, preload, contractility, afterload, Hb, SaO_2 (%). Furthermore, the complex interaction of various factors in maintaining hemodynamics is shown in Fig. 31A.1, with the common goal to constantly maintain and "match"—the supply and demand (the "center" in Fig. 31A.1).

Pathophysiological correlates of neonatal disease states

Using the aforementioned principles and abnormality of each variable, a number of common disease states present in the newborn period. A good understanding/detection of pathophysiological derangement is paramount in trying to reverse the reachieved hemodynamic equilibrium. Tools to assess are described in next section. Most common tool in today's NICU is the use of targeted neonatal echocardiography (TnE) for a real time assessment of CV hemodynamics. A succinct pictorial summary of *pathophysiological* correlates of neonatal disease states is described later (Fig. 31A.2) [5].

What is normal blood pressure in neonate? **Correct answer is**: this question has not been answered by literature, as far as 2018.

There are large variations in NICU practice across the globe in determination as to what is normal BP. Most centers use a simplified "thumb rule." Across the spectrum, there are at least 15 definitions based on various studies. No single definition is widely accepted, but 3–4 are most commonly used and reported in studies. The "thumb rule" of MBP less than GA (gestational age) has no pathophysiologic or evidence basis and based from a consensus of experts for respiratory distress syndrome (RDS) in a Joint Working Group British Association Perinatal Medicine, 1992 [6].

In 2006, a Canadian survey of neonatologist ($n = 95$) was sought, albeit no consensus arrived. Great variation in practice regarding when to intervene and with what agent(s) and at what threshold. Most common BP definition used was the aforesaid thumb rule MBP < GA followed by Watkins et al. [7], Zubrow et al. [8], and Miall-Allen et al. [9]. See later for discussion on various BP criteria. Most common volume expander used in this survey was normal saline. Most common treatment regimen was Volume–Dopamine–Hydrocortisone (32% of responders) next closely followed by regimen Volume–Dopamine–Dobutamine (29% of responders) [10].

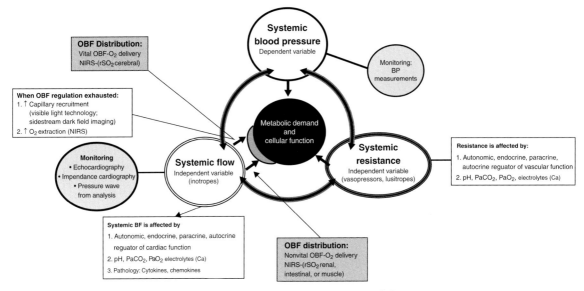

Fig. 31A.1 Hemodynamic Equilibrium and Factors Affecting Each Component [4].

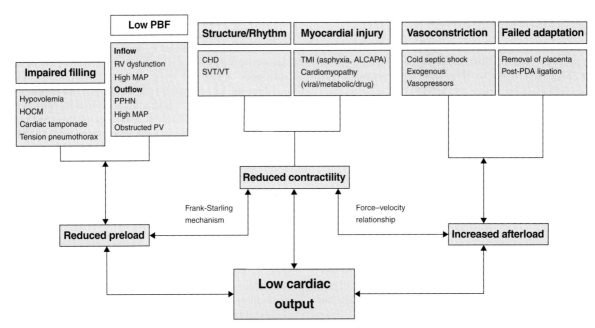

Fig. 31A.2 Factors Contributing to Low Cardiac Output With Clinical Examples [5]. *ALCAPA*, Anomalous left coronary arising from pulmonary artery; *CHD*, congenital heart disease; *HOCM*, hypertrophic obstructive cardiomyopathy; *MAP*, mean airway pressure; *PDA*, patent ductus arteriosus; *PPHN*, persistent pulmonary hypertension; *PV*, pulmonary veins, *RV*, right ventricle; *SVT*, supraventricular tachycardia; *TMI*, transient myocardial ischemia; *VT*, ventricular tachycardia. Modified with permission from Giesinger RE, McNamara PJ. Hemodynamic instability in the critically ill neonate: an approach to cardiovascular support based on disease pathophysiology. Semin Perinatol 2016;40(3):174–188 [5].

Furthermore, in 2014 further exploration led to a larger international survey of about 26,000 very low birth weight (VLBW) infants across 38 countries which was published using a web-based questionnaire [11]. The majority of respondents (73%) used the thumb rule of MBP in mmHg as less than GA in weeks, as the "cut off" to determine hypotension. However, 60% of respondents used additional assessment tools including echocardiography being the most commonly used in about 74% of them. A prospective study by Lee et al. in neonates in first 24 h and by 12–24 h MBP in mmHg was noted to trend toward GA in weeks. The MBP in first 12 h was lower potentially pointing toward a fact that MBP improves on an hourly basis [12]. The specific "normative" data on BP in 23–25 weeks of GA within 7 days of life was published in 2007 [13]. This study further quantified the previous study's [12] principle that BP continuously improves even in absence of intervention in first 48 h. It was noted that MBP improves by 0.3 mm/h in first 24 h, whereas the next 24 h rate of rise slows down to 0.1 mm/h, thereafter stable plateau graph is obtained [13,14].

Interestingly, in the same publication [11] about 80% of neonatologist stated they would consider "permissive hypotension" approach on nonintervention in a clinical setting where a numerical value below the thumb rule but without signs of poor organ perfusion on assessment [11–15]. A detailed subsection on assessment of hemodynamic derangement in organ perfusion follows.

Historically, classical studies like Miall-Allen et al. have shown that preterm neonates <30 weeks with MBP <30 mmHg is associated with an increased incidence of severe neurologic lesions and/or deaths than those infants with a MBP > 30 mmHg ($P < 0.01$) [9]. This abrupt value of 30 mmHg is sometimes informally often referred to as "Allen's" cut off. There is some pathophysiologic argument supporting these numbers (see Section: The Autoregulation).

Watkins et al. [7] also corroborated previous study finding that hypotension (defined < 10th centile) associated with intraventricular hemorrhage ($P < 0.0005$) and mortality. They also arrived at an equation in estimating MBP. The so called *Watkins formula* for (mean) MBP in first 96 h of VLBW infants is ([31.6] + [0.1 × hours of life] + [0.0057 × BW]) [7]. Many authors have used BP curves generated by various authors and common ones include Zubrow et al. [16], Nuntramuit [17], Bada et al. [18], Versmold et al. [19], Goldstein et al. [20], Cunningham et al. [21] (Table 31A.1).

Lastly, despite so many variations in BP definitions, it is clear that no one definition is superior. For purpose of this review we have chosen to use either the northern neonatal initiative (NNI) [23] or the Zubrow's graphs [22]. The Zubrow's graphs were cumulative data of 1–99 days in about 600 infants admitted to 14 NICUs' in the United States and also data generated by Philadelphia [16]. Similarly, the NNI data are robustly collected with ~400 infants in the United Kingdom, and give a comprehensive BP assessment from 3rd centile to 97th centile of SBP, DBP, or MBP (Table 31A.2).

Hence, by choosing hypotension as BP <3rd centile, it allowed us to "correct or reverse" the hemodynamic abnormality based on specific pathophysiology contributing to hypotension.

Lastly, it must be again noted here that simply a BP value <3rd centile for age/GA may not mean the infant is in shock as infant may have minimal to no metabolic supply/demand "mismatch." This phenomenon is further clarified with autoregulation (AR) and NIRS later.

The autoregulation

AR is an inherent vascular property of a vascular bed/tissue where vessel dynamics are altered by neuroendocrine

Table 31A.1 Normative data on blood pressure (BP) commonly quoted in literature and used worldwide [9–23]

Author (year)	Definition BP	Type study and number (n)	References
Miall-Allen et al. (1987)	MBP < 30 mmHg	Prospective ($n = 33$)	[9]
Watkins et al. (1989)	Weight-based criteria	Retrospective ($n = 131$)	[7]
Cunningham et al. (1999)	MBP < 10th centiles	Retrospective ($n = 232$)	[21]
Goldstein et al. (1995)	SBP < 35 mm (<750 g)	Prospective ($n = 191$)	[20]
Lee et al. (1999)	Graphs by lower 95% CI	Prospective ($n = 61$)	[12]
Versmold et al. (1981)	Graphs 1st 12 h	Prospective ($n = 16$)	[19]
Bada et al. (1990)	Graphs 1st 48 h as ±2SD	Prospective ($n = 72$)	[18]
Zubrow et al. (1995)	Graphs > 24 h until 99 days	Prospective ($n = 608$)	[16]
Batton et al. (2007)	Graphs BP 5th–95th centiles	Retrospective ($n = 142$)	[13]
McNamara et al. (2016)	Graphs 3rd–97th centiles	Prospective ($n = 398$)	[23]

Table 31A.2 Normal neonatal BP centiles (northern neonatal nursing initiative) [23]

GA (weeks)	Systolic (mmHg)	Diastolic (mmHg)	Mean (mmHg)
24	32	15	26
25	34	16	26
26	36	17	27
27	38	17	27
28	40	18	28
29	42	19	28
30	43	20	29
31	45	20	30
32	46	21	30
33	47	22	30
34	48	23	31
35	49	24	32
36	50	25	32

Blood pressures thresholds–3rd percentile as per gestational age. *GA*, Gestational age; *mmHg*, Millimeter mercury.

pathways with a goal of preservation of end organ perfusion. This property of the arteries has a limited capacity and as a result blood flow to the tissue will decrease when BP is below a "critical threshold."

AR can be static or dynamic. The dynamic AR (measuring before steady state) seems not to exist in preterm infant [24]. However, the static AR (measuring at steady state) is developed albeit at a lower threshold. AR plateau has a classical relation between MBP and cerebral blood flow (CBF) (Fig. 31A.3).

The AR plateau for CBF and its lower threshold in a preterm newborn is found to be at 30 mmHg while upper threshold is not exactly known. It is reasonable assumption that ischemic threshold is about 50% of resting blood flow. It is assumed in preterm infants that critical closing pressure (CrCP) is near MBP (note: CPP = MBP − CrCP).

Various animal studies have corroborated this AR concept and the CBF–BP interaction. In newborn lambs, AR could be completely abolished for ~7 h with a 20-min hypoxemia [25]. The classical beagle puppy study in 1982 where rapid BP fluctuation induced by hypovolemia/hypotension and volume expansion leads to IVH similar to that seen in premature infants. The plausible explanation was that cerebral circulation had "lost autoregulation" (pressure passive circulation) and was in a compensatory "protective" state, when vessels were maximally dilated while

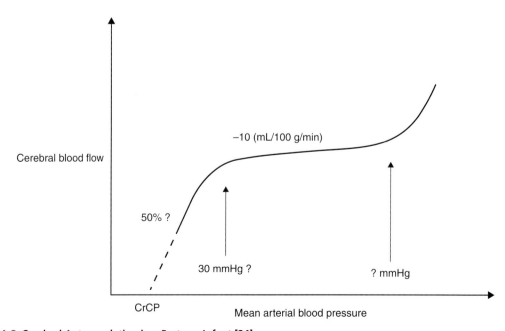

Fig. 31A.3 Cerebral Autoregulation in a Preterm Infant [24].

The perils of rapid volume expansion have been studied and include higher incidence of BPD, increased IVH [53]. Greenough et al. in 2002 have shown consistent association between increased colloid use and poorer long-term neurodevelopmental outcomes [54]. A Cochrane meta-analysis in 2014 overall suggested higher fluid intakes were associated with a trend toward increased mortality but these trends were not statistically significant [55]. Volume expansion has no effect on cerebral oxygen delivery as compared to a cardiotropic medications (e.g., Dopamine) which provide small increase in cerebral oxygen delivery measured by NIRS data [56].

Furthermore, volume expansion at birth or delayed cord clamping or cord milking has regained interest in the neonatal literature in prevention of hypotension and optimization of fetal hemoglobin and its favorable oxygen binding properties. Other maneuvers to improve volume of blood reaching the cardia include weaning excessive mean airway pressure especially while on the oscillation and/or prompt identification and drainage of air leaks.

Hence, currently unless there is an evidence of intravascular volume loss or hypoalbuminemia; initial volume expansion is recommended as empiric normal saline 0.9% or lactated Ringer's solution up to maximum 10–20 mL/kg/dose. Should this be ineffective in correcting hemodynamic derangement then a detailed clinical assessment is mandatory ideally with a TnE to search for the cause. An interesting and extensive review of all studies in this area has been provided by Evans and its summary reemphasizes avoidance of repeated fluid bolus beyond 20 mL/kg/day without an obvious etiology in prevention of the "Michelin Man" appearance (generalized edema) [57].

Dopamine

Dopamine is a sympathomimetic and a naturally occurring precursor of noradrenaline/adrenaline. It is released by stress, the adrenal medulla, and neural tissues endogenously. According to many surveys, Dopamine is the most commonly used inotrope in NICU today; approximately 25% of Dopamine is converted to noradrenaline endogenously [5]. As we note from Tables 31A.3 and 31A.4, relative actions of Dopamine are concentrated on peripheral alpha-1, alpha-2 receptors (++++), and cardiac beta-1 receptors (++++) with reduced peripheral beta-2 action (++) and receptor stimulation of dopaminergic receptors. It exerts CV effects via dose-dependent stimulation of dopaminergic-, alpha-, beta-receptors. Dopamine also has serotonergic actions. In addition, by stimulating epithelial, peripheral neuronal dopaminergic, and adrenergic receptors, Dopamine activates dopaminergic receptors and the resultant renal and endocrinal effects are independent of CV effects [58].

Dopamine affects all three major determinants of CV function (preload, contractility, and afterload). By decreasing venous capacitance improves preload [59]. Contractility and afterload is mediated by beta-receptors and peripheral alpha/beta, respectively [58].

At lower doses (0.5–5 µg/kg/min), dopaminergic receptors are activated potentially stimulating vasodilatation in the renal, mesenteric, and coronary vascular beds [58]. There is, however, considerable controversy regarding the vasodilatory action on renal and coronary beds [60]. At higher doses, beta cardiac inotropic effect followed by peripheral vasoconstriction-mediated alpha-receptors takes over. The dose-dependent effects of dopamine are depicted in Fig. 31A.4.

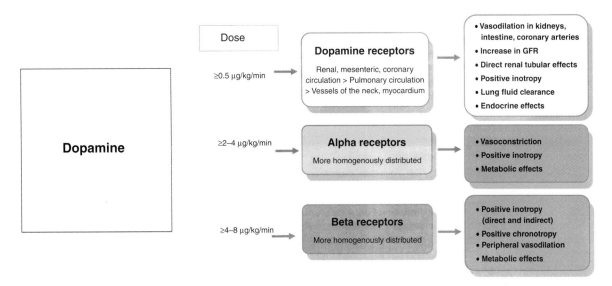

Fig. 31A.4 **Dose-Dependent Effects of Dopamine in Neonates [61].**

However, data from preterm infants suggest that order of receptor sensitivity is different in preterm infants while dopaminergic and alpha-receptors stimulation occur before beta stimulation. Thus, the enhanced responsiveness of the preterm infant to pressor effects of dopamine in the early postnatal period is further complicated by fact that there is decreased clearance of dopamine by sick preterm infants enhancing its pressor effects clinically. It must be emphasized that excess vasoconstriction can further impair end organ perfusion and potentially worsen hemodynamics clinically [62]. A RCT using Dopamine at 5 µg/kg/min versus albumin could not demonstrate improvement in CBF although this study noted significant effects on systemic circulation [63]. The Dopamine group had an effective increase in MBP.

Cochrane meta-analysis in 2003 of five trials suggested superiority of Dopamine over Dobutamine in increasing blood pressure. There was no difference between these two inotropes on overall mortality or brain injury. One trial showed Dobutamine increased LVO. However, they concluded that no firm recommendation could be made to prefer dopamine or dobutamine as the drug of choice [64].

A meta-analysis in 2011 of Dopamine use in hypotensive preterm and cerebral hemodynamic was published including 12 eligible studies. The results showed that Dopamine is associated with significant increases in BP in hypotensive preterm infants. With exception of EPI where BP increase is higher, Dopamine is superior to therapeutic agents in increasing BP. Dopamine also increases CBF in hypotensive infants, however, incidence of adverse neurological outcomes was not increased with Dopamine compared to other agents [59].

In a head-to-head RCT between Dopamine and Hydrocortisone fewer infants were successfully treated with Hydrocortisone (81%), while Dopamine was successful in 100%. Albeit, the magnitude and rapidity of response was similar in both groups in the first 12 h [65].

The European consensus guideline in 2016 suggested [66] that Dopamine is more effective in treating hypotension, although in case of myocardial dysfunction and low CO, Dobutamine can be a rational choice given its pharmacologic property of enhancing contractility while mild peripheral action vasodilatation (reduce afterload) [66]. It is also emphasized that there is no difference between these two drugs in terms of mortality or severe IVH in the longer term.

Adverse effects of Dopamine, especially at higher dosing, include tachyphylaxis, ventricular arrhythmias, excess peripheral vasoconstriction, excess myocardial oxygen consumption, site extravasation, increase Na^+ and bicarbonate losses, pituitary hormonal suppression (hypothyroidism, etc.) [67,68].

Dobutamine

Dobutamine, unlike Dopamine, is not an endogenous hormone and a synthetic drug that closely mimics catecholamine actions. It is a relatively cardioselective sympathomimetic catecholamine with significant alpha and beta effects and limited chronotropy. This drug was initially developed as a short-term i.v. therapy for adults with cardiac failure as the positive inotropy improved ventricular function while decreasing pulmonary arterial pressure [59]. The efficacy of Dobutamine is independent of its affinity for adrenal receptors. Dobutamine has relative affinity for cardiac beta receptors (++++) and peripheral alpha 2 (++). Dobutamine dose-dependent effects are described later (Tables 31A.3 and 31A.4 and Fig. 31A.5) [61].

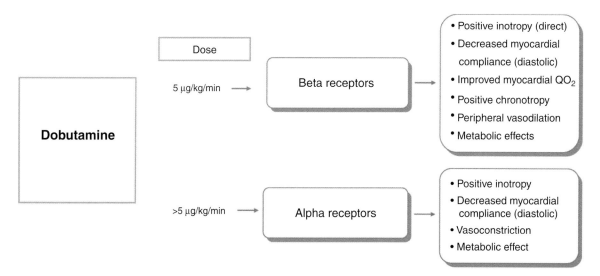

Fig. 31A.5 Dobutamine Dose-Dependent Effects [61].

Dobutamine is suited for myocardial dysfunction with low CO (LCO) and improves left ventricular end-diastolic (LVED) pressures. The CV effects start as low as 3–5 µg/kg/min up to maximum 20 µg/kg/min. It has a dose-dependent increase in CO, SBF, among others [69,70]. Further, Dobutamine does not rely on release of endogenous catecholamines for inotropic effect.

Cochrane review in 2010 concluded that there are no studies with sufficient power to compare inotropes to "no-treatment" in preterm infants with low systemic blood flow [71]. The Osborn trial in 2012 was a head-to-head trial comparing Dobutamine to Dopamine with low systemic blood (SVC) flow normalization as the therapeutic end point. Dobutamine was associated with greater increase in SVC flow and less severe periventricular-IVH [69]. A follow-up study by same author at 3 years noted no significant difference between two groups except surviving infants in Dobutamine group had a higher development quotient [72]. Another RCT performed by Spanish investigators in 2015 concluded that there was a tendency toward improved short-term perfusion and clinical outcomes in infants with low SVC treated with Dobutamine [73]. However, the study was underpowered.

Studies on Dobutamine effects on preterm with cardiac functional parameters have shown that after 20 min of Dobutamine of approximately 8–10 µg/kg/min, cardiac functional parameters improved including SV, ejection fraction, blood velocities of anterior cerebral artery, superior mesenteric artery, and renal artery; and some of these parameters remained improved even 8–10 h later. This establishes the cardiovascular superiority of Dobutamine in preterm infants with myocardial dysfunction [45]. LV dysfunction was defined by echo criteria (LV preejection period [LV PEP]) >80 ms or LV PEP/ET (>0.45). Dobutamine is shown to have a consistent positive inotropic effect but variable peripheral vasodilation [74].

Overall, it appears that Dobutamine may be more effective in asphyxiated hypotensive preterm infants with myocardial dysfunction who are also present with elevated PVR as an adjunct agent [49]. There is indirect evidence from HR variability data with Dobutamine, leading experts to suggest preload optimization prior to initiating Dobutamine to mitigate the potential vasodilator negative effects and drop in BP [73].

Dobutamine's adverse effects include tachycardia, undesirable drop in BP due to variable peripheral vasodilatation. Higher dosing may impair myocardial diastolic performance.

Adrenaline/Epinephrine

EPI is a pan-selective sympathomimetic, hence, is agonist to alpha-1, alpha-2, beta-1, beta-2 receptors. EPI is an endogenous catecholamine released by adrenal gland due to stress stimuli. In Low doses increases myocardial contractility and some peripheral vasodilatation (beta-2 effects); In high doses—alpha effects predominate like peripheral vasoconstriction and increased afterload. Pharmacologic effects of EPI are discussed later. Adrenaline competitively increases cardiac output, SVR, and SBP greater than Dopamine in animal models. (Note: as we recall the VIS scoring EPI is 100 times Dopamine for µg) [46] (Fig. 31A.6).

Further, another study comparing EPI versus Dopamine in VLBW <96 h, in which Dopamine up to 10 µg/kg/min was used and EPI up to 0.5 µg/kg/min. Authors concluded that low-dose EPI is as efficacious as low-moderate dose of Dopamine in increasing MBP in a VLBW population [75].

Further, another retrospective study using EPI for VLBW (when MBP < GA definition for hypotension was used) with BP improved with a dosing >0.05 µg/kg/min, EPI was able to raise BP in all critically ill subjects not responding

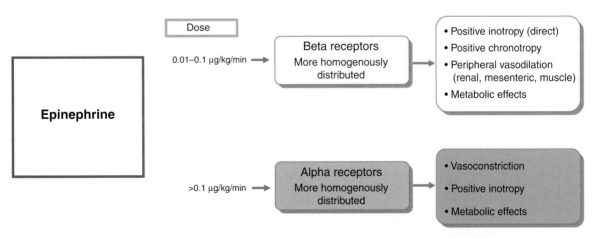

Fig. 31A.6 Adrenaline Dose-Dependent Effects [61].

to Dopamine >15 µg/kg/min. It was presumed that infants must have had sepsis and vasodilatation; and hence, the beneficial effects of alpha effect and UO might be counteracted by due to beta-2 vasodilatation [44].

Epinephrine side effects:Tachycardia, hypertension, decreased systemic perfusion (medium to high doses), lactic acidosis (worsening metabolic acidosis), increased gluconeogenesis, increased insulin need—another concern of EPI is chronic use can lead to myocardial ischemia (increased myocardial oxygen demand) that causes to increase chronotropic/inotrope effect of EPI. Animal models show evidence that prolonged/high dose EPI in piglets is associated with myocardial injury (sarcolemma rupture/ mitochondrial injury) [76].

Overall, although EPI is a potent inotrope with significant cardiovascular actions, there is insufficient evidence about safety, optimal dosage for EPI in sick neonates. Current consensus practice in most NICU is to use EPI in refractory hypotension with a minimal dosage for a minimum time period to restore hemodynamics.

Noradrenaline

Noradrenaline/NE is another sympathomimetic with agonist actions predominant on alpha-1 and alpha-2 receptors with affinity for beta-1 receptors leading to more peripheral vasoconstriction and significant inotropic actions respectively. NE in neonates has been used with success in septic shock and pulmonary hypertension to augment the peripheral vascular resistance and improve PVR, respec-tively. Physiologically attractive, although NE is less commonly used overall as was less well studied in neonates compared to traditional inotropes.

The combined effects of EPI/NE and Dopamine may have advantages of improved renal perfusion and increased renal fraction of CO [49]. Alpha-1 vasoconstriction increases venous return from capacitance vessels and helps optimize preload further indirectly with relatively less tachycardia due to its effect on vagal tone. NE potentially has been implicated to be beneficial due to ventricular–arterial coupling and pulmonary vasodilator effect, especially with data from animal studies.

In a large multicentered RCT with 1600 adult patients with shock comparing head-to-head NE and Dopamine, it was found that there was an increasing trend toward death at 28th day postinotropes in Dopamine arm ($P < 0.07$). Strikingly, the rate of arrhythmias in Dopamine was twice as much as in NE arm ($P < 0.001$) [76].

Other studies of near-term infant (22 newborns) with refractory septic shock (refractory to fluid and Dopamine/ Dobutamine) were treated with NE (median dosing 0.5 µg/ kg/min). NE was effective in increasing SBP, hemodynamic metrics including UO, cardiac function, and tissue perfusion [14].

In 2016, a study of 48 preterm infants with median 27 weeks, NE was found to be effective in treating preterm hypotensive infants associated with sepsis or PH. NE can be used in relatively low dose as first line [77]. Previously, studies have shown physiologic benefit of NE in fluid refractory septic shock in term infants. Recently, similar results have been replicated in preterm infants with septic shock. Whether NE improves long-term outcomes is not certain.

Side effects: Tachycardia, unpredictable total increase in SVR/PVR, relative decrease in CO (due to increased LV afterload), with higher doses can decrease tissue perfusion, hypertension, decreased myocardial oxygen delivery, extravasation necrosis, "accidental" priming and spike in BP especially VLBW < 96 h.

Overall, NE may appear to have some physiological superiority over Dopamine in specific scenarios including septic shock, pulmonary hypertension.More trials are required for recommending NE as first-line shock therapy as is currently emerging in adult literature.

Lastly, American College of Critical Care Medicine (ACCM) in September 2017, published Clinical Practice Parameters for shock recommends NE in its algorithm with warm septic shock especially fluid/Dopamine-resistant hypotension [78].

Vasopressin

Vasopressin (AVP) or antidiuretic hormone (ADH) is a posterior pituitary hormone secreted in response to hyperosmolality. The endogenous receptors leading to peripheral vasoconstriction are mediated by V1a receptors, renal water reabsorption mediated by V2a, and neurotransmitter release of cortisol hormone mediated by V3a. Terlipressin is an analogue of AVP with pronounced V1a constrictor effect; and hence, higher potency with higher likelihood of side effects. The half-life of AVP is 6 min and Terlipressin is 6 h.

The compensated shock neonate is presumed to have adequate AVP levels, however, when infant slips into vasodilator uncompensated shock, it is suggested that there is a relative deficiency of AVP endogenously [79].

There is limited evidence on dosing ranging from RCTs (doses 0.01–0.04 units/kg/h). AVP use has been sporadic in postcardiac bypass and in catecholamine-resistant shock in VLBW preterm infant as case reports [80]. This medication has minimum to no cardiac Inotropic or chronotropic effect with significant vasoconstrictor effect and additional pulmonary vasodilator effect.

A head-to-head trial of AVP to Dopamine in 2015 with 70 VLBW infants on day 1 was done. The group defined hypotension as MBP < GA and symptomatic hypotension or MBP < GA by less than 4 mmHg [81]. Although the arms had no difference in primary outcomes (raising

MBP greater or sooner), the AVP group had secondary benefits from absence of tachycardia seen in Dopamine group, and presence of better pulmonary outcomes in short term (lesser surfactant, normalized pCO_2, reduce RDS most likely secondary to pulmonary vasodilatation). Hence, AVP might have some pulmonary benefits in addition to significant pressor effects with lack of cardiac side effects. Although, this small trial showed a "promise," larger phase 2 or 3 trials are needed. Obvious limitation is that it is a small sample size study and safety cannot be established with such a small study patients [81].

Another study of ELBW infants with median GA of 25 weeks treated refractory shock with AVP at doses (0.01–0.04 units/kg/h) and noted a significant improvement in MBP, UO within 12 h [82].

Side effects: Splanchnic hypoperfusion and potential for NEC, rebound vascular hyporeactivity and recurrent hypotension (postdiscontinuation AVP), oligoanuria, IVH (use within 72 h) [82].

AVP may be viable alternative in intractable shock in face of vasodilatation and acute kidney injury [79]. It may also be a viable rescue in catecholamine-resistant shock especially septic shock. Dosing range (0.01–0.04 units/kg/h). Further, research evaluating this pressor is needed. Liver necrosis noted at higher doses ~0.36 units/kg/h dose [82].

Overall, benefits of AVP definitely seen in vasodilator uncompensated shock, with some pulmonary vasodilator benefits, renal benefits with no cardiac inotropic or chronotropic effect. However, splanchnic or peripheral vasoconstriction at high dose remains a concern. Safety dosing not yet established. Hence, at present, not enough data to recommend its routine use are shock-resistance.

Milrinone

Milrinone is a methylxanthine derivative and a phosphodiesterase type 3 inhibitor. Milrinone is commonly known as inodilator due to its inotropic effect combined with pulmonary and systemic vasodilator effect and is a lusitropic medication. Potentially useful when myocardial dysfunction (especially diastolic dysfunction) and heart needs support as well as needs an afterload reduction agent. Currently, increasingly used in the setting of a postligation cardiogenic shock (PLCS).

Small study in Toronto 24–32 weeks in 2014, showing utility of its use in PLCS especially in low CO (defined as LVO < 200 mL/kg/min), was associated with recovery of LVO, TDI leading to positive inotropic, vasodilation, and afterload reduction [83].

Evidence from an Australian RCT in 90 < 30-week infants within 6 h of life. Milrinone infusion (0.75 µg/kg/min) was compared with placebo with improvement of SVC flow (>45 mL/kg/min) as an outcome measure. The trial showed there was no effect. This is likely due to

decreased effectiveness in a immature myocardium and also need for preceding volume and also possibly due to late start of Milrinone ~4 h after SVC nadir, or lastly possibly due to dosage itself [84].

A large double-blinded RCT (PRIMACORP trial) was a multicenter trial across North America with 238 term neonatal and young children. The trial noted Milrinone (0.75 µg/kg/min) in post-CHD surgery has shown to reduce the postcardiac surgery, LCO syndrome (LCOS) with a RRR 55% (preemies were excluded) [85]. The most likely explanation was that in postcardiac clamping there is a sudden increase in SVR and PVR and increased biventricular afterload and decreased cardiac contractility (cardioplegia). This phenomenon was thought to be somewhat reversed with the Milrinone given for 36 h prior to established LCO. Interestingly, established LCO (cardiac index < 2 L/min) is an exclusion criterion.

However, in a retrospective study in a non-TnE center in the United States could not replicate the risk-reduction effect of Milrinone in PLCS when used in a nontargeted manner at lower doses (0.25 µg/kg/min) [86].

Furthermore, Cochrane has analyzed five studies in neonates and young children and concluded that at this time, there is insufficient evidence of effectiveness of prophylactic Milrinone in preventing PLCS [87].

Side effect: Minimum adverse effects but include variable hypotension, tachycardia among others [84–87].

Overall, it appears that the pharmacology of Milrinone is attractive in specific pathophysiology especially when diastolic dysfunction with high PVR scenario, or postcardiac surgery scenario. However, larger trials need to be performed to clarify exact dose, efficacy, and clinical indications of Milrinone.

Levosimendan

A novel molecule with a mechanism of action of calcium sensitizing inotrope and increases affinity to Troponin C and is a ATP sensitive K channel opener in cardiomyocytes. It also has vasodilator effect and thought to be beneficial in increased afterload scenarios. Hence, considered an inodilator with positive lusitropic effect and induces vascular relaxation in smooth muscle of peripheral and coronaries. It does so without increasing calcium (ICF), thus avoiding well-known catecholamine and phosphodiesterase-related side effects [88–92]. Hence, pharmacologically Levosimendan is close to Milrinone in its therapeutic effect.

Although it is relative new in the neonatal population and less experience in NICU, it has currently been used in 60 countries in adults either to prevent or to treat postcardiac surgery LCOS. However, three large RCTS in adults failed to show a beneficial effect of prophylactic Levosimendan over placebo in this subpopulation [88–90].

Ricci et al. was the first prospective trial to show a cardiovascular benefit (VIS scores with $P < 0.0001$) with Levosimendan over other conventional inotropes in 63 neonates post-CBG [92].

Furthermore, a prospective RCT "pilot" in 2012 had two arms. Postcardiac surgery while weaning CBG, infants were randomized to either of two arms Levosimendan versus Milrinone with prevention of LCO syndrome as an outcome within 90 min. Results noted that prophylactic Levosimendan was superior to Milrinone in raising the CO and CI [93].

Interestingly, a Spanish trial combined VIS with NIRS data while evaluating Levosimendan versus Milrinone as post-CBG. The Milrinone group had higher VIS and more acidosis. Authors concluded that Levosimendan may have advantages over Milrinone as an inodilator [94].

Overall, Levosimendan is an emerging molecule with inodilation properties and further studies are needed to ascertain its role in current day NICI/CICU.

Pentoxifylline

It is a methylxanthine derivative/newer concept is a neonatal sepsis redox cycle involving redox-active agent; it prevents intestinal vasoconstriction and has noted beneficial effect on endothelial cell function and coagulation in sepsis, especially late onset sepsis. Six RCTs suggest PTX given with antibiotics in neonatal sepsis shock reduces mortality and length of stay. The ACCM, in September 2017 recommends a 5-day course of PTX in septic shock [78].

The dilemma of treatments

In spite of multiple studies, in absence of concrete evidence, at this time as of 2018, there is no clarity on the best approach and therapy as guided by the current state of evidence. The best approaches would be a physiological basis and/or an expert consensus basis until more trials are done. There are trials studying this question and hope to have some answers in the next few years (HIPS trial, NICHD–ELGAN trial, TOHOP trial, AHIP trial among others).

The Canadian neonatal database in <29 weeks showed that inotrope use is about 10% (approximately 8000 infants per year). Inotrope use was also associated with use in sicker infants as well as with both higher mortality and morbidity.

Another study in 2013 showed that treating hypotension with definition of MBP. Thirty weeks did not improve regional oxygenation ($RcSCO_2$) potentially, as they were in the autoregulatory zone. Additionally, patients are at higher risk of unnecessary pharmacotherapy without short-term cerebral oxygenation benefits [95] or long-term NDD at 2 years.

Most current NICUs have chosen to approach neonatal shock by specifically reversing the purported pathophysiology and most likely mechanisms (Figs. 31A.2 and 31A.9) [5]. As noted in Fig. 31A.2, broad categories are: (1) optimizing preload, (2) optimizing contractility, or (3) modulating afterload.

It may also be practically argued that currently the management of neonatal shock could be divided into three categories types of NICU centers.

1. The NICU with TnE and NIRS capability in resources and manpower.
2. The NICU with TnE alone capability in resources and manpower.
3. The NICU with clinical facilities and echocardiography as cardiology consult service.

In the NICU A. There is emerging studies that use of advanced hemodynamic tools such as the NIRS monitoring to assess regional organ perfusion and oxygen extraction is common. In these centers it may be best to choose a normative data most representative of their NICU and follow a standardized guideline. A tertiary care center in Canada (Winnipeg, MB) has been able to demonstrate lesser clinical recovery days when previous clinical regimens were now changed to integrated hemodynamics [2,3]. Time to recovery in compromised hemodynamics was 32 h (median) compared to 71 h (median) previously among many other parameters studied. The published guideline is as follows (Figs. 31A.7 and 31A.8):

In the NICU B. The approach here is to choose a more cardiovascular-focused hemodynamic etiopathophysiologic-based approach based on BP 3rd–97th centile, signs of hypoperfusion with the assumption that <3rd centile is hypotension for that GA and chronologic age. The therapy is tailored to the diagnosed pathophysiology which is the best guess from clinical examination, laboratory measures, and TnE findings. A suggested approach is given later and is depicted in standard neonatology textbooks [5] (Fig. 31A.9). A common example is isolated low diastolic BP in otherwise well neonate could be seen in hemodynamic significant PDA (Hs-PDA), and hence, diagnosis and therapy should be directed toward the PDA rather than interventions trying to raise BP beyond a number without attending to pathophysiology (the PDA as diagnosis).

In the NICU C. The approach is traditionally tried and tested with sound clinical acumen using clinical skills and tools to assess shock and hypoperfusion (see section on tools of assessment aforementioned). However, should a septic shock be suspected or confirmed, the American College of Ccritical Medicine has recently published a stepwise time-critical shock guidelines for neonate in September 2017 [78]. Furthermore, in resource limited settings a simplified algorithm has also been published recently [96] (Fig. 31A.10).

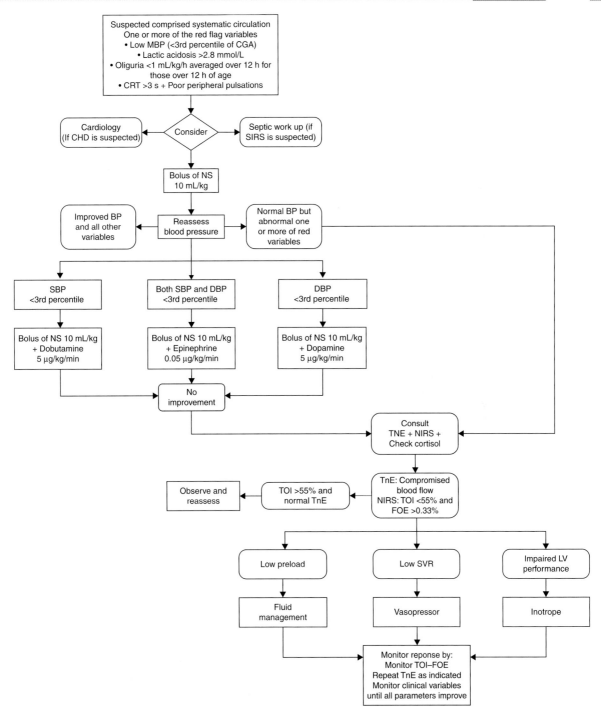

Fig. 31A.7 Integrated Hemodynamics Algorithm as a Suggested Approach [2,3]. *BP*, Blood pressure; *CGA*, corrected gestational age; *CHD*, congenital heart disease; *CRT*, capillary refill time; *DPB*, diastolic blood pressure; *FOE*, fractional oxygen extraction; *LV*, left ventricle; *MBP*, mean blood pressure; *NIRS*, near-infrared spectroscopy; *NS*, normal saline; *SBP*, systolic blood pressure; *SIRS*, systemic inflammatory response syndrome; *SVR*, systemic vascular resistance; *TnE*, targeted neonatal echocardiography; *TOI*, tissue oxygenation index. Adapted with permission from Elsayed YN, Fraser D. Integrated evaluation of neonatal hemodynamics. Part 2: systematic bedside assessment. Neonatal Netw 2016;35(4):192–203 [3].

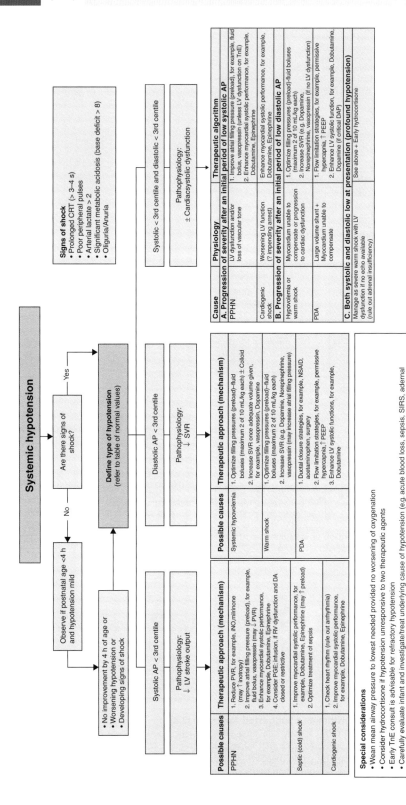

Fig. 31A.8 Algorithm for Assessment and Treatment of Hypotension According to SBP, DBP or MBP [5]. *AP*, Arterial pressure; *CRT*, capillary refill time; *iNO*, inhaled nitricoxide; *LV*, left ventricle; *NSAID*, nonsteroidal antiinflammatory drug; *PDA*, patent ductus arteriosus; *PGE1*, prostaglandinE1; *PPHN*, persistent pulmonary hypertension; *PVR*, pulmonary vascular resistance; *SIRS*, systemic inflammatory response syndrome; *SVR*, systemic vascular resistance; *TnE*, targeted neonatal echocardiography. Reproduced with permission Giesinger RE, McNamara PJ. Hemodynamic instability in the critically ill neonate: an approach to cardiovascular support based on disease pathophysiology. Semin Perinatol 2016;40(3):174–188. [5].

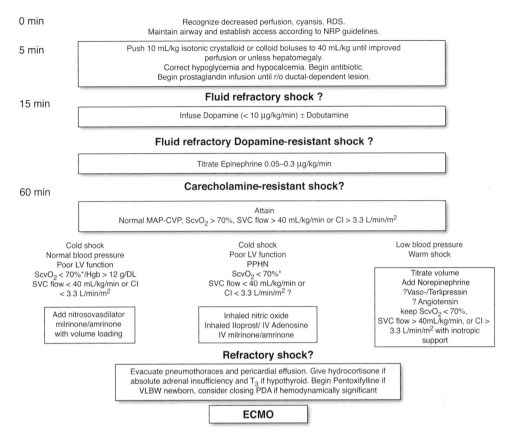

0 min

Recognize decreased perfusion, cyansis, RDS.
Maintain airway and establish access according to NRP guidelines.

5 min

Push 10 mL/kg isotonic crystalloid or colloid boluses to 40 mL/kg until improved
perfusion or unless hepatomegaly.
Correct hypoglycemia and hypocalcemia. Begin antibiotic.
Begin prostaglandin infusion until r/o ductal-dependent lesion.

Fluid refractory shock ?

15 min

Infuse Dopamine (< 10 µg/kg/min) ± Dobutamine

Fluid refractory Dopamine-resistant shock ?

Titrate Epinephrine 0.05–0.3 µg/kg/min

60 min

Carecholamine-resistant shock?

Attain
Normal MAP-CVP, $ScvO_2$ > 70%, SVC flow > 40 mL/kg/min or CI > 3.3 L/min/m^2

Cold shock
Normal blood pressure
Poor LV function
$ScvO_2$ < 70%*/Hgb > 12 g/DL
SVC flow < 40 mL/kg/min or CI
< 3.3 L/min/m^2

Add nitrosovasdilator
milrinone/amrinone
with volume loading

Cold shock
Poor LV function
PPHN
$ScvO_2$ < 70%*
SVC flow < 40 mL/kg/min or
CI < 3.3 L/min/m^2 ?

Inhaled nitric oxide
Inhaled Iloprost/ IV Adenosine
IV milrinone/amrinone

Low blood pressure
Warm shock

Titrate volume
Add Norepinephrine
?Vaso-/Terlipressin
? Angiotensin
keep $ScvO_2$ < 70%,
SVC flow > 40mL/kg/min, or CI >
3.3 L/min/m^2 with inotropic
support

Refractory shock?

Evacuate pneumothoraces and pericardial effusion. Give hydrocortisone if
absolute adrenal insufficiency and T_3 if hypothyroid. Begin Pentoxifylline if
VLBW newborn, consider closing PDA if hemodynamically significant

ECMO

Fig. 31A.9 ACCM 2017 Algorithm for Stepwise Hemodynamic Support in the Newborns [78].

Future directions, trials, and research

As neonatology continues to evolve, newer technologies are becoming available, such as impedance electrical cardiometry, impedance cardiograph among many other technologies. However, the next steps in hemodynamic revolution appear to be the use of simultaneous multimodal channels detecting not only systemic hemodynamic but all vital organ hemodynamic data in real time and dynamic with neurocritical monitoring [97] (Table 31A.5).

Summary and conclusion

In summary, we conclude that "neonatal shock" is a pathophysiological and deranged state of VO and DO_2 mismatch. Hence, therapy must be geared to reverse this pathophysiological derangement.

Indeed, a simple question like: *What is a normal BP has a complex answer*: and at this time the precise answer is unknown.

Hence, recommendation remains that a low BP "number" alone may not be treated. There needs to be more signs of hyoperfusion and or physiologic corroboration data to start therapy. Novel methods of assessing autoregulation, V/Q mismatch may be included in overall hemodynamic assessment and plans to potentially devise a robust treatment plan. Although, these newer metrics are not yet proven in a randomized controlled trial to prevent/treat shock. However, in the interim while trials are still ongoing it may be prudent to continue managing shock based on the best etiopathophysiologic clinical data available including NIRS-/TnE-generated (integrated IEH protocols or TnE algorithms).

It appears that knowing two rules are a paramount before we embark of treating an infant with a pharmacology agent. First, in-depth pathopharmacologic knowledge of inotropes/receptors, and second, in-depth pathophysiology and hemodynamic knowledge of infant's disease in real time.

Lastly, although it appears that multimodal monitoring and NIRS with neurocritical care is heading toward

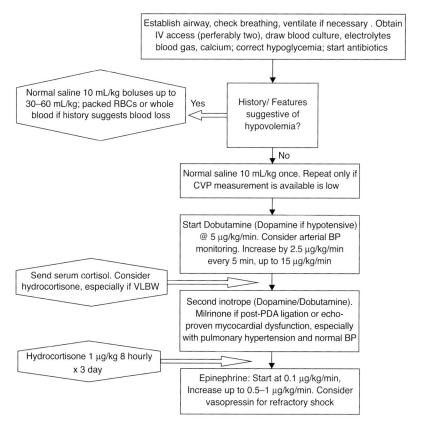

Fig. 31A.10 A Simplified Algorithm for Neonatal Shock (Resource Limited Settings) [96]. Modified with permission from Bhat BV, Plakkal N. Management of shock in neonates. Indian J Pediatr 2015;82(10):923–929 [96].

Table 31A.5 A brief summary of ongoing trials/studies

Sr. no.	Names	Recruit	Results	Condition	Intervention	References
1	Early BP in ELGAN	C	NO	Low BP	Dopamine HC Placebo	[98]
2	HC treatment in HIE	R	NO	Low BP HIE	HC Placebo	[99]
3	HIP trial	R	NO	Low BP IVH	Dopamine Placebo	[22]
4	HC in VLBW	C	NO	Low BP	HC Placebo	[100]
5	TOHOP trial	U	NO	Low BP	Treatment	[101]
6	AHIP trial	C	NO	Low BP	Treatment	[102]
7	NICHD—observational	C	NO	Low BP	HC	[103]
8	Monitoring of systemic perfusion using NIRS	R	NO	Hypoperfusion	NIRS monitoring	[104]

C, Completed; *HC,* hydrocortisone; *HIP,* hypotension in preterm; *NIRS,* near infrared spectroscopy; *R,* recruiting; *VLBW,* very low birth weight.

standard of care in times to come, for now, we have to wait for existing trials to finish and more larger RCTS are needed to answer these complex hemodynamics questions.

To conclude, we remind ourselves that absence of evidence is not evidence of absence. Hence, we continue to practice neonatal medicine in 2018 remembering principles of hippocratic oath of medicine *primum non nocere* (first do no harm!).

References

[1] Weindling AM. Peripheral oxygenation and management in the perinatal period. Semin Fetal Neonatal Med 2010;15(4):208–215.

[2] Elsayed YN, Fraser D. Integrated evaluation of neonatal hemodynamics program optimizing organ perfusion and performance in critically ill neonates. Part 1: understanding physiology of neonatal hemodynamics. Neonatal Netw 2016;35(3):143–150.

[3] Elsayed YN, Fraser. Integrated evaluation of neonatal hemodynamics. Part 2: systematic bedside assessment. Neonatal Netw 2016;35(4):192–203.

[4] Soleymani S, Borzage M, Seri I. Hemodynamic monitoring in neonates: advances and challenges. J Perinatol 2010 Oct;30:S38–S45.

[5] Giesinger RE, McNamara PJ. Hemodynamic instability in the critically ill neonate: an approach to cardiovascular support based on disease pathophysiology. Semin Perinatol 2016;40(3):174–188.

[6] Development of audit measures and guidelines for good practice in the management of neonatal respiratory distress syndrome. Report of a Joint Working Group of the British Association of Perinatal Medicine and the Research Unit of the Royal College of Physicians. Arch Dis Child 1992;67(10 Spec. No.):1221–1227.

[7] Watkins AM, West CR, Cooke RW. Blood pressure and cerebral haemorrhage and ischaemia in very low birthweight infants. Early Hum Dev 1989;19(2):103–110.

[8] Zubrow AB, Hulman S, Kushner H, Falkner B. Determinants of blood pressure in infants admitted to neonatal intensive care units: a prospective multicenter study. Philadelphia Neonatal Blood Pressure Study Group. J Perinatol 1995;15(6):470–479.

[9] Miall-Allen VM, de Vries LS, Whitelaw AG. Mean arterial blood pressure and neonatal cerebral lesions. Arch Dis Child 1987;62(10):1068–1069.

[10] Dempsey EM, Al Hazzani F, Barrington KJ. Permissive hypotension in the extremely low birthweight infant with signs of good perfusion. Arch Dis Child Fetal Neonatal Ed 2009;94(4):F241–F244.

[11] Stranak Z, Semberova J, Barrington K, O'Donnell C, Marlow N, Naulaers G, et al. HIP consortium. International survey on diagnosis and management of hypotension in extremely preterm babies. Eur J Pediatr 2014;173(6):793–798.

[12] Lee J, Rajadurai VS, Tan KW. Blood pressure standards for very low birthweight infants during the first day of life. Arch Dis Child Fetal Neonatal Ed 1999;81(3):F168–F170.

[13] Batton B, Batton D, Riggs T. Blood pressure during the first 7 days in premature infants born at—age 23 to 25 weeks. Am J Perinatol 2007;24(2):107–115.

[14] Tourneux P, Rakza T, Abazine A, et al. Noradrenaline for management of septic shock refractory to fluid loading and dopamine or dobutamine in full-term newborn infants. Acta Paediatr 2008;97(2):177–180.

[15] Logan JW, O'Shea TM, Allred EN, Laughon MM, Bose CL, Dammann O, et al. ELGAN study investigators. Early postnatal hypotension is not associated with indicators of white matter damage or cerebral palsy in extremely low gestational age newborns. J Perinatol 2011;31(8):524–534.

[16] Zubrow AB, Hulman S, Kushner H, Falkner B. Determinants of blood pressure in infants admitted to neonatal intensive care units: a prospective multicenter study. Philadelphia Neonatal Blood Pressure Study Group. J Perinatol 1995;15(6):470–479.

[17] Nuntnarumit P, Yang W, Bada-Ellzey HS. Blood pressure measurements in the newborn. Clin Perinatol 1999;26(4):981–996.

[18] Bada HS, Korones SB, Perry EH, Arheart KL, Ray JD, Pourcyrous M, et al. Mean arterial blood pressure changes in premature infants and those at risk for intraventricular hemorrhage. J Pediatr 1990;117(4):607–614.

[19] Versmold HT, Kitterman JA, Phibbs RH, Gregory GA, Tooley WH. Aortic blood pressure during the first 12 hours of life in infants with birth weight 610 to 4,220 grams. Pediatrics 1981;67(5):607–613.

[20] Goldstein RF, Thompson RJ Jr, Oehler JM, Brazy JE. Influence of acidosis, hypoxemia, and hypotension on neurodevelopmental outcome in very low birth weight infants. Pediatrics 1995;95(2):238–243.

[21] Cunningham S, Symon AG, Elton RA, Zhu C, McIntosh N. Intra-arterial blood pressure reference ranges, death and morbidity in very low birthweight infants during the first seven days of life. Early Hum Dev 1999;56(2–3):151–165.

[22] Available from: https://clinicaltrials.gov/ct2/show/NCT01482559.

[23] McNamara PJ, Weisz DE, Giesinger RE, Jain A. Hemodynamics. In: MacDonald MG, Seshia MMK, editors. Avery's neonatology: pathophysiology and management of the newborn. Philadelphia: Wolters Kluwer; 2016. p. 457–486.

[24] Greisen G. Autoregulation of cerebral blood flow in newborn babies. Early Hum Dev 2005;81(5):423–428.

[25] Tweed A, Cote J, Lou H, Gregory G, Wade J. Impairment of cerebral blood flow autoregulation in the newborn lamb by hypoxia. Pediatr Res 1986;20(6):516–519.

[26] Osborn DA, Evans N. Early volume expansion versus inotrope for prevention of morbidity and mortality in very preterm infants. Cochrane Database Syst Rev 2001;(2):CD002056.

[27] Soul JS, Hammer PE, Tsuji M, Saul JP, Bassan H, Limperopoulos C, et al. Fluctuating pressure-passivity is common in the cerebral circulation of sick premature infants. Pediatr Res 2007;61(4):467–473.

[28] Vesoulis ZA, Liao SM, Trivedi SB, Ters NE, Mathur AM. A novel method for assessing cerebral autoregulation in preterm infants using transfer function analysis. Pediatr Res 2016;79(3): 453–459.

[29] Kluckow M, Evans N. Superior vena cava flow in newborn infants: a novel marker of systemic blood flow. Arch Dis Child Fetal Neonatal Ed 2000;82(3):F182–F187.

[30] Hunt RW, Evans N, Rieger I, Kluckow M. Low superior vena cava flow and neurodevelopment at 3 years in very preterm infants. J Pediatr 2004;145(5):588–592.

[31] Escourrou G, Renesme L, Zana E, Rideau A, Marcoux MO, Lopez E, et al. How to assess hemodynamic status in very preterm newborns in the first week of life? J Perinatol 2017;37(9):987–993.

[32] Hyttel-Sorensen S, Greisen G, Als-Nielsen B, Gluud C. Cerebral near-infrared spectroscopy monitoring for prevention of brain injury in very preterm infants. Cochrane Database Syst Rev 2017;9:CD011506.

[33] Hyttel-Sorensen S, Pellicer A, Alderliesten T, et al. Cerebral near infrared spectroscopy oximetry in extremely preterm infants: phase II randomised clinical trial. BMJ 2015;350:g7635.

[34] Alderliesten T, Dix L, Baerts W, Caicedo A, et al. Reference values of regional cerebral oxygen saturation during the first 3 days of life in preterm neonates. Pediatr Res 2016;79(1–1):55–64.

[35] Pellicer A, Greisen G, Benders M, Claris O, Dempsey E, Fumagalli M, et al. The SafeBoosC phase II randomised clinical trial: a treatment guideline for targeted near-infrared-derived cerebral tissue oxygenation versus standard treatment in extremely preterm infants. Neonatology 2013;104(3):171–178.

[36] Dempsey EM, Al Hazzani F, Barrington KJ. Permissive hypotension in the extremely low birthweight infant with signs of good perfusion. Arch Dis Child Fetal Neonatal Ed 2009;94(4):F241–F244.

[37] Hall RW, Kronsberg SS, Barton BA, NEOPAIN Trial Investigators Group. et al. Morphine, hypotension, and adverse outcomes among preterm neonates: who's to blame? Secondary results from the NEOPAIN trial. Pediatrics 2005;115(5): 1351–1359.

[38] de Boode WP. Clinical monitoring of systemic hemodynamics in critically ill newborns. Early Hum Dev 2010;86(3):137–141.

[39] Dempsey EM, El-Khuffash AF. Objective cardiovascular assessment in the neonatal intensive care unit. Arch Dis Child Fetal Neonatal Ed 2018;103(1):F72–F77.

[40] Akcan-Arikan A, Zappitelli M, Loftis LL, Washburn KK, Jefferson LS, Goldstein SL. Modified RIFLE criteria in critically ill children with acute kidney injury. Kidney Int 2007;71(10):1028–1035.

[41] Bezerra CT, Vaz Cunha LC, Libório AB. Defining reduced urine output in neonatal ICU: importance for mortality and acute kidney injury classification. Nephrol Dial Transplant 2013;28(4):901–909.

[42] Kimble KJ, Darnall RA Jr, Yelderman M, Ariagno RL, Ream AK. An automated oscillometric technique for estimating mean arterial pressure in critically ill newborns. Anesthesiology 1981;54(5):423–425.

[43] Colan SD, Fujii A, Borow KM, MacPherson D, Sanders SP. Noninvasive determination of systolic, diastolic and end-systolic blood pressure in neonates, infants and young children: comparison with central aortic pressure measurements. Am J Cardiol 1983;52(7):867–870.

[44] Heckmann M, Trotter A, Pohlandt f, et al. Epinephrine treatment of hypotension in VLBW. Acta Paediatric 2002;91:566–570.

[45] Robel-Tillig E, Knüpfer M, Pulzer F, Vogtmann C. Cardiovascular impact of dobutamine in neonates with myocardial dysfunction. Early Hum Dev 2007;83(5):307–312.

[46] Gaies MG, Gurney JG, Yen AH, et al. Vasoactive inotropic score as a predictor of morbidity and mortality in infants post cardiopulmonary bypass surgery. Pediatr Crit Care med 2011;234–238.

[47] Rowe H, Jones JG, Quine D, Bhushan SS, Stenson BJ. A simplified method for deriving shunt and reduced VA/Q in infants. Arch Dis Child Fetal Neonatal Ed 2010;95(1):F47–52.

[48] Noori S, Seri I. Neonatal blood pressure support: the use of inotropes, lusitropes, and other vasopressor agents. Clin Perinatol 2012;39(1):221–238.

[49] Seri I. Circulatory support of the sick preterm infant. Semin Neonatol 2001;6(1):85–95.

[50] Wright IM, Goodall SR. Blood pressure and blood volume in preterm infants. Arch Dis Child Fetal Neonatal Ed 1994;70(3):F230–F231.

[51] Ewer AK, Tyler W, Francis A, Drinkall D, Gardosi JO. Excessive volume expansion and neonatal death in preterm infants born at 27-28 weeks gestation. Paediatr Perinat Epidemiol 2003;17(2):180–186.

[52] White P Jr, Sylvester JT, Humphrey RL, Permutt T, Permutt S, Brower R. Effect of hypoxia on lung fluid balance in ferrets. Am J Respir Crit Care Med 1994;149(5):1112–1117.

[53] Dempsey EM, Barrington KJ. Evaluation and treatment of hypotension in the preterm infant. Clin Perinatol 2009;36(1):75–85.

[54] Greenough A, Cheeseman P, Kavvadia V, Dimitriou G, Morton M. Colloid infusion in the perinatal period and abnormal neurodevelopmental outcome in very low birth weight infants. Eur J Pediatr 2002;161(6):319–323.

[55] Bell EF, Acarregui MJ. Restricted versus liberal water intake for preventing morbidity and mortality in preterm infants. Cochrane Database Syst Rev 2014;(12):CD000503.

[56] Kooi EM, van der Laan ME, Verhagen EA, Van Braeckel KN, Bos AF. Volume expansion does not alter cerebral tissue oxygen extraction in preterm infants with clinical signs of poor perfusion. Neonatology 2013;103(4):308–314.

[57] Evans N. Volume expansion during neonatal intensive care: do we know what we are doing? Semin Neonatol 2003 Aug;8(4):315–323.

[58] Schmaltz C. Hypotension and shock in the preterm neonate. Adv Neonatal Care 2009 Aug;9(4):156–162.

[59] Seri I. Cardiovascular, renal, and endocrine actions of dopamine. J Pediatr 1995;126(3):333–344.

[60] Sassano-Higgins S, Friedlich P, Seri I. A meta-analysis of dopamine use in hypotensive preterm infants: blood pressure and cerebral hemodynamics. J Perinatol 2011;31(10):647–655.

[61] Seri I. Management of hypotension and low systemic blood flow in the very low birth weight neonate during the first postnatal week. J Perinatol 2006;26(Suppl. 1):S8–13. discussion S22-3.

[62] Seri I, Rudas G, Bors Z, Kanyicska B, Tulassay T. Effects of low-dose dopamine infusion on cardiovascular and renal functions, cerebral blood

flow, and plasma catecholamine levels in sick preterm neonates. Pediatr Res 1993;34(6):742–749.

[63] Lundstrøm K, Pryds O, Greisen G. The haemodynamic effects of dopamine and volume expansion in sick preterm infants. Early Hum Dev 2000;57(2):157–163.

[64] Subhedar NV, Shaw NJ. Dopamine versus dobutamine for hypotensive preterm infants. Cochrane Database Syst Rev 2003;(3):CD001242.

[65] Bourchier D, Weston PJ. Randomised trial of dopamine compared with hydrocortisone for the treatment of hypotensive very low birthweight infants. Arch Dis Child Fetal Neonatal Ed 1997;76(3):F174–F178.

[66] Sakonidou S, Dhaliwal J. The management of neonatal respiratory distress syndrome in preterm infants (European Consensus Guidelines—2013 update). Arch Dis Child Educ Pract Ed 2015;100(5):257–259.

[67] Filippi L, Pezzati M, Poggi C, Rossi S, Cecchi A, Santoro C. Dopamine versus dobutamine in very low birthweight infants: endocrine effects. Arch Dis Child Fetal Neonatal Ed 2007;92(5):F367–F371.

[68] Furukawa S, Nagashima Y, Hoshi K, Hirao H, Tanaka R, Maruo K, et al. Effects of dopamine infusion on cardiac and renal blood flows in dogs. J Vet Med Sci 2002;64(1):41–44.

[69] Osborn D, Evans N, Kluckow M. Randomized trial of dobutamine versus dopamine in preterm infants with low systemic blood flow. J Pediatr 2002;140(2):183–191.

[70] Stopfkuchen H, Queisser-Luft A, Vogel K. Cardiovascular responses to dobutamine determined by systolic time intervals in preterm infants. Crit Care Med 1990;18(7):722–724.

[71] Osborn DA, Paradisis M, Evans N. The effect of inotropes on morbidity and mortality in preterm infants with low systemic or organ blood flow. Cochrane Database Syst Rev 2007;(1):CD005090.

[72] Osborn DA, Evans N, Kluckow M, Bowen JR, Rieger I. Low superior vena cava flow and effect of inotropes on neurodevelopment to 3 years in preterm infants. Pediatrics 2007;120(2):372–380.

[73] Bravo MC, López-Ortego P, Sánchez L, Riera J, Madero R, Cabañas F, et al. Randomized, pacebo-controlled trial of Dobutamine for low superior vena cava flow in infants. J Pediatr 2015;167(3). 572-8.e1-2.

[74] Caspi J, Coles JG, Benson LN, Herman SL, Diaz RJ, Augustine J, et al. Age-related response to epinephrine-induced myocardial stress. A functional and ultrastructural study. Circulation 1991;84(Suppl. 5):III394–III399.

[75] Valverde E, Pellicer A, Madero R, et al. Dopamine versus epinephrine for cardiovascular support in VLBW infants: analysis of systemic effects and neonatal clinical outcomes. Pediatrics 2006;117(6):1213–1222.

[76] De Backer D, Biston P, Devriendt J, SOAP II Investigators. et al. Comparison of dopamine and norepinephrine in the treatment of shock. N Engl J Med 2010;362(9):779–789.

[77] Rowcliff K, de Waal K, Mohamed AL, Chaudhari T. Noradrenaline in preterm infants with cardiovascular compromise. Eur J Pediatr 2016;175(12):1967–1973.

[78] Davis AL, Carcillo JA, Aneja RK, et al. The American College of Critical Care Medicine Clinical Practice Parameters for Hemodynamic Support of Pediatric and Neonatal Septic Shock: Executive Summary. Pediatr Crit Care Med 2017;18(9):884–890.

[79] Beaulieu MJ. Vasopressin for the treatment of neonatal hypotension. Neonatal Netw 2013;32(2):120–124.

[80] Meyer S, Gottschling S, Baghai A, et al. Arginine-vasopressin in catecholamine-refractory septic versus non-septic shock in extremely low birth weight infants with acute renal injury. Crit Care 2006;10(3):R71.

[81] Rios DR, Kaiser JR. Vasopressin versus dopamine for treatment of hypotension in extremely low birth weight infants: a randomized, blinded pilot study. J Pediatr 2015;166(4):850–855.

[82] Bidegain M, Greenberg R, Simmons C, et al. Vasopressin for refractory hypotension in extremely low birth weight infants. J Pediatr 2010;157(3):502–504.

[83] El-Khuffash AF, Jain A, Weisz D, et al. Assessment and treatment of post patent ductus arteriosus ligation syndrome. J Pediatr 2014;165(1):46–52.e1.

[84] Paradisis M, Evans N, Kluckow M, Osborn D. Randomized trial of milrinone versus placebo for prevention of low systemic blood flow in very preterm infants. J Pediatr 2009;154(2):189–195.

[85] Hoffman TM, Wernovsky G, Atz AM, et al. Efficacy and safety of milrinone in preventing low cardiac output syndrome

in infants and children after corrective surgery for congenital heart disease. Circulation 2003;107(7):996–1002.

[86] Halliday M, Kavarana M, Ebeling M, Kiger J. Milrinone use for hemodynamic instability in patent ductus arteriosus ligation. J Matern Fetal Neonatal Med 2017;30(5):529–533.

[87] Burkhardt BE, Rücker G, Stiller B. Prophylactic milrinone for the prevention of low cardiac output syndrome and mortality in children undergoing surgery for congenital heart disease. Cochrane Database Syst Rev 2015;(3):CD009515.

[88] Cholley B, Caruba T, Grosjean S, et al. Effect of levosimendan on low cardiac output syndrome in patients with low ejection fraction undergoing coronary artery bypass grafting with cardiopulmonary bypass: The LICORN randomized clinical trial. JAMA 2017;318(6):548–556.

[89] Mehta RH, Leimberger JD, van Diepen S, et al. Levosimendan in patients with left ventricular dysfunction undergoing cardiac surgery. LEVO-CTS investigators. N Engl J Med 2017;376(21):2032–2204.

[90] Landoni G, Lomivorotov VV, Alvaro G, A; CHEETAH Study Group. et al. Levosimendan for hemodynamic support after cardiac surgery. N Engl J Med 2017;376(21):2021–2031.

[91] Schumann J, Henrich EC, Strobl H, Prondzinsky R, Weiche S, Thiele H, et al. Inotropic agents and vasodilator strategies for the treatment of cardiogenic shock or low cardiac output syndrome. Cochrane Database Syst Rev 2018;1:CD009669.

[92] Ricci Z, Garisto C, Favia I, et al. Levosimendan infusion in newborns after corrective surgery for congenital heart disease: randomized controlled trial. Intensive Care Med 2012;38(7):1198–1204.

[93] Lechner E, Hofer A, Leitner-Peneder G, et al. Levosimendan versus milrinone in neonates and infants after corrective open-heart surgery: a pilot study. Pediatr Crit Care Med 2012;13(5):542–548.

[94] Pellicer A, Riera J, Lopez-Ortego P, et al. Phase 1 study of two inodilators in neonates undergoing cardiovascular surgery. Pediatr Res 2013;73(1):95–103.

[95] Garner RS, Burchfield DJ. Treatment of presumed hypotension in very low birthweight neonates: effects on regional cerebral oxygenation. Arch Dis Child Fetal Neonatal Ed 2013;98(2):F117–F121.

[96] Bhat BV, Plakkal N. Management of shock in neonates. Indian J Pediatr 2015;82(10):923–929.

[97] Azhibekov T, Soleymani S, Lee BH, Noori S, Seri I. Hemodynamic monitoring of the critically ill neonate: an eye on the future. Semin Fetal Neonatal Med 2015;20(4):246–254.

[98] Available from: https://clinicaltrials.gov/ct2/show/NCT00874393.

[99] Available from: https://clinicaltrials.gov/show/NCT02700828.

[100] Available from: https://clinicaltrials.gov/show/NCT00358748.

[101] Available from: https://clinicaltrials.gov/show/NCT01434251.

[102] Available from: https://clinicaltrials.gov/ct2/show/NCT01910467.

[103] Available from: https://clinicaltrials.gov/show/NCT00882284.

[104] Available from: https://clinicaltrials.gov/show/NCT03136172.

Further reading

[105] da Costa CS, Greisen G, Austin T. Is near-infrared spectroscopy clinically useful in the preterm infant? Arch Dis Child Fetal Neonatal Ed 2015;100(6):F558–F561.

[106] Pellicer A, Valverde E, Elorza MD, Madero R, Gayá F, Quero J, et al. Cardiovascular support for low birth weight infants and cerebral hemodynamics: a randomized, blinded, clinical trial. Pediatrics 2005;115(6):1501–1512.

Chapter | 31B |

Hypotension and Shock in Preterm Newborns

Merlin Pinto, P.K. Rajiv, MBBS, DCH, MD, Jeya Balaji, Thouseef Ahmed

CHAPTER POINTS

1. The newborns with MAP in the hypotension range may have normal blood flow and oxygen delivery.
2. Numerical data suggestive of hypotension should be evaluated for perfusion and cardiovascular dynamics before initiating treatment.
3. Symptomatic hypotension and its management in preterm infants is associated with significant morbidity and mortality. Cautious treatment is advised.
4. The management strategies should be carefully extrapolated from adults due to anatomic and physiologic differences in the cardiovascular system.
5. An individualised comprehensive assessment and management strategy should be devised for every newborn with shock.

Shock is defined as a state of failing circulation characterized by inadequate tissue perfusion resulting in decreased oxygen and nutrient supply combined with decreased clearance of the metabolic by-products from the organ system. The incidence of shock is high in preterm infants compared with term infants and is commonly seen in the first few days after birth [1]. Development of shock serves as an independent predictor of early neonatal mortality, morbidity, and neurological impairment [2].

The recognition of shock in preterm infants is immensely difficult during transitioning circulation. This gray area poses a clinical dilemma for timely diagnosis and effective management. The factors that play into this are uncertain treatment threshold levels, treatment target levels, and appropriate management techniques including medications and the presence of physiological shunts [2].

The unique characteristics of the neonatal cardiovascular system

The basic understanding of the intricacies of the neonatal myocardium is essential in explaining the pathophysiology of shock. The neonatal myocardium operates at a near-maximal capacity [3]. Cardiac myocytes are still in developing phase and contain high proportion of fibrous tissue [4] (not innervated by sympathetic fibers). These more rounded myocytes contain immature T-tubules, sarcoplasmic reticulum [5], and large disorganized mitochondria [6], their contraction is highly dependent on calcium influx. Any changes in ionized calcium level affect myocardial contractility.

Anatomical, physiological, and biochemical differences of the newborn heart are as follows:

1. Newborn myocardium has limited capacity to increase stroke volume (can increase only up to 30%) above the basal level in hyperdynamic circulation states. The increase in heart rate is the major contributor to increased cardiac output compared to adults which are usually a combination of both.
2. The parasympathetic system is fully developed at birth compared to the sympathetic system.

3. The presence of PDA affects circulation by the flow of blood across the defect, depending on the systemic or pulmonary vascular resistance.
4. Lactate is the energy source for neonatal myocardium compared to adults where it is fatty acids [7].

Other parameters which increase the risk for hypotension in preterm infants are as follows:

1. Preterm infants are usually on positive pressure ventilation either through CPAP or mechanical ventilation. Mechanical ventilation increases intrathoracic pressure and decreases venous return, uncommonly seen in spontaneously breathing infants on CPAP, and thereby decreasing the systemic blood flow [8].
2. Relative adrenal insufficiency is a known entity in preterm infants due to immaturity of adrenal glands. This results in suboptimal cortisol production in response to stressful stimuli. The hypothalamic–pituitary axis also remains suppressed transiently due to maternal antenatal steroids [9].

The response to cardiac drugs is different in newborns when compared with children and adults. Most of the vasoactive drugs increase heart rate as well as afterload. Increase in afterload nullifies the positive inotropic effect. Therefore, a greater increase in afterload may negatively impact by decreasing the cardiac output [10] which is called inotropic/afterload imbalance (Table 31B.1).

Hemodynamic monitoring of preterm infants

On admission to NICU, an infant is attached to various types of equipment for continuous hemodynamic monitoring. An ideal method is described as easy, reliable, convenient, painless, effective, and can record real-time measurements, which currently is nonexistent and yet to be developed. In general, the subjective assessment of good circulation is described as well-perfused, pink, good urine output and active infant [11]. However, the objective assessment is essential in monitoring sick infants.

Some of the methods usually used are as follows:

1. Clinical monitoring
   a. Continuous heart rate monitoring: It is routinely practiced in all NICUs. However, the changes in the heart rate depend on various factors such as anemia, drugs, asphyxia, and so on.
   b. *Blood pressure monitoring*: It is done usually by noninvasive method using cuff measurements, intermittently. The accuracy and reliability depend on the usage of appropriate size and application of the cuff. If frequent monitoring is needed, umbilical or peripheral intra-arterial catheter is placed.
   c. *Saturation monitoring*: It is done either by pulse oximeter or by blood gas monitoring which is routinely used in NICU. The detection of fetal hemoglobin, carboxyhemoglobin, and methemoglobin is not possible with clinical oximeter monitoring.
   d. Carbon-dioxide monitoring: It is used by end-tidal capnography in ventilated patients, transcutaneous carbon-dioxide monitoring, or blood gas monitoring. Sudden large variations may reflect the acute changes in the hemodynamic status of the infant.

   The sensitivity of this assessment can be increased by supplementing with biochemical parameters such as lactate, pH, base deficit, and hemoglobin [12].

2. Echocardiography
   This is the objective assessment of the hemodynamic status of the infant. It is indicated when one or multiple of the above parameters are consistently abnormal. The information gathered during this study are cardiac contractility, output, pulmonary hemodynamics, PDA, and shunting across it. It is also used for assessment of the volume status and myocardial dysfunction [13].

3. Assessment of systemic and organ blood flow
   Near-infrared spectroscopy (NIRS) technology records the oxygen delivery and consumption along

Table 31B.1	Factors affecting hemodynamic response to shock and its management in neonates, when compared with older children and adults
1.	Presence of patent ductus arteriosus
2.	Perinatal asphyxia
3.	Developmental differences • Immaturity of cardiomyocyte structure and function • Transition from fetal to neonatal circulation
4.	Persistent pulmonary hypertension
5.	Decreased ability to handle fluid load and contractility of the myocardium
6.	Transient adrenal insufficiency of prematurity

with fractional oxygen extraction by measuring the hemoglobin flow and venous saturation. The pulse oximeter uses the light signal from the arterial pulse. NIRS uses the total light signal from the vascular bed mainly from venous-weighted capillary blood. It was initially used only for the research, and over the course of time it has been used in the monitoring of sick infants in NICUs. It is gaining popularity as an important monitoring tool in hypotensive or shock neonate.

The utilization of NIRS in sepsis/septic shock helps in the early recognition of tissue hypoxia and aids in better management. The values recorded by NIRS have shown good correlation with invasive monitoring techniques [14]. A positive relationship between regional cerebral oxygenation index and venous oxygen saturation has been endorsed by many studies [15–18]. NIRS has been studied in post operative cardiac surgical infants, in a study of 79 neonates with hypoplastic left heart syndrome, in the first 48 hours postoperative period the difference in the body and cerebral oxygen saturation of 10 or more was associated with the increased risk of biochemical shock and postoperative complications [19]. NIRS can assist in the real-time assessment of the tissue perfusion.

The potential uses of NIRS are as follows:
1. Noninvasive monitoring of cardiac output.
2. Noninvasive monitoring of cerebral oxygen saturation.
3. Early recognition of shock.
4. Assessment of response to therapy.
5. Early detection of necrotizing enterocolitis.

Despite this significant correlation, the sensitivity and reliability of NIRS are debated. The lack of standardization across devices, absence of normative data, decrease in reliability with increase in subcutaneous tissue, and unproven cost–benefit analysis [20] are some of the hurdles need to be overcome before accepting NIRS as standard of care across the world (Fig. 31B.1).

Blood pressure and cerebral blood flow

Autoregulation is a type of myogenic reflex. It palys an important role in maintaining blood flow during variations in mean arterial pressure within considerable limits. Extremely preterm infants have immature cerebral autoregulation depending on the gestational age, other factors such as male sex, low birth weight were associated with

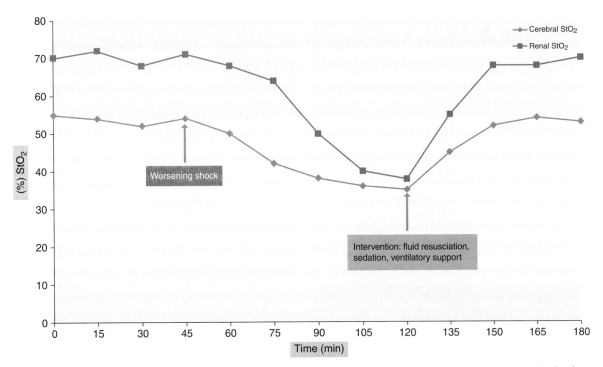

Fig. 31B.1 NIRS demonstrating the decrease in renal and cerebral oxygen saturation, corresponding increase in saturation levels after appropriate intervention. Adapted from Samraj RS, Nicoals L. Near infrared spectroscopy (NIRS) derived tissue oxygenation in critical illness. Clin Invest Med. 2015; 38(5):E285-295 [20].

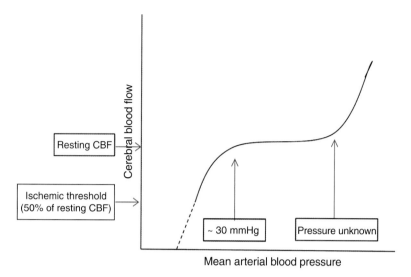

Fig. 31B.2 Autoregulation of Cerebral Blood Flow and its relation to Mean Arterial Blood Pressure. The plateau phase of the curve shows cerebral autoregualtion. Below the threshold of 30 mmHg the the cerebral blood flow falls more than in proportion of pressure and above the upper limit of the MAP the cerebral blood flow increases steeply increasing the risk of cererbal injury. Reproduced with permission from Greison G, Autoregulation of cererbral blood flow in newborn babies. Early Human Development. 2005;81:423-428.

symptomatic hypotension necessitating treatment in NICU [1]. The relationship between mean arterial pressure and autoregulation has been studied for decades. The animal models show, when the cerebral blood flow decreases to 50% of it resting state the brain ischemic injury ensures [21]. Miall-Allen VM [22] et al studied MAP and brain injury in preterm infants between 26-30 weeks of gestation and found that when mean arterial pressure stayed lower than 30 mmHg for at least an hour, it was associated with intracerebral hemorrhage and cerebral ishemic injury.

Greisen G [21] emphasizes that the cerebral blood flow decreases when the MAP is below 30 mmHg and the upper limit of the of the MAP to affect the cerebral blood flow is not known. Adequate cerebral blood flow is maintained during the plateau phase of the curve as shown in Fig. 31B.2. In contrast to this Tyszczuk et al. [23] in preterm infants of gestational age between 24-34 weeks found no correlation between cerebral perfusion and MAP either above or below 30 mmHg. More studies are needed for better understanding this relation.

Hypotension

Hypotension is defined as mean minus 2 standard deviations or <10th centile for the gestational age. The mean arterial blood pressure closely corresponds to the gestational age [24] of the infants and is frequently used in the clinical setting. This definition holds good for the first 48 h of age after which

the age-specific nomograms should be used for the diagnosis (refer to Figs. 31B.3 and 31B.4 for blood pressure values for preterm infants <28 weeks of gestation). Once the hypotension is diagnosed in these tiny infants, the management varies from center to center. In some NICUs, the treatment is initiated based only on numbers, and in others the overall pictures including risk factors, clinical findings, laboratory parameters, and echocardiography findings are considered.

Dempsey et al. [25] describe the concept of permissive hypotension as nontreatment of the blood pressure even if it is below the clinically accepted range till tissue perfusion is maintained.

Some clinicians may disagree not to treat hypotension persisting for >3 h or if the blood pressure values are significantly lower or when there is accompanied low blood flow. In these events, one may feel more compelled to start volume and/or vasopressor therapy immediately. Overzealous management of hypotension results in more harm. Hence, monitoring of tissue perfusion in the hypotensive infant can guide the appropriate management.

The importance of identifying and treating hypotension in preterm infants is to prevent brain injury and impaired neurodevelopment. A recent systematic review showed significant association between hypotension and increase in brain injury diagnosed by head ultrasound [26]. There is a multitude of research supporting this association, but the threshold at which blood pressure causes the brain injury, whether low/high blood pressure with or without treatment, or a combination of both increase the risk is still debatable.

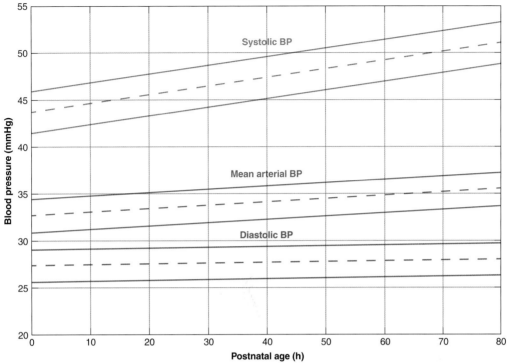

Fig. 31B.3 Blood Pressure Values in Extremely Premature Infants by Postgestational Hours. *Dashed line* represents the blood pressure estimate, while *solid line* represents the boundaries of the 95% confidence interval. Reprinted with permission from Macmillan Publishers Ltd., *Journal of Perinatology*; Vesoulis ZA, El Ters NM, Wallendorf M, Mathur AM. Empirical estimation of the normative blood pressure in infants <28 weeks of gestation using a massive data approach. J Perinatol 2016;36:291.

The studies by Fanaroff and Fanaroff [27] and Batton et al. [28] showed treated symptomatic hypotension in ELBW infants in first 72 h of life is associated with significant short-term and long-term morbidity, delayed motor development, hearing loss, and death. Batton et al. [29] in preterm infants between 23 and 26 weeks of gestation found that hypotension with treatment was associated with severe retinopathy of prematurity, severe intraventricular hemorrhage, and mortality. However, the regression analysis found there was no significant difference in survival or in hospital morbidity rates among the treated and untreated groups. On the contrary, the EPIPAGE 2 [30] study showed a significantly higher survival rate with no major morbidity in preterm infants <29 weeks treated for isolated hypotension in less than 72 h. Due to these conflicting findings, further large randomized control trials are needed to arrive at a definitive conclusion. Untill then antihypotensives should be cautiously used in ELBW infants.

Low cerebral oxygenation is shown to be associated with lower neurodevelopmental outcomes. Alderliesten et al. [31] showed that the mean arterial blood pressure lower than the gestational age need not correspond to low cerebral oxygenation and low neurodevelopmental outcomes. Hence, in an infant with a low MAP, it may be worthwhile to check the cerebral oxygenation by NIRS, before initiating treatment. In most of the hypotensive studies, the treatment threshold considered is low blood pressure values rather than low blood flow or cardiac output affecting the mortality and morbidity [32].

Alternatively, the superior vena cava (SVC) flow has been of interest in predicting intraventricular hemorrhage (IVH). Cerebral venous returns constitutes 80% of Superior vena caval blood. Decrease in superior vena caval blood to <40–41 ml/kg/ min is significantly associated with IVH and mortality [33–35]. On the contrary, recent studies argue the interobserver reliability and reproducibility of the test and inconclusiveness of SVC flow in predicting IVH [36].

Pathophysiology of hypotension

Blood pressure is a product of cardiac output and systemic vascular resistance. Increase or decrease in one or both can affect blood pressure [15].

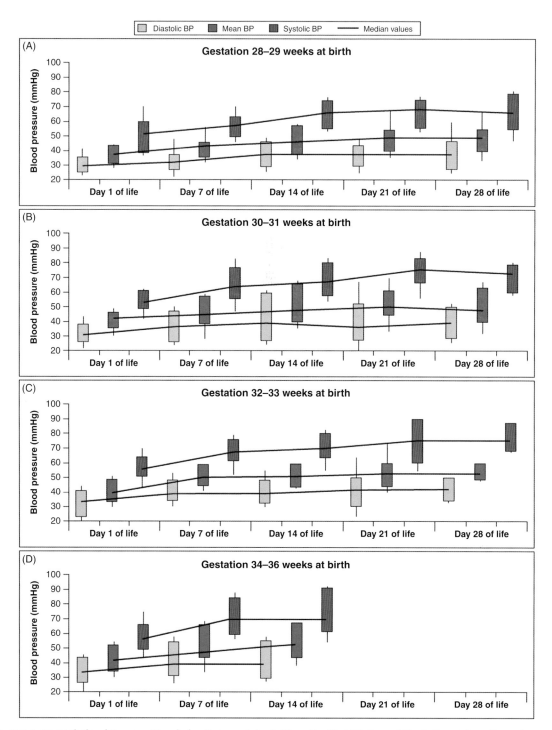

Fig. 31B.4 Normal Blood Pressure Trends for Preterm Infants Over the First 28 days of Gestational Age. *Boxes* show the 10th–90th percentiles and the *vertical line* shows the delineating range. Reproduced with permission from Springer. Pediatr Nephrol. Kent L, Meskell S, Falk MC, Shadbolt B. Normative blood pressure data in non ventilated premature neonates from 28–36 weeks of gestation. Pedatric Neohrology. 2009;24(1):141–146.

1. Hypovolemia: Absolute hypovolemia is a loss of circulating blood volume either internally due to bleeding into internal organs/third space loss or externally such as abruption of the placenta and many other causes. Relative hypovolemia is vasodilation with resultant inadequate filling of vascular bed with existing blood volume [37]. This results in inadequate filling pressure leading to decreased cardiac output and hypotension.
2. Myocardial dysfunction

Myocardial contraction is an energy-dependent process. In preterm infants, as mentioned earlier, it is still in the process of maturation. It mainly depends on extracellular calcium for contraction rather than the calcium from the sarcoplasmic reticulum. The preterm hypotensive infants do not respond appropriately to volume or medications. In addition to this, the preterm infants are highly sensitive to increased afterload and this further decreases the cardiac output and worsens blood pressure and systemic blood flow.

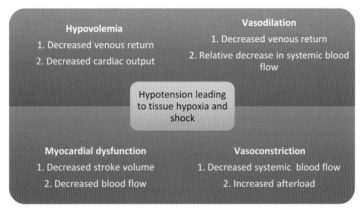

Hypovolemia
1. Decreased venous return
2. Decreased cardiac output

Vasodilation
1. Decreased venous return
2. Relative decrease in systemic blood flow

Hypotension leading to tissue hypoxia and shock

Myocardial dysfunction
1. Decreased stroke volume
2. Decreased blood flow

Vasoconstriction
1. Decreased systemic blood flow
2. Increased afterload

Shock

Shock is a pathophysiologic state characterized by an imbalance between oxygen delivery and oxygen demand in the tissues leading to tissue hypoxia [38]. Prime determinants of the shock are systemic blood flow, blood oxygen content, oxygen demand, and oxygen extraction by the organ systems. However, measuring all or any of these in a clinical setting is extremely challenging and impossible. The oxygen delivery to the organs is best reflected by the mixed venous partial pressure of oxygen (PO_2). In preterm neonates, this value is compromised by the presence of shunt at atrial and at patent ductus arterial level.

Shock without hypotension

The primordial aspect of treatment of shock in term/preterm neonates is recognizing shock in its early phase. Identifying the cause, initiation of management strategies timely is essential to improve outcomes. In compensated shock, which is also called early or reversible shock, various neuroendocrine mechanisms are at play to maintain normal blood pressure and this normal blood pressure does not translate into normal flow. The flow could be normal or high depending on the degree of peripheral vascular resistance

with variable blood pressure. In preterm newborns, there is poor correlation between the blood pressure and blood flow especially in first few days after birth [39–41].

Normotensive shock is usually seen in septicemia. In a study done on newborn piglets by inducing GBS sepsis [42], the cardiac output is decreased in the early phase of sepsis with increasing pulmonary hypertension and normal blood pressure was sustained by vigorous peripheral constriction. As the course of sepsis progresses, the blood pressure falls contrary to adults which results in warm shock (increased cardiac output with vasodilation-induced hypotension).

The adult literature shows treatment of shock with goal-directed therapy, where the goal is to achieve mixed venous saturation of more than 70% and involves use of vasopressors, early volume therapy, and blood and blood products transfusion as needed. However, in neonates, there is a lack of this approach due to difficulty in obtaining mixed venous saturation.

Treatment of normotensive shock in preterm neonates should be directed toward normalizing cardiac output and optimizing systemic and pulmonary vascular resistance. Dobutamine with or without low-dose epinephrine can be rightly used. Dobutamine at dose of 2–5 µg/kg/min increases myocardial contractility by direct stimulation of myocardial adrenergic receptors. At higher doses, dobutamine increases heart rate and increases the tissue metabolic rate. Administration of the fluid bolus should be considered depending on the pathophysiology.

685

1. In compensated shock, if the clinical and echo findings are consistent with pulmonary hypertension, inhaled nitric oxide can be used to improve right ventricular output [42].
2. If decreased intravascular status due to leaky blood vessels or loss of blood either due to IVH or NEC is suspected, fluid boluses are to be considered before commencing dobutamine/low-dose epinephrine.

Shock with hypotension

The nonavailability of identifying shock in its early phase and lack of instituting timely management leads to the irreversible phase of shock. Hypotension develops when shock starts rolling from reversible to irreversible phase. The morbidity and mortality of newborn with low blood pressure and shock is very high [42]. When the diagnosis of hypotension is made based on the numerical data, a thorough evaluation of the clinical, laboratory, and echocardiography with or without NIRS data should be obtained. The etiological cause of the hypotension should be explored to better aid in the treatment.

The hemodynamic management of shock with hypotension mainly involves three strategies:
1. Fluid boluses
2. Vasopressor medications
3. Inotropic medications

Refer to the chapter 31A. Neonatal Shock Management, for a detailed description of the aforementioned strategies in treatment of hypotension with shock (Fig. 31B.5).

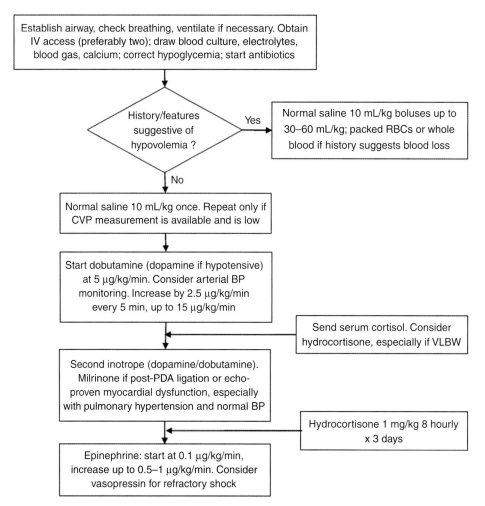

Fig. 31B.5 A Simplified Algorithm for Management of Neonatal Shock. Reproduced with permission. Bhat BV, Plakkal N. Management of shock in neonates. Indian J Pediatr. 2015;82(10):923–929

The challenges unique to the fluid and medication administration in the preterm infants compared with adult and pediatric population are as follows:

1. The absence of knowledge about the maturity of the receptors for the effective functioning of administered medications.
2. The long lag times/dead space through the long catheters, as the infusion rates are low.
3. Use of multiple medications can leave a meager room for parenteral nutrition, thereby increasing the risk of metabolic complications.
4. The is a dearth of literature/studies regarding the safety of many drugs and their adverse effects, especially when used in preterm infants.

Key learning points

1. The management strategies of shock should be carefully extrapolated from adults due to anatomic and physiologic differences in the cardiovascular system.
2. The newborns with mean arterial blood pressure values in the hypotension range may have normal blood flow and oxygen delivery.
3. Mere numerical data suggestive of hypotension should not lead to the initiation of treatment. The overall perfusion and cardiovascular dynamics should be assessed before treating. Persistently low numbers for >3 h after first 24–48 h of birth may warrant investigations and initiation of the treatment early.
4. An individualized comprehensive assessment and management strategy should be devised for every newborn with shock.

References

[1] Laughon M, Bose C, Allred E, et al. ELGAN Study Investigators. Factors associated with treatment for hypotension in extremely low gestational age newborns during the first postnatal week. Pediatrics 2007;119:273–280.

[2] Al-Aweel I, Pursley DM, Rubin LP, Shah B, Weisberger S, Richardson DK. Variations in prevalence of hypotension, hypertension, and vasopressor use in NICUs. J Perinatol 2001;21:272–278.

[3] Teitel DF, Sidi D. Developmental changes in myocardial contractile reserve in the lamb. Pediatr Res 1985;119:948–955.

[4] Friedman WF. The intrinsic physiologic properties of the developing heart. Prog Cardiovasc Dis 1972;15:87–111.

[5] Walker AM. Developmental aspects of cardiac physiology and morphology. In: Lipshitz J, Maloney J, Nimrod C, Nimrold G, editors. Perinatal development of the heart and lung. Perinatology Press; 1987. p. 73–82.

[6] Anderson PAW. Maturation and cardiac contractility. Cardio Clin 1989;7:209–225.

[7] Baum VC, Yuki K, de Souza DG. Cardiaovascular Physiology. In: Smith's anesthesia for infants and children. 9th ed. p. 429–437.

[8] Kluckow M. Low systemic blood flow and pathophysiology of the preterm transitional circulation. Early Hum Dev 2005;81(5):429–437.

[9] Fernandez EF, Watterberg KL. Relative adrenal insufficiency in the preterm and term infant. J Perinatol 2009;29(Suppl. 2):S44–S49.

[10] Belik J, Light RB. Effect of increased afterload on right ventricular function in newborn pigs. J Appl Physiol 1989;66:863–869.

[11] Dempsey EM. Challenges in treating low blood pressure in preterm infants. Children (Basel) 2015;2(2):272–288.

[12] Dempsey EM, Al Hazzani F, Barrington KJ. Permissive hypotension in the extremely low birthweight infant with signs of good perfusion. Arch Dis Child Fetal Neonatal Ed 2009;94(4):F241–F244.

[13] Kluckow M, Seri I, Evans N. Functional echocardiography: an emerging clinical tool for the neonatologist. J Pediatr 2007;150(2):125–130.

[14] Mulier KE, Skarda DE, Taylor JH, Myers DE, McGraw MK, Gallea BL, et al. Near-infrared spectroscopy in patients with severe sepsis: correlation with invasive hemodynamic measurements. Surg Infect (Larchmt) 2008;9(5):515–519.

[15] Noori S, Seri I. Pathophysiology of newborn hypotension outside the transitional period. Early Hum Dev 2005;81(5):399–404.

[16] Abdul-Khaliq H, Troitzsch D, Berger F, Lange PE. Regional transcranial oximetry with near-infrared spectroscopy (NIRS) in comparison with measuring oxygen saturation in the jugular bulb in infants and children for monitoring cerebral oxygenation. Biomed Tech (Berl) 2000;45(11):328–332.

[17] Ranucci M, IsgrO G, De La Torre T, Romitti F, Conti D, Carlucci C. Near infrared spectroscopy correlates with continuous superior vena cava oxygen saturation in pediatric cardiac surgery patients. Pediatr Anesth 2008;18(12):1163–1169.

[18] Ricci Z, Garisto C, Favia I, Schloderer U, Giorni C, Fragasso T, et al. Cerebral NIRS as a marker of superior vena cava oxygen saturation in neonates with congenital heart disease. Pediatr Anesth 2010;20(11):1040–1045.

[19] Hoffman GM, Ghanayem NS, Mussatto KA, Berens RJ, Tweddell JS. Postoperative two sites NIRS predicts complications and mortality after stage 1 palliation of HLHS. Ann Thorac Surg 2000;70:1515–1521.

[20] Samraj RS, Nicoals L. Near infrared spectroscopy (NIRS) derived tissue oxygenation in critical illness. Clin Invest Med 2015;38(5):E285–E295.

[21] Greisen G. Autoregulation of cerebral blood flow in newborn babies. Early Hum Dev 2005;81(5):423–428.

[22] Miall-Allen VM, De Vries LS, Whitelaw AGL. Mean arterial blood pressure and neonatal cerebral lesions. Arch Dis Child 1998;62:1068–1069.

[23] Tyszczuk L, Meek J, Elwell C, Wyatt JS. Cerebral blood flow is independent of mean arterial blood pressure in preterm infants undergoing intensive care. Pediatrics 1998;102: 337–341.

[24] Cunningham S, Symon AG, Elton RA, Zhu C, McIntosh N. Intra-arterial blood pressure reference ranges, death and morbidity in very low birthweight infants during the first seven days of life. Early Hum Dev 1999;56:151–165.

[25] Dempsey EM, Al Hazzani F, Barrington KJ. Permissive hypotension in the extremely low birthweight infant with signs of good perfusion. Arch Dis Child Fetal Neonatal Ed 2009;94(4):F241–F244.

[26] Dempsey EM, Barrington KJ. Treating hypotension in the preterm infant: when and with what: a critical and systematic review. J Perinatol 2007;27:469–478.

[27] Fanaroff AA, Fanaroff JM, et al. Short- and long-term consequences of hypotension in ELBW infants. Semin Perinatol 2006;30(3):151.

[28] Batton B, Li L, Newman N, Das A, et al. Eunice Kennedy Shriver National Institute of Child Health and Human Development Neonatal Research Network. Early blood pressure, anti-hypotensive therapy and outcomes at 18–22 months corrected age in extremely preterm infants. Arch Dis Child Fetal Neonatal Ed 2016;101(3):F201–F206.

[29] Batton B, Li L, Newman NS, Walsh MC, et al. Eunice Kennedy Shriver National Institute of Child Health and Human Development Neonatal Research Network. Use of antihypotensive therapies in extremely preterm infants. Pediatrics 2013;131(6):e1865–e1873.

[30] Durrmeyer X, Marchand-Martin L, Porcher R, Gascoin G, Roze JC, Storme L, et al. Abstention or intervention for isolated hypotension in the first 3 days of life in extremely preterm infants: association with short-term outcomes in the EPIPAGE 2 cohort study. Arch Dis Child Fetal Neonatal Ed 2017;102:F490–F496.

[31] Alderliesten T, Lemmers PM, van Haastert IC, de Vries LS, Bonestroo HJ, Baerts W, et al. Hypotension in preterm neonates: low blood pressure alone does not affect neurodevelopmental outcome. J Pediatr 2014;164:986–991.

[32] Joynt C, Cheung PY. Treating Hypotension in Preterm neonates with vasoactive medications. Front Pediatr 2018;6:86.

[33] Hunt RW, Evans N, Rieger I, Kluckow M. Low superior vena cava flow and neurodevelopment at 3 years in very preterm infants. J Pediatr 2004;145:588–592.

[34] Osborn DA, Evans N, Kluckow M, Bowen JR, Rieger I. Low superior vena cava flow and effect of inotropes on neurodevelopment to 3 years in preterm infants. Pediatrics 2007;120:372–380.

[35] Cerbo RM, Scudeller L, Maragliano R, Cabano R, et al. Cerebral oxygenation, Superior vena cava flow, severe intraventricular hemorrhage and mortality in 60 very low birth infants. Neonatology 2015;108:246–252.

[36] Bates S, Odd D, Luyt K, Mannix P, Wach R, Evans D, et al. Superior vena cava flow and intraventricular haemorrhage in extremely preterm infants. J Matern Fetal Neonatal Med 2016;29:1581–1587.

[37] Ezaki S, Tamura M. Evaluation and treatment of hypotension in premature infants. D. Gaze (Ed.), The Cardiovascular System—Physiology, Diagnostics and Clinical Implications. In Tech, China; 2012: pp. 419–444.

[38] Singh Y, Katheria AC, Vora F, et al. Advances in diagnosis and management of hemodynamic instability in neonatal shock. Front Pediatr 2018;6:2.

[39] Groves AM, Kuschel CA, Knight DB, Skinner JR. Echocardiographic assessment of blood flow volume in the superior vena cava and descending aorta in the newborn infant. Arch Dis Child Fetal Neonatal Ed 2008;93(1):F24–F28.

[40] Shah DM, Condò M, Bowen J, Kluckow MJ. Blood pressure or blood flow: which is important in the preterm infant? A case report of twins. Paediatr Child Health 2012;48(3):E144–E146.

[41] Miletin J, Pichova K, Dempsey EM. Bedside detection of low systemic flow in the very low birth weight infant on day 1 of life. Eur J Pediatr 2009;168(7):809–813.

[42] Barrington KJ, Etches PC, Schulz R, et al. The hemodynamic effects of inhaled nitric oxide and endogenous nitric oxide synthesis blockade in newborn piglets during infusion of heat killed group B streptococci. Crit Care Med 2000;28:800–808.

Further reading

[42] Hegyi T, Carbone MT, Anwar M, et al. Blood pressure ranges in premature infants. I. The first hours of life. J Pediatr 1994;124:627–633.

[43] Dempsey EM. What should we do about hypotension in preterm infants? Neonatology 2017;111(4):402–407.

[44] Barrington KJ. Hypotension and shock in the preterm infant. Semin Fetal Neonatal Med 2008;13(1):6–23.

Chapter | **31C**

Hypotension and Poor Circulation in Neonates

Koert de Waal, MD, PhD

CHAPTER POINTS

- Assessment of perfusion in newborns can be difficult.
- Adding blood flow measures to clinical assessment can help support targeted treatment.

Introduction

Neonatal hypotension is ideally defined as a clinical condition of abnormally low arterial blood pressure affecting perfusion [1]. Newborns in the neonatal intensive care are of variable gestation, weight, and postnatal age, hence one accepted cut point of low blood pressure in mmHg is not available. Furthermore, the clinical diagnosis of poor perfusion is also not without difficulties, making the diagnosis and treatment of hypotension in neonates complex [2]. There is little disagreement that inadequate perfusion or poor circulation should be treated. However, it is still unknown what standards or thresholds should be used to trigger treatment, and which agents should be used [3].

The causes of neonatal hypotension vary from immature myocardium, ischemic myocardial damage after hypoxic injury, loss of blood, loss of vascular tone as seen in sepsis, to underlying structural heart diseases (Fig. 31C.1) [4]. Therapies for complications of prematurity can cause low blood pressure, with medications such as sedatives, opioids, or antiepileptics reducing vascular tone, and high intrathoracic pressures with mechanical ventilation reducing preload and lower blood pressure. It is not possible to treat all of the above utilizing the same approach, and hence the selection of specific cardiovascular support often requires more information than just a blood pressure reading to target the therapy to the underlying problem. Hypotension as a new clinical feature in a previously stable baby requires immediate attention and investigations, and cardiovascular supportive treatment will often be needed. However, very preterm infants with transitional hypotension (low blood pressure in the first few hours after birth) pose a specific problem as to when and how to treat [5]. Currently, there is no known blood pressure threshold below which very preterm infants are at an increased risk for a poor outcome. Although short-term outcomes might be improved, there is little evidence that antihypotensive therapy improves long-term outcomes for infants with low blood pressure, however defined [6–8].

Hemodynamic assessment of the newborn

Perfusion is defined as the balance between energy and nutrient delivery to meet cellular demand. The physiology behind adequate perfusion is complex, and requires many

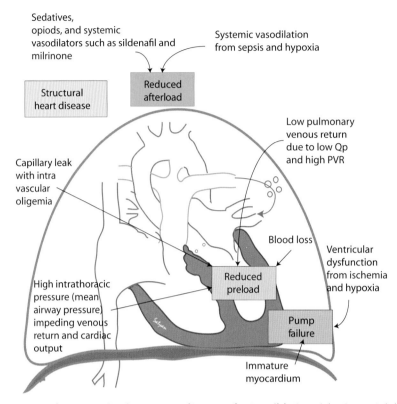

Sedatives, opiods, and systemic vasodilators such as sildenafil and milrinone

Systemic vasodilation from sepsis and hypoxia

Structural heart disease

Reduced afterload

Low pulmonary venous return due to low Qp and high PVR

Capillary leak with intra vascular oligemia

Blood loss

Ventricular dysfunction from ischemia and hypoxia

High intrathoracic pressure (mean airway pressure) impeding venous return and cardiac output

Reduced preload

Pump failure

Immature myocardium

Fig. 31C.1 Common Causes of Hypotension in Neonates (See Text for Details). Copyright: Satyan Lakshminrusimha.

functions of the body to work together [9]. Arterial oxygen content has to be delivered to organs and tissues using the heart as pump (contractility), sufficient volume to pump around (preload), and a driving pressure difference. Basic physiological principles, pressure = flow × resistance, are neatly tailored to local needs with large variations depending on wherein the cardiovascular system is measured (Fig. 31C.2).

An "ideal" tool for the assessment of perfusion would provide continuous, noninvasive parameters of cellular and organ energy balance. As such a measurement does not exist, we have to rely on alternatives summarized in Table 31C.1. Each diagnostic tool provides unique information on part of the physiological process as described earlier, but none of them can describe all.

Clinical assessment

Clinical examination is essential in detecting poor perfusion. However, all current clinical parameters have significant

limitations in predicting stroke volume [10]. Normal capillary refill in newborn infants is generally less than 3 s. However, the diagnostic accuracy of this clinical test to predict low blood flow is limited to significantly increased refill times (>5 s. There is no association between heart rate and cardiac output or clinical perfusion. Urine output is low in all newborns in the first day, making interpretation difficult and there are no studies correlating urine output (and cutoff) and cardiac output. A serum lactate >2.8 mmol/L can reasonably predict low blood flow on day 1, and persistent high values (>5.6 mmol/L) are associated with morbidity and mortality [11,12].

Blood pressure

Because of the limited techniques and skills available for bedside hemodynamic assessment, blood pressure remains the most used diagnostic tool to establish perfusion. The accuracy of blood pressure measurements is dependent on technique (location of measurement, device used) and this aspect deserves attention when considering treatment [13,14]. The systolic pressure is the amount of pressure

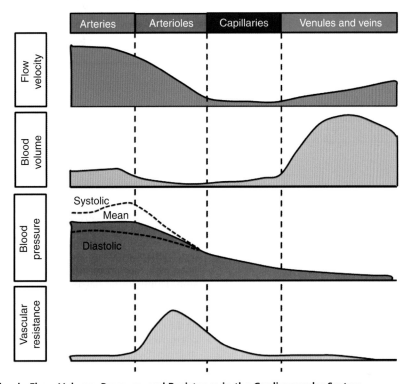

Fig. 31C.2 Variation in Flow, Volume, Pressure, and Resistance in the Cardiovascular System.

Table 31C.1 Hemodynamic assessment tools [3]

	Clinical	Noninvasive	Invasive
Cardiac function	Heart rate	Echocardiogram	Catheterization
Artery	Pulse volume	Noninvasive blood pressure (NIBD)	Arterial blood pressure
Peripheral blood flow	Capillary refill	Pulse oximetry, laser Doppler	
End organ perfusion	Organ function; urine output, K+, lactate	Near-infrared spectroscopy, aEEG (brain)	Arterial blood gas, mixed venous saturation
Veins	Jugular venous pressure	Echocardiography	Central venous pressure

that blood exerts on arteries and vessels while the heart is beating, whereas the mean pressure is the average arterial pressure during a single cardiac cycle. Determinants of blood pressure are stroke volume and arterial wall compliance (stiffness), and interactions between the two can vary depending on the physiological situation. Mean blood pressure does not provide information about pulse pressure (systolic pressure − diastolic pressure), and might not reveal clues to certain underlying pathology.

Normal blood pressure values are not easy to obtain in very preterm infants, as many would receive therapies that could influence cardiovascular function. Blood pressure is dependent on gestational age, and gradually increases over the first days of life. Table 31C.2 provides a guide to the lowest centiles of blood pressure values found in newborn infants [15]. The established rule of thumb "mean blood pressure < gestational age" is not supported by any evidence, but can help guide the

Table 31C.2 Estimated lowest percentiles of blood pressure (mmHg) in newborn infants

Gestation (week)	Systolic	Mean	Diastolic
23–28	36–38	23–28	—
28–29	40	33	25
30–35	45	35	28
≥36	50	40	30

clinician as to indicate what blood pressure is low and if further action is needed.

Blood flow

Adding blood flow measurements to the hemodynamic assessment can significantly increase insight into the physiology and pathophysiology at hand. Echocardiography provides detail on cardiac function, volume status, and shunts through the ductus arteriosus and the foramen ovale [16]. Vascular resistance can be calculated and help provide further insight into the cause of the hypotension and poor perfusion. Blood flow is the blood velocity (mL/min) in a vessel, stroke volume is blood volume (mL) per single heart beat, and cardiac output is stroke volume × heart rate (mL/min), usually indexed on weight. The most common used blood flow parameters are right ventricular output (RVO), left ventricular output (LVO), and flow in the vena cava superior (SVC flow) [17]. Although no studies explored the absolute threshold of low systemic blood flow and whether treatment improves outcome (similar to the situation with hypotension), an SVC flow less than 30 mL/kg/min at 5 h of age and less than 45 mL/kg/min thereafter or a ventricular output (RVO or LVO) less than 150 mL/kg/min is associated with increased morbidity and mortality [18–20].

Cardiovascular support therapies

Hypotension and poor perfusion can be supported with volume, inotropes, lusitropes, and vasopressors [21]. It is important to understand the estimated relative cardiovascular receptor stimulatory effects of each individual cardiovascular support medication, as receptor number, binding capacity and stimulatory effect changes with increasing gestational age and postnatal age [22,23].

Dopamine is the most commonly used cardiovascular support therapy in neonatology, mostly having a vasopressor effect with minimal or no increase in blood flow. There is accumulating evidence that dopamine in higher doses (>10 mcg/kg/min) increases the pulmonary vascular resistance to the same or even higher extent as it increases the systemic vascular resistance, especially during hypoxia [24,25]. Dopamine should be used with caution in infants with pulmonary hypertension. Dobutamine has inotropic effects, as do epinephrine and norepinephrine. Before prescribing any drug, it is important to consider the underlying pathophysiology of the cardiovascular compromise as well as the pharmacokinetics and pharmacodynamics of the drug you want to prescribe (Table 31C.3).

Although much supportive data on pharmacodynamics are available from animal and adult studies, limited data are available on cardiovascular action in newborn infants, and even less on actions in very preterm infants [21]. The expected action (e.g., vasoconstriction with dopamine) is not always happening, and this is reflected in a 10%–20% nonresponder rate of commonly used cardiovascular support medications. Careful titration of these medications is fundamental to decrease the chances of side effects and enhance drug effectiveness. Catecholamine overload should be avoided, but an appropriate starting dose could improve response rates. Many available clinical guidelines would recommend to start norepinephrine at a dose of 0.05 mcg/kg/min, but the available clinical evidence shows that this dose is not sufficient for newborn infants. Effective doses in term and preterm infants were 10× higher at a median dose of 0.5 mcg/kg/min [26,27]. Continuous monitoring, including echocardiography, and adjustment of therapy if the patient does not respond are needed to optimize cardiovascular support. Some neonatal units, including our own, have changed the choice of first-line vasoactive drug from dopamine to epinephrine or norepinephrine depending on the clinical findings (presence of PPHN) and the findings on echocardiography. The risk of tachycardia might be reduced by replacing one vasopressor–inotrope for another (epinephrine for dopamine or norepinephrine for epinephrine) instead of adding them all together.

Table 31C.3 Cardiovascular support agents, mechanism of action, and physiological targets

Cardiovascular support agent	Expected actions	Comments	Physiological target
Volume	Improves cardiac input		Low preload, collapsed systemic veins
Dopamine	Pressor	Increases afterload May increase PAP/SAP ratio	Systemic hypotension, normal blood flow
Dobutamine	Pressor, improves contractility	Tachycardia May decrease PAP/SAP ratio	Low contractility, low blood flow
Epinephrine	Pressor, improves contractility	Tachycardia Beta-adrenergic stimulation with hyperglycemia and increased lactate May decrease PAP/SAP ratio	Low contractility, low blood flow, systemic hypotension
Norepinephrine	Pressor, improves contractility	Increases afterload Can decrease PAP/SAP ratio	Low contractility, systemic hypotension with PPHN
Milrinone	Phosphodiesterase inhibitor, improves contractility	Reduces afterload Tachycardia, systemic hypotension May exacerbate right-to-left shunting	Low contractility, low blood flow, high afterload
Vasopressin	Pressor, no effect on contractility	Increases afterload	Systemic hypotension refractory to catecholamine

PAP/SAP, Pulmonary to systemic pressure ratio.

Stepwise approach to cardiovascular support

Hypotension and/or poor perfusion are clinical signs due to an underlying disease processes and pathology, so the primary goal would be to treat the underlying cause and to restore tissue perfusion. Cardiovascular supportive treatment might be needed until the underlying cause has been controlled, and should be targeted toward the pathophysiology found on clinical examination and additional assessments. Review and document all clinical and available physiological parameters such as clinical appearance, mental state, capillary refill, blood pressure (including how and where measured), current respiratory support and settings, (changes in) oxygenation, lactate, pH, and echocardiography findings if available. Document your initial working diagnosis (the most likely cause of the hypotension and/or poor perfusion) and describe the expected underlying physiology. Choose your cardiovascular supportive treatment, and document your expected actions. Predefining "success" can help guide escalation of therapy. If the chosen treatment is not successful, consider changing drug dose or type and repeat your diagnostic assessment. Common clinical situations with cardiovascular compromise are detailed below with a suggested stepwise approach to treatment.

The treatment suggestions are based on the limited available clinical studies, animal data, and unpublished personal case series data.

Transitional hypotension in the very preterm infant

If low blood pressure is the only sign (i.e., normal clinical assessment of perfusion, normal lactate, normal urine output) and there are no significant risk factors for the immediate development of poor perfusion (peripartum hemorrhage, sepsis, significant perinatal hypoxia), current evidence does not support the use of cardiovascular support therapies as this does not improve short-term (cerebral perfusion) or long-term (neurodevelopment) outcomes. However, with persistent (>3 h) or very low blood pressure or associated low blood flow, many clinicians feel increasingly obliged to start supportive measures. There is considerable debate whether to start dopamine or dobutamine, and targeted treatment could be directed by adding measurements of blood flow. If no echocardiography is available, one could direct treatment based on the prevalence of the presence of low blood flow. In ventilated preterm infants, the prevalence is estimated at 30%, but this is significantly lower if the infant is on nasal CPAP [28,29].

- Step 1. Fluid expansion (10 mL/kg bolus over 60 min, up to 20 mL/kg). Generally, the most accepted first intervention, although with very limited supportive evidence.

- Step 2. If normal blood flow or blood flow is unknown, start dopamine 5 mcg/kg/min and increase with 5 mcg/kg/min until effect. If low blood flow, start dobutamine 10 mcg/kg/min.
- Step 3. If dopamine >10 mcg/kg/min is needed, consider echocardiography to evaluate blood flow, preload, contractility, and blood flow distribution. If low blood flow, start dobutamine 10 mcg/kg/min. Consider hydrocortisone 1 mg/kg/dose every 8 h.
- Additional steps. Epinephrine can be considered for refractory hypotension and persistent acidosis. There is no clinical data available on the use of norepinephrine in this clinical situation.

Sepsis with cardiovascular compromise, or systemic inflammatory response syndrome after major surgery

- Step 1. Early fluid expansion (20 ml/kg bolus in 30 min, up to 60 mL/kg).
- Step 2. If unsuccessful to restore blood pressure, start norepinephrine 0.3–0.5 mcg/kg/min and increase with 0.1 mcg/kg/min until effect. Alternatively and if no PPHN is present, start dopamine 5 mcg/kg/min and increase with 5 mcg/kg/min until effect.
- Step 3. If norepinephrine >0.5 mcg/kg/min or dopamine >10 mcg/kg/min is needed, consider echocardiography to evaluate blood flow, preload, contractility, and blood flow distribution. Consider hydrocortisone 1 mg/kg/dose every 8 h.
- Additional steps. Preterm infants with sepsis often present with high central blood flow and (initial) good contractility. Persistent acidosis might change cardiac function that can respond to dobutamine. Dopamine can increase the splanchnic circulation and might be beneficial when NEC is suspected. Epinephrine and/or vasopressin as rescue therapy should be considered for refractory hypotension and persistent acidosis.

Cardiovascular support in infants with pulmonary hypertension

- Step 1. Lowering pulmonary pressures with inhaled nitric oxide reduces right ventricular afterload, and should be started early in the disease process, preferably after confirmation with echocardiography. Inhaled nitric oxide is contraindicated when pulmonary venous pressure is significantly increased (as seen with severe left ventricular dysfunction).
- Step 2. Cardiovascular support can be indicated for left ventricular dysfunction (often early) and/or right ventricular dysfunction (often later, after ductal constriction). Norepinephrine as first-line drug has the best pharmacodynamics for the treatment of low blood pressure (inotropy, increasing systemic vascular resistance > pulmonary vascular resistance) and left ventricular dysfunction in term and preterm infants with PPHN. Dopamine has the worst pharmacodynamics, and should be avoided when possible. Increasing inotropic support until so-called "supra-systemic pressures" are reached is not recommended, as this will increase the pulmonary pressure as well and does not restore the systemic to pulmonary pressure imbalance.
- Additional steps. Milrinone can be used to treat low systemic blood flow due to cardiac dysfunction, but can cause significant systemic hypotension in preterm infants. Low-dose vasopressin as additive has been shown to be effective in improving oxygenation in small cohort studies. Careful management of mean airway pressure can assist in optimizing cardiac function. Continuous distending pressure can significantly increase right atrial pressure. Pump function can be optimized with conventional ventilation strategies if lung parenchymal disease allows.

Cardiovascular support after significant perinatal hypoxia

- Step 1. Fluid expansion (10 mL/kg bolus over 60 min, up to 20 mL/kg).
- Step 2. If significant cardiovascular compromise is present, obtain a cardiac ultrasound to determine cardiac function and target treatment appropriately. Hypotension due to depressed cardiac function with low blood flow will respond best to dobutamine, hypotension due to loss of vascular tone, and normal blood flow to dopamine.
- Additional steps. Pulmonary hypertension after hypoxic ischemia responds to normalizing pCO_2, acidosis, and blood pressure.

References

[1] Short BL, Van Meurs K, Evans JR. Cardiology G. Summary proceedings from the cardiology group on cardiovascular instability in preterm infants. Pediatrics 2006;117:S34–S39.

[2] Stranak Z, Semberova J, Barrington K, O'Donnell C, Marlow N, Naulaers G, et al. International survey on diagnosis and management of hypotension in extremely preterm babies. Eur J Pediatr 2014;173(6):793–798.

[3] Gupta S, Donn SM. Neonatal hypotension: dopamine or dobutamine? Semin Fetal Neonatal Med 2014;19(1):54–59.

[4] Noori S, Seri I. Pathophysiology of newborn hypotension outside the transitional period. Early Hum Dev 2005;81(5):399–404.

[5] Seri I. Management of hypotension and low systemic blood flow in the very low birth weight neonate during the first postnatal week. J Perinatol 2006;26(Suppl. 1):S8–S13.

[6] Faust K, Hartel C, Preuss M, Rabe H, Roll C, Emeis M, et al. Short-term outcome of very-low-birthweight infants with arterial hypotension in the first 24 h of life. Arch Dis Child Fetal Neonatal Ed 2015;100(5):F388–F392.

[7] Batton B, Li L, Newman NS, Das A, Watterberg KL, Yoder BA, et al. Early blood pressure, antihypotensive therapy and outcomes at 18–22 months' corrected age in extremely preterm infants. Arch Dis Child Fetal Neonatal Ed 2016;101(3):F201–F206.

[8] Durrmeyer X, Marchand-Martin L, Porcher R, Gascoin G, Roze JC, Storme L, et al. Abstention or intervention for isolated hypotension in the first 3 days of life in extremely preterm infants: association with short-term outcomes in the EPIPAGE 2 cohort study. Arch Dis Child Fetal Neonatal Ed 2017;102(6):490–496.

[9] Andersen CC, Hodyl NA, Kirpalani HM, Stark MJ. A theoretical and practical approach to defining "adequate oxygenation" in the preterm newborn. Pediatrics 2017;139(4). pii: e20161117.

[10] de Boode WP. Clinical monitoring of systemic hemodynamics in critically ill newborns. Early Hum Dev 2010;86(3):137–141.

[11] Miletin J, Pichova K, Dempsey EM. Bedside detection of low systemic flow in the very low birth weight infant on day 1 of life. Eur J Pediatr 2009;168(7):809–813.

[12] Nadeem M, Clarke A, Dempsey EM. Day 1 serum lactate values in preterm infants less than 32 weeks gestation. Eur J Pediatr 2010;169(6):667–670.

[13] O'Shea J, Dempsey EM. A comparison of blood pressure measurements in newborns. Am J Perinatol 2009;26(2):113–116.

[14] Dannevig I, Dale HC, Liestol K, Lindemann R. Blood pressure in the neonate: three non-invasive oscillometric pressure monitors compared with invasively measured blood pressure. Acta Paediatr 2005;94(2):191–196.

[15] Kent AL, Chaudhari T. Determinants of neonatal blood pressure. Curr Hypertens Rep 2013;15(5):426–432.

[16] de Waal K, Kluckow M. Functional echocardiography; from physiology to treatment. Early Hum Dev 2010;86(3):149–154.

[17] de Waal KA. The methodology of Doppler-derived central blood flow measurements in newborn infants. Int J Pediatr 2012;2012:680162.

[18] Osborn DA, Evans N, Kluckow M. Hemodynamic and antecedent risk factors of early and late periventricular/intraventricular hemorrhage in premature infants. Pediatrics 2003;112(1 Pt. 1):33–39.

[19] Kluckow M, Evans N. Low superior vena cava flow and intraventricular haemorrhage in preterm infants. Arch Dis Child Fetal Neonatal Ed 2000;82(3):F188–F194.

[20] Hunt RW, Evans N, Rieger I, Kluckow M. Low superior vena cava flow and neurodevelopment at 3 years in very preterm infants. J Pediatr 2004;145(5):588–592.

[21] Noori S, Seri I. Neonatal blood pressure support: the use of inotropes, lusitropes, and other vasopressor agents. Clin Perinatol 2012;39(1):221–238.

[22] Buckley NM, Gootman PM, Yellin EL, Brazeau P. Age-related cardiovascular effects of catecholamines in anesthetized piglets. Circ Res 1979;45(2):282–292.

[23] Kim MY, Finch AM, Lumbers ER, Boyce AC, Gibson KJ, Eiby YA, et al. Expression of adrenoceptor subtypes in preterm piglet heart is different to term heart. PLoS One 2014;9(3):e92167.

[24] Cheung PY, Barrington KJ. The effects of dopamine and epinephrine on hemodynamics and oxygen metabolism in hypoxic anesthetized piglets. Crit Care 2001;5(3):158–166.

[25] Barrington KJ, Finer NN, Chan WK. A blind, randomized comparison of the circulatory effects of dopamine and epinephrine infusions in the newborn piglet during normoxia and hypoxia. Crit Care Med 1995;23(4):740–748.

[26] Tourneux P, Rakza T, Bouissou A, Krim G, Storme L. Pulmonary circulatory effects of norepinephrine in newborn infants with persistent pulmonary hypertension. J Pediatr 2008;153(3):345–349.

[27] Rowcliff K, de Waal K, Mohamed AL, Chaudhari T. Noradrenaline in preterm infants with cardiovascular compromise. Eur J Pediatr 2016;175(12):1967–1973.

[28] Kluckow M. Low systemic blood flow and pathophysiology of the preterm transitional circulation. Early Hum Dev 2005;81(5):429–437.

[29] Lakkundi A, Wright I, de Waal K. Transitional hemodynamics in preterm infants with a respiratory management strategy directed at avoidance of mechanical ventilation. Early Hum Dev 2014;90(8):409–412.

Section | VII |

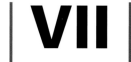

Ancillary Services

Chapter | **32** |

Monitoring of Gas Exchange in the NICU

Bobby Mathew, MBBS, MRCP, Junaid Muhib Khan, MD, FAAP, FAAF, Satyan Lakshminrusimha, MD

CHAPTER POINTS

- Gas exchange is often compromised in preterm and sick term newborns in the NICU and needs close monitoring.
- Neonatal respiratory conditions and their management can result in hypoxemia, hyperoxemia, hypocarbia and hypercarbia and can potentially have deleterious effects on morbidity, mortality and neurodevelopmental outcomes.
- Arterial blood gas analysis provides information on gas exchange in the lungs and metabolism at the tissue level and is the gold standard; however, it is invasive, requires a blood sample and assesses gas exchange on an intermittent basis only.
- Noninvasive monitoring using pulse oximetry, transcutaneous oxygen saturation and carbon dioxide monitoring, capnography and near infrared spectroscopy provide continuous assessment and have decreased the need for frequent blood gas analysis.

The lung is the organ of gas exchange in mammals. Gas exchange is a complex process involving dynamic interactions between the respiratory, cardiovascular, and central nervous systems. In healthy individuals breathing room air, the blood gases are maintained in a narrow normal range. However, in premature infants and sick newborns receiving supplemental oxygen or assisted ventilation, gas exchange may be compromised. The deleterious effects of hypoxia, hyperoxia, hypocarbia, and hypercarbia on morbidity, mortality, and neurodevelopmental outcomes have been well documented [1–4]. Hence close frequent monitoring of blood gases is needed to optimize respiratory and cardiovascular support and maintain homeostasis. Analysis of arterial blood gas (ABG) is the gold standard for assessment of gas exchange. However, blood gas analysis provides only a snapshot of a very dynamic process, and often there is a delay unless performed using a point-of-care device. Arterial access is also associated with inherent risks such as vasospasm, thrombosis, ischemic injury (see Chapter 37 B on limb ischemia), blood loss, and resulting anemia. Noninvasive methods confer minimal risk to the patient and do not require a specimen and provide continuous measurement. Various modalities such as pulse oximetry, transcutaneous monitoring of oxygen and carbon dioxide tension, end-tidal carbon dioxide monitoring, and near-infrared spectroscopy (NIRS) allow less invasive and more continuous assessment of gas exchange and are being used in the neonatal intensive care unit (NICU). This chapter describes the various modalities of monitoring of gas exchange, the indications, strengths, and limitations as it relates to infants receiving neonatal intensive care. A brief review of the physiology of acid-base balance, gas exchange and transport, and the technical aspects of blood gas measurement is included.

Physiology of gas exchange

The blood gas analysis provides information about gas exchange in the lungs and oxygen extraction and utilization at the tissue level. As the blood passes the pulmonary capillaries, oxygen diffuses from the alveolus into the pulmonary capillary and carbon dioxide from the blood into the alveolus. In an individual with normal lung function, the hemoglobin is fully saturated with oxygen in the blood that returns to the left atrium. In conditions that allow blood from the right ventricle to the left atrium, bypassing the gas exchange processes in the lung, leads to a decrease in arterial oxygen content. This may be due to ventilation perfusion mismatch with pulmonary blood flow through atelectatic or underventilated alveoli (intrapulmonary shunt) or through an anatomic right-to-left shunt as in cyanotic congenital heart disease (CHD) (extrapulmonary shunt, Fig. 32.1). The carbon dioxide level in the arterial blood is the measure of the adequacy of alveolar ventilation. As minute ventilation decreases or with perfusion to atelectatic areas of the lungs the $PaCO_2$ in the arterial blood increases. ABGs provide information about adequacy of alveolar ventilation and ventilation–perfusion matching.

Oxygen transport

The gas tension is the partial pressure of a gas in the blood. The partial pressure of a gas is the pressure exerted by the gas in a mixture of gases. It is related to the concentration of the gas to the total pressure of the mixture. Oxygen diffuses into the pulmonary capillary from the alveolus down its concentration gradient. Gas exchange in the lungs occurs as a function of partial pressure differences in oxygen and carbon dioxide between the alveoli and the blood in the pulmonary capillaries. Although the solubility of oxygen in blood is not high, the difference in the partial pressure of oxygen in the alveoli (PAO_2, approximately 100 mmHg) versus in the blood of the pulmonary capillaries (40 mmHg, usually the same as mixed venous PvO_2) is high (about 60 mmHg). This large difference in partial pressure creates a very strong pressure gradient that causes oxygen to rapidly cross the respiratory membrane from the alveoli into the blood. The partial pressure of oxygen in the arterial blood in a newborn is between 55 and 90 mmHg. Most of the oxygen (approximately 97%) is bound to the hemoglobin and the rest 3% is dissolved in plasma. Although only a small fraction of oxygen is dissolved in the plasma, this is physiologically very important as this is the fraction that is available for diffusion to the tissue.

The oxygen delivery to the tissues is dependent on the cardiac output and the oxygen content of the blood. The oxygen content of the arterial blood is the sum of the oxygen bound to hemoglobin and the dissolved fraction. The amount of oxygen carried by the hemoglobin-bound fraction depends on the hemoglobin concentration and the percent saturation of hemoglobin. The oxyhemoglobin dissociation curve depicts the relationship between PaO_2 and the oxygen saturation. It is sigmoidal over the physiological range with the hemoglobin almost fully saturated at PaO_2

between 80 and 100 mmHg. The amount of oxygen bound to hemoglobin at any given pO_2 depends upon the position on the hemoglobin–oxygen dissociation curve. The position of the oxyhemoglobin dissociation curve depends on the type of hemoglobin, adult hemoglobin (HbA) versus fetal hemoglobin (HbF), the concentration of red blood cell 2,3-diphosphoglycerate (2,3-DPG), temperature, and pH. Higher levels of HbA, 2,3-DPG, temperature, and hydrogen ions concentration shift the curve to the right which favors the release of oxygen from the hemoglobin. The amount of dissolved oxygen is directly proportional to the PaO_2 and at normal body temperature is about 0.3 mL dissolved in 100 mL of plasma for 100 mmHg of oxygen. The oxygen content in the blood can be mathematically expressed as:

$$CaO_2 \text{ (in mL / dL of blood)}$$
$$= Hb\,(g\%) \times \text{Oxygen capacity}$$
$$\times\% \text{ saturation} + 0.003 \times PaO_2 \text{ (in mmHg)}$$

Oxygen capacity is the maximum amount of oxygen that can be carried by a gram of hemoglobin that is fully saturated and is 1.34 mL oxygen per gram of 100% saturated hemoglobin.

In a normal newborn infant with hemoglobin of 15 mg/dL with oxyhemoglobin saturation of 100% and the PaO_2 of 100 mmHg the oxygen content of the arterial blood is approximately equal to

$$15 \times 1.34 \times 1 + 0.003 \times 100 = 20.3 \text{ mL O}_2 \text{ / 100 mL}$$

of arterial blood or 0.2 mL O_2 per mL of arterial blood.

Assuming that the normal newborn cardiac output is approximately 120 mL/kg/min, the systemic oxygen delivery may be calculated approximately to be:

$$\text{Cardiac output (Qs)} \times \text{Oxygen content (CaO}_2)$$
$$= 120 \text{ mL / kg / min} \times 0.2 \text{ mL O}_2 \text{ / mL of blood}$$
$$= 24 \text{ mL O}_2 \text{ / kg / min}$$

In the resting state, oxygen consumption in a neonate is approximately 6 mL/kg/min. The body extracts 6 mL/kg/min oxygen from the 24 mL/kg/min of oxygen delivered within extraction rate of approximately 25% of the delivered oxygen. The blood that is returning to the heart would therefore be approximately 75% saturated. The mixed venous saturation of the blood is an indication of the adequacy of tissue perfusion and oxygen delivery. In most cases, in neonates, mixed venous saturation monitoring is not performed and other indirect indicators of anaerobic metabolism such as lactic acid levels are relied upon as indicators of adequate tissue oxygen delivery.

Carbon dioxide transport

The $PaCO_2$ in the arterial blood reflects the balance between metabolic production of carbon dioxide and its excretion by ventilation through the lungs. Although the

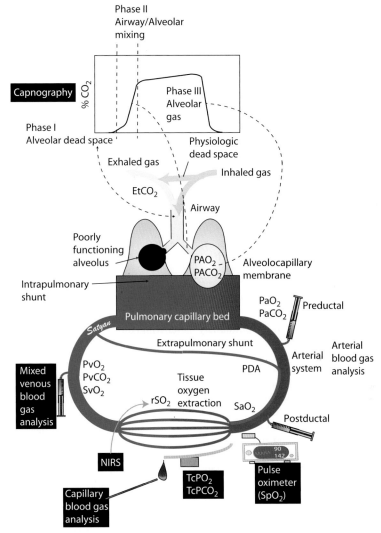

Fig. 32.1 Invasive and Noninvasive Assessment of Gas Exchange in Neonates. Gas exchange in the lung occurs at the alveolocapillary membrane. Oxygen and CO_2 diffuse from and to the alveolus. The $PACO_2$ and PAO_2 are in equilibration with pulmonary blood. During exhalation, the initial part of exhaled gas (phase I) is predominantly from the airway and has minimal CO_2. During phase II, a mixture of airway and alveolar gas is exhaled resulting in increase in CO_2. During phase III, alveolar gas is exhaled and the $EtCO_2$ evaluated by capnography. The physiologic dead space "dilutes" exhaled gas and increased dead space increases the difference between $PACO_2$ and $EtCO_2$. Arterial blood gas analysis is the gold standard invasive assessment of gas exchange and measures partial pressure of arterial oxygen, CO_2, and arterial oxygen saturation (PaO_2, $PaCO_2$, and SaO_2). Increasing venous shunt (either due to pulmonary hypertension, congenital heart disease, or ventilation–perfusion mismatch) can decrease PaO_2. A pulse oximeter measures oxygen saturation (SpO_2) and is a reliable estimate of SaO_2. Transcutaneous sensors heat the cutaneous capillary bed and measure CO_2 and O_2 tension ($TcPCO_2$ and $TcPO_2$). A capillary blood sample obtained after warming the heel ("arterialized" sample) is commonly used in neonates. NIRS can measure tissue oxygen saturation (rSO_2). Mixed venous blood gas analysis provides partial pressure of CO_2 and O_2 and oxygen saturation ($PvCO_2$, PvO_2 and SvO_2). *EtCO_2,* End-tidal CO_2; *NIRS,* near-infrared spectroscopy; *PACO_2,* alveolar tension of CO_2; *PAO_2,* alveolar tension of O_2. Modified from Assisted Ventilation of the Neonate. 6th ed. Copyright: Satyan Lakshminrusimha.

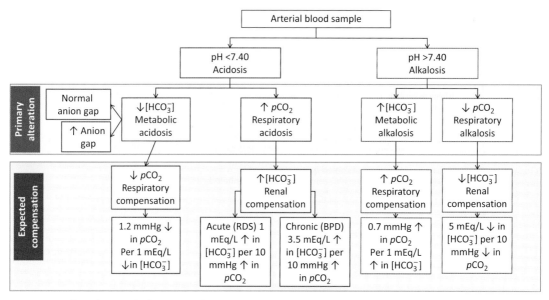

Fig. 32.2 Basics of Acidosis and Alkalosis and Compensatory Mechanisms.

partial pressure difference of CO_2 between the pulmonary capillary (46 mmHg) and the alveolus (40 mmHg) is lower, the high solubility of CO_2 (about 20 times greater than that to O_2) allows for the rapid equilibration of the CO_2 tension between the pulmonary capillary blood and alveolar compartments, which occurs within a fraction of the transit time of the red blood cells along the pulmonary capillaries. Carbon dioxide is carried in the blood as carbonic acid (85%), carbaminohemoglobin (10%), and the rest as dissolved in the plasma. During maximal exercise, CO_2 production increases by as much as 20-fold of the basal rate, but the associated hyperventilation keeps the CO_2 tension in body fluids relatively constant.

Assessment of acid-base balance (Fig. 32.2)

To analyze the acid–base status from a blood gas, three questions must be addressed:
1. Is there acidosis/alkalosis?
   a. Is the pH <7.4 or >7.4
2. What is the primary cause of the disturbance?
   a. Respiratory acidosis if $PaCO_2$ is elevated, respiratory alkalosis if $PaCO_2$ is low.
   b. Metabolic acidosis if bicarbonate is low or metabolic alkalosis if bicarbonate is high
3. Is it compensated? And is the compensation appropriate?
   An acute increase of $PaCO_2$ (as in the acute phase of RDS) by 10 mmHg is expected to drop the pH by 0.08 and increase the HCO_3 by 1 mEq/L. A chronic increase of $PaCO_2$ by 10 mmHg (as in infants with BPD) decreases the pH by 0.03

units and increases the HCO_3 by 3.5 mEq/L. This magnitude of compensation is true up to 70 mmHg $PaCO_2$.

Blood gas analysis

The traditional blood gas analysis provides values for the pH, the partial pressure of oxygen, and carbon dioxide, bicarbonate, and the base excess. The pH is the measure of acidity or alkalinity of a solution and is the negative logarithm of the hydrogen ion concentration in the solution. The blood is slightly alkaline (compared to water) with a pH of 7.35–7.45. When the pH drops from 7.4 to 7 the hydrogen ion concentration increases 2.5-fold. The enzymes catalyzing different reactions within the body work at an optimal level in the physiological range of pH and become nonfunctional below a critical range. The body has an elaborate mechanism to keep the pH within the physiological range under varying levels of exercise/stress. These mechanisms include the different buffer systems in the blood, the lungs and the kidneys. The predominant buffer system in the body is bicarbonate in the plasma. Hemoglobin, plasma phosphate, and plasma proteins also play important role to buffer the extracellular compartment.

Measurement of pH

The first pH electrode was discovered in 1906 by Max Cremer. The pH electrode is based on the principle that an electrical potential develops when two liquids of different pH come in contact at opposite sides of a thin glass membrane. The pH electrode in the blood gas analyzers consists of a glass measuring electrode and a reference electrode. The tip of the measuring electrode is a thin glass membrane that is capable of ion exchange which senses the hydrogen ion concentration of the test solution. The reference electrode potential is produced by the reference electrode internal element which is in contact with the reference fluid solution kept at a pH of 7. The voltage output produced is linearly dependent upon the pH of the solution being measured. The pH is determined by measuring the potential difference between these two electrodes which is converted to and displayed as the pH. The pH electrode's sensitivity increases linearly with temperature and hence it is important to input the temperature of the solution being measured.

Measurement of $PaCO_2$

The $PaCO_2$ sensor is a modification of the pH electrode by Stowe and Severinghaus. The electrode has an outer Silastic semipermeable membrane through which CO_2 diffuses into the bicarbonate buffer. CO_2 reacts with the buffer forming carbonic acid which then dissociates into bicarbonate ion and hydrogen ions.

$$CO_2 + H_2O \rightarrow H_2CO_3 \rightarrow H^+ + HCO_3^-$$

The hydrogen ion diffuses across the glass electrode and this change is measured as it is with the pH electrode. The $PaCO_2$ is determined from the change in pH using the Henderson–Hasselbalch equation.

Measurement of PaO_2

The partial pressure of oxygen is measured using the Clark electrode. It consists of a platinum cathode and the silver chloride anode immersed in phosphate buffer. The platinum electrode is covered with a small lipophilic plate and a gas permeable membrane that separates the test specimen from the electrode and is selectively permeable to oxygen. Oxygen diffuses into the electrolyte to contact the cathode. Electrons are drawn from the anode surface to the cathode to reduce the oxygen. The current produced is proportional to the PaO_2 of the test solution.

Measurement of bicarbonate

Bicarbonate is the principal buffer in the plasma and the predominant form of carbon dioxide transport in the blood. Bicarbonate is a calculated value from the measured values of pH and $PaCO_2$ using the Henderson–Hasselbalch equation. *Actual* bicarbonate is calculated from the pH and pCO_2 of an aerobically drawn arterial specimen. As the pH is affected by the $PaCO_2$ and to eliminate the effect of the

respiratory component, the *standard* bicarbonate is calculated with standard values of $PaCO_2$ of 40 mmHg, PaO_2 100 mmHg, and temperature at 37 °C. Standard bicarbonate is hence a more precise measure of the metabolic component of acidosis. Bicarbonate levels may be decreased due to loss of HCO_3 from the kidneys or the intestines, consumption from need for buffering of excessive acid in the body, or from failure to regenerate bicarbonate. Bicarbonate levels may be elevated due to increased generation of HCO_3 or excessive loss of hydrogen or chloride ions as occurs with loss of acid from the stomach or with diuretic use or with excessive administration of base.

Measurement of base excess

The base excess is defined as the concentration of titratable base when a fluid is titrated to a pH of 7.4 at a pCO_2 of 40 mmHg or it is the number of millimoles of strong acid needed to titrate a blood sample to pH of 7.4 at pCO_2 of 40 mmHg. It can be calculated using the Van Slyke equation or using a nomogram [5]. The base excess is positive if there is a surplus and negative when there is a deficit of bicarbonate. The base excess is calculated using the values of hemoglobin, $PaCO_2$ and bicarbonate.

Base excess reflects the metabolic component of acid-base balance. Two values of BE are provided by the blood gas analyzer. Base excess in whole blood BE(B) and the in extracellular fluid BE(ECF). The BE(ECF) is independent of the effects of $PaCO_2$ and is hence the recommended parameter to use clinically.

Direct measurements are more accurate and reliable; the parameters that are automatically calculated by the analyzer may be subject variables that are not accounted for, contributing to error.

Common acid–base disturbances in the NICU

Respiratory acidosis

Carbon dioxide is the product of aerobic metabolism of glucose in the tissues. It is transported in the blood as bicarbonate (85%), carbaminohemoglobin (10%), and dissolved carbon dioxide (5%) and excreted through the lungs. Respiratory acidosis is due to carbon dioxide retention from impaired excretion through the lungs. Common causes of hypercarbia include atelectasis (ventilation–perfusion mismatch), decreased surface area for gas exchange as in pulmonary hypoplasia and bronchopulmonary dysplasia (BPD), decreased alveolar ventilation as occurs either during mechanical ventilation with inadequate minute ventilation or in spontaneously ventilating infants with decreased respiratory drive, or muscle weakness. Hypercarbia also occurs with airway obstruction and with obstruction of endotracheal tube in mechanically ventilated infants. Restriction of the chest wall as in thoracic dystrophies or severe scoliosis also leads to hypercarbia. Imbalance in the carbohydrate to fat and protein balance can lead to greater CO_2 load and lead to CO_2 retention in the acute phase of RDS or in infants with BPD. Hypercarbia or fluctuation in $PaCO_2$ impairs cerebral autoregulation and increases the risk of intraventricular hemorrhage [4]. Acidosis also increases pulmonary vascular resistance (PVR) and worsens oxygenation in infants with hypoxemic respiratory failure and persistent pulmonary hypertension of the newborn.

Respiratory alkalosis

Respiratory alkalosis is rare as a primary acid–base abnormality. In infants on mechanical ventilation, respiratory alkalosis is often secondary to excessive ventilation. It occurs commonly in infants with hypoxic-ischemic encephalopathy (HIE) related to metabolic acidosis and the attendant increase in respiratory drive. Induced respiratory alkalosis by hyperventilation had been used as a therapeutic strategy in infants with PPHN. Respiratory alkalosis promotes pulmonary vasodilation. However, it also causes cerebral vasoconstriction and is associated with periventricular leukomalacia in premature infants and increased risk of deafness and neurodevelopmental disabilities in infants with PPHN. Recent studies in infants with HIE, it has been shown that hypocapnia is associated with worse neurodevelopmental outcomes.

Metabolic acidosis

Renal bicarbonate wasting is the commonest cause of metabolic acidosis in premature infants. Impaired oxygen delivery leads to tissue hypoxia and anaerobic metabolism resulting in increased production of lactic acid resulting in metabolic acidosis. Other causes of metabolic acidosis include sepsis, inborn errors of metabolism, and iatrogenic as in increased protein load in total parenteral nutrition. The anion gap is useful in evaluation of the etiology and severity in acid-base balance disturbances.

The anion gap is calculated as:

$$Na - [Cl + HCO_3]$$

An elevated serum anion gap is associated with elevated levels of an unmeasured anion such as lactate (lactic acidosis due to anaerobic metabolism), beta hydroxybutyrate and acetoacetate (diabetic ketoacidosis), sulfates and phosphates (renal failure), or an inborn error of metabolism such as organic acidemia. The use of sodium acetate in TPN can often compensate for the renal bicarbonate

loss in premature infants to maintain pH in the normal range. However, the increased CO_2 load may overwhelm the immature lung resulting in hypercapnia and respiratory acidosis.

Metabolic alkalosis

Common causes of metabolic alkalosis in infants include diuretic use and loss of gastric secretions. Hypochloremia and the ensuing metabolic alkalosis during diuretic therapy may be mitigated by supplementation of oral potassium chloride or by decreasing the dose of the diuretic or the use of acetazolamide. Loss of gastric secretions (due to pyloric stenosis or gastric suction) can lead to hypokalemic, hypochloremic metabolic alkalosis. However, in order to conserve vital potassium, the renal tubule may exchange hydrogen ions for potassium resulting in paradoxical aciduria.

Combined metabolic and respiratory acidosis may occur in the setting of HIE or infants with BPD with acute metabolic acidosis superimposed on chronic respiratory acidosis.

Sampling sites for blood gas analysis

Arterial blood gas

Blood gas analysis can be performed on a variety of specimen types including arterial, venous, and capillary samples depending on patient's condition and availability of access. Although the ABG provides the most comprehensive information of gas exchange and acid–base status, it may not be possible or even needed in many clinical scenarios. In addition, indwelling arterial catheters provide continuous assessment of blood pressure. In the newborn, umbilical artery catheters are the preferred route for arterial access for their ease of placement, relative low-risk of complications as compared to peripheral arterial access. Two different sizes (3.5 and 5 Fr) of single lumen arterial catheters are available and the choice is mainly dictated by the size of the infant. Although their relative merits have not been studied, theoretically smaller catheters minimize the disturbance in blood flow in the aorta but may lead to dampening of the arterial pressure wave tracing and may also have a higher risk of failure from clot formation within the lumen of the catheter. Umbilical arterial blood is postductal and this fact has to be considered while assessing oxygenation in newborn infants with hypoxemic respiratory failure and persistent pulmonary hypertension with significant pulmonary artery to systemic shunting of desaturated blood at the level of patent ductus arteriosus

(PDA, Fig. 32.1). Complications associated with umbilical arterial cannulation include those related to vascular compromise, embolization, catheter malposition, infection, thrombosis, and malfunction. Vascular compromise commonly presents with duskiness/pallor of the lower limbs which may be due to vasospasm or due to microemboli and may lead to ischemic necrosis of the limb or the digits. Malpositioning of the tip of the catheter at or near major branches of the aorta can lead to compromised blood supply to the intestines or to the kidneys. Thrombus formation is very common following umbilical catheterization but is usually not clinically evident as in most cases it is nonobstructive and usually presents with thrombocytopenia due to platelet consumption. Bleeding from accidental catheter disconnection or vascular perforation during catheter insertion is rare but can be life threatening. Sterile precautions should be ensured during placement and while accessing these lines to reduce the risk of central line-associated sepsis. Studies using NIRS and ultrasound have shown alterations in cerebral blood flow and oxygenation during blood sampling from umbilical catheters. Although it is unclear whether these changes in cerebral hemodynamics leads to complications, smaller volumes and slower rate of withdrawal may reduce the magnitude of these changes.

In older infants and in infants in whom umbilical arterial catheterization is unsuccessful, cannulation of a peripheral artery such as radial, ulnar, posterior tibial, or dorsalis pedis may be an option. It is important to assess and document adequacy of collateral circulation by physical examination or by Doppler study prior to cannulating the vessel. Close monitoring for signs of vascular compromise should be ensured as ischemic necrosis of the digits is a known complication associated with peripheral arterial catheters.

Percutaneous puncture of one of the peripheral arteries may be performed in less ill infants in whom the need for ABG analysis is infrequent and do not justify the risks associated with an indwelling line. The main disadvantage of arterial puncture is the discomfort associated with the procedure frequently causes agitation enough to disrupt the steady state and blood gas results may not be reflective of the infants cardiorespiratory status.

Venous blood gas

Venous blood gas (VBG) analysis provides reliable estimates of the pH, $PaCO_2$, and bicarbonate levels. Results obtained from VBGs are affected by tissue metabolism and effects from peripheral circulation. Multiple studies in adult patients have validated the correlation between arterial and central VBG for pH, $PaCO_2$, and bicarbonate levels [6,7]. In general, central venous pH is on average 0.03 units lower, $PaCO_2$ 5–6 mmHg higher, and bicarbonate similar to arterial samples. Calculations using the regression equations

that have been developed from studies comparing ABGs versus Central VBGs provide more precise estimates of pH and $PaCO_2$ and bicarbonate values. With noninvasive monitoring using pulse oximetry being standard in most NICUs, a combination of SpO_2 monitoring with intermittent VBGs may provide the information needed to make treatment decisions in most clinical situations. However, it is important to bear in mind that these studies were all performed in adult patients and central venous blood samples were used in these studies.

Capillary blood gas

The concept of arterialized capillary blood gas (CBG) is based on the premise that blood flowing through a dilated capillary bed approximates that of the arterial blood as there is little time for O_2 and CO_2 exchange to occur. CBG is obtained by arterializing the capillary blood by warming the extremity. During collection as the blood is exposed to the atmosphere, PaO_2 and to a lesser extent the $PaCO_2$ values are subject to error. CBG analysis is often used to follow trends in $PaCO_2$ and pH in chronically ventilated infants.

Fiber-optic catheters may be used for invasive inline analysis of pH, pCO_2, and pO_2. In dwelling catheters and analysis systems allow for continuous blood gas and blood pressure monitoring with minimal blood loss. However, the use of this technology has not gained widespread application in the NICU.

Details of indications, technique of insertion, positioning of catheters, and complications are explained in the chapter on Procedures (Chapter 37 A).

Temperature correction

The solubility of a gas in a liquid increases with a decrease in temperature (Henry's law). The partial pressure of the gas decreases as the solubility increases. Hence, hypothermia is associated with decreased $PaCO_2$ and PaO_2 due to increased solubility and hyperthermia with increased $PaCO_2$ and PaO_2. This temperature-dependent change in $PaCO_2$ affects blood pH. Hence hypothermia causes an increase and hyperthermia a decrease in pH [8]. Change in body temperature shifts in the oxyhemoglobin dissociation curve and changes oxygen consumption and carbon dioxide production (Fig. 32.3). Decrease in body temperature causes a leftward shift in the oxyhemoglobin dissociation curve with increased hemoglobin affinity for oxygen. The change in hemoglobin affinity for oxygen induced by change in body temperature has the potential of decreasing oxygen delivery to tissues in hypothermia and decrease binding of oxygen to hemoglobin at the lungs in normothermia. Due to the sigmoidal shape of the oxyhemoglobin curve, the potential for these body temperature effects is exaggerated in conditions of hypoxemia [9]. Hypothermia

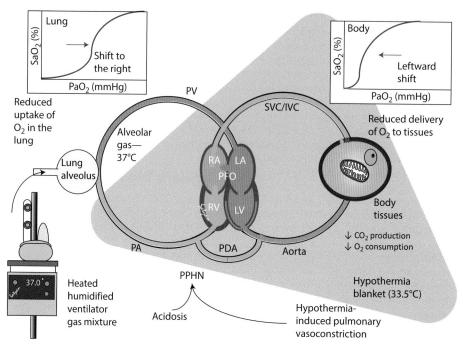

Fig. 32.3 The Influence of Whole Body Hypothermia on Gas Exchange in a Patient With PPHN on Mechanical Ventilation. The lung is ventilated with humidified, heated gas usually at approximately 37°C. During whole body hypothermia, the body is cooled to 33.5°C. During hypothermia, the oxygen–hemoglobin dissociation curve shifts to the left increasing hemoglobin's affinity for oxygen. This phenomenon results in reduced delivery of oxygen to the tissues. During hypothermia, the metabolism is lower and there is reduced demand for oxygen. In the lungs, the alveolar gas temperature is normal at 37°C. Here the oxygen–hemoglobin dissociation curve is shifted to the right resulting in reduced uptake of oxygen. Copyright: Satyan Lakshminrusimha.

is associated with reduced oxygen consumption and carbon dioxide production. Design of blood gas analyzers only allows for samples to be prewarmed to 37°C prior to measurement. The temperature-corrected values, which can be obtained by inputting the patient's temperature to the analyzer, are the true in vivo values of the patient and are calculated using formulas and algorithms. The formulas used for correction for pH and PaCO$_2$ are as follows.

$$pH(T) = pH(37) - [0.0146 + 0.065 \times (pH(37) - 7.40)][T-37]$$

$$pCO_2(T) = pCO_2(37) \times 10^{[0.021 \times (T-37)]}$$

where pH (T) = patient's temperature-corrected pH
  pH (37) = patient's pH measured at 37°C
  pCO_2 (T) = patient's temperature-corrected pCO_2
  pCO_2 (37) = patient's pCO_2 measured at 37°C
  T = patient's core temperature (°C)
PaO$_2$ changes approximately 7% for each 1°C deviation from 37°C (Fig. 32.4).

The pulmonary and cerebral blood flows are sensitive to changes in pH, PaCO$_2$, and PaO$_2$. These differences within physiological range of temperature may not cause discernible changes in homeostasis due to the ability of the body

to compensate. However, in pathological states where the ability of the body is compromised due to illness or stress these may lead to disruptions in homeostasis. With the clinical use of hypothermia treatment for HIE and during cardiopulmonary bypass, the higher degrees of deviation of temperature from the normal lead to physiologically significant changes in pH and PaCO$_2$. For example, an arterial sample drawn on an infant during cardiac surgery while undergoing hypothermia to 20°C and analyzed at that temperature with pH 7.65 and pCO_2 18 mmHg, when analyzed at 37°C the values would be pH 7.4 and pCO_2 40 mmHg.

With decreasing temperature, more gas is dissolved in plasma, and the partial pressure of CO_2 and O_2 decreases [10]. Maintenance of the same pCO_2 or pO_2 under hypothermic conditions will require greater CO_2 or O_2 content. Two acid–base management approaches during hypothermia are described in the literature in reference to pediatric cardiac anesthesia management and profound hypothermia (usually 18–20°C) for brief periods of time [11]. However, no studies have evaluated the optimal approach during mild hypothermia (33–34°C) for HIE [12].

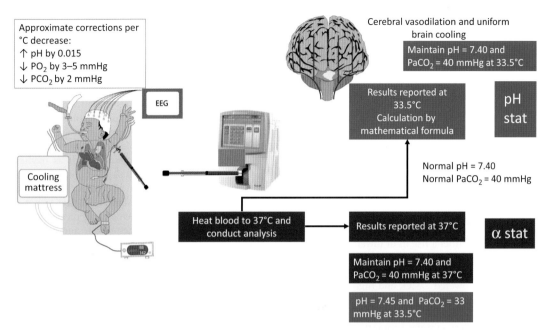

Fig. 32.4 The Differences Between pH-Stat and α-Stat Approaches to Blood Gas Management During Hypothermia.
All blood samples are warmed to 37°C during measurement in the blood gas analyzer. Subsequently, the gases may be reported at patient's body temperature (pH-stat method) and attempts are made to maintain normal pH and $PaCO_2$ at patient's body temperature (33.5°C). In the α-stat method, blood gases are reported at 37°C and attempts are made to normalize pH and $PaCO_2$ at 37°C. The main difference with the two approaches is that pH-stat method results in slightly higher $PaCO_2$ levels leading to cerebral vasodilation and uniform brain cooling. Copyright: Satyan Lakshminrusimha.

Management by the *α-stat technique* is focused on maintaining a normal pH and $PaCO_2$ at 37°C and not at the current body temperature. As the temperature falls during induced hypothermia, $PaCO_2$ measured at the patient's temperature decreases and pH increases. Ventilation is adjusted to maintain normal $PaCO_2$ at 37°C. This approach is based on the fact that as temperature decreases, blood and tissue pH rise but the dissociative state of α-imidazole, and thus protein function, remains close to normal. In the *pH-stat technique*, $PaCO_2$ in the blood gas drawn from a hypothermic patient is measured after warming the blood to 37°C but is mathematically corrected to the patient's temperature (Fig. 32.4). Ventilation is then adjusted to achieve a normal pH and $PaCO_2$ at patient's temperature. This results in higher CO_2 content (as compared to the α-stat method), and leads to concurrent cerebral vasodilation and pulmonary vasoconstriction, resulting in higher cerebral blood flow and more effective and homogenous brain cooling [11]. Thus, most studies evaluating hypothermia for HIE have adapted pH-stat method for acid–base management [13–15]. In addition, animal studies with hypothermia demonstrate better suppression of cerebral metabolic rate with pH-stat method [11]. Maintaining high $PaCO_2$ values

(>50 mmHg, when corrected for body temperature) can theoretically be associated with high dissolved CO_2 levels and exacerbate pulmonary vasoconstriction.

The optimal range of $PaCO_2$ and PaO_2 during whole-body hypothermia for HIE are not known. The cerebral and pulmonary circulations respond to changes in pH, pCO_2, and pO_2 in opposite ways. Low $PaCO_2$ (<35 mmHg) [2] and high PaO_2 (>100 mmHg) [16] during the immediate postnatal period are associated with poor outcomes in neonates with HIE undergoing whole-body hypothermia [17]. In contrast, animal studies have demonstrated that hypercarbia, acidosis (pH <7.25), and hypoxemia (PaO_2 <50 mmHg) increase PVR [18] leading to PPHN. Hence, we recommend adopting the pH-stat method and maintaining corrected $PaCO_2$ in the mid-40s and corrected PaO_2 in the 50–80 mmHg range to optimize cerebral and pulmonary circulations [19]. These guidelines for corrected $PaCO_2$ are similar to those recommended by Chakkarapani and Thoresen (corrected $PaCO_2$: 41–50 mmHg) [20].

Although it is unclear at this time as to the relative merits of either methodology in clinical management of the neonate, it is important that each facility has a consistent approach to avoid inconsistencies with interpretation of blood gases and decision making in treatment. The authors prefer the use of pH-stat method during management of infants with respiratory disease and PPHN associated with HIE undergoing moderate hypothermia.

Errors in blood gas monitoring

Sources of error in blood gas monitoring can occur during collection, analysis, or reporting. Errors in collection include mislabeling of specimens, suboptimal technique, exposure of the sample to air, inadequate mixing of the sample, delay and improper storage of sample during transit, dilution of sample from inadequate "waste," and clotting of specimen. The room air has PaO_2 of approximately 150 mmHg and $PaCO_2$ close to 0. Exposure to ambient air/contamination with air bubbles results in lowering of $PaCO_2$ and either a rise in or lowering of the PaO_2 depending on whether the PaO_2 of the sample is greater or less than 150 mmHg. Dilution of the sample with IV fluids typically results in lowered $PaCO_2$ and higher base deficit. Delay in processing of the sample can result in increase in $PaCO_2$ as the metabolism continues in the cells. Hence, it is important to process samples promptly or to transport the sample on ice if there will be a delay in processing the sample.

Errors in analysis include errors associated with inadequate instrument maintenance, quality control, failure to run calibration or inaccurate calibration set points, analyzing insufficient samples, and temperature control errors. Errors in the reporting stage include failure to recognize and interpret flags, instrument errors, and transcription errors. Coordinated efforts from phlebotomists, nursing, medical, and laboratory staff; biomedical engineering; and IT team managing electronic medical records is needed to reduce/prevent these errors that have serious impact on patient care.

Noninvasive monitoring of oxygenation—pulse oximetry

Supplemental oxygen has been widely used in the neonatal intensive care for over the last 60 years. Large gaps in knowledge exist regarding the indications, optimal dose, and monitoring of oxygen use in the NICU. The epidemic of retinopathy of prematurity in the 1940s is well documented in the neonatal literature. Controversy surrounding the target saturation during intensive care of preterm infants continues despite multiple large randomized controlled trials done specifically to address this question [21–25]. Clinically cyanosis is detectable by visual examination only when deoxyhemoglobin is above 5 g/dL and this corresponds to saturations in the low 70% range

depending on the hematocrit and is an unreliable assessment of oxygenation. Hence, continuous monitoring of hemoglobin oxygen saturation is imperative to provide optimal care.

Pulse oximetry measures the percentage of hemoglobin saturated with oxygen. It is a transcutaneous, noninvasive estimate of SaO_2 and displays a plethysmographic waveform and provides a continuous recording of the heart rate (Fig. 32.5). The monitoring of hemoglobin saturation by pulse oximetry is possible due to the distinct absorption spectra of the chromophores such as oxyhemoglobin and deoxyhemoglobin and the transparency of tissue to light in the near-infrared spectrum. Pulse oximetry is based on the Beer–Lambert law which states that absorption of light of a given wavelength is proportional to the product of the solute concentration and the light path length [26,27]. Pulse oximetry is based on the principles of (1) spectrophotometry—oxygenated hemoglobin and reduced hemoglobin have different absorption spectra at different wavelengths of light (red and near infrared) and (2) photoplethysmography—the amount of light absorbed by blood in the tissue changes with the arterial pulse. The pulse oximeter probe consists of two light-emitting diodes and a photo detector that are positioned facing each other with the light passing intermittently at very high frequency through the interposed tissue. Absorption during pulsatile flow is due to the arterial blood, venous blood, and the interposed tissue whereas absorption during nonpulsatile flow is due to the venous blood and tissue. Saturation is calculated from the relative absorption of the two wavelengths during pulsatile flow (due to arterial blood—AC) divided by absorption during nonpulsatile flow (venous and tissue absorption—DC).

$$SpO_2 = f(AC_{red} / DC_{red}) / (AC_{infrared} / DC_{infrared})$$

where f is the calibration constant.

Calibration algorithm for pulse oximetry is generated by subjecting healthy volunteers to varying inspired oxygen concentrations and correlating the arterial SaO_2 estimated by cooximetry with the ratio of absorption ratios over a range of saturation values [28]. Due to ethical concerns from exposing healthy volunteers to hazardously low saturations, readings below 75% are based on data extrapolated from calibration values obtained between 100% and 75%. "Blue" (Masimo, Irvine, CA, USA) sensors calibrated for 60%–80% range are being used in neonates with cyanotic CHD (http://www.masimo.com/sensors/specialty.htm). These sensors are more accurate in the 75%–85% range with 86% of samples being within 5% of values obtained by cooximetry with a decrease in accuracy for SaO_2 values less than 75%.

Although pulse oximetry is now standard of care in NICUs, there are no established normal values in newborns. Pulse oximetry studies in healthy term infants and

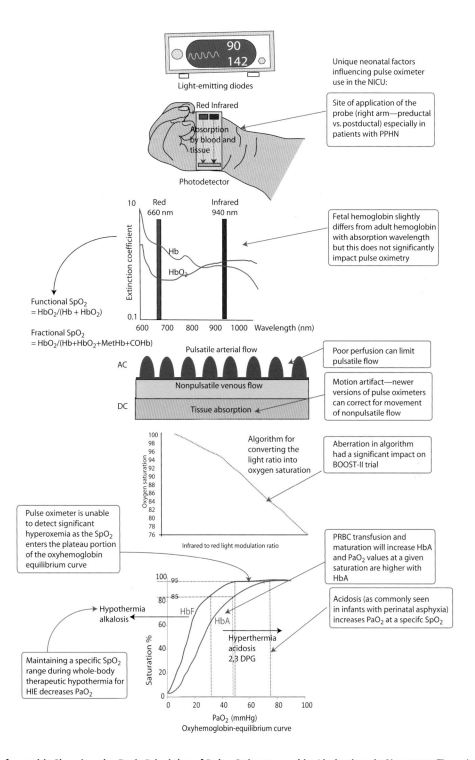

Fig. 32.5 Infographic Showing the Basic Principles of Pulse Oximetry and its Limitations in Neonates. The pulse oximeter probe has diodes that emit light in the red and infrared spectrum. After absorption of this light by pulsatile arterial blood, venous blood, and tissue, it is detected by photodetectors in the pulse oximeter probe. The extinction coefficient for Hb and HbO_2 are different at red and infrared spectra. The infrared to red light modulation ratio is converted to a SpO_2 number using an algorithm. The SpO_2 is usually within ±3% of SaO_2. The relationship between PaO_2 and SaO_2 is the oxyhemoglobin–equilibrium curve. Limitations of pulse oximetry are shown in red boxes. *Hb*, Hemoglobin. Modified from Assisted Ventilation of the Neonate. 6th ed.

preterm infants have shown average saturations to be 97% and 95%, respectively [29–31]. The controversies regarding the target range of saturations for premature infants receiving respiratory support/supplemental oxygen or term infants with persistent pulmonary hypertension remain unresolved [32,33]. Arterial oxygen saturation measured by pulse oximetry accounts for approximately 98% of arterial oxygen content. In the presence of normal hematocrit and perfusion, saturations over 90% ensure adequate tissue oxygen delivery. Some of the limitations are outlined in Fig. 32.6.

Indications of pulse oximetry

Pulse oximetry is considered as the fifth vital sign and has become the standard of care in NICUs. In the NICU, pulse oximetry is used to:

1. titrate inspired oxygen concentration in infants receiving supplemental oxygen;

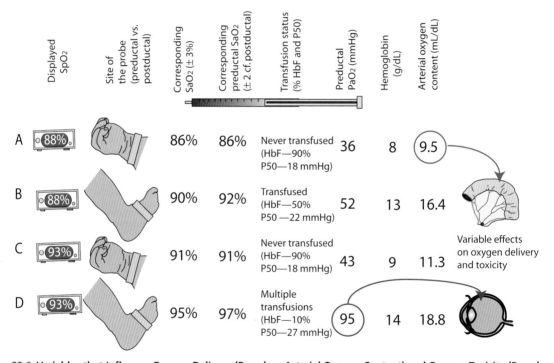

Fig. 32.6 Variables that Influence Oxygen Delivery (Based on Arterial Oxygen Content) and Oxygen Toxicity (Based on PaO₂). This figure illustrates the variation in the arterial oxygen content compared to pulse oximetry based on factors such as site of probe placement, hemoglobin type, and content. Each row represents an infant with a specific combination of variables. The oxygen content can vary twofold with a 5% difference in SpO$_2$ on the pulse oximeter, and an infant with a lower SpO$_2$ (88%) can actually have higher oxygen content than the one with a higher SpO$_2$ (93%). Infant A has a preductal SpO$_2$ of 88%, which can correspond to SaO$_2$ range of 85%–91% in approximately two-third of subjects (±3% variation with pulse oximeters). If the corresponding preductal SaO$_2$ is assumed to be 86%, and she has never received a transfusion, her HbF concentration is ~90%. The corresponding preductal PaO$_2$ is 36 mmHg. If this infant has Hb concentration of 8 g/dL, her arterial oxygen content will be approximately 9.5 mL/dL. Infant B has a postductal SpO$_2$ of 88%, which can correspond to a SaO$_2$ range of 85%–91% in approximately two-third of subjects. If postductal SaO$_2$ is assumed to be 90%, the corresponding preductal SaO$_2$ may be 92%. If this baby had received two transfusions, her HbF concentration is approximately 50% and the corresponding preductal PaO$_2$ is 52 mmHg. If this infant's Hb concentration is 13 g/dL, her arterial oxygen content will be approximately 16.4 mL/dL. Infant C who has never been transfused with blood and with a preductal SpO$_2$ of 93% and a PaO$_2$ of 43 mmHg is at significantly reduced risk of oxygen toxicity compared with infant B in spite of a higher displayed SpO$_2$. Infant D has the same displayed SpO$_2$ as infant C (93%). However, his pulse oximeter is located on his left foot (postductal), and he has received blood transfusions. His PaO$_2$ is considerably higher (95 mmHg) compared with infant C (43 mmHg) placing him at risk for oxygen toxicity. A higher Hb concentration results in higher arterial oxygen content. *Hb*, Hemoglobin; *HbF*, hemoglobin F; *SaO$_2$*, arterial oxygen saturation; *SpO$_2$*, displayed oxygen saturation. Modified from Assisted Ventilation of the Neonate. 6th ed; Lakshminrusimha et al. J Perinatol (2015) [32]. Copyright: Satyan Lakshminrusimha.

2. monitor stable growing premature infants for bradycardia and desaturation spells for fitness for discharge;
3. define BPD with the oxygen reduction test;
4. monitor supplemental oxygen therapy during delivery room resuscitation and stabilization;
5. screen for critical CHD in the newborn period;
6. diagnose and manage PPHN by pre- and postductal saturation monitoring;
7. monitor cardiorespiratory status during transport of critically ill newborns and premature infants; and
8. perform car seat testing prior to discharge of at-risk infants.

Delivery room

With increasing awareness of the dangers of oxidative stress associated with hyperoxia in the immediate newborn period, the use of oxygen blenders and pulse oximetry is recommended for resuscitation and stabilization of newborn infants in the delivery room. Pulse oximetry is used to gauge response to resuscitation (improvement in saturation and heart rate) and to titrate supplemental oxygen therapy. The Neonatal Resuscitation Program 2015 guidelines provide target saturations for time after birth to guide oxygen therapy for newborn infants in the delivery room [34–37]. The delivery room presents unique challenges from other settings in which pulse oximetry is routinely used. Delay in obtaining stable tracing and read out of saturations and heart rate is common in the delivery room setting. The average time to detect reliable signal on pulse oximetry in the delivery room has been estimated to be between 1 and 2 min [35,38,39]. The probe should be applied to the right wrist as there is a substantial pre- and postductal saturation difference in the immediate newborn period and the nomograms for delivery room target saturations have been created using preductal oxygen saturations. Also signal detection has been shown to be sooner with the pulse oximetry probe applied to the hand as compared to the foot [40]. Difficulties with probe placement, movement, poor perfusion, and high ambient light can all interfere with obtaining reliable pulse oximetry signal.

CHD screening

Pulse oximetry is being used as newborn screening test for critical CHD, between 24 and 48 h of postnatal age and prior to discharge. A positive screen is defined as having SpO_2 reading of less than 95% in either pre- or postductal sites or difference of greater than 3% between pre- and postductal values. The sensitivity of detecting CHD with the screen is around 75% with a very low false positive rate of less than 0.1%. There is currently no recommendation for screening infants admitted to the NICU [41].

Limitations of pulse oximetry

Due to the sigmoid shape of the oxygen dissociation curve, pulse oximetry is unable to detect significant hyperoxia and is slow to detect acute hypoxemia. In infants receiving supplemental oxygen, even large changes in PaO_2 result in minimal changes in SpO_2 if the saturation is close to 100%. Alveolar hypoventilation may also be missed in infants on supplemental oxygen monitored solely with pulse oximetry and can lead to significant hypercarbia without an appreciable change in SpO_2. Hence, patients on supplemental oxygen at risk of hyperoxia/hypoxemia/hypercapnia should have intermittent PaO_2 and $PaCO_2$ measured by ABGs.

Anemia, unless severe <5 g/dL, and polycythemia do not affect pulse oximetry readings [42].

Hypoperfusion and hypothermia

Pulse oximetry relies on normal pulsatile flow for its signal and hence can be falsely low in the setting of impaired perfusion or vasoconstriction associated with hypothermia, vasopressor treatment, tourniquet effect from blood pressure cuff, etc. [43]. Sensor placement over a more central location such as the earlobe or forehead in these situations can improve signal detection and provide reliable readings. Care should be taken not to apply the sensor too tightly around the finger, hand, or foot.

Movement artifact

Conventional pulse oximetry is based on pulsatile flow of blood and calculates saturation based on the assumption that arterial blood is the only component that moves at the site of measurement. During periods of movement of the monitoring site, the blood in the venous and tissue compartment also moves and interferes with the SpO_2 reading or causes a signal dropout. This can disrupt monitoring during periods of spontaneous activity and during transport. Newer pulse oximeters with signal extraction technology (SET) use adaptive filtering that is able to separate the components of the data and filter noise from the signal and are less prone to motion artifact [44,45].

Signal averaging time

The stability of the pulse oximeter reading depends on the signal averaging time. The longer the averaging time the more stable the reading with lesser false alarms, but this causes delay in response time of the oximeter and can result in significant underestimation of true desaturation episodes [31]. The signal averaging time can be optimized based on the indication for which monitoring is being undertaken.

Hemoglobin variants—functional versus fractional saturation

Functional saturation refers to the percentage of hemoglobin that is saturated with oxygen to the amount of hemoglobin that is capable of transporting oxygen: $HbO_2/(HbO_2 + Hb)$. Fractional saturation is the percentage of oxygenated hemoglobin to the total hemoglobin, which includes variant hemoglobin molecules such as methemoglobin (MetHb) or carboxyhemoglobin (COHb) that are incapable of binding oxygen. Conventional oximeters do not distinguish the variant hemoglobins from HbO_2 and provide functional saturation readings that are higher than the fractional saturations in patients with dyshemoglobinemia. High levels of COHb cause an increase in the SpO_2 approximately equal to the amount of COHb that is present [46]. In presence of high levels of MetHb, the SpO_2 reading is decreased approximately by about half of the MetHb percentage concentration [47]. New generation oximeters by using additional wavelength of light detect COHb and MetHb and provide saturation readings that are more appropriate in the clinical setting. In instances where there is a greater than 5% discrepancy between the oxygen saturation by cooximetry and pulse oximetry then the presence of variant hemoglobin has to be considered.

Additional considerations

HbF and HbA have light absorption characteristics that are similar and hence the presence of HbF does not affect pulse oximetry readings [48]. However, one has to be cognizant of the effect of HbF on the oxygen dissociation curve and on the tissue oxygenation at the displayed SpO_2 values (Fig. 32.6). Indirect bilirubin has a different light absorption spectrum at 450 nm and hence does not affect pulse oximetry readings [49]. However, interference from ambient light from phototherapy and elevated of COHb levels from hemolysis can alter pulse oximetry readings in neonates with hyperbilirubinemia.

Perfusion index and plethysmographic variability index

Perfusion index (PI) and plethysmographic variability index (PVI) are measures derived from pulse oximetry (Fig. 32.7). PI, by comparing the pulsatile to the nonpulsatile signal, gives an indication of the perfusion at the monitored site. The value of PI is being investigated for detection of CHD (left obstructive heart diseases that are missed on pulse oximetry-based screening), subclinical chorioamnionitis, assessing severity of illness, and evaluation of intravascular volume status [50,51].

The arterial pulse volume changes during phases of the respiratory cycle and this is more pronounced when the preload is inadequate. PVI measures the change in PI during a respiratory cycle and is expressed as a percentage. The role of PVI in assessing hemodynamic significance of PDA in preterm infants and intravascular volume status both in adult and neonatal patients is being studied and the early results are promising [51,52].

Transcutaneous oxygen saturation monitoring

Transcutaneous PaO_2 (TcO_2) monitoring is being used in NICUs as an alternative to arterial PaO_2 measurements in infants with poor arterial access or in cases in which the risks of arterial line placement are not justified. TcO_2 monitoring is also useful in acutely ill infants at risk of wide fluctuations in PaO_2 is anticipated and is deemed to be in need of continuous monitoring of PaO_2. It is a direct polarographic measurement based on an electrochemical electrode chain with a platinum cathode (sensor) and a silver reference anode. The electrode is separated from the skin surface by a thin membrane through which the oxygen diffuses. The reduction of oxygen at the cathode generates a current that is processed to PaO_2 readout. Studies comparing arterial PaO_2 with TcO_2 in infants have shown good correlation [53]. However, sensors need frequent repositioning and recalibration with ABGs. The need for higher operating temperature is associated with risk of thermal burns in preterm infants. With oxygenation being routinely monitored by pulse oximetry, transcutaneous oxygen monitoring is becoming less common.

Noninvasive assessment of $PaCO_2$

The $PaCO_2$ is a reflection of the interaction of CO_2 production in the body (metabolism), transport (systemic and pulmonary perfusion), and elimination (ventilation). Capnography provides instantaneous breath-to-breath analysis of exhaled CO_2 and has become an integral part of monitoring during anesthesia and intensive care. $PaCO_2$ in normal healthy infants ranges between 35 and 45 mmHg. Cerebral blood flow is dependent on the arterial $PaCO_2$ [50]. Cerebral blood flow increases with hypercapnia and decreases with hypocapnia. In mechanically ventilated extremely preterm infants, fluctuations of $PaCO_2$ are common and predispose infants to intraventricular hemorrhage (with hypercapnia) and periventricular leukomalacia and BPD (with hypocapnia) [4,54,55]. Also, decisions for adjustment of ventilator settings are frequently made based on assessment of $PaCO_2$. At the present time, assessment

$$PI = (AC/DC) \times 100\%$$

$$PVI = [(PI_{max} - PI_{min})/PI_{max}] \times 100\%$$

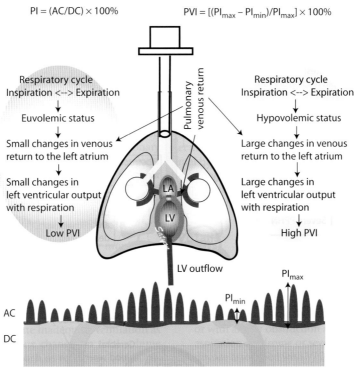

Fig. 32.7 Pulsatility Index (PI) and Plethysmographic Variability Index (PVI) and Changes With Hypovolemia. Changes in intrathoracic pressure with respiration alter venous return to the LA and influence LV preload and LV output and PI. These changes in LV output and PI with respiration (PVI) are more marked in the presence of hypovolemia and can predict response to a fluid bolus. *LA*, left atrium; *LV*, left ventricular; *PI*, pulsatility index; *PVI*, plethysmographic variability index. Modified from Assisted Ventilation of the Neonate. 6th ed. Copyright: Satyan Lakshminrusimha.

of $PaCO_2$ for most of these infants is intermittent with ABG measurements. This can lead to unrecognized periods of hypercapnia and hypocapnia and missed opportunities for ventilator weaning and prolongation of duration of mechanical ventilation. The continuous noninvasive assessment of $PaCO_2$ may be achieved using end-tidal CO_2 ($EtCO_2$) or transcutaneous CO_2 ($TcCO_2$).

Capnography and end-tidal CO_2 monitoring (Fig. 32.8)

Capnography is based on the principle that due to the very high diffusibility of carbon dioxide, the CO_2 from the pulmonary capillary diffuses into the alveolus and rapidly equilibrates with the alveolar pCO_2 ($PaCO_2$). Hence the $PACO_2$ is an indirect measure of the $PaCO_2$ in the blood reaching the lungs. The capnogram is a graphical display of levels of carbon dioxide in the conducting airways during a respiratory cycle. In a respiratory cycle, during inspiration, pCO_2 on the capnogram is zero as the atmospheric

air contains very little carbon dioxide (Fig. 32.1). At the beginning of exhalation, it is the gas from the anatomical dead space that is exhaled and has minimal amount of CO_2 (phase 1, Fig. 32.1). In phase II there is a sharp increase in the slope of the capnogram, as the gas from the alveoli rich in CO_2, mixes in with gas in the dead space. This reaches a peak and then plateaus as all of the expired gas is from the alveoli (phase III).

Measurement

The CO_2 level in the sampled gas is measured using infrared spectroscopy. CO_2 absorbs infrared light of a specific wavelength (426 μm) and this is used to calculate the amount of CO_2 in the sample.

Mainstream and sidestream capnography

$EtCO_2$ monitors based on the position of the measurement device with respect to the infant's airway, fall into two categories.

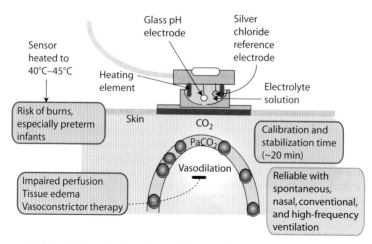

Fig. 32.9 Transcutaneous CO$_2$ Monitoring. The benefits are shown in the green box and limitations are shown in the red box (see text for details). Modified from Assisted Ventilation of the Neonate. 6th ed.

Transcutaneous CO$_2$ monitoring (Fig. 32.9)

Severinghaus in 1960 first described the method for transcutaneous measurement of CO$_2$ in skin capillaries that are arterialized by application of heat [61]. The Stowe–Severinghaus electrode in use at present consists of two electrodes—a glass pH electrode and a silver chloride reference electrode; a heating element; a temperature sensor; and an electrolyte reservoir. The electrodes are separated from the surface of the skin by a membrane. When the sensor is attached to the skin, the generated heat causes local vasodilation and increases the permeability of the skin to CO$_2$. The CO$_2$ diffuses through the membrane and reacts with water to form carbonic acid which dissociates to hydrogen and bicarbonate ions. The change in pH causes a potential difference between the electrodes. This is converted to a pCO$_2$ reading based on the linear relationship between pH and log pCO$_2$. Johns et al. have shown linear correlation of TcCO$_2$ with PaCO$_2$ in the range of 20–74 mmHg [62]. It is important to recognize that the measured value is the gas tension in the cutaneous tissue. Under stable hemodynamic conditions these correlate closely with the ABG values. As the electrodes operate at an elevated temperature, tissue metabolism at the site increases elevating local CO$_2$ production. Hence the value is corrected to the body temperature. Calibration of TcCO$_2$ monitor can be performed by gas calibration using mixtures of known CO$_2$ concentration or may be done by calibrating using the patient's ABG sample. The in vivo calibration has been shown to align more closely with the ABG CO$_2$ tension as it eliminates many of the patient-related factors that influence TcPCO$_2$ measurements. The commercially

available monitors have a measurement range of TcCO$_2$ between 0–200 mmHg and accuracy within ±4.5 mmHg. Following application of the sensor to the patient it takes approximately 20 min for stabilization and to obtain a reliable measurement of the TcCO$_2$. Also the response time to changes in TcCO$_2$ is in the range of 60 s and it increases with decrease in temperature setting of the electrode. Therefore, transcutaneous monitoring is used more for following TcCO$_2$ over periods of time. In settings such as during anesthesia, or intubation where a more rapid response time is needed, capnography and EtCO$_2$ monitoring may be more appropriate.

There have been many studies evaluating the correlation of TcCO$_2$ with arterial PaCO$_2$. Studies by Hand et al., Given et al., and Binder et al. showed good correlation of TcCO$_2$ with PaCO$_2$ [52,63,64]. A prospective study of premature infants of less than 28 weeks gestation by Aliwalas et al. had showed poor correlation [65]. This discrepancy in results may be due to differences in monitors, methodologies, and patient characteristics between studies.

Both patient and instrument-related factors can cause erroneous estimation of TcCO$_2$ levels. Improper placement, trapped air bubbles, membrane, and calibration errors can lead to inaccurate readings (for patient-related factors see Table 32.1).

There are many commercially available monitors that combine electrodes for TcCO$_2$/TcO$_2$ into a single sensor. Sensors with electrodes measuring pO$_2$ need higher temperature at the site than pCO$_2$ sensors and this may be a drawback of the combined sensor especially in preterm infants. Manufacturers recommend changing the position of the sensors every 4–12 h of monitoring depending on the operating temperature of the electrode.

Table 32.1 Advantages and disadvantages of capnographic and transcutaneous measurement of carbon dioxide in the NICU

Parameter	Capnography/end-tidal CO_2	Transcutaneous CO_2
Site of measurement	Measures CO_2 in expired gas	Measures CO_2 at the skin surface
Calibration	Does not need calibration	Needs frequent calibration
Rapidity of response to change	Responds instantaneously to change in $PACO_2$	Slower response to change of $PaCO_2$
Rapidity of result following initial application	Reads instantaneously	Stabilization time of 20 min prior to obtaining reading
Accuracy	Often under reads $PaCO_2$	Better correlation to $PaCO_2$
Limitations	Unreliable in infants with lung disease, shunts or VQ mismatch, or with large leak around ETT	Unreliable in infants with impaired perfusion, acidosis, edema, or on vasoconstrictors
Concerns	May increase dead space in ELBW infants	Risk of skin burns, need for changing sensor position
Mode of ventilation	Cannot be used with HFOV, limited with spontaneous breathing	Can be used in spontaneously breathing, conventional ventilation, or HFOV

$TcCO_2$ versus capnography

Many head to head comparisons of $tcCO_2$ and $EtCO_2$ in different patient groups have been done to study the correlation of each to the $PaCO_2$. In general, $tcCO_2$ correlates better than $EtCO_2$ with $PaCO_2$ in most studies and especially so in infants with lung disease. $EtCO_2$ generally underestimates $PaCO_2$. Both of these technologies should be seen as complimentary and one has to be aware of the strengths and limitations of each modality and chose the appropriate technique based on the clinical situation. For monitoring infants requiring mechanical ventilation, both these monitors provide reliable trends of CO_2 levels that enable the clinician to make decisions on ventilator support and are likely to decrease the need for ABG monitoring.

Near-infrared spectroscopy (Fig. 32.10)

Oxygen delivery to the tissue is dependent on the hemoglobin oxygen saturation and cardiac output. When oxygen demand (VO_2) exceeds the oxygen delivery (DO_2) a state of oxygen debt is created and energy is derived from inefficient anaerobic metabolic pathway. Prompt recognition and institution of therapy to correct oxygen debt is associated with improved outcomes. The parameters currently in use for monitoring of perfusion, such as blood pressure, capillary refill time, urine output, and lactate levels lacks

sensitivity, specificity, and are lagging indicators. At present there is no reliable way of monitoring the oxygenation status of the tissue in newborns as catheterization for mixed venous oxygen saturation is not possible in these infants due to size limitation.

Franz Jobosis in 1977 first described the use of NIRS in the human brain. Much like pulse oximetry, NIRS is based on the modified Beer–Lambert law. Light of specific wavelengths are generated by light emitting diodes and passed through the interposed tissue in an arc-like configuration. The depth of penetration of the transmitted light is proportional to the distance between the transmitting optode and receiving optode. The reflected light is detected by the receiving optode and this is measured and processed to estimate the amount of oxygenated hemoglobin and deoxyhemoglobin in the interposed tissue (Fig. 32.10). NIR oximetry measures a weighted average of arterial capillary and venous compartments and a fixed ratio of venous to arterial blood volume is assumed, usually 70:30. There are different methodologies used by manufacturers of NIRS devices but the most commonly used in commercially available devices is the spatially resolved spectroscopy.

Tissue oxygen saturation
$$rSO_2 = SaO_2 - VO_2 / DO_2$$

The arteriovenous oxygen difference is measured as:
$$\Delta arSO_2 = SaO_2 - rSO_2$$

Fractional oxygen extraction is measured as:
$$fOE = (SaO_2 - rSO_2) / SaO_2$$

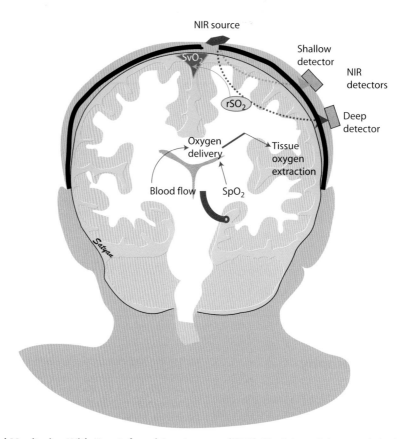

Fig. 32.10 Cerebral Monitoring With Near-Infrared Spectroscopy (NIRS). The light emitting optode is placed over the scalp. Two detectors—shallow detector and a deep detector; are placed a short distance from the emitting optode. The rSO$_2$ depends on oxygen delivery and tissue oxygen extraction. Low oxygen delivery or high oxygen extraction can decrease rSO$_2$. *rSO$_2$*, Regional oxygen saturation. Modified from Assisted Ventilation of the Neonate. 6th ed. Copyright: Satyan Lakshminrusimha.

NIRS can be considered as the pulse oximetry equivalent for the circulatory system. It provides continuous noninvasive monitoring of the venous side of the vascular beds of various organs and provides information in real time of the balance between oxygen supply and demand. NIRS is very well suited for application in newborns and infants due to the decreased thickness of the scalp and skull and smaller amount of fat in the abdominal wall. NIRS has been applied mainly in assessing regional cerebral and splanchnic saturation in the neonatal population. There have been many studies that have demonstrated good correlation between cerebral oxygenation measured by NIRS and jugular venous saturation [66]. Cerebral oximetry has also been validated using correlation with levels of tissue adenosine triphosphate and phosphocreatine in the brain [67]. Studies of gastric tonometry have been shown to correlate with mesenteric rSO$_2$.

Normal values—In infants breathing room air the cerebral rSO$_2$ is around 60%–70% and the splanchnic rSO$_2$ is about 80%. rSO$_2$ also depends on the metabolic state of the tissue and is elevated in brain tissue following ischemic damage and during treatment with therapeutic hypothermia. It is decreased during increased metabolic activity as in seizures despite normal oxygen delivery. The utility of tissue oximetry at this time is as a trend monitor with a baseline for the individual patient and a percentage below this baseline chosen for intervention.

Application of NIRS in newborns—The clinical utility of NIRS monitoring in infants and newborns have been studied mainly in cardiac surgery. In infants undergoing surgery for CHD, low cerebral oximetry readings during surgery and in the postoperative period have been shown to be associated with increase in abnormalities on neuroimaging, seizures, prolonged length of stay, need for ECMO, and death [68–70].

Management of hypotension—In hypotensive newborns impaired cerebral autoregulation increases the risk of adverse neurodevelopmental outcomes. Autoregulation can be presumed to be intact when low blood pressure is not associated with a decrease in cerebral oxygenation by NIRS. NIRS by providing information on the oxygen supply and demand can guide therapy to the need for and choice of inotropes/vasopressors and monitoring response to treatment [71,72].

Patent ductus arteriosus—Impairment of cerebral blood flow and oxygenation due to diastolic runoff occurs in hemodynamically significant PDA. Changes in rSO_2 and fractional extraction of oxygen by NIRS in combination with echocardiography may be used to monitor status of the ductus arteriosus and response to pharmacological treatment for PDA [73].

Cerebral perfusion with changes in mean airway pressure and ventilation—Preterm infants who are mechanically ventilated for respiratory distress syndrome are at high risk for intraventricular hemorrhage. Increased intrathoracic pressure associated with high mean airway pressure may decrease preload and cardiac output and cause impairment of cerebral blood flow [74]. Changes in cerebral rSO_2 and FTOE by NIRS can lead to early recognition and timely intervention to prevent related complications. Cerebral blood flow is very sensitive to changes in $PaCO_2$ and rapid fluctuations in $PaCO_2$ may occur especially in infants on high-frequency ventilation. NIRS by providing real-time information of changes in cerebral oxygenation can alert the clinician to monitor $PaCO_2$ more closely in these infants.

Mesenteric Ischemia—Necrotizing enterocolitis. The cerebrosplanchnic oxygenation ratio (CSOR), splanchnic NIRS/cerebral NIRS less than 0.75 is indicative of splanchnic ischemia and it may be possible to identify infants at risk of necrotizing enterocolitis [75,76].

Transfusion—A body of literature on transfusion-associated necrotizing enterocolitis and mesenteric blood flow and oxygenation during transfusion of packed red blood cells and changes associated with feeding using NIRS is emerging in neonatology [77–79].

Limitations of NIRS

There are no well-established norms for normal values of rSO2 or thresholds for intervention and there is wide intra- and interpatient variability in rSO2 values with a coefficient of variation for absolute baseline values of approximately 10%. The reading obtained is site specific and is not possible to exclude abnormalities in other areas of the brain. In order to be able to obtain reliable readings over periods of monitoring, nursing and medical staff need training and experience in the correct placement and fixation of optodes and shielding from ambient light. The response to an abnormal reading needs evaluation of gas exchange, oxygen transport, hemodynamics, and regional perfusion.

Conclusions

Monitoring of gas exchange remains a cornerstone of management of premature and critically ill newborns in the delivery room, NICU, operating rooms, and during inter- and intrahospital transfers. Early recognition of impairment and institution of corrective measures in a timely manner prevents deterioration in clinical status, and reduces morbidity and mortality. The wide array of modalities are routinely used in neonatal units that are described in this chapter and emerging technologies such as NIRS have helped improve outcomes in these most vulnerable infants.

References

[1] Silverman W. A cautionary tale about supplemental oxygen: the albatross of neonatal medicine. Pediatrics 2004;113:394–396.

[2] Pappas A, Shankaran S, Laptook AR, Langer JC, Bara R, Ehrenkranz RA, et al. Eunice Kennedy Shriver National Institute of Child Health and Human Development Neonatal Research Network. Hypocarbia and adverse outcome in neonatal hypoxic-ischemic encephalopathy. J Pediatr 2011;158(5). 752.e1–758.e1.

[3] Carlo WA, Finer NN, Walsh MC, Rich W, Gantz MG, Laptook AR, et al. Target ranges of oxygen saturation in extremely preterm infants. N Engl J Med 2010;362(21): 1959–1969.

[4] Kaiser JR, Gauss CH, Pont MM, Williams DK. Hypercapnia during the first 3 days of life is associated with severe intraventricular hemorrhage in very low birth weight infants. J Perinatol 2006;26(5):279–285.

[5] Siggaard-Andersen O. The van Slyke equation. Scand J Clin Lab Invest Suppl 1977;146:15–20.

[6] Malatesha G, Singh NK, Bharija A, Rehani B, Goel A. Comparison of arterial and venous pH, bicarbonate, PCO_2 and PO_2 in initial emergency department assessment. Emerg Med J 2007;24(8):569–571.

[7] Treger R, Pirouz S, Kamangar N, Corry D. Agreement between central venous and arterial blood gas measurements

in the intensive care unit. Clin J Am Soc Nephrol 2010;5(3):390–394.

[8] Alston TA. Blood gases and pH during hypothermia: the "-stats". Int Anesthesiol Clin 2004;42(4): 73–80.

[9] Bisson J, Younker J. Correcting arterial blood gases for temperature: (when) is it clinically significant? Nurs Crit Care 2006;11(5):232–238.

[10] Lumb AB. Nunn's applied respiratory physiology. Philadelphia PA, USA: Elsevier Health Sciences; 2016.

[11] Lake CL, Booker PD. Pediatric cardiac anesthesia. Philadelphia PA, USA: Lippincott Williams & Wilkins; 2005.

[12] Groenendaal F, De Vooght KM, van Bel F. Blood gas values during hypothermia in asphyxiated term

neonates. Pediatrics 2009;123(1): 170–172.

[13] Gluckman PD, Wyatt JS, Azzopardi D, Ballard R, Edwards AD, Ferriero DM, et al. Selective head cooling with mild systemic hypothermia after neonatal encephalopathy: multicentre randomised trial. Lancet 2005;365(9460):663–670.

[14] Shankaran S, Laptook AR, Ehrenkranz RA, Tyson JE, McDonald SA, Donovan EF, et al. National Institute of Child Health and Human Development Neonatal Research Network. Whole-body hypothermia for neonates with hypoxic-ischemic encephalopathy. N Engl J Med 2005;353(15):1574–1584.

[15] Shankaran S, Laptook AR, Pappas A, McDonald SA, Das A, Tyson JE, et al. Eunice Kennedy Shriver National Institute of Child Health and Human Development Neonatal Research Network. Effect of depth and duration of cooling on deaths in the NICU among neonates with hypoxic ischemic encephalopathy: a randomized clinical trial. JAMA 2014;312(24):2629–2639.

[16] Kapadia VS, Chalak LF, DuPont TL, Rollins NK, Brion LP, Wyckoff MH. Perinatal asphyxia with hyperoxemia within the first hour of life is associated with moderate to severe hypoxic-ischemic encephalopathy. J Pediatr 2013;163(4):949–954.

[17] Klinger G, Beyene J, Shah P, Perlman M. Do hyperoxaemia and hypocapnia add to the risk of brain injury after intrapartum asphyxia? Arch Dis Child Fetal Neonatal Ed 2005;90(1): F49–F52.

[18] Rudolph AM, Yuan S. Response of the pulmonary vasculature to hypoxia and H+ ion concentration changes. J Clin Investig 1966;45(3):399–411.

[19] Peeters LL, Sheldon RE, Jones MD Jr, Makowski EL, Meschia G. Blood flow to fetal organs as a function of arterial oxygen content. Am J Obstet Gynecol 1979;135(5):637–646.

[20] Chakkarapani E, Thoresen M. Use of hypothermia in the asphyxiated infant. Perinatology 2010;3:20–29.

[21] Silverman WA. Retrolental fibroplasia: a modern parable. Cambridge University Press, UK: Grune & Stratton; 1980.

[22] Carlo WA, Finer NN, Walsh MC, Rich W, Gantz MG, Laptook AR, et al. SUPPORT Study Group of the Eunice Kennedy Shriver NICHD Neonatal Research Network. Target ranges of oxygen saturation in extremely preterm infants. N Engl J Med 2010;362(21):1959–1969.

[23] Avery ME. Recent increase in mortality from hyaline membrane disease. J Pediatr 1960;57:553–559.

[24] Stenson BJ, Tarnow-Mordi WO, Darlow BA, Simes J, Juszczak E, Askie L, et al. BOOST II United Kingdom Collaborative Group; BOOST II Australia Collaborative Group; BOOST II New Zealand Collaborative Group. Oxygen saturation and outcomes in preterm infants. N Engl J Med 2013;368(22):2094–2104.

[25] Schmidt B, Whyte RK, Asztalos EV, Moddemann D, Poets C, Rabi Y, et al. Canadian Oxygen Trial (COT) Group. Effects of targeting higher vs lower arterial oxygen saturations on death or disability in extremely preterm infants: a randomized clinical trial. JAMA 2013;309(20):2111–2120.

[26] Aoyagi T. Pulse oximetry: its invention, theory, and future. J Anesth 2003;17(4):259–266.

[27] Mannheimer PD. The light-tissue interaction of pulse oximetry. Anesth Analg 2007;105(6 Suppl):S10–S17.

[28] Batchelder PB, Raley DM. Maximizing the laboratory setting for testing devices and understanding statistical output in pulse oximetry. Anesth Analg 2007;105(Suppl. 6):S85–S94.

[29] Brockmann PE, Poets A, Urschitz MS, Sokollik C, Poets CF. Reference values for pulse oximetry recordings in healthy term neonates during their first 5 days of life. Arch Dis Child Fetal Neonatal Ed 2011;96(5):F335–F338.

[30] Levesque BM, Pollack P, Griffin BE, Nielsen HC. Pulse oximetry: what's normal in the newborn nursery? Pediatr Pulmonol 2000;30(5):406–412.

[31] Harigopal S, Satish HP, Taktak AF, Southern KW, Shaw NJ. Oxygen saturation profile in healthy preterm infants. Arch Dis Child Fetal Neonatal Ed 2011;96(5):F339–F342.

[32] Lakshminrusimha S, Manja V, Mathew B, Suresh GK. Oxygen targeting in preterm infants: a physiological interpretation. J Perinatol 2015;35(1):8–15.

[33] Sola A, Golombek SG, Montes Bueno MT, Lemus-Varela L, Zuluaga C, Dominguez F, et al. Safe oxygen saturation targeting and monitoring in preterm infants: can we avoid hypoxia and hyperoxia? Acta Paediatr 2014;103(10):1009–1018.

[34] Pediatrics AAo, Association AH. Neonatal Resuscitation Textbook Plus: Amer Academy of Pediatrics; 2011

[35] Kamlin CO, O'Donnell CP, Davis PG, Morley CJ. Oxygen saturation in healthy infants immediately after birth. J Pediatr 2006;148(5): 585–589.

[36] Mariani G, Dik PB, Ezquer A, Aguirre A, Esteban ML, Perez C, et al. Pre-ductal and post-ductal O2 saturation in healthy term neonates after birth. J Pediatr 2007;150(4):418–421.

[37] Gandhi B, Rich W, Finer N. Achieving targeted pulse oximetry values in preterm infants in the delivery room. J Pediatr 2013;163(2):412–415.

[38] Gandhi B, Rich W, Finer N. Time to achieve stable pulse oximetry values in VLBW infants in the delivery room. Resuscitation 2013;84(7):970–973.

[39] O'Donnell CP, Kamlin CO, Davis PG, Morley CJ. Obtaining pulse oximetry data in neonates: a randomised crossover study of sensor application techniques. Arch Dis Child Fetal Neonatal Ed 2005;90(1):F84–F85.

[40] Meier-Stauss P, Bucher HU, Hurlimann R, Konig V, Huch R. Pulse oximetry used for documenting oxygen saturation and right-to-left shunting immediately after birth. Eur J Pediatr 1990;149(12):851–855.

[41] Manja V, Mathew B, Carrion V, Lakshminrusimha S. Critical congenital heart disease screening by pulse oximetry in a neonatal intensive care unit. J Perinatol 2015;35(1): 67–71.

[42] Perkins GD, McAuley DF, Giles S, Routledge H, Gao F. Do changes in pulse oximeter oxygen saturation predict equivalent changes in arterial oxygen saturation? Crit Care 2003;7(4):R67.

[43] Talke P, Stapelfeldt C. Effect of peripheral vasoconstriction on pulse oximetry. J Clin Monit Comput 2006;20(5):305–309.

[44] Goldman JM, Petterson MT, Kopotic RJ, Barker SJ. Masimo signal extraction pulse oximetry. J Clin Monit Comput 2000;16(7):475–483.

[45] Workie FA, Rais-Bahrami K, Short BL. Clinical use of new-generation pulse oximeters in the neonatal intensive care unit. Am J Perinatol 2005;22(7):357–360.

[46] Barker SJ, Tremper KK. The effect of carbon monoxide inhalation on pulse oximetry and transcutaneous PO_2. Anesthesiology 1987;66(5):677–679.

[47] Barker SJ, Tremper KK, Hyatt J. Effects of methemoglobinemia on pulse oximetry and mixed venous oximetry. Anesthesiology 1989;70(1):112–117.

[48] Rajadurai VS, Walker AM, Yu VY, Oates A. Effect of fetal haemoglobin on the accuracy of pulse oximetry in preterm infants. J Paediatr Child Health 1992;28(1):43–46.

[49] Veyckemans F, Baele P, Guillaume JE, Willems E, Robert A, Clerbaux T. Hyperbilirubinemia does not interfere with hemoglobin saturation measured by pulse oximetry. Anesthesiology 1989;70(1):118–122.

[50] Leahy FA, Cates D, MacCallum M, Rigatto H. Effect of CO2 and 100% O2 on cerebral blood flow in preterm infants. J Appl Physiol Respir Environ Exerc Physiol 1980;48(3):468–472.

[51] Piasek CZ, Van Bel F, Sola A. Perfusion index in newborn infants: a noninvasive tool for neonatal monitoring. Acta Paediatr 2014;103(5):468–473.

[52] Hand IL, Shepard EK, Krauss AN, Auld PA. Discrepancies between transcutaneous and end-tidal carbon dioxide monitoring in the critically ill neonate with respiratory distress syndrome. Crit Care Med 1989;17(6):556–559.

[53] Lewallen PK, Mammel MC, Coleman JM, Boros SJ. Neonatal transcutaneous arterial oxygen saturation monitoring. J Perinatol 1987;7(1):8–10.

[54] Wiswell TE, Graziani LJ, Kornhauser MS, Stanley C, Merton DA, McKee L, et al. Effects of hypocarbia on the development of cystic periventricular leukomalacia in premature infants treated with high-frequency jet ventilation. Pediatrics 1996;98(5):918–924.

[55] Erickson SJ, Grauaug A, Gurrin L, Swaminathan M. Hypocarbia in the ventilated preterm infant and its effect on intraventricular haemorrhage and bronchopulmonary dysplasia. J Paediatr Child Health 2002;38(6):560–562.

[56] Falk JL, Rackow EC, Weil MH. End-tidal carbon dioxide concentration during cardiopulmonary resuscitation. N Engl J Med 1988;318(10):607–611.

[57] Garnett AR, Ornato JP, Gonzalez ER, Johnson EB. End-tidal carbon dioxide monitoring during cardiopulmonary resuscitation. JAMA 1987;257(4):512–515.

[58] Sanders AB, Kern KB, Otto CW, Milander MM, Ewy GA. End-tidal carbon dioxide monitoring during cardiopulmonary resuscitation. A prognostic indicator for survival. JAMA 1989;262(10):1347–1351.

[59] Tai CC, Lu FL, Chen PC, Jeng SF, Chou HC, Chen CY, et al. Noninvasive capnometry for end-tidal carbon dioxide monitoring via nasal cannula in nonintubated neonates. Pediatr Neonatol 2010;51(6):330–335.

[60] Lopez E, Mathlouthi J, Lescure S, Krauss B, Jarreau PH, Moriette G. Capnography in spontaneously breathing preterm infants with bronchopulmonary dysplasia. Pediatr Pulmonol 2011;46(9):896–902.

[61] Severinghaus JW. Methods of measurement of blood and gas carbon dioxide during anesthesia. Anesthesiology 1960;21:717–726.

[62] Johns RJ, Lindsay WJ, Shepard RH. A system for monitoring pulmonary ventilation. Biomed Sci Instrum 1969;5:119–121.

[63] Geven WB, Nagler E, de Boo T, Lemmens W. Combined transcutaneous oxygen, carbon dioxide tensions and end-expired CO2 levels in severely ill newborns. Adv Exp Med Biol 1987;220:115–120.

[64] Binder N, Atherton H, Thorkelsson T, Hoath SB. Measurement of transcutaneous carbon dioxide in low birthweight infants during the first two weeks of life. Am J Perinatol 1994;11(3):237–241.

[65] Aliwalas LL, Noble L, Nesbitt K, Fallah S, Shah V, Shah PS. Agreement of carbon dioxide levels measured by arterial, transcutaneous and end tidal methods in preterm infants < or = 28 weeks gestation. J Perinatol 2005;25(1):26–29.

[66] Bhutta AT, Ford JW, Parker JG, Prodhan P, Fontenot EE, Seib PM, et al. Noninvasive cerebral oximeter as a surrogate for mixed venous saturation in children. Pediatr Cardiol 2007;28(1):34–41.

[67] Nollert G, Jonas RA, Reichart B. Optimizing cerebral oxygenation during cardiac surgery: a review of experimental and clinical investigations with near infrared spectrophotometry. Thorac Cardiovasc Surg 2000;48(4):247–253.

[68] Dent CL, Spaeth JP, Jones BV, Schwartz SM, Glauser TA, Hallinan B, et al. Brain magnetic resonance imaging abnormalities after the Norwood procedure using regional cerebral perfusion. Thorac Cardiovasc Surg 2006;131(1):190–197.

[69] Kurth CD, Steven JM, Nicolson SC. Cerebral oxygenation during pediatric cardiac surgery using deep hypothermic circulatory arrest. Anesthesiology 1995;82(1):74–82.

[70] Andropoulos DB, Stayer SA, Diaz LK, Ramamoorthy C. Neurological monitoring for congenital heart surgery. Anesth Analg 2004;99(5):1365–1375.

[71] Wong FY, Leung TS, Austin T, Wilkinson M, Meek JH, Wyatt JS, et al. Impaired autoregulation in preterm infants identified by using spatially resolved spectroscopy. Pediatrics 2008;121(3):e604–e611.

[72] Brady KM, Mytar JO, Lee JK, Cameron DE, Vricella LA, Thompson WR, et al. Monitoring cerebral blood flow pressure autoregulation in pediatric patients during cardiac surgery. Stroke 2010;41(9):1957–1962.

[73] Lemmers PM, Toet MC, van Bel F. Impact of patent ductus arteriosus and subsequent therapy with indomethacin on cerebral oxygenation in preterm infants. Pediatrics 2008;121(1):142–147.

[74] Lemmers PM, Toet M, van Schelven LJ, van Bel F. Cerebral oxygenation and cerebral oxygen extraction in the preterm infant: the impact of respiratory distress syndrome. Exp Brain Res 2006;173(3):458–467.

[75] Fortune PM, Wagstaff M, Petros AJ. Cerebro-splanchnic oxygenation ratio (CSOR) using near infrared spectroscopy may be able to predict splanchnic ischaemia in neonates. Intensive Care Med 2001;27(8):1401–1407.

[76] Cortez J, Gupta M, Amaram A, Pizzino J, Sawhney M, Sood BG. Noninvasive evaluation of splanchnic tissue oxygenation using near-infrared spectroscopy in preterm neonates. J Matern Fetal Neonatal Med 2011;24(4):574–582.

[77] Bailey SM, Hendricks-Munoz KD, Mally P. Splanchnic-cerebral oxygenation ratio as a marker of preterm infant blood transfusion needs. Transfusion 2012;52(2):252–260.

[78] Christensen RD, Lambert DK, Henry E, Wiedmeier SE, Snow GL, Baer VL, et al. Is "transfusion-associated necrotizing enterocolitis" an authentic pathogenic entity? Transfusion 2010;50(5):1106–1112.

[79] Krimmel GA, Baker R, Yanowitz TD. Blood transfusion alters the superior mesenteric artery blood flow velocity response to feeding in premature infants. Am J Perinatol 2009;26(2):99–105.

Chapter 33

Nursing Care and Endotracheal Suction

Prakash Manikoth, MBBS, MRCP (UK), FRCPCH, Manoj N. Malviya, MBBS, MRCP (UK), Said A Al-Kindi, MD, MRCPCH, FRACP

CHAPTER CONTENTS HD

CHAPTER POINTS

- Neonates admitted with respiratory illness require a detailed maternal and neonatal history, clinical examination and ongoing assessment.
- The selection of equipment and the type of respiratory support provided depend on pulmonary pathology, gestation, the age of the infant, and availability.
- Meticulous nursing care as well as close monitoring of infant and equipment are essential to detect any deterioration or improvement.
- Establishing patency of the airways and general supportive care are essential requirements for an infant on invasive or noninvasive respiratory support.

Introduction

Despite all the advances in the science and technology of neonatology, nursing care alone delivers the art of neonatal care. The need for respiratory support is one of the major reasons for admission of neonates to the neonatal intensive

care unit (NICU) [1] and nursing care constitutes one of the most important operational fulcrums of the unit. Nurses are the eyes and ears of the unit who provide a bridge between the neonate and the multidisciplinary team caring for the infant and can never be replaced by machines. The vast majority of neonatal care is driven by established protocols and due diligence in following them as well as auditing outcomes ensure a better quality of care. The NICU staffing levels dictate outcomes especially for the survival of very low birth weight and preterm infants [2,3] but in reality, most units do not receive the recommended levels of nursing care worldwide. The assessment system of the British Association of Perinatal Medicine (BAPM) includes four categories of neonates with varying nursing requirements [4]. The BAPM recommends a nurse-to-patient ratio of 1:1 for NICU, 1:2 for high dependency care, and 1:4 for neonates requiring special care [5]. The American Academy of Pediatrics (AAP) and the American College of Obstetricians and Gynecologists (ACOG) guidelines for perinatal care relating to NICU nurse-to-patient ratios call for assessment of infant, nursing staff, and nursing unit factors into consideration [6]. This chapter covers neonatal history, assessment of neonate and equipment, nursing care of the neonate, monitoring of equipment, and management strategies including endotracheal suctioning and chest physiotherapy of neonates receiving respiratory support.

Neonatal history

The neonatal period extends from birth to 28 days of life. Maternal history is an integral part of neonatal history. Hence great importance should be given to reviewing in detail the maternal history as well as the birth history, which together forms the complete neonatal history. A detailed perinatal history helps in identifying the risk factors associated with respiratory distress in neonates (Table 33.1).

Table 33.1 Perinatal history relevant to respiratory distress in the newborn

Condition	Perinatal history
Transient tachypnea of newborn	Cesarean section, fetal distress, gestational diabetes mellitus, late preterm, early term gestation, maternal sedation
Respiratory distress syndrome	Prematurity, gestational diabetes mellitus, multiple gestation
Meconium aspiration syndrome	Fetal distress, meconium-stained amniotic fluid, post-term gestation, perinatal depression
Neonatal pneumonia	Maternal fever, chorioamnionitis, group B streptococcus carrier, prematurity, prolonged rupture of membranes, perinatal depression
Pulmonary hypoplasia	Anhydramnios, oligohydramnios, dysplastic or absent kidneys, obstructive uropathy, premature prolonged rupture of membranes

Maternal history

Age and details of previous pregnancies with complications, if any

Blood type and history of blood group sensitization and transfusions

Status of: Group B Streptococcus, HIV, hepatitis B, VDRL, and herpes simplex

Maternal illness: diabetes mellitus; hypertension; cardiac, endocrine, or renal diseases, and bleeding disorders

Recent infections or exposure to alcohol, drugs, tobacco, and teratogens

Consanguinity and genetic disorders in family members

Occupation and socioeconomic status

Complications of pregnancy

Antenatal steroids

Birth history

Presentation (normal or abnormal)

Onset of labor (premature, spontaneous, or induced)

Rupture of membranes (premature or prolonged)

Amniotic fluid volume and presence of blood or meconium

Complications during labor (maternal fever, bleeding, or fetal distress)

Time of membrane rupture, amniotic fluid quantity, and quality

Medications during labor (magnesium sulfate or narcotics within 4 h of delivery)

Duration of labor; anesthesia (epidural, spinal, or general)

Method of delivery (spontaneous vaginal, assisted breech, forceps, vacuum, or cesarean section)

Resuscitation required and Apgar scores

Methods of placental transfusion (delayed cord clamping, umbilical cord milking), if any

Cord gas results (pH, hematocrit, base deficit and lactate)

Assessment of neonate

All health care providers should have a thorough understanding of developmental pulmonary physiology, pathophysiology, and the requirements of the neonate and family. Neonates who require respiratory support need meticulous medical and nursing care as well as close monitoring to detect early deterioration or improvement so that remedial action can be taken. Assessment of the neonate with respiratory distress should begin by observation without disturbing, and followed by palpation and auscultation.

Observation

1. General observation: Level of activity (awake, alert, crying, or sleeping) and tone. Term infants are alert and active with a flexed posture, while preterm infants have decreased tone and activity.
2. Color: Cyanosis is caused by an increase in the deoxygenated hemoglobin level to above 5 g/dL. Central cyanosis is caused by diseases of the heart or lungs and seen over the tongue and mucous membranes of the mouth. Peripheral cyanosis (acrocyanosis) is a normal finding in the first few hours after birth and seen over hands and feet (nail beds) and occasionally around the lips. Cyanosis that improves with crying may be due to choanal atresia/stenosis or hypoventilation.
3. Mouth and nose: Note the amount, color, and consistency of secretions; copious nasal secretions are seen in congenital syphilis and oral secretions with tracheoesophageal fistula. Nasal flaring helps to reduce the resistance in upper airways; nasal stuffiness may occur with maternal substance abuse.
4. Chest:
   a. Size and shape: Examine the size, shape, and symmetry of the chest. In a term infant, the chest size is wider than long and its diameter is 2 cm lesser than the head circumference. A barrel-shaped chest with an increase in anteroposterior diameter results from increased intrathoracic volume; it

may occur with meconium aspiration syndrome (MAS), pneumothorax, or transient tachypnea of the newborn. A bell-shaped chest may be seen in neonates with pulmonary hypoplasia or neuromuscular disease. In pectus carinatum or pigeon chest the sternum is protuberant and in pectus excavatum or funnel chest, it is depressed. The symmetry of chest is assessed at the nipple line and an asymmetric shape can be observed with unilateral pneumothorax.

b. Respiratory rate: The normal respiratory rate is 30–60 breaths/min at rest and counted for a full minute. Apnea refers to the cessation of breathing for 20 s or longer and/or is accompanied by hypoxia or bradycardia. Tachypnea refers to a respiratory rate of more than 60 per minute.

c. Movement: The normal breathing pattern is characterized by predominantly diaphragmatic movements, as result of which the abdomen expands with inspiration while the chest moves inward. Chest movements are reduced in the presence of air or fluid in the pleural cavity. In an infant with respiratory distress, retractions occur due to the soft cartilage and muscle groups; these may be intercostal, subcostal, sternal, and suprasternal. In neonates with muscle weakness, "seesaw pattern" of the chest and abdominal breathing may be observed. With conventional synchronized ventilation, the chest rises with ventilator-delivered breaths and in high-frequency ventilation, chest vibration or wiggle is observed.

5. Pain: Assessment of neonatal pain, agitation, and sedation can be made by using any of the pain scales. The Neonatal Pain, Agitation, and Sedation Scale (N-PASS) is a valid and reliable tool for assessing pain/agitation and sedation in ventilated and/or postoperative infants of 0–100 days of age and 23 weeks gestation and above [7]. The N-PASS consists of five indicators such as crying or irritability, behavior state, facial expression, extremities tone, and vital signs (Table 33.2). Sedation is scored from 0 to –2 for each behavioral and physiological criteria, then summed and noted as a negative score (0 → –10). Pain is scored from 0 to +2 for each behavioral and physiological criteria, then summed and documented as a positive number (0 → +10). A high pain/agitation

Table 33.2 Neonatal Pain, Agitation, and Sedation Scale (N-PASS) [7]

Assessment criteria	Sedation		Normal	Pain/Agitation	
	−2	−1	0	1	2
Crying irritability	No cry with painful stimuli	Moans or cries minimally with painful stimuli	Appropriate crying Not irritable	Irritable or crying at intervals Consolable	High-pitched or silent-continuous cry. Inconsolable
Behavior state	No arousal to any stimuli No spontaneous movement	Arouses minimally to stimuli. Little spontaneous movement	Appropriate for gestational age	Restless, squirming Awakens frequently	Arching, kicking Constantly awake or arouses minimally/no movement (not sedated)
Facial expression	Mouth is lax No expression	Minimal expression with stimuli	Relaxed Appropriate	Any pain expression intermittent	Any pain expression continual
Extremities tone	No grasp reflex Flaccid tone	Weak grasp reflex ↓ Muscle tone	Relaxed hands and feet Normal tone	Intermittent clenched toes, fists/finger splay Body is not tense	Continual clenched toes, fists, or finger splay Body is tense
Vital signs: HR, RR, BP, SaO$_2$	No variability with stimuli Hypoventilation or apnea	<10% variability from baseline with stimuli	Within baseline or normal for gestational age	↑ 10%–20% from baseline; SaO$_2$ 76%–85% with stimulation—quick ↑	↑ >20% from baseline; SaO$_2$ ≤75% with stimulation—slow ↑. Out of sync with ventilator

BP, Blood pressure; HR, heart rate; RR, respiratory rate; SaO$_2$, arterial saturation of oxygen.

score indicates more frequent or intense behaviors, and a low sedation score indicates a decreased response to stimulation, or a deeper level of sedation. The Premature Infant Pain Profile-Revised (PIPP-R) is another tool found to be useful in infants of varying gestational ages, diagnoses, and procedures [8].

Palpation and percussion

Chest palpation reveals crepitus or conducted sounds in the presence of airway secretions and crepitus with subcutaneous emphysema. The cardiac apex beat is shifted with pleural effusion, pneumothorax, and congenital diaphragmatic hernia. The percussion note will be dull with pleural effusion and hyperresonant with pneumothorax.

Auscultation

Airway secretions and nasal congestion can produce audible sounds. Grunting is an audible sound heard without a stethoscope and present with moderate to severe respiratory distress syndrome. It is produced by exhaling against a partially closed glottis in order to maintain a higher functional residual capacity. Stridor is a high-pitched sound produced by partial obstruction of the upper airway and may be inspiratory or expiratory. It may occur in laryngomalacia, post-extubation due to edema, or due to neurological damage to the vocal cords. Audible sound of an air leak is often heard in neonates with undersized endotracheal tube (ETT) and with high ventilation settings.

A clean and warm neonatal stethoscope which has both a bell and a diaphragm should be used for auscultation of breath sounds. Prior to auscultating a neonate who is either intubated or has a tracheostomy, remove water from the corrugated ventilator tubing, since it can mimic adventitious sounds. Auscultate over both the anterior and the posterior surfaces and the sides of the chest and compare one side to the other. Listen for normal and abnormal breath sounds, as well as for adventitious sounds. The breath sounds are reduced in respiratory distress syndrome, collapse, air leak syndrome, and pleural effusion. Breath sounds are increased in pneumonia due to the presence of consolidation. Unequal breath sounds may occur with mainstem bronchial intubation, collapse, pneumothorax, or pleural effusion. Crackles are produced by the movement of air or fluid in the small or large airways; it may be fine, medium, or coarse. Fine crackles in the first few hours after birth are a normal finding as fetal lung fluid is cleared; subsequently, it may be heard in neonates with respiratory distress syndrome (RDS) or bronchopulmonary dysplasia (BPD). Wheezes can be heard in infants with MAS or BPD. High-pitched and vibratory sounds are heard in neonates receiving high-frequency ventilation. Complete the auscultation of the chest by assessment of

heart sounds and irregular beats or murmurs, if any. In an infant on high-frequency ventilation, it is easier to listen to heart sounds by switching transiently to standby or continuous positive airway pressure (CPAP) mode of ventilation.

Newborn respiratory distress score

Neonates presenting with severe respiratory distress have increased morbidity and mortality. Based on clinical assessment, a modified Downes Scoring system [9] has been established to identify those infants at significant risk (Table 33.3). The sum of all the individual scores gives the total score based on which respiratory distress (RD) can be classified into mild, moderate, and severe.

1. Mild (RD score <5): requires close monitoring with or without oxygen
2. Moderate (RD score 5–8): requires some form of respiratory support (CPAP) or even mechanical ventilation to prevent further deterioration
3. Severe (RD score >8): requires immediate intubation for assisted ventilation

Table 33.3 Newborn respiratory distress score (RD score) [9]

RD score	0	1	2
Cyanosis	None	In room air	In 40% FiO_2
Retractions	None	Mild	Severe
Grunting	None	Audible with stethoscope	Audible without stethoscope
Air entry (midaxillary line)	Clear	Delayed or decreased	Barely audible
Respiratory rate (per min)	60	60–80	>80 or apneic episodes

Selection and set up of equipment for respiratory support

The aim of respiratory support is to maintain adequate gas exchange while causing the least amount of lung damage. The selection of equipment and level of respiratory support required depend on pulmonary pathology, gestation, the age of the infant, and availability. The current emphasis is to reduce the risk of ventilator-induced lung injury, especially in preterm infants. Noninvasive respiratory support is increasingly used in preterm infants, either as the primary

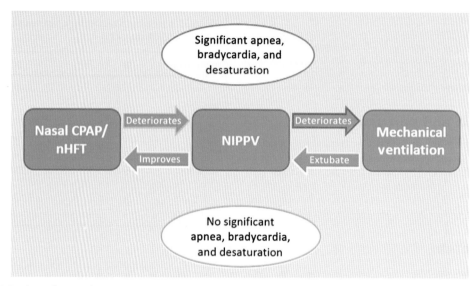

Fig. 33.1 Selection of Type of Respiratory Support. *CPAP*, Continuous positive airway pressure; *nHFT*, nasal high-flow therapy; and *NIPPV*, nasal intermittent positive pressure ventilation.

mode of respiratory support or following extubation to avoid reintubation. Infants who develop significant respiratory distress while on noninvasive respiratory support will require positive-pressure ventilation (PPV). Fig. 33.1 provides a route map for the health care provider to choose the type of respiratory support.

Essential equipment for each infant care area

Each patient space shall contain a minimum of 120 ft² and have the following essential equipment:
1. Oxygen supply with blender and flow meter
2. Pulse oximeter with neonatal probe
3. Wall suction with different sizes of catheters
4. Respiratory and ECG module, cable, and leads
5. Invasive or noninvasive blood pressure module and cable
6. Transcutaneous module and probe
7. Resuscitation equipment
8. Ventilator setup: ventilator circuit with humidification cartridge, water bag, temperature probe, flow sensor, and artificial lung
9. Infant care setup: equipment for intravenous and arterial lines and syringe driver pump

Supplemental oxygen

Oxygen given to prevent hypoxia can be delivered via nasal cannula (NC), mask, oxygen hood, or ambient in the

incubator (Table 33.4) [10]. A blender is used to mix air and oxygen and the gas is warmed and humidified before passing through a flow meter. The oxygen delivered to the infant via a NC varies based on the gas flow rate, FiO_2 set on the air-oxygen blender, inspiratory time, variations in inspiratory flows, and nasal versus oral breathing (Table 33.5) [10,14]. A web-based calculator from NICU tools makes it easy to calculate the effective FiO_2 delivered by low-flow NC, by entering the infant's weight (in kg), respiratory rate, the current oxygen flow rate, and oxygen percent at the blender [11].

The use of low-flow NC with 100% FiO_2 results in stable delivery of oxygen, as it minimises the contribution of variations in nasal breathing. The predicted hypo pharyngeal delivery of oxygen based on infant weight and oxygen flow rate, when 100% FiO_2 is given through NC is listed in Table 33.6 [12,13]. However, it must be noted that providing low-flow/high oxygen concentration will expose extreme preterm infants to unnecessarily high oxygen, unlike the use of pressure support which leads to reduced oxygen requirement. Support of these infants with flow/pressure only can prevent the microatelectasis that contributes to inflammation and ultimately chronic lung disease, besides avoiding the oxygen exposure that leads to BPD as well as retinopathy of prematurity [15]. The administered oxygen must always be regulated by measuring the oxygen saturation of the infant using a pulse oximeter. Hypoxia can lead to brain damage, while hyperoxia leads to tissue damage due to the release of oxygen-free radicals and result in retinopathy of prematurity

Table 33.4 Oxygen-delivery devices for neonates [10]

Device	Advantages	Disadvantages	FiO$_2$ range
Nasal cannula	• Provides tactile stimulation while delivering oxygen • Can feed and care for patient without interrupting oxygen • Allows patient greater mobility	• FiO$_2$ varies with changes in inspiratory flow and tidal volume • Cannula prongs can become occluded by secretions	0.21–0.70 at flows of 0.25–2 L/min
High-flow nasal cannula	• Delivers accurate FiO$_2$ at higher flows (>6.0 L/min) • Keeps patient comfortable • Delivers gas at body temperature, 100% relative humidity	• Incorrect cannula size can provide inadvertent positive distending pressure, similar to CPAP	0.21–1, at flows of 1–8 L/min
Face mask	• Can provide moderate concentrations of oxygen • Provides oxygen to nose and mouth	• FiO$_2$ can vary significantly • Must be removed for feeding • Can cause skin irritation	0.35–0.50 (FiO$_2$ data from studies in children) at flows of 5–10 L/min
Oxygen hood	• Maintains a relatively constant FiO$_2$ • Does not need to be attached to patient's skin	• Higher FiO$_2$ may be found at bottom of hood • High noise levels inside • Must be set at 5–10 L/min to flush out exhaled CO$_2$ • Baby unable to be held or nursed when hood in place	0.21–1
Incubator	• Requires no additional device to attach to patient • Displays set and measured FiO$_2$ continuously on new model incubators	When care ports are open, FiO$_2$ may vary widely	0.21–0.65

FiO$_2$, Fraction of inspired oxygen.

Table 33.5 FiO$_2$ levels delivered to the neonatal airway via nasal cannula [10,14]

FiO$_2$ (set on air oxygen blender)	Delivered FiO$_2$ by flow rate (L/min)			
	0.25	0.50	0.75	1.0
0.40	0.22	0.23	0.25	0.26
0.60	0.26	0.31	0.35	0.37
0.80	0.31	0.36	0.41	0.49
1.0	0.35	0.45	0.61	0.66

FiO$_2$, Fraction of inspired oxygen.

in preterm infants. The future lies in the successful clinical application of an automated closed-loop control of inspired oxygen concentration [16]. The system consist of an oxygenation monitoring device (pulse oximeter), gas delivery device (ventilator or cannula), and an algorithm that determines the timing and magnitude of the FiO$_2$ adjustments.

Continuous positive airway pressure

CPAP is the application of positive pressure to the airways of a spontaneously breathing patient throughout the respiratory cycle, and resulting in improvement of oxygenation and ventilation. CPAP reduces upper airway obstruction and upper airway resistance by mechanically splinting the

Table 33.6 Predicted patient FHO$_2$ on 100% FiO$_2$ nasal cannula [12,13]

Weight (g)	FHO$_2$				
	0.1 L	0.2 L	0.3 L	0.4 L	0.5 L
700	0.32	0.44	0.55	0.66	0.77
800	0.31	0.41	0.51	0.61	0.70
900	0.30	0.39	0.47	0.56	0.65
1000	0.29	0.37	0.45	0.53	0.61
1100	0.28	0.35	0.43	0.50	0.57
1200	0.28	0.34	0.41	0.47	0.54
1300	0.27	0.33	0.39	0.45	0.51
1400	0.27	0.32	0.38	0.44	0.49
1500	0.26	0.32	0.37	0.42	0.47
1600	0.26	0.31	0.36	0.41	0.46
1700	0.26	0.30	0.35	0.40	0.44
1800	0.25	0.30	0.34	0.39	0.43
1900	0.25	0.29	0.33	0.38	0.42

FHO$_2$, Hypopharyngeal oxygen concentration; *FiO$_2$*, fraction of inspired oxygen.

airways open. This improves ventilation by recruiting collapsed alveoli and increasing the functional residual capacity and the surface area available for gas exchange. It also splints the chest wall, airways, and pharynx and reduces the work of breathing. It regularizes the breathing pattern, reduces mechanical obstruction (with meconium if applied early), and promotes lung growth. Three components are required to deliver CPAP: a flow circuit, an airway interface, and positive-pressure system. The various airway interfaces are single nasal prong, bi-nasal prongs (short and long), nasal cannula, face masks, and nasopharyngeal tube. Short bi-nasal prongs with the largest internal diameters have the lowest resistance and are the most effective and least invasive [17].

Nasal CPAP can be delivered by any of the following devices: bubble CPAP (continuous flow CPAP, oscillatory vibrations), Infant Flow SiPAP (variable flow CPAP, unique fluid mechanics), infant ventilators (continuous flow CPAP), or nasal cannula (high flow or low flow). A gas flow of 5–10 L/min and CPAP of 5–8 cm H$_2$O are commonly used, with minimal air leak around the nasal prongs or mask. The success of nasal CPAP depends on three factors: the underlying lung disease, the tolerance of the neonate, and the meticulous nursing experience in delivering it. Complications of nasal CPAP include nasal trauma causing nasal septum breakdown or erosion and nasal deformity, obstruction of prongs due to mucus plugging or tube displacement leading to impaired ventilation/oxygenation, air leak syndromes, feeding intolerance due to gaseous distension of the stomach, and infection.

Bubble CPAP

It consists of three major components (Fig. 33.2):
1. Gas source: An oxygen blender connected to a source of oxygen and compressed air and flow meter delivers the desired fraction of inspired oxygen (FiO$_2$). The warmed, humidified, and blended oxygen is driven through the inspiratory tubing.
2. Pressure generator: Pressure in the bubble CPAP system is generated by keeping the distal expiratory tubing under water. The depth of immersion of the tubing under water determines the CPAP pressure.
3. Infant interface: Hudson nasal prongs (short and wide) or INCA nasal cannula provides the nasal interface between the infant's airway and the gas flow circuit.

Bubble CPAP setup and nursing care

The following steps explain how to set it up (Fig. 33.3) [18]:
1. Position the baby in the supine position with the head elevated ~30 degrees and place a small roll under

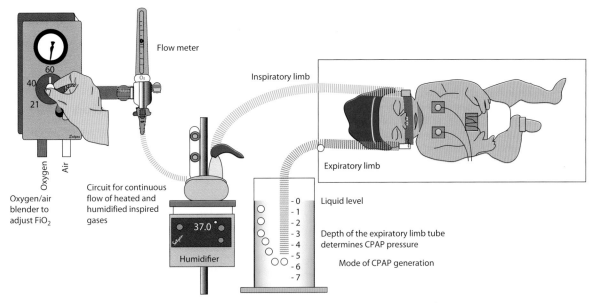

Fig. 33.2 Bubble CPAP Circuit Using INCA Nasal Cannula. Copyright: Satyan Lakshminrusimha.

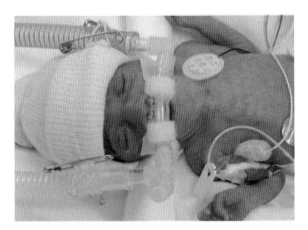

Fig. 33.3 Bubble CPAP Setup Using Hudson Nasal Prongs.

the baby's neck. Wear a pre-made hat or stockinette on the baby's head to hold the CPAP tube and insert an 8-F orogastric (OG) tube with its free end kept open.

2. Choose FiO_2 to keep PaO_2 at 60s or pre-ductal O_2 saturation at 90%–95%.

3. Adjust a flow rate of 5–10 L/min. Keep inspired gas temperature at $37\,^\circ$C in the humidifier.

4. Insert the expiratory tubing in a bottle of sterile water filled up to a height of 7 cm. The tube is immersed to a depth of 5 cm to create 5 cm H_2O CPAP as long as air is bubbling out of solution.

5. Choose proper size of the nasal cannula (Hudson) and attach to corrugated tubing (size 0 for <700 g; 1, ~1000 g; 2, ~2000 g; 3, ~3000 g; 4, ~4000 g; and 5, infant).

6. Lubricate the nasal CPAP prongs with saline and place the prongs' curved side down and direct into nasal cavities.

7. Secure tubing on both sides of the hat with safety pins and rubber band or Velcro.

8. Bubble CPAP maintenance:
   a. Observe baby's vital signs, oxygenation, and activity.
   b. Check CPAP systems, inspired gas temperature, air bubbling out of solution, and empty condensed water in the circuit; aspirate gastric air before feeding.
   c. Check position of CPAP prongs and keep them away from the septum at all times.
   d. Suction nasal cavities, mouth, pharynx, and stomach 4 hourly and p.r.n.; watch for nasal erythema.
   e. Change the baby's position 4 hourly; watch for humidification water condensation or visible soiling of tube; change CPAP circuit once a week.

Infant Flow SiPAP

1. It is a variation of the variable flow CPAP system that can deliver synchronized pressure support breaths triggered by an abdominal wall Grasby capsule.

2. It provides bi-level nasal CPAP for the spontaneously breathing neonate through the delivery of sighs above a baseline CPAP pressure. These sighs may be timed, at a rate specified by clinicians, or "triggered" by patients own inspiratory efforts.

Nasal high-flow therapy

Adequately warmed and humidified gas mixture of air and oxygen, delivered at a high flow rate (2–8 L/min) via nasal cannula is getting more popular as an alternative to CPAP or for post-extubation from invasive ventilation. The advantages claimed for nasal high-flow therapy (nHFT) include ease of setting it up, less nasal trauma, better patient comfort [19], provision of positive airway pressure [20], and improved gas exchange through wash-out of dead space [21]. A recent Cochrane meta-analysis has shown similar rates of the efficacy of high-flow nasal cannula (HFNC) to other forms of noninvasive respiratory support in preterm infants for preventing treatment failure, death, and chronic lung disease [22]. Current evidence favors CPAP over HFNC since latter has no titration/measurement of delivered pressures. However, the ease of use and less risk of nasal trauma have increased the use of HFNC. Two common devices used for delivering nHFT are Precision Flow (Vapotherm) and Optiflow Junior (Fisher and Paykel Healthcare). Based on current evidence a consensus approach to initiation, escalation, weaning, and discontinuation of nHFT has been outlined [23]. It is safe and effective for post-extubation respiratory support of most neonates (≥28 weeks) and for weaning from nasal CPAP. The gas must be adequately heated, well humidified, and with some leak from the nostrils. All of the currently available devices (Vapotherm, Optiflow Junior, and bubble CPAP) generate similar noise levels and much above the current AAP recommendation of 45 dB [24].

Noninvasive mechanical ventilation (NIMV/NIPPV)

Nasal intermittent mandatory ventilation (NIMV) and nasal intermittent positive pressure ventilation (NIPPV) are often used interchangeably for respiratory support provided without an ETT. NIMV/NIPPV delivers intermittent peak inspiratory pressure (PIP), either mandatory or triggered, besides positive end-expiratory pressure (PEEP), through nasal prongs. It may provide better oxygenation and ventilation than CPAP and deliver assisted ventilation during apneic spells, as long as the airway is patent. It can be used as a primary mode of respiratory support soon after birth and as a secondary mode after extubation from invasive ventilation, to prevent reintubation. NIPPV may reduce apnea frequency better than NCPAP and may augment the beneficial effects of NCPAP in preterm infants with frequent and severe apnea [25]. NIPPV and CPAP have similar overall survival and rates of BPD in extremely low birth weight infants [26]. NIPPV is associated with reduced incidence of extubation failure and the need for reintubation within 48 h to 1 week when compared to NCPAP [27]. NIPPV is delivered using the same components required for CPAP and has been listed earlier. Contraindications for NIPPV include upper airway abnormalities (choanal atresia, cleft lip and palate, and tracheoesophageal fistula), necrotizing enterocolitis, and severe cardiovascular instability.

Positive-pressure ventilation

This respiratory support is provided by a mechanical ventilator through an ETT. In conventional ventilation, intermittent positive-pressure ventilator breaths are given on a background of PEEP. Minute ventilation (CO_2 removal) is determined by the product of tidal volume and respiratory rate. Oxygenation is determined by the mean airway pressure (MAP) and the fraction of inspired oxygen concentration (FiO_2). The care provider should be familiar with the type of ventilator and the airway interface. Conventional mechanical ventilation is commonly pressure limited and time cycled. PIP is set by the physician and tidal volume varies from breath to breath, based on airway resistance and lung compliance. In patient-triggered ventilation (PTV), also known as assist control (AC) or synchronized intermittent positive-pressure ventilation (SIPPV), each breath is supported by the ventilator. With synchronized intermittent mandatory ventilation (SIMV), only a set number of breaths are supported by the ventilator and the remaining breaths are unsupported. In both modes, if the infant becomes apneic, there is a backup ventilation rate. To reduce the risk of volutrauma and atelectotrauma, volume-targeted ventilation is often used. In this mode, a desired tidal volume (usually 4–6 mL/kg) is set and the PIP will automatically adjust to achieve the desired tidal volume. It helps in auto-weaning and results in reduced incidence of air leak syndromes and chronic lung disease. It is less effective in the presence of a large leak around the ETT. Disease-specific lung protective ventilator strategies are helpful to minimize lung damage in extremely preterm infants, by using the lowest possible pressure, volume, and oxygen [28].

High-frequency oscillatory ventilation

This mode of ventilation achieves gas exchange by the use of tiny tidal volumes at supraphysiological rates (10 Hz = 600 per minute). It improves ventilation at lower MAP, reduces volutrauma, and produces uniform lung inflation which can reduce air leaks. Carbon dioxide elimination is dependent on the oscillatory amplitude (delta P) and frequency. Oxygenation is dependent on the MAP and FiO_2. Based on the level of MAP, two strategies can be used to deliver HFOV. A high-volume strategy is used for infants' with homogeneous lung disease (RDS). A low-volume strategy is used for infants with nonhomogeneous lung disease especially when associated with lung hypoplasia and/or air leak syndromes (pneumothorax with active air leak, congenital diaphragmatic hernia, pulmonary hypoplasia, and idiopathic or black-lung PPHN). Studies have not revealed any short- or long-term benefits with the use of HFOV over conventional ventilation in either term or preterm infants [29].

Endotracheal intubation

It is often required for airway management in neonates with respiratory failure or who require resuscitation. Intubation can be done orally or nasally and non-cuffed ETTs are commonly used in neonates. The rates of ETT malposition and blockage, accidental extubation, septicemia, clinical infection, and local trauma have been found to be similar in both nasal and oral intubation [30]. In very low birth weight infants, post-extubation atelectasis has been observed to be more frequent after nasal intubation.

1. Intubation equipment:
   a. ETTs: sizes 2.5, 3.0, 3.5, and 4.0 mm; stylet and Magill neonatal forceps
   b. Laryngoscope with straight blade: infant (Miller No. 1), premature (Miller No. 0), and extremely premature (Miller No. 00) blades; additional bulbs and batteries
   c. Carbon dioxide detector, stethoscope (neonatal)
   d. Suction apparatus and catheters: 5.0, 6.0, 8.0, and 10.0 F
   e. Self-inflating bag (0.5 L) bag with reservoir, or a flow-inflating bag or a T-piece resuscitator, and ETT fixation materials
   f. Compressed air and oxygen with blender, humidifier, warmer, and flow meter
2. ETT:
   a. Size of tube and suction catheter: Table 33.7 provides guidance on choosing the correct size of ETT and suction catheter, based on birth weight and gestational age of the infant [31]

b. Correct tube placement: Correct placement of the tube inside mid-trachea is ensured both clinically and by chest radiography. Clinical indicators include a rise in heart rate, bilateral chest wall movement with respiration, breath sounds heard better over the lung fields than stomach, the presence of vapor in the tube during expiration and change in color of CO_2 detector to yellow

c. Depth of tube insertion: The correct position for the tip of an ETT is below the larynx and above the carina (approximately T2). For orotracheal intubation a common rule of thumb is to add six to the birth weight, to get the initial depth of insertion of the tracheal tube; for nasotracheal intubation, add 1 cm more to this number. The aforementioned rule may be incorrect for infants with micrognathia, short neck, and weighing <750 g. A chest X-ray should be taken to confirm the tip, and special care should be taken to keep the infant's head in a "neutral" position and to avoid extension or flexion of the neck during this procedure. The tip of the ETT follows the movement of the tip of the nose. Neck extension displaces the tube away from the carina, whereas neck flexion moves the tube toward the carina [32]. Rotation of the neck also causes the tube to move away from the carina. Neck extension causes greater ETT displacement in orotracheal intubation when compared to the nasotracheal route. The size and position of the ETT should be clearly documented in the infant's notes

d. Tube fixation: Failure to fix the tube securely is the commonest cause for accidental extubation. A secure tube is essential during the administration of surfactant, airway suctioning, and chest physiotherapy. There are a variety of methods for tube fixation and these include the conventional adhesive tape applied to the tube from the upper lip/cheek, the umbilical clamp method, or by the use of various commercially available fixation

Table 33.7 Size of endotracheal tube, length of insertion, and size of suction catheter based on body weight and gestational age [31]

Tube size (internal diameter in mm)	Weight (g)	Gestational age (week)	Length (oral) (cm)	Suction catheter size (F)
2.5	<1000	<28	7	5 or 6
3.0	1000–2000	28–34	7–8	6 or 8
3.5	2000–3000	34–38	8–9	8
3.5–4.0	>3000	>38	9–10	8 or 10

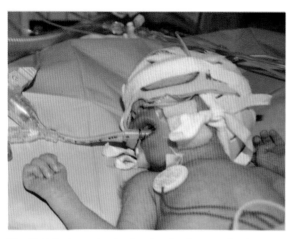

Fig. 33.4 Endotracheal Tube Fixation by Suturing it to a Portex Sleeve Tied to a Hat.

devices. A simple and secure practice without using an adhesive tape, is to stitch the ETT to a Portex sleeve tied to a hat (Fig. 33.4). Plastic locking clips can also be used instead of sutures to hold the tube tightly inside the Portex sleeve (Fig. 33.5). There is lack of evidence to show the most effective and safe method to stabilize the ETT in the ventilated neonate [33]

e. Tube suctioning: There is an absence of the normal mucociliary clearance of the airways with an ETT in situ and hence mechanical removal of secretions will be required to maintain patency of the ETT and for optimal ventilation. This is explained in detail in section: Airway Patency and Suction

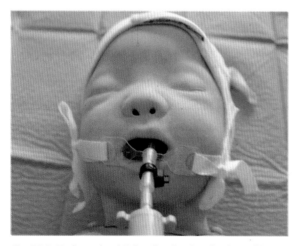

Fig. 33.5 Endotracheal Tube Fixation by Plastic Locking Clip Around a Portex Sleeve Tied to a Hat.

f. Tube complications: Acute complications of endotracheal intubation include malposition, displacement or obstruction, perforation (pharyngeal, esophageal, tracheal), hemorrhage, and vocal cord injuries. Chronic complications include glottic or subglottic stenosis, granuloma or cyst, and hoarseness, stridor, or wheezing. Systemic side effects include infection, oropharyngeal aspiration, apnea, bradycardia, and hypoxia. Nasotracheal tubes can cause nasal septal erosion and stricture of the nasal vestibule. Orotracheal tubes can cause alveolar and palatal grooves, dentition defects, and speech abnormalities

g. Unplanned extubation (UE): It denotes premature removal of an ETT by the patient or the health care provider. Despite lack of a standardized definition and classification of UE in neonates, it is a major patient safety issue and can lead to significant morbidity and mortality. It can result in sudden cardiorespiratory collapse, trauma to the airway, intracranial hemorrhage in extremely preterm infants, and ventilator-associated pneumonia (VAP). Factors associated with UE in neonates include excessive secretions, unsupported ventilator tubing, patient procedure, sedation-related, loose tape, blocked ETT, and loose skin-protective barrier [34]. A suggested benchmark to achieve is an UE rate <1 per 100 patient-intubated days [35]. A quality improvement initiative has recommended the following guidelines to reduce UE in the NICU [36]:
   - Establish a standardized airway management guideline detailing ETT and tracheostomy best practices
   - Require at least two providers when moving patients
   - Define standards for head and airway position during chest radiograph
   - Define ETT securing method and depth
   - Establish a postoperative handoff to address airway concerns
   - Utilize an unplanned extubation huddle assessment tool to identify contributing factors

Ventilator-associated pneumonia

It is a preventable nosocomial infection in the NICU and is discussed in great detail in chapter 35 (Ventilator-Associated Pneumonia and Infection Control). Despite lack of objective criteria specific to VAP in neonates, a VAP prevention bundle is suggested for neonates on assisted ventilation [37].

Nursing care of the neonate and monitoring of equipment

Hand hygiene

Use strict hand hygiene before and after patient contact and while handling equipment for respiratory support. Observe universal precautions and wear gloves when at risk of contact with secretions.

Clinical evaluation and ongoing assessment

Clinical evaluation of the cardiorespiratory system should focus on general physical signs, severity of respiratory distress (by assessment of respiratory rate, respiratory effort, recession, grunting, nasal flaring, oxygen saturation, and FiO_2), chest wall movement, air entry (by auscultation of both axillae), and the presence of adventitious sounds and murmurs.

Assessment of blood gases

The interpretation of blood gases and acid–base balance should always be made in a clinical context. The pH of arterial blood is dependent on $PaCO_2$, lactate, and bicarbonate. Capillary venous sampling can be considered for all values (pH, CO_2, base, and bicarbonate) but arterial sampling is required for assessment of oxygenation status. A stepwise approach to evaluate blood gases is as follows:

Step 1: Assess the pH as normal (7.35–7.45), acidotic (<7.35), or alkalotic (>7.45).

Step 2: Assess the respiratory (normal CO_2 = 35–45 mmHg) component and metabolic (normal HCO_3 = 22–26 mEq./L) component.

Step 3: Assess the compensation status. When the pH becomes normal, by correction of both acid–base components (PCO_2 and HCO_3) in opposite directions, the gas is said to be compensated.

Step 4: Assess oxygenation by measuring PaO_2 from arterial blood or from a preductal pulse oximeter. The normal PaO_2 values in the term infant are 50–80 mmHg and in the preterm infant, 45–65 mmHg.

Step 5: Make a plan to correct the acid–base imbalance by treating the underlying cause.

Respiratory acidosis: for non-ventilated infants, apply nasal CPAP or provide invasive ventilation. For ventilated infants, increase alveolar ventilation by increasing tidal volume, respiratory rate, PIP, or PEEP (if the lungs have low inflation).

Respiratory alkalosis: For ventilated infants, decrease tidal volume, respiratory rate, or PIP.

Metabolic acidosis: Treat the underlying cause of the acidosis (e.g., correction of hypovolemia, the addition of acetate, and reduction of protein load in total parenteral nutrition).

Metabolic alkalosis: Treat the underlying cause by discontinuing diuretics, correcting electrolyte imbalances (hyponatremia, hypokalemia, and hypochloremia), and replacing gastrointestinal losses.

Hypoxemia can be corrected by administering supplemental oxygen and increasing the MAP for an infant on mechanical ventilation.

Noninvasive respiratory monitoring

1. Transcutaneous PO_2 ($TcPO_2$): It is measured using an electrode placed over the skin and heated to 42–44 °C; it measures skin PO_2 and not arterial PO_2. Underestimation of PO_2 occurs with poor perfusion of skin and inadequate heating and calibration of the electrode. Calibrate the sensor as per the recommendation of the manufacturer, change its location every 4 h with repeat calibration and observe for signs of thermal injury at the sensor site (e.g., erythema, blisters, burns, skin tears).

2. Pulse oximetry: Continuous arterial oxygen saturation is calculated from differential absorption of emitted red and infrared light. The pulse oximeter probe (disposable or reusable) is attached to a finger or toe in term infants or to a hand or foot in small premature infants. Unlike $TcPO_2$, pulse oximetry does not require skin warming or calibration, has no time delay, and does not require its position to be changed. Its accuracy is affected by motion artifacts, hypotension, poor perfusion, and phototherapy. Oxygen saturation measured by pulse oximetry (SpO_2) is usually a good indicator of hypoxemia but not hyperoxemia, due to the shape of the oxyhemoglobin dissociation curve (Fig. 33.6). On the flat upper portion of the curve, PaO_2 values above 100 mmHg commonly occur and are harmful.

The optimal values for arterial oxygen tension (PaO_2) and saturation (SpO_2) vary between preterm and term infants. In preterm infants, PaO_2 is maintained at 45–80 mmHg with oxygen saturation at 91%–95% [38]; fetal hemoglobin results in higher saturations at lower oxygen levels. Lower oxygen saturations have been associated with increased mortality but less retinopathy of prematurity. In infants receiving supplemental oxygen, saturation above 95% may denote very high oxygen tensions (any

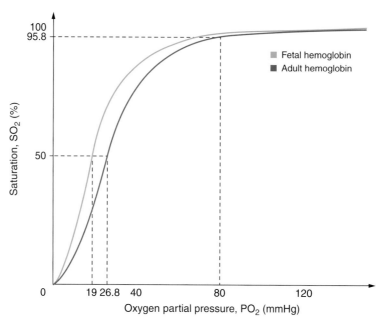

Fetal hemoglobin
Adult hemoglobin

Fig. 33.6 Oxyhemoglobin Dissociation Curve.

value >80 mmHg). This can cause tissue damage due to the release of oxygen free radicals and lead to retinopathy of prematurity in preterm infants and further brain damage in term infants with birth asphyxia.

3. Transcutaneous PCO_2 ($TcPCO_2$): It is measured with a glass electrode that is pH-sensitive and its response time is slower than that of $TcPO_2$. The measured value is electronically corrected for skin production of carbon dioxide and is quite useful for monitoring chronically ventilated patients. Similar precautions as mentioned under $TcPO_2$ measurement are necessary to avoid skin damage.

4. End-tidal carbon dioxide: It gives a continuous measure of expired CO_2 in ventilated infants and shows good correlation with PCO_2. The end-tidal device is positioned between the infant's ETT and the ventilator flow sensor and is of two types: side stream and in line. It is mainly used to detect trends in $PaCO_2$ and for immediate detection of extubation. The device should not be used for 4 h after surfactant administration. $ETCO_2$ monitoring is not useful in presence of significant leak around ETT and with HFOV. $TcCO_2$ monitoring is more precise than $ETCO_2$, but both require regular correlation with $PaCO_2$. Increased physiological dead space and/or V/Q mismatch increases the difference between $ETCO_2$ and $PaCO_2$.

Ventilator settings

Oxygenation depends on ventilation and perfusion, while removal of CO_2 is based on minute ventilation (tidal volume × respiratory rate). Changes in the ventilator parameters of FiO_2, MAP (derived from PIP, PEEP, and inspiratory time), tidal volume, and bias flow rate affect oxygenation. It is very important to be familiar with the type of ventilator, mode of ventilation as well as its settings. Before making any changes to the settings of ventilator, you need to know the current clinical status and result of blood gas analysis. Besides target oxygen saturation, there should be clarity in what is to be achieved, changes in oxygenation, ventilation, or both. Useful gentle strategies to protect the infant lung during invasive ventilation include optimizing lung volume, limiting excessive lung expansion, appropriate PEEP, shorter inspiratory time, smaller tidal volume, and permissive hypercapnia [39]. Table 33.8 provides general guidelines while making changes in ventilation [40].

Imaging

1. Chest radiography: Anteroposterior projection from a supine position is used to evaluate the infant's heart, lung fields, ETT, the course of long lines, and umbilical catheters. It gives an idea about lung volume and helps in early detection of pulmonary air leaks. The cross-table view helps visualization of pleural chest

Table 33.8 Guidelines for making changes in ventilation [40]

Aim	Action	Evaluation
Conventional ventilation		
Increase oxygenation	Increase FiO_2 in increments of 5%–10% Increase MAP by increasing PIP or PEEP in increments of 1–2 cm H_2O Keep inspiratory time of 0.35–0.40 s for preterm infants	Observe for chest expansion Observe oxygen requirement Observe pulmonary graphic analysis of pressure, volume, and airflow
Decrease oxygenation	Decrease FiO_2 in decrements of 5%–10% Decrease MAP by reducing PIP or PEEP in decrements of 1–2 cm H_2O Keep inspiratory time of 0.35–0.40 s for preterm infants	Same as previous Aim for SpO_2 target of 91%–95% for preterm infants
Increase CO_2 elimination	Increase rate (in increments of 5 per min) Increase PIP (in increments of 1–2 cm H_2O) In volume guarantee mode of ventilation, increase set or desired tidal volume	Observe minute ventilation on the ventilator Check CO_2 by blood gas analysis or transcutaneous monitoring
Decrease CO_2 elimination	Reduce rate (in decrements of 5 per min) Reduce PIP (in decrements of 1–2 cm H_2O) Decrease PEEP while the PIP is reduced. In volume guarantee mode of ventilation, decrease set or desired tidal volume	Same as previous
High-frequency oscillatory ventilation		
Increase oxygenation	Increase FiO_2 in increments of 5%–10% Increase MAP in increments of 1–2 cm H_2O	Observe for chest expansion and oxygen requirement Obtain an early blood gas Initial chest radiograph at 1–2 h to determine the baseline lung volume on HFOV (aim for eight ribs); repeat chest radiography with changes in patient condition
Decrease oxygenation	Decrease FiO_2 in increments of 5%–10% Decrease MAP in increments of 1–2 cm H_2O	Same as previous Aim for SpO_2 target of 91%–95% for preterm infants
Increase CO_2 elimination	Increase amplitude (delta P) by 2–5 cm H_2O based on chest wiggle Decrease frequency (1–2 Hz)	Observe for good chest wiggle Observe tidal volume and DCO_2; check CO_2 by blood gas analysis or transcutaneous monitoring
Decrease CO_2 elimination	Decrease amplitude in increments of 1–2 cm H_2O according to CO_2 and chest wiggle	Same as previous

tube being placed anteriorly or posteriorly. The lateral decubitus view is ideal to reveal a small pneumothorax or minimal pleural effusion. Care should be taken to position the infant well and keep the head in neutral position before imaging. Expose the area of interest, after removal of unnecessary things from the chest and moving aside the monitor leads and tubes. The gonads of the infant should be shielded if they are within 5 cm of the primary X-ray beam. The nursing staff holding the infant for the exposure should wear a lead apron and gloves. Proper immobilization improves image quality, shortens the examination time, and eliminates repeat imaging. Avoid routine chest X-rays after a change of ETT, before and after extubation, and on a stable ventilated infant. With clinical deterioration and in HFOV, more frequent radiographs are required.

2. Ultrasound: is useful for detecting pleural effusion and diaphragmatic palsy, and in screening for intraventricular hemorrhage and periventricular leukomalacia. Lung ultrasound is radiation free and may complement chest radiography in determining which neonates admitted with respiratory distress will require mechanical ventilation [41].

3. Functional echocardiography (fECHO): is a novel method of assessment of the hemodynamic status of a sick neonate by measuring left ventricular cardiac output and superior vena cava flow. It is quite useful in classifying a patent ductus arterious as hemodynamically significant and in the management of persistent pulmonary hypertension of the newborn.

Real-time pulmonary graphics [42]

Real-time pulmonary graphic analysis helps to understand lung mechanics and interactions between patient and ventilator. It displays pressure, volume, and flow waveforms as well as pressure–volume and flow–volume loops. It enables to customize ventilation based on the underlying pathophysiology and requirement of the infant and facilitates early weaning from ventilation.

1. Pressure–volume (P–V) loops: demonstrate the relationship of pressure to volume. It is useful to evaluate lung compliance after surfactant administration. A flattened loop indicates poor compliance and an upright loop indicates improved compliance. The P–V loops are also useful to reduce volutrauma by correcting overdistension.

2. Flow–volume loops: display the relationship between volume and flow and are useful in evaluating airway resistance in conditions like MAS and BPD.

Airway patency and suction

Noninvasive nasal and nasopharyngeal suction

Patency of the upper airways is an essential requirement for an infant on noninvasive respiratory support. Airway secretions can cause obstruction during or after administration of nasal CPAP/nasal IMV in preterm infants. The common practice of intermittent suctioning by insertion of a catheter into the nose and nasopharynx can result in bradycardia, laryngospasm, cardiac dysrhythmias, nasal mucosal injury, edema, and bleeding. Oral suctioning should always precede nasal suction. A noninvasive method of nasopharyngeal suctioning has been found to be very effective and without side effects [43]. Sterile 0.9% saline solution is instilled drop wise into one nostril from a 5-mL syringe

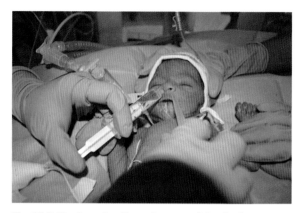

Fig. 33.7 Noninvasive Nasopharyngeal Suctioning.

and suctioned from the other nostril using a Neotech little sucker (Fig. 33.7) or De Lee suction catheter, attached to a central vacuum source (suction pressure of 100 mmHg). This results in passage of fluid and sticky secretions from one nostril and nasopharynx to the other nostril which gets aspirated. It is then repeated on the other side (Video 33.1). Saline should never be pushed rapidly into the nostril, for fear of aspiration or injury to the middle ear. To keep the upper airway open at all times, it is advisable to do suctioning 4–6 hourly and whenever indicated.

Endotracheal suction

Infants on assisted ventilation require patency of the ETT for effective ventilation and oxygenation. An ETT in situ impairs airway clearance of secretions by preventing the cough reflex and the normal physiological mucociliary clearance mechanism; it can also result in increased secretion of mucus. Though endotracheal suction is a common procedure performed to remove secretions, there are only limited studies and scientific evidence in the neonatal population to guide practice. The smaller diameter of the neonatal ETT not only makes the procedure difficult but also results in more complications. Adequate humidity (maintained at 100% with the gas warmed to 32–34°C) makes the secretions loose, lubricates the ETT, and protects the surrounding tracheal tissue from dehydration. The various aspects of endotracheal suctioning in intubated neonates can be discussed as follows, in order to improve patient care and potentially avoid adverse events resulting from the inappropriate nursing action:

1. Assessment of patient: An individualized clinical assessment of the neonate should form the basis for endotracheal suction and the following parameters need to be closely monitored before, during, and after the procedure.

   a. Breath sounds, respiratory rate, and pattern.

b. Oxygen saturation, heart rate, and blood pressure.
c. ETT CO_2 or transcutaneous CO_2.
d. Sputum characteristics: Color, volume, consistency, and odor.
e. Ventilator parameters: PIP and plateau pressure, tidal volume, FiO_2, pressure, flow, and volume graphics, if available.

2. Indications for endotracheal suction: Endotracheal suctioning should not be performed as a routine ritual but according to the need and clinical status of the baby.
   a. To maintain the patency and integrity of the artificial airway and obtain a sputum specimen for laboratory analysis.
   b. To remove accumulated pulmonary secretions as evidenced by one of the following:
      • Deteriorating oxygen saturation levels or arterial blood gases.
      • Bradycardia or tachycardia.
      • Absent or decreased chest movement.
      • Reduced chest wall vibration for patients on HFOV.
      • Audible or visible secretions in ETT.
      • Increased $ETCO_2$ or transcutaneous CO_2.
      • Coarse or decreased breath sounds.
      • Increased work of breathing and irritability.
      • Blood pressure fluctuations.
      • Saw tooth pattern on the flow–volume loop on the monitor screen of the ventilator.
      • Increased PIP during volume-controlled mechanical ventilation or decreased tidal volume during pressure-controlled ventilation.
      • Recent history of large amounts of thick/tenacious secretions in the past 12 h.
      • Suspected aspiration of meconium or gastric contents.

3. Assessment of successful outcome of endotracheal suction:
   a. Improvement in chest movement, breath sounds, and ventilator graphics.
   b. Removal of airway secretions.
   c. Improved oxygen saturation, transcutaneous CO_2, heart rate, blood pressure, and respiratory rate.
   d. Decreased work of breathing, PIP and airway resistance.
   e. Increased tidal volume delivery during pressure-limited ventilation.

4. Methods of endotracheal suctioning:
   a. Open and closed techniques: The open suctioning technique requires disconnecting the infant from the ventilator to insert the suction catheter into the ETT. After suctioning, manual breaths are given with the use of a resuscitation bag or the infant placed back on the ventilator. The closed suctioning technique involves attachment of a closed, in-line,

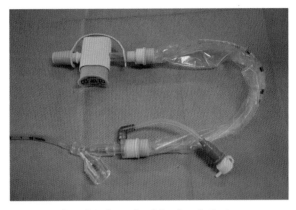

Fig. 33.8 Closed Endotracheal Suction Catheter.

sterile suction catheter to the ventilator circuit, which allows passage of a suction catheter through the ETT without disconnecting the infant from the ventilator (Fig. 33.8). The Cochrane review of suctioning without disconnection from the ventilator shows some evidence of improvement in short-term outcomes [44]. Closed suctioning uses less nursing time compared to open suctioning and may limit aerosolization of infectious mucus particles and prevent the spread of infection between patients and from patients to staff.
   b. Shallow and deep suctioning: These two methods of suctioning differ on the depth of insertion of the suction catheter during the procedure. In shallow suctioning, the suction catheter is inserted to a predetermined depth which is usually the length of the ETT plus the adapter. In deep suctioning the catheter is inserted into the ETT until resistance is felt, withdrawn by 1 cm and suction applied to remove secretions. The Cochrane review of randomized controlled trials found no evidence concerning the benefits or risks of deep versus shallow suctioning of ETTs in ventilated neonates and infants [45]. Deep suctioning can cause mucosal damage to the carina and surrounding tissues and a vagal response from tracheal stimulation. This damage can be due to contact of the suction catheter with the mucosa and from the negative pressure applied. We recommend shallow suctioning over deep suctioning since it maintains better physiologic stability in intubated neonates [46,47].

5. Suctioning procedure [48]:
   a. Closed suctioning procedure (Video 33.2):
      • Perform hand hygiene and use personal protective equipment (PPE). Adjust wall suction pressure of 80–100 mmHg.

- Monitor patient for dysrhythmias, changes in heart rate, or SpO_2 while suctioning.
- Preoxygenate if hypoxemic before suctioning by increasing FiO_2 0.1–0.2 above baseline for 1 min.
- Determine correct color or number for suction depth and unlock in-line suction.
- Stabilize the catheter and endotracheal or tracheostomy tube with the nondominant hand.
- Advance catheter to the premeasured depth within the plastic sheath without suction.
- Depress the control valve to apply continuous suction and withdraw the suction catheter fully, while stabilizing ETT to prevent dislodgement. The duration of suction should not exceed 5 s.
- When suction is complete, ensure catheter tip fully retracted from ETT.
- Check viewing port for secretions and assess patient. If further suctioning is required, repeat the procedure as before. Allow the infant to rest and reoxygenate between suction passes.
- Clean the catheter off debris by flushing sterile 0.9% saline via the irrigation port while simultaneously applying suction. Close suction control valve.
- Return ventilator to baseline parameters, decreasing FiO_2 according to SpO_2 and clinical status.
- Cap the irrigation port, disconnect suctioning from in-line suction catheter and re-cap in-line catheter end. Provide mouth care as per unit policy.
- Auscultate chest to determine the effectiveness of suctioning and ensure patient's stability, comfort, and safety.

b. Open suctioning procedure (Video 33.3):
  - Perform hand hygiene and use PPE for open suctioning.
  - Set up sterile 0.9% saline for instillation and for flushing of the catheter between catheter passes.
  - Open suction catheter package maintaining the sterility of catheter. Attach catheter end to the connection tubing from the suction apparatus. Adjust wall suction pressure of 80–100 mmHg. Cleanse hands and put on sterile gloves.
  - Disconnect the patient from the ventilator ensuring ventilator connections are kept clean. Preoxygenate infant if hypoxemic before suctioning by hyperventilating for 3–5 breaths using a manual resuscitation bag, at a rate 10%–20% above baseline and increasing FiO_2 0.1–0.2 above baseline.
  - With sterile gloved hand, advance catheter to the pre-measured depth without applying suction.

- Apply intermittent suction while withdrawing the catheter in a slow, rotating manner (up to 360 degree) with the help of thumb and finger, to minimize effects of negative pressures caused by suctioning. Continuous suction may be required for thick, copious secretions or meconium aspiration. The duration of suction should not exceed 5 s.
- Reoxygenate with the manual resuscitation bag for a minimum of 3–5 breaths at a rate 10%–20% above baseline and with FiO_2 to keep oxygen saturation within ordered parameters between suction passes.
- If further suctioning is required, repeat the procedure as before. Allow the infant to rest and reoxygenate as necessary.
- Clear the catheter and connecting tubing with sterile normal saline as needed before reinserting catheter and at the end of the procedure.
- Reconnect patient to the ventilator when suctioning is completed.
- After tracheal suctioning, the mouth/nose may be suctioned with the same catheter.
- Auscultate the chest to determine the effectiveness of suctioning and ensure patient's comfort, stability, and safety.

c. Suctioning patients on high-frequency ventilation: oscillating (HFOV) or jet (HFJV).
  - Cues for suctioning are based on visualization of secretions in the ETT, changes in vital signs, and reduced chest vibrations. With HFOV the frequency of suctioning should be minimized, based on decreased chest wiggle. With HFJV a decrease in servo pressure may indicate the need for suction.
  - Preoxygenation should be based on patient's needs and suctioning is done utilizing pre-measured suction depth.
  - HFOV:
    - In-line suction (closed suction technique) should always be used. Avoid disconnecting the ventilator to prevent derecruitment of alveoli.
    - Stop oscillations while maintaining MAP during suction passes. HFOV is turned back on by pressing the "Reset" button between suction passes to restart ventilator to oxygenate patient.
    - Follow the in-line suction procedure as mentioned earlier and apply suction both during insertion and withdrawal of the suction catheter. Withdraw the catheter in a slow, rotating manner (5–10 s) to minimize

effects of negative pressures caused by suctioning.

- HFJV:
  - In-line suction (closed suction technique) should always be used. Avoid disconnecting the ventilator to prevent derecruitment of alveoli.
  - HFJV with nitric oxide: The jet must be put into "Standby" when suctioning to minimize bolus delivery of nitric oxide that can occur.

6. Complications:
   a. Decrease in dynamic lung compliance and functional residual capacity.
   b. Hypoxemia, bronchospasm, and atelectasis.
   c. Tissue trauma to the tracheal and/or bronchial mucosa.
   d. Increased microbial colonization of lower airway.
   e. Changes in cerebral blood flow and increased intracranial pressure.
   f. Hypertension/hypotension and cardiac dysrhythmias.
   g. Routine use of normal saline instillation may be associated with: desaturation, bronchospasm, and dislodgement of the bacterial biofilm that colonizes the ETT into the lower airway.

7. Infection control:
   a. Centers for Disease Control guidelines for standard precautions should be followed. If manual ventilation is used, care must be taken not to contaminate the airway. Sterile technique is encouraged during the entire suctioning event.
   b. All equipment and supplies should be appropriately disposed of or disinfected.
   c. Disinfection of fomites associated with ventilation.

8. Pain assessment and management: Assessment of pain and adoption of non-pharmacologic measures, such as facilitated tucking [49] and developmentally supportive care may help to modulate the stressful responses of neonates. In a four-handed endotracheal suctioning strategy, person 1 supports the infant's efforts at self-regulation, such as promoting flexion, allowing finger grasp, or touching the infant gently, while person 2 performs the suctioning procedure [50]. The parent of the infant can replace person 1 as the caregiver providing support.

9. Evidence-based recommendations for endotracheal suctioning in neonates (Table 33.9): The following recommendations [51,52] are made based on the Grading of Recommendations Assessment, Development and Evaluation (GRADE) system for

Table 33.9 Recommendations for endotracheal suctioning in neonates [51–53]

Clinical procedure	Recommendation	Evidence level
Frequency of suctioning	Suctioning should only be performed when clinically indicated and not routinely	1C
Preoxygenation	Preoxygenation may be considered if the patient has a clinically important reduction in oxygen saturation with suctioning	2B
Closed versus open suctioning	Closed in-line suctioning without disconnecting the infant from the ventilator is preferred	2B
Depth of catheter insertion	Shallow suction is preferred instead of deep suction	2B
Saline instillation	Should not routinely use normal saline prior to suction	2C
Diameter of suction catheter	Suction catheter diameter must not exceed 50% of ETT diameter	2C
Duration of suctioning	Should not exceed 15 s	2C
Suction pressure	Negative suction pressure should be between 80 and 100 mmHg	2C
Saline instillation	Should not be performed routinely	2C
Number of repetitions	Should not exceed three per suctioning procedure	
Monitoring	Adequate monitoring prior to, during, and after the procedure	
Biosafety standards	CDC guidelines for standard precautions should be followed	

grading evidence [53]. The grading system classifies recommendations as strong (Grade 1) or weak (Grade 2), based on the balance between benefits, risks, burden, and cost and the degree of confidence in estimates of benefits, risks, and burden. It classifies the quality of evidence as high (Grade A), moderate (Grade B), or low (Grade C) according to factors that include the risk of bias, the precision of estimates, the consistency of the results, and the directness of the evidence.

Chest physiotherapy

The aim of chest physiotherapy (CPT) is to improve the clearance of lung secretions and maintain lung expansion, which, in turn, will lead to better oxygenation and ventilation. It also aims to prevent endotracheal tube obstruction and failure of extubation by the use of methods such as percussion, vibration, postural drainage, and suctioning. Despite widespread practice, there is lack of high-quality evidence to prove its efficacy and it has the potential to cause a range of serious complications. Hence, it should not be a routine practice in ventilated neonates and performed only when atelectasis or obstructive secretions are present and impacting on lung mechanics and gaseous exchange.

A 2008 Cochrane review of the literature on "chest physiotherapy for reducing respiratory morbidity in infants requiring ventilatory support" analyzed the results of three trials that studied 106 infants and found no evidence to guide present-day clinical practice [54]. Two of the three included trials were conducted over 30 years ago, and hence the applicability of the results to current neonatal practice may be limited due to changes in population characteristics and interventions; these include antenatal steroids, postnatal surfactant, gentle ventilation, and changes in the delivery of CPT. A 2010 Cochrane review of the literature on "chest physiotherapy for preventing morbidity in babies being extubated from mechanical ventilation" found no clear benefit in the use of postextubation active CPT [55]. Two of the four included trials were conducted over 30 years ago, and hence the applicability of the results to current neonatal practice may be limited due to changes in population characteristics and interventions. These changes include better humidification of inspired gases, exogenous surfactant, gentle ventilation, less endotracheal suctioning, and the use of postextubation nasal continuous positive airway pressure (NCPAP). This review did not find any evidence of harm for babies receiving a short course of CPT following extubation. A 2016 Cochrane review of the literature on "chest physiotherapy for acute bronchiolitis in pediatric patients between 0 and 24 months old" revealed no reduction in the severity of disease by the any of the CPT techniques analyzed (conventional, slow passive expiratory techniques, or forced expiratory techniques). This review found high-quality evidence that forced expiratory techniques in severe patients do not improve their health status and can lead to severe adverse events [56].

Indications

CPT should be provided only to those neonates considered most likely to benefit with significant respiratory distress and thick tenacious secretions. The potential risk of intraventricular hemorrhage in extremely preterm infants prevents its use in them unless the benefit is considered to outweigh any potential harm. Neonatal CPT may be considered in the presence of

- significant atelectasis;
- thick and/or copious secretions;
- pneumonia/aspiration;
- infants who require muscle relaxation and ventilatory support;
- recently extubated infants at risk for deterioration; and
- significant bronchopulmonary dysplasia with secondary atelectasis ± secretions.

Contraindications

- Extremely low birth weight (<1000 g) and <26 weeks' gestation
- Coagulopathy or severe thrombocytopenia ($<50 \times 10^9$/L)
- Recent (within 48 h) intraventricular hemorrhage (IVH)
- Pulmonary hemorrhage, undrained pneumothorax, pulmonary interstitial emphysema (PIE)
- Cardiovascular instability, increased intracranial pressure
- Metabolic bone disease/rib fracture
- Following thoracic, cardiac, and abdominal surgeries—withheld for 24 h

Precautions

- Poor skin integrity
- Platelet count $<100 \times 10^9$/L
- Avoid near sites of chest drain, Broviac lines, wounds, and stomas
- Effectiveness reduced with edema of the chest wall
- Distended abdomen, suspected necrotizing enterocolitis

Procedure

1. Assessment: Confirm physician's order, review recent chest X-rays, nursing, and respiratory therapy flow sheets, and assess the chest of the neonate. Before commencing active CPT, the physiotherapist must

note the baseline heart rate, mean blood pressure, oxygen saturation, as well as the ventilator mode, rate, pressures, and FiO_2. Do not disconnect the baby from the ventilator for turning and reduce the sensitivity of trigger from 1.0 to 1.6 to avoid triggering due to artifacts like manual vibration [57].

2. Treatment: Neonatal CPT includes gentle percussions, gentle active vibrations, positioning, and suctioning. It is given according to individual need and assessment may be done 4, 6, 8, or 12 hourly. The infant's head must be fully supported, never kept down, and excessive neck flexion/extension should be avoided during the whole procedure. The positions should be based on chest X-ray findings and auscultation and selected from the positioning chart. A maximum of two positions may be used, but in unstable or very small babies only one position is appropriate.
   a. Neonates <1000 g: 2 min per position or 2 finger percussions; approximately 60/min
   b. Neonates 1000–3500 g: Mask percussions × 3 min per position followed by 5 spaced vibrations
   c. Neonates >3500 g: Hand or mask percussions × 3 min per position followed by 5 spaced vibrations

3. Suctioning: It is performed after the use of active gentle vibrations. The endotracheal tube may be suctioned using a 6–8 F suction catheter with up to 100 mmHg low-flow suction. If secretions are excessively tenacious, consider saline instillation (0.2–0.5 mL) and repeat suction as tolerated by the infant until clear return. Neonates on nasal CPAP should be suctioned nasally after CPT. Nonventilated infants should be suctioned orally with size 8 or 10 F catheter, in a side lying position to reduce the risk of aspiration if the infant vomits.

4. Documentation: The details of treatment given should be documented on the physiotherapy chart and the time of the next physiotherapy session should also be noted. Mention any changes in the infant's condition or management after every treatment session.

5. Cessation of physiotherapy: CPT should be discontinued when there is evidence of re-expansion of collapsed/consolidated lung associated with significant reduction in the production of excessive or thick secretions.

Monitoring for complications

Mechanical ventilation saves many lives but can also result in pulmonary and non-pulmonary complications in a few infants.

1. BPD and ventilator-induced lung injury can result from the following:
   a. Volutrauma: Overdistension of the lung tissue caused by excessive delivery of tidal volume (>6 mL/kg).
   b. Atelectotrauma: Insufficient end-expiratory pressure leading to excessive shearing forces caused by the repeated collapse and reinflation of lung.
   c. Barotrauma: Excessive PIPs leading to overdistension and damage of compliant lung tissue.
   d. Biotrauma: Damage to lung tissue caused by inflammatory mediators, triggered by direct lung injury or infection.
   BPD is multi-factorial in origin and can potentially be reduced by volume controlled ventilation (targeting tidal volume in the normal range of 4–6 mL/kg), pulmonary graphics monitoring, and use of gentle ventilation by allowing permissive hypercapnia in appropriate conditions.

2. Pulmonary air leak syndrome: It includes pneumothorax, pulmonary interstitial emphysema, pneumomediastinum, pneumopericardium, pneumoperitoneum, and subcutaneous emphysema. Pneumothorax can be the result of high MAP, high inspiratory flow, prolonged inspiratory time, and asynchrony between patient and ventilator. Preventive measures can minimize the incidence of this life-threatening complication.

3. Sudden deterioration of infant on the ventilator can result from **DOPPIE**:
   a. **D**isplaced ETT
   b. **O**bstructed ETT
   c. **P**neumothorax
   d. **P**ulmonary hemorrhage
   e. **I**ntraventricular hemorrhage (IVH)
   f. **E**quipment failure

4. Gradual deterioration of infant on the ventilator can result from:
   a. Infection
   b. IVH
   c. Patent ductus arteriosus
   d. Partial blockage of the ETT
   e. Anemia/hypotension
   f. Slowly evolving air leak syndrome

5. VAP: It is discussed in great detail in chapter 36.

6. Airway injury and subglottic stenosis: It can result from prolonged and repeated endotracheal intubation, deep suctioning, and infection.

7. Retinopathy of prematurity: It is associated with hyperoxia, hypoxia, and fluctuations of arterial oxygen in preterm infants (<32 weeks) who require prolonged mechanical ventilation with supplemental oxygen. Its incidence can be reduced by maintaining PaO_2 between 60 and 80 mmHg and SpO_2 between 91% and 95%.

8. Neurological complications: Premature babies who require mechanical ventilation are prone to develop neurological complications, such as IVH and periventricular leukomalacia. Its incidence and severity can be minimized by avoiding hyper/hypocapnia, pneumothorax, and systemic hypo/hypertension. This can be achieved by synchronized ventilation and judicious use of ventilatory parameters and sedation.

General supportive care

Minimal handling

Neonatal care is unique, sensitive, complex, and shared. It should be based on the concept of minimal handling, which gives the care in the least invasive and disruptive way. With excessive handling and distressing procedures, the neonate deteriorates rapidly leading to hypoxia. Invasive procedures should only be done by experienced caregivers and no more than two attempts should be allowed per person. Avoid unnecessary interventions and based on the tolerance of the infant, practice grouping of care. Abrupt flexion or extension of head should be avoided. Support shoulder and head within one palm and finger grasp during caring while stabilizing the ETT.

Positioning

Proper positioning is important to optimize ventilation and oxygenation. There are differences in lung function between infants who are spontaneously breathing and those who are on a ventilator support [58] and also among infants with healthy and diseased lungs. Recent studies reveal that distribution of ventilation in neonates is less dependent on gravity [59]. Infants on noninvasive respiratory support need to be placed in any position that provides optimal airway positioning and gives comfort. The prone position is often preferred to improve oxygenation and reduce the episodes of apnea and bradycardia. The Cochrane review on infant position in neonates receiving mechanical ventilation found evidence of low to moderate quality favoring the prone position for slightly improved oxygenation. However, there was no specific body position during mechanical ventilation that was effective in producing sustained and clinically relevant improvement [60]. For prevention of VAP, it is advisable to keep the side-lying position, elevate the head of the bed by 15–30 degrees, and keep left lateral positioning after feedings [61]. Change position from supine, right or left lateral, and prone, if feasible, every 2–4 hourly. Infants in any position need to be supported with appropriate rolls and must have the developmental boundaries while in the supine and side-lying positions to facilitate flexion, containment, and comfort.

Oral care procedure for ventilated neonate

The immature immune system of neonates makes them highly susceptible to develop nosocomial infections. Oral care has been recommended as one of the components of a neonatal VAP prevention bundle [62]. Provide oral care within 24 h after intubation, every 3–4 h, and prior to OG tube insertion or reintubation. Use fresh colostrum, mother's milk, or sterile water. The procedure involves gently cleaning the gums and inside of the cheeks using q-tip or folded gauze. Avoid frequent and prolonged oral suctioning, as it can lead to the development of oral-tactile hypersensitivity. Do not place oral suction equipment where it can become contaminated and change it every 24 h. The Canadian Evidence-Based Practice for Improving Quality (EPIQ-II) network has recommended oral immune therapy (OIT) with colostrum to reduce the incidence of NEC and nosocomial infection in critically ill newborns [63]. Studies have shown OIT to be safe, feasible, and well tolerated by even the smallest, critically ill infants. Every infant (preterm or term) who is not feeding by mouth should receive OIT unless breast milk is contraindicated. The procedure involves administering one drop of fresh colostrum (0.05 mL) from a 1-mL syringe between the cheek and gum, every 2–4 h. OIT should continue till the infant is able to feed by mouth (breast or bottle) at least twice a day.

Sedation and pain management

Mechanical ventilation is a stressful experience for sick neonates and untreated pain can lead to negative consequences on long-term neurodevelopment [64]. Current evidence does not support the routine use of sedation and pain medications. However when clinically indicated it can be used along with a scoring tool, such as the Premature Infant Pain Profile to quantify and qualify discomfort and pain (Table 33.2) [7]. A high pain/agitation score indicates more frequent or intense behaviors, and a low sedation score indicates a decreased response to stimulation, or a deeper level of sedation. The use of the scale also ensures appropriate use and weaning of medications. Due to the potential for harm with the use of these medications, non-pharmacologic methods like skin-to-skin care, facilitated tucking, swaddling, minimal handling, clustered care, non-nutritive sucking (NNS), and oral sucrose are often used to reduce distress.

Medications

Nurses should have thorough knowledge about the commonly used medications in the NICU, despite most units having clear guidelines regarding their use. Therapeutic drug monitoring is required for drugs with a narrow therapeutic index (gentamicin, amikacin, vancomycin, phenobarbital, and phenytoin). Incompatible drugs should never be given through the same intravenous infusate. Concentrated dextrose solutions (>12.5%) and total parenteral nutrition must not be given via a peripheral cannula, as it carries a greater risk of thrombophlebitis and extravasation injury due to the increased osmolarity of the solution. The appropriate use of sedation and analgesia in ventilated infants using drugs like morphine, fentanyl, or midazolam is an accepted practice. The early use of methylxanthines (caffeine or theophylline) has been found to reduce the duration of ventilation by facilitating early extubation and the incidence of BPD. It is effective for the treatment of apnea of prematurity. Corticosteroids in low doses have been given systemically or by inhalation to extreme preterm and chronically ventilated infants to prevent or treat BPD, despite its concern for causing cerebral palsy when given early in life.

Nutrition

Sick infants on ventilator support suffer from malnutrition due to increased caloric requirement coupled with poor nutritional intake and intolerance to enteral feeding. Growth failure is common in infants with BPD, and likely to have a major adverse effect on their subsequent growth and development. Stable infant on ventilator support requires a caloric intake of 90–100 kcal/kg/day, while a rapidly growing preterm infant will require 120 kcal/kg/day. The energy requirements of long-term ventilated infants with chronic lung disease are further increased by 25%–30%. Early introduction of enteral feeds with expressed breast milk, even as trophic feeds (10–20 mL/kg/day) is essential for growth, development, and normal function of the gastrointestinal and hepatobiliary systems. Parenteral nutrition should be discontinued, once the infant tolerates 100–120 mL/kg/day of enteral feeds.

Developmental care [65]

It is an essential philosophy of neonatal care that integrates the developmental needs of each individual infant and their family within a medical framework. The aims of developmental care are to reduce stress and pain, conserve energy and promote physiological stability, recognize and support infants emerging neurodevelopment maturity, and to provide support and encouragement to their parents or caregivers. Developmental care can be considered under the following categories:

1. Sound: The background noise in the nursery should be quiet, an average of 45 dB, with peak noises up to 65 dB according to AAP committee on environmental health [66]. Care interventions to help reduce noise include:
   a. Education of staff and parents about effects of sound and need for quiet hours.
   b. Close incubator doors softly and avoid placing objects on top of the incubator.
   c. Silence alarms as soon as practicable and set alarms and phones at lowest safe level.
   d. Consider ear muffs during excessively noisy procedures—MRI.

2. Light and vision: Ambient lighting should vary from 10 to 600 lux and the lighting levels should be adjustable, allowing dimming and increased levels for safe working. Aim to keep lighting levels below 300 lux and use dim lighting whenever possible. Care interventions include:
   a. Protect infants from light with levels below 25 lux until 32/34 weeks corrected gestational age (CGA); use incubator cover or canopy with an open cot.
   b. From 32 weeks CGA begin to introduce moderate light exposure—2 h/day—canopy or incubator cover reduced, while still shielding baby from bright overhead lights or sunlight.
   c. Gradually build up to "cycled lighting," which reflects day/night lighting when infant is approaching term (35–37 weeks CGA).
   d. Protect infants from focused lighting during medical procedures/examinations.

3. Smell and taste: Support early exposure to parent's odor and opportunities for positive taste and oral sensory experiences. Exposure of babies to noxious odors and unpleasant tastes should be minimized. Care interventions include:
   a. Encourage the mother to leave a small piece of clothing with her odor next to her baby.
   b. Babies will experience their parent's odor through the regular skin to skin contact.
   c. Educate staff and parents about the need to avoid introducing noxious smell when handling infants and allow alcohol hand gel to dry before handling babies.

4. Postural support/positioning: Infants should be supported in comfortable positions which help to protect their postural and movement development, behavioral organization, and stability. Their needs will change depending on their gestational age, movement maturity, and clinical condition. Positioning should not compromise an infant's

medical care or stability. Infants less than 34 weeks should be nested, aiming to provide containment and a supportive boundary. Older infants who are unable to maintain or change their head position, due to tone or instability will benefit from appropriate sized gel pillow and boundaries. Promotion of flexed symmetrical postures helps the infant conserve body temperature and energy, promoting growth and weight.

5. Cue-based cares and handling: Cares, handling, and interventions should be adapted and delivered following observation of an infant's behavioral cues and physiological responses.
   a. Prior to any intervention, consider and prepare environmental needs (lighting/noise, etc.).
   b. Parent participation: Encourage and involve parents from early on to recognize their baby's behavioral patterns.
   c. Positive touch: Let the infant know before an intervention is about to happen and after it is completed.
   d. Move and turn infants slowly, keeping part of their trunk in contact with the mattress or base of support. Sudden turning will stimulate a startle reflex and extensor postures.
   e. Pace caregiving according to an infant's cues and pause when they show signs of stress/avoidance.

6. Kangaroo mother care/skin-to-skin contact: Kangaroo care (KC) is a care intervention where an infant is held in "skin-to-skin" contact in an upright prone position on a parent's chest. The infant is covered in a blanket or enclosed within the parents clothing or KC wrap to maintain temperature stability. KC should be considered for all medically stable infants, including those receiving respiratory support.

7. Developmentally supportive measures to minimize pain/stress: Use the following measures to help minimize pain and stress responses prior to, during, and once procedures are completed with the infant:
   a. Timing: Consider medical need but try to fit in with infant's sleep pattern.
   b. Environmental: Minimize infant's exposure to bright light and reduce noise levels.
   c. Comfort: Provide nesting and support in flexed posture.

d. Offer and facilitate NNS: prior to, during, and following an intervention.
e. Facilitate baby to self-comfort: hands to face/grasping/able to brace feet.
f. Assess infant's behavior/stability/posture prior and on completion of procedure or care.
g. Pace intervention in response to infant's responses and stability.

Documentation

Nursing documentation helps in good clinical communication and provides a higher quality of care based on the effect of audited interventions. It should have a structured and standardized approach and may be in a format which is written, electronic, or a combination of both. It must include patient assessment, plan of care, and real-time progress notes. The structure of each progress note entry should follow the Identification, Situation, Background, Assessment, and Recommendation (ISBAR) format. All entries should be accurate and relevant to the patient and only standard abbreviations should be used. Medicolegally if any given nursing care was not documented, it was not done and can be subject to litigation.

Summary

The need for respiratory support is one of the major reasons for admission of neonates to the NICU. Neonatal care is unique, sensitive, complex, and shared and is best provided in the least invasive and disruptive way. Infants who require respiratory support require meticulous medical and nursing care, as well as close monitoring of patient and equipment to detect early deterioration or improvement. Nurses who provide ventilator support for infants must know how the equipment works and must be able to set it up properly and troubleshoot problems. The neonatal nurse must be familiar with all aspects of airway management and possess the skills to assist with intubation. The nursing care provided within the medical framework must also meet the developmental needs of each individual infant and their family.

References

[1] Edwards MO, Kotecha SJ, Kotecha S. Respiratory distress of the term newborn infant. Paediatr Respir Rev 2013;14(1):29–36.

[2] Hamilton KESC, Redshaw ME, Tarnow-Mordi W. Nurse staffing in relation to risk-adjusted mortality in neonatal care. Arch Dis Child Fetal Neonatal Ed 2007;92:F99–F103.

[3] Watson SI, Arulampalam W, Petrou S, et al. The effects of a one-to-one nurse-to-patient ratio on the mortality rate in neonatal intensive care: a retrospective, longitudinal, population-based study. Arch Dis Child Fetal Neonatal Ed 2016;101:F195–F200.

[4] British Association of Perinatal Medicine (BAPM). Categories of care 2011, https://www.bapm.org/resources/categories-care-2011.

[5] British Association of Perinatal Medicine (BAPM). Service standards for hospitals providing neonatal care. 3rd ed. London: BAPM; 2010. https://www.bapm.org/resources/service-standards-hospitals-providing-neonatal-care-3rd-edition-2010.

[6] American Academy of Pediatrics Committee on Fetus and Newborn, American College of Obstetricians and Gynecologists Committee on Obstetric Practice. Guidelines for Perinatal Care. 7th ed. Elk Grove Village, IL: AAP; 2012.

[7] Hummel P, Puchalski M, Creech SD, et al. Clinical reliability and validity of the N-PASS: neonatal pain, agitation and sedation scale with prolonged pain. J Perinatol 2008;28:55–60.

[8] Gibbins BJ, Stevens J, Yamada, et al. Validation of the premature infant pain profile–revised (PIPP–R). Early Hum Dev 2014;90(4):189–193.

[9] Downes JJ, Vidyasagar D, et al. Respiratory distress syndrome of newborn infants. Clin Pediatr 1970;9:325–331.

[10] Perretta Julianne S. Neonatal and pediatric respiratory care: a patient case method. F. A. Davis Company; 2014.

[11] Available from: http://www.nicutools.org/default.html?./MediCalcs/ActualO2.php3

[12] Jackson JK, Ford SP, Meinert KA, et al. Standardizing nasal cannula oxygen administration in the neonatal intensive care unit. Pediatrics 2006;118(S2):S187–S196.

[13] Benaron DA, Benitz WE. Maximizing the stability of oxygen delivered via nasal cannula. Arch Pediatr Adolesc Med 1994;148:294–300.

[14] Vain NE, Prudent LM, Stevens DP, et al. Regulation of oxygen concentrations delivered to infants by nasal cannulas. Am J Dis Child 1989;143(12):1458–1460.

[15] Chow L, Wright KW, Sola A. the CSMC Oxygen Administration Study Group. Can changes in clinical practice decrease the incidence of severe retinopathy of prematurity in very low birth weight infants? Pediatrics 2003;111:339–345.

[16] Claure N, Bancalari E. Automated closed loop control of inspired oxygen concentration. Respir Care 2013;58(1):151–161.

[17] De Paoli AG, Davis PG, Faber B, et al. Devices and pressure sources for administration of nasal continuous positive airway pressure (NCPAP) in preterm neonates. Cochrane Database Syst Rev 2008;1:CD002977.

[18] Bonner KM, Mainous RO. The nursing care of the infant receiving bubble CPAP therapy. Adv Neonatal Care 2008;8(2):78–95.

[19] Klingenberg C, Pettersen M, Hansen EA, et al. Patient comfort during treatment with heated humidified high flow nasal cannulae versus nasal continuous positive airway pressure: a randomised cross-over trial. Arch Dis Child Fetal Neonatal Ed 2014;99:F134–F137.

[20] Al-Alaiyan S, Dawoud M, Al-Hazzani F. Positive distending pressure produced by heated, humidified high flow nasal cannula as compared to nasal continuous positive airway pressure in premature infants. J Neonatal Perinatal Med 2014;7(2):119–124.

[21] Möller W, Celik G, Feng S, et al. Nasal high flow clears anatomical dead space in upper airway models. J Appl Physiol 2015;118:1525–1532.

[22] Wilkinson D, Andersen C, O'Donnell CPF, et al. High flow nasal cannula for respiratory support in preterm infants. Cochrane Database Syst Rev 2016;2:CD00645.

[23] Yoder BA, Manley B, Collins C, et al. Consensus approach to nasal high-flow therapy in neonates. J Perinatol 2017;37:1–5.

[24] Roberts CT, Dawson JA, Alquoka, et al. Are high flow nasal cannulae noisier than bubble CPAP for preterm infants? Arch Dis Child Fetal Neonatal Ed 2014;99(4):F291–F295.

[25] Lemyre B, Davis PG, de Paoli AG. Nasal intermittent positive pressure ventilation (NIPPV) versus nasal continuous positive airway pressure (NCPAP) for apnea of prematurity. Cochrane Database Syst Rev 2002;1:CD002272.

[26] Kirpalani H, Millar D, Lemyre B, et al. A trial comparing noninvasive ventilation strategies in preterm infants. N Engl J Med 2013;369:611–620.

[27] Lemyre B, Davis PG, de Paoli AG, Kirpalani H. Nasal intermittent positive pressure ventilation (NIPPV) versus nasal continuous positive airway pressure (NCPAP) for preterm neonates after extubation. Cochrane Database Syst Rev 2017;1:CD003212.

[28] Dargaville PA1, Tingay DG. Lung protective ventilation in extremely preterm infants. J Paediatr Child Health 2012;48(9):740–746.

[29] Cools F, Offringa M, Askie LM. Elective high frequency oscillatory ventilation versus conventional ventilation for acute pulmonary dysfunction in preterm infants. Cochrane Database Syst Rev 2015;3:CD000104.

[30] Spence K, Barr P. Nasal versus oral intubation for mechanical ventilation of newborn infants. Cochrane Database Syst Rev 2000;2:CD000948.

[31] Weiner GM, editor. Textbook of neonatal resuscitation. 7th ed. Elk Grove Village, IL: American Academy of Pediatrics; 2016.

[32] Donn SM, Kuhns LR. Mechanism of endotracheal tube movement with change of head position in the neonate. Pediatr Radiol 1980;9(1):37–40.

[33] Lai M, Inglis GD, Hose K, et al. Methods for securing endotracheal tubes in newborn infants. Cochrane Database Syst Rev 2014;7:CD007805.

[34] Merkel L, Beers K, Lewis MM, et al. Reducing unplanned extubations in the NICU. Pediatrics 2014;133(5):e1367–e1372.

[35] Loughead JL, Brennan RA, DeJuilio P, et al. Reducing accidental extubation in neonates. Jt Comm J Qual Patient Saf 2008;34(3):164–170.

[36] Crezeé KL, DiGeronimo RJ, Rigby MJ, et al. Reducing unplanned extubations in the NICU following implementation of a standardized approach. Respir Care 2017;62(8):1030–1035.

[37] Weber CD. Applying adult ventilator-associated pneumonia bundle evidence to the ventilated neonate. Adv Neonatal Care 2016;16(3):178–190.

[38] Saugstad OD, Aune D. Optimal oxygenation of extremely low birth weight infants: a meta-analysis and systematic review of the oxygen saturation target studies. Neonatology 2014;105(1):55–63.

[39] Brown MK, DiBlasi RM. Mechanical ventilation of the premature neonate. Respir Care 2011;56(9):1298–1313.

[40] Petty J. Understanding neonatal ventilation: strategies for decision making in the NICU. Neonatal Netw 2013;32(4):246–261.

[41] Rodríguez-Fanjul J, Balcells C, Aldecoa-Bilbao V, et al. Lung ultrasound as a predictor of mechanical ventilation in neonates older than 32 weeks. Neonatology 2016;110(3):198–203.

[42] Mammel MC, Donn SM. Real-time pulmonary graphics. Semin Fetal Neonatal Med 2015;20(3):181–191.

[43] Waisman D. Non-traumatic nasopharyngeal suction in premature newborn infants with upper airway obstruction from secretions following nasal CPAP. J Pediatr 2006;149(2):279.

[44] Taylor JE, Hawley G, Flenady V, Woodgate PG. Tracheal suctioning without disconnection in intubated ventilated neonates. Cochrane Database Syst Rev 2011;12:CD003065.

[45] Gillies D, Spence K. Deep versus shallow suction of endotracheal tubes in ventilated neonates and young infants. Cochrane Database Syst Rev 2011;7:CD003309.

[46] Kalyn A, Blatz S, Sandra F, et al. Closed suctioning of intubated neonates maintains better physiologic stability: a randomized trial. J Perinatol 2003;23(3):218–222.

[47] Gardner DL, Shirland L. Evidenced-based guideline for suctioning the intubated neonate and infant. Neonatal Netw 2009;28(5):281–302.

[48] Suctioning—pediatric/neonate patients ventilated (conventional and high frequency) via artificial airways, https://www.saskatoonhealthregion.ca/about/NursingManual/1056.pdf

[49] Hartley KA, Miller CS, Gephart SM. Facilitated tucking to reduce pain in neonates: evidence for best practice. Adv Neonatal Care 2015;15(3):201–208.

[50] Cone S, Pickler RH, Grap MJ, et al. Endotracheal suctioning in preterm infants using four-handed versus routine care. J Obstet Gynecol Neonatal Nurs 2013;42(1):92–104.

[51] American Associaton for Respiratory Care. AARC clinical practice guidelines: endotracheal suctioning of mechanically ventilated patients with artificial airways 2010. Respir Care 2010;55(6):758–764.

[52] Gonçalves RL, Tsuzuki LM, Carvalho MG. Endotracheal suctioning in intubated newborns: an integrative literature review. Rev Bras Ter Intensiva 2015;27(3):284–292.

[53] Available from: https://www.uptodate.com/home/grading-guide

[54] Hough JL, Flenady V, Johnston L, Woodgate PG. Chest physiotherapy for reducing respiratory morbidity in infants requiring ventilatory support. Cochrane Database Syst Rev 2008;3:CD006445.

[55] Flenady V, Gray PH. Chest physiotherapy for preventing morbidity in babies being extubated from mechanical ventilation. Cochrane Database of Syst Rev 2002;2:CD000283.

[56] Roqué i Figuls M, Giné-Garriga M, Granados Rugeles C, et al. Chest physiotherapy for acute bronchiolitis in paediatric patients between 0 and 24 months old. Cochrane Database Syst Rev 2016;2:CD004873.

[57] Chest Physiotherapy in NICU. BCCH child & youth health policy and procedure manual (Policy # PT.08.04); 2000.

[58] Hough J, Trojman A, Schibler A. Effect of time and body position on ventilation in premature infants. Pediatr Res 2016;80(4):499–504.

[59] Hough JL, Johnston L, Brauer S, Woodgate P, Schibler A. Effect of body position on ventilation distribution in ventilated preterm infants. Pediatr Crit Care Med 2013;14:171–177.

[60] Rivas-Fernandez M, Roqué i Figuls M, Diez-Izquierdo A, et al. Infant position in neonates receiving mechanical ventilation. Cochrane Database Syst Rev 2016;11:CD003668.

[61] Hooven TA, Polin RA. Pneumonia. Semin Fetal Neonatal Med 2017;22(4):206–213.

[62] Weber CD. Applying adult ventilator-associated pneumonia bundle evidence to the ventilated neonate. Adv Neonatal Care 2016;16(3):178e90.

[63] Pletsch D, Ulrich C, Angelini M, et al. 'Mothers' "liquid gold": a quality improvement initiative to support early colostrum delivery via oral immune therapy (OIT) to premature and critically ill newborns. Nurs Leadersh (Tor Ont) 2013;26:34–42.

[64] Kesavan K. Neurodevelopmental implications of neonatal pain and morphine exposure. Pediatr Ann 2015;44(11):e260–e264.

[65] Developmental Care Guideline. 2014. Available from: https://nornet.org.uk/professionals.

[66] American Academy of Pediatrics, Committee on Environmental Health. Noise: a hazard for the fetus and newborn. Pediatrics 1997;100(4):724–727.

Online supplementary materials

Please visit MedEnact to access the following videos:

▶ Video 33.1 **Noninvasive Nasopharyngeal Suctioning.**

▶ Video 33.2 **Closed Endotracheal Suctioning.**

▶ Video 33.3 **Open Endotracheal Suctioning.**

Chapter | **34**

Neonatal Airway Management

Vikrum A. Thimmappa, MD, Ramasubbareddy Dhanireddy, MD, RoseMary S. Stocks, MD, PharmD, Jerome W. Thompson, MD, MBA

CHAPTER CONTENTS HD

CHAPTER POINTS

- Understand normal anatomy and physiology of the neonatal airway as a basis for understanding pathologic states
- Review pathologies of the neonatal airway
- Discuss common otolaryngology airway procedures from a diagnostic and therapeutic perspective

Introduction

In order to discuss neonatal airway management, it is important to have a strong anatomic foundation in understanding the form of the airway and its relation to overall physiologic function. It has oft been noted that children and particularly neonates cannot be viewed as small adults [1]. There are variations in their mechanics that end up changing over time with growth and development.

Some of the difference relates to relative size of structures. Taking a global view, the head is larger with a more prominent occiput tending toward a baseline flexion of the neck in neutral positioning [2], leading to more difficult airway accessibility. The tongue is relatively larger in the mouth [2] and can more easily tend toward obstruction falling into the back of the oropharynx. However, there is also a role played by increased amounts of connective tissue and weaker rigid

structural support [2,3]. Per Bluestone, the trachea of the newborn collapses with compliance 3 times that of a 1-year old and 6 times that of adult cartilage [1]. The cartilage of the larynx and trachea do not begin to ossify until later in life and the initial flexibility of the structures can lead to collapse, particularly in dynamic settings [3].

In terms of airway variations, starting cranially and working caudally, the discussion begins with the nasal cavity and nasopharynx. Infants are known to be preferential nasal breathers, under normal conditions using the nasal passage for primary airflow [2]. Conditions that interfere with this breathing pattern, ranging from intranasal inflammation to a more severe choanal atresia, can put neonates into a clinical picture of respiratory distress, which would not be an expected adult physiological response to nasal obstruction.

The vertical height of the pharynx is much shorter in newborns leading to a relatively smaller oropharynx and a tongue, which takes up more space. There are also frequently seen prominent tonsillar and adenoidal tissues that are space consuming [3]. Also seen is the abutment of the epiglottis to the soft palate with a significant elevation of associated structures high in the neck. This is thought to contribute to the ability of the neonate to simultaneously swallow and breath, a characteristic lacked by their adult counterparts [1]. Vertical growth occurs in the infant face extending the length of the pharynx and separating the distance between the epiglottis and soft palate, occurring during the first 6 months and then in spurts throughout childhood [4]. Compounding this increase in oropharyngeal space is the descent of the pediatric larynx with age, as the infant organ is very compact. The thyroid cartilage, which can initially be found within the hyoid arch, descends to create a separation between the two and a more prominent thyrohyoid membrane. During the first 3 years, the growth of the cartilage is most rapid and equivalent between genders. In the neonatal period, the inferior

747

margin of the cricoid is at the vertebral level of C3–C4; at age 5, approximately C5; and by age 15 at C6–C7 [1]. (Fig. 34.1) The initial elevation of the larynx also makes it more difficult to directly visualize the airway during direct laryngoscopy as the angle to visualize the vocal cords over the plane of the tongue becomes more acute [5].

There is also a change in the internal structure and particularly the view of the neonatal airway during laryngoscopy. The airway has a curved epiglottis with anterior displacement, more prominent aryepiglottic folds, coupled with bulkier arytenoids, and a comparatively shorter membranous portion of vocal cords (Fig. 34.2) [1]. As the infant

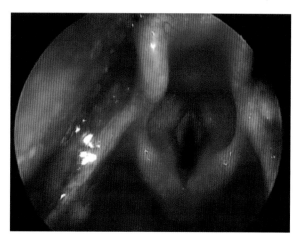

Fig. 34.2 Neonatal Larynx With Bulky Arytenoids, Curved Epiglottis, and Relatively Shorter Membranous Vocal Folds as Compared to an Adult Larynx .

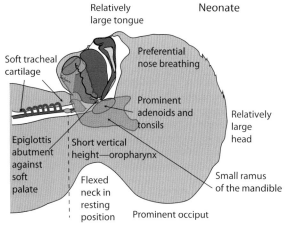

Inferior margin of the cricoid at C3–4

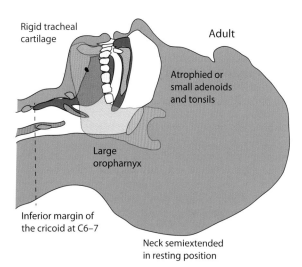

Fig. 34.1 Comparison Between Neonatal Airway and Adult Airway (see text for details). Copyright: Satyan Lakshminrusimha.

ages, the epiglottis flattens out and the vocal cords lengthen [1]. The arytenoids become less prominent and the trilaminar structure of the human vocal cord begins to develop that increases capabilities of phonation [1].

The pediatric larynx is often described as having the narrowest part of the airway at the cricoid ring in contrast to the adult where it is located at the glottis [1,2]. This makes it a more frequent site of injury and can lead to difficulty in passing an endotracheal tube further into the airway despite being past the vocal cords. There is, however, data in the anesthesiology literature [6,7] of direct and radiologic studies of airway dimensions in a sedated pediatric population being more consistent with the narrowest portion of the childhood airway being located at the glottis, like in adults. Although, the functionally narrowest portion is likely still at the level of the cricoid secondary to it being a complete ring and its associated lack of distensibility as compared to glottic tissue [3]. The neonatal trachea and lower airways are known to be more collapsible as well as shorter and more compact than their adult counterparts.

Additionally, due to the significantly smaller caliber of the pediatric airway, it is useful to understand the mathematical relationship of airflow to diameter of the airway. This is seen by Poiseuille's law, which is described as

$$Q \propto \frac{\Delta P r^4}{\mu L}$$

where Q is flow rate of air, P is change in pressure, r is radius of the airway, μ is viscosity of air, and L is length of the airway. In the setting of laminar flow, even a small decrease in the radius of the of the airway leads to a proportional drop in the flow rate to the fourth power, which in turbulent flow is to the fifth power [2,8]. As even small anatomic changes can have a relatively drastic effect on airway caliber in a smaller airway, the physiologic impact is vital for appropriate clinical management.

While there are structural and physiologic changes that occur with growth and development, there are also abnormalities of the neonatal airway. Those pathologies and their resultant management are the further focus of this chapter. It is also important to realize that airway abnormalities are not always isolated and patients present with synchronous lesions. The overall discussion will follow an anatomic pathway starting with the airway proximally and traveling distally.

Airway pathology

Nose

Regarding nasal airway obstruction in the neonatal period, the initial dichotomy that develops is one of an anatomic abnormality versus physiologic. A complete history and physical exam are integral in determining root cause of the obstruction.

Signs and symptoms described by family members of nasal obstruction, but also particularly, the timing and onset of the obstruction in relation to patient's birth are important factors to consider as a complete obstruction is going to be more temporally associated with birth as is any birth trauma. A description of the sounds associated with breathing pattern, namely the difference between stridor and stertor needs to be identified. Stertor is a partial obstruction of the airway above the larynx and sounds more akin to snoring and is lower pitched [1]. Often accompanying respiratory complaints are swallowing issues, particularly in the neonate, manifested with dysphagia and failure to thrive [2]. Medication history of the neonate as well as of the mother can also play a role in the development of obstruction of the nasal airway as it can affect physiologic responses and characteristics [9].

As previously discussed, in the neonatal period the child is a preferential nasal breather, and nasal obstruction, particularly if complete, can put them into a clinical picture of cyclic respiratory distress punctuated by crying which allows for oropharyngeal airflow [2]. Thus, upon initial observation, the neonatal respiratory status needs to be evaluated, and if is one of concern with associated tachypnea, retractions, altered mental status, or cyanosis the possibility for immediate airway intervention arises.

If the patient's clinical status allows time for complete assessment, the external nose should first be visualized to see if there are any visible deformities present that would prevent appropriate nasal airflow, followed by evaluation of airway patency. This can be done by a number of methods.

A strip of paper or gauze can be placed below each nostril, with movement indicating airflow. Fogging of a mirror placed sequentially below each naris can also identify the sidedness of airflow presence [9]. A more invasive, yet vital, evaluation involves passage of an 8 Fr catheter, 2.5 mm endotracheal tube, or pediatric flexible laryngoscope to assess if there is structural patency. On examination of the nasal cavity, if there is bony obstruction anteriorly, consider congenital pyriform aperture stenosis. However, if the obstruction is posteriorly, this opens up the possibility of choanal stenosis/atresia [2,9,10]. Flexible laryngoscopy is a commonly done procedure at bedside without sedation or NPO requirements. If unable to obtain an adequate exam, there is a role for nasal endoscopy in the operating room. Use of a topical nasal decongestant can help identify whether obstruction exists due to a structural abnormality or mucosal edema. The adequate intranasal exam also allows for evaluation of presence of a nasal mass or septal deviation from birth trauma that may cause obstruction [2]. Important to note, there must be cognizance that an intranasal mass may originate intracranially and would call for imaging studies prior biopsy or significant manipulation.

Imaging studies to identify nasal cavity abnormalities can be undertaken and are more frequently CT and MRI scans due to easy availability and generally poorer resolution of plain films [9]. CT scans have the best bony definition and are going to provide the best evidence for congenital nasal pyriform aperture stenosis (CNPAS) or bony choanal atresia. MRI will be more useful for the evaluation of intranasal masses and defining the presence of intracranial extension.

Congenital nasal pyriform aperture stenosis (CNPAS)

Pyriform aperture stenosis causes nasal obstruction due to bony overgrowth of the medial nasal process of the maxilla, narrowing the anterior entrance of the nasal cavity. This can occur in isolated cases or in conjunction with other craniofacial abnormalities such as holoprosencephaly, or presence of solitary central incisor (Fig. 34.3) [10]. Clinically, CNPAS will present similarly to choanal atresia as there is nasal obstruction, just at a more proximal point in the airway. The history and physical exam, particularly inability to pass catheter or scope through the anterior nasal cavity will direct the provider toward this diagnosis. The pyriform aperture will measure less than 11 mm in width on confirmatory imaging study, which is ideally a noncontrast, fine-cut CT with the axial plane parallel to the hard palate (Fig. 34.4) [1,11].

The degree of nasal obstruction will determine the treatment that is required. If in respiratory distress, oral intubation is necessary. If the patient has a stable airway and is not encountering feeding difficulties they can often be managed

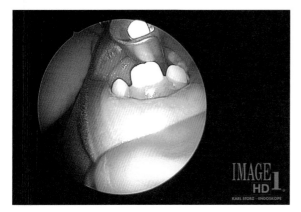

Fig. 34.3 Solitary Central Incisor Associated With CNPAS.
CNPAS, Congenital nasal pyriform aperture stenosis.

conservatively with nasal decongestant and humidification coupled with close observation [1]. Symptoms will improve as the neonate ages due to enlargement of the nasal cavity with craniofacial growth [10,12]. Surgery is indicated in cases of failure of medical therapy or a clinical picture consistent cyclic cyanosis, obstructive apneas, supplemental oxygen requirements, or failure to thrive [10,12,13]. For surgical management, a sublabial approach to the pyriform aperture with use of a diamond burr to widen the nasal inlet is the most frequently used technique [10,13,14]. Postoperative stenting is often used to prevent restenosis and this can be done with 3.5 mm endotracheal tube, silastic stents [10], or even steroid eluting stent [13]. Surgical risks include damage to tooth buds, nasolacrimal duct injury, and midface hypoplasia [10]. Overall prognosis is very good

with both medical and surgical management and decision-making is dependent on overall clinical presentation.

Choanal atresia

The choana, the region that separates nasal cavity from nasopharynx, can be stenosed or atretic in either a unilateral or bilateral manner with a soft tissue membrane and/or bone. It is always clinically significant in the neonate if bilateral but has been identified in older children if solely unilateral, as they are able to maintain an airflow pathway [2,9,14]. Choanal atresia is more frequently found in females and is more often unilateral in nature. In bilateral cases, 50% are displays of a clinical syndrome, most frequently CHARGE syndrome (~30%) and genetic evaluation, as well as further workup for other manifestations should be considered [9,15]. Like CNPAS, presentation is often with respiratory distress and cyclical cyanosis that improves with crying. On exam, once again there will be inability to pass 8 Fr catheter, but this time through the distal portion of the nasal cavity. On visualization with a flexible laryngoscope, a blind sac will be encountered. A CT scan is integral for confirmation and can help identify if the atretic segment is membranous or bony in nature and whether there is also concomitant medialization of the medial pterygoids or a thickened vomer (Fig. 34.5). In terms of management, intubation may be required depending on clinical status but there may also be an initial role for an oral airway that separates the apposition of the neonatal tongue to the soft palate allowing for airflow [1]. Repair is surgical in nature and can take multiple approaches, transnasal, transpalatal, or endo-

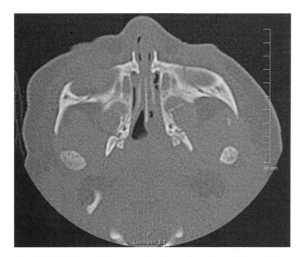

Fig. 34.4 CT Scan Showing Pyriform Aperture Stenosis in CNPAS. *CNPAS, Congenital nasal pyriform aperture stenosis.*

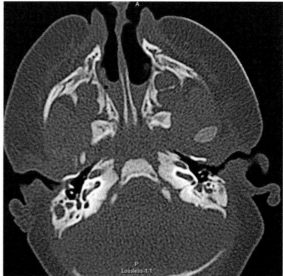

Fig. 34.5 Bilateral Membranous Choanal Atresia.

scopic transnasal. It is usually completed within a couple weeks of birth [2,14]. In the current surgical clime, with the advent of easily accessible high-resolution camera equipment, the endoscopic method is the most favored. There is controversy again on the need for postoperative stenting, with some advocating endotracheal tubes and others using steroid-eluting stents [15–17]. In any scenario, there is significant rate of restenosis after surgery with recent literature indicating approximately 65%–85% primary success rate with choanal atresia repair [18,19].

Nasal masses

Congenital nasal masses are a rare cause of neonatal nasal airway obstruction. There are a variety of etiologies but presentations are often similar. Often described are encephaloceles, gliomas, and nasal dermoids, which are the most common of this uncommon family, while vascular lesions and other benign and malignant masses do occur but are much less encountered [20]. Due to the reliance of the neonates on the nasal air passageway until 3–6 months of age, any of these masses, if large enough, can result in respiratory distress and require intubation to protect the airway. If diagnosed in utero, it may require the neonate to be delivered through an ex utero intrapartum treatment (EXIT) procedure [1,2], which will be discussed further, later in the chapter.

Encephaloceles are neural tube malformations where cranial contents have herniated through a midline congenital skull defect. The description can be changed depending on the contents within the herniated sac, and can include meninges, neural tissue, or even a portion of the ventricular system [1,20]. They can be found intra- and/or extranasally depending on path of growth. If externally located, it is much easier to identify than a lesion that is contained in the nasal cavity that would need to be identified by a nasopharyngoscopy, where a compressible, bluish lesion with possible pulsation and enlargement with venous compression could be seen [20]. Imaging is always required with nasal masses prior to biopsy or manipulation as these can have communication intracranially, as is the case with the CSF continuity associated with encephaloceles. CT and MRI are indicated, as it is necessary to evaluate the bone of the anterior skull base for dehiscence as well as the soft tissue continuity of intracranial contents [1,9].

Gliomas can be considered in the same spectrum of disease as encephaloceles, but without the intracranial continuity. It is formed of tissue of neural origin and 10%–15% of cases have a noncommunicating fibrous "stalk" connection to the subarachnoid space [1]. On exam they are firm, reddish, and noncompressible.

Nasal dermoids are the most common congenital nasal midline mass. It contains mesodermal and ectodermal components and can present as a pit, sinus tract, or cyst extending to the glabellar region or further inferior on the dorsum of the nose [9]. There is also a high rate of associated congenital anomalies [1]. Complete removal is vital to prevent recurrence and fistulization [1]. It can again, depending on size, compromise the nasal airway of the neonate. The time frame for surgery is dependent on the overall clinical context of the patient including airway stability, size of mass, and distortion of nasal framework, extent, and rate of growth.

These nasal masses are being discussed in the context of the neonatal airway and their surgical management is out of the scope of this chapter but frequently involves a multidisciplinary approach with neurosurgical and plastic surgery support for definitive treatment.

Oral cavity/oropharynx

Oropharyngeal causes of neonatal airway obstruction most often lie with tongue-based obstruction of the oropharynx. This can take a couple forms, often micrognathia/retrognathia or oropharyngeal mass, which will be the discussion of this segment. An oropharyngeal mass can cause airway obstruction in the neonate and similar to the enlarged nasal mass, and may be an indication to consider an EXIT procedure.

Micrognathia

Anatomically, the neonatal mandible has a much smaller ramus and is less developed as compared to an adult, leading to a smaller pharyngeal space with a tendency for the mandible to be posteriorly positioned [2]. The tongue base is attached to the mandible and in cases of micrognathia the tongue displaces into the airway causing obstruction. This constellation of symptoms is called the Pierre Robin sequence (PRS), and is described by hypoplasia of the mandible leading to glossoptosis and supraglottic airway obstruction (Fig. 34.6). These are also often associated

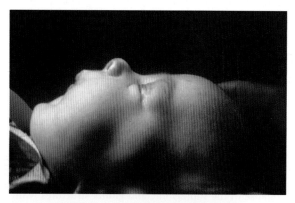

Fig. 34.6 Profile View of Patient With Pierre Robin Sequence Demonstrating Hypoplastic Mandible.

with a wide U-shaped cleft in the palate due to failure of palatal fusion secondary to obstruction by the tongue from its abnormal posterior positioning in the hypoplastic mandible [1,2]. There are multiple syndromes accompanied by solely congenital micrognathia, while PRS, with its associated airway obstruction, is seen in isolated cases as well as part of syndromes. Stickler syndrome is an autosomal dominant disorder that despite its rarity of 1 in 8000 live births, is present in 30% of patients with PRS [1,2]. Craniofacial abnormalities as a whole are abound with multiple different types of airway obstruction issues, but this is out of the scope of this chapter as each presents with its own unique challenges.

The evaluation of micrognathia is to assess the degree of obstruction that is being caused to the neonatal airway and to determine if there is need for surgical intervention. Patients can present with respiratory distress in the most severe cases that can require emergent management, but in less severe situations patients may only display increased work of breathing and obstruction, particularly with reduced tone during sleep, respiratory improvement with prone positioning, significant gastroesophageal reflux (GERD), or even failure to thrive secondary to abnormalities with oxygenation and ventilation [2].

Along with a full history and physical exam, special attention should be paid to appropriate weight gain, feeding ability, oxygen requirements, polysomnogram, presence of syndromic features, and having a thorough airway evaluation with a direct laryngoscopy [2]. Management options include conservative measures such as positioning, and nasopharyngeal airway, to surgical methods such as a tongue–lip adhesion, mandibular distraction, or tracheostomy [2,21,22]. A tool to evaluate if a neonate is likely to require further surgical intervention after a tongue–lip adhesion is the GILLS criteria [21]. A five-point scoring system evaluating for the presence of gastroesophageal reflux, preoperative intubation, surgical intervention after 2 weeks, low birth weight, and presence of a syndrome. A score of ≤2 was predictive of success with a tongue–lip adhesion, while those with a score of 3 or greater had a 5 times greater chance to fail the initial surgical procedure and require further intervention such as mandibular distraction or the "gold standard" tracheostomy [21,22].

Larynx

In a child presenting with elements of airway obstruction, a frequent sign is stridor, and it is vital to localize the site. Depending on the degree of obstruction and site of the lesion, the stridor has distinct characteristics [1]. Collapse of the supraglottic and glottis structures while breathing in leads to inspiratory stridor. Intrathoracic lesions can lead to expiratory stridor, while fixed lesions

in the cervical trachea and subglottis can present as biphasic stridor [1].

Laryngomalacia

The most common congenital laryngeal anomaly, laryngomalacia, is responsible for ~70% of cases of stridor in infants and neonates [23–25]. Inspiratory stridor is the hallmark finding secondary to collapse of the supraglottic airway, but also frequently seen are feeding difficulties such as coughing, aspiration, and slow intake. Often presenting within the first couple weeks, it usually worsens with agitation and feeding, and improves with prone positioning. The current leading theory as to the etiology of laryngomalacia relates to neuromuscular discoordination. There is decreased laryngeal tone thought to be related to neurosensory dysfunction of the larynx leading to the signs that are seen, namely the apneas, aspirations, and feeding difficulties [2,24]. Closely associated, is GERD, which is seen in 65%–100% of patients with laryngomalacia [2]. No causal relationship has been identified, but they are thought to be involved in a positive feedback cycle where airway obstruction creates a larger negative intrathoracic pressure, worsening GERD, and worsening GERD causes edema and inflammation of supraglottic structures with chronic acid exposure resulting in a less robust neurosensory functionality, all of which contribute to the overall worsening airway obstruction [2,24]. Diagnosis is made with a dynamic exam, awake flexible fiberoptic laryngoscopy, to determine the collapsibility of the supraglottic structures with inspiration, an omega-shaped epiglottis, shortened aryepiglottic folds, and posterior displacement of the epiglottis (Fig. 34.7). There are multiple mentions in the literature of the presence of synchronous airway lesions

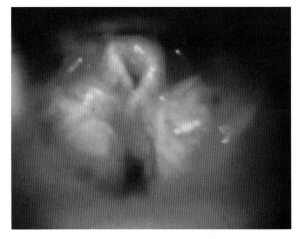

Fig. 34.7 **Severe Laryngomalacia With Tubular Epiglottis.**

in those with laryngomalacia, likely in those with more severe disease, multiple sites of obstruction, or nonresolving stridor [1,2].

As with many of the causes of airway obstruction, there is continuum related to severity and on presentation 40% are seen to have mild disease, 40% moderate, and 20% more severe [2]. Infants can progress to worsening degrees of laryngomalacia if not appropriately treated. Worse severity entails increased baseline respiratory distress, lower resting oxygen saturation, recurrent cyanosis, aspiration, and failure to thrive.

For the majority of mild and moderate laryngomalacia (~80%) cases, particularly without any feeding difficulties, conservative medical therapy is the best option. Ensuring the patient is on adequate medication for GERD, if that is a diagnosis that has been made, helps to break the positive feedback cycle with the redundant mucosa of the supraglottis [2,24]. Laryngomalacia is typically self-limited, and resolves by ~1 year of age. Those with severe or worsening disease trend toward needing surgical intervention [14]. Indications are severe stridor with any of the following, largely indicating chronic airway obstruction.

- Failure to thrive
- Obstructive apnea
- Hypoxia
- Pectus excavatum
- Pulmonary hypertension
- Cor pulmonale

An endoscopic supraglottoplasty is the current primary surgical treatment with incision and release of the aryepiglottic fold as well as removal of supraglottic prolapsing tissue with cold steel or CO_2 laser [26]. Overall success in the literature is greater than 90% with significant symptom improvement [2,23]. As laryngomalacia is exceedingly common, it is important to not become complacent with treatment and realize that timely surgical intervention is vital in patients with more severe disease.

Laryngeal cyst

Whilst relatively uncommon, another neonatal cause of stridor is the laryngeal cyst. These come in two forms, ductal and saccular cysts based on the work of DeSanto in the 1970s [27]. Ductal cysts are relatively more common, frequently found in the vallecula, and thought to be related to blockage of submucosal glands (Fig. 34.8). The saccule is the region that communicates anteriorly with the laryngeal ventricle and has many mucous glands that assist in keeping the larynx lubricated. If there is outflow obstruction of the saccular opening into the ventricle, either from lack of congenital patency or other causes such as infection or trauma, there can be submucosal fluid accumulations, which are termed saccular cysts [1,14,26]. Saccular cysts come in two types, lateral and anterior, depending on

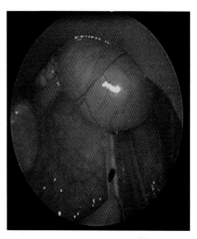

Fig. 34.8 Fluid-Filled Vallecular Cyst.

their anatomic locations. The lateral can be seen protruding superiorly into the false cords and aryepiglottic folds, while the anterior saccular cyst will emerge from between the true and false vocal cords [1].

Often clinically difficult to distinguish, but important to mention, is the laryngocele. It is described as dilation and/or herniation of the saccule, usually filled with air. It is pathologically different than a saccular cyst as it is in communication with the laryngeal lumen and not submucosal. Depending on the pathway of herniation, it can be internal, into the laryngeal lumen; external, into the neck via the thyrohyoid membrane; or a combined entity [1,14].

It can be noted that the exact prevalence of any of these entities may be underestimated as they can be present but not clinically relevant as there are studies showing their presence during autopsies or radiographically in otherwise asymptomatic patients [1]. Symptoms depend on location and most frequently, proximity to the glottic opening, and often present earlier if a saccular cyst [27]. With increased obstruction of the laryngeal lumen, worsening inspiratory stridor, a muffled cry and respiratory distress are more likely. Less severe symptoms, again depending on location, would be the more insidious dysphagia and failure to thrive. Diagnosis is made with laryngoscopy, either flexible or rigid, and can be confirmed radiographically to reveal extent of the lesion. Laryngoceles can be made more prominent with a Valsalva maneuver. Treatment is frequently endoscopic in nature with marsupialization, particularly if only endolaryngeal. It is important to monitor for recurrence and in those cases or cases of extralaryngeal extension, an external neck approach may be warranted [1,14,27]. Tracheostomy is usually not warranted; however, patients may require short-term intubation postoperatively until edema resolves.

Laryngeal cleft

During development, initially the lung buds and foregut are in direct communication, but tracheoesophageal ridges develop and fuse to form the septum [28]. Congenital clefting of the larynx is a rare condition with a midline defect in the posterior larynx that can stretch from the hypopharynx through the intrathoracic trachea. These defects may be isolated or associated with other anomalies, such as tracheoesophageal fistulas (TEFs), or other syndromes, like Pallister–Hall or Opitz–Frias [1,26,29]. The Benjamin–Inglis classification of the laryngeal cleft is dependent on the length. Type I is supraglottic with an interarytenoid defect, type II presents with a partial cricoid defect, type III with complete posterior cricoid defect into cervical trachea, and type IV with cleft extending into thoracic trachea (Fig. 34.9) [30]. Minor cases where there is only an interarytenoid defect may be minimally symptomatic and present much later than more extensive clefting. The presenting symptoms can be respiratory in nature, but are frequently closely related to feeding. Patients can have cyanotic episodes with feeding, aspiration, and chronic pulmonary infections [1,29]. These can be subtle in type I and type II, but can be marked respiratory distress with a more severe lesion. For diagnostic purposes, it is difficult to evaluate the presence of a laryngeal cleft with flexible laryngoscopy as there is much redundant mucosal tissue that will obscure visualization. Rigid laryngoscopy and bronchoscopy is vital to accurate diagnosis, as an instrument is needed to separate the interarytenoid mucosa to palpate the cricoid cartilage and feel if a defect extends below level of the true vocal cords [1]. Additionally, it is important to also evaluate for a TEF, as they may be cosynchronous lesions. A modified barium swallow study is also useful to determine if there is aspiration; however, it is not specific for laryngeal cleft and there may be other underlying neurologic abnormalities [2].

Treatment is dependent on the extent of the cleft. Type I and some type II clefts can be managed with upright positioning, thickened food, and reflux medication to reduce inflammatory changes to cleft site. However, there is also evidence to support an endoscopic injection laryngoplasty with resorbable gel or calcium hydroxylapatite at the site of the cleft to bulk up the region and prevent aspiration, particularly in the cases of minor laryngeal clefts [31]. For more extensive clefts, an endoscopic multilayer repair is indicated, but in some situations, particularly with larger type III and type IV clefts, as well as some revision cases, an open approach is recommended, again with the principle of a multilayer closure [2].

Prognosis with type I and type II laryngeal clefts is good with ability to manage aspiration and feeding problems; however, as clefting is more extensive, there is a much higher morbidity and mortality associated because there are frequently other associated anomalies as well. In the situation of requiring intubation and an urgent airway for these patients, the endotracheal tube can easily pass into the esophagus distal to the vocal cords as would be expected from an anatomical cleft. Thus, it is particularly vital to ensure proper positioning and appropriate end-tidal CO_2.

Laryngeal web

During the formation of the laryngeal cartilage there is also propagation of internal laryngeal epithelium during the 10th week of embryogenesis. During this process, there is a time point in which the laryngeal lumen is fully occluded by soft tissue, which then undergoes recanalization [28]. If only partially recanalized, the patient is left with an obstruction of an anterior glottic web versus no recanalization and the presence of laryngeal atresia [26]. Laryngeal atresia is very rare (Fig. 34.10), and it is imperative it is identified prenatally by ultrasonography, as after birth, it is

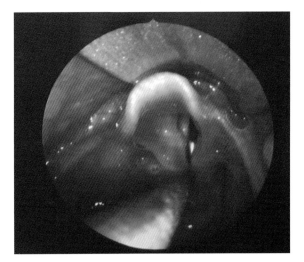

Fig. 34.9 Direct Laryngoscopy Demonstrating Extension of Laryngeal Cleft Below True Vocal Cords.

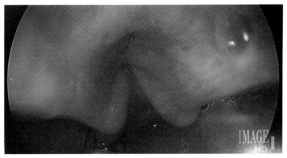

Fig. 34.10 Laryngeal Agenesis.

incompatible with life without an emergent tracheostomy, ideally carried out via an EXIT procedure. Ultrasound signs of CHAOS (congenital high airway obstruction syndrome) include hyperechogenic lungs due to inability of formed fluid to exit the obstructed airway, flattened diaphragm, polyhydramnios, and fetal hydrops [1,2].

Alternatively, a glottic web is usually not identified prenatally, and can have tissue across the anterior third of the vocal cords with extent into the subglottis. 65% of patients with a glottic web have evidence of velocardiofacial syndrome or a 22q11 microdeletion by genetic testing, but otherwise may have very minor other manifestations [2,26]. Symptoms depend on severity of the obstruction. There may be respiratory distress, associated with aphonia, requiring urgent intervention, or be as mild as a slight hoarseness depending on the thickness and extent of the web [1,26].

Diagnostically, flexible laryngoscopy should be able to identify glottic webs, but the gold standard of visualization is rigid laryngoscopy in the operating room. Additional physical signs to evaluate for in these patients include palatal abnormalities, medialized carotids, and in an overall exam, cardiac defects, as well as pharyngeal arch abnormalities that all point toward velocardiofacial syndrome [2]. Treatment is based on separating the glottic web, largely done endoscopically, especially with thinner webs. However, if there is extension into the subglottis, this may require much more extensive surgery, such as an external approach with placement of a laryngeal keel and concomitant tracheostomy [1,2,26]. Timing of surgery is again dependent on severity and degree of associated respiratory dysfunction. Treatment failures may occur with anterior scar band reformation and cause long-term functional voice deficits.

Vocal cord paralysis

Another glottic airway obstruction cause is vocal fold immobility. It is second only to laryngomalacia in terms of prevalence in congenital laryngeal anomalies, coming in at 15%–20%. Of those, 48% are unilateral and 52% are bilateral [32]. Causes are either neurologic or mechanical in nature. Neurologic causes can occur anywhere from the central nervous system to the level of the laryngeal musculature. These include such congenital situations, such as Arnold–Chiari malformations, hydrocephalus, or their associated neurosurgical treatments [1]. In unilateral cases, etiologies are more frequently peripheral with birth trauma or iatrogenic origins. It is frequently associated with cardiovascular or mediastinal surgery, particularly in relation to the aortic arch, putting the left recurrent laryngeal nerve and left true vocal cord more frequently at risk [2,32].

Symptoms associated with vocal fold immobility are once again, on a spectrum. It depends on the degree of airway obstruction and for those with a unilaterally malfunc-

tioning vocal cord, symptoms are much less prominent. In unilateral immobility, a mild stridor or weak cry can be seen, hoarseness, and signs of aspiration such as chronic cough or recurrent pneumonia may also be present. If time has passed and the child has compensated for the lack of movement in one cord with past midline excursion in the other cord, there may be minimal persistent symptoms [2,26]. Symptoms of bilateral vocal cord paralysis can be much more emergent and frequently present with respiratory distress, high pitched stridor, apneic spells, cyanosis and aspiration concerns, and an approximately 50% of patients requiring tracheostomy [2].

In order to appropriately identify the immobility of the vocal cord, either unilateral or bilateral, awake flexible laryngoscopy is the ideal study. It is important to note that bilateral vocal-fold immobility can be difficult to identify due to minor passive motion that is seen adducting the cords with inspiration. This is paradoxical motion and not indicative of vocal cords working appropriately [1]. General anesthesia and direct laryngoscopy and bronchoscopy are important to identify if there is any mechanical obstruction such as posterior glottic scarring (Fig. 34.11), which can occur with a prolonged intubation, or cricoarytenoid dislocation both of which, among others need to be differentiated from neurologic causes of paralysis [32]. There are also studies that advocate ultrasound as a useful tool to evaluate vocal cord immobility, but flexible laryngoscopy remains the gold standard [33]. However, once the diagnosis is made, it is important to find the root cause, which involves imaging from the head through the chest following the vagus nerve through recurrent laryngeal to assess neurologic or cardiovascular pathologies [1].

For cases of unilateral paralysis, most do not require surgical intervention and improve given time and development, particularly with only mild to moderate respiratory distress. The most frequent complaint of feeding issues and aspiration need to be observed and alleviated with thickener as able. In those instances when that does not work,

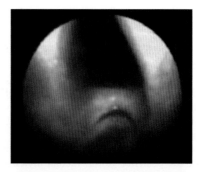

Fig. 34.11 Posterior Glottic Scarring, Which can Cause Bilateral Vocal-Fold Immobility Secondary to Mechanical Obstruction.

there are medialization procedures of the errant vocal cord. In 8% of the population, a tracheostomy is required if feeding issues are intractable [26,32]. Bilateral cord dysfunction on the other hand, with a much more significant likelihood of respiratory distress, most importantly requires the airway to be secured, either with temporary endotracheal tube or tracheostomy, if needed. It is known that there is high rate of spontaneous resolution of bilateral cord paralysis in the neonate population, particularly if of idiopathic origin or with management of the primary insult if known, which is why more extensive surgery is not undertaken until a 2-year period of watchful waiting has occurred [1,2,14,26]. There are other surgical procedures that can be undertaken to widen the glottic aperture and to reinnervate vocal cords, which will be discussed later. The best time for surgical intervention is patient specific and contingent upon patient and family goals, as waiting longer for definitive surgery may prolong tracheostomy dependence, but allows more time for spontaneous recovery. Additionally, most surgery that can be completed will sacrifice voice for improvement to the airway, which is an outcome that families should expect [32].

Subglottic stenosis

Subglottic stenosis (SGS) is narrowing of the airway below the vocal cords to less than 4.0 mm in the full-term neonate and less than 3.0 mm in a premature infant [2,32]. In 5% of cases, the etiology is congenital and akin to the formation of laryngeal atresia, a lack of recanalization of the airway during development. This is usually cartilaginous in nature [32]. In 95% of cases, the cause is acquired and while in the past this was rare, after the 1960s, with more frequent episodes of endotracheal intubation, this became the leading etiology [34]. In acquired cases, it is theorized that risk factors are length of intubation, size of endotracheal tube, traumatic intubation, multiple intubations, presence of GERD, systemic hypoperfusion, low body weight of the child, and concurrent infection with intubation; however, there has not necessarily been definitive support in the literature [2]. It is important to note that clinical guidelines, particularly in the neonate, that may be intubated for longer periods of time, are to use the smallest endotracheal tube that allows adequate ventilation and to keep balloon pressures less than 20–25 cm of H_2O to limit trauma to the overlying mucosa and reduce remodeling of the underlying cartilage with associated granulation tissue [34]. At pressures exceeding this level, there is risk of overwhelming mucosal perfusion pressure and restricting local blood flow. The most frequent sites of damage are the posterior glottis, medial arytenoids, and the cricoid ring, largely due the predetermined curvature of the endotracheal tube [32]. Particularly at risk for acquired stenosis are those with any degree of congenital subglottic narrowing due to needing a smaller size endotracheal tube than would be expected [2].

A hallmark symptom of SGS is biphasic stridor, due to the fixed lesion in the airway. There may also be retractions and an associated barking cough reminiscent of croup. Depending on degree of obstruction there may be respiratory distress and need for endotracheal intubation and possible tracheostomy. In more significant cases of obstruction, exclusively of the congenital variety, this may be identified prenatally and require an EXIT procedure at birth. Patients are also identified due to having suspicious episodes of prolonged or multiply recurrent "croup," which may be a SGS that is exacerbated by viral respiratory illnesses [2]. In other neonates, SGS needs to be considered when there is a prolonged failure to wean off the ventilator, multiple failed extubations, or if there is inability to pass the appropriate size endotracheal tube during intubation despite adequate visualization [2].

The best method of evaluation is rigid laryngoscopy and bronchoscopy to directly visualize the airway and to determine the degree of narrowing as well as the exact location and length of stenosis (Fig. 34.12). A common parlance is vital for communication amongst clinicians about the severity of disease. The Cotton–Myer grading scale is one such system [1]. Grade I stenosis is less than 50%, grade II is 50%–70%, grade III is 71%–99%, and grade IV is 100% stenosis [1,2]. This is determined in the operating room by assessing the expected endotracheal tube size with the tube that is able to fit with a cuff pressure of 10–20 cmH_2O [1]. For a complete stenosis, it may be necessary to determine length with a CT scan due to the inability to assess in the operating room.

Treatment options depend on degree of stenosis, with grade I lesions rarely requiring significant intervention and often managed with observation. Surgical options are utilized after there has been a failure of medical therapy, with the goals to reduce localized inflammation, edema, and

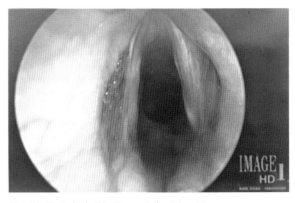

Fig. 34.12 Subglottic Stenosis by Direct Laryngoscopy.

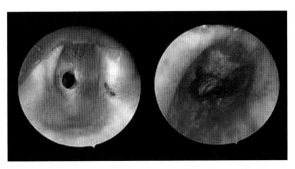

Fig. 34.13 Before and After Picture of Balloon Dilation to Address Subglottic Stenosis.

infection. To this end, corticosteroids, racemic epinephrine, proton pump inhibitors, and antibiotics are necessary as the mainstay of treatment. The intricacies of decision making in terms of the surgical management of SGS are a complicated one that is beyond the scope of this chapter. However, in general, initial procedures for grade II and some of grade III stenoses are endoscopic procedures, namely resection with cold steel and/or CO_2 Laser and balloon angioplasty (Fig. 34.13) [1,32]. Adjunct tools of injecting corticosteroids and mitomycin C can also be used to limit scarring and restenosis [14]. There is high likelihood of restenosis and multiple procedures may be required. For higher grade and more extensive stenosis, an external approach may be required. In the very small neonate and early infant an anterior cricoid split can be performed. Laryngotracheal reconstruction (LTR) via an anterior approach, to widen the subglottis, can be completed in single or double stages, with or without cartilage grafts and/or stents and this will be discussed further in the procedures section [2,14,32,34]. For timing of an LTR, allowing for the airway to mature to older than 2 years of age allows for a larger airway, better tolerance of postsurgical recovery, and larger allowance of autogenous rib cartilage graft; however, a bridging tracheostomy will be required. There has been some data that earlier procedures may be associated with improved speech and language outcomes [2]. Additionally, for high grade III and grade IV stenotic regions another option is a cricotracheal resection (CTR), which is a more extensive surgery requiring airway reanastomosis [2,32].

SGS is a complicated disease entity to address as there can be many morbidities and recurrences. It is thus vital, particularly in the critical care setting, to be cognizant about preventing acute intubation lesions that can later develop into acquired SGS. This is done through good intubation technique, choosing the smallest endotracheal tube to adequately ventilate the patient, minimizing intubation time and good communication with nursing support for atraumatic suctioning, and adequate sedation to prevent tube/patient movement. Close, multidisciplinary vigilance

is required to appropriately choose the management pathway that best maximizes outcomes and quality of life.

Trachea and bronchi

Airway compromise from a trachea and bronchus origin in neonates is a much less frequent entity than that of laryngeal origin; however, cases do arise, and the ones that do, often require significant multidisciplinary communication to appropriately manage. Pathologies can be divided into tracheal stenoses and deformation, airway obstruction without stenosis, and several externally compressive etiologies. Tracheal stenosis, tracheomalacia, TEFs, and necrotizing tracheobronchitis will be discussed in this section. Cardiovascular abnormalities will be discussed in the vascular abnormalities section, but it is known that the persistent external compression by these entities can contribute to long-term tracheobronchomalacia.

Tracheobronchomalacia

Tracheomalacia can be isolated or associated with bronchomalacia depending on the length of collapse. It is a dynamic process, similar to laryngomalacia, where there are differences in the patency of the airway depending on phase of respiratory cycle. Physiologically during inspiration, in the thoracic cavity, the negative pressure increases airway diameter during inspiration and decreases it during expiration. This pattern is reversed in the extrathoracic trachea [1]. Mild movement is the normal pattern, but with tracheomalacia, the collapsibility of the trachea and/or bronchi due to weaker structural support is much greater and can lead to respiratory symptomatology [2]. Primary tracheomalacia is seen secondary to weakened tracheal cartilage often due to developmental immaturity or those with congenital structural cartilage abnormalities and diffusely affect the trachea. Secondary tracheomalacia is an acquired weakness to the tracheal cartilage caused by degeneration of normal supportive structures and is usually localized. There are a number of causes, such as tracheostomy tubes, chronic tracheal infections, and prolonged intubations, that weaken the tracheal wall internally, but also compressive causes like vascular, skeletal, and cardiac malformations or mediastinal masses that compress externally and cause weakening of the associated segments.

Symptoms are often not specific for tracheobronchomalacia. The time frame to presentation is variable, and based on history and physical exam, a confusing picture can arise, leading to alternate, incorrect diagnoses such as asthma or suspicion of foreign body aspiration. Expiratory stridor is commonly seen in thoracic tracheal stenosis as this is the region that collapses on expiration, while there may be inspiratory stridor associated with malacia of the cervical trachea. Wheezing may also be present, but in more

757

severe situations, respiratory distress, exertional dyspnea, cyanosis, and desaturations can occur. Symptoms may be position-dependent and improved while prone. Feeding difficulties, like dysphagia, regurgitation, and cough can also occur, similar to many other airway issues and if respiratory compromise is great enough there can be secondary failure to thrive due to inability to meet metabolic demands [1,2].

Diagnosis is based on operative bronchoscopy and dynamic visualization of the tracheobronchial tree. It is necessary to have the patient spontaneously ventilating as positive pressure will obscure the collapsibility of the airway, and is one of the treatment modalities that is utilized. Compromise of the tracheal lumen more than 50% is likely to be symptomatic. Imaging is indicated for concern of external tracheal compression leading to secondary tracheomalacia. CT scan with contrast is used for compressing masses and MRI is more useful for vascular abnormalities [1].

Treatment of primary tracheomalacia largely involves temporizing airway status until the child grows and develops, as there is usually resolution by 2 years of age. In more severe cases, positive pressure ventilation with a tracheostomy may be indicated, or even a longer tracheostomy to stent opens the collapsible segment. Secondary tracheomalacia is managed by identifying and treating the underlying cause that is reducing the integrity of the tracheal wall [1,2].

Tracheoesophageal fistula

TEF can occur in conjunction with esophageal atresia (EA) and classification schemes involve five subtypes. The most common subtype is type III with a blind proximal pouch of the esophagus and a distal TEF. At the fistula site, the common wall is not adequately supportive, this can allow for posterior distension into the tracheal lumen, narrowing the airway. Additionally, the adjacent cartilaginous rings are weakened. Localized tracheomalacia is seen in 75% of this patient population, but is not always symptomatic [1,32]. Presenting symptoms are found early as the majority of cases have an element of EA. Only one subtype, type V, the "H-type," named for its TEF without EA has an esophagus in continuity and this occurs in 4% of the population. Feeding problems, chronic aspiration, and inability to pass a nasogastric tube are hallmarks, in conjunction with signs of tracheomalacia. Rigid bronchoscopy and esophagoscopy is important to identify TEF and to determine the level of the blind pouch of the atretic esophagus. Barium esophagram can also be completed to identify fistula site. Treatment is dictated by recognizing if there are synchronous anomalies of the airway that need to be addressed, as this is a not infrequent finding. Surgical repair involves reestablishing continuity of the esophagus, closing fistula with the trachea, and supporting malacic segments of the

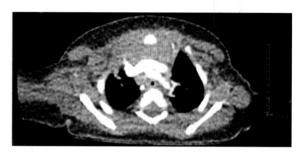

Fig. 34.14 Complete Tracheal Ring Causing Narrowed and Circular Airway by CT Scan.

airway with autologous cartilage or periosteum grafts [32]. The Spitz classification is used to assess survival rates and is influenced by low birth weight and concurrent cardiac defects. Without either of these, survival is >95%, while with both, it falls to approximately 30%–50% [1].

Tracheal stenosis

Structural tracheal stenosis or narrowing can come in a couple of forms. There can be congenital narrowing related to a cartilaginous structural abnormality with a variety of lengths, and formulations. Complete tracheal rings (Fig. 34.14), disorganized plates of cartilage, or even entire sleeves. Lack of the posterior membrane of tracheal wall leads to fixed diameters that are frequently stenotic and manifest with respiratory symptoms, particularly, if there is greater than 50% luminal narrowing. Children with these anomalies are usually identified during infancy and there are frequently other associated congenital abnormalities. It is more likely to need surgical intervention to correct the airway if identified at a younger age. Symptoms are dependent on degree of narrowing, rather than length of stenosis. Symptoms can include a biphasic stridor, cyanosis, exertional dyspnea, and manifest more profoundly during respiratory infections. Diagnosis is based on rigid bronchoscopy (Fig. 34.15); however, depending on the degree of stenosis, it may be difficult to fully evaluate the lesion. It is important to minimize instrumentation of the stenotic region as with any swelling, airway obstruction will get markedly worse. Imaging, such as a CT scan with 3D reconstruction, may be required to evaluate the length of the lesion for surgical planning, and also the presence of any cardiovascular congenital anomalies as they are present in approximately 50% of cases of complete tracheal rings [2,32].

Treatment is dependent on severity of symptoms and length of stenosis. Endoscopic treatment with balloon dilation has not been shown to be the optimal route of management. For short segments (3–4 rings), tracheal resection and primary anastomosis can be completed. However, if segments are longer, a slide tracheoplasty is the intervention of choice.

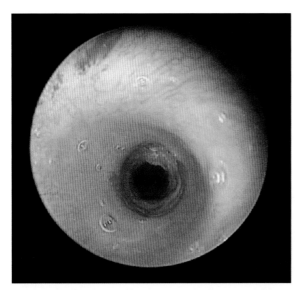

Fig. 34.15 Bronchoscopic Image of Complete Tracheal Rings.

Although it shortens the overall tracheal length, requires extensive mobilization of the tracheobronchial tree, and often requires cardiopulmonary bypass or extracorporeal membrane oxygenation (ECMO), it has become the procedure of choice for these difficult cases in enlarging airway diameter.

Necrotizing tracheobronchitis

Necrotizing tracheobronchitis is an infrequently encountered pathology but should be mentioned to be complete, particularly in the overall discussion of neonatal ventilation strategies. This is considered an iatrogenic etiology most frequently seen in intubated and ventilated premature infants. The clinical presentation is of sudden difficulty in ventilation and persistent hypercarbia in the setting of an intubated infant. This is after obstruction of the endotracheal tube as well as worsening pulmonary parenchymal disease has been ruled out [35]. While etiology of the pathology is unclear, what is clear that there is desquamation of the tracheal mucosa at a point distal to the tip of the endotracheal tube. It is not thought to be related to direct mechanical forces. A possible etiology is considered to be secondary to ischemic causes and interruption in blood flow to the mucosa and submucosa [36]. The most frequently affected region of the airway is the thoracic trachea, which also has the least robust perfusion, but more distal airways can also be affected. Often these infants also suffer concomitant hemodynamic instability and are on vasoactive medications, making them more prone to vascular insult [36].

Diagnostically, there are not always significant changes that are seen on a plain X-ray. However, there can be regions of atelectasis and irregular narrowing of the airway that can be more clearly seen in a CT, with regions of soft tissue obstruction in the tracheobronchial tree. Flexible tracheoscopy via the endotracheal tube would also be a useful method to assess obstruction status but in terms of diagnostic and therapeutic capabilities, rigid bronchoscopy would be the gold standard. Bronchoscopic findings include plugs of necrotic tissue and exfoliated tracheal mucosa as well as mucous plugs, which are removed with a combination of suction and optical forceps.

In the past, this pathology was more often diagnosed histologically on autopsy as it is acutely life threatening. However, with prompt recognition, treatment can be undertaken, which involves emergent rigid bronchoscopy to remove the obstructing debris. Another option would be the use of ECMO to provide adequate oxygenation while allowing for better endoscopic debridement of the airway and the opportunity to reduce ventilator settings [36]. If the initial insult is survived there is a risk of granulation tissue and cicatricial stenosis at these desquamated sites.

Vascular abnormalities

Vascular anomalies are generally divided into two subgroups, those of vascular tumors and that of vascular malformation. The tumor distinction is given based on hyperproliferation of cell types, while a malformation does not have excessive propagation or turnover but a developmental error leading to expanding networks of vessels. The name of the malformation is dependent on its most prominent involved vessel type. While vascular tumors or malformations are frequently cutaneous based, they do occur in the airway with hemangiomas being more common. Additionally, with size of cervicofacial lesions, there can be concern for airway compromise secondary to compression [29].

Hemangioma

Overall, hemangiomas are a benign vascular tumor and the most common tumor affecting the pediatric population, with the majority occurring in the head and neck. When there are cutaneous hemangiomas identified, the practitioner must be vigilant for associated visceral lesions such as in the subglottis, liver, or gastrointestinal tract [1]. Infantile hemangiomas of the larynx, while a rare entity, accounting for 1.5% congenital laryngeal anomalies, have a predilection for being found in the subglottis, are female predominant, 2:1, and more often encountered in premature infants than the general population [2,32]. There is an association with PHACES syndrome (posterior fossa, hemangioma, cerebrovascular aArterial anomalies, cardiovascular anomalies, eye abnormalities), where approximately 50% of these patients have airway hemangiomas

[2,26]. In the initial weeks of life, neonates are usually not symptomatic from a subglottic hemangioma, but the lesion frequently begins undergoing rapid proliferation of endothelial cells after 4–6 weeks and respiratory difficulties may develop. 80–90% of neonates will become symptomatic with this type of lesion within 6 months, and on average 3–4 months [2]. Progressive involution and resolution will begin after 1–1.5 years and often full resolution by 5–12 years of age [32].

Presentation occurs with biphasic stridor, barking cough, and worsening symptoms associated with upper respiratory infections. Identification is often difficult because presentation is frequently mistaken for laryngotracheobronchitis that is recurrent or prolonged [2,32]. The gold standard for examining the subglottis is a direct laryngoscopy and bronchoscopy in the operating room, but also useful for diagnosis is flexible laryngoscopy to ensure no other dynamic airway lesion such as vocal cord paresis exist. Particularly with larger lesions, imaging studies, such as MRI, are used to evaluate range of the lesion and to identify if there are extensions into the mediastinum. If seen on laryngoscopy, lesion is often described as a round, reddish/bluish mass, compressible, and often on the left side posterolaterally [2,32]. The mass is often not biopsied for risk of bleeding.

Management has undergone some changes over the years, but the mainstay is again dependent on the degree of respiratory dysfunction. In scenarios where there is minimal respiratory distress, watchful waiting is a valid option, as the lesion is known to resolve given enough time [2,32]. In the past, the medical management included interferon α-2a, which is no longer used. Also, more frequently used in the past were systemic steroids, which have largely been supplanted with propranolol. Propranolol (2 mg/kg/day) has shown significant success with cutaneous hemangiomas and in many places, has become first-line medical treatment for subglottic hemangiomas [37,38] However, there is still a surgical role as there is not an insignificant population that does not respond to propranolol or if they require more urgent surgical intervention based on overall airway status 5 [2,39]. Surgical options include endoscopic resection with CO_2 laser or microdebrider, adjuvant lesion injection with corticosteroids, or the more invasive methods of open excision through a laryngofissure. Tracheostomy used to be the gold standard for treatment, particularly as the disease resolves on its own given time, but it has its own comorbidities and there is a more modern arsenal of tools available for treatment.

Vascular compression

Compression of the trachea and/or esophagus externally by abnormal vascular development is termed a vascular

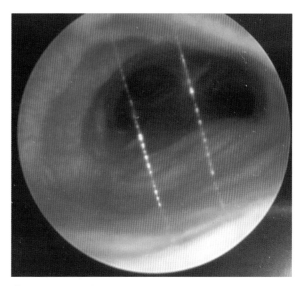

Fig. 34.16 **Vascular Compression Narrowing the Lumen of the Trachea.**

ring. These can take the form of complete or incomplete depending on degree of encirclement. Abnormalities of branchial arch vessels result in vascular anomalies such as double aortic arch, right aortic arch, Innominate artery compression, pulmonary artery sling, or aberrant subclavian vessels (Fig. 34.16). Those with more complete encirclement around trachea and esophagus, namely double aortic arch, are likely to present with symptoms earlier, within the first 3 months of life. Biphasic stridor, dysphagia, cyanosis, and wheezing are seen, secondary to compression of both trachea and esophagus. On diagnostic bronchoscopy for these lesions, a pulsatile compression is seen on the anterior wall and if there is full encirclement, on the posterior wall of the trachea as well. Imaging studies of barium esophagram to examine esophageal compression and MRI to trace vasculature to identify tracheal compression are needed to confirm diagnosis [1]. Treatment consists of alleviating the compression on the trachea by these vascular rings if patients are symptomatic. If asymptomatic a "watchful waiting" policy is valid. Surgical correction involves either division and reimplantation or suspension of the offending vessel by cardiothoracic surgery. In terms of specific entities, pulmonary artery slings are frequently associated with complete tracheal rings and may need concurrent slide tracheoplasty. Many of these vascular rings despite repair can still be symptomatic and that is due to a secondary tracheomalacia from the chronic tracheal compression. These segments may need to be bolstered with grafts or supports depending on degree of collapse or patient's symptoms.

Procedures

Diagnostic and therapeutic procedures concerning the neonatal airway are an extensive topic. As a medical pediatric provider, it may not be vital to know the procedural ins and outs of each of these interventions, as that would be the role of the surgeon. However, it is necessary to have a basis for understanding when they are indicated, types of postoperative complications, and other management pearls from a surgical viewpoint. We will discuss a selection of different case types.

Flexible fiberoptic laryngoscopy

Diagnostic flexible fiberoptic laryngoscopy is the mainstay of otolaryngology evaluation of the airway and allows for the screening of the anatomy and functionality of the nasal cavity, nasopharynx, oropharynx, and larynx. It is done in an awake population, without regard to age, is usually well tolerated, and allows the practitioner to assess the mobility of the vocal cords and patency of the upper airway in a dynamic setting. In neonates, the scope can also be passed orally. It is important to realize that the provider is not able to well visualize the airway below the vocal cords, particularly in the neonatal and pediatric population, as they are more likely to laryngospasm with minor mechanical stimuli to the larynx [14]. This is a bedside procedure and there is no need to be NPO, or a requirement to have sedative or pain medications.

Direct laryngoscopy and bronchoscopy

A direct laryngoscopy and bronchoscopy is completed in the operating room or similarly monitored setting, with the aid of anesthesia, to allow for a thorough airway examination as well as ability to therapeutically intervene. There are a number of laryngoscopes, bronchoscopes, rigid telescopes, and laryngeal instruments that are used to examine for the pathologies previously discussed (Fig. 34.17). Additionally, a dynamic assessment is possible as the patient is awakening from anesthesia. Using a bronchoscope allows for ventilation during evaluation and intervention of the airway below the vocal cords. The main risks associated with rigid laryngoscopy and bronchoscopy is damage to the teeth, laryngospasm, arytenoid dislocation, or perforation [14].

Tracheostomy

Tracheostomy is a common procedure, but the decision to undertake one, should not be taken lightly (Fig. 34.18).

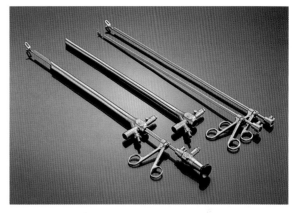

Fig. 34.17 Rigid Bronchoscopic Instrumentation.

Its complexity requires close discussion with family, critical care providers, and pediatric airway specialists. There is nonnegligible rate of tracheostomy related mortality related to blockage of tube or accidental decannulation, ranging from 0.5%–2% [1]. There are of course indications for tracheostomy in which it is life saving, with near complete upper airway obstructions that allow the pathology to be bypassed, but the most frequent reasons for tracheostomy are prolonged intubation, airway maintenance, and pulmonary toilet with the most common diagnosis being bronchopulmonary dysplasia.

For timing of a tracheostomy, it can be an emergent tracheostomy that is required, for example, if the patient is in respiratory distress and unable to be intubated orally, or it could be for prolonged intubation, where the time frame is age dependent. In neonates and premature infants requiring chronic ventilation, they can tolerate intubation for months without significant laryngeal edema or ill effects. As children age, their airway loses its compliance, becoming more structurally firm, and prolonged intubation will

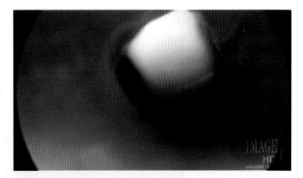

Fig. 34.18 Endoscopic View of Tracheostomy Tube in the Trachea.

cause more laryngeal trauma, resulting in the recommendation for tracheostomy after 2–3 weeks.

In choosing the right tracheostomy tube for the patient, it is important to consider length and diameter. In first discussion about length, too short and there will be more frequent accidental decannulation, too long and it may rest on the carina and cause vagal effects, such as bradycardia and cough, as this is a very sensitive region. There are shorter neonatal tubes for this reason and the end of the tube should be at least 1–2 cm from the carina. For tube diameter, the reason for the tracheostomy tube needs to be addressed. If expected to have some translaryngeal airflow, a narrower tube should be chosen to allow air to pass around the tube, while a wider tube should be chosen if all airflow is expected to travel through tracheostomy site. A diameter that is too large should not be chosen that would cause trauma to the luminal mucosa. A cuff, if present, should be filled to minimal occlusive volume and not overfilled. More modern cuff balloons on pediatric tracheostomy tubes are of a high volume low pressure (HVLP) type to try and minimize pressure necrosis of tracheal mucosa. The provider must be aware that these tend to allow air leak at pressure greater than 35 cmH$_2$O, which can make it a challenge to positive pressure ventilate a neonate with poorly compliant lungs.

Postoperative complications to be wary of include significant bleeding from within the tracheostomy tube. There may be sentinel bleeding for a trachea-innominate fistula arising from erosion of the tracheostomy tube through the anterior tracheal wall. This is an acutely life-threatening emergency. Attempts at tamponade must be made, either with a cuffed endotracheal tube or digital occlusion from the pretracheal region to compress onto the posterior sternum, followed by emergent trip to the operating room and possible median sternotomy. There is frequent development of granulation tissue at the tip of the tracheostomy tube, which is exacerbated by mucosal trauma from the tracheostomy tube as well as by suctioning past the end of the tracheostomy tube. This can cause luminal obstruction if not addressed. There

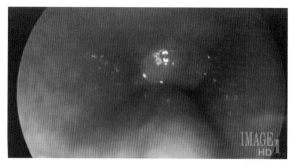

Fig. 34.19 **Luminal Obstruction From Suprastomal Fibroma Superior to Tracheostomy Tube.**

can also be granulation tissue that forms above the tracheostomy tube that can delay decannulation due to suprastomal obstruction (Fig. 34.19). In the early perioperative period, also to be monitored for is pulmonary edema, particularly after bypassing a chronic airway obstruction, and the other is possible pneumothorax. Accidental decannulation is also a significant risk but one that is persistent, as it can quickly lead to mortality, especially if the tracheostomy is the only route of ventilation. To address this issue at our institution we create a superior and inferior Bjork flap during the tracheostomy and suture those edges to the skin to make replacement of the tube as easy as possible. After the first tracheostomy change, there should be well-healed tract allowing for easy replacement of the tube during future changes.

Supraglottoplasty

For severe laryngomalacia for which medical management as failed, a supraglottoplasty is considered in the operating room. Multiple instruments can be used, but the goal is to widen the supraglottic airway. This is done by incising the shortened aryepiglottic folds, reducing the length of the epiglottis, or removing redundant mucosa surround the arytenoid (Fig. 34.20). Depending on extent of surgery,

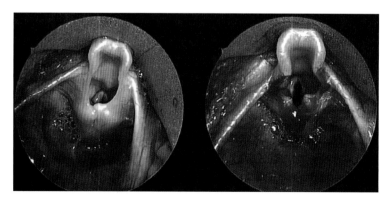

Fig. 34.20 **Preoperative and Postoperative Supraglottoplasty.**

there is risk of supraglottic swelling in the postoperative period and at our institution, these patients are given steroids and are extubated on the following day. Complications other than airway swelling include the possibility of impaired laryngeal sensation and increased risk for aspiration. Supraglottic stenosis is also a possibility, but rare, as is the need for revision surgery.

EXIT procedure

The need for an EXIT procedure is identified prenatally, usually with polyhydramnios on ultrasound and then with further delineation with MRI (Fig. 34.21). Fig. 34.22 shows a patient with a congenitally obstructed upper airway who would not be able to successfully ventilate at birth (Fig. 34.21). A multidisciplinary team is organized with pediatric otolaryngology, anesthesiology, neonatology, pediatric surgery, fetal cardiology, and high-risk obstetrics. The crux of the procedure is keeping the mother under deep sedation and paralysis, delivering

the fetal head and neck via cesarean section, ensuring the infant is paralyzed so as not to draw breath, and to remain on maternal circulation. The airway is secured at this point by the pediatric otolaryngologist either by direct visualization and intubation or transitioning to a surgical airway with a tracheostomy. If still unable to secure the airway, ECMO is an option if infant is older than 35 weeks. Once the airway is secure, the infant can be delivered and removed from maternal circulation. There is high risk for adverse events, the main ones being loss of neonatal airway and significant postpartum hemorrhage. (Video 34.1)

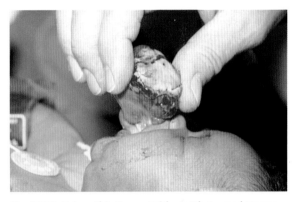

Fig. 34.22 Epignathic Tumor With an Obstructed Upper Airway that Required an EXIT Procedure. *EXIT*, Ex utero intrapartum treatment.

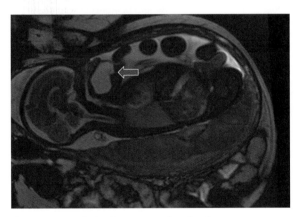

Fig. 34.21 Fetal MRI Demonstrating Cystic Oropharyngeal Mass.

Online supplementary material

Please visit MedEnact to access the following video:

▶ **Video 34.1** Neonatal Airway Pathology.

References

[1] Bluestone CD. Pediatric otolaryngology. 4th ed. Philadelphia: Saunders; 2003.

[2] Sobol SE, Lioy J. Disorders of the neonatal airway: fundamentals for practice. New York, NY: Springer; 2015.

[3] Harless J, Ramaiah R, Bhananker SM. Pediatric airway management. Int J Crit Illn Inj Sci 2014;4(1):65–70.

[4] Burdi AR, Huelke DF, Snyder RG, Lowrey GH. Infants and children in the adult world of automobile safety design: pediatric and anatomical considerations

for design of child restraints. J Biomech 1969;2(3):267–280.

[5] Coté CJ, Lerman J, Todres ID. A practice of anesthesia for infants and children [electronic resource]. 4th ed. Philadelphia, PA: Saunders/Elsevier; 2009. [chapter 12]. p. 237–278. c2009.

[6] Dalal PG, Murray D, Messner AH, Feng A, McAllister J, Molter D. Pediatric laryngeal dimensions: an age-based analysis. Anesth Analg 2009;108(5):1475–1479.

[7] Litman RS, Weissend EE, Shibata D, Westesson PL. Developmental

changes of laryngeal dimensions in unparalyzed, sedated children. Anesthesiology 2003;98(1):41–45.

[8] Strohl KP, Butler JP, Malhotra A. Mechanical properties of the upper airway. Compr Physiol 2012;2(3):1853–1872.

[9] Gnagi SH, Schraff SA. Nasal obstruction in newborns. Pediatr Clin North Am 2013;60(4):903–922.

[10] Tate JR, Sykes J. Congenital nasal pyriform aperture stenosis. Otolaryngol Clin North Am 2009;42(3):521–525.

[11] Belden CJ, Mancuso AA, Schmalfuss IM. CT features of congenital nasal piriform aperture stenosis: initial experience. Radiology 1999;213(2):495–501.

[12] Moreddu E, Le Treut-Gay C, Triglia JM, Nicollas R. Congenital nasal pyriform aperture stenosis: elaboration of a management algorithm from 25 years of experience. Int J Pediatr Otorhinolaryngol 2016;83:7–11.

[13] Smith A, Kull A, Thottam P, Sheyn A. Pyriform aperture stenosis: a novel approach to stenting. Ann Otol Rhinol Laryngol 2017;126(6):451–454.

[14] Thompson JW, Vieira FOM, Rutter MJ. Management of the difficult airway: a handbook for surgeons. London, UK: JP Medical Ltd; 2016.

[15] Eladl HM, Khafagy YW. Endoscopic bilateral congenital choanal atresia repair of 112 cases, evolving concept and technical experience. Int J Pediatr Otorhinolaryngol 2016;85:40–45.

[16] Bangiyev JN, Govil N, Sheyn A, Haupert M, Thottam PJ. Novel application of steroid eluting stents in choanal atresia repair: a case series. Ann Otol Rhinol Laryngol 2017;126(1):79–82.

[17] Riepl R, Scheithauer M, Hoffmann TK, Rotter N. Transnasal endoscopic treatment of bilateral choanal atresia in newborns using balloon dilatation: own results and review of literature. Int J Pediatr Otorhinolaryngol 2014;78(3):459–464.

[18] Strychowsky JE, Kawai K, Moritz E, Rahbar R, Adil EA. To stent or not to stent? A meta-analysis of endonasal congenital bilateral choanal atresia repair. Laryngoscope 2016;126(1):218–227.

[19] Durmaz A, Tosun F, Yldrm N, Sahan M, Kvrakdal C, Gerek M. Transnasal endoscopic repair of choanal atresia: results of 13 cases

[20] Losee JE, Kirschner RE, Whitaker LA, Bartlett SP. Congenital nasal anomalies: a classification scheme. Plast Reconstr Surg 2004;113(2):676–689.

[21] Abramowicz S, Bacic JD, Mulliken JB, Rogers GF. Validation of the GILLS score for tongue-lip adhesion in Robin sequence patients. J Craniofac Surg 2012;23(2):382–386.

[22] Schaefer RB, Stadler JA 3rd, Gosain AK. To distract or not to distract: an algorithm for airway management in isolated Pierre Robin sequence. Plast Reconstr Surg 2004;113(4):1113–1125.

[23] Ayari S, Aubertin G, Girschig H, et al. Management of laryngomalacia. Eur Ann Otorhinolaryngol Head Neck Dis 2013;130(1):15–21.

[24] Dobbie AM, White DR. Laryngomalacia. Pediatr Clin North Am 2013;60(4):893–902.

[25] Thorne MC, Garetz SL. Laryngomalacia: review and summary of current clinical practice in 2015. Paediatr Respir Rev 2016;17:3–8.

[26] Parkes WJ, Propst EJ. Advances in the diagnosis, management, and treatment of neonates with laryngeal disorders. Semin Fetal Neonatal Med 2016;21(4):270–276.

[27] Prowse S, Knight L. Congenital cysts of the infant larynx. Int J Pediatr Otorhinolaryngol 2012;76(5):708–711.

[28] Sadler TW. Langman's medical embryology. 10th ed. Baltimore, MD: Lippincott Williams & Wilkins; 2006.

[29] Evans KL, Courteney-Harris R, Bailey CM, Evans JN, Parsons DS. Management of posterior laryngeal and laryngotracheoesophageal clefts. Arch Otolaryngol Head Neck Surg 1995;121(12):1380–1385.

[30] Benjamin B, Inglis A. Minor congenital laryngeal clefts: diagnosis and classification. Ann Otol Rhinol Laryngol 1989;98:417–420.

[31] Cohen MS, Zhuang L, Simons JP, Chi DH, Maguire RC, Mehta DK. Injection laryngoplasty for type 1 laryngeal cleft in children. Otolaryngol Head Neck Surg 2011;144(5):789–793.

[32] Monnier P. Pediatric airway surgery. Berlin: Springer; 2010.

[33] Wang LM, Zhu Q, Ma T, et al. Value of ultrasonography in diagnosis of pediatric vocal fold paralysis. Int J Pediatr Otorhinolaryngol 2011;75(9):1186–1190.

[34] Jefferson ND, Cohen AP, Rutter MJ. Subglottic stenosis. Semin Pediatr Surg 2016;25(3):138–143.

[35] Bua J, Trappan A, Demarini S, Grasso D, Schleef J, Zennaro F. Neonatal necrotizing tracheobronchitis. J Pediatr 2011;159(4). 699.e1–699.e1.

[36] Gaugler C, Astruc D, Donato L, Rivera S, Langlet C, Messer J. Neonatal necrotizing tracheobronchitis: three case reports. J Perinatol 2004;24(4):259–260.

[37] Hardison SA, Wan W, Dodson KM. The use of propranolol in the treatment of subglottic hemangiomas: A literature review and meta-analysis. International Journal of Pediatric Otorhinolaryngology. 2016; 90: 175–180.

[38] Elluru RG, Friess MR, Richter GT, et al. Multicenter evaluation of the effectiveness of systemic propranolol in the treatment of airway hemangiomas. Otolaryngol Head Neck Surg 2015;153(3):452–460.

[39] Siegel B, Mehta D. Open airway surgery for subglottic hemangioma in the era of propranolol: is it still indicated? Int J Pediatr Otorhinolaryngol 2015;79(7):1124–1127.

Chapter | 35 |

Ventilator-Associated Pneumonia and Infection Control

Manoj N. Malviya, MBBS, DCH, MRCP (UK), Prakash Manikoth, MBBS, DCH, MRCP (UK), FRCPCH, Hakam Yaseen, MD, CES (Paed), DUN (Neonat), CCST (UK), FRCPCH (UK)

CHAPTER POINTS

- VAP is the second most common cause of healthcare-associated infection and can be prevented by the use of VAP prevention bundles.
- Diagnosis of VAP specific to neonates is imprecise and based on CDC criteria which includes clinical, laboratory, and imaging findings.
- A variety of host, microbial, therapeutic, and environmental risk factors contribute to its pathogenesis; microbes causing VAP are acquired from endogenous or exogenous sources.
- Audit and surveillance of VAP, CLABSI and HAI are the major pillars of an effective infection prevention and control program.

Introduction

Advances in neonatal intensive health care delivery have resulted in improved survival for both sick term and extreme preterm infants and increased incidence of complications, such as health care-associated infections (HAI) and ventilator-associated pneumonia (VAP). The complexity of care in neonatal intensive care has exponentially increased with widespread use of invasive devices like central lines, and mechanical ventilation has further promoted VAP and HAI. Both HAI and VAP result in prolonged hospital stay, long-term disability, waste of human and financial resources, and death in many cases [1]. Many of the microorganisms causing VAP are resistant to currently used antibiotics. The situation has become grave with emerging antibiotic resistance and lack of new antibiotics in the research pipeline. It is speculated in future that there will be no effective infection control due to pan-antibiotic resistance. Hence, the only remedy left with us to deal with multidrug-resistant microorganisms is infection prevention.

The paradigm of health care-associated infection including VAP has changed recently from being considered as an inevitable complication associated with intensive care therapy to a preventable harm. The expectation from health policy makers, managers, patients, and society is to provide high-quality care at low cost coupled with less preventable harm. More recently, most health care facilities are expected to report HAI and VAP as quality indicators of their health care delivery system.

between the two, refer Table 35.4 [7,8]. Isolation of microorganism from TA helps in early initiation of specific antimicrobial therapy for true infection, which may translate into improved patient survival. However, there is a risk that the isolate from TA may represent colonization, and treating it as pneumonia with antibiotics may result in development of multidrug-resistant bacteria.

In addition to early initiation of specific antimicrobial therapy, other advantages of isolating microorganisms from ETA are: it allows record of local antibiotics resistance trend, permits microbial specific prognosis, and early detection and implementation of infection-control measures for local VAP outbreaks.

Pathogenesis of VAP (Fig. 35.1)

A sound understanding of the pathogenesis and risk factors is essential for prevention and adequate treatment of VAP. In a mechanically ventilated infant, VAP is the end result

Table 35.4 Tracheal aspirate: colonization versus true infection [7,8]

	Colonization	True infection/VAP
Tracheal aspirate	Defined as two positive samples 1 week apart	Positive for microorganism
Clinical signs and symptoms	Absent	Present
Radiological signs	No changes in X-ray	Recent changes in X-ray
Gram-staining of TA—intracellular bacteria in polymorphoneuclear cell [7]	<2%	>2% suggestive of true infection
TA—CFU [8]	CFU $\leq 10^5$	CFU $\geq 10^5$

CFU, Colony forming unit; *TA*, Tracheal aspirate.

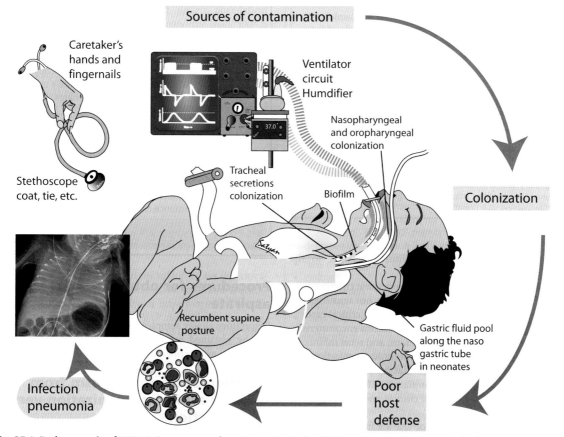

Sources of contamination

Caretaker's hands and fingernails

Ventilator circuit Humdifier

Nasopharyngeal and oropharyngeal colonization

Stethoscope coat, tie, etc.

Tracheal secretions colonization

Biofilm

Colonization

Recumbent supine posture

Gastric fluid pool along the naso gastric tube in neonates

Infection pneumonia

Poor host defense

Fig. 35.1 Pathogenesis of VAP. Various sources of contamination in the NICU environment lead to colonization. Due to poor host defense, especially in preterm infants, infection can spread leading to pneumonia. Copyright: Satyan Lakshminrusimha.

Table 35.5 Risk factors for VAP

Host factors	Environmental factors	Therapeutic factors
Low birth weight infant (OR 1.37; 95% CI, 1.01–1.85)	Design of neonatal intensive care unit	Previous antibiotic therapy (OR, 2.89; 95% CI, 1.41–5.94)
MV (OR 9.7; 95% CI, 4.6–20.4)	Contamination of respiratory devices and circuit	Histamine-2 antagonist, antacid
Duration of MV reintubation (OR 5.3; 95% CI, 2.0–14.0)	Frequent endotracheal suctioning (OR 3.5; 95% CI, 1.6–7.4)	Total parenteral nutrition
Congenital airway malformation (OR, 2.04; 95% CI, 1.08–3.86)	Duration of ventilator circuit	Opiate sedation (OR 3.8; 95% CI, 1.8–8.5)
	Overcrowding	Neuromuscular blockade
Extra uterine growth failure	Nursing–patient ratio	
Gastro esophageal reflux		
Blood infection (OR 3.5; 95% CI, 1.2–10.8)		

CI, Confidence interval; *MV*, mechanical ventilation; *OR*, odds ratio, provided where information available in the literature.

Table 35.6 Layers of natural defenses against microbial invasion

Anatomical and physiological integrity prevents microbial acquisition and colonization
- Glottis and larynx
- Saliva
- Mucociliary apparatus
- Cough reflex
- Aerodynamic of airways
  - Turbulent airflow
  - Humidification
- Defensins (antimicrobial)
- Mucosal turnover

Immunological integrity promotes microbial containment or killing
- Secretory IgA
- Macrophages
- Immunoglobulin

Table 35.7 Effect of mechanical ventilation on natural defense system

Presence of ETT
- Gives direct access for microbes to sterile lower airways
- Promotes biofilm formation
- Injures epithelial surface
- Uncuffed ETT, supine and constant recumbency position promotes microaspirate

Abolish
- Mucociliary clearance
- Cough reflex
- Upper airway humidification

Prematurity-related immunocompromise
- Salivary IgA
- Macrophages
- Immunoglobulin
- Defensin (antimicrobial)

of a complex interplay between the strength and integrity of the host defense system versus the virulence and magnitude of potential pathogenic microorganisms (PPM), in the context of complex neonatal intensive care environment. PPM causing VAP are usually acquired from an endogenous source (patient's own flora) or exogenous source (patient's environment). Pathogenesis of VAP is extensively studied in adult and pediatric patients but only limited data are available for newborns. A variety of host, microbial, therapeutic, and environmental risk factors play a causative role (Table 35.5) [3,4,9–11] .

Susceptible host with compromised defense system

Microbiologically, the human lower respiratory system is considered sterile and in possession of layers of anatomical, physiological, and immunological natural defense systems (Table 35.6) that prevent microbial invasion, limit microbial proliferation within the host and ultimately contain or eradicate the potential pathogenic microorganisms. Newborn infants admitted to NICU for critical illness have multiple host factors that make them vulnerable to acquisition of VAP. There is an inverse relationship between birth weight and gestational age relating to frequency of VAP and nosocomial infection [9]. An infant with low birth weight has a greater likelihood of requiring mechanical ventilation for prolonged period, compromising natural defense systems (Table 35.7) [4,12,13]. Data from the National Institute of Child Health and Human Development (NICHD) showed that 82%–90% of VLBW (birth weight ≤ 1500 g) infants who survived beyond 3 days required conventional mechanical ventilation [14]. Other systemic host factors specific to neonatal patients like extra uterine malnutrition secondary to poor enteral nutrition with breast milk, dependence on total parental nutrition, associated critical illness requiring invasive monitoring and procedures, further compromise host defense, making them vulnerable to the development of VAP. The skin of extreme premature is deficient in stratum corneum before 26 weeks of gestation, allowing easy microbial access by an invasive procedure.

Microbial causes and sources

Understanding the types and sources of microbes responsible for VAP will guide in formulating preventive and treatment strategies. The various microbes causing VAP are listed in Table 35.8. The endogenous source comes from patient's own flora and the exogenous source from the environment. Major endogenous sources for microorganisms include secretions from oral, nasopharyngeal, and stomach and from hematogenous spread (sepsis or infections from other organs). Exogenous sources for microorganism are hands of health care personnel and patient environments (respiratory and other monitoring and therapeutic equipment).

Endogenous sources of microbes

Role of Naso-oro-pharyngeal and stomach microbes in causing VAP

Traditionally, newborn lungs were pursued to be sterile; however, a recent study showed that bacterial DNA was detected in the tracheal aspirate collected immediately after intubation on day 1 of life in 25 preterm infant of less than 32 weeks gestation [15]. In term infant, the microbial communities were detected in the upper airway (nasopharynx and oral cavity) within 5 min of birth [16]. From this, it seems that colonization of newborn's airways begins very early in life, at birth or possibly in utero.

Microbial flora of mouth, nasopharynx, and stomach of NICU patients constantly changes during their stay in NICU and are influenced by underlying illness, days of mechanical ventilation, antibiotics treatment, and feeding choices. Evidence from adult literature show that oropharyngeal flora are dynamic and change to a predominance of aerobic Gram-negative bacilli and *Staphylococcus aureus* during ICU stay [12]. A study compared microbial communities between 10 preterm infants with RDS and VAP with 15 infants with RDS without VAP. Tracheal aspirate collected within 1, 3, and 5 days of ventilation revealed decreased microbial diversity on day 3 in infants with VAP. The greater constituent ratios of *Klebsiella* sp., *Acinetobacter* sp., and *Streptococcus* sp. in the aspirate may be indicators of VAP [17]. The major limitations to study include small sample size, lack of control group that was not treated with antibiotics and not ventilated.

Microbes causing VAP [2–4]	Antibiotics resistance (%) [2]	Region [3]
Gram-negative microorganism • *Pseudomonas aeruginosa* • *Escherichia coli* • *Klebsiella pneumoniae* • *Enterobacter* sp. • *Acinetobacter* sp.	Carbapenem-resistant microbes [3] • *Pseudomonas aeruginosa* (43.5%), *Escherichia coli* (11.7%), • *Klebsiella pneumoniae* (35.7%), and *Acinetobacter* sp. (90.1%)	Common in Asia
Gram-positive • *Staphylococcus aureus*	Methicillin resistant staphylococcus aureus (MRSA)	Common in North America and Europe

Table 35.8 Microbes causing VAP

Microbes causing VAP may originate from stomach. Data from 92% of tracheal aspirate from preterm infants who were ventilated in the first 28 days of life showed the presence of pepsin indicative of chronic aspiration of gastric material [18]. Gastric microbe's access to lungs in NICU patients is abetted by recurrent microaspiration caused by ever recumbency position of neonates, the constant presence of naso- or orogastric tube, methylxanthine therapy, and in some infants with impaired swallowing or anatomical abnormalities. The most concerning issue is that the gut microbes are the epicenter of antibiotic resistance [19], and when excreted in stool, will act as a source for cross transmission by hands of health care workers.

Early life colonization of gut is influenced by multiple factors, including the type of delivery (vaginal versus cesarean section), antibiotics use (perinatal and postnatal), type of feeding (breast milk vs. formula feed), and medications, for example, H2 blocker [20]. The influence of these factors on airways colonization in early life has not been fully examined. Evidence suggest that neonates skin, oral mucosa, and nasopharynx acquire bacterial communities (dominated by *Lactobacillus*, *Prevotella*, or *Sneathia* spp.) similar to maternal vaginal microbial flora if born by vaginal delivery and also acquire similar flora (dominated by *Staphylococcus*, *Corynebacterium*, and *Propionibacterium* spp.) of mother's skin if born by cesarean section [16]. A strong association has been observed between breastfeeding and microbial community composition in the upper respiratory tract of 6-week-old infants, which may offer protective effect for wheezing and the number of mild respiratory tract infections [21]. Breastfed infant showed increased presence and abundance of the lactic acid bacterium *Dolosigranulum* and *Corynebacterium* and decreased abundance of *Staphylococcus* and anaerobic bacteria, such as *Prevotella* and *Veillonella* when compared to formula-fed infants.

Exogenous sources of microbes

Exogenous microbes causing VAP can be acquired from: patient and hospital environment, health care worker's apparel, hand and equipment, invasive monitoring and therapy equipment (Fig. 35.1). Exogenous sources of microbes-responsible epidemics of VAP can be traced to various environment sources as shown in Table 35.9.

Biofilm formation and VAP

Biofilms are the houses or colonies of microorganisms formed by both Gram-positive and Gram-negative bacteria within 48 h of intubation on the inner and outer surfaces of ETT, from microbes-produced extracellular matrix substance called slime. It has been demonstrated that microorganisms hide in these biofilms and communicates with each other with much sophisticated chemical communication system called "quorum sensing" [22]. Evidence suggests that biofilms over ETT act as significant and constant reservoirs of microorganism causing VAP. Emerging data suggest that diversity of microbes in the biofilm is different in patients with VAP and non-VAP. A study evaluating the diversity of bacterial communities in the biofilm of ETT of 29 mechanically ventilated newborns after extubation found *Klebsiella* spp., *Streptococcus* spp., and *Pseudomonas* spp., the most frequent microbes on the surface ETT [23]. A recent study provided new insight by comparing microbial biodiversity in 49 ventilated newborns with or without VAP by newer nonculture-independent technique. The study found that Streptococci facilitate biofilm formation of the common nosocomial pathogen *Pseudomonas aeruginosa* PAO1 and decreased IL-8 expression of airway epithelial cells exposed to the biofilm-conditioned medium of PAO1 [24].

Pathogenic sequential evolution of microbes in NICU and development of VAP

The first step in causation of VAP in the complex environment of NICU is virulent microorganisms getting acquisition or colonization into a normally sterile lower respiratory tract of newborn, whose natural defense system is compromised because of comorbid illness (prematurity or other critical illnesses) and the presence of ETT abolishing local immunity. Critical illness, requiring multiple invasive monitoring and therapies like TPN with inadequate hand hygiene practices, encourages entry of exogenous bacteria into airways via hematogenous or local route. Misuse of antibiotics (overuse or inappropriate use) will change internal milieu and dynamics of protective versus pathogenic microbial colonies,

Table 35.9 Source of exogenous microbes and reported epidemic* of VAP

Source of exogenous microbes	Microorganisms
ETT—biofilm	
Ventilator circuit*, sensor*, humidifier*, nebulized medication*	*Burkholderia cepacia* *Stenotrophomonas maltophilia* *Acinetobacter calcoaceticus*
Monitoring devices	
Health worker hands* and finger nails*	*Pseudomonas aeruginosa* *Klebsiella pneumoniae*
Stethoscope/Doctors apron	
Infected patient* and health care worker*	Respiratory syncytial virus *Mycobacterium tuberculosis* Methicillin-resistant *Staphylococcus aureus*
Water* and ice*	*Legionella pneumophila* *Pseudomonas aeruginosa* Nontuberculous mycobacteria
Ambient air*	*Aspergillus*, zygomycetes
Miscellaneous—milk bank*, breast milk pump, blood gas analyzer*	*Pseudomonas aeruginosa*

*Reported source from epidemic
Source: Adopted and modified from Safdar N, Crnich CJ, Maki DG. The pathogenesis of ventilator-associated pneumonia: its relevance to developing effective strategies for prevention. Respir Care 2005;50(6):725–739 [12].

allowing pathogenic microbes to multiply resulting into VAP. Suboptimal infection control practices like hand hygiene and noncompliance with VAP bundle promote cross infection.

VAP treatment and prevention

VAP treatment

Key principles guiding the empirical treatment of VAP are knowledge of most likely microbes present, local antibiotics resistance patterns within NICU, and previous antibiotics exposure. Empirical antibiotic coverage should be broad enough to cover both Gram-positive and Gram-negative microbes including those that are resistant. Based on unit bacterial surveillance, antibiotic coverage should

---

Table 35.10 Bedside action when VAP is suspected or confirmed

---

Begin empirical antibiotics (combination therapy preferred)

Blood culture (two sets if PICC line)
Tracheal aspirate culture

Deescalate or narrow antibiotics according to culture sensitivity pattern after 48–72 h
• Monotherapy preferred if no systemic signs and blood culture is negative

---

Monitor response to therapy: Clinical, laboratory, and radiological response

---

Duration:
• 7–14 days or longer in severe persistent cases with MDROs
• In culture negative (blood or tracheal aspirate) follow biomarkers (such as C-reactive protein or procalcitonin), clinical and radiological response

---

Isolation of microbes from tracheal aspirate: (CDC recommendations with level of evidence)*
Personal protective equipment
• *Follow contact precautions*: Before direct contact with patients or surfaces and articles in close proximity to a NICU patient with any respiratory infection, including rhinovirus, human metapneumovirus, bocavirus, undifferentiated suspected viral illness, influenza, parainfluenza, adenovirus infection, pertussis, and varicella. (Category IB)
• Wear a gown whenever anticipating that clothing will have direct contact with the infected patient or potentially contaminated environmental surfaces or equipment. Remove gown and gloves and observe hand hygiene before leaving the patient-care environment. (Category IB)
• Maintain isolation precautions for the duration of illness for patients known or suspected to be infected with pathogens. (Category IB)
• *Droplet precautions:* Wear a facemask upon entry into the room or cubicle of patients. (Category I)
  Further research is needed on the benefit of routinely wearing eye protection. (No recommendation, unresolved issue)
• *Cohorting of health care personnel*
  During outbreaks: Assign dedicated health care personnel to care for one patient cohort and not to move between patient cohorts (e.g., restrict personnel who give care to infected or exposed patients from giving care to uninfected or unexposed patients). (Category II)
  In a nonoutbreak setting, assign dedicated health care personnel based primarily in the NICU to care for one patient cohort and not to move between patient cohorts when feasible assessing the risks and benefits (e.g., restrict personnel who give care to infected or exposed patients from giving care to uninfected or unexposed patients). (Category II)
Prevent cross-transmission: (Refer VAP prevention)
• Strict hand hygiene
• Identify microbial source if more than one case in the nursery with the same microorganism

---

*CDC level of evidence:
Category IA: A strong recommendation supported by high-to-moderate quality evidence suggesting net clinical benefits or harms.
Category IB: A strong recommendation supported by low-quality evidence.
Category IC: A strong recommendation required by state or federal regulation.
Category II: A weak recommendation supported by any quality evidence suggesting a trade-off between clinical benefits and harms.
No recommendation: An unresolved issue for which there is low to very low-quality evidence with uncertain trade-offs between benefits and harms.

---

be narrowed or deescalated once the culture and sensitivity results from blood or airway secretions are available. Evidence suggests that appropriate empirical treatment reduces mortality [25]. Tables 35.10 and 35.11 provide bedside action and the choices of empirical antibiotics combinations to be considered when VAP is suspected or VAP confirmed.

VAP prevention

The "all or none" or bundle-care concept of the quality process has been utilized in the prevention of various health care-associated infections, including VAP and CLABSI, both in adults and children [27]. VAP is usually multifactorial and needs multipronged preventive strategies. VAP "bundles" are multiple evidence-based care practices when implemented together will have a synergistic effect and shown to improve outcomes. VAP bundles are well standardized for adult patients; however, most of these practices are not relevant for neonatal population. VAP preventive practices customized to neonatal population based on pathophysiology have been suggested. The corner stone of prevention is early extubation to noninvasive mode

Table 35.11 Empirical therapy of VAP

Potential pathogen	Combination antibiotic therapy
Multidrug-resistant pathogens *Pseudomonas aeruginosa* *Klebsiella* spp. *Acinetobacter* spp.	Antipseudomonal cephalosporin (cefepime, ceftazidime) or antipseudomonal carbapenem (imipenem or meropenem) or β-lactam/β-lactamase inhibitor (Piperacillin/tazobactam) plus antipseudomonal fluoroquinolone (Ciprofloxacin or Levofloxacin) or aminoglycoside (Amikacin, Gentamicin, or Tobramycin)
Methicillin-resistant *Staphylococcus aureus*	Linezolid or vancomycin
Fungi	Fluconazole or Amphotericin

Source: Adapted and modified from Hooven TA, Polin RA. Pneumonia. Semi Fetal Neonatal Med 2017;22(4):206–213 [26].

of ventilation, which protects natural respiratory airway defense system and prevents access of potential pathogenic exogenous and endogenous microbes to airways and lung parenchyma, by strictly following VAP bundles and infection control practices (Table 35.12).

Health care-associated infection and central line-associated bloodstream infection

Background

HAIs are serious health hazards for patients admitted to NICU. The data from the NICHD Neonatal Network showed that 32% of VLBW (birth weight ≤1500 g) infants who survived beyond 3 days developed late-onset sepsis [14]. Detailed information about pathophysiology and preventive strategies of HAI are beyond the scope of this textbook, and readers are advised to refer to CDC guidelines. This section will cover measures to reduce central line-associated bloodstream infection (CLABSI).

Table 35.12 VAP prevention bundle

Neonatal practices	Rationale	Level of evidence
Education and implementation of VAP bundle • Nurse and respiratory therapist led implementation VAP bundle program	Educational program of VAP and nurse-led implementation showed 71% reduction of VAP [28]	IIB
Promote noninvasive ventilation • Noninvasive ventilation like NIPPV or CPAP or high flow	Studies showed that VAP rates are lower in neonates undergoing nasal continuous positive airway pressure compared to the use of mechanical ventilation [5,29]	IIA
Early weaning and rapid extubation • Assess readiness of extubation daily on round	VAP reduced from 3.3 to 1.0/1000 ventilation days in study after aggressive weaning and early extubation [30,31]	IIA
Nasal versus oral intubation	No comparative data for VAP Nasal intubation gives stability but nasal cavity is common site for MRSA colonization	Unresolved
Hand hygiene • Meticulous hand hygiene before and after patient contact and handling respiratory equipment • Wear gloves when handling ventilator condensate and other respiratory/oral secretions	Hand hygiene practices reduced VAP rate by 38% [32]	IIA
ET intubation • Use a new, sterile ETT for each intubation attempt • Ensure that the ETT does not contact environmental surfaces before insertion • Use a sterilized laryngoscope	Cross-contamination risk can be reduced by using an aseptic technique and a sterile or disinfected equipment	IIB

(Continued)

Table 35.12 VAP prevention bundle (*cont.*)

Neonatal practices	Rationale	Level of evidence
Measures to prevent oropharyngeal colonization and aspiration		

Suction practice
• Suction an ET tube on an "as-needed" basis and avoid using normal saline
• Clear secretions from the posterior oropharynx prior to:
  • ET tube manipulation (i.e., retaping) or suctioning
  • Repositioning patient
  • Extubation
  • Reintubation
	Normal saline does not thin or mobilize mucous, can adversely affect arterial and global tissue oxygenation, and can dislodge bacterial colonies [33]	IIB

	Secretions forming in the subglottic area are rapidly colonized with pathogenic bacteria [34,35]	IIIB
	Hypopharyngeal suctioning before suctioning or repositioning the ET tube and/or the patient reduces risk of aspirating-pooled oropharyngeal and nasopharyngeal secretions	IIB
Closed versus open suction Closed suction system recommended	Closed suction system is easier, faster to use, and better tolerated by patients. Open system may cause environment contamination and has concern for losing lung volume. However, study examining two systems found no difference in incidence of VAP or mortality between groups [36]	IIIB
Positioning • Use side-lying position as tolerated • Keep the head of bed elevated 15–30 degree as tolerated • Use left lateral positioning after feedings, as tolerated	Neonatal tracheal colonization from oropharyngeal contamination has shown to be reduced from 87% in the supine position to 30% in the lateral position [37,38]	IA
	Maintaining at least 15 degree head elevation in neonates after ventilation correlates with less microaspiration of stomach contents [39]	IIIB
Oral care Provide oral care: • Within 24 h after intubation; every 3–4 h • Prior to reintubation as time allows • Prior to orogastric tube insertion • Use sterile water, mother's milk, or approved pharmaceutical oral care solution	Intubated patients become colonized with oral pathogenic bacteria within 24 h of intubation [34]	IIB, IIIB
Safe respiratory equipment • Use a separate suction catheter, connection tubing, and canister for oral and tracheal suction • Drain ventilator condensate away from the patient every 2–4 h and before repositioning • Avoid unnecessary disconnection of the ventilator circuit • Change ventilator equipment when visibly soiled or mechanically malfunctioning • Use heated ventilator circuits	Respiratory equipment can become colonized with pathogens that cause VAP and should avoid direct contact with the patient's bed to prevent environment contamination [34,40] To avoid equipment contamination [40]: • Keep the ventilator circuit closed and free from condensate by draining water away from the patient and before repositioning every 2–4 h • Avoid manipulation and routine ventilator circuit changes • Heated ventilator circuits decrease the occurrence of condensate	IIB, IIIB
Feeding • Prevent gastric distention • Monitor gastric residuals if other signs of feeding intolerance • Adjust feeding to prevent large residuals and/or distention	Avoid gastric distention, it may increase risk of aspiration Routine monitoring of gastric residual is not recommended in asymptomatic infant	IIIB

Table 35.12 VAP prevention bundle (*cont.*)

Neonatal practices	Rationale	Level of evidence
Medication not recommended • Use of histamine-2 receptor antagonists or antacids • Selective digestive tract decontamination with nonabsorbable antimicrobials • Silver-coated ETT • Chlorhexidine mouth wash • Probiotics	The use of H2-blockers is associated with increased risk of late-onset fungal infection and necrotizing enterocolitis among very low birth weight NICU infants [41]	H2 blocker = IIB
	Suppression of acid–gastric content may promote colonization with pathogenic organisms and will increased the risk of VAP	Probiotics = Unresolved
Safe environment: Safe air, safe water	Reports of outbreaks of VAP with pseudomonas and other microbes with contaminated water and equipment	
Audit and surveillance	Monitoring of practices and processes of VAP bundle is essential	

Level of evidence: I, demonstrated by at least one RCT or meta-analysis; II, demonstrated by a comparative study that is not an RCT or by a cohort study; III, a case series study or an expert opinion. Ranking of recommendation: A, strongly recommended or strongly advised against; B, generally recommended or generally advised against; C, optional, the effect of it is unclear, there is no evidence or unresolved.
Source: Adapted and modified from Hooven TA, Polin RA. Pneumonia. Semi Fetal Neonatal Med 2017;22(4):206–213 [26]; Weber CD. Applying adult ventilator-associated pneumonia bundle evidence to the ventilated neonate. Adv Neonatal Care 2016;16(3):178e90 [42].

The use of central lines (UVC, UAC, PICC, and CVL) is common in NICU and is considered to be the most stable and reliable way of providing intravenous access for sick neonates. CLABSIs are the commonest type of HAI in NICU. Both HAI and CLABSI are associated with increased morbidity and mortality. CLABSI results in prolonged hospital stay and drains the financial and human resources of the health care system. The multinational surveillance data from the International Nosocomial Infection Control Consortium (INICC) reported the incidence of CLABSI per 1000 central line days as 10.5 for the infant weighing more than 2500 g to 20.9 for the infant weighing less than 750 g [2]. The most common pathogens responsible for causing CLABSI are Gram-positive cocci (mainly coagulase-negative staphylococci and *S. aureus*), Gram-negative bacilli (particularly Enterobacteriaceae), and *Candida* species. The emergence of extended spectrum β-lactamases (ESBL) and carbapenemases producing Gram-negative bacteria and Methicillin-resistant *Staphylococcus aureus* (MRSA) is a cause for concern due to the paucity of effective antibiotics to treat these infections.

CLABSI definition

To diagnose a bloodstream infection as CLABSI, CDC criteria to be satisfied are as follows:
1. At least one positive culture of noncommensal organism or two blood culture positives from two separate sites if it is a commensal organism like CONS.
2. Catheter in place for more than 2 days before the event or removed 2 days prior to the event.
3. No other documented primary site of infection.

CLABSI prevention

Implementing an evidence-based CLABSI bundle (Table 35.13) [43,44] results in the reduction of CLABSI. Studies reported a decrease in CLABSI rate from 4.9 to 1.5 per 1000 central line days and even zero rates in some centers by strictly adhering to the CDC CLABSI bundle [45,46].

Audit and surveillance of VAP, CLABSI and HAI

Auditing and surveillance are the major pillars of an effective infection prevention and control (IPC) program of any hospital. It is a systemic way of collecting, analyzing, and interpreting the data of effectiveness of infection-control processes, practices, and outcomes. It provides distribution and determinants of various health care-associated adverse events. It measures care system performance and allows comparison nationally or internationally. HAI, CLABSI and VAP surveillance should be a part of any IPC program. The major components of surveillance are mentioned in Table 35.14.

Table 35.13 CLABSI prevention

Neonatal practices	Rationale and level of evidence*
Education and implementation of CLABSI bundle: • Staff education and efforts to promote adherence to recommended practices (e.g., checklist)	• Low-quality evidence from 10 studies evaluated the use of "bundled interventions" to prevent CLABSI among neonates and suggested reduction in CLABSI rate. (IB)
CLABSI bundle	• Site selection • Catheter type and duration • Insertion bundle • Maintenance and care bundle • Miscellaneous
Optimum site selection: • Peripheral veins versus central veins: Peripheral veins are preferred than femoral • Upper extremity versus lower extremity: No difference in CLABSI rate • Long-term surgically implanted central line (SICL): Consider using subclavian or femoral and avoid internal jugular • Risk for CLABSI among different central lines (UVC, PICC, SICL) • Central line tip placement for lower extremity PICC	• Low-quality evidence suggested an increase in CLABSIs in neonates with a PICC placed directly into the femoral vein compared to those placed peripherally (nonfemoral) (II) • No difference in CLABSI rate between PICC in the lower extremity peripheral sites (generally saphenous veins) versus upper extremity peripheral sites (antecubital) (unresolved issue) • Increase in the risk for CLABSIs with internal jugular in two low-quality studies (II) • Unresolved issue • There were no differences in catheter complications between catheters that terminated in the upper vena cava (T8–T10) compared to those that terminated in the lower vena cava (around L2) (II)
Catheter type: • Use single lumen or double lumen UVC Catheter duration: • UAC: Short duration (maximum 5 days) • UVC: Short duration (<7 days) preferred, maximum 14 days • PICC: Intermediate duration: weeks • SICL: Weeks to months	Low-quality evidence suggested that there was no difference in sepsis rate between single- or double-lumen catheters Duration: • UAC should not be left in place for >5 days • UVC can be used up to 14 days if managed aseptically; study comparing UVC for >10 days versus ≤7 days, found 20% increase in the odds of a CLABSI for each day of UVC in situ • Discontinue PICC as soon as they are no longer needed. Low-quality evidence suggested that the longer a PICC was in place, the higher the odds or risk of CLABSI (IB)
Insertion bundle: • Perform hand hygiene before insertion • Adhere to aseptic technique • Use maximal sterile barrier precautions (i.e., mask, cap, gown, sterile gloves, and sterile full body drape) • Perform skin antisepsis with >0.5% chlorhexidine with alcohol • Choose the best site to minimize infections (as mentioned above) • Cover the site with sterile gauze or sterile, transparent, semipermeable dressings	• Promote adherence to hand hygiene to prevent health care-associated infections. Hand hygiene adherence programs should include education of health care personnel about the importance of hand hygiene for infection prevention, reminders, and adherence to surveillance with feedback of results to frontline providers (IB) • Do not use topical antibiotic ointment or creams on insertion sites because of potential to promote fungal infections and antimicrobial resistance

Table 35.13 CLABSI prevention (*cont.*)

Neonatal practices	Rationale and level of evidence*
Maintenance and care bundle: • Remove nonessential catheters. Assess the need for continued intravascular access on a daily basis during multidisciplinary rounds. Remove catheters when not required for patient care • Comply with hand hygiene requirements • Scrub the access port or hub immediately prior to each use with an appropriate antiseptic (e.g., chlorhexidine, povidone iodine, an iodophor, or 70% alcohol) • Access catheters only with sterile devices. Replace dressings that are wet, soiled, or dislodged • Perform dressing changes under aseptic technique using clean or sterile gloves • Use the minimum number of ports or lumens essential for management of the patient	Hub cleaning/catheter manipulations/blood draws • Frequent central line hub manipulations requiring disinfection (e.g., disconnection of the infusion set from a central line) or drawing blood through a central line increases the risk of CLABSIs (IB) • Minimize the number of times central line hubs are accessed and minimize blood sampling through central lines to decrease the risk for CLABSI
Miscellaneous: • *Dedicated central line insertion and care team*: It is desirable • *Systemic antimicrobial prophylaxis:* Before insertion or during use of central line is not indicated • *In-line filter:* Not indicated • Central line antimicrobial locks: Consider in setting of high CLABSI rate when other recommendation failed • Heparin infusion: For prevention of CLABSI: not indicated Change of IV sets for central line infusion: • IV infusion of dextrose 5% with 0.45% saline: 72 h • IV infusion blood, blood products lipid solution, and IV amino acid solution: 24 h	• The use of teams for central line insertion and care resulted in lower number of CLABSIs (IA) • Although studies on prophylactic vancomycin did appear to result in a decrease in CLABSIs due to coagulase-negative *Staphylococci*, the development of antimicrobial resistance was not adequately evaluated in these studies (IB) • Do not use in-line filters solely for the prevention of CLABSIs (IA) • Central line antimicrobial locks: Three studies showed that the use of catheter locks prevented CLABSIs (II) • Do not use heparin infusions solely for the purpose of preventing CLABSIs (IA)

CLABSI, Central line-associated bloodstream infection; *PICC*, percutaneous inserted central catheter; *SICL*, surgically implanted central line; *UAC*, umbilical arterial catheter; *UVC*, umbilical venous catheter.
*CDC level of evidence:
Category IA: A strong recommendation supported by high-to-moderate quality evidence suggesting net clinical benefits or harms.
Category IB: A strong recommendation supported by low-quality evidence.
Category IC: A strong recommendation required by state or federal regulation.
Category II: A weak recommendation supported by any quality evidence suggesting a trade-off between clinical benefits and harms.
No recommendation: An unresolved issue for which there is low to very low-quality evidence with uncertain trade-offs between benefits and harms.
Source: Adopted and modified from Marschall J, Mermel LA, Fakih M, et al. Strategies to prevent central line associated bloodstream infections in acute care hospitals. Infection Cont Hosp Epidemiol 2014;35:753–771 [43] and from https://www.cdc.gov/infectioncontrol/guidelines/bsi/index.html [44].

Cleaning, disinfection, and sterilization in NICU

1. **Cleaning** is the removal of visible organic and inorganic material from objects and surfaces before disinfection and sterilization; it is done manually or mechanically using water with detergents or enzymatic products.

2. **Disinfection** is a process that eliminates many or all pathogenic microorganisms, except bacterial spores, on inanimate objects; it is done using liquid chemicals or wet pasteurization.

3. **Sterilization** is a process that destroys or eliminates all forms of microbial life and is carried out by physical or chemical methods; these include steam under pressure, dry heat, ethylene oxide (EO) gas, hydrogen peroxide gas plasma, and liquid chemicals.

Table 35.14 Surveillance of VAP, CLABSI and HAI

Surveillance	Details
Measure outcomes	Monitor the incidence density by calculating rates of major HAI (CLABSI, VAP, UTI, SSI) as per CDC guidelines
Measure processes and practices	Monitor the compliance with various infection control practices and bundles such as CLABSI bundles, VAP bundles, UTI bundles, and SSI bundles
Environment and equipment	Monitor and evaluates the state of contamination of the hospital environment and equipment, determine sources and routes of infections, identify the carriers
Microorganisms and MDROs	Monitor growth of various microorganisms and their sensitivity. Identify MDROs and establish hospital isolation policy
Antibiotics stewardship	Monitor antibiotics consumption; establish disease and department-specific antibiotics policy, as per local flora and sensitivity pattern
VAP, CLABSI, HAI specific surveillance	• VAP rate: Number of VAPs per 1000 ventilation days • Ventilation device utilization ratio: Ratio of ventilation days to patient days • CLABSI rate: Number of blood stream infection per 1000 central line days
Audit and feedback	• Provide feedback to the facility staff about the VAP rates and compliance with bundles. Education and reminders to health care personnel to adhere to infection-control practices and VAP-preventive bundles

CLABSI, central line associated blood stream infection; *HAI*, health care associated infection; *MDRO*, multi-drug resistant organism; *SSI*, surgical site infection; *UTI*, urinary tract infection; *VAP*, ventilator associated pneumonia.

Table 35.15 Spaulding's classification of medical devices [47]

Classification	Definition	Processing level	Examples
Critical device	Device that enters into sterile tissues, including the vascular system	Cleaning followed by sterilization	Laryngoscope blades, surgical instruments, cardiac catheters, cystoscopes
Semicritical device	Device that comes in contact with nonintact skin or mucous membranes but does not penetrate them	Cleaning followed by high-level disinfection with germicides; sterilization is preferred	Respiratory circuits, self-inflating bags and masks; reusable enteral feeding equipment
Noncritical device	Device that comes in contact with intact skin	Cleaning followed by low-level disinfection; cleaning alone is required for some	Stethoscopes, thermometers, pulse oximeter and cardiorespiratory leads, ultrasound probes, phototherapy mats, incubators, cots, and mattresses

4. **Spaulding's classification of medical devices [47,48]:**
The level of terminal processing required for medical devices is based on the classification system developed by Spaulding in 1970. It divides medical devices into three categories, based on the risk of infection resulting from contact with various types of devices (Table 35.15).

5. **Resistance of microorganisms to disinfection and sterilization [48]:** Fig. 35.2 outlines the variable order of resistance of microorganisms to disinfection and sterilization (with the disinfection levels indicated). The recommendations for cleaning, disinfection and sterilization in NICU are listed in Table 35.16. The indications and directions for

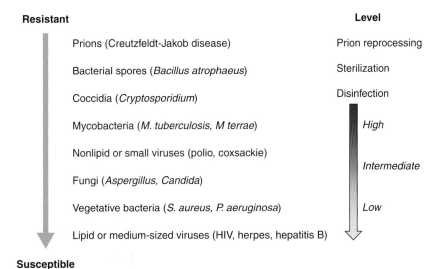

Fig. 35.2 Decreasing Order of Resistance of Microorganisms to Disinfection and Sterilization [48].

use of disinfectants and germicides are outlined in Table 35.17.

6. **Hand hygiene** should be performed before patient contact, before any aseptic task, after exposure risk to body fluids, after patient contact, and after contact with patient surroundings. Hand washing should be performed by first wetting the skin with tepid water, then adding the soap or cleansing agent. The hands should be vigorously rubbed together for at least 40–60 s, covering and generating friction on all surfaces, then thoroughly dried. When using an alcohol-based rub, rubbing should be continued for 20–30 s or until the hands are dry.

7. **Prevention of needle stick injuries**: Percutaneous injury with a hollow injection needle is associated with the risk of transmitting blood-borne infection. Used needles should not be recapped, bent, or broken by hand. If it is necessary to recap needles, a single-handed technique should be used in which the needle is not directed toward the unprotected hand. Puncture-resistant sharps containers must be available closely in all work areas.

8. **Surface disinfection**: Most nosocomial pathogens can survive on surfaces of health care facilities for weeks or months (Table 35.18) and can be a continuous source of transmission [50]. Hence it is advisable to control the spread of nosocomial pathogens by routine surface disinfection.

9. **Safe disposal of hospital waste**: Proper disposal of hospital waste is essential to keep a clean environment. The following are different color drums with different color polythene for different types of waste, to be disposed of in a different way.

   a. Black drums/bags: Left over food, fruits, feeds, vegetables, waste paper, packing material, empty box, bags, and so on. This waste is disposed by the local municipality.
   b. Yellow drums/bags: Infected nonplastic waste, for example, human anatomical waste, blood, body fluids, placenta, diapers, and so on. This type of waste requires incineration.
   c. Blue drums/bags: Infected plastic waste such as used disposable syringes, needles, and soiled gloves. Patients' IV set, blood transfusion set, endotracheal tube, catheter, urine bag, and so on should be cut into pieces. This waste will be autoclaved to make it noninfectious.
   d. Red drums/bags: Used sharps, blade, and broken glass should be discarded in puncture proof containers before discarding.

Implications for practice

- VAP is a preventable harm common in preterm infants requiring prolonged mechanical ventilation.
- Diagnosis of VAP in neonates is not precise. Commonly used CDC criteria for infants less than 1 year are not VAP-specific and overlap with other neonatal conditions, resulting in over- or underdiagnosis and treatment of VAP.

Table 35.16 Recommendations for cleaning, disinfection, and sterilization in NICU [49]

Object	Disinfection method	Frequency and other considerations
Stethoscope, thermometer, BP cuffs, probes of radiant warmer/pulse oximeter	Clean with spirit swab	Daily, before and after use Dedicate stethoscope to single patient
Oxygen hood	Wash with soap and water and dry with clean linen	Daily
Weighing machine	Wipe with surface disinfectant	Daily
Face mask	Clean with soap and water, immerse in glutaraldehyde for 20 min, rinse in distilled water, dry and wrap in autoclaved linen	Daily and after each use
Resuscitation bag and reservoir mask, oxygen tubing, bottle, and tubing of suction machine	Clean with soap and water, immerse in glutaraldehyde for 4–6 h, rinse in distilled water, dry and wrap in autoclaved linen and put a date	Weekly for resuscitation bag and reservoir Daily for others
Laryngoscope	Clean with spirit swabs thoroughly daily and after each use. Wrap in autoclaved cloth and put a date on cover	Daily and after each use If used for an infected baby, wash with soap and water. Put the blade in 2% glutaraldehyde after removing the bulb and wash thoroughly with distilled water
Syringe pumps	Clean with wet clean cloth. If blood stained, use soap and water	Daily and if possible in each shift
Swab container, injection, and medicine tray	Wash with soap and water/autoclave	Daily morning; use separate swab containers for each baby
Feeding utensils	Wash with soap and water and then boil for 10 min	Before each use; use disposable feeding cups if available
Cheatle Forceps	Autoclave	Daily
Sets for procedures	Autoclave	After each use; every 72 h if not used
Radiant warmer, Bassinet and Incubator, dressing trolley, crash trolley, infusion pump	Clean with soap water daily, if occupied. If not occupied, clean with 2% Bacillocid	Daily and between patients

- Microorganisms causing VAP originate either from the patient environment or patient's own flora from oropharyngeal and gastric secretion. Inappropriate use of antibiotics promotes selection of highly resistant microorganism (MDROs), resulting in severe lung injury and death.
- Prevention of VAP is achieved by early removal of the endotracheal tube to minimize the duration of mechanical ventilation and by strictly implementing the VAP prevention bundle.

- The use of central lines is common in NICU, and CLABSIs are associated with increased morbidity and mortality. Implementing an evidence-based CLABSI bundle results in its reduction.
- Hand hygiene should be performed before patient contact, before any aseptic task, after exposure risk to body fluids, after patient contact, and after contact with patient surroundings.
- Audit and surveillance of HAI, CLABSI, and VAP are the major pillars of an effective infection prevention and control program of any hospital.

Table 35.17 Disinfectants and germicides [49]

Name	Indication for use	Direction for use and special considerations
Bacillocid spray (2%)	Walls of nursery Incubators and warmers (not in use) Surface of weighing machine	Switch off air conditioners at the time of spray
2% Glutaraldehyde (Cidex)	Face mask and Ambu bag Reservoir	Before immersing into Cidex, clean thoroughly with soap and water; duration of contact: • for disinfection, 15–20 min • for sterilization, 4–6 h
EcoShield (H_2O_2 11% w/v, 0.01% w/v silver nitrate)	Fumigation of NICU	Routine fumigation: 200 mL of EcoShield in 800 mL of water, 1 L/1000 ft³ for aerial fumigation
Sodium hypocholorite (bleach)	Sharps/needles and disposables	Keep the solution covered, change it every 24 h
Spirit	Skin preparation, cleaning laryngoscope blades, tape measure, and stethoscope	Do not use to clean incubators and warmers
Soap and water	Oxygen hood, feeding utensils, swab containers, injection tray, face mask, buckets	After washing in soap and water, boil the feeding utensils for 20 min
Povidone-iodine	Skin preparation Urinary catheterization	Use with caution in extremely preterm babies
Chlorhexidine 2%	Skin preparation	Infants <29 weeks and less than 3 weeks of age, use without alcohol

Table 35.18 Persistence of clinically relevant pathogens on dry inanimate surfaces [50]

Persistence of clinically relevant bacteria	
Acinetobacter spp.	3 days to 5 months
Bordetella pertussis	3–5 days
Campylobacter jejuni	up to 6 days
Clostridium difficile (spores)	5 months
Chlamydia pneumoniae, C. trachomatis	≤30 h
Chlamydia psittaci	15 days
Corynebacterium diphtheriae	7 days to 6 months
Corynebacterium pseudotuberculosis	1–8 days
Escherichia coli	1.5 h to 16 months
Enterococcus spp. including VRE and VSE	5 days to 4 months
Haemophilus influenzae	12 days
Helicobacter pylori	≤90 min
Klebsiella spp.	2 h to >30 months
Listeria spp.	1 day to months

(Continued)

Table 35.18 Persistence of clinically relevant pathogens on dry inanimate surfaces [50] (*cont.*)

Persistence of clinically relevant bacteria

Mycobacterium bovis	>2 months
Mycobacterium tuberculosis	1 day to 4 months
Neisseria gonorrhoeae	1–3 days
Proteus vulgaris	1–2 days
Pseudomonas aeruginosa	6 h to 16 months; on dry floor: 5 weeks
Salmonella typhi	6 h to 4 weeks
Salmonella typhimurium	10 days to 4.2 years
Salmonella spp.	1 day
Serratia marcescens	3 days to 2 months; on dry floor: 5 weeks
Shigella spp.	2 days to 5 months
Staphylococcus aureus, including MRSA	7 days to 7 months
Streptococcus pneumoniae	1–20 days
Streptococcus pyogenes	3 days to 6.5 months
Vibrio cholerae	1–7 days

Persistence of clinically relevant fungi

Candida albicans	1–120 days
Candida parapsilosis	14 days
Torulopsis glabrata	102–150 days

References

[1] Centers for Disease Control and Prevention. Criteria for defining nosocomial pneumonia. Available from: http://www.cdc.gov/nhsn/PDFs/pscManual/6pscVAPcurrent.pdf.

[2] Rosenthal VD, Al-Abdely HM, El-Kholy AA, AlKhawaja SA, Leblebicioglu H, Mehta Y, et al. International nosocomial infection control consortium report, data summary of 50 countries for 2010–2015: device-associated module. Am J Infect Control 2016;44(12):1495–1504.

[3] Aelami MH, Lotfi M, Zingg W. Ventilator-associated pneumonia in neonates, infants and children. Antimicrob Resist Infect Control 2014;3:30.

[4] Garland JS. Strategies to prevent ventilator associated pneumonia in neonates. Clin Perinatol 2010;37:629–643.

[5] Geffers C, Baerwolff S, Schwab F, Gastmeier P. Incidence of healthcare associated infections in high-risk neonates: results from the German surveillance system for very-low-birthweight infants. J Hosp Infect 2008;68:214–221.

[6] Wiener-Kronish JP. Ventilator-associated pneumonia: problems with diagnosis and therapy. Best Pract Res Clin Anaesthesiol 2008;22(3):437–449.

[7] Köksal N, Hacimustafaoğlul M, Çelebi S, Ozakin C. Non bronchoscopic bronchoalveolar lavage for diagnosing ventilator associated pneumonia in newborns. Turk J Pediatr 2006;48(3):213–220.

[8] Cernada M, Aguar M, Brugada M, Gutierrez A, Lopez JL, et al. Ventilator-associated pneumonia in newborn infants diagnosed with an invasive bronchoalveolar lavage technique: a prospective observational study. Pediatr Crit Care Med 2013;14(1):55–61.

[9] Apisarnthanarak A, Holzmann-Pazgal G, Hamvas A, Olsen MA, Fraser VJ. Ventilator-associated pneumonia in extremely preterm neonates in a neonatal intensive care unit: characteristics, risk factors, and outcomes. Pediatrics 2003;112:1283–1289.

[10] Lee P-L, Lee W-T, Chen H-L. Ventilator-associated pneumonia in low birth weight neonates at a neonatal intensive care unit: a retrospective observational study. Pediatr Neonatol 2017;58:16e21.

[11] Foglia E, Meier MD, Elward A. Ventilator-associated pneumonia in neonatal and pediatric intensive care unit patients. Clin Microbiol Rev 2007;20(3):409–425.

[12] Safdar N, Crnich CJ, Maki DG. The pathogenesis of ventilator-associated pneumonia: its relevance to developing effective strategies for prevention. Respir Care 2005;50(6):725–739.

[13] Kohler PF, Farr RS. Elevation of cord over maternal IgG immunoglobulin: evidence for an active placental IgG transport. Nature 1966;210: 1070–1071.

[14] Stoll BJ, Hansen NI, Bell EF, et al. Trends in care practices, morbidity and mortality of extremely preterm neonates, 1993–2012. JAMA 2015;314:1039–1051.

[15] Lohmann P, Luna RA, Hollister EB, Devaraj S, Mistretta T-A, Welty SE, et al. The airway microbiome of intubated premature infants: characteristics and changes that predict the development of bronchopulmonary dysplasia. Pediatr Res 2014;76(3):294–301.

[16] Dominguez-Bello MG, Costello EK, Contreras M, Magris M, Hidalgo G, Fierer N, et al. Delivery mode shapes the acquisition and structure of the initial microbiota across multiple body habitats in newborns. Proc Natl Acad Sci USA 2010;107(26): 11971–11975.

[17] Lu W, Yu J, Ai Q, Liu D, Song C, Li L. Increased constituent ratios of Klebsiella sp.; Acinetobacter sp., and Streptococcus sp. and a decrease in microflora diversity may be indicators of ventilator-associated pneumonia: a prospective study in the respiratory tracts of neonates. PLoS One 2014;9(2):e87504.

[18] Farhath S, He Z, Nakhla T, et al. Pepsin, a marker of gastric contents, is increased in tracheal aspirates from preterm infants who develop bronchopulmonary dysplasia. Pediatrics 2008;121(2): e253–e259.

[19] Carlet J. The gut is the epicentre of antibiotic resistance. Antimicrob Resist Infect Control 2012;1:39.

[20] Gallacher DJ, Kotecha S. Respiratory microbiome of new-born infants. Front Pediatr 2016;4:10.

[21] Biesbroek G, Bosch AA, Wang X, Keijser BJ, Veenhoven RH, Sanders EA, et al. The impact of breastfeeding on nasopharyngeal microbial communities in infants. Am J Respir Crit Care Med 2014;190(3):298–308.

[22] Jamal M, Tasneem U, Hussain T, Andleeb S. Bacterial biofilm: its composition, formation and role in human infections. Res Rev 2015;4(3):1–14.

[23] Li H, Song C, Liu D, Ai Q, Yu J. Molecular analysis of biofilms on the surface of neonatal endotracheal tubes based on 16S rRNA PCR-DGGE and species-specific PCR. Int J Clin Exp Med 2015;8(7):11075–11084.

[24] Pan Y, Song S, Tang X, Qing Ai Q, Danping Zhu, et al. Streptococcus sp. in neonatal endotracheal tube biofilms is associated with ventilator associated pneumonia and enhanced biofilm formation of Pseudomonas aeruginosa PAO1. Sci Rep 2017;7:3423.

[25] Luna CM, Vujacich P, Niederman MS, Vay C, Gherardi C, Matera J, Jolly EC. Impact of BAL data on the therapy and outcome of ventilator-associated pneumonia. Chest 1997;111:676–685.

[26] Hooven TA, Polin RA. Pneumonia. Semi Fetal Neonatal Med 2017;22(4):206–213.

[27] Nolan T, Berwick DM. All or none measurement raises the bar on performance. JAMA 2006;295: 1168–1170.

[28] Ceballos K, Waterman K, Hulett T, Makic MB. Nurse-driven quality improvement interventions to reduce hospital-acquired infection in the NICU. Adv Neonat Care 2013;13: 154–163.

[29] Rosenthal VD, Rodriguez-Calderon ME, Rodriguez-Ferrer M, Singhal T, Pawar M, et al. Findings of the international nosocomial infection control consortium (INICC). Part II: impact of a multidimensional strategy to reduce ventilator-associated pneumonia in neonatal intensive care units in 10 developing countries. Infect Control Hosp Epidemiol 2012;33:704–710.

[30] Hentschel J, Brungger B, Studi K, Muhlemann K. Prospective surveillance of nosocomial infections in a Swiss NICU: low risk of pneumonia on nasal continuous positive airway pressure? Infection 2005;33:350–355.

[31] Ng SP, Gomez JM, Lim SH, Ho NK. Reduction of nosocomial infection in a neonatal intensive care unit (NICU). Singapore Med J 1998;39: 319–323.

[32] Won SP, Chou HC, Hsieh WS, et al. Handwashing program for the prevention of nosocomial infections in a neonatal intensive care unit. Infect Control Hosp Epidemiol 2004;25:742–746.

[33] Halm M, Krisko-Hagel K. Instilling normal saline with suctioning: beneficial technique or potentially harmful sacred cow? Am J Crit Care 2008;17:469–472.

[34] Sole M, Poalillo F, Byers J, Ludy J. Bacterial growth in secretions and on suctioning equipment of orally intubated patients: a pilot study. Am J Crit Care 2002;11:141–149.

[35] Dezfulian C, Shojania K, Collard H, Kim HM, Matthay MA, Saint S. Subglottic secretion drainage for preventing ventilator-associated pneumonia: a meta-analysis. Am J Med 2005;118:11–18.

[36] Cordero L, Sananes M, Ayers LW. Comparison of a closed (Trach Care MAC) with an open endotracheal suction system in small premature infants. J Perinatol 2000;20: 151–156.

[37] Aly H, Badawy M, El-Kholy A, Nabil R, Mohamed A. Randomized, controlled trial on tracheal colonization of ventilated infants: can gravity prevent ventilator-associated pneumonia? Pediatrics 2008;122:770–777.

[38] Drakulovic M, Torres A, Bauer T, Nicolas JM, Nogué S, Ferrer M. Supine body position as a risk factor for nosocomial pneumonia in mechanically ventilated patients: a randomized trial. Lancet 1999;354:1851–1858.

[39] Garland J, Alex C, Johnston N, Yan J, Werlin S. Association between tracheal pepsin, a reliable marker of gastric aspiration, and head of bed elevation among ventilated neonates. J Neonatal Perinatal Med 2014;7(3): 185–192.

[40] Institute for Healthcare Improvement. How-to guide: prevent ventilator-associated pneumonia. Cambridge, MA: Institute for Healthcare Improvement; 2012.

[41] Terrin G, Passariello A, De Curtis M, et al. Ranitidine is associated with infections, necrotizing enterocolitis, and fatal outcome in newborns. Pediatrics 2012;129(1):e40–e45.

[42] Weber CD. Applying adult ventilator-associated pneumonia bundle evidence to the ventilated neonate. Adv Neonatal Care 2016;16(3):178e90.

[43] Marschall J, Mermel LA, Fakih M, et al. Strategies to prevent central line-associated bloodstream infections in acute care hospitals: 2014 update. Infect Control Hosp Epidemiol 2014;35:753–771.

[44] Available from: https://www.cdc.gov/infectioncontrol/guidelines/bsi/index.html.

[45] Patrick SW, Kawai AT, Kleinman K, et al. Health care-associated infections among critically ill children in the US, 2007–2012. Pediatrics 2014;134:705–712.

[46] Erdei C, MacAvoy LL, Gupta M, Pereira S, McGowan EC. Is zero central line associated bloodstream infection rate sustainable? A 5 year perspective. Pediatrics 2015;135:e1485–e1493.

[47] British Columbia Ministry of Health. Best practice guidelines for cleaning, disinfection and sterilization in health authorities. British Columbia Ministry of Health Ontario, Canada; 2011.

[48] Available from: https://www.cdc.gov/infectioncontrol/pdf/guidelines/disinfection-guidelines.pdf.

[49] Available from: https://www.newbornwhocc.org/Dec2014_pdf/Prvention-of-infection-house-keeping-in-facilty-2014.pdf.

[50] Kramer A, Schwebke I, Kampf G. How long do nosocomial pathogens persist on inanimate surfaces? A systematic review. BMC Infect Dis 2006;6:130.

Chapter | 36 |

Nutrition in the Preterm Neonate Requiring Respiratory Support

Mahmoud Saleh Elhalik, MD, DCH, ABP, FAAP, FRCPCH, Josef Neu, MD, Abrar Ahmed Khan, MD, Swarup Kumar Dash, MD, DNB

CHAPTER POINTS

- Postnatal or extrauterine growth restriction is common among preterm infants on respiratory support and can be prevented by judicious fluid and nutritional management.
- Human milk (with fortification for preterm infants) is preferred for all infants.
- Protein intake as high as 4.5 g/kg/d may be required in extremely preterm infants to compensate for accumulated protein deficit and achieve adequate linear growth.
- Lipids have high caloric density and are an important source of calories in ventilated infants on fluid-restriction.
- High rates of glucose delivery in parenteral nutrition (> 12.5 mg/kg/min) increases CO_2 production as it has a high respiratory quotient (RQ).

Introduction

Over the last several decades, neonatal intensive care for preterm infants has resulted in major improvement in their survival. Unfortunately, there is still major room for improvement in the physical as well as neurodevelopmental

outcome of these survivors. Preterm infants receiving respiratory support such as mechanical ventilation, continuous positive airway pressure (CPAP), and supplemental oxygen present challenges in terms of both intravenous and enteral nutritional support. Concerns about metabolic imbalances, especially in terms of intravenous nutritional support, have precluded in many cases the resumption of the same level of nutritional support these babies would be otherwise achieving in utero had they not been born preterm. Furthermore, concerns about maturity of the gastrointestinal tract and necrotizing enterocolitis (NEC) have led to prolonged periods prior to initiation of enteral feedings as well as prolonged periods of placing babies nil per orally (NPO).

In this chapter, we will present information about nutritional requirements for preterm infants, especially those requiring additional respiratory support. We will discuss macronutrients as well as several important micronutrients that are important in maintenance of health, growth, prevention of further damage to the lungs and other tissues, as well as promotion of optimal neurodevelopment.

Several controversial areas will be discussed, which include enteral feeding while on CPAP, mechanical ventilation, progression of enteral feedings, the relative value of mother's milk versus formula feeding for these infants, composition of parenteral nutrition (PN), and safety of PO feeding while on CPAP and high-flow nasal cannula treatment.

Nutritional goals

Preterm infants are at increased risk for potential nutritional compromise as they are born with limited nutrient reserves, immature metabolic pathways, and have increased nutrient demands. Prematurity-associated medical and surgical conditions contribute to altered nutrient requirements. There are several reasonable goals for nutritional support of these infants:

1. The goal of preterm neonatal nutrition is to mimic intrauterine growth rates and later to imitate growth rates of term breastfed infants [1].

2. We should aim to limit the degree and duration of initial weight loss in preterm infants, to support their nutritional needs, and to facilitate regain of birth weight within 7–14 days of life.

3. Approximate target weight gain considered is 10–20 g/kg/day [2].

4. Energy needs are dependent on age, weight, rate of growth, thermal environment, activity, hormonal activity, organ size, and maturation. The metabolic rate increases during the first week of life from a resting metabolic rate (RMR) of 40–41 kcal/kg/day during the first week to 62–64 kcal/kg/day by the third week of life [3].

5. Judicious nutritional support to maintain lean body mass and bone density, prevention of complications (e.g., chronic lung disease [CLD], NEC, infection), optimization of neurodevelopment growth, and consideration of its impact on adult health [2].

6. Infants receiving respiratory support and especially those with increased work of breathing require specialized nutritional support beyond that required by healthy preterm infants. The nutritional support to maintain safe metabolic balance, growth, and optimization of neurodevelopment is a special challenge of these infants with respiratory problems.

Fluids

Maintenance of fluid and electrolyte balance is essential for normal cell and organ function during intrauterine development and throughout extrauterine life. Requirements are based on gestational age, postnatal age, illness, and environmental conditions [4]. Preterm infants have immature skin, and renal function coupled with environmental factors such as use of radiant warmers and phototherapy increases water loss [5]. Table 36.1 and Table 36.2 show the insensible water losses (IWLs).

Increased fluid administration may lead to complications such as intraventricular hemorrhage (IVH), patent ductus arteriosus (PDA), bronchopulmonary dysplasia (BPD), and NEC. During the immediate postnatal period, critically ill premature infants may require volume resuscitation for shock or acidosis, which should be considered when planning subsequent fluid management [6].

Table 36.1 Sources of water loss

Renal	Immature renal functions (↓ GFR, ↓ Na reabsorption, ↓ capacity to concentrate urine, ↓ bicarbonate, K, and hydrogen ion secretion)
Extra renal	Environmental Skin breakdown and immaturity ↑ Respiratory rate Insensible water loss is inversely related to gestational age Ventilation (e.g., ↓ humidification of inspired gas) Losses in stools, NG tube drainage, intercostal drainage

Insensible water loss = fluid intake – urine output + weight change

Table 36.2 Factors influencing insensible water loss

Increased loss	Decreased loss	Incubator
Lower gestational age	Clothing	Body box
Lower postnatal age	High humidity	Plastic blanket
Denuded/broken skin		Good skin care
Increased skin temperature		Topical ointments and emollients
Increased activity		Humidification of inspired gases
Increased environmental temperature		High humidity
Radiant heat sources		
Radiant warmers		
Phototherapy units		
Draughts		
Excessive crying		

Source: Reprinted from Modi N, Fluid and electrolyte balance. In: Rennie JM, Roberton NRC, editors. Textbook of neonatology, 5th ed. Table no. 18.1 (factors influencing insensible water loss), p. 333. Copyright © 2012, Elsevier Limited, with permission from Elsevier.

Preterm infants with surfactant deficiency have low lung compliance [4]. These fragile lungs have higher tendency for barotrauma and other injuries. Also, there are chances of pulmonary capillary endothelial injury due to underlying elements of perinatal hypoxia, mechanical ventilation, and oxygen administration [7]. This damage leads to capillary leak and formation of interstitial edema which further compromises pulmonary functions [4].

RDS may lead to hypoxia and acidosis, which further compromises renal function [8]. With the gradual improvement of pulmonary function, there was noticed to be improvement in renal perfusion and diuresis which typically occurs on 3rd to 4th postnatal days (especially in presurfactant era) [4]. Further water retention may occur owing to increased secretion of aldosterone and ADH related to positive pressure ventilation [9]. Restriction of fluids in the first couple of postnatal days is still required to allow the contraction of extracellular volume [4]. If fluid restriction is not followed then fluid over load may lead to complications like PDA, IVH, NEC and BPD etc [4]. Studies on restricted water intake showed the trend toward decreased severity of complications, but increased risk of dehydration and weight loss. But these values were not statistically significant [10]. A careful fluid restriction to meet the physiological needs without allowing significant dehydration is advocated [10]. Restricted fluid demonstrated no adverse effect on the urine specific gravity or weight loss. In uncomplicated cases such as TTNB, mild fluid restriction is proved to be beneficial [11,12]. Complications like hypernatremia and dehydration should be kept in mind upon fluid restriction [13]. Fluid intake must be reassessed frequently in preterm infants requiring respiratory support. IWL for the infants in incubators during the first week of life is estimated to be higher for babies between 750 and 1000 g birth weight at approximately 80–85 mL/kg/day and is lower for more mature babies [3].

Total fluid requirements

Total fluid requirements = maintenance of fluids (IWL + urine + stool water) + growth requirements [13] (Tables 36.3 and 36.4).

IWL is greater in early days of life, whereas later the renal loss increases to compensate for the increased solute load. Stool loss is usually 5–10 mL/kg/day.

The fluid and electrolyte requirements are as follows:
- Expected weight loss of 10%–15% of birth weight during the initial 3–5 days
- Maintenance of electrolytes
- Avoidance of oliguria
- Transition to enteral intake
- Avoidance of fluid overload
- Input and output calculations

Term infants

On subsequent days, increments of 10–20 mL/kg/day may be considered based upon the tolerance of the previous

Table 36.3 Fluid requirement on day 1 of life

60–70 mL/kg/day	For urine output—50 mL/kg/day (to excrete a solute load of about 15 mosm/kg/day at a urine osmolarity of 300 mosm/kg) + IWL of 20 mL/kg

The initial fluids should be 10% dextrose in order to maintain a glucose infusion rate (GIR) of 4–6 mg/kg/min [5]

Table 36.4 Estimated starting intravenous intake, at an ambient humidity of 50%*

Gestational age (weeks)	Birth weight (kg)	Approximate transepidermal water loss (mL/kg/24 h)	Allowance for urine output (mL/kg/24 h)	Estimated intake range (mL/kg/24 h)	Suggested starting volume (mL/kg/24 h)[†]
<27	<1.0	120	30–60	150–180	150[‡]
27–30	1.0–1.5	40	30–60	70–100	90
31–36	1.5–2.5	15	30–60	45–75	60
>36	>2.5	10	30–60	40–70	60

*At higher ambient humidity, transepidermal water losses will be reduced and requirements will be lower.
[†]Once sustained weight loss of at least 5% is achieved, proceed to the intravenous volume necessary to support nutritional goals without stepwise increments.
[‡]A cautious approach, commencing at the lower end of the estimated requirement, is recommended.
Source: Reprinted from Modi N, Fluid and electrolyte balance. In: Rennie JM, Roberton NRC, editors. Textbook of neonatology, 5th ed. Table no. 18.3 (estimated starting intravenous intake, at an ambient humidity of 50%*), p. 334. Copyright © 2012, Elsevier Limited, with permission from Elsevier.

day's fluid therapy, estimations of IWL, and clinical status [5,6]. Electrolytes should be added.

Preterm infants

Extreme preterm infants require more fluids and are less tolerant of glucose [5,6]. They have increased IWL owing to skin immaturity and more weight loss compared with term babies and hence the fluid requirement will be higher during the initial 5–7 days.

Dextrose 5% provides a more suitable glucose load at these increased rates, and insulin infusions may be needed in ELBW infants. Fluids need to be increased at 10–15 mL/kg/day till a maximum of 150–160 mL/kg/day.

Monitoring and considerations

Morbidities caused by hypervolemia and hypovolemia can be prevented by proper fluid management [6,13]. After birth, the infant undergoes an isotonic contraction of the ECF compartment, with excretion of excess water, which attributes to initial weight loss. Transitional phase of volume contraction is followed by a maintenance phase, and fluid administration can then be decreased as the skin becomes more mature and IWL through the skin decreases [6].

- **Sodium:** Requirements 2–5 mEq/kg/day; to target sodium levels of 135–145 mEq/L. Sodium and potassium should be added after 48 h. Serum sodium levels can serve as a "proxy" for hydration status, and in the absence of rapidly rising sodium, fluid adequacy can be ensured.
- **Potassium:** Requirements 1–3 mEq/kg/day, administered after urine output is established.
- **Calcium:** Supplemented in preterm infants because their low body stores.
- **Nutrition:** Enteral feedings should be started as soon as possible. Intravenous fluids are simultaneously decreased as enteral fluid intake is increased.
- **Body weight:** For ELBW infants, body weights should be checked 2 or more times daily to more closely monitor fluid status. Uncompensated IWL is indicated by a cumulative weight loss of >20% in the first week. Excessive fluid administration is manifested by <2% per day of weight loss. Due to "severity of illness" many clinicians use birth weight in order to design fluid therapy until the infant is stable enough to be safely weighed. Inbuilt weighing scales in incubators may be used and fluid calculations are estimated based on gestational age, day of life, IWL, and clinical condition.
- **Blood levels:** Tests for hematocrit (HCT), sodium, potassium, blood urea nitrogen (BUN), creatinine, acidosis, and base deficit should be performed on a regular basis to monitor the hydration status and fluid adjustment to be done accordingly. Increases in any of these parameters may indicate inadequate fluid therapy. Overhydration is indicated by low sodium, a falling HCT, or a low BUN.
- **Glucose to be administered to maintain a GIR of** 5–8 mg/kg/min: Further glucose adjustments are based upon blood glucose values; up to 12–15 mg/kg/min as tolerated.
- **Fluid intake and output:** Fluid administration should be optimized to maintain a urine output of 1–3 mL/kg/h. Oliguria warrants increasing the fluids and polyuria indicates overhydration and needs fluid restriction. However, in the presence of renal failure fluid restriction might be needed in the presence of decreasing urine output. In infants without urinary catheters or urine bags, diapers need to be weighed soon after voiding to reduce errors due to evaporation [13,14].
- **General appearance and vital signs:** Hypotension, poor perfusion, tachycardia, and poor pulses may all be signs of hypovolemia.
- **Environmental factors:** The causes of increased IWL include immature skin, environmental temperature, radiant warmers, and phototherapy. Polythene wrap as heat shield may decrease IWL by 10%–30%. Optimal humidification of the isolette can decrease IWL by up to 30% [13].

Summary

1. The goal of preterm neonatal nutrition is to mimic intrauterine growth rates and later to imitate growth rates of term breastfed infants.
2. We should aim to limit the degree and duration of initial weight loss in preterm infants, to support their nutritional needs, and to facilitate regain of birth weight.
3. During the immediate postnatal period, critically ill premature infants may require volume resuscitation for shock or acidosis, which should be considered when planning subsequent fluid management.
4. Excessive fluid administration may lead to complications such as IVH, PDA, BPD, and NEC.
5. A careful fluid restriction to meet the physiological needs without allowing significant dehydration is advocated.
6. Initial fluid requirement and its subsequent increments depend on the gestational age, birth weight, postnatal age, and clinical assessment. As a general rule, preterm infants require more fluids than term infants.
7. Sodium requirements 2–5 mEq/kg/day; to target sodium levels of 135–145 mEq/L.
8. Potassium requirements 1–3 mEq/kg/day, administered after urine output is established.

9. Calcium—supplemented in preterm infants because their low body stores.
10. Fluid administration should be optimized to maintain a urine output of 1–3 mL/kg/h.

Enteral nutrition

Human milk is preferred for feeding to all newborn babies. Term healthy infants should be breastfed as soon as possible. Preterm birth survivors are at a higher risk of growth and developmental disabilities. Early administration of optimal nutrition to these babies lowers the risk of adverse health outcomes and improves cognition in adulthood [15]. Very low birth weight (VLBW) infants, growing along the lower quartiles during neonatal period, are at higher risk for neurodevelopmental damage as well as chronic pulmonary complications [16].

Infants with RDS have high work of breathing, increased oxygen consumption, and increased energy expenditure, which may lead to growth impairment. Infants on mechanical ventilation are at risk of growth delay. The causes include increased calorie requirement, prolonged PN, restricted fluid intake, and associated feed intolerance. Some infants may need exogenous steroids which further interfere with growth [17,18].

Neonates with respiratory problems often experience poor growth and delayed development. It has been shown that adequate nutrition is crucial in reducing the risk and severity of BPD and plays a major role in lung growth, lung alveolar development, and lung function including surfactant production, lung repair, and defense against infection and therefore optimizing the growth [19–21]. Therefore, inadequate early nutrition interferes with lung repair and plays an important role in pathogenesis of BPD [22].

It has been observed that CPAP may interfere with physiological increase in postnatal superior mesenteric artery blood flow [23,24] which deranges intestinal motility and leads to feed intolerance [25,26]. The CPAP may exert pressure on the diaphragm, thus increasing velocity of gastric emptying [27].

Energy intake

Denne estimated that the energy needs of infants with BPD are 15%–25% above healthy controls. An energy intake of 140–150 kcal/kg/day may be required during active periods of disease [18,28]. Weight and length gains must be strictly monitored as the energy needs differ depending upon the clinical condition and respiratory status [29].

According to the European Society of Pediatric Gastroenterology, Hepatology and Nutrition (ESPGHAN) Committee on Nutrition recommendations, the daily energy intake for healthy growing preterm infants is 110–135 kcal/kg, and higher calorie intake may be beneficial for infants with BPD [30,31].

The following criteria are assessed prior to initiating infant feeding [6]:
1. Respiratory rate <60 breaths/min for oral feeding and <80 breaths/min for gavage feeding.
2. No history of excessive oral secretions, vomiting, or bile-stained gastric aspirate.
3. Nondistended, soft abdomen, with normal bowel sounds. If the abdominal examination is abnormal, evaluation is warranted.
4. Prematurity: Trophic feeds should be started as soon as possible depending on clinical status. Delayed feeding may lead to morphologic and functional changes in the intestine with a significant decrease in gut enzyme activity, and an increase in gut permeability [32].

Initial feedings

In order of preference, mother's milk should be considered for initiating feeding and if it is not available then donor breast milk should be considered after screening and obtaining consent if the center policy permits [33]. Minimal enteral feedings (trophic feeding) are subnutritional quantities of milk, also called as hypocaloric feeds, characterized by a small-volume feeding to prime the gut. Trophic feeding has been shown to be beneficial in facilitating the gastrointestinal tract maturation, better tolerance of feeds which leads to faster attainment of full enteral feeding and decreased duration of PN [34] (Table 36.5).

Table 36.5 Volume of feeding according to birth weight

Day of feeding	<750 g	>750 to <1250 g	>1250 to <1500 g
1	0.5 mL 6 qh	0.5 mL 6 qh	1 mL 3 qh
2	1 mL 6 qh	1 mL 6 qh	Increase by 1 mL 3 qh every 12 h from day 2 until reaching full enteral
3	1 mL 3 qh	1 mL 3 qh	
4	1 mL 3 qh	1 mL 3 qh	
5	1.5 mL 3 qh for 12 h, then increase by 0.5 mL per feed every 12 h until reaching full enteral	Increase by 1 mL 3 qh every 12 h until reaching full enteral	

Minimal enteral nutrition can be started as early as the first day if there are no contraindications [6]. Early trophic feeds are known to facilitate release of endogenous agents which decrease the effects of cytokines and other inflammatory mediators [35,36]. It also helps in early establishment of gut microbiota (*Bifidobacterium* and *Lactobacillus* strains), which prevents NEC and infection [37–39].

Omega-3 and omega-6 fatty acids are concentrated in the infant brain during the last trimester and they are present in breast milk [40,41]. As per the American Society for Parenteral and Enteral Nutrition recommendations in 2009, trophic feeds can be started with a volume of 0.5–1 mL/kg/day and increased gradually by 20 mL/kg/day [42]. 0.5–1 mL/kg/h volume may be used if giving as continuous feeds [6,43]. Evidence shows that early introduction of feeding in babies with invasive or noninvasive respiratory support was not associated with increased risk of feed intolerance and NEC [44,45].

Hence it is advised that the feeding schedule for the preterm babies on respiratory support can be same as the babies without RDS [46]. Infants on CPAP manifesting as CPAP belly syndrome are shown to have no association with NEC and the feeding method does not contribute to CPAP belly [47].

If expressed breast milk is not available, special premature formula (24 kcal/oz) can be used. Formula milk should contain all essential nutrients including docosahexaenoic acid (DHA) and is specifically designed to meet the requirements of LBW infants [15,48].

Advancement of enteral feeds

Feedings should be advanced as tolerated once to twice a day and a safe rate of advancement is 10–30 mL/kg/day [6]. A study comparing fast versus slow advancement of feeds in <1250 g neonates revealed that neonates in fast feeding group attained full feeds faster than the slow feeding group. Incidence of feed intolerance and NEC were similar in both the group. The babies in fast feeding groups discharged home earlier [44]. In intrauterine growth restriction (IUGR) infants with antenatal Doppler ultrasound showing absent end-diastolic flow are of increased risk of NEC [49]. Feeding in such situations depends on clinical status of babies. However, the available evidence regarding starting early versus late feeding is not conclusive. Growth-restricted infants born <29 weeks' gestation with abnormal antenatal Doppler failed to tolerate even the careful feeding regimen of Abnormal Doppler Enteral Prescription Trial (ADEPT). A slower advancement of feeds may be required for these infants [50].

Feeding method

Routine use of nasogastric tube is not recommended in preterm infants because it may increase airway resistance by 30%–50% and may interfere with breathing [51,52]. Current evidence is insufficient to recommend any particular type of feeding method. A systematic review compares continuous versus bolus feeding method in preterm infants with birth weight <1500 g revealed better weight gain and shorter hospital stay for babies on continuous feeding [53]. Bolus feeding was associated with deranged pulmonary function and altered cerebral blood flow [54,55].

Feeding intolerance

Episodes of feeding intolerance are common in preterm infants with poor peristalsis. A small volume of altered milk is usually benign, while significant and frequent vomiting, bile- or blood-stained vomitus should be assessed. According to Ziegler et al., gastric residuals (GRs) are very frequent in the early neonatal period and are virtually always benign, for example, not associated with NEC [56].

Clearly defining feeding intolerance can lead to dramatic improvements in nutritional outcomes [57]. GR in the absence of other clinical signs and symptoms during trophic feed may not be considered as a significant sign of feeding intolerance. Feed intolerance is characterized by significant vomiting, color of aspirates, blood in stool, abdominal distension, tenderness or discoloration, and increasing abdominal girth or a combination of any of the above features [58]. Some of these may be manifested in healthy preterm so careful clinical judgment is required to prevent unnecessary interruption of feeding [59].

Gastric motility changes more rapidly to a normal pattern if feeds are started early and offered frequently rather than being withheld [60]. Routine gastric aspiration is not recommended as it may cause damage to gastric mucosa and delay enteral feeding [61,62]. In the absence of any clinical signs, <1.5 cm increase in abdominal girth may occur normally [63]. Check pre-feed gastric residual volume (GRV) only after a minimum feed volume (per feed) is attained. Use the smallest volume syringe for checking residuals. GRs are considered significant if it is greater than 30% of the previous feed, blood- or bile-stained or associated with significant systemic manifestations [64]. In infants <750 g, <2 mL of gastric aspirate and in infants 750–1500 g aspirates up to 3 mL were considered normal [65,66].

Evidence shows that there is no correlation between GR volume and attainment of full enteral nutrition [67,68]. Gastric aspirates should only be considered in the presence of abnormal gastrointestinal signs and symptoms [69]. Voidance of gastric residues may lead to loss of hydrochloric acid and pepsin resulting in intestinal bacterial overgrowth and increase the risk of late-onset sepsis and NEC [70,71]. A recent study done by Neu and colleagues on 'the value of routine evaluation of GRs in VLBW infants' concluded that routine evaluation of GRs may not improve nutritional outcomes in premature infants [67].

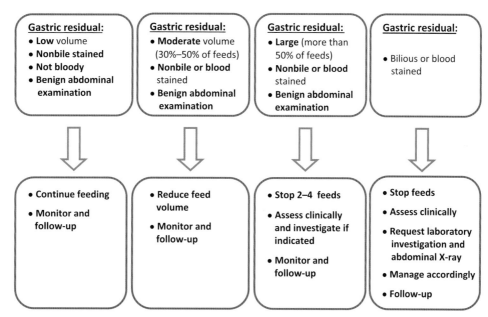

Fig. 36.1 Example Scenarios of Feeding Intolerance.

Re-feeding aspirates

Push back GR volume of up to 50% of the previous feed volume (Cobb et al.) [72]. If it recurs, subtract the residual volume from the current feed. If the GRV is >50% of the previous feed volume, and if the clinical status of the baby allows, push back the residue up to 50% of the feed volume and skip the current feed. One may consider slow bolus feeds or withholding feeds if >50% GRV persists, depending on the clinical condition (Fig. 36.1).

Considerations

If the problem of residual volumes persists despite slow bolus feeds, consider decreasing the feed volume to the last well-tolerated feed volume [6]. Vomiting bile may indicate an intestinal obstruction or ileus. Withhold feeds in case of hemorrhagic residuals, as hemorrhagic residuals are significant.

If feeding is initiated but not tolerated, a complete abdominal examination should be performed. If the abdominal evaluation is normal, we can attempt continuous feedings with a nasogastric or orogastric tube. Check the gastric aspirate and follow as per tolerance. Use breast milk preferably or special formula because they may be better tolerated.

Nutritional supplements

Extrauterine growth restriction (EUGR) is a major clinical problem in VLBW infants [73–76]. Nutritional supplements

are added to feedings, primarily to increase caloric intake with no concomitant increase in fluid volume. Nutritional supplements are often used in infants with BPD who are not gaining weight and need additional calories with no increase in protein, fat, or water intake [6].

The AAP Committee on Nutrition recommends to provide nutrients so as to achieve comparable postnatal growth rate and weight gain to that of a normal fetus of the same PMA [77].

Proteins

Supplementation with proteins results in increase in short-term weight gain, linear growth, and head growth. Protein supplement can be increased to as high as 4.5 g/kg/day in extremely preterm babies to compensate for accumulated protein deficit [21].

Term milk approximates to 0.9–1.2 g/dL for protein [78]. The recommended range of protein intake is therefore 3.5–4.5 g/kg/day [30]. Macronutrient composition differs between preterm and term milk, with preterm milk tending to be higher in protein and fat [78].

Carbohydrates

The main carbohydrate in the term human milk is lactose −6.7 to 7.8 g/dL [78]. Glucose polymers have an advantage in that they increase caloric density without a rise in osmolality. In preterm formulas, part of the carbohydrate is in the form of glucose polymers. Recommended carbohydrate intakes for premature infants are 11.6–13.2 g/kg/day [79].

Lesser amounts of carbohydrates should provide total energy requirements in infants with CLD [6].

Lipids

Ventilated infants with restricted fluid and feed intakes due to feeding intolerance may need high-fat intakes to meet energy needs. Moreover, due to the high caloric density of lipids emulsion, these are a good energy source in clinical conditions requiring fluid restriction [21].

Energy estimates range from 65 to 70 kcal/dL and are highly correlated with the fat content of human milk [78]. Term human milk content of fat is 3.2–3.6 g/dL [78]. The absorption of fatty acids increases with decreasing chain length and with the degree of unsaturation. Consequently, medium-chain triglycerides are hydrolyzed more rapidly than long-chain triglycerides. Human milk supplies 8%–12% of fat as medium-chain triglycerides. Recommended intake for preterm infants is in a range of 4.8–6.6 g/kg/day [79,80].

Calcium

Studies showed that calcium absorption depends on calcium and vitamin D intakes, and that calcium retention is additionally related to absorbed phosphorus [81]. With an intake of 120–140 mg/kg/day and at calcium absorption rate of 50%–65%, calcium retention will be approximately 60–90 mg/kg/day. In addition, 60–90 mg/kg/day (55–80 mg/100 kcal) of phosphate is recommended which can diminish the clinical symptoms of osteopenia and ensures appropriate mineralization in VLBW infants [30].

Vitamin D

A vitamin D intake of 800–1000 IU/day is recommended [30].

Iron

Daily recommended intake of iron is 2–3 mg/kg/day. Prophylactic enteral iron can be started at 2–4 weeks of age, and depending upon the postdischarge diet, it can be continued at least until 6–12 months of age [30].

Other supplements

Various nutritional supplements that may be used to maximize enteral nutrition are as follows: carbohydrate (polycose and infant rice cereal), fat (medium-chain triglyceride, vegetable oil, and micro-lipid), protein, and human milk fortifier.

Human milk fortification

Human milk fortifiers are the most efficient way to supplement protein, calcium, phosphorus, and micronutrients when premature infants are fed with human milk [82], though some studies demonstrated that the addition of HMF may temporarily delay gastric emptying and cause a short-term increase in GRs and emesis [83].

Fortification should begin when the infant is tolerating at least 50–100 mL/kg/day enteral feeds and gradually increased to achieve 24 kcal/oz [15,84]. It is advisable to start at a concentration of 1 packet/sachet:50 mL of EBM and if this is tolerated for 48 h, it can be increased to 1:25 mL of EBM [85]. For infants with fluid restriction, consider dose 1 pkg fortifier per 20 mL EBM [86].

HMF increases osmolarity of breast milk [87]. Some evidence shows increased incidence of infections and NEC in babies who received cow's milk-based fortifier versus nonfortified human milk. However, the infants in the study received >50% of their feeds from formula [88].

Fortification should continue until the infant reaches at least 1.8–2.0 kg or is established at breastfeeding [89]. Fortification may be used for longer periods of time in nutritionally compromised infants [90].

Probiotics

Definitions

- **Probiotic:** These are live selected microorganism strains, when administered in appropriate quantity confers a health benefit to the host (WHO).
- **Prebiotic:** These are nondigestible ingredients of food, which have a beneficial effect on the health of the host by selectively activating the growth and/or activity of beneficial microorganism species in the gut.
- **Symbiotic:** This a mixture of both prebiotics and probiotics.
- **Functional food:** A modified nutrition that has potential beneficial effect on health other than providing basic nutrition. Foods with probiotics or prebiotics fall in this categories [91].

Probiotics are microbial strains of human origin, are nonpathogenic, adhere to gut epithelium, colonize the intestinal tract, produce antimicrobial substances, and modulate immune responses [92]. Probiotics act on mucosal immune system and alter the gut permeability by interacting with commensal microorganisms and pathogenic organisms [93].

Breast milk contains various probiotic strains like *Bifidobacteria* (primarily *Bifidobacterium longum* subsp. *infantis*) and also oligosaccharides that act as prebiotics; hence, it is considered as functional food [94].

Probiotics inhibit growth of pathogenic microorganisms and decrease gut inflammation. In preterm neonates, there is less colonization of commensals in gut which increases the risk of NEC [92,95]. Probiotics are Gram-positive nonpathogenic and nontoxigenic live microbes, and colonization with these organisms is thought to protect the gut from colonization by more pathogenic species [96]. Probiotic products contain lactobacilli and *Bifidobacterium*, the predominant organisms found in the GI tract of healthy breastfed infants.

As evidenced in Cochrane review, probiotics decrease the incidence of NEC and death in VLBW infants [97]. But the data on protective effect of probiotics in ELBW babies are limited.

Summary

1. Human milk is preferred for feeding to term, preterm, and sick infants.
2. Term healthy infants should be breastfed as soon as possible.
3. It is important that early aggressive nutritional strategy should be used so as to ensure smooth transition from the intrauterine to the extrauterine life.
4. Nutrition and pulmonary function in VLBWIs are closely interrelated.
5. It has been shown that adequate nutrition is crucial in reducing the risk and severity of BPD and plays a major role in lung growth, lung alveolar development, and lung function including surfactant production, lung repair, and defense against infection.
6. According to the European Society of Pediatric Gastroenterology, Hepatology and Nutrition (ESPGHAN) Committee on Nutrition recommendations, the daily energy intake for healthy growing preterm infants is 110–135 kcal/kg, and higher calorie intake may be beneficial for infants with BPD.
7. Minimal enteral nutrition can be started as early as the first day when there are no contraindications.
8. Ventilator or CPAP treatment should not serve as a hindrance to enteral feeding.
9. A systematic review compares continuous versus bolus feeding method in preterm infants with birth weight <1500 g revealed better weight gain and shorter hospital stay for babies on continuous feeding.
10. Enteral feedings should be advanced as clinically tolerated.
11. A small volume of altered milk is usually benign, while significant and frequent vomiting, bile- or blood-stained vomitus should be assessed.
12. If the problem of residual volumes persists despite slow bolus feeds, consider decreasing the feed volume to the last well-tolerated feed volume.
13. Extra uterine growth restriction (EUGR) is a major clinical problem in VLBW infants; hence, nutrient supplementation needs meticulous care.
14. Human milk fortifiers are the most efficient way to supplement protein, calcium, phosphorus, and micronutrients when premature infants are fed with human milk.
15. Probiotics inhibit growth of pathogenic microorganisms and decrease gut inflammation. In preterm neonates, there is less colonization of commensals in gut, which increases the risk of NEC.

Parenteral nutrition

Intravenous administration of all nutrients in sufficient amounts is necessary for metabolic requirements and adequate growth. The components of the PN are protein, carbohydrates, lipids, minerals, vitamins, and trace elements. It is a substitute for enteral feeding in circumstances where the initiation and establishment of full enteral feeds will be delayed or inadequate.

There is growing evidence that inadequate nutrition early in life delays the time to regain birth weight and subsequently leads to extrauterine growth restriction [98]. Inadequate supplementation of early nutrition to ELBW infants is associated with critical illness in the first week of life and later growth. This is also associated with worsening BPD, late-onset sepsis, prolonged hospital stays, neurodevelopmental impairment, cognition, and death [99,100].

To prevent the growth failure, avoid early malnutrition and in order to enhance neurodevelopment in ELBW babies, administrating TPN early in the initial postnatal hours is very important [101].

PN for the premature infant is classified as follows [102]:
- Administration of adequate calories for optimal growth.
- To satisfy the energy requirement, carbohydrates in combination with lipids can be administered. Positive nitrogen balance required for optimal growth can be attained by providing sufficient protein intake, which includes essential amino acids.
- Minerals, electrolytes, vitamins, and trace elements are also supplemented.

PN is classified as follows [98]:
- Total when all the energy/nutrition is administered parenterally.
- Partial or supplemental when used along with enteral nutrition.

Indications

Medical

- Prematurity
- Ileus
- Hypoxic-ischemic encephalopathy
- Cooling
- Feeding intolerance
- Short gut syndrome
- Failure to thrive secondary to cardiac/renal/pulmonary diseases [98]

Surgical

- Hirschsprung disease
- Intestinal atresias
- Surgical NEC/bowel perforation
- Gastrointestinal malformations (e.g., gastroschisis, omphalocele, imperforate anus, esophageal atresia/tracheoesophageal fistula)
- Diaphragmatic hernia

Routes

The following two routes are commonly used for administration [6,79,103]:

- **Central PN:** It is used in babies requiring long-term administration of nutrients and calories. It involves infusion of a hypertonic nutrient solution (up to 15%–25% dextrose) into a catheter with tip in a central position.
- **Peripheral PN:** It is indicated in the neonates who require short-term infusion of nutrients and is used as a route for partial PN or supplemental PN in situations where full feeds are likely to be achieved relatively soon. The maximum concentration of dextrose that can be administered is 12.5%.

Fluids and energy

"Water—the major nutrient" is the title of a review illustrating that water represents the major component of the human body as well as of enteral and PN [104]. In fetuses, water content decreases from 95% initially to 85% by 8 months of gestation and downs to 75% at term [105]. In neonates who are parenterally fed and are stabilized in a thermoneutral environment have a RMR of 40–60 kcal/kg/day.

For every gram of gain in weight, 3–4.5 kcal of energy is utilized [106]; 50 kcal/kg/day is optimal for ongoing expenditure, but for optimal growth an additional of 70 kcal/kg/day is required. Energy needs may need to be identified and optimized for a rapidly growing preterm baby. Some

hypermetabolic infants and infants with CLD may require ≥ 120 kcal/kg/day [6,107].

The energy sources available to the neonate are carbohydrates and fat, which provide 4 and 9 kcal/g, respectively [108]. Ideal distribution of calories should be 60% carbohydrate, 10%–15% protein, and 30% (25%–40%) fat [6]. Protein, which can provide approximately 4 kcal/g, is not typically used unless total energy expenditure exceeds total energy intake [108].

Term infants require a minimum of 60 mL/kg/day on day 1 of life and subsequently intake can be increased as per tolerance to reach a total of 120–150 mL/kg/day [105]. In preterm neonates, fluid needs are higher. They need up to 80–100 mL/kg/day on day 1 of life and required to be increased by 10–20 mL/kg/day to reach a total of 130 to 180 mL/kg/day [105].

An account of total daily intake (including other infusions, e.g., UAC/UVC fluid, inotropes, drugs) is important and it may warrant the need of checking the concentration of solution for nutrition. Studies show that there is increased risk of death, BPD, and PDA with fluid overload and reduced incidence with restricted intake [19,109–111]. Therefore, a "prudent prescription" of water intake for preterm infants so that physiological needs can be met without causing significant dehydration is advised [111].

Extrauterine growth restriction is difficult to overcome, and poorer growth during the neonatal period is associated with long-term adverse neurocognitive effects [98]. Up to 4.6-point increase in Bayley Mental Development Index (MDI) was observed in babies who received higher energy supply during their first postnatal week [103].

Nutrients and respiratory diseases

Carbohydrates

High rate of carbohydrate delivery (>12.5 mg/kg/min) increases carbon dioxide production as it has a high respiratory quotient (RQ). To excrete the built-up CO_2, there is increase in work of breathing and increased ventilator requirements, thereby exposing the infants to ventilator-associated injuries. Infants on mechanical ventilation may benefit by receiving lipids as they have lower RQ and are energy dense [108].

Lipids

Lipid emulsions produce vasoactive metabolites, increase ventilation/perfusion mismatch, and effect pulmonary functions by impairing gas exchange. Early initiation of lipids is advantageous despite its effects on lung ventilation as significant growth failure is associated with severe lung disease [108].

Protein

Negative nitrogen balance and undernutrition lead to delayed structural and functional maturation of lungs, which escalates risk of hyperoxia, barotrauma, and infection. Low oncotic pressure in protein-deficient infants can lead to pulmonary edema. A lower incidence of CLD has been reported in infants receiving higher protein intakes (4 g/kg/day) than in those receiving 3 g/kg/day [98].

Protein intolerance in babies receiving amino acid intakes of up to 2.9 g/kg/day was not evidenced in ventilated babies in their first week of life [112]. Evidence suggest that infants can be started at or close to the maximal protein dose and gradual increments is not necessary [108].

It was demonstrated that high-dose dexamethasone for BPD reduces linear growth and weight gain by markedly increasing protein breakdown without affecting rates of protein synthesis [113].

Minerals

Transient neonatal hypocalcemia often is exacerbated by acute respiratory disease. Infants whose mothers have received magnesium sulfate have higher risk of having hypermagnesemia which may lead to apnea [108].

Vitamins

Studies showed that early vitamin A supplementation during the time of acute pulmonary disease can decrease the risk of BPD [108].

Composition of parenteral nutrition solutions

Carbohydrates

The endogenous glucose production is estimated to be 8 mg/kg/min in term and 6 mg/kg/min in preterm infants, and these rates can be used as starting points [114,115]. Excess glucose administration results in its conversion to lipids which have clinical effects on exacerbation of lung diseases [116,117].

In infants receiving long-term PN, maximum glucose oxidation capacity is 12 mg/kg/min and, therefore, should not exceed this concentration generally [118]. Glucose oxidative capacity is affected by gestational age and clinical status. The minimum recommended blood glucose concentration is 45 mg/dL [119,120].

ELBW infants sometimes have hyperglycemia in initial days because of their limited glycogen storage capacity and they also fail to respond to exogenous supply by inability to suppress endogenous production. It can be managed by decreasing glucose infusion rate or using intravenous insulin [121,122].

A suggested range of hyperglycemia in ELBW babies is 150–220 mg/dL [122]. Higher glucose infusion rates >5 to 8 mg/kg/min may hamper endogenous insulin response and may potentially lead to osmotic diuresis [6]. Hyperglycemia may also be stabilized by administering amino acids early as it stimulates endogenous insulin secretion [121]. Infusion rates can be increased gradually by 0.5–2 mg/kg/min/day as per tolerance to achieve adequate caloric intake [6]. The presence of glucose in urine needs to be monitored.

Proteins

Protein accretion rates by fetuses demonstrates a declining trend from 4.0, 3.6, and 3.3 g/kg/day at 24–25, 27–28, and 30–32 weeks' gestation, respectively [123,124]. Net protein accretion in babies can be enhanced by infusing amino acids with glucose from the first postnatal day as it serves a substrate and prevents protein catabolism [125,126]. It is important to the reduce number of hours an infant is receiving in suboptimal nutrition, that is, without amino acids [127].

Nitrogen retention and growth may correspond to the intrauterine rate when amino acid intake is 2.7–3.5 g/kg/day and nonprotein energy intake is 80–85 kcal/kg/day [19]. Older practice of commencing amino acids at 0.5–1 g/kg/day and increasing it gradually is challenged, and a regimen maximizing protein intake (at least 3 g/kg/day) from day 1 of life in VLBW infants is associated with shorted time of PN and better weight gain [125–130].

With the use of current crystalline solutions of amino acids, the complications such as metabolic acidosis, azotemia, and hyperammonemia are minimized [131–133]. The current recommendations for preterm infants are to start amino acids at minimum 2.5–3 g/kg/day in the first day of life and advance to 3.5 g/kg/day and adequate nonprotein energy meets requirements for anabolism [98]. Protein should provide 8%–10% of total calories, and should not exceed 12% [1]. Inadequate protein intake may result in failure to thrive, hypoalbuminemia, and edema [6].

Cysteine hydrochloride and glutamine

Cysteine is often considered a semiessential AA in the newborn period, as the premature infants are unable to convert methionine to cysteine [6]; hence, it is added routinely to AA preparations [134]. Cysteine is a major substrate for glutathione, an antioxidant important in maintaining redox potential and calcium homeostasis [134]. Cysteine prevents the precipitation of calcium and phosphorous and increases its bioavailability by reducing the PH of solution. As cysteine demonstrates lower solubility, it is added last to the solution at a dose of 30–40 mg/g AA [6,135]. It may also decrease hepatic cholestasis [6].

Glutamine, the most abundant amino acid in plasma and human milk, is not included in PN solutions owing to decreased solubility [98].

Lipids

Lipids acts as a high energy source with low osmolarity [103]. Lipid emulsions are available in 10, 20, and 30% concentrations. For infants, the 20% concentration is preferred because of the lower phospholipid content and more rapid clearance than 10% emulsions [98]. Lipids should provide 40%–50% of the daily energy intake [98].

Essential fatty acids cannot be synthesized endogenously by infants [103]. Therefore, specifically ω-6 and ω-3 fatty acids or their precursors (i.e., linoleic acid [LA] and alpha-linolenic acid [ALA]) must be provided in PN [124].

There is no strong evidence to support low initial dose of lipids (as traditionally practiced) and its gradual increment versus staring higher doses (2–3 g/kg/day) on day 1 of life [136–138]. Evidence reflects that administration of higher lipid doses of 0.2 g/kg/h and 4 g/kg/day in VLBW infants has no deleterious effects on blood pH and alveolar–arteriolar oxygen diffusion gradient [136]. Evidence shows that optimizing nutrition (use of 3–3.5 g/kg/day of proteins and 3g/kg/day of lipids) from day 1 of life (even during 1 to 2 hours of age) in VLBW infants is well tolerated without any adverse effects or increase in duration of mechanical ventilation [139,140].

The inhibitions and dogmas related to the early use of intravenous lipids have either been disproved, not based on fact, or weak. Salama et al. recommended to start intravenous lipids on day 1 of life at 2–3 g/kg/day. Lipid should be given as a continuous infusion over 24 hours at a rate not exceeding 0.15 g/kg/h [136].

Carnitine

Carnitine is a carrier molecule necessary for oxidation of long-chain fatty acids and its synthesis, and storage is not well developed in infants <34 weeks of gestation [6,141]. However, a meta-analysis does not show beneficial effect of carnitine on ketogenesis and lipid tolerance [142].

Carnitine-deficient infants may experience hypotonia, nonketotic hypoglycemia, cardiomyopathy, encephalopathy, and recurrent infections [6]. Nonetheless, carnitine supplementation at 2–10 mg/kg is recommended in infants exclusively receiving PN for more than 4 weeks [130].

Vitamins

Preterm infants are especially at risk for vitamin deficiency due to their poor vitamin stores and increased requirement for rapid growth [103]. Both fat and water-soluble vitamins should be given within 48 h of commencing PN. Vitamins are added to intravenous solutions as water-soluble vitamins and fat-soluble vitamins, available as pediatric multivitamin suspension/reconstituted from sterile lyophilized powder.

Table 36.6 Vitamins

Recommendations		Composition of Vitlipid (per mL)
Vitamin A	700–1500 IU	230 units
Vitamin D	40–160 IU	40 units
Vitamin E	2.8–3.5 IU	0.7 units
Vitamin K	10 μg	20 μg

Source: Reprinted from Cairns P. Parenteral nutrition. In: Rennie JM, Roberton NRC, editors. Textbook of neonatology, 5th ed. Table no. 17.3 (Vitamins), p. 324. Copyright © 2012, Elsevier Limited, with permission from Elsevier.

Various formulations are available with different recommendations.

Examples: Water-soluble vitamins are supplied as solution (Soluvit) containing thiamine, riboflavin, nicotinamide, pyridoxine, sodium pantothenate, vitamin C, biotin, folic acid, and cyanocobalamin (Table 36.6).

Dose of Soluvit: 1 mL/kg/day. Fat-soluble vitamins are given along with intralipids. (Up to maximum of 10 mL) which is available as Vitalipid. Dose of Vitalipid: 4 mL/kg/day [143].

Trace elements

Trace elements are a very important constitute of prolonged TPN [6]. Zinc, copper, manganese, chromium, selenium, and molybdenum are currently recommended for neonatal PN [103] (Table 36.7).

Electrolytes

Sodium, potassium, chloride, calcium, magnesium, and phosphorus levels need to be closely monitored and the infusion needs to be prescribed accordingly (Table 36.7). Sodium and potassium are generally not required in the first 24 h until natriuresis is started and are needed to be monitored on at least daily basis, but smaller babies may require more frequent monitoring [144]. Restricted sodium intake in VLBW infants is shown to have a beneficial effect on oxygen requirement and risk of BPD [145].

Maximum fetal accretion of calcium (140 mg/kg/day) and phosphorous (75 mg/kg/day) occurs in third trimester of pregnancy, hence the goal of PN in PT babies should be to achieve these intrauterine rates [130].

Heparin

To prevent catheter occlusion and thrombosis, prophylactic heparin at a dose of 0.25–1 U/mL of PN solution is used [146–149]. Heparin has been shown to increase lipoprotein lipase levels and lipolytic activity, thereby stabilizing triglyceride levels [147].

Table 36.7 Recommendations for intravenous mineral, trace elements, and vitamins in very low birth weight infants (amount per kilogram per day)

Sodium	3–5 mmol
Chloride	3–7 mmol
Potassium	2–3 mmol
Calcium	1.5–2.0 mmol
Phosphorus	1.5–1.9 mmol
Magnesium	0.2–0.3 mmol
Zinc	6.1 µmol
Copper	0.3 µmol
Selenium	19–57 nmol
Manganese	18.2 nmol
Iodine	7.9 nmol
Chromium	1–5.8 nmol
Molybdenum	2.6 nmol

Source: Reprinted from Cairns P. Parenteral nutrition. In: Rennie JM, Roberton NRC, editors. Textbook of neonatology, 5th ed. Table no. 17.2 (recommendations for intravenous mineral, trace elements and vitamins in very low birthweight infants (amount per kilogram per day), p. 324. Copyright © 2012, Elsevier Limited, with permission from Elsevier.

Table 36.8 Risks associated with total parenteral nutrition

Metabolic

Hyperglycaemia
Hyperchloraemic acidosis
Metabolic bone disease of prematurity
Abnormal aminogram
Hyperlipidaemia

Line-related

Infection

Atrial or superior venocaval thrombus
Pleural effusions
Pericardial tamponade, peritoneal extravasation
Tissue necrosis from extravasation injury

General

Cholestasis
Gut mucosal atrophy

Source: Reprinted from Cairns P. Parenteral nutrition. In: Rennie JM, Roberton NRC, editors. Textbook of neonatology, 5th ed. Table no. 17.1 (risks associated with total parenteral nutrition), p. 322., Copyright © 2012, Elsevier Limited, with permission from Elsevier.

Complications of parenteral nutrition

Most of the metabolic complications can be prevented using a stepwise advancement in the constituents and careful monitoring (Table 36.8). Infectious complications can be prevented by aseptic line insertion and careful maintenance, including sterile change of infusion solutions, minimizing access to the line for administering other medications or blood products, and removing the catheters when enteral feeds are progressing well and have reached 80–100 mL/kg/day.

Monitoring of parenteral nutrition

At least daily or more frequent monitoring of fluid intake, glucose, electrolytes, blood gas and urine output is advocated till stabilization of acutely ill newborns [103]. Monitoring the infant and adjusting the PN to his or her needs is of paramount importance to prevent complications and achieve the desired growth and development.

Once the baby is stable, the pricks can be optimized and collaborated with other collections.

Following is the suggested monitoring plan as described in PN chapter in workbook in practical neonatology (Table 36.9).

Table 36.9 Monitoring during parenteral nutrition

Daily body weight and weekly body length and head circumference
Initially during grading-up of parenteral nutrients or during periods of metabolic instability: Strict fluid balance
• 6–12-hourly blood glucose
• Daily plasma sodium, potassium, calcium, urea, and acid–base
• Twice-weekly triglycerides
When on full parenteral nutrition and during metabolic steady state:
• Strict fluid balance
• 12–24-hourly blood glucose
• Twice-weekly plasma sodium, potassium, calcium, urea, and acid–base
Plasma magnesium, phosphorus, alkaline phosphatase, albumin, transaminases, triglycerides, and bilirubin (total and conjugated) weekly
Plasma amino acids and ammonia not usually routinely monitored
Trace elements and fat-soluble vitamins should be monitored monthly

Source: Reprinted from Cairns P. Parenteral nutrition. In: Rennie JM, Roberton NRC, editors. Textbook of neonatology, 5th ed. Table no. 17.3 (monitoring during parenteral nutrition), p. 325. Copyright © 2012, Elsevier Limited, with permission from Elsevier.

Weaning parenteral nutrition

- Planning of weaning should be simultaneously started from the inception TPN.
- Weaning of PN should be considered once the baby is able to tolerate some enteral feed which should be initiated as early as possible.
- Newborns may need frequent monitoring of glucose after the solution has been stopped.
- PN should generally be continued until at least 75% or 120 mL/kg/day of nutritional requirement is tolerated enterally.

Summary

1. To prevent the growth failure, avoid early malnutrition, and to enhance neurodevelopment in ELBW babies, administrating TPN from the initial postnatal hours is very important.
2. PN is a substitute for enteral feeding in circumstances where the establishment of full enteral feeds will be delayed or inadequate owing to the associated clinical condition of the baby.
3. Inadequate supplementation of early nutrition to ELBW infants is associated with critical illness in the first week of life and later growth and outcomes such as BPD, late-onset sepsis, hospital stays, neurodevelopmental impairment, cognition, and death.
4. Each gram of weight gain for growth, including the stored energy and the energy costs of component synthesis, requires between 3 and 4.5 kcal.
5. 50 kcal/kg/day is optimal for ongoing expenditure but for optimal growth an additional 70 kcal/kg/day is required.
6. Energy needs may need to be identified and optimized for a rapidly growing preterm baby. Some hypermetabolic infants and infants with CLD may require ≥120 kcal/kg/day.
7. Studies show that there is increased risk of death, BPD, and PDA with fluid overload and reduced incidence with restricted intake.
8. High rates of carbohydrate delivery (>12.5 mg/kg/min) increases carbon dioxide production as it has a high respiratory quotient (RQ). To excrete the built-up CO_2, there is increase in work of breathing and increased ventilator requirements, thereby exposing the infants to the risk of ventilator-associated injuries. Infants on mechanical ventilation may be benefited by receiving lipids as they have lower RQ and are energy dense.
9. The current recommendations for preterm infants are to start amino acids at minimum 2.5–3 g/kg/day in the first day of life and advance to 3.5 g/kg/day and adequate nonprotein energy meets requirements for anabolism.
10. Evidence shows starting 2–3 g/kg/day of intravenous lipids to be given at a rate not exceeding 0.15 g/kg/h as an infusion over 24 h starting on day 1.

References

[1] American Academy of Pediatrics. Pediatric nutrition handbook. 6th ed. Elk Grove Village, IL: American Academy of Pediatrics; 2009.

[2] desRobert C, Lane R, Li N, Neu J. Neonatal nutrition and consequences on adult health. NeoReviews 2005;6(5):e211–e219.

[3] Ellard DM, Anderson DM. Nutrition. In: Cloherty JP, Eichenwald EC, editors. Manual of neonatal care. 7th ed. Wolters Kluwer/Lippincott Williams & Williams; 2012.

[4] Michael AP, Jacquelyn RE. Avery's disease of the newborn. 9th ed. Elsevier; 2011.

[5] Aggarwal R, Deorari A, Paul VK. Fluid and electrolyte management in term and preterm neonates. Division of Neonatology, Department of Pediatrics; All India Institute of Medical Sciences; India.

[6] Gomella LT, Cunningham D, Fabien E. Fluid and electrolytes. In: Neonatology: management, procedures, on-call problems, diseases, and drugs. 7th ed. McGraw-Hill Education/LANGE; 2013.

[7] Zwer-Aleka FK. Pulmonary injury, oxidant stress, and gap junctional communication. Acute lung injury and acute respiratory distress syndrome—part II (applied physiology) [extensive basic and clinical study]. MedCrave Group LLC Publishing; 2016. p. 43–46.

[8] Bell EF, Acarregui MJ. Restricted versus liberal water intake for preventing morbidity and mortality in preterm infants. Cochrane Database Syst Rev 2000;2:CD000503.

[9] Koyner Jay L, Murray Patrick T. Mechanical ventilation and the kidney. Blood Purif 2010;29(1):52–68.

[10] Bell EF, Acarregui MJ. Restricted versus liberal water intake for preventing morbidity and mortality in preterm infants. Cochrane Database Syst Rev 2014;12:CD000503.

[11] Dehdashtian M, Aramesh MR, Melekian A, Aletayeb MH, Ghaemmaghami A. Restricted versus standard maintenance fluid volume in management of transient tachypnea of newborn: a clinical trial. Iran J Pediatr 2014;24(5):575–580.

[12] Stroustrup A, Trasande L, Holzman IR. Randomized controlled trial of restrictive fluid management in transient tachypnea of the newborn. J Pediatr 2012;160(1). 38.e1–43.e1.

[13] Namasivayam A, Rosenkrantz T. Fluid, electrolyte, and nutrition management of the newborn; 2014; Medscape articles on pediatrics: cardiac disease and critical care medicine; Medscape. Available from: http://emedicine.medscape.com/article/976386-overview.

[14] Hermansen MC, Buches M. Urine output determination from superabsorbent and regular diapers under radiant heat. Pediatrics 1988;81(3):428–431.

[15] Kumar RK, et al. Optimizing nutrition in preterm low birth weight infants—consensus summary. Front Nutr 2017;4:20.

[16] Ehrenkranz RA, Dusick AM, Vohr BR, Wright LL, Wrage LA, Poole WK. Growth in the neonatal intensive care unit influences neurodevelopmental and growth outcomes of extremely low birth weight infants. Pediatrics 2006;117:1253–1261.

[17] Kurzner SI, Garg M, Bautista DB, Bader D, Merritt RJ, Warburton D, et al. Growth failure in infants with bronchopulmonary dysplasia: nutrition and elevated resting metabolic expenditure. Pediatrics 1988;81:379–384.

[18] Dani C, Poggi C. Nutrition and bronchopulmonary dysplasia. J Matern Fetal Neonatal Med 2012;25(Suppl. 3):37–40.

[19] Stephens BE, Gargus RA, Walden RV, Mance M, Nye J, McKinley L, et al. Fluid regimens in the first week of life may increase risk of patent ductus arteriosus in extremely low birth weight infants. J Perinatol 2008;28:123–128.

[20] Davidson S, Schrayer A, Wielunsky E, Krikler R, Lilos P, Reisner SH. Energy intake, growth, and development in ventilated very-low-birth-weight infants with and without bronchopulmonary dysplasia. Am J Dis Child 1990;144:553–559.

[21] Bozzetti V, et al. Nutritional approach to preterm infants on noninvasive ventilation: an update. Nutrition 2017;37:14–17.

[22] deRegnier RA, Guilbert TW, Mills MM, Georgieff MK. Growth failure and altered body composition are established by one month of age in infants with bronchopulmonary dysplasia. J Nutr 1996;126:168–175.

[23] Havranek T, Thompson Z, Carver JD. Factors that influence mesenteric artery blood flow velocity in newborn preterm infants. J Perinatol 2006;26:493–497.

[24] Robel-Tillig E, Knupfer M, Pulzer F, Vogtmann C. Blood flow parameters of the superior mesenteric artery as an early predictor of intestinal dysmotility in preterm infants. Pediatr Radiol 2004;34:958–962.

[25] Bozzetti V, Paterlini G, De Lorenzo P, Gazzolo D, Valsecchi MG, Tagliabue PE. Impact of continuous vs bolus feeding on splanchnic perfusion in very low birth weight infants: a randomized trial. J Pediatr 2016;176. 86.e2–92.e2.

[26] Fang S, Kempley ST, Gamsu HR. Prediction of early tolerance to enteral feeding in preterm infants by measurement of superior mesenteric artery blood flow velocity. Arch Dis Child Fetal Neonatal Ed 2001;85:F42–F45.

[27] Gounaris A, Costalos C, Varchalama L, Kokori P, Kolovou E, Alexiou N. Gastric emptying in very-low-birth-weight infants treated with nasal continuous positive airway pressure. J Pediatr 2004;145:508–510.

[28] Denne SC. Energy expenditure in infants with pulmonary insufficiency: is there evidence for increased energy needs? J Nutr 2001;131:935S–937S.

[29] Carlson SJ. Current nutrition management of infants with chronic lung disease. Nutr Clin Pract 2004;19:581–586.

[30] Agostoni C, Buonocore G, Carnielli VP, De Curtis M, Darmaun D, Decsi T, et al. Enteral nutrient supply for preterm infants: commentary from the European Society of Paediatric Gastroenterology, Hepatology and Nutrition Committee on Nutrition. J Pediatr Gastroenterol Nutr 2010;50:85–91.

[31] Yunis KA, Oh W. Effects of intravenous glucose loading on oxygen consumption, carbon dioxide production, and resting energy expenditure in infants with bronchopulmonary dysplasia. J Pediatr 1989;115:127–132.

[32] Adamkin DH. Nutritional strategies for the very low birth weight infant. Cambridge University press; 2009.

[33] Ho MY, Yen YH. Trend of nutritional support in preterm infants. Pediatr Neonatol 2016;57:365–370.

[34] Morgan J, Young L, McGuire W. Delayed introduction of progressive enteral feeds to prevent necrotising enterocolitis in very low birth weight infants. Cochrane Database Syst Rev 2014;12:CD001970.

[35] Marik PE, Zaloga GP. Early enteral nutrition in acutely ill patients: a systematic review. Crit Care Med 2001;29:2264–2270.

[36] Sánchez C, López-Herce J, Carrillo A, Mencía S, Vigil D. Early transpyloric enteral nutrition in critically ill children. Nutrition 2007;23:16–22.

[37] Berseth CL, Nordyke C. Enteral nutrients promote postnatal maturation of intestinal motor activity in preterm infants. Am J Physiol 1993;264:G1046–G1051.

[38] Leaf A, Dorling J, Kempley S, McCormick K, Mannix P, Linsell L, et al. Early or delayed enteral feeding for preterm growth restricted infants: a randomized trial. Pediatrics 2012;129:e1260–e1268.

[39] Henderson G, Anthony MY, McGuire W. Formula milk versus maternal breast milk for feeding preterm or low birth weight infants. Cochrane Database Syst Rev 2007;4:CD002972.

[40] Helland IB, Smith L, Saarem K, Saugstad OD, Drevon CA. Maternal supplementation with very-long-chain n-3 fatty acids during pregnancy and lactation augments children's IQ at 4 years of age. Pediatrics 2003;111:e39–e44.

[41] Innis SM. Human milk: maternal dietary lipids and infant development. Proc Nutr Soc 2007;66:397–404.

[42] Bankhead R, Boullata J, Brantley S, Corkins M, Guenter P, Krenitsky J, et al. Enteral nutrition practice recommendations. JPEN J Parenter Enteral Nutr 2009;33:122–167.

[43] Morgan J, Bombell S, McGuire W. Early trophic feeding versus enteral fasting for very preterm or very low birth weight infants. Cochrane Database Syst Rev 2013;3:CD000504.

[44] Salhotra A, Ramji S. Slow versus fast enteral feed advancement in very low birth weight infants: a randomized control trial. Indian Pediatr 2004;41(5):435–441.

[45] Morgan J, Young L, McGuire W. Slow advancement of enteral feed volumes to prevent necrotising enterocolitis in very low birth weight infants. Cochrane Database Syst Rev 2014;12:CD001241.

[46] Newell SJ, Morgan ME, Durbin GM, Booth IW, McNeish AS. Does mechanical ventilation precipitate gastro-oesophageal reflux during enteral feeding? Arch Dis Child 1989;64:1352–1355.

[47] Jaile JC, Levin T, Wung JT, Abramson SJ, Ruzal-Shapiro C, Berdon WE. Benign gaseous distension of the bowel in premature infants treated with nasal continuous airway pressure: a study of contributing factors. AJR Am J Roentgenol 1992;158:125–127.

[48] Bentley D, Aubrey S, Bentley M. Infant feeding and nutrition for primary care: preterm and low birth weight babies. Radcliffe Medical Press Ltd; 2004. p. 47–51.

[49] Dorling J, Kempley S, Leaf A. Feeding growth restricted preterm infants with abnormal antenatal Doppler results. Arch Dis Child Fetal Neonatal Ed 2005;90(5):F359–F363.

[50] Kempley S, Gupta N, Lindsell L, Dorling J. ADEPT Trial Collaborative Group. Feeding infants below 29 weeks' gestation with abnormal antenatal Doppler: analysis from a randomised trial. Arch Dis Child Fetal Neonatal Ed 2014;99(1):F6–F11.

[51] Stocks J. Effect of nasogastric tubes on nasal resistance during infancy. Arch Dis Child 1980;55:17.

[52] van Someren V, Linnett SJ, Stothers JK, Sullivan PG. An investigation into the benefits of resiting nasoenteric feeding tubes. Pediatrics 1984;74:379–383.

[53] Premji SS, Chessell L. Continuous nasogastric milk feeding versus intermittent bolus milk feeding for premature infants less than 1500 grams. Cochrane Database Syst Rev 2011;11:CD001819.

[54] Blondheim O, Abbasi S, Fox WW, Bhutani VK. Effect of enteral gavage feeding rate on pulmonary functions of very low birth weight infants. J Pediatr 1993;122:751–755.

[55] Nelle M, Hoecker C, Linderkamp O. Effects of bolus tube feeding on cerebral blood flow velocity in neonates. Arch Dis Child Fetal Neonatal Ed 1997;76:F54–F56.

[56] Adamkin DH, Ziegler EE, et al. Aggressive nutrition of the very low birth weight infant. Clin Periatol 2002;29:225–244.

[57] Schanler RJ. The low birth weight infant. In: Walker, Watkins, Duggan, editors. Nutrition in pediatrics: basic science and clinical applications. 3rd ed. Hamilton, Ontario: BC Decker, Inc; 2003.

[58] Nutritional Support of the Very Low Birth Weight Infant; Quality Improvement Toolkit; California Perinatal Quality Care Collaborative; CPQCC Toolkit Rev. 2008.

[59] Quigley MA, et al. Formula milk versus donor breast milk for feeding preterm or low birth weight infants. Cochrane Database Syst Rev 2007;4:CD002971.

[60] Berseth CL, et al. Prolonges small feeding volumes early in life decreases the incidence of necrotising enterocolitis in very low birht weight infants. Pediatrics 2003;111:529–534.

[61] McClave SA, Snider HL. Clinical use of gastric residual volumes as a monitor for patients on enteral tube feeding. JPEN J Parenter Enteral Nutr 2002;26:S43–S48.

[62] Parker L, Torrazza RM, Li Y, Talaga E, Shuster J, Neu J. Aspiration and evaluation of gastric residuals in the neonatal intensive care unit: state of the science. J Perinat Neonatal Nurs 2015;29:51–59.

[63] Bhatia P, Johnson KJ, Bell EF. Variability of abdominal circumference of premature infants. J Pediatr Surg 1990;25:543–544.

[64] Fanaro S. Feeding intolerance in the preterm infant. Early Hum Dev 2013;89(Suppl. 2):S13–S20.

[65] Mihatsch WA, et al. The significance of gastric residuals in the early enteral feeding advancement of extremely low birth weight infants. Pediatrics 2002;109:457–459.

[66] Bertino E, et al. Necrotising enterocolitis: risk factor analysis and role of gastric residuals in very low birth weight infants. J Pediatr Gastroenterol Nutr 2009;48(4):437–442.

[67] Torrazza RM, Parker LA, Li Y, Talaga E, Shuster J, Neu J. The value of routine evaluation of gastric residuals in very low birth weight infants. J Perinatol 2015;35(1):57–60.

[68] Shulman RJ, Ou CN, Smith E.O. Evaluation of potential factors predicting attainment of full gavage feedings in preterm infants. Neonatology 2011;99(1):38–44.

[69] Berman L, Moss RL. Necrotizing enterocolitis: an update. Semin Fetal Neonatal Med 2011;16(3):145–150.

[70] Basaran UN, Celayir S, Eray N, Ozturk R, Senyuz OF. The effect of an H2-receptor antagonist on small-bowel colonization and bacterial translocation in newborn rats. Pediatr Surg Int 1998;13(2–3):118–120.

[71] Graham PL 3rd, Begg MD, Larson E, Della-Latta P, Allen A, Saiman L. Risk factors for late onset gram-negative sepsis in low birth weight infants hospitalized in the neonatal intensive care unit. Pediatr Infect Dis J 2006;25(2):113–117.

[72] Cobb BA, Carlo WA, Ambalavanan N. Gastric residuals and their relationship to necrotizing enterocolitis in very low birth weight infants. Pediatrics 2004;113(1 Pt. 1):50–53.

[73] Clark RH, Thomas P, Peabody J. Extrauterine growth restriction remains a serious problem in prematurely born neonates. Pediatrics 2003;111:986–990.

[74] American Academy of Pediatrics. Pediatric nutrition handbook. 6th ed. Elk Grove Village, IL: American Academy of Pediatrics; 2009.

[75] Tsang RC, Uauy R, Koletzko B, Zlotkin S. Nutrition of the pre-term infant: scientific basis and practical guidelines. Cincinnati, OH: Digital Educational Publishing, Inc; 2005. p. iii.

[76] Lynne Radbone. East of England Perinatal Networks. Clinical guideline: enteral feeding of preterm infants on the neonatal unit. NHS; 2013.

[77] American Academy of Pediatrics. Committee on nutrition. Nutritional needs of preterm infants. In: Kleinman RE, editor. Pediatric nutrition handbook. 5th ed. Elk Grove Village, IL: American Academy of Pediatrics; 2004. p. 23–54.

[78] Ballard O, Morrow AL. Human milk composition: nutrients and bioactive factors. Pediatr Clin North Am 2013;60(1):49–74.

[79] Suraj G, Pankaj B, Satish T. Recent advances in pediatrics: perspectives in neonatology: nutrition in newborn: an overview, vol. 25. Jaypee Brothers Medical Publishers; 2014.

[80] Lindquist S, Hernell O. Lipid digestion and absorption in early life: an update. Curr Opin Clin Nutr Metab Care 2010;13:314–320.

[81] Rigo J, Senterre J. Nutritional needs of premature infants: current issues. J Pediatr 2006;149:s80–s88.

[82] Thoene M, Hanson C, Lyden E, Dugick L, Ruybal L, Anderson-Berry A. Comparison of the effect of two human milk fortifiers on clinical outcomes in premature infants. Nutrients 2014;6:261–275.

[83] Martins EC, Krebs VL. Effects of the use of fortified raw maternal milk on very low birth weight infants. J Pediatr (Rio J) 2009;85:157–162.

[84] Di Natale C, Coclite E, Di Ventura L, et al. Fortification of maternal milk for preterm infants. J Matern Fetal Neonatal Med 2011;24(Suppl. 1):41–43.

[85] Su B-H. Optimizing nutrition in preterm infants. Pediatr Neonatol 2014;55:5–13.

[86] McMaster Children's Hospital. NICU Nutrition; Summary Guidelines July 2012. Available from: https://www.macpeds.com/documents/NICUnutritionattachment.pdf.

[87] De Curtis M, Candusso M, Pieltain C, Rigo J. Effect of fortification on the osmolality of human milk. Arch Dis Child Fetal Neonatal Ed 1999;81:F141–F143.

[88] Lucas A, Fewtrell MS, Morley R, Lucas PJ, Baker BA, Lister G, et al. Randomized outcome trial of human milk fortification and developmental outcome in preterm infants. Am J Clin Nutr 1996;64:142–151.

[89] Di Natale C. Fortification of maternal milk. J Pediatr Neonatal Individualized Med 2013;2(2):e020224.

[90] Kuschel CA, Harding JE. Multicomponent fortified human milk for promoting growth in preterm infants. Cochrane Database Syst Rev 2004;1:CD000343.

[91] Barnes D, Yeh AM. Bugs and guts: practical applications of probiotics for gastrointestinal disorders in children. Nutr Clin Pract 2015;30(6):747–759.

[92] Indrio F, Neu J. The intestinal microbiome of infants and the use of probiotics. Curr Opin Pediatr 2011;23(2):145–150.

[93] Butel M-J, Waligora-Dupriet A-J, Aires J. Usefulness of probiotics for neonates? Intech; 2012.

[94] Underwood MA, German JB, Lebrilla CB, Mills DA. Bifidobacterium longum subspecies infantis: champion colonizer of the infant gut. Pediatr Res 2015;77(1–2):229–235.

[95] Caplan MS. Probiotic and prebiotic supplementation for the prevention of neonatal necrotizing enterocolitis. J Perinatol 2009 May;29:S2–S6.

[96] Bartle D, Knight C, Cairns P. The use of probiotics in preterm babies. South West Neonatal Network Guideline Working Group; version 1; NHS; 2016.

[97] AlFaleh K, Anabrees J. Probiotics for prevention of necrotizing enterocolitis in preterm infants. Cochrane Database Syst Rev 2014;4:CD005496.

[98] Bazacliu C, Bhatia JS. Parenteral nutrition. In: Polin R, Yoder M, editors. Workbook in practical neonatology. 5th ed. Saunders; 2015.

[99] Ehrenkranz RA, Das A, Wrage LA, Poindexter BB, Higgins RD, Stoll BJ, et al. Early nutrition mediates the influence of severity of illness on extremely LBW infants. Pediatr Res 2011;69:522–529.

[100] Radmacher PG, Rafail ST, Adamkin DH. Nutrition and growth in VVLBW infants with and without bronchopulmonary dysplasia. Neonatal Intensive Care 2004;16:22–26.

[101] Adamkin DH. Early total parenteral nutrition in very low birthweight infants: is it safe? Is it worth it? J Pediatr 2013;163(3):622–624.

[102] Schanler RJ. Parenteral nutrition in premature infants UpToDate; 2017. Available from: https://www.uptodate.com/contents/parenteral-nutrition-in-premature-infants.

[103] El Hassan NO. Parenteral nutrition in the neonatal intensive care unit. NeoReviews 2011;12(3).

[104] Friis-Hansen B. Water—the major nutrient. Acta Paediatr Scand Suppl 1982;299:11–16.

[105] Bhatia J. Fluid and electrolyte management in the very low birth weight neonate. J Perinatol 2006;26(Suppl. 1):S19–S21.

[106] Committee on Nutrition. Nutritional needs of the preterm infant. In: Kleinman RE, editor. Pediatric nutrition handbook. 6th ed. Elk Grove Village, IL: American Academy of Pediatrics; 2009. p. 79–104.

[107] Ben XM. Nutritional management of newborn infants: practical guidelines. World J Gastroenterol 2008;14(40):6133–6139.

[108] Premer DM, Georgieff MK. Nutrition for ill neonates. Pediatr Rev 1999;20(9):e56–e62.

[109] Bell EF, Warburton D, Stonestreet BS, Oh W. Effect of fluid administration on the development of symptomatic patent ductus arteriosus and congestive heart failure in premature infants. N Engl J Med 1980;302:598–604.

[110] Oh W, Poindexter BB, Perritt R, Lemons JA, Bauer CR, Ehrenkranz RA, Stoll BJ, Neonatal Research Network. et al. Association between fluid intake and weight loss during the first ten days of life and risk of bronchopulmonary dysplasia in extremely low birth weight infants. J Pediatr 2005;147:786–790.

[111] Bell EF, Acarregui MJ. Restricted versus liberal water intake for preventing morbidity and mortality in preterm infants. Cochrane Database Syst Rev 2008;1:CD000503.

[112] Thureen PJ. Protein balance in the first week of life in ventilated neonates receiving parenteral nutrition. Am J Clin Nutr 1998;68:1128–1135.

[113] van Goudoever JV, Wattimena J, Carnielli V, Sulkers E, Degenhart H, Sauer P. Effect of dexamethasone on protein metabolism in infants with bronchopulmonary dysplasia. J Pediatr 1994;124:112–118.

[114] Kalhan SC, Kilic I. Carbohydrate as nutrient in the infant and child: range of acceptable intake. Eur J Clin Nutr 1999;53:S94–S100.

[115] Sunehag A, Ewald U, Larsson A, Gustafsson J. Glucose production rate in extremely immature neonates (28 weeks) studied by use of deuterated glucose. Pediatr Res 1993;33:97–100.

[116] Nose O, Tipton JR, Ament ME. Effect of the energy source on changes in energy expenditure, respiratory quotient, and nitrogen balance during total parenteral nutrition in children. Pediatr Res 1987;21:538–541.

[117] Forsyth JS, Murdock N, Crighton A. Low birthweight infants and total parenteral nutrition immediately after birth. III. Randomized study of energy substrate utilisation, nitrogen balance, and carbon dioxide production. Arch Dis Child Fetal Neonatal Ed 1995;73:F13–F16.

[118] Jones MO, Pierro A, Hammond P, Nunn A, Lloyd DA. Glucose utilization in the surgical newborn infant receiving total parenteral nutrition. J Pediatr Surg 1993;28:1121–1125.

[119] Lafeber HN, Sulkers EJ, Chapman TE, Sauer PJ. Glucose production and oxidation in preterm infants during total parenteral nutrition. Pediatr Res 1990;28:153–157.

[120] Valentine C, Puthoff T. Enhancing parenteral nutrition therapy for the neonate. Nutr Clin Pract 2007;22:183–193.

[121] Hay WW Jr. Intravenous nutrition of the very preterm infant. Acta Paediatr Suppl 2005;94:47–56.

[122] Bottino M, Cowett RM, Sinclair JC. Interventions for treatment of neonatal hyperglycemia in very low birth weight infants. Cochrane Database Syst Rev 2009;21:CD007453.

[123] Pediatric Nutrition Practice Guide. Parenteral nutrition. In: Groh-Wargo S, Thompson M, Cox JH, editors. ADA pocket guide to neonatal nutrition. Chicago, IL: Precept Press, Inc; 2009. p. 29–63.

[124] Anderson D, Pittard WB. Parenteral nutrition for neonates. In: Baker R, Baker S, Cavis A, editors. Pediatric parenteral nutrition. New York, NY: International Thompson Publishing; 1997. p. 301–314.

[125] Valentine CJ, Fernandez S, Rogers LK, et al. Early amino acid administration improves preterm infant weight. J Perinatol 2009;29:428–432.

[126] Thureen PJ, Hay WW Jr. Early aggressive nutrition in preterm infants. Semin Neonatol 2001;6:403–415.

[127] Ziegler EE, Carlson SJ. Early nutrition of very low birth weight infants. J Matern Fetal Neonatal Med 2009;22:191–197.

[128] te Braake FW, van den Akker CH, Wattimena DJ, Huijmans JG, van Goudoever JB. Amino acid administration to premature infants directly after birth. J Pediatr 2005;147:457–461.

[129] Saini J, MacMahon P, Morgan JB, Kovar IZ. Early parenteral feeding of amino acids. Arch Dis Child 1989;64:1362–1366.

[130] Koletzko B, Goulet O, Hunt J, Krohn K, Shamir R. Parenteral Nutrition Guidelines Working Group; European Society for Clinical Nutrition and Metabolism; European Society of Paediatric Gastroenterology, Hepatology and Nutrition (ESPGHAN); European Society of Paediatric Research (ESPR). Guidelines on Paediatric Parenteral Nutrition of the European Society of Paediatric Gastroenterology, Hepatology and Nutrition (ESPGHAN) and the European Society for Clinical Nutrition and Metabolism (ESPEN), Supported by the European Society of Paediatric Research (ESPR). J Pediatr Gastroenterol Nutr 2005;41:S1–S87.

[131] Ridout E, Melara D, Rottinghaus S, Thureen PJ. Blood urea nitrogen concentration as a marker of amino-acid intolerance in neonates with birthweight less than 1250 g. J Perinatol 2005;25:130–133.

[132] Radmacher PG, Lewis SL, Adamkin DH. Early amino acids and the metabolic response of ELBW infants (1000 g) in three time periods. J Perinatol 2009;29:433–437.

[133] Roggero P, Gianni ML, Morlacchi L, et al. Blood urea nitrogen concentrations in low-birth-weight preterm infants during parenteral and enteral nutrition. J Pediatr Gastroenterol Nutr 2010;51: 213–215.

[134] Van Goudoever JB, Sulkers FJ, Timmerman N, et al. Amino acid solutions for premature neonates during the first week of life: the role of N-acetyl-L-cysteine and N-acetyl-L-tyrosine. JPEN J Parenter Enteral Nutr 1994;18:404–408.

[135] Fitzgerald KA, Mackay MW. Calcium and phosphate solubility in neonatal parenteral nutrient solutions containing TrophAmine. Am J Hosp Pharm 1986;43:88–93.

[136] Salama GS, et al. Intravenous lipids for preterm infants: a review. Clin Med Insights Pediatr 2015;9: 25–36.

[137] Auestad N, Halter R, Hall RT, et al. Growth and development in term infants fed long-chain polyunsaturated fatty acids: a double-masked, randomized, parallel, prospective, multivariate study. Pediatrics 2001;108:372–381.

[138] Auestad N, Scott DT, Janowsky JS, et al. Visual, cognitive, and language assessments at 39 months: a follow-up study of children fed formulas containing long-chain polyunsaturated fatty acids to 1 year of age. Pediatrics 2003;112:e177–e183.

[139] Ibrahim HM, Jeroudi MA, Baier RJ, Dhanireddy R, Krouskop RW. Aggressive early total parenteral nutrition in low-birth-weight infants. J Perinatol 2004;24:482–486.

[140] Simmer K, Rao SC. Early introduction of lipids to parenterallyfed preterm infants. Cochrane Database Syst Rev 2005;18:CD005256.

[141] Peterson J, Bihain BE, Bengtsson-Olivecrona G, Deckelbaum RJ, Carpentier YA, Olivecrona T. Fatty acid control of lipoprotein lipase: a link between energy metabolism and lipid transport. Proc Natl Acad Sci USA 1990;87:909–913.

[142] Cairns PA, Stalker DJ. Carnitine supplementation of parenterally fed neonates. Cochrane Database Syst Rev 2000;4:CD000950.

[143] Clinical practice guideline. Guidelines for babies requiring total parenteral nutrition in NICU, Latifa Hospital, Dubai; 2016.

[144] Aggarwal R, et al. Fluid and electrolyte management in term and preterm neonates. AIIMS, india.

[145] Hartnoll G, Betremieux P, Modi N. Randomised controlled trial of postnatal sodium supplementation on body composition in 25 to 30 week gestational age infants. Arch Dis Child Fetal Neonatal Ed 2000;82:F24–F28.

[146] Shah PS, Shah VS. Continuous heparin infusion to prevent thrombosis and catheter occlusion in neonates with peripherally placed percutaneous central venous catheters (review). Cochrane Database Syst Rev 2008;2:CD002772.

[147] August D, Teitelbaum D, Albina J, et al. Guidelines for the use of parenteral and enteral nutrition in adult and pediatric patients. JPEN J Parenter Enteral Nutr 2002;26(1):S1–S137.

[148] Moreno Villares JM, Fernandez Shaw TC, Munoz Garcia MJ, Gomis Munoz P. Survey on parenteral nutrition preparation variability in pediatrics. Nutr Hosp 2002;17(5):251–255.

[149] Ankola PA, Atakent YS. Effect of adding heparin in very low concentration to the infusate to prolong the patency of umbilical artery catheters. Am J Perinatol 1993;10(3):229–232.

Further reading

[150] Neonatology clinical guidelines. Nutrition: parenteral and enteral King Edward Memorial/Princess Margaret Hospitals, Perth, Western Australia; 2013.

[151] Feeding and Enteral Nutrition Protocol; clinical practice guideline; Latifa Women and Children Hospital, Dubai; 2016.

[152] British Association of Perinatal Medicine; The Provision of Parenteral Nutrition within Neonatal Services—A Framework for Practice; BAPM; 2016.

Chapter |37A|

Neonatal Procedures Involving Catheters and Tubes

Khaled El-Atawi, Mb.Bch, M.Sc., Ph.D., iFAAP, FRCPCH (Pediatrics) & M.Sc. (HCM),
Swarup Kumar Dash, MD (Pediatrics), DNB (Neonatology), Ahmed Zakaria Elmorsy, Mb.Bch, M.Sc. (Pediatrics)

CHAPTER CONTENTS HD

CHAPTER POINTS

- Umbilical arterial lines are placed in a "high" position (between T6 to T9 vertebrae) or "low" position (L3 to L4). Common complications include lower limb ischemia and renovascular hypertension.

- Umbilical venous lines are placed with the tip in the inferior vena cava just below the right atrium (typically T9-10 vertebral level).

- Peripherally inserted central catheters (PICC) are placed at the superior vena cava – right atrial junction (from upper extremity, head and neck region) or in the inferior vena cava (from lower extremity). Occlusions, infections and pericardial/pleural effusions are common complications.

- Peripheral arterial cannulation should only be performed after confirming adequate collateral flow by modified Allen test.

- Premedication with a sedative (atropine and paralytics are optional) is standard prior to non-emergent intubation in the NICU

Abbreviations

ETT	Endotracheal intubation tube
ICD	Intercostal chest drain
LMA	Laryngeal mask airway
NICU	Neonatal intensive care unit
PAC	Peripheral arterial catheters
PICC	Peripherally inserted central catheters
UAC	Umbilical arterial catheters
UVC	Umbilical venous catheters

Introduction

Neonatal procedures involving catheters and tubes are essential components in the care of critically ill infants in neonatal intensive care units. These are used for critical neonates; for blood pressure monitoring, arterial blood gas collection, infusion of medications, and total parenteral nutrition.

This chapter reviews the indications, techniques, complications and their treatment, care, surveillance, and evidence-based recommendations of various catheters and invasive tubes. Catheters discussed in this chapter include venous catheters, such as umbilical venous catheters (UVCs), peripherally placed central catheters, and arterial catheters, such as peripheral arterial catheters (PACs) and umbilical arterial catheters (UACs). In addition, intercostal chest drain (ICD) tubes (thoracostomy tubes) and endotracheal intubation are also discussed.

Umbilical arterial catheters

UACs are frequently used in the neonatal intensive care units for the purpose of blood sampling, continuous monitoring of systemic blood pressure, and measurement of arterial blood gases [1]. The contraindications include omphalitis, omphalocele, necrotizing enterocolitis, peritonitis, and when there is an evidence of vascular compromise in lower limbs.

Insertion of the UAC is an urgent procedure in critically ill preterm neonates as the catheter insertion becomes difficult if umbilical arteries start constricting. According to a comparative cohort study published in 2014, early insertion of UAC in the first 30 min of life is associated with more success rates than late insertion in the NICU [2].

There are two positions in which the tip of the UAC can be located; at a "high" position between thoracic vertebrae T6 to T9 with the catheter tip above celiac axis or at a "low" position between lumbar vertebrae L3 to L4 with the tip above the aortic bifurcation but below the renal arteries (Figs. 37A.1 and 37A.2) [1]. However, the current body of evidence does not support the use of low-placed UAC [1].

Procedure (Fig. 37A.3)

The first step to be considered for UAC insertion is selection of appropriate sized catheter and estimation of the expected depth of insertion by measuring the shoulder-to-umbilical length and weight of the infant. Depending upon the shoulder-to-umbilical length nomograms, the position of catheter insertion is decided either as high or low. To date, there is no guidance regarding the proper estimation of the length of catheter to be inserted (Table 37A.1). After proper sterilization, umbilical tie should be placed at the base of umbilical cord and incised perpendicular leaving 1 cm of the umbilical stump. The umbilical stump should be held with the toothed forceps and the umbilical artery should be dilated with iris forceps. Before placement, UAC should be primed with heparinized saline (1 unit/mL), and then the catheter should be introduced into the lumen without any force to the required length. The position of the catheter should be confirmed with the help of ultrasound or X-ray. The catheter should be sutured and secured. The area should be further observed for any signs of bleeding. The entire procedure of catheter insertion should be carried out aseptically. To facilitate the blood pressure monitoring, transducer must be placed [1].

Complications

The common side effects of UAC placement are vasospasm or thromboembolic phenomena leading to cold lower extremities and pallor or discoloration. Occasionally,

renovascular hypertension is associated with microscopic hematuria and can potentially lead to renal failure which is observed more commonly with low-placed UAC [3]. The material of catheter has been shown to influence the extent of thromboembolic events, although conclusive evidence is not available. Silicone rubber catheters were shown to be associated with outcomes that are more favorable. Use of heparinized fluids in the catheters was shown to reduce the mechanical occlusion of UAC [4]. Treatment of catheter-associated thromboembolism includes use of anticoagulation, fibrinolytic therapy, and rarely surgical excision, if necessary.

UACs are also associated with potentially life-threatening complications, such as umbilical artery perforation [5] and pseudoaneurysm formation [3], rare complications, such as scrotal hypoperfusion [6] and flaccid paraplegia [7], and known complications, such as catheter-associated infections, bleeding, thromboembolism, and persistent hypoglycemia.

Several studies have shown that high-placed catheters are associated with fewer complications than low-placed ones [1]. However, high-placed catheters are associated with hypoglycemia as streaming of glucose occurs to superior mesenteric and celiac arteries [8]. However, the recently published literature discouraged the use of UAC to provide glucose-containing solutions.

Malpositioning of catheters have been implicated in vascular complications, such as umbilical artery perforation and pseudoaneurysm formation. Molanus et al. (2017) have reported a case of umbilical artery perforation leading to hemorrhagic shock, renal failure, and death of the preterm infant [5]. Hence, neonatologists should be aware of this life-threatening complication while using UAC. Straight forward placement of the UAC has been implicated in the formation of pseudoaneurysm in the presence of coagulopathy in an infant [3].

Muñoz et al. (1993) reported flaccid paraplegia as a complication of UAC in two patients, where it was presumed to be triggered by the spasm of Adamkiewicz artery during the movement of the catheter [7].

Care and surveillance

Strict aseptic technique must be maintained while inserting the UAC in order to prevent catheter-associated infections. The catheter should not be forced into the umbilical artery if spasm is noted. Instead, it should be inserted after sometime when spasm is relieved. The malpositioned lines need to be removed immediately to avoid vascular complications. Surveillance needs to be in line with the recommended guidelines to watch for the signs of catheter-related infections, bleeding, thromboembolic events, and effusion. Thromboembolism can be identified by cyanosed and cold extremities. The catheter needs to be removed when thromboembolism is

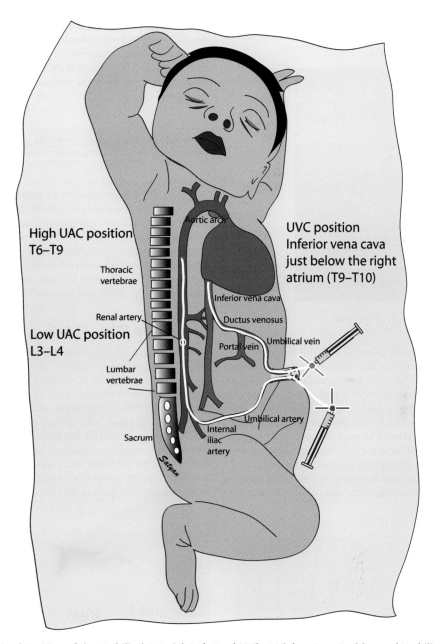

Fig. 37A.1 Optimal Position of the Umbilical Arterial Catheter (UAC) at High or Low Position and Umbilical Venous Catheter (UVC). High position for UAC is between T6 and T9 thoracic vertebrae and low position is below the renal arteries at L3–L4 lumbar vertebrae. Copyright: Satyan Lakshminrusimha.

suspected. Treatment options include anticoagulant therapy, fibrinolytic agents, surgical intervention, and supportive care, such as restoring the fluids and electrolytes, blood transfusion to correct anemia and thrombocytopenia, and administration of antibiotics to treat sepsis [1].

Recommendations

According to CDC guidelines, the UAC should be removed (and not replaced) when the signs of infection, cyanosis, or thrombosis are observed [9]. The catheter insertion site must be cleaned with the antiseptic solution. However,

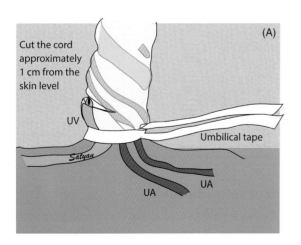

Fig. 37A.2 Optimal Path of the UVC.

tincture of iodine should be avoided for this purpose as this has a detrimental effect on the thyroid gland of the infant. Instead, povidone-iodine is recommended [10]. Topical antimicrobial agents should not be applied over the catheter insertion site as this may lead to the development of antimicrobial resistance and further promote the fungal infections [11]. Heparin should be used in low doses (typically 0.5–1 unit/cc of normal saline or ½ normal saline infusing at 0.25–1 mL/h) in the catheter to avoid occlusion [12].

Infants who show mild ischemia or cyanosis of the toes may be treated by warming of the toes or catheter removal,

in case of no improvement after toes warming; while UAC needs to be removed immediately if any sign of vascular insufficiency in the extremities is seen [6]. The optimal time to retain UAC is less than 5 days or when frequent arterial blood gas or blood pressure monitoring is no longer needed [9].

Umbilical venous catheters

UVCs may be used in preterm infants who require vascular access and resuscitation, as a lifesaving technique. This catheter can be inserted up to 1 week of birth as the umbilical vein remains open and possibly patent for this period. After the placement of the catheter, the parenteral nutrition and emergency medications, such as inotropes can be administered in these preterm infants [12]. The contraindications for UVC placement are presence of local infections, omphalitis, peritonitis, and necrotizing enterocolitis [12].

Procedure (Fig. 37A.4)

The first step to be considered for UVC insertion is selection of appropriate sized catheter (3.5 F for <1500 g infant and 5 F for >1500 g infant) by measuring the shoulder-to-umbilical length and weight of the infant. The umbilical vein should be identified. The length of catheter to be inserted should be estimated. After proper sterilization, umbilical tape should be placed at the base of umbilical cord and incised. The umbilical cord should be held with the toothed forceps and the umbilical artery should be dilated with iris forceps. Then the catheter should be introduced into the lumen without any force to the required length. The catheter

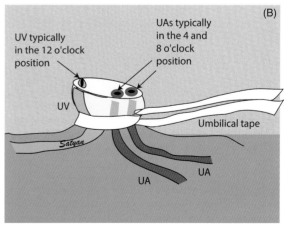

Fig. 37A.3 (A–D) Steps involving the insertion of the UAC. Copyright: Satyan Lakshminrusimha.

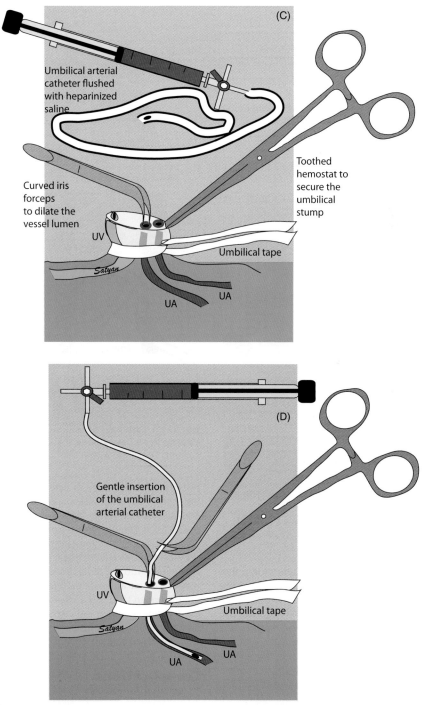

Fig. 37A.3 *(cont.)*

Table 37A.1 UAC catheter size based upon birth weight	
Birth weight (g)	**UAC catheter size (F)**
<1200	3.5
>1200	5

Source: Fletcher MA, MacDonald MG, Avery GB. Atlas of procedures in neonatology. Philadelphia, PA: JB Lippincott Co.; 1983.

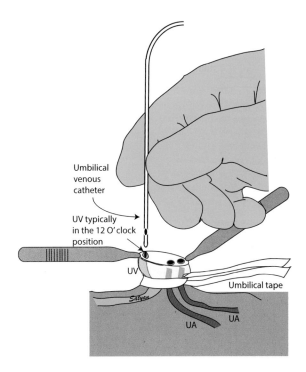

Fig. 37A.4 Insertion of the Umbilical Venous Line. Copyright: Satyan Lakshminrusimha.

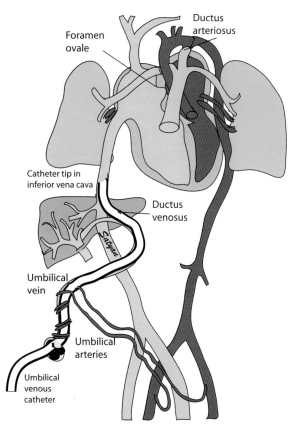

Fig. 37A.5 Optimal Positioning of a Central UVC in the Inferior Vena Cava Above the Liver But Below the Right Atrium. Copyright: Satyan Lakshminrusimha.

should be sutured. The entire procedure of catheter insertion should be carried out aseptically. According to a prospective observational study published in 2017, the position of the UVC should be determined by the anatomical structures like diaphragm, cardiac silhouette, and vertebrae. Further, the position of the catheter tip needs to be confirmed by echocardiography [13]. The ideal position of UVC is in the inferior vena cava and was identified as catheter tip being in between 9th and 10th thoracic vertebrae, which lies just above liver and below the right atrium (Fig. 37A.5). If the catheter tip is higher than the 9th vertebra, then the position of UVC is considered as too high. If the catheter tip is below than the 10th vertebra, then the position of UVC is considered as too low. Mutlu et al. (2017) have conducted a prospec-

tive observational study to determine the accurate method for appropriate UVC catheter insertion. It was observed that Shukla–Ferrara formula [(9 + weight in kg × 3)/2 + 1 cm] or modified Shukla–Ferrara formula [(9 + weight in kg × 3)/2 cm] was more accurate than Dunn method (using shoulder–umbilical length and the Dunn nomogram) [14]. For infants who are term or near-term and sick enough to require central access (e.g., sepsis, MAS, or PPHN), a 5-F double-lumen UVC should be inserted. For infants <1000 g, a 3.5-F double-lumen catheter should be considered if the infant is likely to need inotropes or multiple infusions. This will be decided on an individual basis.

Complications

UVC are often associated with complications, such as bleeding, malposition of catheters, catheter-related bloodstream infections, presence of catheter remnants in umbilicus, catheter-related thrombosis, hepatic complications, such as hepatic hematoma and hepatic laceration, and cardiac tamponade. Mutlu et al. (2016) have conducted a retrospective observational study over a period of 6 years in a hospital setting and identified that 198 out of 974 neonates developed UVC complications; 189 of 198 patients developed complications due to malpositioning of UVC and remaining infants developed complications due to catheter-related infections and presence of catheter remnants in umbilicus [15]. Therefore, this study highlights that extreme care should be taken while insertion and removal of UVC in neonates to avoid the complications.

Abiramalatha et al. (2016) demonstrated that even appropriately placed UVC could lead to life-threatening complications, such as hepatic hematoma, cardiac tamponade resulting from pericardial effusion, and atrial thrombosis. It is recommended that regular echocardiographic examination is required in neonates with UVCs for early detection of such life-threatening UVC-related complications [16].

Pericardial tamponade is another life-threatening complication due to UVC in neonates. This may be caused due to high glucose concentration in the pericardial fluid due to administration of parenteral nutrition through UVC. This condition can be treated by pericardiocentesis [17].

Care and surveillance

Strict asepsis must be maintained while inserting the UVC in order to prevent catheter-associated infections. Malpositioned catheters need to be immediately removed or repositioned to avoid complications. The physicians need to be vigilant and observe for the signs of complications caused by malpositioning of catheter with the help of echocardiographic examination.

An observational study published in 2017 demonstrated that chest radiography along with echocardiographic visualization helps in proper positing of UVC, which thereby reduces the complications of malpositioned catheter [13].

Recommendations

According to CDC guidelines, the UVC should be removed if there is no need but can be used for a maximum duration of 14 days with aseptic technique [9]. Tincture of iodine should be avoided for the cleaning of catheter insertion as this has a detrimental effect on the thyroid gland of the infant. Instead, povidone-iodine is recommended [10]. Topical antimicrobial agents should not be applied over the catheter insertion site as this may lead to the development of antimicrobial resistance and further promote the fungal infections [11]. Heparin should be used in low doses (typically 0.5–1 unit/cc at 0.25–1 mL/h) in the catheter to avoid occlusion [12].

UVC needs to be removed immediately if any complications are seen due to malpositioning or presence of catheter remnants in the umbilicus. The optimal time to retain UVC is less than 14 days or when no longer needed [9]. Early planned removal of UVC is recommended to prevent the catheter-related bloodstream infections. However, a recently published Cochrane review found that the current evidence is insufficient to show a significant difference in infection rates between early planned and longer duration removal of the catheter [18].

Peripherally inserted central catheters

Peripherally inserted central catheters (PICCs) have been most commonly used rather than surgical procedures as the insertion procedure is simple without any surgical incisions, comparatively rapid, less expensive, and requires only mild sedation or pain relief. PICCs are available in various sizes to facilitate their insertion in micro preemies with weight less than 1 lb. These are mostly made of materials like silicone, polyurethane, or polyethylene [1].

PICCs are routinely inserted through basilic, brachial, or cephalic veins. The indications of PICC include neonates needing vascular access for more than 1 week, antimicrobial agents, and analgesics [19]. PICCs are contraindicated in micro preemies with anatomical asymmetry in the extremities or with infection or broken skin at the insertion site [20].

Procedure (Fig. 37A.6)

PICC is first inserted in the larger peripheral vein and later it is passed through the further larger veins until the catheter tip reaches distal superior or inferior vena cava. The ideal position for the catheter tip is parallel to vessel wall in the superior vena cava or inferior vena cava, proximal to right atrial junction. It is 1 cm outside the heart in a premature infant and 2 cm outside in a full-term neonate [21]. The length of the inserted catheter may be around 20–60 cm. The insertable length should be estimated by measuring the distance from insertion site to xiphisternum for long lines inserted via the leg, and from insertion site to sterna notch for long lines inserted via the arm. Then the PICC is passed till the appropriate length and without resistance. In case of joints resistance, the joint must be straightened, and heparinized solution should be passed through the catheter. The catheter tip should not be in the heart as there is a risk of heart tamponade and arrhythmias. Appropriate

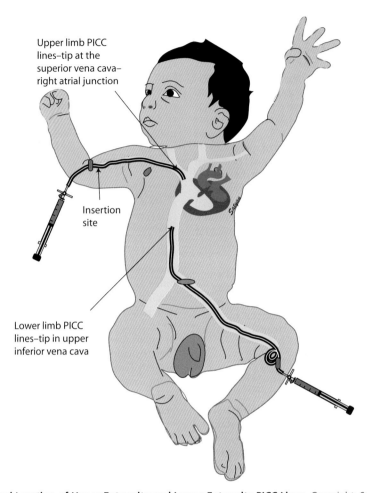

Upper limb PICC
lines–tip at the
superior vena cava–
right atrial junction

Insertion
site

Lower limb PICC
lines–tip in upper
inferior vena cava

Fig. 37A.6 Insertion and Location of Upper Extremity and Lower Extremity PICC Lines. Copyright: Satyan Lakshminrusimha.

positioning of PICC must be ensured with the diagnostic methods, such as chest radiography and ultrasound. An X-ray should be taken with infant positioned in anatomical position with arms by their side for upper limb lines or legs with hips slightly flexed for lower limb lines. If the position of the catheter tip is not clear, a subsequent X-ray with contrast is advised.

Care should be taken that the dressing at the site of insertion should be transparent to make it visible. The intravenous fluid should be always passed through PICC as there are chances of blockade due to small lumen [20].

Complications

The most common complications associated with PICC are occlusion of catheter, phlebitis, and thrombosis. PICCs are believed to have lower rate of catheter-related infections

than other centrally inserted catheters. However, no conclusive evidence is available yet to substantiate that PICCs have lower rate of infections [19].

Sertic et al. (2017) conducted a retrospective case control study to identify the risk factors for the PICC-associated perforations, a devastating complication resulting in pericardial and pleural effusion. Lower birth weight was identified as a risk factor for pericardial effusion. Catheter tip position, more proximal to the heart at the time of insertion resulted in higher pericardial effusions. Whereas, catheter tip position more distal from the heart at the time of insertion resulted in higher pleural effusions. Mild oozing of blood from the insertion site may occur for up to 24 h. This can be stopped with mild pressure. If the oozing of blood continues, thrombin foam can be applied over the area and under the dressing immediately after insertion [22]. Early recognition and being vigilant about these complications may help in avoiding and treating them. A recently published prospective cohort study identified the caliber thickness and age as the risk factors for the development of complication in neonates with inserted PICC [23].

Care and surveillance

Heparinized solution (0.5 units/mL) should be passed through the catheter to avoid the complications, such as occlusion of catheter. The number of connections should be kept low. PICCs may require flushing and if there is a sign of inflammation or bleeding then the dressing needs to be changed. Care should be taken that the insertion site does not get wet [19]. Closed medication system is preferred due to lower rate of bloodstream infection [8].

Recommendations

The PICCs should not be replaced routinely to prevent catheter-related infections. This is substantiated by the evidence that routine catheter replacement did not result in lower infection rates. The PICC should not be removed on the basis of fever alone. Instead, the cause of fever needs to be determined if it is related or not to PICCs [24]. Strict aseptic precautions should be maintained while inserting the catheters.

Peripheral artery catheterization

Peripheral artery catheterization is a common procedure used in the neonatal intensive care unit. PAC helps in sampling of arterial blood for the analysis where insertion of UAC is not possible, invasive arterial BP monitoring, and during exchange transfusion to remove the blood.

The contraindications to PAC usage are if there is an insufficient blood circulation to the extremities, localized skin infection at the insertion site, malformation of limbs, and uncontrolled coagulopathy.

The preferred arteries for insertion of PAC are radial artery, posterior tibial artery, and dorsalis pedis artery. Most common primary sites are radial artery and posterior tibial artery as dorsalis pedis artery is absent in some neonates. Brachial artery should not be used for peripheral cannulation as the collateral circulation is absent [25].

Procedure

Allen's test

The first step in peripheral artery catheterization is to check for collateral circulation. This can be performed by the Allen's test (Fig. 37A.7). This test is used to determine the patency of

(A)

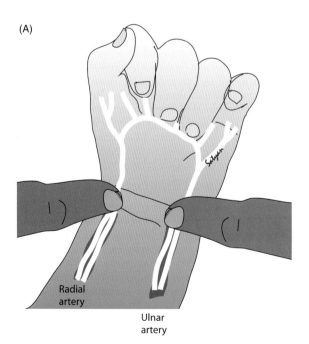

(B)

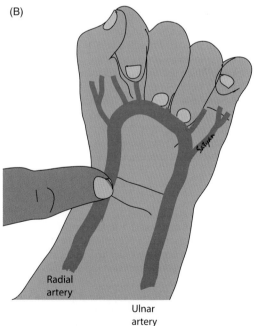

Fig. 37A.7 Modified Allen Test for Neonates. (A) Occlusion of both radial and ulnar arteries results in blanching of the hand. (B) Releasing pressure over the ulnar artery results in reperfusion of the hand suggesting collateral flow. (C) Persistent blanching of the hand after releasing pressure over the ulnar artery indicates poor collateral perfusion. Copyright: Satyan Lakshminrusimha.

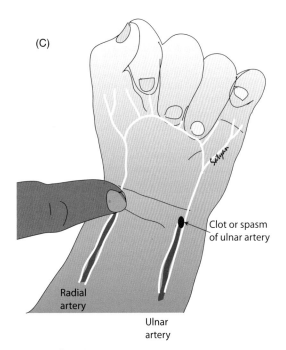

(C)

Clot or spasm
of ulnar artery

Radial
artery

Ulnar
artery

Fig. 37A.7 (cont.)

radial or ulnar arteries. The arm of the neonate is elevated and the radial and ulnar arteries at the wrist are simultaneously compressed for 30 s; the palm of the infant is rubbed in order to cause blanching (transient ischemia in the hand). Then, the ulnar artery is released and the hand of the neonate is relaxed. The time taken to see the normal color that is, sufficient perfusion of blood to tips of thumb and fingers of the hand is noted. If the time taken is less than 5 s, then test is said to be positive. If the time taken is between 6 and 10 s, it is equivocal. If time taken is more than 10 s, then the test failed. The artery can be cannulated if the time taken is less than 10 s, as it indicates adequate collateral circulation [25].

Technique

Transillumination can be tried to locate the artery. The entire procedure of peripheral arterial cannulation must be done under strictly aseptic conditions. The wrist of the neonate is hyperextended in order to expose it. According to Mitchell and Welsby (2004), appropriate position of the arm is the most important part as it helps in surfacing the radial artery to more superficial position which thereby improves the success of peripheral arterial cannulation [26]. Chlorhexidine is used to wash the skin and a sterile drape is applied over a larger area of the skin. Then the radial artery is palpated using the first and second fingers. A 24-gauge angiocath is used at an angle of 30–45

degrees, and when the blood flow is noted the catheter should be placed slowly into the artery with the needle in a still position. Cannulate the vessel percutaneously and secure the catheter with a tape. A subcutaneous tunnel made with a wider gauge needle prior to the arterial cannulation will facilitate procedure in larger babies; however, it is not routinely done in NICU. According to CDC guidelines, the catheter should not be sutured and should be continuously infused with heparinized normal saline (1 unit/mL).

Complications

The most common complications of PAC are occlusion of the radial artery, catheter-related infections, bleeding, ischemic injury, hematoma, and rarely pseudoaneurysm. Even if the catheterization is for a shorter duration, local injury and scarring have been noted. Radial artery occlusion may not always appear immediately; it can occur several days after the cannulation or even after the removal of the catheter [25].

Very rare complications of PAC include median nerve paralysis and presence of catheter remnants intravascularly [27]. The ischemic complications of PAC can be attributed to some risk factors, such as presence of vasospasm, smaller vessel diameter in female neonates, and larger diameter of the catheter. Technical risk factors including more number of attempts in insertion and hematoma formation due to more number of arterial pricks may increase the complications. For ischemic injury, apply warm towel or cloth on opposite unaffected leg to induce reflex vasodilatation of the affected leg and maintain neutral thermal environment for the affected extremity [25]. However, if there is no improvement after 20 min of warming, the catheter should be removed; while UAC needs to be removed immediately if the limb becomes pale. (Please see chapter Neonatal Limb Ischemia Due to Arterial Catheters for further management.)

Care and surveillance

Heparinized solution should be used to prevent the occlusion of catheter. After the catheter is inserted, asepsis must be maintained. PAC must be removed when it is no longer needed or if any signs of cyanosis are seen. Slight discoloration of fingers should be watched carefully; if there is no improvement after 20 min, remove the catheter. If complications arise due to heparin solution, then the treatment with topical nitroglycerin ointment is required. Cases of cerebral embolization were noted because of vigorous flushing of PAC, hence flushing should be avoided. To achieve hemostasis after catheter removal, simple compression of insertion site with gauze is enough instead of using compression devices [28].

Recommendations

Strict asepsis should be maintained while inserting the catheters. According to CDC guidelines, the catheter should not be sutured and should be continuously infused with heparinized normal saline. The heparin infusion should be stopped before removing the catheter. The removal site should be pressed for 3–5 min and checked for adequate limb perfusion and bleeding. PAC must be removed when it is no longer needed or if any signs of cyanosis are seen [29].

Thoracocentesis and intercostal chest drain placement

The most common indications of ICD in neonates are pneumothorax, pleural effusions, hemothorax, chylothorax, empyema, and postoperative drainage after the thoracic procedures.

Pneumothorax

Pneumothorax can be an emergency life-threatening condition, if the air collection is under pressure. This is commonly called tension pneumothorax. The diagnosis of pneumothorax can be suspected if there are reduced chest movements, diminished air entry, compromised circulation, and desaturation. The arterial blood gas analysis reveals hypoxia or respiratory acidosis and signs of respiratory distress are seen in the neonates. The clinical signs which can be seen in the presence of pneumothorax are asymmetrical chest movements, sudden deterioration of blood pressure in invasive monitoring, and tachycardia.

If the pneumothorax is smaller in size, it may resolve spontaneously without any treatment. However, larger pneumothorax results in severe complications as it starts pushing other organs (e.g., heart) in the chest to the other side. This is called tension pneumothorax. If blood starts accumulating in the pleural space instead of air, it is known as hemopneumothorax. Both these conditions require chest drainage [30]. In such cases, transillumination test will be usually positive in preterm infants. However, the results of transillumination may occasionally be false positive due to subcutaneous air and false negative due to small pneumothorax or thick folds of skin in the neonate [31].

Pneumopericardium

Pneumopericardium is a life-threatening condition in which there is a collection of air in the pericardial cavity. This condition in neonates mostly occurs due to respiratory distress syndrome or mechanical ventilation. Even though this is a rare condition, it can result in fatal outcomes in the neonates. It can occur in association with other related conditions, such as pneumothorax, pneumomediastinum, pneumoperitoneum, and emphysema [32].

The diagnosis can be made based on both clinical signs and diagnostic examination. Heart sounds with metallic tinkling sometimes called as "the mill wheel murmur" can be heard. Excessive air or gas in the pericardial cavity can cause pericardial tamponade, which may be serious. A high index of suspicion should be maintained especially with dampening of arterial waveform to the possibility of pericardial tamponade. Accurate diagnosis is made through chest X-ray, ultrasound, and CT scan. Immediate treatment includes needle aspiration and pericardial drainage [33].

Procedure (Fig. 37A.8)

ICD insertion is an emergency lifesaving procedure. In cases of severe emergency of tension pneumothorax, insertion of a simple needle can be lifesaving. However, needle aspiration is an emergency procedure only. Avoiding laceration of lung or puncturing of blood vessels should be taken care of while using needle aspiration. The neonate should be placed in a supine position and the area should be prepared with alcohol wipes. Insert needle into the pleural space (directly over the top of the rib in the 2nd or 3rd intercostal space in the midclavicular line) until air is aspirated into the syringe, then expel air through the three-way stop cock. After this procedure, further management is done by insertion of an intercostal catheter.

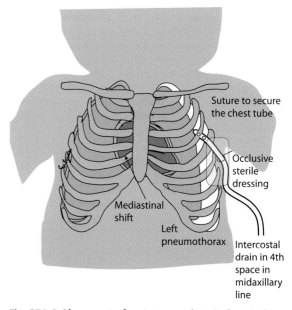

Fig. 37A.8 Placement of an Intercostal Drain for a Left Pneumothorax. Copyright: Satyan Lakshminrusimha.

Even though clinical signs of pneumothorax are seen, it must be confirmed with a chest X-ray. ICDs are commonly inserted between 3rd and 4th intercostal space in the midaxillary line. The tube is inserted in midaxillary line between 1st and 3rd intercostal space and directed anteriorly for anterior pneumothorax. It is placed in midaxillary line between 4th and 5th intercostal space for effusion and directed posteriorly. The drain is placed above the rib to avoid injury to the intercostal vessels located under the ribs. In smaller neonates, the ribs can be counted with the help of transillumination.

ICD can be of following types: a polyvinyl chloride chest tube with or without trocar, in various sizes like 8, 10, and 12 F or pigtail catheter (Table 37A.2).

ICD insertion is usually carried out under the local anesthesia as this can be a painful procedure. If the procedure is preplanned, then pre-insertion pain relief agents need to be administered in the neonates; intravenous pain relief with fentanyl or morphine can be provided, if baby is on respiratory support. Sterilize the insertion area to avoid any infectious complications. At the midclavicular line, insert a scalp vein and drain through a three-way tap. Before insertion of ICD in mid-axillary line, lidocaine (Local anesthesia) to be infiltrated. Make an incision of 3–4 mm with the sterile surgical blade and the tissues need to be spread using a hemostat. Insert the ICD between the spaces of rib, placing it above the rib and directing it to opposite shoulder for tension pneumothorax. Remove the stilette and connect it to the assembly arranged. ICD should be inserted for about 2–3 cm in a preterm neonate whereas; in a term neonate it can be up to 3–4 cm. Connect to closed drainage system at vacuum of 5 cm H_2O and increase to 10 cm H_2O, if necessary [34]. For the drainage of air and fluid, the column movement needs to be observed. This fluid can be collected simultaneously for investigation. Appropriate negative suction pressure must be used from the beginning. Then, suture ICD to the skin and secure it with a tape. A positive improvement in oxygen saturation can be seen if the ICD insertion is successful [31].

Table 37A.2 Intercostal chest drains

ICD	Infant weight (g)	Catheter size
PVC chest tube	>1500	10 or 12 F
	<1500	8 or 10 F
	<1000	8 F
Pigtail catheter	>1501	6.0 F/15 cm
	<1500	5.0 F/15 cm

Complications

The most common complications associated with ICD are bleeding, intercostal nerve damage, formation of fistula, malpositioning of the tube, occlusion of the drain tube, subcutaneous emphysema, chylothorax, heart tamponade, and perforation. A multicentric case series identified thoracic organ injury due to chest tubes, the common sites being mediastinum and pericardium [35].

Care and surveillance

Care must be taken that the height of ICD should always be lower than the patient's position to avoid backflow of fluid into neonate's chest wall. After the ICD insertion, regular monitoring of breath sounds and chest movements need to be performed. Large amounts of dressing material should not be placed at the ICD insertion site as this can inhibit proper chest movements. Transilluminate periodically for re-accumulation that could be silent. Water column must move with respiratory movement [36].

Recommendations

ICD insertion must be carried out under the local anesthesia as this can be a painful procedure. If the procedure is preplanned, then pre-insertion pain relief agents need to be administered in the neonates. Sterilize the insertion area to avoid any infectious complications. When the air or the fluid is completely drained, it is confirmed with chest X-ray showing clearing of pneumothorax or pleural effusion. Then, a trial must be conducted for about 24 h without suction to observe for collection of any fluid. If no fluid or air is seen, then ICD can be removed immediately, and the insertion site must be dressed immediately to avoid any air entering the chest. Further monitoring for tachypnea and arterial blood gases must be carried out. ICD must be removed in spontaneously breathed baby [37].

Pericardiocentesis (Fig. 37A.9)

The primary indication for pericardiocentesis is cardiac tamponade. This is not indicated when the effusion is self-resolving or if the effusion can be diagnosed and treated with a less invasive procedure, the underlying pathology can be determined through another noninvasive test, in case of viral pericarditis which can be treated with anti-inflammatory agents, and when there is more risk with less diagnostic benefit [38,39].

Complications

The contraindications for this procedure are myocardial rupture, aortic dissection, uncorrected coagulopathy,

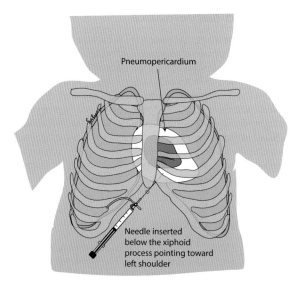

Fig. 37A.9 Emergency Pericardiocentesis for Cardiac Tamponade Due to Pneumopericardium. Ultrasound guidance, if available, is recommended. Copyright: Satyan Lakshminrusimha.

thrombocytopenia, and traumatic effusion with hemodynamic instability [40].

Procedure

There are three approaches for performing pericardiocentesis as explained in following sections.

Apical. The needle is inserted 1–2 cm lateral to the apex beat within the 5th, 6th, or 7th intercostal space. The needle must be advanced over the superior border of the rib to avoid intercostal nerves and vessels. Risks with this approach include ventricular puncture and pneumothorax [41].

Parasternal. The needle is inserted in the 5th left intercostal space, close to the sternal margin. The needle must be directed perpendicularly to the skin at the level of the cardiac notch of the left lung. The risks with this approach are pneumothorax and puncture of internal thoracic vessels [41].

Subxiphoid. The needle must be inserted between the xiphisternum and left costal margin. Once it is beneath the cartilage cage, the needle should be lowered to a 15- to 30-degree angle with the abdominal wall directed toward the left shoulder. ECG monitoring must be maintained throughout the procedure. Ultrasound guidance is helpful; however, the procedure may be performed without it in emergency situations. The major risk involved with this approach is right atrial puncture. This approach has a lower

risk of pneumothorax compared to the other approaches [41]. Thus, this is the recommended approach for pericardiocentesis.

Care and surveillance

Once the drainage has reduced to less than 30 mL in 24 h, the catheter can be removed, and aspiration must be provided every 6 h. Pericardial catheter care is the same as central venous catheter care. To exclude the presence of pneumothorax, chest radiography has to be performed after the procedure [41].

Endotracheal intubation

Endotracheal intubation is an obligatory procedure in the newborn to provide an efficient airway in order to deliver positive pressure ventilation. It is important for the administration of surfactant, medications such as tolazoline, aerosols with antibiotics, inhaled nitric oxide, and for clearing the trachea of meconium.

ET intubation is a lifesaving procedure in the micro preemie. Micro preemie is an infant born before 26 weeks of gestation or weighing less than 1 lb. There are two main types of intubation namely orotracheal intubation and nasotracheal intubation. Orotracheal intubation is most commonly performed than nasotracheal intubation as it is easier and quicker. Nasotracheal intubation is a difficult procedure to be performed electively.

Premedication

ET intubation is a painful procedure. Premedication reduces the pain and discomfort experienced during intubation. All the neonates undergoing intubation must receive premedication. Exceptional cases are neonates undergoing emergency intubation [42].

The standard protocol for premedication in neonates undergoing nonemergent intubation is as follows:
- Oxygen may be required before and during the procedure to maintain target saturation and prevent hypoxic episodes. In term neonates FiO_2 of 21% may be sufficient. For preterm neonates start FiO_2 between 21% and 30% and adjust to maintain target saturation
- Administration of a vagolytic agent, atropine (0.01–0.03 mg/kg IV) in order to prevent bradycardia
- A rapid acting analgesic/sedative/hypnotic, fentanyl (2–3 mcg/kg/dose)
- Muscle relaxant like vecuronium (0.1 mg/kg/dose) or succinylcholine (2 mg/kg) may be needed only in selective cases, as they may cause higher mortality in neonates

Administering the premedication is ethically important in neonates as intubation is a painful procedure. Even though, there is a risk of complications associated with the premedication, no conclusive evidence is present [42].

Procedure

Prepare the neonate and place in the sniffing position. Hyperextension should not be done as it can collapse the trachea. Suction the oropharynx and nasopharynx. If not an emergency, ventilate and oxygenate for 60 s to prevent hypoxia to less than 20 s. The blade attached to laryngoscope must be held in left hand and the mouth should be opened with the fingers. Now, introduce the blade into the right side of the mouth and move it to center. Lift the epiglottis until larynx is seen. Press the thyroid cartilage gently to properly visualize the glottis. When the glottis is visible, insert the appropriate size of endotracheal intubation tube (ETT) in the opening. Initially insert 1–2 cm of the tube while maintaining direct vision. Then, insert 2–2.5 cm into the trachea; the depth of insertion is determined according to infant size. Hold the ETT and withdraw the laryngoscope gently. After confirming the air entry, fix the ETT and secure with a tape. The position of ETT must be confirmed with chest X-ray and it should be 1 cm above carina. In micro preemie, it should be in between carina and clavicle [43]. The ETT insertion length must be 6 + weight in kg for orotracheal tube and 6 + weight in kg + 1 for nasotracheal tube (Table 37A.3).

Complications

The common complications associated with intubation are accidental extubations, hypoxia, bradycardia or apnea, pneumothorax, bronchial intubation, esophageal intubation, tracheal and esophageal perforation, ETT occlusion, infections associated with the inserted tube, bleeding, local injury, and subglottic stenosis on prolonged intubation. Hypoxia can result from multiple prolonged attempts of intubation, which can be reduced by providing ventilation through bag mask. Bronchial and esophageal complications arise due to malpositioning of the ETT [44].

Care and surveillance

Care and surveillance is required to minimize the complications arising due to endotracheal intubation as it is a difficult procedure in neonates. Pre-oxygenation should be provided when required to maintain target oxygen saturation and prevent hypoxic episodes. Number of attempts of ETT insertion should be reduced. ETT must be placed appropriately by trained staff and should be confirmed by the detection of exhaled carbon dioxide. Strict hand hygiene must be maintained while placing the endotracheal tube to minimize the infections associated with the procedure. Watch for humidified air column coming from endotracheal tube. It must be checked through CO_2 detectors [39].

Recommendations

Trained staff should insert the ETT in neonates to avoid the malposition-related complications. The neonate should be regularly monitored with the help of pulse oximetry. All the neonates undergoing intubation must receive appropriate premedication, such as vagolytic agent, rapidly acting analgesic, or hypnotic and fentanyl. The ETT must be removed as soon as possible at an appropriate time when they are no longer required [45].

Laryngeal mask airway (Fig. 37A.10)

Laryngeal mask airway (LMA) can be used in emergencies where ventilation and intubations are not feasible. The most common indications of LMA include as a rescue in providing emergency airway when intubation fails. For short-term resuscitation in the delivery, these can be used. LMA is less invasive to the respiratory tract and results in lesser hemodynamic stress response when compared with an endotracheal tube [46]. Conditions, such as cerebral hemorrhage and tracheal edema can be avoided with LMA, which generally are seen with endotracheal intubation. In the neonates with respiratory tract malformations, LMA can be lifesaving where endotracheal intubation fails. Regarding

Table 37A.3 Endotracheal tube size, suction catheter size, laryngoscope blade, and distance for orotracheal insertion

Weight (kg)	Gestational age (weeks)	Laryngoscope blade	Endotracheal tube size (inner diameter mm)	Suction catheter size (F)	Insertion depth at lips (cm)
Below 1	<28	00 or 0	2.5	5 or 6	5.5–6.5
1–2	28–34	0	3.0	6 or 8	7–8
>2	>34	1 or 0	3.5	8	8–9

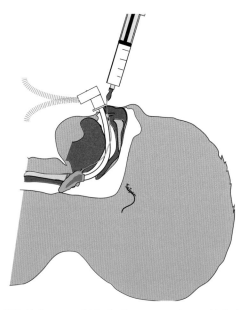

the insertion technique, endotracheal tube requires multiple attempts for successful intubation, whereas LMA can be easily inserted by non-anesthetist personnel. LMA insertion does not require the use of neuromuscular blocking agents, further diminishing pharmacological risk in neonates [47].

The most common complications associated with LMA are laryngospasm, bronchospasm, abdominal distension, aspiration, and tongue edema. LMA can be removed when ETT can be inserted successfully and in cases where spontaneous respiration can be seen.

Conclusions

Catheters and tubes remain indispensable in the neonatal intensive care units. However, many complications are associated with the use of these invasive catheters and tubes. Being vigilant about the complications and handling by well-trained staff are the important prerequisites for the success of these procedures, which may be lifesaving procedures in critically ill neonates. Guidelines have been presented in this review based on the currently available evidence.

Fig. 37A.10 Laryngeal Mask Airway. Insertion and inflation of the cuff to secure position. Copyright: Satyan Lakshminrusimha.

References

[1] Ramasethu J. Complications of vascular catheters in the neonatal intensive care unit. Clin Perinatol 2008;35(1):199–222.

[2] Fontana M, Morgillo D, Stocker M, Berger TM. The golden first 30 minutes of the umbilical artery catheter. Pediatr Crit Care Med 2014;15(4_Suppl.):175.

[3] So MJ, Kobayashi D, Anthony E, Singh J. Pseudoaneurysm formation after umbilical arterial catheterization: an uncommon but potentially life-threatening complication. J Perinatol 2012;32(2):147–149.

[4] Barrington KJ. Umbilical artery catheters in the newborn: effects of catheter materials. Cochrane Database Syst Rev 2000;2:CD000949.

[5] Molanus D, van Scherpenzeel M, Derikx J, van den Dungen F. Umbilical artery perforation: a potentially life-threatening complication of umbilical artery catheterisation. BMJ Case Rep 2017;2017. bcr-2017-222664.

[6] Chaaya SB, Al Zidgali F, Ofoegbu BN. Scrotal hypoperfusion: a rare complication of umbilical artery catheterisation. Arch Dis Child 2016;101(6):F561.

[7] Muñoz ME, Roche C, Escribá R, Martínez-Bermejo A, Pascual-Castroviejo I. Flaccid paraplegia as complication of umbilical artery catheterization. Pediatr Neurol 1993;9(5):401–403.

[8] Takci S, Esenboga S, Gonc N, Yigit S. Persistent hypoglycemia caused by umbilical arterial catheterization. J Pediatr Endocrinol Metab 2011;24 (11–12):1081–1083.

[9] Boo NY, Wong NC, Zulkifli SZ, Lye MS. Risk factors associated with umbilical vascular catheter-associated thrombosis in newborn infants. J Paediatr Child Health 1999;35(5):460–465.

[10] Garland JS, Buck RK, Maloney P, Durkin DM, Toth-Lloyd S, Duffy M, et al. Comparison of 10% povidone-iodine and 0.5% chlorhexidine gluconate for the prevention of peripheral intravenous catheter colonization in neonates: a prospective trial. Pediatr Infect Dis J 1995;14(6):510–516.

[11] Zakrzewska-Bode A, Muytjens HL, Liem KD, Hoogkamp-Korstanje JAA. Mupirocin resistance in coagulase-negative staphylococci,

after topical prophylaxis for the reduction of colonization of central venous catheters. J Hosp Infect 1995;31(3):189–193.

[12] Butler-O'Hara M, Buzzard CJ, Reubens L, McDermott MP, DiGrazio W, D'Angio CT. A randomized trial comparing long-term and short-term use of umbilical venous catheters in premature infants with birth weights of less than 1251 grams. Pediatrics 2006;118(1):e25–e35.

[13] Guimarães AF, De Souza AA, Bouzada MCF, Meira Z. Accuracy of chest radiography for positioning of the umbilical venous catheter. J Pediatr 2017;93(2):172–178.

[14] Mutlu M, Parıltan BK, Aslan Y, Eyüpoğlu , Kader , Aktürk FA. Comparison of methods and formulas used in umbilical venous catheter placement. Turk Arch Pediatr 2017;52(1):35.

[15] Mutlu M, Aslan Y, Kul S, Yılmaz G. Umbilical venous catheter complications in newborns: a 6-year single-center experience. J Matern Fetal Neonatal Med 2016;29(17):2817–2822.

[16] Abiramalatha T, Kumar M, Shabeer MP, Thomas N. Advantages of

being diligent: lessons learnt from umbilical venous catheterisation in neonates. BMJ Case Rep 2016;2016. bcr2015214073.

[17] Erolu Gunay E, Memisoglu A, Altinyuva Usta S, Tosun Ö, Ak K, Akalin F. High glucose concentration in pericardial fluid: an indication for iatrogenic cardiac tamponade in a neonate. Marmara Med J 2016;29:189–191.

[18] Gordon A, Greenhalgh M, McGuire W. Early planned removal of umbilical venous catheters to prevent infection in newborn infants. Cochrane Database Syst Rev 2017;10:CD012142.

[19] Tariq M, Huang DT. PICCing the best access for your patient. Crit Care 2006;10(5):315.

[20] Jain P, Pant D, Sood J. Atlas of practical neonatal and pediatric procedures. JP Medical Ltd.; 2012.

[21] Nowlen TT, Rosenthal GL, Johnson GL, Tom DJ, Vargo TA. Pericardial effusion and tamponade in infants with central catheters. Pediatrics 2002;110(1):137–142.

[22] Sertic AJ, Connolly BL, Temple MJ, Parra DA, Amaral JG, Lee KS. Perforations associated with peripherally inserted central catheters in a neonatal population. Pediatr Radiol 2018;48:109–119.

[23] Flores Moreno M, Pueblas Bedoy KS, Ojeda Sánchez A, Zurita-Cruz J. Risk factors associated with complications that required the removal of peripherally inserted central venous catheters in a tertiary pediatric hospital. Bol Med Hosp Infant Mex 2017;74(4):289–294.

[24] Maki DG, Goldmnan DA, Rhame FS. Infection control in intravenous therapy. Ann Intern Med 1973;79(6):86.

[25] Tiru B, Bloomstone JA, McGee WT. Radial artery cannulation: a review article. J Anesth Clin Res 2012;3(5):1000209.

[26] Mitchell JD, Welsby IJ. Techniques of arterial access. Surgery 2004;22(1):3–4.

[27] Shah US, Downing R, Davis I. An iatrogenic arterial foreign body. Br J Anaesth 1996;77(3):430–431.

[28] Murphy GS, Szokol JW, Marymont JH, Avram MJ, Vender JS. Retrograde air embolization during routine radial artery catheter flushing in adult cardiac surgical patients: an ultrasound study. Anesthesiology 2004;101(3):614–619.

[29] Abubakar M. . In: MacDonald M, Ramasthu J, editors. Atlas of procedures in noenatology. Wolters Kluwer/Lippincott Williams & Wilkins; 2007.

[30] Carroll P. Chest tubes made easy. RN 1995;58(12):46–54.

[31] Mehrabani D, Kopelman AE. Chest tube insertion: a simplified technique. Pediatrics 1989;83(5):784–785.

[32] Karadžić R, Antović A, Ilić G, Kostić-Banović L. Pneumopericardium: a possible rare cause of neonatal death. Facta Universitatis 2007;14(2):98–100.

[33] Cummings RG, Wesly RL, Adams DH, Lowe JE. Pneumopericardium resulting in cardiac tamponade. Ann Thorac Surg 1984;37(6):511–518.

[34] MacDonald MG, Ramasethu J. Atlas of procedures in neonatology. 5th ed. Lippincott Williams & Wilkins, Wolters Kluwer; 2012. p. 271.

[35] Reed RC, Waters BL, Siebert JR. Complications of percutaneous thoracostomy in neonates and infants. J Perinatol 2016;36(4):296–299.

[36] Hyde J, Sykes T, Graham T. Reducing morbidity from chest drains. Br Med J 1997;314(7085):914.

[37] Lazzara D. Eliminate the air of mystery from chest tubes. Nursing 2002;32(6):36–45.

[38] Kumar R, Sinha A, Lin MJ, Uchino R, Butryn T, O'Mara MS, et al.

Complications of pericardiocentesis: a clinical synopsis. Int J Crit Illn Inj Sci 2015;5(3):206.

[39] Maggiolini S, Osculati G, Vitale G. Utility and safety of diagnostic pericardiocentesis. Eur Heart J 2005;26(10):1046–1047.

[40] Maisch B, Seferović PM, Ristić AD, Erbel R, Rienmüller R, Adler Y, et al. Guidelines on the diagnosis and management of pericardial diseases executive summary: the Task Force on the Diagnosis and Management of Pericardial Diseases of the European Society of Cardiology. Eur Heart J 2004;25(7):587–610.

[41] De Carlini CC, Maggiolini S. Pericardiocentesis in cardiac tamponade: indications and practical aspects. J Cardiol Pract 2017; 15:19.

[42] Barrington K. Premedication for endotracheal intubation in the newborn infant. Paediatr Child Health 2011;16(3):159–164.

[43] Donn SM, Kuhns LR. Mechanism of endotracheal tube movement with change of head position in the neonate. Pediatr Radiol 1980;9(1):37–40.

[44] Khatami SF, Parvaresh P, Behjati S. Common complications of endotracheal intubation in newborns. Iran J Neonatol 2011;2(1):12–17.

[45] Australian Resuscitation Council. Paediatric advanced life support: Australian Resuscitation Council Guidelines 2006. Emerg Med Australas 2006;18(4):357–371.

[46] Tanaka A, Isono S, Ishikawa T, Sato J, Nishino T. Laryngeal resistance before and after minor surgery endotracheal tube versus Laryngeal Mask Airway™. Anesthesiology 2003;99(2):252–258.

[47] Lavies NG. Use of the laryngeal mask airway in neonatal resuscitation. Anaesthesia 1993;48(4):352–1352.

Further reading

[48] Murki S, Kumar P. Blood exchange transfusion for infants with severe neonatal hyperbilirubinemia. Semin Perinatol 2011;35(3):175–184.

[49] Erdei C, McAvoy LL, Gupta M, Pereira S, McGowan EC. Is zero central line-associated bloodstream infection rate sustainable? A

5-year perspective. Pediatrics 2015;135(6):e1485–e1493.

Chapter |37B|

Neonatal Limb Ischemia Due to Arterial Catheters

Catherine C. Beaullieu, MD, Suzanne M. Lopez, MD, P. Syamasundar Rao, MD, FAAP, FACC, FASCAI

CHAPTER POINTS

- Umbilical (UACs) or peripheral arterial catheters are often used in the neonates and premature infants for hemodynamic monitoring and access for frequent blood sampling.
- Neonates are at a risk for development of blood vessel occlusion and limb ischemia, secondary to small size of the arteries relative to size of the catheters and immature anti-coagulation system.
- Pallor of the affected extremity with discoloration and mottling along with diminished or absent pulse may be seen with limb ischemia which, if untreated, may evolve into irreversible necrosis.
- Strategies to prevent limb ischemia include: 1. Development of guidelines standardizing the use of umbilical and peripheral arterial catheters at each institution and 2. Removal the UACs and peripheral arterial lines as soon as the need for close monitoring is reduced or if less invasive monitoring methods become available.
- Steps in the management of limb ischemia: 1. Conservative management including removal of the catheter and warm compresses to the contralateral limb to facilitate reflex vasodilatation in the affected limb, 2. Medical management with drug therapy with a nitroglycerin patch, a combination of nitroglycerin patch with papaverine infusion, thrombolytic therapy with heparin and tissue plasminogen activator (tPA), in that order, and 3. When medical management fails to improve limb perfusion, surgical thrombectomy along with reconstructive vascular surgery may have to be undertaken.

Introduction

The use of arterial catheters is common in the neonatal population given the need for invasive hemodynamic monitoring in addition to easy access for blood sampling in critically ill infants. However, neonates are at a higher risk for developing thrombosis and catheter-induced ischemia due to the small size of the arterial diameter relative to size of the catheters likely to be used and owing to their immature anticoagulation system [1].

There are multiple abnormalities of the coagulation factors in the neonates and premature infants. At birth, the plasma concentrations of vitamin-K-dependent factors, contact factors, and direct inhibitors of thrombin are only 50% of adult values. In addition, α2-macroglobulin; factors V, VIII, and XIII; and von Willebrand factor are elevated. In the premature infant, the aforementioned factors attain adult values by the age of 6 months. In addition, any illness that may arise further disrupts normal hemostasis.

Postnatal limb ischemia is most commonly iatrogenic in origin and is often due to the presence of umbilical or peripheral arterial catheters. The catheters cause an additive damage of the vascular endothelium, triggering inflammatory cascade, which increases adhesion and aggregation of platelets. This results in local stasis, reduced blood flow, and consequent thrombosis [2].

The objective of this chapter is to discuss the diagnosis and management of limb ischemia related to arterial catheters in neonates. Discussion of prenatal limb ischemia will not be included in this review.

Umbilical arterial catheterization

Umbilical arterial catheters (UACs) are commonly used in the neonate to monitor blood pressure and for ease of blood sampling. Because of availability of pulse oximeters, UACs are no longer used just for monitoring oxygenation. The earlier the catheters are inserted, the better is the probability of successful catheterization. Indwelling UACs have been shown to be an independent risk factor for limb ischemia in the neonate [3]. Thrombus formation with resulting ischemia is the second most common complication associated with UACs; the first being hemorrhage [4]. Nearly 20% of babies with UACs may have thrombus formation [5]; however, the complications rates vary markedly, between 1.5% and 95%, depending upon the method (clinical, sonography, angiography, or autopsy) used for detection of thrombi [4]. The mechanism of ischemia is from vasospasm, thrombus formation, or emboli arising from the distal aorta and its branches [4]. Complications occur less often when UACs are positioned high (tip in the descending aorta above the level of the diaphragm and below the left subclavian artery—usually corresponding to thoracic vertebral level T6–T9) [6]. Continuous heparin infusion at 0.25–1 unit/mL is recommended by Centers for Disease Control (CDC) and is thought to lengthen catheter patency rates, but may not reduce the risk for thrombosis [7]. It would appear that longer a UAC is left in place, the higher the chance of thrombus formation (80% prevalence if the catheter is in place for >21 days) [8]. The CDC recommends <5 days as optimal duration of use for UAC and <14 days for UVC.

Peripheral arterial catheterization

When umbilical arterial catheterization is not feasible, cannulation of radial, dorsalis pedis, posterior tibial arteries, and less commonly, ulnar and temporal arteries are undertaken [9]. In order to minimize risk associated with occlusion, it is recommended that peripheral arterial catheters are placed in locations with potential collateral circulation. The adequacy of collateral circulation may be tested by Allen's test [10]. The neonate's arm is elevated, the radial and ulnar arteries are occluded simultaneously by digital pressure, and

the arm rubbed to produce blanching of the palm. Releasing the digital pressure on the ulnar artery should result in return of normal color to the palm in less than 10 s if there is adequate collateral circulation from the ulnar artery. Conversely, release of digital pressure on the radial artery would verify adequacy of the ulnar artery (refer to procedures chapter for a figure and more details on Allen's test).

At the present time, brachial and femoral arteries are rarely used in the neonatal intensive care units (NICUs) because of significant complications associated with use of these sites in both the term and preterm infants. However, femoral arteries are used for cardiac catheterization, but the catheters are removed after the study. Sometimes, the femoral arterial lines may be used for monitoring blood pressures in postoperative cardiac patients, especially when umbilical arterial access is not feasible (Fig. 37B.1).

Complications associated with peripheral arterial catheterization include vasospasm, thrombus formation, embolism, ischemia, and tissue necrosis. Hematoma, infection, peripheral nerve damage, and other complications may also occur. Incidence of complications with the use of peripheral arterial catheterization appears to be low, although nearly 50% of the catheters had to be removed because of the lack of blood return, ischemia, thrombosis, or a combination of these adverse consequences [9,11–13].

Clinical presentation of limb ischemia associated with arterial catheters

Neonates affected by limb ischemia often present with pallor of the affected extremity followed by discoloration and mottling with diminished or absent pulse which may evolve to irreversible necrosis, if untreated. Upon detection of limb perfusion abnormality, detailed clinical evaluation along with ankle/brachial blood pressure index and Doppler assessment should be undertaken. Audible Doppler signals at a location distal to the site of presumed obstruction are absent (portable Doppler probes are likely to be available at most nursing stations—SonoSite X-Porte point-of-care ultrasound system is one such machine). Formal duplex and color Doppler studies from Radiology/Ultrasound Department are useful in confirming the site of obstruction and for detecting the presence of collateral flow. If there is a clinical evidence for ischemia as stated in the first sentence of this paragraph, the management, as discussed in the next section, should begin immediately without waiting for confirmation by formal Doppler study.

It is frequently difficult to distinguish between thrombus formation, embolus from a remote site, or vascular spasm as a cause of limb perfusion deficiency. Improved perfusion following warming of contalateral extremity, causing vasodilatation, may indicate vasospasm. Development of

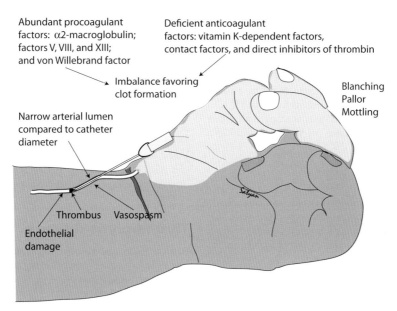

Fig. 37B.1 Factors Contributing to Limb Ischemia in Neonates Undergoing Intensive Care. The presence of an arterial catheter, small arterial lumen compared to the catheter size, endothelial damage, and imbalance between procoagulant and anticoagulant factors predispose to limb ischemia. Copyright: Satyan Lakshminrusimha.

perfusion deficit in close proximity to the indwelling catheter is likely to be due to thrombus formation. Limb ischemia remote from the location of the catheter (for example, compromised circulation in the femoral or popliteal artery distribution in the presence of an umbilical artery catheter) is probably an embolus. Irrespective of the possible etiology, the approach to the management and the algorithm used, as detailed later, are similar.

Prevention

If the UACs and peripheral arterial lines are not inserted, the limb ischemia complications are unlikely to occur. It was shown that adopting guidelines standardizing the use of umbilical catheters in the preterm infants resulted in reduction of UAC use from 42.3% to 23.6% ($P < 0.001$) without increase in the use of peripheral arterial lines [14]. In addition, inappropriate use of UACs was reduced from 8% to 1% ($P = 0.01$) concurrently. Consequently, we would suggest that strict guidelines for UAC usage should be developed in all NICUs. Similar guidelines for insertion of peripheral arterial lines should also be developed.

Additionally, the UACs and peripheral arterial lines should be removed as soon as the need for close monitoring has decreased or if less invasive monitoring methods become available.

Management

If ischemia, thrombosis, or any other limb perfusion abnormalities are detected, catheter removal is indicated along with conservative measures, anticoagulants, thrombolytic agents, and/or surgery as deemed appropriate. However, unfortunately, there are no randomized, controlled, clinical trials to demonstrate efficacy of one method over the other [13,15,16]; therefore, the decision to use a given treatment modality is largely based on local institution experience. We will review each of these treatment options.

Conservative management

Once an infant develops symptoms of limb ischemia associated with an arterial catheter, the catheter should be removed. The only exception to this recommendation is the need for immediate volume expansion in babies with shock and/or hypovolemia. Imaging with Doppler ultrasound should be performed before catheter removal and consideration should be given to whether local thrombolysis via catheter is indicated [17]. The affected limb should be elevated and warm compresses should be applied to the contralateral limb, a technique that facilitates reflex vasodilatation in the affected limb.

Medical management (drug therapy)

If limb ischemia is unresponsive to catheter removal and other conservative measures, the next step is medical management with drugs. Options for management are a nitroglycerin patch, a combination of nitroglycerin patch with papaverine infusion, or thrombolytic therapy with either heparin, streptokinase/urokinase, or tissue plasminogen activator (tPA).

Nitroglycerin patch

Nitroglycerin is known to be a vascular smooth muscle relaxant that is readily absorbed through intact skin. It is indicated in the setting of acute vasospasm related to both umbilical and peripheral arterial catheters for symptoms unresponsive to conservative measures. The amount of absorbed nitroglycerin and systemic levels (of the drug) attained are likely related directly to the amount of ointment and dimension of the area of application [18]. The initial dose of 2% nitroglycerin ointment is 4 mm/kg (1.22 mg/kg) [19]. It is typically applied 1–2 cm proximal to the line of pallor, and the vasodilator effect usually manifests within 15–30 min of application. Dose frequency has varied; it is most frequently applied every 6–8 h. The duration of application of nitroglycerin patch also varied, ranging from 1—27 days, which was typically dependent upon improvement on clinical examination [20]. In considering the use of topical application, preterm babies have an undeveloped epidermal permeability barrier, which may increase absorption of the drug [21]. Infants should be monitored for hemodynamic instability during drug application especially within the first 6 h of administration when the drug reaches its peak plasma concentration [18]. Systemic complications that may occur in neonates include: hypotension, tachycardia, flushing, and rarely methemoglobinemia, which warrants close monitoring of heart rate and blood pressure in addition to daily methemoglobin levels while the drug is being administered [20].

Nitroglycerin patch and Papaverine

Papaverine is an opium alkaloid with vasodilator and spasmolytic action due to its inhibition of oxidative phosphorylation and calcium flux during muscle contraction. It has been used to prolong the patency of arterial catheters of preterm neonates without evidence of associated hypotension or intraventricular hemorrhage (IVH) [22]. Some studies have shown that administration of intraarterial papaverine before removal of the arterial line combined with subsequent placement of a nitroglycerin patch can also be effective in preventing residual damage in arterial catheter-induced ischemia secondary to vascular spasm [23].

Thrombolytic therapy

If there is no discernible clinical improvement following institution of conservative therapy and nitroglycerin patch with or without papaverine, a consideration for thrombolysis should be given. Prior to initiation of thrombolytic therapy, it is generally recommended that pediatric hematology consultation is sought to obtain their input in the management of thromboembolism [17].

Heparin

Low-molecular-weight heparin, specifically enoxaparin, is the most commonly used anticoagulant in the pediatric patient given demonstration of fewer bleeding complications in clinical trials, the longer half-life and most consistent pharmacokinetics and pharmacodynamics [24–30]. But, it should be noted that there are higher rates of heparin clearance and lower levels of antithrombin in neonates when compared with those of adults; therefore, neonates often require higher doses of anticoagulants to achieve therapeutic levels [31,32].

Anticoagulation with heparin is indicated in the setting of definite occlusive nonlimb-threatening asymptomatic or symptomatic thrombosis [33]. Dosing of both unfractionated and low molecular weight heparin is based on gestational age (Tables 37B.1 and 37B.2, respectively) [34].

Table 37B.1 Unfractionated Heparin (UFH) Dosing*	
Gestational Age	**Doses**
<28 weeks of gestational age	25 u/kg IV bolus, 15 u/kg/h IV infusion
28–37 weeks of gestational age	50 u/kg IV bolus, 15 u/kg/h IV infusion
>37 weeks of gestational age	100 u/kg IV bolus, 28 u/kg/h IV infusion
*Goal anti-Xa levels of 0.3–0.7.	

Table 37B.2 Low Molecular Weight Heparin Dosing*

Gestational Age	Doses
<28 weeks of gestational age	1.25 mg/kg SQ q12
28–37 weeks of gestational age	1.5 mg/kg SQ q12
>37 weeks of gestational age	1.625 mg/kg SQ q12
*Goal anti-Xa levels of 0.5–1 U/mL (blood sample obtained 4–6 h after last dose).	

Babies receiving heparin should have their anti-Xa activity monitored. The recommended target value anti-Xa activity for unfractionated heparin use is 0.35–0.7 units/mL and for low molecular-weight heparin use, the target values is 0.5–1.0 units/mL. For further details regarding monitoring, the reader referred to the recommendations proposed by 9th edition of the American College of Chest Physicians' guidelines [17].

Streptokinase (SK) and urokinase (UK)

Streptokinase (SK) and urokinase (UK) have been used in the past to dissolve thrombotic arterial occlusions [35]. A study of 182 infants (analysis of reports from the literature) comparing SK and UK with tissue tPA revealed no significant difference ($P > 0.05$) in the efficacy rates of the three agents. Effective thrombolysis varied from 39% to 86% in different studies evaluated in this paper. Bleeding complications including IVH were low. The authors recommended controlled prospective multicenter studies to evaluate patency and adverse event rates with the use of these thrombolytic agents [35]. While SK and UK were used extensively in the past, they are largely replaced by tPA at the present [17].

Tissue plasminogen activator

Thrombolysis with tPA is reserved for limb- or life-threatening thrombosis. Dosing of tPA is determined by gestational age (Table 37B.3) [34]. Senior author's (PSR) prior experience is suggestive of favorable outcome of thrombolytic therapy (with tPA) of thrombus/embolus at other locations in the cardiovascular system [36].

Imaging with Doppler ultrasound is indicated prior to treatment and every 12–24 h during treatment. Cranial ultrasound is also indicated prior to initiation of therapy to detect IVH. Recommended laboratory studies to follow include fibrinogen, platelets, coagulation factors, and plasminogen prior to treatment and every 12–24 h during treatment [14,16]. Because of the concern for associated adverse events with tPA use in the neonate, the tPA should be used only when thrombosis is life-threatening or is likely to result in limb loss.

Surgical management

When medical management fails to improve limb perfusion, surgical thrombectomy or embolectomy should be considered. Additional surgical indications include: total limb ischemia, evidence of compartment syndrome, pregangrenous tissue evolution, documented absence of arterial blood flow by Doppler ultrasound or angiography for longer than 24 h, and extremely high bleeding risk for thrombolysis (recent cardiovascular surgery or cerebral hemorrhage) [37]. One study reported good outcomes following embolectomy and reconstructive vascular surgery in a group of 11 children including premature infants [38].

Amputation should be delayed for as long as possible given that eventual demarcation may lie distal to the original line of ischemia. Consideration must also be given for

Table 37B.3 Tissue Plasminogen Activator (tPA) Dosing

Gestational Age	Doses
<28 weeks of gestational age	0.03 or 0.06 mg/kg/h (Infuse UFH at 10 u/kg/h)
>28 weeks gestationl age	0.1–0.5 mg/kg/h for 6–12 h, repeat daily for up to 3 days (infuse UFH at 10 u/kg/h)
UFH, Unfractionated heparin.	

ALGORITHM 37B.1 MANAGEMENT OF LIMB ISCHEMIA

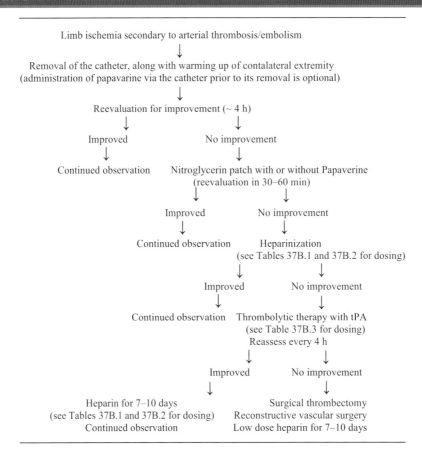

Limb ischemia secondary to arterial thrombosis/embolism
↓
Removal of the catheter, along with warming up of contalateral extremity
(administration of papavarine via the catheter prior to its removal is optional)
↓
Reevaluation for improvement (~ 4 h)
↓   ↓
Improved   No improvement
↓   ↓
Continued observation   Nitroglycerin patch with or without Papaverine
(reevaluation in 30–60 min)
↓   ↓
Improved   No improvement
↓   ↓
Continued observation   Heparinization
(see Tables 37B.1 and 37B.2 for dosing)
↓   ↓
Improved   No improvement
↓   ↓
Continued observation   Thrombolytic therapy with tPA
(see Table 37B.3 for dosing)
Reassess every 4 h
↓   ↓
Improved   No improvement
↓   ↓
Heparin for 7–10 days   Surgical thrombectomy
(see Tables 37B.1 and 37B.2 for dosing)   Reconstructive vascular surgery
Continued observation   Low dose heparin for 7–10 days

tPA, Tissue plasminogen activator.

future prosthetic limb application and prevention of joint contracture [39].

We would recommend the below proposed algorithm for management of babies with limb ischemia (Algorithm 37B.1).

Ultimately, successful outcome of management of limb ischemia secondary to arterial catheterization is dependent upon early recognition, diagnosis of etiology, and prompt treatment.

References

[1] Mosalli R, Elbaz M, Paes B. Topical nitroglycerine for neonatal arterial associated peripheral ischemia following cannulation: a case report and comprehensive literature review. Case Rep Pediatr 2013;2013:1–7.

[2] Stump DC, Mann KG. Mechanisms of thrombus formation and lysis. Ann Emerg Med 1988;17:1138–1147.

[3] Alpert J, O'Donnell JA, Parsonnet V, et al. Clinically recognized limb ischemia in the neonate after umbilical artery catheterization. Am J Surg 1980;140:413–418.

[4] Arshad A, McCarthy MJ. Management of limb ischemia in the neonate. Eur J Vasc Endovasc Surg 2009;38: 61–65.

[5] Joseph R, Chong A, Teh M, et al. Thrombotic complication of umbilical arterial catheterization and its sequelae. Ann Acad Med Singapore 1985;14:576–582.

[6] Barrington K. Umbilical artery catheters in the newborn: effects of position of the catheter tip. Cochrane Database of Syst Rev 2000;(2):CD000505.

[7] Barrington K. Umbilical artery catheters in the newborn: effects of heparin. Cochrane Database Syst Rev 2000;(2):CD000507.

[8] McAdams RM, Winter VT, McCurnin DC, et al. Complications of umbilical artery catheterization in a model of extreme prematurity. J Perinatol 2009;29:685–692.

[9] Randel SN, Tsang BH, Wung JT, et al. Experience with percutaneous indwelling peripheral arterial catheterization in neonates. Am J Dis Child 1987;141:848–851.

[10] Available from: https://www2.health. vic.gov.au/hospitals-and../neonatal../ peripheral-arterial-access.

[11] Aldridge SA, Gupta JM. Peripheral artery cannulation in newborns. J Singapore Paediatr Soc 1992;34:11–14.

[12] Spahr RC, MacDonald HM, Holzman IR. Catheterization of the posterior tibial artery in the neonate. Am J Dis Child 1979;133:945–946.

[13] Monagle P, Chan AK, Goldenberg NA, et al. Antithrombotic therapy in neonates and children: antithrombotic therapy and prevention of thrombosis, American College of Chest Physicians Evidence based Clinical Practice Guidelines 9th ed. Chest 2012;141:e737S–e801S.

[14] Shahid S, Dutta S, Symington A, Shivananda S. McMaster University NICU. Standardizing umbilical catheter usage in preterm infants. Pediatrics 2014;133:e1742–e1752.

[15] Saxonhouse MA. Management of neonatal thrombosis. Clin Perinatol 2012;39:191–208.

[16] Saxonhouse MA. Thrombosis in the neonatal intensive care unit. Clin Perinatol 2015;42:651–673.

[17] Monagle P, Chan AKC, Goldenberg NA, et al. Antithrombotic therapy in neonates and children.

[18] Bogaert MG. Clinical pharmacokinetics of glyceryl trinitrate following the use of systemic and topical preparations. Clin Pharmacokinet 1987;12:1–11.

[19] Guran P, Beal GN, Brion, et al. Topical nitroglycerin as an aid to insertion of peripheral venous catheters in neonates. J Pediatr 1989;115:1025.

[20] Samiee-Zafarghandy S, van den Anker JN, Ben Fadel N. Topical nitroglycerin in neonates with tissue injury: a case report and review of the literature. Paediatr Child Health 2014;19:9–12.

[21] Rutter N. Percutaneous drug absorption in the newborn: hazards and uses. Clin Perinatol 1987;14: 911–930.

[22] Griffin MP, Siadaty MS. Papaverine prolongs patency of peripheral arterial catheters in neonates. J Pediatr 2005;146:62–65.

[23] Panigrahy N, Kumar PP, Chirla DK, Vennapusa SR. Papaverine for ischemia following peripheral arterial catheterization in neonates. Indian Pediatr 2016;53:169.

[24] Bounameaux H. Unfractionated versus low-molecular-weight heparin in the treatment of venous thromboembolism. Vasc Med 1998;3:41–46.

[25] Chan AK, Monagle P. Updates in thrombosis in pediatrics: where are we after 20 years? Hematology Am Soc Hematol Educ Program 2012;2012:439–443.

[26] Kerlin BA, Blatt NB, Fuh B, et al. Epidemiology and risk factors for thromboembolic complications of childhood nephrotic syndrome: a Midwest Pediatric Nephrology Consortium (MWPNC) study. J Pediatr 2009;155:105–110.e1.

[27] Molinari AC, Banov L, Bertamino M, et al. A practical approach to the use of low molecular weight heparins in VTE treatment and prophylaxis in children and newborns. Pediatr Hematol Oncol 2015;32:1–10.

[28] Raffini L, Huang YS, Witmer C, et al. Dramatic increase in venous

thromboembolism in children's hospitals in the United States from 2001 to 2007. Pediatr 2009;124:1001– 1008.

[29] Samama MM, Gerotziafas GT. Comparative pharmacokinetics of LMWHS. Semin Thromb Hemost 2000;26(Suppl. 1):31–38.

[30] Young G. Old and new antithrombotic drugs in neonates and infants. Semin Fetal Neonatal Med 2011;16:349–354.

[31] Andrew M, Paes B, Johnston M. Development of the hemostatic system in the neonate and young infant. Am J Pediatr Hematol Oncol 1990;12:95–104.

[32] Berfelo FJ, Kersbergen KJ, van Ommen CH, et al. Neonatal cerebral sinovenous thrombosis from symptom to outcome. Stroke 2010;41:1382–1388.

[33] Manco-Johnson MJ. Diagnosis and management of thromboses in the neonatal period. Semin Perinatol 1990;14:393–402.

[34] Armstrong-Wells JL, Manco-Johnson MJ. Neonatal thrombosis. In: de Alarcon P, Werner EJ, Christensen RD, editors. Neonatal hematology. New York, NY: Cambridge University Press; 2013. p. 282.

[35] Nowak-Gottl U, Auberger K, Halimeh S, et al. Thrombolysis in newborns and infants. Thromb Haemost 1999;82(Suppl. 1):112–116.

[36] Pugh KJ, Jureidini SB, Ream R, Rao PS, Dossier J. Successful thrombolytic therapy of pulmonary embolism associated with urosepsis in an infant. Pediatr Cardiol 2002;23:77–79.

[37] Rashish G, Paes BA, Nagel K, et al. Thrombosis and hemostasis in newborns (THiN) group. Spontaneous neonatal arterial thromboembolism: infants at risk, diagnosis, treatment, and outcomes. Blood Coagul Fibrinolysis 2013;24:787–797.

[38] Coombs CJ, Richardson PW, Dowling GJ, Johnstone BR, Monagle P. Brachial artery thrombosis in infants: an algorithm for limb salvage. Plast Reconstr Surg 2006;117:1481–1488.

[39] Blank JE, Dormans JP, Davidson RS. Perinatal limb ischemia: orthopaedic implications. J Paediatr Orthop 1996;16:90–96.

Section $|$VIII$|$

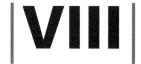

General Issues

Chapter | **38** |

Neonatal Developmental Follow-Up Program

Nagamani Beligere, MD, MPH

CHAPTER POINTS

- As the survival of premature infants are increasing, the morbidity is replacing the mortality.

- The need for establishing the Developmental follow up programs, at centers providing ventilatory care.

- The importance of required multidisciplinary approach, correction of age for prematurity, recommended schedule for standard evaluation and tools used at different ages for follow up care.

- The chapter emphasizes the importance of on going research, and quality improvement.

Introduction

During the last 3 decades, neonatal and perinatal technologies have improved the survival of preterm as well as term infants. Although the neonatal intensive care improves the survival, there has been increased morbidity among these surviving very low birth weight infants. With transfer of technology to middle-income countries, the survival has improved with similar results, but morbidity is reported to be higher. This suggests that neonatal follow-up care is not uniform due to variation in perinatal and neonatal care practices. There is a need for uniform data collection and long-term follow-up of the survivors is essential. The Eunice Kennedy Shriver National Institute of Child Health and Human Development (NICHD) and AAP have well-established protocols for follow-up care [1]. This chapter describes the organization and the follow-up of these high-risk graduates of neonatal intensive care units.

Programs, criteria, its objectives, and benefits

Objectives of the follow-up program:
1. To define the type of high-risk infants who are prone to develop neurodevelopmental disabilities.
2. To define the ages at which the children need appropriate evaluations and develop plans for interventions to minimize the long-term untoward effects on growth and development of motor, cognitive, language, vision, hearing, and behavior.
3. To develop standard method of assessment for optimal ages.
4. To provide proper information to parents and families, to care for their infants.
5. To facilitate early therapeutic intervention to those affected children and minimize the disabilities.
6. To further advance the research and uniform data collection system and to define the long-term outcomes.
7. To influence the health care policies of the country from information on long-term outcomes of the high-risk infants.

Primary responsibilities of the follow-up programs:

- **Infant Surveillance**: Surveillance establishes the pattern of systematic monitoring of all the high-risk infants [2].
- **Intervention programs**: Intervention programs help to prevent further developmental delay and improve the habilitation programs in each community.
- **Family counseling and guidance**: follow-up information facilitates counseling of parents and families with regard to prognosis of the infant and also teaching the parents to care for the child.
- It is necessary for each neonatal center to establish appropriate data collection system, get involved in the collaborative research, and publish results of outcomes. Such information can be useful in establishing proper therapeutic interventions and can influence the public policy of the nation.

Specialists in the follow-up programs:

It is essential to have multidisciplinary approach.

The disciplines required for a standard follow-up program are as follows:

- Developmental and behavioral pediatrician
- Physical therapist
- Occupational therapist
- Developmental specialist with special educational teacher
- Speech pathologist
- Clinic nurse and intake coordinator
- Family counselor or a social worker

AAP recommends few conditions to be followed up as high-risk infants.

Table 38.1 summarizes the type of infants that need to be followed up.

1. Respiratory distress at birth (5 min Apgar score <4)
2. Birth weight <1500 g with GA 23–32 weeks and late premature neonates (GA 34–37 weeks)
3. Small for gestational age infants (SGA)
4. Infants with intraventricular hemorrhage (all grades)
5. Abnormal head ultrasound (PVL, infarcts, hydrocephalus)
6. Recurrent and severe hypoglycemia–infants of diabetic mothers
7. Premature infants with hydrocephalus and seizure disorder
8. Neonatal hyperbilirubinemia and infants who required exchange transfusions

Table 38.1 AAP recommended criteria for follow-up of high-risk infants.

Risk factors	Preterm infants	Term infants
Biologic risk factors	VLBW < 1500 g birth weight, ELBW < 1000 g birth weight infants, RDS, IVH, BPD, ROP, PVL, NEC, sepsis, seizures, higher order multiple twins, triplet infants of assisted reproductive technology; infants who are treated with postnatal corticosteroids; prolonged ventilated infants; abnormal ultrasound exam in the nursery; male gender Small for gestation, failure to thrive in nursery, restricted growth (IUGR), abnormal neurologic exam at discharge	Full term infants with encephalopathy, HIE, meningitis, complex medical problems, congenital malformations (CNS, cardiac), any surgical interventions for NEC, gastroschisis, TEF, poor feeding, and GT-tubes Infants with cleft lip and palate
Interventions	Resuscitation at birth for those who required ventilation at birth with Apgar score <4; use of postnatal steroids, prolonged ventilation, ECMO in infants; high-frequency ventilated infants; prolonged O_2-dependent infants, CLD; recurrent apnea, infants with hypoglycemia, IDM, treated with ACTH; infants with hyperbilirubinemia and exchange transfusions; surgically treated infants with PDA ligation, NEC, shunt, etc.; and nutritional support	Resuscitated infants with Apgar score <4; infants were ventilated where interventions are used postnatal steroids, prolonged ventilation, ECMO, recurrent apnea, O_2-dependent infants, IDM, treated with ACTH, exchange transfusion in hyperbilirubinemia, and nutritional support; infants requiring surgical treatment
Social and environmental	Low socioeconomic status, minority status, single or teen age mothers; prenatally exposed to drugs, alcohol, and no prenatal care; environmental influence on life and stress (poor accommodation and need for food and shelter)	Low socioeconomic status, minority status, single/teen mother; low income mothers and with low maternal education; infants prenatally exposed to drugs, alcohol, and poor prenatal care; environmental influence on life and stress (poor accommodation and need for food and shelter)

Source: Modified from Follow up care of high risk infants. Pediatric 2004;114(5) [1].

9. Chronic illness, such as concurrent cardiac and renal or GI conditions
10. Abnormal neurologic evaluation at the time of discharge
11. Infant with poor nutrition with feeding difficulties and not gaining weight
12. Any infant who is showing developmental delay with no apparent neonatal complications
13. Maternal factors, such as postpartum depression, substance abuse including alcohol dependency
14. Poverty and poor maternal education
15. All infants who received invasive mechanical ventilation

Recommended follow-up schedule

- Ideally the infant should be examined at 2, 4, 6, 8, and 12 months of corrected age (CA) during the 1st year, at 15, 18, and 24 months of CA during 2nd year, and at 30 and 36 months of chronological age during the 3rd year; also can be followed up to chronologic ages of 3–8 years.
- Beyond this age, school system evaluates children.
- Correction of age for prematurity before administering any tool from 0–2 years of age. Correction of age is not recommended beyond 2 years of age. Evaluation continues at chronological age after 2 years [3].
- Most children are evaluated for learning disability in the school system for behavior and learning disorder. Intervention at school age focuses on occupational therapy and day-to-day function and behavior, reading math social behavior. Some of the evaluations are described in Table 38.2. Based on the results of the test, school system places the children in the classroom for individualized educational plan (IEP).

Calculation of the corrected age

- Mother's EDD was 3/16/2015. The infant's birth date is 1/13/2015. Child is evaluated on 12/15/2015.
- The chronologic age of the child on the day of evaluation is 11 months and 2 days.
- For correcting the age, one has to adjust for the prematurity of 2 months or 8 weeks (considering 40 weeks GA as full term). Now correction is performed by subtracting the number of months from chronological age.
- Subtraction can be done as 11 months and 2 days − 2 months = 9 months and 2 days.
- Child is evaluated as 9 months and 2 days CA.

When Bayley-III is used, the evaluation can be started at point H which is appropriate for the infant between 9 and 10 months of age.

The tools used in newborn to 12 months

1. Amiel-Tison neurologic evaluation of the newborn and infant [4]
2. Brazelton neurobehavior screening [5]
3. Bayley-III infant motor assessment scale [6]
4. Test of infant motor performance [7]
1. **Amiel-Tison scale can be used even in the nursery before discharge for continuity of care:**
   a. Growth parameter of the head, motor function, vision and hearing
   b. Axis: if infant's central axis is deviated from the central axis of spine, it determines the case of monoplegia, diplegia, or quadriplegia
   c. Motor tone: for hypertonicity or hypotonicity
   d. Angle: determines the limitation of movement of muscle and joint, the flexor and extensor angles of the extremities, and neck
   e. Primitive reflexes: persistence of reflexes even at later age
   f. Head circumference for head growth: microcephaly/macrocephaly
   g. Visual fields: esotropia, exotropia, visual following
   h. Hearing: basic response to sound
   i. Final impression of diagnosis
2. **Brazelton neurobehavioral screening is done at birth and at 72 h to evaluate the alertness of the infant [5]. This test is used in the term infant for maturity as well as behavior response.**
3. **Bayley-III infant and toddler motor assessment: evaluates in ages from 16 days to 42 months at intervals of 15 days. Bayley scale evaluates the status of gross motor, fine motor, cognitive, receptive, and behavior performance.**
   What does Bayley test determine?
   a. Gross motor: large muscle movement
   b. Fine motor: small muscle movements
   c. Cognitive: looks at how the child thinks, reacts, understands, and learns the environment around him/her by accommodation and assimilation
   d. Receptive language: how the child recognizes the sound of environment, such as toys, people, mother's, etc., and understands the words and directions
   e. Expressive: how well the child responds and communicates using gestures, sounds, or words

Table 38.2 The recommended assessment tools and appropriate ages [1]

Areas of assessment	2, 4, 6, 9, and 12 months, CA	12–14 months, CA	18–24 months, CA	36–60 months (5 years), chronological age	6–8 years, chronological age
Growth and nutrition	Ht, WT, HC, BMI*, caloric intake, nutrition	Ht, WT, HC, nutrition	Ht, WT, HC, BMI, caloric intake, nutrition	Ht, WT, HC, BMI, caloric intake, nutrition, skin fold	Ht, WT, nutrition, counseling
Neurologic assessment	Amiel-Tison*, EEG*, or MRI when indicated, such as seizures, CP*, etc. Metabolic studies when unknown neurologic diagnosis, such as SMA, PKU, or cretinism, etc.	Amiel-Tison, EEG, or MRI when necessary	Amiel-Tison, EEG, or MRI when necessary	Amiel-Tison, EEG, or MRI when necessary; for 4 years and older, MRI or functional MRI when indicated, CT*, IQ test Wechsler intelligence (WPPSI, WISC)	Neurologic assessment, metabolic screen, genetic screen; Gait, coordination; balance, EEG, MRI
Gross motor, fine motor, cognitive, language and behavior	Bayley-III infant motor development; NIDCAP* neonatal infant, developmental care program in the nursery; Brazelton behavior screening within first 72 h; may go up to 2 months	Bayley-III infant motor development; establish cognitive, motor, language and adaptive and social, emotional composite scores, and functional status	Bayley-III infant motor development	Bayley-III infant motor development; GMFCS for CP; Peabody gross motor; IQ visual motor skills; PPVT*, TEGI* for speech impairment; functional independence measure for CP in children (Wee-FIM)*	GMFCS, Wee-FIM; language, pediatric behavior symptom checklist, CBCL; Vanderbilt Checklist for ADHD, executive function; high functional autism screen for pragmatic speech, speech and language testing; WPPSI and WISC for IQ test for childhood
Vision	Vision by ophthalmologist	Vision by ophthalmologist, fundoscopic evaluation and charts	Vision charts by ophthalmologist Beery-Buketencia, developmental test for VMI* skills inventory: Oregon Project for Visually Impaired and Blind pre school and primary school children. (6th) edition	Tumble-E chart, and VMI, skills inventory, Oregon Project for visually blind and impaired children	Vision screening, EYE chart, Snellen's chart, ophthalmologist fundal examination
Hearing	OAE* at birth, and up to 3 months; ABR* when OAE is abnormal even at birth	Behavior hearing by audiometry, and ABR*	Audiometry, ABR	Sound booth audiometry, auditory CPT, and verbal IQ	Sound booth, audiometry, verbal IQ; temporal bone CT and cochlear functional evaluation, hearing aid requirement

Table 38.2 The recommended assessment tools and appropriate ages [1] *(cont.)*

Areas of assessment	2, 4, 6, 9, and 12 months, CA	12–14 months, CA	18–24 months, CA	36–60 months (5 years), chronological age	6–8 years, chronological age
Functional behavior	Brazelton newborn behavior screening test, newborn up to 2 months	CBCL*, Ages and Stages social and emotional checklist (ASQ-SE), Wee-FIM, Vineland Social Maturity scale	Parent behavior checklist, CHAT, and MCHAT-R, CBCL, ASQ-SE*, Wee-FIM*, Vineland Social Maturity scale	Parent behavior checklist, ASQ-SE, CBCL	GMFCS, Wee-FIM, Wechsler IQ, behavior checklist, CDI* screen, learning disability, ADHD, autistic observation
Language	Young children's parent checklist	Parent checklist	Parent checklist	PPVT, TEGI	Speech and language test for early grammar impairment, IQ test for learning disability
QOL and research		HRQL*, QOL, and health status	HRQL, QOL, and health status	HRQL, QOL, and health status	HRQL, QOL, and health status

ABR*, Auditory Brain wave Response; *Amiel-Tison**, Neurologic Evaluation of the Newborn and the Infant; *ASQ**, Ages and Stages Questionnaires; *ASQ-SE**, Ages and Stages social and Emotional Questionnaire; *BIND**, Bayley-III scale of Infant and toddler development; *BMI**, Body Mass Index; *CA**, corrected age; *CBCL**, Child Behavior Check List; *CDI**, Child Depression Inventory, *CT**, Cerebral Tomography; *CHAT**, Checklist for Autism in Toddlers; *EEG**, Electro Encephalogram; *GMFCS**, Gross motor Functional Classification; *HC**, Head circumference; *HRQL**, Health Related Quality of Life; *HT**, Height; *MCHAT_R**, Modified checklist for Autism in toddlers; *NIDCAP**, Newborn and infant Developmental care program; *OAE*, Acoustics auditory emission; *OPSI**, Oregon Project for Visual acuity; *PPVT**, Peabody Picture Vocabulary Test; *QOL**, Quality of life; *SMA**, Spinal Muscular Atrophy; *TEGI**, Test of Early Grammatical Impairment; *MI**, Visual Motor Integration Test; *Wee-FIM**, Functional Independence Measure for Children; *WPPSI**, Wechsler Preschool Premature Independence scale; *WISC**, Wechsler Intelligence scale for Children; *WT**, Weight.

f. Emotional and social development: how the child responds to getting along with people, skills to use manners recognizing emotions at age, appropriately at different ages

g. General adaptive behavior (GAC), such as self-care, learning, eating, toileting, bathing, locomotion, dressing self, following the rules and directions, home living, taking care of the personal possessions, such as his toys, school books, pencils, etc; able to communicate with his parents, siblings, and the community, etc.; and again making simple decisions, such as to play, or to go outside, or to help others if needed

The standardized scores are compared to the child's performance.

Bayley-III scores are presented in composite scores.

Interpretation of composite score determines whether the child requires early intervention or further evaluation. This will enable the physician to counsel parents with regard to developmental function. Scores are explained as follows:

- 130 and above is very superior
- 120–129, superior
- 110–119, high average
- 90–109, normal
- 70–89, mild moderate delay
- <69, severe delay

Based on the scores and information, the need for therapy is determined. Therapy depends on that particular parameter the child is scoring at 25%–30% less than the optimum score. Intervention is provided in that particular area. The percentile delay is important to determine whether the child requires early intervention or further investigations. The results of the score help to counsel the parents, with regard to child's functional ability and developmental age, and plan for therapy.

4. Test of infant motor performance: is a standardized test. It can evaluate infants from 34 weeks of GA to 16–17 months post-term. It evaluates motor functions of the infant in the nursery as well as after discharge from the nursery. It is well correlated with BSID–II up to 4 months of age [7,8].

If gross motor function is delayed or suspected, Peabody gross motor evaluation is indicated [9]. It is a standardized test that can evaluate infants from 34 weeks of GA to 16–17 months post-term and up to 8 years.

When motor function is compromised severely, cerebral palsy is suspected. Gross motor functional classification (GMFCS) for CP is indicated when the children [10–12] need mobility for attending school and community events.

GMFC is available for age-adjusted variations in five levels. Here the description is referred to toddlers and older group of 4–8 years. This classification is based on the functional limitation and quality of movement with supportive devices.

GMFC classification:
- For toddlers (palisano)
  - Level-1: child can walk without any assistance for about 10 steps. With symmetrical gait, child sits, creeps, and crawls
  - Level-2: uses hands for support in sitting posture
  - Level-3: sits with external assistance
  - Level-4: has good head control but needs assistance for mobility
  - Level-5: poor head control, no truncal balance, and no voluntary movement.
- Levels in older age group of cerebral palsy are described as:
  - Level-1: walks without any restrictions with tip-toe
  - Level-2: walks without any support, but limits walking in the community
  - Level-3: walks with assistive device like indoor walker, crutches, etc. but limited mobility outside in the community
  - Level-4: mobility is more limited; need powered assistive devices for transportation in the community
  - Level-5 self-mobility is severely affected even with the use of assistive technology

Speech and language evaluation

Infant/toddler checklist can be evaluated by parent questionnaire for speech and language evaluation. Bayley-III evaluates speech and language in children less than 42 months. Communication and Symbolic Behavior Scales-Developmental Profile (CSBS-DP) developed by Weatherby and Prizant (2001) [13] can be used as first step in routine developmental behavior testing for children between 6 and 24 months, which identifies following language predictors:
1. Emotion and use of eye gaze
2. Use of communication
3. Use of gestures
4. Use of sounds
5. Use of words
6. Understanding of words
7. Use of objects
   This is scored and standardized for older children.

Test of Early Grammatical Impairment (TEGI*) can be used for speech impairment. It is used in children who have speech impairment after 6 years [14].

Peabody Picture Vocabulary Test (PPVT) can be used for children with language impairment [15].

Emotional and social behavior and adaptation

Social and emotional behavior screening for autism is recommended for all toddlers at 18–24 months. Recommended tools are modified checklist for autism in toddlers, revised (M-CHAT) [16] screening by AAP, or checklist for autism in toddlers [17] (CHAT) (UK).

Bayley-III evaluates social and emotional behavior from 42 months.

Childhood Behavior Checklist (CBCL) by Achenbach for children 2–4 years evaluates for functional assessment [18,19].

Pediatric behavior checklist by Michael Jellinek: is a behavior checklist for children 4 years and older and consists of 35 questions [20].

Ages and Stages Questionnaire-Social Emotional Questionnaire (ASQ-SE) [21] is another evaluation tool.

Hearing evaluation [22,23]: Universal screening test for hearing of the newborn is recommended. Otoacoustic emission (OAE) is used in newborn period and up to 2 months and it evaluates tympanic membrane and middle ear. It does not give the status of auditory nerve response. OAE response is only pass or fail unequivocal or failed response.

Audiometry [brainstem-evoked response audiometry (BERA)] is recommended. BERA is a gold standard measure for auditory nerve evaluation.

Vision evaluation by ophthalmologist for ROP [24]: Visual acuity is evaluated in infants using teller acuity cards under 3 years of age. If the child is able to match pictures, Lee symbols chart is used. If the children are uncooperative or suspected with amblyopia, electrophysiologic testing known as visually evoked potential (VEP) is used. It involves invasive test by placing the electrodes closer to the eye. Electrical impulses, as they are transmitted from eye to the visual part of the brain, are recorded.

Binocular vision is tested by covering one eye with cooperative children. Ocular motility testing is done by observing the child's ability to fixate on the moving objects. Refractive error is evaluated by retinoscopy. Fundoscopic examination of the retina is performed by ophthalmoscope or retinoscopy (specifically for ROP). Intraocular pressure is measured after dilatation of the eyes.

Other evaluation tools recommended for research purposes

1. Vineland Social Maturity Scale Test
2. Visual motor integration (VMI) test (K. Beery, N Beery): For children with visual impairment, to assess the visual perception and motor coordination
3. Oregon Project: for visually impaired and blind preschool and primary school children for skill inventory
4. QOL: Quality of life assessment
5. HRQOL: health-related quality of life

References

[1] Follow up care of high risk infants. Pediatrics 2004;114(5):1377–1397.
[2] Developmental surveillance and screening of infants and children. Pediatrics 2001;108(1):192–196.
[3] Lems W, Hopkins B, Smson JF. Mental and motor development in preterm infants: the issue of corrected age. Early Hum Dev 1993;34:113–123.
[4] Amiel-Tison C. Neurologic evaluation of the newborn and the infant. Neuromotor status. USA: Masson Publishing USA Inc.; 1983.
[5] Brazelton B, Nugent, K. Neonatal behavioral assessment scale. 4th ed. London: McKeith/Blackwell Press; 2011.
[6] Bayley N. Bayley scales of infant and toddler development® 3rd ed. USA; 2005. Available from: https://www.pearsonclinical.com/.
[7] Campbell SK. The test of infant motor performance (TIMP), http://www.thetimp.com; 2005.
[8] Barbosa VM, Campbell SK, Sheftel D, Singh J, Beligere N. Longitudinal performance of infants with cerebral palsy on the Test of Infant Motor Performance and on the Alberta Infant Motor Scale. Phys Occup Ther Pediatr 2003;23(3):7–29.
[9] Folio MR, Fewell R. Peabody developmental and motor scale (PDMS-2). 2nd ed. USA: Pearson; 2000.

[10] Wood E, Rosenbaum P. The gross motor functional classification for cerebral palsy: a study of reliability and stability over time. Dev Med Child Neurol 2000;42:292–296.
[11] Palisano RJ. Developmental and reliability of a system to classify gross motor functional classification in children with cerebral palsy. Dev Med Child Neurol 1997;39:214.
[12] Palisano RJ. Validity of goal attainment scaling in infants with motor delays. Phys Ther 1993;73: 651–658. discussion 658–660.
[13] Wetherby AM, Prizant BM. Communication and symbolic behavior scales–developmental profile (CSBS-DP). Baltimore, MD: Paul A. Brookes Publishing; 2001.
[14] Dunn M, Dunn LM. Peabody picture vocabulary test-III. Circle pines, MN: American Guidance Service; 1997.
[15] Rice M, Wexler K. The test of early grammatical impairment (TEGI). USA: Psychological Corporation; 2001.
[16] Robins D, Fein D, Barton M. Modified checklist for autism in toddlers, revised (M-CHAT-R™). 1999. Available from: https://www.autismspeaks.org/.
[17] CHAT (Checklist for autism in toddlers)-help autism now society. Available from: www.helpautismnow.com/CHAT_Checklist_English.pdf.

[18] Achenbach TM. CBCL 2–3 yrs. Burlington, VT: University of Vermont, Department of psychiatry; 1992.
[19] Achenbach TM. Integrative guide for the 1991, CBCL/4-18, YSR, and TRF profiles. Burlington, VT: University of Vermont, Department of Psychiatry; 1991.
[20] Jellinek MS. Pediatric behavior symptom check list for 3-16 yrs. Arch Pediatr Adolesc Med 1999;153(3):254–260.
[21] Squires J, Bricker D. Ages & Stages Questionnaires® (ASQ-3™): ASQ parent questionnaire. 3rd ed. Baltimore, MD: Brookes Publishing, www.brookespublishing.com/resource-center/screening-and-asse; 2009.
[22] Vohr BR, Widen JE, Cone-Wesson B, Siniger YS, Gorga MP, Folsom RC, et al. Identification of neonatal hearing impairment: characteristics of infants in the neonatal intensive care unit and well-baby nursery. Ear Hear 2002;2(5):373–382.
[23] Erenberg A, Lemons J, Sia C, Trunkel D, Ziring P. New born and infant hearing loss: detection and intervention. Task Force on Newborn and Infant Hearing screening. Pediatrics 1999;(2)103:527–530. http://www.aappublications.org.
[24] American Academy of Pediatrics Policy Statement. Screening examination of premature infants for retinopathy of prematurity. Pediatrics 2013;131(1):189–195. Available from: http://www.aappublications.org.

Chapter 39

Management of Ethical Challenges in Neonatal Intensive Care

Gautham Suresh, MD, DM, MS, FAAP

CHAPTER POINTS

- Ventilator support is one of the main life-sustaining therapies used in neonatal care. In selected situations, it is appropriate to withdraw, withhold, or not escalate such therapy.

- Conflicts between the family and health professionals about such decisions are common, can be ethically challenging, and lead to moral distress.

- Physicians should consider anticipated outcome of individual patients, and clarify whether the family's request is obligatory, impermissible, or permissible prior to making decisions about withdrawal or continuation of life-sustaining therapy.

- Options for the provider when there is disagreement with the family include communication and persuasion, agreeing to provide intensive care, request a second opinion, transfer care, or seek legal advice from a court or child protective services.

Ethical dilemmas are common in neonatal intensive care. Since respiratory support is one of the cornerstones of intensive care, these ethical dilemmas often involve the provision, escalation, or withdrawal of respiratory support (Fig. 39.1). In the neonatal intensive care unit (NICU), many deaths follow withdrawal or limitation of life-sustaining treatments (LSTs). Therefore, clinicians working in neonatal intensive care should have a clear understanding of the principles and frameworks of ethics and apply them to the challenging cases they encounter.

The foundational principles of ethics in the NICU are as follows:

1. Clinicians providing neonatal intensive care should always act in the best interests of the infant. They have an individual as well as a collective obligation to act in the neonate's best interests. While the term "best interests" is admittedly subjective and hard to define objectively, clinicians should keep the interests of the patient central to all decisions.

2. The parents or legal guardians are the default surrogate decision-makers for the child.

3. Parental decisions and preferences should be respected and accommodated in most situations, but if they are not in the best interest of the child, they should be challenged and occasionally overturned.

4. For certain diagnoses and categories of patients that are considered to have poor outcomes, interventions that may extend life and decrease morbidity may not be provided by clinicians in one era but may be offered in a subsequent era due to a change in social and medical attitudes.

5. Ethically and morally there is no difference between withholding and withdrawing life-sustaining therapy but in reality, withdrawing such therapy is often more difficult.

Anticipated outcome	Clinician determination: is life-sustaining therapy	Clinician-family discussion	Final decision about life-sustaining therapy

Life limited in quantity despite maximal intensive care
• NEC-totalis with shock
• Inoperable congenital heart disease in cardiogenic shock
• Severe perinatal asphyxia with no response to resuscitation
 	
Life limited in quality
• Grade IV IVH
• Trisomy 18
• Severe brain injury from hypoxic ischemic encephalopathy
	• Obligatory?
	
	• Permissible?
	  • Advisable?
	  • Inadvisable?
	
	• Impermissible?
		Incorporating medical facts, values of family, and uncertainty of prediction	• Initiate or withhold?
			• If already initiated:
			  • Withdraw or continue?
			• If continue:
			  • Escalate or not?

Fig. 39.1 Management of Ethical Challenges in Neonatal Intensive Care.

6. In settings where resources are generally not constrained, concerns about appropriate use of health care resources and about excessive health care costs should not influence decisions about individual patients, but should be a factor in institutional or regional policies and guidelines.

7. Physicians are not obligated to provide care that is not expected to benefit the patient.

8. While making decisions about withholding, withdrawing, or limiting life-sustaining therapy, clinicians should adhere to (and not violate) local institutional policies, and to local, state, and national laws.

9. Physicians should help the family make decisions about the best choices of care for their infant and should not hesitate to provide recommendations, but should not be too directive and should not impose their own values and opinions about treatment choices for the infant. They should also not function as mere technicians who provide any intervention that the family requests.

10. All decisions about withholding or withdrawing LST should be made after a careful review of all the medical facts, and after discussions have been completed within the health care team and with the parents or surrogate decision-makers. If a clinician is suddenly and unexpectedly faced with a decision about initiating LST (e.g., in the delivery room), he or she should initiate the LST and attempt to preserve life, and reassess the situation after the infant is stabilized. A decision about withholding LST should not be made "in the moment"–snap judgments should be avoided.

11. Potential or emerging ethical challenges in the NICU should be identified early and preventive or early actions should be taken to prevent the situation from becoming severe. Plans of care should be put in place well before any acute clinical deterioration occurs.

12. A decision about withholding, withdrawal, or non-escalation of LST is not permanent and can be rescinded or modified if the patient's clinical condition or course changes, or if the parents change their opinions or perspective.

Common ethically challenging questions in the NICU

1. In which patients, should life-sustaining therapy be offered, not offered, or considered optional? For example, infants who were born at very early gestation, who have major birth defects, such as trisomy 13 or trisomy 18.

2. How should disagreement between the parents and the clinicians about initiation or continuation of life-sustaining therapy be handled? In such situations, parents may request or insist upon life-sustaining therapy while clinicians feel that this is not in the child's best interest; or parents may request withholding or discontinuation of life-sustaining therapy, while clinicians feel that such therapy is in the child's best interest.

3. How should decisions about life-sustaining therapy be made when resources are limited?

In which patients, should life-sustaining therapy not offered or considered optional?

Over the past few decades, advances in technology, development of new medications, and increasing refinements in the delivery of neonatal intensive care have led to increasing survival and improved clinical outcomes for neonatal patients. Over this period, there has been a trend for neonatologists to provide interventions and intensive care support to categories of infants for whom such interventions were previously not offered, such as extremely preterm neonates and neonates with birth defects. These treatments can sustain life in circumstances where this was previously impossible, but carry a risk of causing pain, suffering, and a poor quality of life in the long term. Therefore in modern neonatal intensive care, it is common for clinicians to encounter ethical dilemmas and moral distress about the management of infants with a low likelihood of a good clinical outcome, and about whether an intervention should be provided just because it is technically feasible to provide it. While many of the situations described next can be handled by the NICU health professionals themselves, in some situations an Ethics Committee consultation may have to be obtained.

Intensive care is usually provided with the default presumption of treating to sustain life. Questions about the appropriateness of life-sustaining therapy might arise about several medical or surgical interventions that are components of such therapy. These include chest compressions, medications to stimulate the heart, vasoactive infusions, mechanical ventilation, thoracentesis, thoracostomy, vascular access, antibiotics for infection, transfusion of blood or blood products, supplemental oxygen, renal replacement therapy, extracorporeal membrane oxygenation, implanted medical devices, and surgery. Any of these may be withheld or withdrawn if it is in the infant's best interests to do so. Rarely, medically provided nutrition and hydration may be withheld as well.

The first step in making any decision about LST is to confirm the diagnosis and prognosis of the infant. Until these are confirmed, LST should be continued. Ultimately, decisions to withhold or withdraw certain treatments are based on probabilities rather than certainties, and a decision to forgo LST should be considered only when the probability of a poor outcome is high enough (i.e., it exceeds a certain threshold of likelihood). Before considering forgoing LST, all remediable causes for the child's condition must be excluded, for example, drugs and metabolic encephalopathy.

There are two sets of circumstances when treatment (LST) limitation can be considered based on the rationale that LST is unlikely to provide overall benefit, and is therefore not in the infant's best interest:

When the anticipated life in spite of maximal treatment is limited in quantity: Imminent death, where physiological deterioration is occurring irrespective of treatment; and inevitable death, where death is not immediately imminent but will follow and where prolongation of life by LST confers no overall benefit.

When the anticipated life in spite of maximal treatment is limited in quality: This includes situations where treatment may be able to prolong life significantly but will not alleviate the burdens associated with illness or treatment itself. These comprise: burdens of treatments, where the treatments themselves (e.g., surgery or invasive procedures) produce sufficient pain and suffering so as to outweigh any potential or actual benefits (i.e., there is net harm rather than net benefit); burdens of the infant's underlying condition, where the severity and impact of the child's underlying condition is in itself sufficient to produce such pain and distress in spite of maximal palliative care as to overcome any potential or actual benefits in sustaining life; and inability to benefit, where the infant's underlying condition (e.g., severe cognitive impairment) makes it extremely unlikely that she will enjoy the benefits of a continued life.

A useful framework for classifying LST, described by Mercurio, is for clinicians to themselves first clarify, before communicating with the infant's family, whether the treatment being considered or requested is: *(1) obligatory to provide; (2) impermissible; or (3) permissible*. Permissible interventions can further be categorized as *advisable* or *inadvisable* (Fig. 39.1).

Decisions to limit treatments—or what treatments should be given—should be made by clinical teams in partnership with, and with the agreement of the parents. They should be based on shared knowledge and mutual respect, using the principles of shared decision-making. It is preferable for both parents to be fully involved in decision-making as far as possible, whether or not the father has parental responsibility. Although the infant's family is granted a key role in making decisions about the neonate's treatment, they may not always want to make those decisions themselves. They may be unable or unwilling to make decisions or prefer to abdicate this responsibility to health care professionals. However, the presumption should be that parents will always want to take part in discussion about limiting LST and that they should always be invited to do so. Parental interests may overlap with the interests of the child and are difficult to separate. An approach that considers family welfare rather than purely best interests of an individual child is a model that is used by the majority of neonatologists.

Wherever possible, discussions between the clinical team and the family should occur early in the patient's course, and all decisions about withholding or withdrawing LST should be made in advance of acute events in the form of care plans, and should be available for all relevant parties.

How should disagreement between the parents and the clinicians about initiation, continuation, or escalation of life-sustaining therapy be handled?

In the context of life-limiting illness, it is often possible for health care teams, parents, and children to reach agreement as to whether LST should be provided, withheld, or withdrawn. In these situations the interests of the child and family are likely to coincide.

Due to the sensitive nature of the discussions to limit treatment, differences of opinion, often based on sincerely held beliefs and values, may occur between the parents or legal guardians of the neonate and the health care team. A family's view of their child's best interests is influenced by their own system of values and their degree of trust in the health care system and in the health professionals. A family's collective value system is influenced by religious beliefs, political and cultural attitudes, and life experiences. These parental values may not coincide with those of professionals. The parents may feel a certain therapy is obligatory or impermissible while the clinicians may feel that it is not, or vice versa. Disagreements may be aggravated by the power gradient that exists inherently in the health care professional/family relationship. Ultimately all decisions about withholding or withdrawing LST are based on probabilities, and there is often uncertainty about the anticipated poor outcomes. Most such decisions have to be made in a context where absolute certainty over outcomes does not exist. This uncertainty may aggravate clinician–parent differences. In addition, there may be legal uncertainty about what is permissible and impermissible. Finally there are often differences of opinion and beliefs among different members of the clinical team, or among the family members. Therefore, decisions about forgoing LST often entail conflicts over what constitutes a child's best interests, and who decides them. In such conflicts, an independent Ethics Committee review may be helpful.

Conflicts about LST between health professionals and families may be of two types (Fig. 39.2):

1. Parents may request or insist upon life-sustaining therapy (i.e., they feel it is obligatory or permissible and advisable) while clinicians feel that forgoing LST is in the child's best interest (i.e., it is, or has become impermissible). This is the more common situation. Parental wishes and interests are important but not necessarily determinative; parents' wishes may be allowed to drive decisions about LST if its burdens

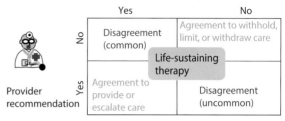

Fig. 39.2 **Types of Conflicts Between Health Care Professionals and Families.** Copyright: Satyan Lakshminrusimha.

to the infant are sufficiently small, or uncertain. Nevertheless, the interests of the infant should remain the primary guiding factor in treatment decisions. Referral to social work and legal intervention should be considered when there is justifiable concern that parental decisions would pose a significant risk of serious harm to the child.

2. Parents may request withholding, limitation, or discontinuation of LST (i.e., they feel it is or has become impermissible) while clinicians feel that such therapy is in the child's best interest, that is, obligatory, or permissible and advisable. This situation is rare, but if it arises, the parents' understanding of the relevant facts and the reason for their judgment should be explored. If the benefits of continuing treatment are sufficiently small or uncertain, the parents' views about the best interests of the child should be given serious consideration. Where the benefit to the child is clear, the presumption should be to provide treatment to the child.

When there is disagreement or conflict, four options are available to arrive at a decision about LST (Fig. 39.3):

1. Communication and persuasion: Good clinical practice at the end of life entails some way of resolving potential conflicts over what constitutes a child's best interests and who decides them. Potential conflicts between clinicians and family members can be avoided by frank, open, and considerate dialogue, by involving supportive personnel from the hospital, such as social workers, patient advocates, chaplains, and clinical ethics consultants and by involving the extended family and members of the community. The goals of care and the likelihood of these goals being achieved with various treatment options should be explicitly discussed and clarified.

2. Provisional intensive care: A time-limited trial of LST can be initiated and withdrawn after a pre-specified

839

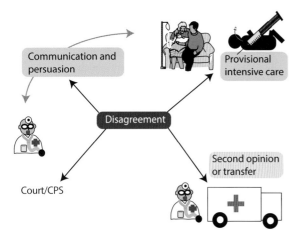

Fig. 39.3 Options Available When There are Disagreements and Conflicts. Copyright: Satyan Lakshminrusimha.

period if the patient does not improve or if the burden outweighs the benefit.

3. Second opinion or transfer to another institution.
4. Seeking a decision from a court of law or from child protective services or both: It may be necessary to refer the case to the court for an independent judgment to resolve matters. In cases where differences cannot be resolved by the previously mentioned means, legal intervention may be necessary with courts as the ultimate arbiter of best interests.

When there is disagreement or conflict between the family and the clinicians about the best management option for the infant, the institutional Risk Management Department should be informed.

How should decisions about life-sustaining therapy be made when resources are limited?

In settings where resources are generally not constrained, such as high-income countries, particularly those with single-payer systems that offer universal health care, decisions about LST are driven primarily by the child's best interests. However, in certain settings in the world, LST resources, such as mechanical ventilation might not be available to all patients who require such therapy, and even if available, might not be affordable to families of neonates who have to pay out of pocket for such care. In such situations, clinicians are often forced to offer LST only to those patients whose families can afford to pay for care, or to those patients who are anticipated to have a good outcome (to make best use of scarce resources), or to those infants who need LST only at times when such LST is available.

Clinicians may be justified in withholding treatments that are highly expensive or of limited availability and that appear to offer little benefit to the child. Such decisions should be based on clear and consistently applied policies developed at institutional, local, or national levels. Even in countries and institutions with plentiful resources, such triaging decisions about which patients receive LST may have to be made during times of natural disaster, accidents, epidemics, or an unexpected surge in the volume of patients that exceeds the institution's capacity to provide LST.

A framework for ethical analysis

The best safeguard for the vulnerable patient is always a combination of a virtuous physician dedicated to the patient's welfare and an explicit and orderly system of ethical analysis.

—E. Pellegrino

1. Collect all the relevant medical facts and the opinions, attitudes, and emotions of the key stakeholders (including parents, extended family, NICU staff, and sub-specialists involved in the baby's care).
2. Identify the sources of the ethical dilemma or conflict or distress.
3. Clarify the goals of care.
4. Use team discussions to arrive at a consensus about the best management options.
5. Communicate clearly and repeatedly with the family to discuss the infant's condition, the anticipate prognosis, and the options for further care.
6. Be clear about the legal, social, and media ramifications about the decisions and actions proposed.

Preventive ethics and advance planning

Many clinical situations that result in ethical dilemmas, conflict, and moral distress can be identified early in the course of the patient before they escalate. Every NICU should have a system of surveillance where existing patients are reviewed periodically to identify such emerging situations early and to intervene before they develop into major problems. These patients should be proactively discussed by the leaders of the NICU and by the team members caring for the patients to identify actions that can be taken to prevent an ethical dilemma, to avoid conflict between the family and the health care team, and to avoid any moral distress that team members may experience. Such advance planning is particularly important in the context of chronic life-limiting or life-shortening conditions, before acute episodes occur or they become life-threatening conditions and before acute situations arise. Such advance planning should include an assessment of all matters related to ethical decision-making, including determination of best interests. Advance planning allows clinicians to discuss potential adverse outcomes in a sensitive manner, ascertain the views of the family, develop appropriate care plans, and ultimately ensure that professional guidance is communicated and implemented well.

Brain death

A process that is very similar to forgoing LST, involves similar discussions, and is prone to similar conflicts is that of managing neonatal patients with brain death. Neonates are infrequently diagnosed with brain death. However clinicians in neonatology should be familiar with the current criteria to diagnose death by neurologic criteria and be prepared to explain to families in such cases that their child meets the legal criteria for death. Clinicians should educate themselves about the institutional policies and regional laws about brain death and exemptions to the determination of brain death. Such infants are often candidates for organ donation and neonatology clinicians should work in coordination with the organ donation professionals to sustain organ function until organ harvesting is performed.

Palliative care

All critically ill neonates and those with life-limiting or life-threatening conditions should receive palliative care, provided either by the NICU staff or by palliative care specialists. Palliative care is an active and total approach to care that continues from the point of diagnosis or recognition throughout the infant's life, death, and beyond. It includes physical, emotional, social, and spiritual elements and focuses on relief of symptoms so as to maximize the quality of life that remains; the provision of psychological, social, and spiritual support for families; provision of respite care for siblings and families; and care through death and bereavement. Palliative care can be given alongside active interventions; it is not confined to situations where a decision to withhold or withdraw active treatment has been made.

Care after LST has been withheld, withdrawn, or limited

Whatever the outcome of the decision-making process, neonatal patients and their families should always receive high-quality expertly delivered care that provides them with comfort and support. Decisions to limit LST do not constitute "withdrawal of care." Decisions to withhold, withdraw, or limit LST involve a change in the goal of care from cure to symptom relief. Treatments that are intended to relieve suffering of the infant and the family, produced by illnesses and their treatments or by disability, are ethically justified. They should be offered early in the course of life-limiting or life-threatening illness. In situations where treatment is withheld or withdrawn, the health care team should be flexible to face the changing circumstances, as the primary intention of limiting treatment is not the death of the child. Sometimes children, in whom LST is withheld or withdrawn, may survive. In these circumstances continuing support and palliative care should be provided.

Communication skills and language in ethically challenging situations

Communication, within health care teams and with parents and children, is important and should also include those in the community who also have a duty of care to the child. Communication of information should be in a form and given at a pace that is appropriate for children and families and takes account of any special needs they have. All clinical staff should have access to continuing professional training and education in communication skills, ethics, and the issues raised by decisions to limit treatments. The process should be audited to ensure that the physical and emotional needs of children and their families facing such decisions are met. Parental decision-making should be properly informed by providing the best information available and by presenting it in a format and at a pace that they can comprehend. Parents whose understanding is limited by cognitive or communication difficulties should receive appropriate services to ameliorate or overcome these difficulties. Clinicians should communicate with families with limited English proficiency using a qualified interpreter. An advocate, for example, from Patient Advocacy or Social Work may help the family to present their views and wishes to the clinical team.

The following terms and phrases should be avoided. Instead, the preferred alternate terminology described next should be used.

841

- "Withdrawal of care." Care is always provided, although the type of care provided might change, based on the goals of care. Use "withdrawal of LST" or "redirection of care" or "comfort measures only."
- "Nothing more can be done." As mentioned earlier, comfort care, pain relief, and emotional support can always be provided even if the infant is likely to die soon. Instead, in an infant who is anticipated to die in spite of maximal intensive care, emphasize that continued intensive care or further escalation is unlikely to prolong life or ensure survival, and that further care should consist of comfort measures only.
- "Futile" and "futility." These are poorly defined and subjective terms. Instead, phrases, such as "the proposed treatment is unlikely to achieve the goals of care," or "potentially inappropriate treatment."
- "The parents want everything done." "Everything" is poorly defined, and this phrase is subject to misinterpretation. Instead use phrases, such as "a trial of intensive care" and describe whether the interventions being proposed are likely to achieve the goals of care.
- "Heroic measures" or "full court-press." These terms are poorly defined and subjective. Instead, use terms, such as "life-sustaining therapy" or specify

interventions, such as intubation, chest compressions, ECMO, or dialysis.

- "Lethal anomaly." Such terminology can cause clinicians to become negatively biased and become overly pessimistic about the outcome of the baby. If they then withhold LST and the baby dies, lethality then becomes a self-fulfilling prophecy. Instead, use specific language based on probability, such as "survival unlikely in spite of maximal intensive care."

Care after death

Professional duties and responsibilities do not cease when a child dies and the provision of bereavement support services for families and support for staff are increasingly recognized as necessary parts of the grieving process for all involved. Clinicians should routinely offer to meet with the families of NICU infants who pass away a few months after the death, to provide bereavement support, discuss the grieving process, discuss the findings of an autopsy if one was conducted, and answer any lingering medical questions the family might have.

Chapter | **40** |

Normal Reference Values

K. Shreedhara Avabratha, MD, DNB (Pediatrics), P.K. Rajiv, MD, Mohamed Soliman M, MBBS, MSc, MRCP, MRCPH, Marwa al Sayyed, MBBS, MSc, Rafique Memon, MBBS, MD, Karunakar Vadlamudi, MD

CHAPTER POINTS

- Normal reference values help to interpret results of laboratory tests. It is always advisable to use reference ranges from one's own laboratory. If it is not available the following may be helpful which are compiled from various sources.

Hematological parameters

Hemoglobin

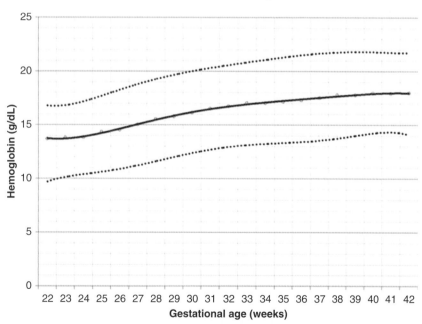

Fig. 40.1 Blood Hemoglobin Concentration on the Day of Birth, According to Gestational Age. Henry E, Christensen RD. Reference intervals in neonatal hematology. Clin Perinatol 2015; 42(3):483–497.

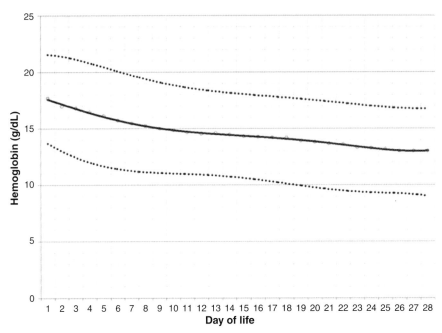

Fig. 40.2 Blood Hemoglobin Concentrations Over the First 28 days of Life for Neonates Born at 35–42 weeks of Gestation. Henry E, Christensen RD. Reference intervals in neonatal hematology. Clin Perinatol 2015; 42(3):483–497.

Hematocrit

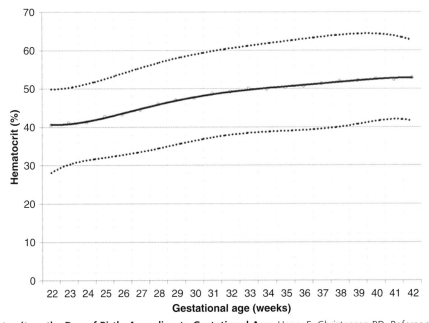

Fig. 40.3 Hematocrit on the Day of Birth, According to Gestational Age. Henry E, Christensen RD. Reference intervals in neonatal hematology. Clin Perinatol 2015; 42(3):483–497.

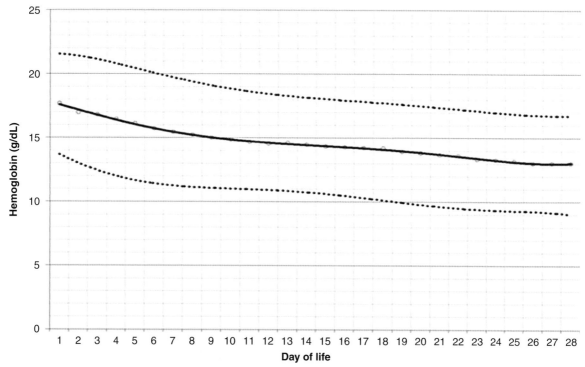

Fig. 40.4 Hematocrit over the First 28 days of Life for Neonates Born at 35–42 weeks of Gestation. Henry E, Christensen RD. Reference intervals in neonatal hematology. Clin Perinatol 2015; 42(3):483–497.

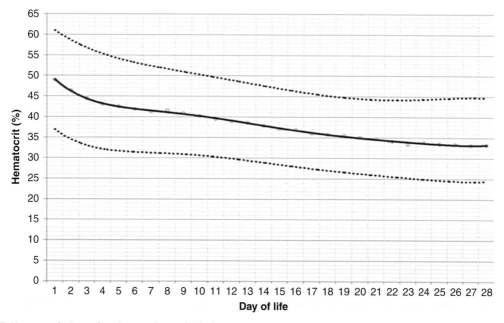

Fig. 40.5 Hematocrit Over the First 28 days of Life for Neonates Born at 29–34 weeks of Gestation.

Table 40.1 Mean haematocrit by postnatal age in hours and gestational age

	Gestational age (weeks)		
Age (h)	35–42	29–34	22–28
0	51	50	45
1	52	50	44
2	54	50	42
3	53	50	41
4	53	48	39

Source: Fanaroff AA, Fanaroff MJ. Klaus and Fanaroff's care of the high risk neonate. 6th ed. Philadelphia, PA: Elsevier; 2013. p. 573.

Nucleated red blood cell (nRBC)

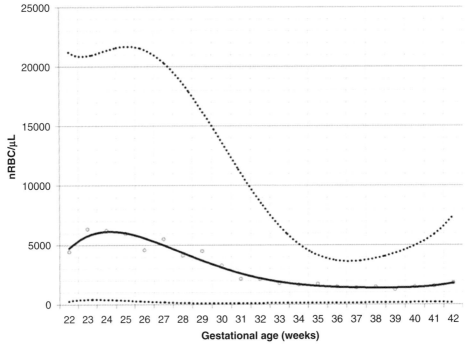

Fig. 40.6 Nucleated Red Blood Cell (nrbc) Levels on the Day of Birth, According to Gestational Age. Henry E, Christensen RD. Reference intervals in neonatal hematology. Clin Perinatol 2015; 42(3):483–497.

Total count and differential count

Table 40.2 Total count and differential count in premature infants

	Birth weight <1500 g			Birth weight 1500–2500 g		
	Age in weeks			Age in weeks		
	1	2	4	1	2	4
Total count (×10³/mm³)						
Mean	16.8	15.4	12.1	13.0	10.0	8.4
Range	6.1–32.8	10.4–21.3	8.7–17.2	6.7–14.7	7.0–14.1	5.8–12.4
Percentage of total polymorphs						
Segmented	54	45	40	55	43	41
Unsegmented	7	6	5	8	8	6
Eosinophils	2	3	3	2	3	3
Basophils	1	1	1	1	1	1
Monocytes	6	10	10	5	9	11
Lymphocytes	30	35	41	9	36	38

Source: Fanaroff AA, Fanaroff MJ. Klaus and Fanaroff's care of the high risk neonate. 6th ed. Philadelphia, PA: Elsevier; 2013. p. 574.

Platelet counts

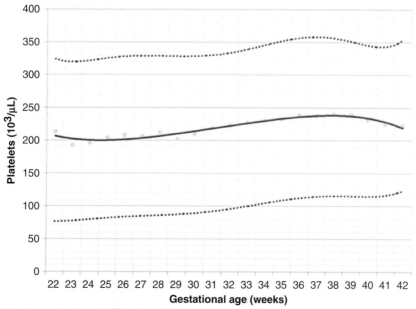

Fig. 40.7 Platelet Counts on the Day of Birth, According to Gestational Age. Henry E, Christensen RD. Reference intervals in neonatal hematology. Clin Perinatol 2015; 42(3):483–497.

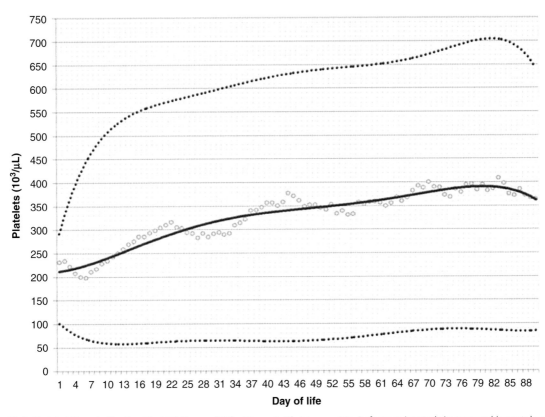

Fig. 40.8 Platelet Counts During First 90 Days of Life. Henry E, Christensen RD. Reference intervals in neonatal hematology. Clin Perinatol 2015; 42(3):483–497.

Biochemistry values

Table 40.3 Values during 1st week in preterms

Blood chemistry values in premature infants during the 1st week of life		
Age: 1 week		
Constituent	Mean ± SD	Range
Na (mEq/L)	139.6 ± 3.2	133–146
K (mEq/L)	5.6 ± 0.5	4.6–6.7
Cl (mEq/L)	108.2 ± 3.7	100–117
CO_2 (mmol/L)	20.3 ± 2.8	13.8–27.1
Ca (mg/dL)	9.2 ± 1.1	6.1–11.6
P (mg/dL)	7.6 ± 1.1	5.4–10.9
BUN (mg/dL)	9.3 ± 5.2	3.1–25.5
Total protein (g/dL)	5.49 ± 0.42	4.40–6.26
Albumin (g/dL)	3.85 ± 0.30	3.28–4.50
Globulin (g/dL)	1.58 ± 0.33	0.88–2.20
Hb (g/dL)	17.8 ± 2.7	11.4–24.8

Source: Fanaroff AA, Fanaroff MJ. Klaus and Fanaroff's care of the high risk neonate. 6th ed. Philadelphia, PA: Elsevier; 2013. p. 566.

Table 40.4 Electrolytes—preterm by postnatal day

Electrolytes—preterm infants (<37 weeks) (by postnatal day)						
Value	Day 1	Day 3	Day 7	Day 21	Day 35	Day 49
Na (mEq/L)	140 (133–146)	140 (133–146)	140 (133–146)	136 (129–142)	137 (133–148)	137(133–142)
K (mEq/L)	5.6 (4.6–6.7)	5.6 (4.6–6.7)	5.6 (4.6–6.7)	5.8 (4.5–7.1)	5.5 (4.5–6.6)	5.7 (4.6–7.1)
Cl (mEq/L)	108 (100–117)	108 (100–117)	108 (100–117)	108 (102–116)	107 (100–115)	107 (101–115)
Ca (mm/L)	2.3 (1.5–2.9)	2.3 (1.5–2.9)	2.3 (1.5–2.9)	2.4 (2.0–2.8)	2.4 (2.2–2.6)	2.4 (2.2–2.7)
Ca (I) (mm/L)	0.81–1.41	0.72–1.44	1.04–1.52 (d5)	1.04–1.52	1.04–1.52	1.04–1.52
PO4 (mm/L)	2.5 (1.7–3.5)	2.5 (1.7–3.5)	2.5 (1.7–3.5)	2.4 (2.0–2.8)	2.3 (1.8–2.6)	2.2 (1.4–2.7)
Mg (mm/L)	0.62–1.02	0.66–1.10	0.75–1.00	0.75–1.00	0.75–1.00	0.75–1.00
Urea (mm/L)	3.3 (1.1–9.1)	3.3 (1.1–9.1)	3.3 (1.1–9.1)	4.8 (0.8–11.2)	4.8 (0.7–9.5)	4.8 (0.9–10.9)

Source: Renni JM, Roberton NRC, editors. Textbook of neonatology. 3rd ed. Edinburgh: Churchill Livingstone; 1999.

Table 40.5 Biochemistry by gestational age

Other biochemistry—preterm infants (by gestation)					
Value	27 weeks	29 weeks	31 weeks	33 weeks	35 weeks
Alb (g/L)	21–33	23–34	22–35	22–35	22–36
ALP	35–604	119–465	112–450	110–398	113–360
Creat (mm/L) day 2	0.08–0.16	0.07–0.14	0.07–0.14	0.05–0.13	0.05–0.13
Creat (mm/L) day 7	0.05–0.11	0.04–0.12	0.04–0.12	0.02–0.11	0.02–0.11
Creat (mm/L) day 14	0.04–0.10	0.04–0.10	0.04–0.10	0.02–0.09	0.02–0.09
Creat (mm/L) day 21	0.03–0.09	0.03–0.09	0.03–0.09	0.02–0.09	0.02–0.09
Creat (mm/L) day 28	0.03–0.08	0.02–0.09	0.02–0.09	0.01–0.06	0.01–0.06

Source: Renni JM, Roberton NRC, editors. Textbook of neonatology. 3rd ed. Edinburgh: Churchill Livingstone; 1999.

Table 40.6 Biochemistry values term babies

Term Infants (postnatal age)						
Value	Cord	1–12 h	12–24 h	24–48 h	48–72 h	3–10 day
Na (mEq/L)	147 (126–166)	143 (124–156)	145 (132–159)	148 (134–160)	149(139–162)	
K (mEq/L)	7.8 (5.6–12)	6.4 (5.3–7.3)	6.3 (5.3–8.9)	6.0 (5.2–7.3)	5.9 (5.0–7.7)	
Cl (mEq/L)	103(98–110)	101(80–111)	103(87–114)	102(92–114)	103(93–112)	
Ca (mm/L)	2.33(2.1–2.8)	2.1(1.8–2.3)	1.95(1.7–2.4)	2.0(1.5–2.5)	1.98(1.5–2.4)	
Ca (I) (mm/L)		1.05–1.37	1.05–1.37	1.05–1.37	1.10–1.44	1.20–1.48
PO4 (mm/L)	1.8(1.2–2.6)	1.97(1.1–2.8)	1.84(0.9–2.6)	1.91(1.0–2.8)	1.87(0.9–2.5)	
Mg (mm/L)			0.72–1.00		0.81–1.05	0.78–1.02
Urea (mm/L)	10.4(7.5–14.3)	9.6(2.9–12.1)	11.8(3.2–22.5)	11.4(4.6–27.5)	11.1(5.4–24.3)	
Creat (mm/L)				0.04–0.11		0.01–0.09
CRP (mg/L)	<7	<7	<7	<7	<7	<7
Lactate (mm/L)	1.5–4.5	0.9–2.7	0.8–1.2			0.5–1.4
Albumin (g/L)	28–43	28–43	28–43	28–43	28–43	30–43
ALP (IU/L)	28–300	28–300	28–300	28–300	28–300	28–300
T4 (microgram/dL)	8.2 (±1.8)	8.2 (±1.8)	19.0 (±2.1)	19.0 (±2.1)	19.0 (±2.1)	15.9 (±3.0)
TSH (U/mL)			3.0–120	3.0–30		0.3–10
Cortisol (nm/L)	200–700	200–700	200–700	200–700	200–700	
17-OHP (nm/L)					0.7–12.4	0.7–12.4

Source: Renni JM, Roberton NRC, editors. Textbook of neonatology. 3rd ed. Edinburgh: Churchill Livingstone; 1999.

Coagulation parameters

Table 40.7 Normal values for coagulation

Normal values for coagulation tests in healthy full-term and premature infants

Coagulation test	Full-term infant	Premature infant	Older child
Platelet (per μL)	150,000–400,000	150,000–400,000	150,000–400,000
Prothrombin time (s)	10.1–15.9	10.6–16.2	10.6–11.4
Partial thromboplastin time (s)	31.3–54.5	27.5–79.4	24–36
Thrombin clotting time (s)	19–28.3	19.2–30.4	19.8–31.2
Fibrinogen (mg/dL)	167–399	150–373	170–405
Fibrin degradation products (μg/mL)	<10	<10	<10
Factor VIII (U/mL)	0.50–1.78	0.50–2.13	0.59–1.42
Factor IX (U/mL)	0.15–0.91	0.19–0.65	0.47–1.04
Von Willebrand factor (U/mL)	0.50–2.87	0.78–2.10	0.60–1.20

Source: Fanaroff AA, Fanaroff MJ. Klaus and Fanaroff's care of the high risk neonate. 6th ed. Philadelphia, PA: Elsevier; 2013. p. 464.

Blood gas

Table 40.8 Acid base values by postnatal age

Acid base values—term and preterm infants (by postnatal age)*

Value	Cord	1–12 h	12–24 h	24–48 h	Range**
pH	7.33 (UV)	7.30 (art)	7.30 (art)	7.39	7.25–7.45
PCO_2 (mmHg)	43 (UV)	39	33	34	35–50
HCO_3 (mEq/L)	21.6(UV)	18.8	19.5	20	17–28
PO_2 (mmHg)	±28 (UV)	62 (±13.8)	68	63–87	60–80
Anion gap	<20	<20	<20	<20	8–16

*Capillary ranges similar except PO_2.
**Very difficult to define, wide variation within/between level III units.
Source: Renni JM, Roberton NRC, editors. Textbook of neonatology. 3rd ed. Edinburgh: Churchill Livingstone; 1999.

CSF values

Table 40.9 Normal CSF values

Type of baby	White cell count (count/mm³)	Protein (g/L)	Glucose (mmol/L)
Preterm (<28 days)	9 (0–30)	1 (0.5–2.5)	3 (1.5–5.5)
Term (<28 days)	6 (0–21)	0.6 (0.3–2.0)	3 (1.5–5.5)

Source: Renni JM. Normal cerebrospinal fluid values. In: Rennie and Roberton's textbook of neonatology. 5th ed. Edinburgh: Churchill Livingstone Elsevier; 2012. p. 1321–22.

Urine

Table 40.10 Urine—term and preterms

Value	Term < 7 days	Term > 7 days	Preterm < 7 days	Preterm > 7 days
WBC (per HPF)	<5	<5	<5	<5
RBC (per HPF)	0–2	0–2	0–2	0–2
Squames (per HPF)	<5	<5	<5	<5
Organisms	Nil	Nil	Nil	Nil

HPF, High power field; *RBC*, red blood cells; *WBC*, white blood cells.
Source: Appedix 2: Illustrative forms and Normal values: Blood, CSF, Urine. Avery's Disease of the newborn 8th ed.

Blood pressure

Table 40.11 Mean arterial BP (mmHg) by birth weight

Birth weight (g)	Mean MAP ± SD		
	Day 3	Day 17	Day 31
501–750	38 ± 8	44 ± 8	46 ± 11
751–1000	43 ± 9	45 ± 7	47 ± 9
1001–1250	43 ± 8	46 ± 9	48 ± 8
1251–1500	45 ± 8	47 ± 8	47 ± 9

Source: Fanaroff AA, Fanaroff MJ. Klaus and Fanaroff's care of the high risk neonate. 6th ed. Philadelphia, PA: Elsevier; 2013. p. 585.

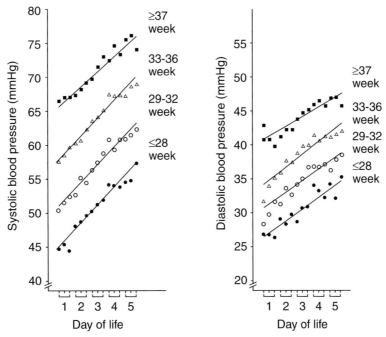

Fig. 40.9 Systolic Blood Pressure and Diastolic Blood Pressure in the First 5 days of Life, With Each Day Subdivided Into 8 h Periods. Fanaroff AA, Fanaroff MJ. Klaus and Fanaroff's care of the high risk neonate. 6th ed. Philadelphia, PA: Elsevier; 2013. p. 587.

Growth charts (Fenton for girls and boys)

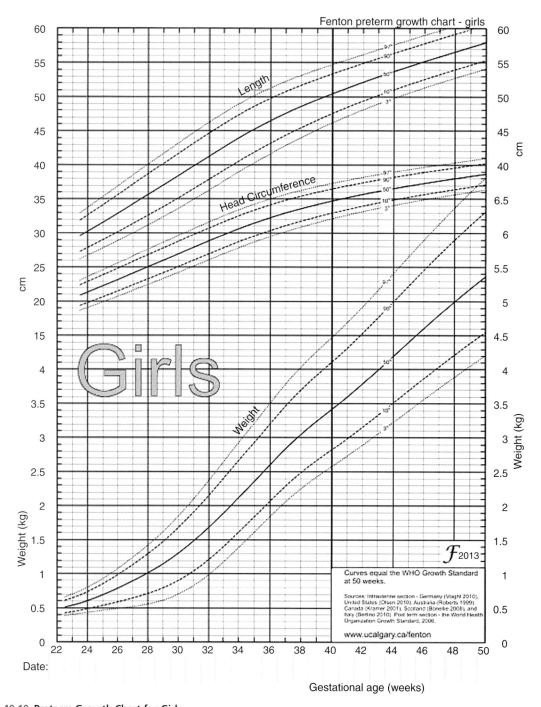

Fenton preterm growth chart - girls

Length

Head Circumference

Girls

Weight

$\mathcal{F}$2013

Curves equal the WHO Growth Standard at 50 weeks.

Sources: Intrauterine section - Germany (Voigt 2010), United States (Olsen 2010), Australia (Roberts 1999), Canada (Kramer 2001), Scotland (Bonellie 2008), and Italy (Bertino 2010). Post term section - the World Health Organization Growth Standard, 2006.

www.ucalgary.ca/fenton

Date:

Gestational age (weeks)

Fig. 40.10 Preterm Growth Chart for Girls.

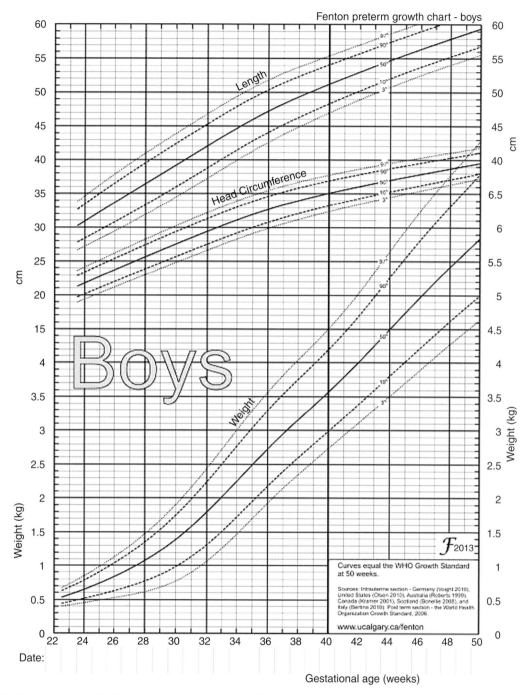

Fig. 40.11 Preterm Growth Chart for Boys. Fenton TR, Kim JH. A systematic review and meta-analysis to revise the Fenton growth chart for preterm infants. BMC Pediatr 2013;13:59.

Index

859

Index